WITHDRAWN

SCHIZOPHRENIA

WITHDRAWN

SCHIZOPHRENIA

EDITED BY

STEVEN R. HIRSCH
MD, FRCP, FRCPsych
Department of Psychiatry
Charing Cross Medical School
London

AND

DANIEL R. WEINBERGER MD
Clinical Brain Disorders Branch
Intramural Research Program
National Institute of Mental Health
Washington DC, USA

FOREWORD BY
TIMOTHY J. CROW
PhD, FRCP, FRCPsych

b
Blackwell
Science

© 1995 by
Blackwell Science Ltd
Editorial Offices:
Osney Mead, Oxford OX2 0EL
25 John Street, London WC1N 2BL
23 Ainslie Place, Edinburgh EH3 6AJ
238 Main Street, Cambridge
  Massachusetts 02142, USA
54 University Street, Carlton
  Victoria 3053, Australia

Other Editorial Offices:
Arnette Blackwell SA
  1, rue de Lille, 75007 Paris
  France

Blackwell Wissenschafts-Verlag GmbH
  Kurfürstendamm 57
  10707 Berlin, Germany

  Zehetnergasse 6, A-1140 Wien
  Austria

First published 1995
Reprinted 1996

Set by Setrite Typesetters, Hong Kong
Printed and bound in Great Britain
at the University Press, Cambridge

DISTRIBUTORS

Marston Book Services Ltd
PO Box 87
Oxford OX2 0DT
(*Orders*: Tel: 01865 791155
        Fax: 01865 791927
        Telex: 837515)

North America
  Blackwell Science, Inc.
  238 Main Street
  Cambridge, MA 02142
  (*Orders*: Tel: 800 215-1000
              617 876-7000
          Fax: 617 492-5263)

Australia
  Blackwell Science Pty Ltd
  54 University Street
  Carlton, Victoria 3053
  (*Orders*: Tel: 03 9347-0300
          Fax: 03 9349-3016)

A catalogue record for his title
is available from the British Library
ISBN 0-632-03276-6

Library of Congress
Cataloging in Publication Data

Schizophrenia/edited by Steven R. Hirsch
and Daniel R. Weinberger.
        p.   cm.
    Includes bibliographical references and index.
    ISBN 0-632-03276-6
    1. Schizophrenia. I. Hirsch, Steven R.
  II. Weinberger, Daniel R. (Daniel Roy)
    [DNLM: 1. Schizophrenia. WM 203 1995]
  RC514.S33413 1995
  616.89'82 – dc20

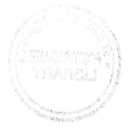

Contents

List of Contributors

NANCY C. ANDREASEN MD PhD, *Department of Psychiatry, The University of Iowa, College of Medicine, MHCRC 2911 JPP, 200 Hawkins Drive, Iowa City IA 52242, USA*

P. ASHERSON MB BS MRCPsych, *Department of Psychological Medicine and Institute of Medical Genetics, University of Wales College of Medicine, Heath Park, Cardiff CF4 4XN, UK*

T.R.E. BARNES MD FRCPsych, *Professor of Clinical Psychiatry, Department of Psychiatry, Charing Cross Medical School, The Reynolds Building, St. Dunstans Road, London W8 8RP, UK*

P.E. BEBBINGTON, *MRC Social and Community Psychiatry Unit, Institute of Psychiatry, De Crespigny Park, London SE5 8AF, UK*

A.S. BELLACK PhD, *Department of Psychiatry, Medical College of Pennsylvania at Eastern Pennsylvania Psychiatric Institute, 3200 Henry Avenue, Philadelphia PA 19129, USA*

A.J. BERGMAN PhD, *Department of Psychology, St John's University, 8000 Utopia Parkway, Jamaica and Mount Sinai School of Medicine, New York, NY, USA*

B. BOGERTS, *Department of Psychiatry, University of Magdeburg, Leipziger Str. 44, 39120 Magdeburg, Germany*

J. BOWEN, *MRC Social and Community Psychiatry Unit, Institute of Psychiatry, De Crespigny Park, London SE5 8AF, UK*

P.F. BUCKLEY, *Department of Psychiatry, Case Western Reserve University, 2040 Abington Road, Cleveland, OH 44106, USA*

A. CARLSSON, *Department of Pharmacology, University of Goteborg, Medicinaregatan 7, S-41390 Goteborg, Sweden*

D.E. CASEY MD, *Psychiatry Service (116A), VA Medical Center, 3710 SW US Veterans Hospital Road, Portland OR 97207, USA*

P.W. CORRIGAN PsyD, *Department of Psychiatry, University of Chicago, Center for Psychiatric Rehabilitation, 7230 Arbor Drive, Tinley Park IL 60477, USA*

B. COSTALL, *Postgraduate Studies in Pharmacology, The School of Pharmacy, University of Bradford, Bradford, West Yorkshire BD7 1DP, UK*

T.K.J. CRAIG PhD FRCPsych, *Professor of Community Psychiatry, United Medical and Dental Schools of Guys and St Thomas' Hospitals, St Thomas Hospital, Lambeth Palace Road, London SE1, UK*

J. CUTTING MD FRCP FRCPsych, *Consultant Psychiatrist, 7 Devonshire Place, London W1N 1PA, UK*

P. FALKAI MD, *Department of Psychiatry, University of Dusseldorf, Bergische Landstrasse 2, 40629 Dusseldorf, Germany*

M. FLAUM MD, *Department of Psychiatry, The University of Iowa, College of Medicine, 200 Hawkins Drive, Iowa City IA 52242, USA*

PATRICIA L. GILBERT MD, *Department of Psychiatry, University of California, San Diego, San Diego VA Medical Center (116A), 3350 La Jolla Village Drive, San Diego CA 92161, USA*

D.C. GOFF, *Department of Psychiatry, Harvard Medical School, Freedom Trail Clinic, 25 Staniford Street, Boston MA 02114, USA*

J.M. GOLD PhD, *Clinical and Research Services Branch, Intramural Research Programs, NIMH Neurosciences Center at St Elizabeths, 2700 Martin Luther King Avenue SE, Washington DC 20032, USA*

T.E. GOLDBERG PhD, *Clinical Brain Disorders Branch, Intramural Research Programs, NIMH Neurosciences Center at St Elizabeths, 2700 Martin Luther King Avenue SE, Washington DC 20032, USA*

T. HADLEY, *Department of Psychiatry, Center for Mental Health Policy, University of Pennsylvania, Philadelphia, PA, USA*

S.C. HEATON, *Geriatric Psychiatry Clinical Research Center, University of California, San Diego, San Diego VA Medical Center (116A), 3350 La Jolla Village Drive, San Diego CA 92161, USA*

S.R. HIRSCH MD FRCP FRCPsych, *Department of Psychiatry, Charing Cross Medical School, The Reynolds Building, St Dunstans Road, London W8 8RP, UK*

A. JABLENSKY MD DMSc FRCPsych, *Department of Psychiatry and Behavioural Science, University of Western Australia, MRF Building, 50 Murray Street, Perth, WA 6000, Australia*

D.V. JESTE MD, *Professor of Psychiatry and Neurosciences, Geriatric Psychiatry Clinical Research Center, University of California, San Diego, San Diego VA Medical Center (116A), 3350 La Jolla Village Drive, San Diego CA 92161, USA*

R.S.E. KEEFE PhD, *Mount Sinai School of Medicine, New York, NY, USA*

ANGELA KODSI PharmD, *Geriatric Psychiatry Clinical Research Center, University of California, San Diego, San Diego VA Medical Center (116A), 3350 La Jolla Village Drive, San Diego CA 92161, USA*

R.B. KRUEGER, *Department of Biological Psychiatry, 722 West 168th Street, New York NY 10032, USA*

ELIZABETH A. KUIPERS, *Department of Psychology, Institute of Psychiatry, De Crespigny Park, London SE5 8AF, UK*

J.P. LACRO PharmD, *Geriatric Psychiatry Clinical Research Center, University of California, San Diego, San Diego VA Medical Center (116A), 3350 La Jolla Village Drive, San Diego CA 92161, USA*

J.J. LEVITT MD, *Department of Psychiatry, Harvard Medical School at the Brockton/West Roxbury VA Medical Center, 940 Belmont Street, Brockton MA 02401, USA*

S.W. LEWIS MD MRCPsych, *Department of Psychiatry, School of Psychiatry and Behavioural Sciences, Withington Hospital, West Didsbury, Manchester M20 8LR, UK*

R.P. LIBERMAN, *Camarillo–UCLA Research Center, PO Box 6022, Camarillo CA 93011-6022, USA*

P.F. LIDDLE, *Hammersmith Hospital, Du Cane Road, London W12 OHS, UK*

J. McGRATH MBBS FRAN ZCP, *Clinical Studies Unit, Wolston Park Hospital, Wacol, Q4076, Australia*

P. McGUFFIN MB PhD FRCP FRCPsych, *Department of Psychological Medicine, University of Wales College of Medicine, Heath Park, Cardiff CF4 4XN, UK*

REBECCA MANT BSc, *Institute of Medical Genetics, University of Wales College of Medicine, Heath Park, Cardiff CF4 4XN, UK*

H.Y. MELTZER, *Laboratory of Biological Psychiatry, Department of Psychiatry, Case Western Reserve University, School of Medicine, Cleveland OH 44106, USA*

H.-J. MÖLLER, *Psychiatric Department of the University München, Nußbaumstrasse 7, D-80336 München, Germany*

K.T. MUESER PhD, *New Hampshire-Dartmouth Psychiatric Research Center, State Office Park South, 105 Pleasant Street, Concord NH 03301, USA*

M. MUIJEN, *Director, The Sainsbury Centre for Mental Health, 134/138 Borough High Street, London SE1 1LB, UK*

R. MURRAY MD DSc FRCP FRCPsych, *King's College Hospital and Institute of Psychiatry, De Crespigny Park, London SE5 8AF, UK*

R.J. NAYLOR, *Postgraduate Studies in Pharmacology, The School of Pharmacy, University of Bradford, Bradford, West Yorkshire BD7 1DP, UK*

F. OWEN, *Division of Neuroscience, University of Manchester, 1.124 Stopford Building, Oxford Road, Manchester M13 9PT, UK*

C.B. PULL, *Department of Psychiatry, Centre Hospitalier de Luxembourg, 4 Rue Barble, 1210 Luxembourg*

M.-A. ROY MD, *Departments of Psychiatry and Human Genetics, Medical College of Virginia, VA Commonwealth University, PO Box 710, Richmond VA 23298, USA*

H.A. SACKEIM PhD, *Department of Biological Psychiatry, New York State Psychiatric Institute, 722 West 168th Street, New York NY 10032, USA*

S.C. SCHULZ, *Department of Psychiatry, Case Western Reserve University, 2040 Abington Road, Cleveland OH 44106, USA*

D.D. SEWELL MD, *Geriatric Psychiatry Clinical Research Center, University of California, San Diego, San Diego VA Medical Center (116A) 3350 La Jolla Village Drive, San Diego CA 92161, USA*

R.I. SHADER MD, *Tufts University, 136 Harrison Avenue, Room 208, Boston, MA 02111, USA*

L.J. SIEVER, *Department of Psychiatry, Bronx VA Medical Center, 130 Kingsbridge Road, Bronx NY10468, USA*

J.C. SIMPSON PhD, *Department of Psychiatry, Harvard Medical School at the Brockton/West Roxbury VA Medical Center, 940 Belmont Street, Brockton MA 02401, USA*

M.D.C. SIMPSON, *Division of Neuroscience, University of Manchester, 1.124 Stopford Building, Oxford Road, Manchester M13 9PT, UK*

S.G. SIRIS MD, *Hillside Hospital, 75–59 263rd Street, Glen Oaks, NY 11004, USA*

W.D. SPAULDING PhD, *Department of Psychology, University of Nebraska, 209 Burnett Hall, Lincoln NE68588-0308, USA*

P.J. TAYLOR MBBS MRCP FRCPsych, *Broadmoor Hospital and Department of Forensic Psychiatry, Institute of Psychiatry, London SE5 8AF, UK*

P.W. TIMMS MRCPsych, *Department of Psychiatry, United Medical and Dental Schools of Guys and St Thomas' Hospitals, Guys Hospital, London Bridge SE1, UK*

M.T. TSUANG MD PhD DSc FRCPsych, *Harvard Department of Psychiatry at Massachusetts Mental Health Center, 74 Fenwood Road, Boston MA 02115, USA*

J.L. WADDINGTON, PhD DSc, *Department of Clinical Pharmacology, Royal College of Surgeons in Ireland, St Stephen's Green, Dublin 2, Ireland*

D.R. WEINBERGER MD, *Clinical Brain Disorders Branch, Intramural Research Program, National Institute of Mental Health, NIMH Neuroscience Center at St Elizabeths, Washington DC 20032, USA*

J.K. WING MD PLD, *Research Unit, Royal College of Psychiatrists, 11 Grosvenor Crescent, London SW1X 7EE, UK*

D. VON ZERSSEN, *Max-Planck-Institute for Psychiatry, Kraepelinstrasse 2, D-80804 München, Germany*

Foreword

I am honoured to be asked to write a foreword to Hirsch and Weinberger's *Schizophrenia*. This timely volume covers a large number of issues which seem to me to be central to understanding the nature of psychiatric disease. As we approach the end of the century it summarizes our knowledge on the concept which crystallized at the beginning of the twentieth century in the writings of E. Kraepelin and E. Bleuler.

Some questions which were asked then remain as major problems today. Is this a single disease entity? Can it be reliably demarcated from other disease states or personality deviations? Is the concept of 'disease' viable at all in the context of mental disturbance? This volume overviews much that we have learned.

I read the first four chapters with particular interest. How does John Wing now view the development of concepts of schizophrenia, to which he has contributed so much? What is the present formulation of Nancy Andreasen, with whom I have had so many fruitful interactions, and her colleagues of the syndrome structure of schizophrenia and its meaning? How does John Cutting attempt to answer the question first addressed by E. Bleuler of the psychological meaning of the symptoms and their relationship to the underlying disease process? Can Ming Tsuang mount a cogent defence of the proposition that schizo-affective disorder is a disease entity, and can be reliably demarcated from 'true' schizophrenia on the one hand, and 'true' manic-depressive disorder on the other? Much of one's thinking on the nature of psychotic disorder hinges on the answer to this question, and here Ming and colleagues have assembled their case.

The diversity and range of conditions related to the term schizophrenia is illustrated by chapter titles on atypical psychotic disorders, late-life schizophrenia and the spectrum disorders. One is tempted to conclude that there is no entity, but rather, as Bleuler suggested, a variety of schizophrenias. But there is also homogeneity — for example of brain changes — as demonstrated in radiological studies, in incidence across cultures as demonstrated in the WHO surveys, and arguably in the relationship between sex, age of onset and outcome. There are underlying consistencies. It is not yet clear that 'schizophrenia' can be fragmented. Indeed it is possible that it is but a part of a larger problem.

Whether or not schizophrenia itself is a true entity, the concept has served as a framework for discussion and research on what are (as the editors emphasize in their Preface) undoubtedly the most serious realms of psychiatric pathology. The extent and severity of the manifestations of these disturbances is well-documented in this volume, for example in terms of the risk of violence (by Pamela Taylor), chronic impairment and hospitalization (by Moller and van Zerssen), and homelessness (by Craig and Timms). These, like other chapters, accurately delineate the boundary between what we have learned and have yet to learn.

In two areas concepts are in a state of particular flux. There is no doubt (as Weinberger cogently argues) that the seeds of psychosis are present early — in some sense it is a developmental disorder. But there is also no question that there is a progressive element — psychotic symptoms appear when they were absent before and they, and other sequelae, so often persist and sometimes even deteriorate. The relationship between the developmental and progressive components is problematic, and at the heart of the problem. One might well conclude that these issues can only be clarified by direct examination of the disease process, and in recent years post-mortem brain studies, here critically evaluated by Bogerts and Falkai, two of the leading exponents, have made a series of decisive contributions.

But what of aetiology, the most fundamental question? Assen Jablensky, a principal contributor to the WHO studies, illustrates how profound and peculiar, considered in an epidemiological context, is the problem. Maybe we should conclude that no parallels can be drawn; that schizophrenia, a specifically human problem, has its origins in the evolution of homo-sapiens and his singular capacity for language.

Given that we understand so little of its origins the surprise is that effective treatments are available at all. But, as well-documented in Part 3, not only do we have moderately effective treatments of acute episodes, but also the means of diminishing the likelihood of relapse. There is even, as Hirsch and Barnes discuss, a question of whether adequate treatment can prevent deterioration.

In this single volume is represented a concensus of what we know about the nature and manifestations of the disorders referred to as schizophrenia; most, if not all, of the major conceptual issues are discussed, and a reliable guide to the use and effectiveness of treatment is provided. I can warmly commend it as a compendium of knowledge in these fields.

T.J. Crow

Preface

Schizophrenia has been a controversial topic since the term was first proposed by Eugen Bleuler to describe a uniquely human syndrome of profoundly disturbed behaviour. In the years following Bleuler's original work the controversies have continued at least as vigorously, but their content has changed. The debate is no longer about the nature of intra-psychic mechanisms, or whether schizophrenia really exists, or whether it is an illness as opposed to a life choice, or whether it is an important public health concern. Indeed, a recent editorial in *Nature* reified the current status of schizophrenia in the biomedical research establishment by declaring, 'Schizophrenia is arguably the worst disease affecting mankind, even AIDS not excepted' (*Nature* Editorial, 1988). In the United States alone it is estimated to cost over $40 billion each year in economic terms: the price that is paid by affected individuals and their families is inestimable.

The debate has shifted away from the view that schizophrenia is caused by a fault in the infant–mother psychological relationship. This had gained the status of orthodoxy during the late/middle part of this century and has been radically revised. Early parenting as a aetiologic factor never stood up to scientific scrutiny (Hirsch & Leff, 1975). The evidence that schizophrenia is associated with objective changes in the anatomy and function of the brain and has a genetic predisposition is incorporated in a major revision of the concept of schizophrenia encompassed in this book.

Schizophrenia has assumed an increasingly important place in neuroscience and molecular biological research programs around the world. Provocative evidence has suggested that aberrations of complex molecular processes responsible for the development of the human brain may be responsible for this illness. The possibility of finding a specific genetic defect that may participate in the liability to develop this disease has never seemed brighter. At the same time, the pharmaceutical industry has revitalized the search for effective new medical treatments. Where it was believed for almost three decades that all antipsychotic drugs were equally effective, it has now been shown that this is not the case. Moreover, it is clear that more effective drugs can be developed which are safer and have fewer side effects.

This textbook of schizophrenia represents a major shift of thinking influenced by the recent changes in our understanding of the brain, the developments in methodology which have influenced scientifically informed notions of our clinical practice, and the changes in our culture which have led to new concepts of management and treatment and a new understanding of the factors which are likely to affect relapse.

While we have asked the authors to make their chapters up to date and comprehensive, we have also worked with them to maintain a 'textbook' orientation so that students and researchers from other disciplines, as well as clinical and research specialists in the field, may be intelligibly informed about schizophrenia.

Promising as some of the basic science may seem, schizophrenia is still a disease whose diagnosis depends on clinical acumen and careful assessment. Therefore all the traditional subject areas are covered. This includes a series of chapters that discuss current issues in the phenomenological characterization of the illness, from its history to the ongoing debate about clinical sub-types, modifying factors, spectrum disorders, and the very nature and prognostic implications of the fundamental symptoms. The increased recognition of the importance of neuropsychological deficits in the chronic disability and outcome of this illness is highlighted by several contributors.

The series of chapters focused around the theme of aetiological factors emphasizes the dramatic shift in thinking on the medical aspects of schizo-phrenia. The application of new methods for studying the brain during life and at post-mortem examination has provided compelling data that subtle abnormalities are associated with the illness. The precise nature of the fundamental pathologi-cal process is unknown, and many uncertainties about it need to be answered. Is brain development disturbed in a characteristic way? Is there a com-mon aetiology, or can schizophrenia arise from a myriad of causes, any of which affect a final common path of brain disturbance? Could the developmental abnormality result solely from environmental causes, or is a genetic factor essen-tial? What is the correspondence between patho-logical changes and clinical manifestations? Does everyone with the pathological change manifest the illness, or is it possible to have the defect but compensate for it? What makes decompensation happen? What factors encourage clinical recovery?

The application of recombinant DNA tech-nology involves a new language in asking the old question of how and what genetic factors play a role in the illness. While it is widely believed that a simple Mendelian genetic defect does not account for schizophrenia, what does it take in genetic terms? How many genes could be involved in liability? Are the genes likely to be recognizable as having anything to do with the phenotype as we have traditionally perceived it? What should rela-tives of a patient be advised about genetic risk? The straightforward dopamine hypothesis that had guided most researchers for the seventies and eighties has become much more sophisticated and enlightened. It is still important in understanding

how the illness is treated, but it clearly has much less explanatory power than it seemed to have in the past. Is dopamine really involved in schizo-phrenia, or is it simply a way of modulating symp-toms by affecting neurotransmission in a relatively unimportant but peripherally connected brain system? Can the illness be treated with drugs that do not touch the dopamine system?

Intensive, insight oriented psychotherapy on an individual basis is no longer used to treat patients with schizophrenia. Indeed, controlled outcome studies indicate that doing so is potentially harm-ful. However, more rationally based cognitive behavioural methods have shown real gains in symptom control and are becoming increasingly important in modern management. There is solid evidence that therapy aimed at altering the family environment significantly reduces the risk of re-lapse. The value of community rather than hospi-tal based treatment is a modern trend, but the evidence from carefully controlled research leaves many questions ananswered: yet, a consensus is beginning to emerge on several of the basic issues.

We have invited leading experts to review estab-lished knowledge of the major fields of study in schizophrenia. This inevitably leads us to include new topical areas of interest including homeless-ness, the risk of violence and the relationship of depression to schizophrenia, as well as brain imaging studies and the treatment of refractory states which would not have appeared in texts a decade ago. The result is a radical revision of our concepts and understanding which we believe justifies the effort of our authors whom we grate-fully thank for their contribution.

Steven R. Hirsch
Daniel R. Weinberger

References

Editorial. (1988) Where next with psychiatric illness? *Nature*, **336**, 95–96.

Hirsch, S.R. & Leff, J. (1975) *Abnormalities in Parents of Schizophrenics: Review of the Literature and an Investigation of Communication Defects and Deviances.* Maudsley Monograph Services, No. 22 (Oxford University Press)

PART 1
DESCRIPTIVE ASPECTS

Chapter 1
Concepts of Schizophrenia

J. K. WING

Introduction

Each historical account of the concepts of schizophrenia, whatever its merits, reaches into the past from a point of view in a temporary 'present'. Berrios and Hauser (1988) commented that such accounts were unhistorical because we still live in a Kraepelinian world. That is fair comment. But it is also true that most people who have been concerned with such concepts over a professional lifetime have found that as their vantage point changes they look back along different sightlines. They find new meanings in old ideas that they thought they had understood. Even to the sceptical eye of the present author, there has been sufficient advance in knowledge during the past decade to make another look backward well worthwhile.

The beginnings

Griesinger and Kraepelin

There has been no time since attempts at classification began when controversy about the nature of 'schizophrenia' was absent. However, there have been periods when a sort of orthodoxy was accepted. One of these was based on Griesinger's teaching, that only what we would now call affective and schizoaffective disorders constituted a 'primary' disease process (Griesinger, 1861). What we would call chronic schizophrenic impairments could develop secondarily, but only after earlier affective episodes.

Griesinger eventually came to agree that there could be a primary psychosis even in the absence of these preliminaries and thus 'abandoned the classification system of mental disorders hitherto traditional for him and his time' (Janzarik, 1987). Thirty years of confusion about the relationships between a multiplicity of syndromes followed. It was not until the publication of the fifth edition of Kraepelin's textbook (1896) that a firm line of demarcation was drawn between dementia praecox and affective psychosis, and a sort of consensus was again achieved.

Both Griesinger's and Kraepelin's concepts were couched in terms of disease entities, following the lines of successful developments in medicine at that time. The discovery of the anatomical and physiological concomitants of clinically identified syndromes, often with a 'natural' history and a pathology, and sometimes with what appeared to be a single causal agent, such as the tubercle

3

bacillus or the cholera vibrio, proved irresistible to the neuropsychiatrists who were also carving more specific syndromes out of the global concepts of dementia, delirium and insanity that preceded them. Since cause was unknown, though variously postulated, classification depended largely on the course and outcome of groups of symptoms.

Kraepelin introduced a simple distinction between conditions characterized by mental deterioration, such as the catatonia and hebephrenia described by his contemporary Kahlbaum (1874), which with paranoid deterioration became subdivisions of the disease, and more periodic forms of mania and melancholia, such as the *folie circulaire* of Falret (1854). His follow-up data suggested a mental-state profile recognizable at the time of presentation and a 'generally regular and progressive' course. The chief symptoms were auditory and tactile hallucinations, delusions, thought disorder, incoherence, blunted affect, negativism, stereotypies and lack of insight. The phenomena were expressed as psychological rather than physical abnormalities; catatonic symptoms, for example, were described in terms of disorders of the will. Paranoia was regarded as a separate disorder, characterized by incorrigible delusions, often circumscribed in topic, a general absence of hallucinations and a chronic but non-deteriorating course.

Kraepelin adopted Kahlbaum's model, general paralysis of the insane, as his prototype for a disease based on unity of cause, course and outcome. The nature of the disease was obscure, though probably related to 'a tangible morbid process in the brain'.

A sympathetic and illuminating account of the development of Kraepelin's ideas up to 1913 has been provided by Berrios and Hauser (1988). They point out that his concept was neither as simple nor as rigid as is generally assumed and that it continued to develop. Indeed, Kraepelin (1920) eventually came to agree that dementia praecox and manic-depressive psychosis could coexist and, thus, a unitary psychosis could not be ruled out.

This fragment of history should be recalled when it is suggested that the Kraepelinian dichotomy has dominated psychiatric thinking during much of the twentieth century. Controversy has continued unabated and recent suggestions concerning a 'unitary psychosis' have brought the wheel full circle (Crow, 1980, 1985, 1987). Moreover, both types of theory have long been under challenge because of their use of an underlying concept, that of disease entity.

Eugen Bleuler

The term 'schizophrenia' stems from work by Eugen Bleuler (1911), who acknowledged in his preface his indebtedness to Kraepelin for 'grouping and description of the separate symptoms' and to Freud, whose ideas Bleuler used to 'advance and enlarge the concepts of psychopathology'. He retained the separation from manic depressive psychosis while pointing out that affective symptoms could coexist. His concept was based on an assumption that the manifold external clinical manifestations masked an inner clinical unity that 'clearly marked [them] off from other types of disease'. Moreover, he argued that 'each case nevertheless reveals some significant residual symptoms common to all'. The end results were identical, 'not quantitatively but qualitatively'.

The primary symptom characterized by Bleuler was cognitive: a form of 'thought disorder', a loosening of the associations. It provided links to Kraepelin's 'dementia' and to the biological origins of the disease, but also, through 'psychic complexes' to disorders of affectivity, ambivalence, autism, attention and will. These essential symptoms could be observed in every case. Catatonia, delusions, hallucinations and behavioural problems he regarded as accessory psychological reactions and not caused by the biological process or processes.

A substantial subgroup was designated 'simple schizophrenia', in which no accessory symptoms (the most easy to recognize) need be present. Diem (1903), who worked with Bleuler, gave a description of two cases that he thought were due to simple dementing forms of dementia praecox. Both individuals were apparently normal as children but as young men began inexplicably to lose volition and purpose, ending up as vagrants. Delusions and hallucinations were absent. Although no early developmental history was available, these two people certainly became severely impaired in psychological and personal functioning and fitted Bleuler's description of simple schizophrenia. Bleuler's own examples are less easy to recognize. Among the lower classes, they 'vegetate as day laborers, peddlars, even as servants'. At higher levels, 'the most common type is the wife . . ., who is unbearable, constantly scolding, nagging, always making demands but never recognising duties'. Beyond this simple form, the largest subgroup was labelled 'latent schizophrenia': 'irritable, odd, moody, withdrawn or exaggerately punctual people'. Bleuler thought it 'not necessary to give a detailed description' of the manifestations in this group but there is a clear merger with subsequent concepts of schizoid and schizotypal personality (e.g. Kendler, 1985).

This is in contrast to the view of Kraepelin, whose account even of the 'mild' form of the course sounds severe. Thus, although Bleuler separated those with the disease from those without, the concept was in effect dimensional. While accepting much of Kraepelin's formulation, Bleuler substantially widened the concept, while continuing to describe his concept as a disease entity. The simple and latent forms, whose vaguely defined primary symptoms could be elaborated through psychic complexes, were thus able to carry the weight and power of a widely recognized diagnosis. Under the influence of contrasting types of theory, one psychoanalytical, the other biological, Bleuler's least differentiated subgroups came to exert an undue influence on the way that diagnoses were made and used in the USA and former USSR (Wing, 1978).

The phenomena of schizophrenia

Many attempts have been made to carry forward, refine, or break up the syndromes described by the two conceptual giants. One motive was to improve earlier formulations of the fundamental characteristics that might underlie all the others. Berze (1914), for example, drew on Griesinger's lowered mental energy to postulate a basic factor, described in terms of a primary insufficiency of mental activity. This negative factor was responsible for the secondary positive phenomena as in Bleuler's theory, but without the psychic complexes. The mechanism was similar to that in Jackson's (1869) theory of a hierarchy of levels of functional organization in the nervous system. A (negative) loss of function higher up can result in a (positive) disturbance of functions lower down. Gruhle (1929) pointed to the difficulty of applying such explanations to the phenomena of schizophrenia. He also made the unexceptionable, but rarely heeded, comment that some experiences and behaviours in schizophrenia cannot easily be fitted into either category. Gruhle distinguished between sets of primary negative and primary positive features, each specifiable descriptively.

Thus, issues connected with theories of 'negative' and 'positive' abnormalities have been hotly debated since at least the time of Griesinger. A post-war attempt (Wing, 1961) to examine the relationships between symptoms in long-term schizophrenia used a profile of four measures: flatness of affect; poverty of quantity or content of speech; incoherence of speech; and coherently expressed delusions and hallucinations. Affective flattening was particularly associated with poverty of speech, less so with incoherence, and least with coherently expressed delusions. There was no evidence that the three types of speech abnormality were mutually exclusive categories.

In a study comparing three hospitals with different social environments, the poverty of content and quantity of speech were classified together with social withdrawal, flat affect, slowness, underactivity and low motivation as 'negative' aspects. Incoherence of speech was included with delusions, hallucinations, overactivity and socially embarrassing behaviour as 'positive' abnormality (Wing & Brown, 1961, 1970).

Crow (1985) gave added point to the descriptive separation by suggesting that different neural mechanisms underlie the two syndromes, which he designated types I and II. Whether there are two, three or more syndromes has continued to be strongly debated, but with fresh impetus to validate such clinical constructions by demonstrating biological differences, as described in later chapters in this volume.

Positive symptoms

In the preface to the second edition, published in 1919, of his book on general psychopathology, Karl Jaspers wrote:

> We trail around with us a great number of vague generalities. I have tried to clarify them as far as possible. But the deep intentions, which sometimes find expression through them, should not simply be set aside and let fall, because full clarification has not been attained . . . .

Jaspers did indeed provide illumination at both levels (1946). In order to clarify the key problem of delusion formation he discriminated between phenomena that can be understood in terms of some antecedent factor, such as social beliefs or abnormal affect (overvalued and delusion-like ideas), and those that are based on irreducible experiences, incomprehensible in such terms. 'There is an immediate intrusive knowledge of the meaning and it is this which is itself the delusional experience'. In the examples he quotes, Jaspers makes it clear that such experiences are direct and sudden in onset, and not congruent with affect.

Jaspers and Kurt Schneider kept up a regular correspondence during the years 1921–55 (Janzarik, 1984). Schneider (1959, 1976) composed a list of experiences that could, in practice, be used to differentiate schizophrenia from manic-depressive psychosis with reasonable reliability. His 'first-rank' symptoms included: thoughts experienced as spoken aloud or echoed or removed or broadcast or alien; voices heard commenting on the patient's thoughts or making references in the third person; experiencing bodily functions, movements, emotions or will as under the control of some external force or agency; delusional atmosphere and delusional perception. Any of these experiences could be elaborated according to the personal preoccupations of the individual

concerned, including those that were socially shared. Schneider did not suggest that the first-rank symptoms carried any special theoretical or prognostic significance but did think (correctly: WHO, 1973) that most clinicians would make a diagnosis of schizophrenia if the symptoms were present in the absence of evident brain disease.

This still left the problem of delusions that seem inexplicable even on the basis of such primary experiences. Kraepelin had regarded paranoia as a separate category. In 1918, Kretschmer (1966) published a monograph on a group of disorders characterized by delusions that developed following a specific stress occurring to someone with a sensitive personality. These conditions could become chronic but were not accompanied by deterioration. Other, usually monothematic, delusional disorders have often been separated from schizophrenia; for example, a single delusion that other people think the individual smells, or that some part of the anatomy is distorted or missing, in the absence of any apparent basis in affective disorder. This one symptom can ruin the sufferer's life. Acute delusional or hallucinatory states of brief duration, with no subsequent development of schizophrenic symptoms, were classified by French psychiatrists as *bouffées délirantes*, following Magnan (1893).

This rich vein of clinical description facilitated subsequent attempts to operationalize the concepts.

Negative symptoms

Another line of development followed the ideas of Kahlbaum (1874), who had been the first to describe both hebephrenia and catatonia, and Kraepelin, who included catatonia as a form of dementia praecox. Bleuler gave a detailed description of catatonic signs but regarded them as 'accessory' phenomena and tended to interpret them in psychoanalytic terms.

Fisher (1983) noted that, 'prior to 1900, when neurological and psychiatric syndromes were being delineated, the symptoms of psychomotor retardation, slowness, apathy and lack of spontaneity were universally regarded as manifestations of abulia'. Much of the literature was concerned with the most severe state, akinetic mutism. Kleist (1960) and Leonhard (1972; Fish, 1958) delineated narrow clinical syndromes intended to serve as indicators of equally specific brain abnormalities, but were unable to convince sceptics who pointed to the lack of evidence of pathology.

More recently, there has been a recrudescence of interest in motor disorders associated with psychological abnormalities. Rogers (1992) has reviewed the history of the concept of catatonia and its long-standing separation from neurological disorders such as dyskinesias and parkinsonism. He points to the occurrence of both kinds of symptom in schizophrenia, affective disorders, obsessive–compulsive disorder and learning disability.

The motor phenomena observed in schizophrenia before the advent of psychotropic medication included reduced and increased speech and behaviour, abnormalities of non-verbal means of communication, symptoms such as negativism, ambitendence, forced grasping, echopraxia and echolalia, opposition, automatic obedience, mannerisms, posturing and stereotypies. This list is taken from the 10th edition of the *Present State Examination* (PSE) (Wing *et al.*, in press). Some of these, such as automatic obedience, forced grasping and negativism, can be interpreted as disturbances of volition. Extrapyramidal and catatonic signs were highly correlated in a sample of patients with schizophrenia examined by McKenna *et al.* (1991). More specifically, there were 'independent associations between tardive dyskinesia and 'positive' catatonic phenomena (i.e. those distinguished by the presence of an abnormality), and between parkinsonism and 'negative' catatonic phenomena (i.e. those featuring the absence/diminution of a normal function.'

The concept of autism

Bleuler (1919) singled out autism as one of the fundamental features of schizophrenia. He regarded it as an active withdrawal from contact with reality in order to live in an inner world of fantasy. Gruhle (1929) pointed out that it was just as likely to be forced on the patient by the cognitive disorder. Kanner (1943) recognized, in a flash of genius, a syndrome worth separating from the then amorphous mass of subnormality and psychosis. His observations were exact and brilliant. At the same time, he adopted the much less exact term 'autism' to describe it, thus linking it to Bleuler's concept. At virtually the same time, Asperger (1944) described, with similar precision, an 'autistic psychopathy in childhood' that is clearly part of the same spectrum because it shares a similar developmental history (Wing, 1981; Tantam, 1988), although after adolescence it shares some features with schizoid personality (Wolff & Chick, 1980).

The diagnosis of autism depends on characteristics of early development that are rarely considered by psychiatrists taking a history from adult patients. People with such disorders who have understandable, if odd, speech are often called 'schizophrenic'. Orton (1930, 1937) discussed aphasic speech disorders in children in terms that were closely similar to those described in autistic children (Wing, 1966, 1976). A further point of confusion in diagnosis is that motor disorder is ubiquitous in autistic conditions, and includes severe catatonia in people with Asperger's syndrome. Case histories indicate associations with other conditions characterized by motor disorders, such as Tourette's syndrome (e.g. Sverd *et al.*, 1993).

A large proportion of those with early childhood autism are also severely retarded intellectually, although the profile of deficits tends to be uneven. Part, perhaps most, of the motor disorders found by Rogers among mentally handicapped people can probably be explained in this way. However, motor disorders are not necessarily associated with other features of autism; much depends on the age of onset.

The concept of 'social impairment' is at the centre of the observable clinical manifestations of Kanner's, Asperger's and a number of other eponymous syndromes that lie within an autistic spectrum (Wing, 1982). Social impairment is not just social withdrawal. It is technically specifiable in terms of a triad of difficulties affecting recipro-

Chapter 1

cal social interaction, verbal and non-verbal language and imaginative activities (Wing & Gould, 1979; Wing, 1993). The spectrum is usefully described in terms of three clinical subgroups:

1 those who are aloof and indifferent to others, and avoid contact except for simple physical needs or pleasures (such as tickling);

2 those who make no spontaneous social contacts but passively accept the approaches of others; and

3 those who initiate contacts but in an odd, one-sided way, unaffected by the reaction of the person approached. This last 'active but odd' pattern is particularly likely to be confused with schizophrenia.

These types could also be divided into positive and negative, but it is clear that one person could manifest all of them at different points of development. In a population survey, the three patterns of behaviour were associated with increasing severity of intellectual, behavioural and language disability, and with associated pathologies. The aloof group is most severely impaired and most likely to have an associated gross pathology; the passive group is intermediate; and the odd group has less global impairment, but behaviour is still markedly abnormal. The central abnormality underlying all the manifestations appears to be an absence of attribution of significance to experience. 'For the child with early childhood psychosis, experiences seem to be wholly or partially devoid of meaning' (Wing, 1982).

The contrast between this formulation and Jaspers' description of the intrusion of abnormal meaning in the primary delusional experience is striking. Taken together with the fact that most of the behavioural and language disorders in childhood autism are also catatonic signs, and that Kraepelin regarded catatonia as a disorder of the will, it is clear that the boundaries between psychological and motor disorders, conventionally regarded as separate, must be reconsidered.

Empirical approaches to classification

The clinical concepts summarized so far, selected from a range that could be broadened to include dozens more authors, have been unsatisfactory in several ways:

their symptomatic and syndromic components overlap but are not identical;

they cannot be stated in precisely reproducible terms;

the weights given to individual symptoms when formulating a diagnosis are not specified but left to clinical interpretation;

other criteria, such as course, are of uncertain value for classification; and

until recently there has been little convincing evidence for specific pathologies or physical causes in the large majority of cases.

One obvious line of development, therefore, has been to try to provide comprehensive, accurate and technically specifiable means of describing and classifying the component concepts (phenomena) in order to allow more meaningful comparisons between clinicians, academic schools, research laboratories and public health statistics.

Standards for symptom definition

The first essential is to provide differential definitions of the symptoms and signs, based as far as possible on deviations from normal psychological functioning. The descriptions of Jaspers and Schneider are well suited to such an exercise. The 10th edition of the PSE (Wing *et al.*, in press) and Rogers' motor scales (McKenna *et al.*, 1991; Rogers, 1992) are examples of such clinical standardization. Such definitions are more likely to approximate to a deviation from normal biological functioning (Lewis, 1953). This basic step should be differentiated from the application of classifying algorithms.

Excluding clinical concepts that cannot be expressed clearly does not mean they are clinically valueless. Some may in time prove to be significant, but they have to wait until someone with the clinical intuition of a Schneider or a Kanner clarifies them.

Some critics of formulations such as schizophrenia (e.g. Bentall *et al.*, 1988) have suggested that there is no need to do more than study symptoms, pointing to evidence that symptom-based therapies can provide relief and greater autonomy to sufferers and their families. It has yet to be demonstrated how far control of one symptom will generalize to others, how long relief lasts and what proportion of sufferers can benefit. A more specific disadvantage is that concentrating on single symptoms instead of (rather than as well as) syndromes may divert attention from the clinical context of the symptoms, to the detriment of those whose underlying problems are multifaceted and interconnected.

Operational criteria for classification

Whether the disorders recognized by applying the criteria laid down in the *Diagnostic and Statistical Manual* DSM-III, and its successors DSM-III-R and DSM-IV (APA, 1993), or in the *International Classification of Disease* (ICD)-10 (WHO, 1993) can be described as concepts is a moot point. Certainly, the rules for schizophrenia laid down in the 'Diagnostic Criteria for Research' in subchapter F20 of ICD-10 are far from describing a disease concept. They do list most of the symptoms described by Kraepelin, but do not include a long-term course or a particular outcome, or refer to a pathology or a cause. The distinction from bipolar disorder, when both are present, is limited to a clinical judgement as to which type of symptom occurs first. In ICD-10 schizophrenia is not a disease but a disorder. The introduction explains that this terminology is adopted:

> ... so as to avoid even greater problems inherent in the use of terms such as 'disease' and 'illness'. 'Disorder' is not an exact term, but it is used here to imply the existence of a clinically recognisable set of symptoms or behaviour that in most cases is associated with distress and with interference with functions ....

An article in the *Schizophrenia Bulletin* illustrates the position clearly (Flaum & Andreasen, 1991). The authors listed DSM-III-R and ICD-10 criteria, and three further versions under consideration for DSM-IV. It is unlikely that a disease concept will change its nature by choosing two of one kind of item and three of another, rather than

three of the first kind and two of the second. In fact, in the version eventually adopted (APA, 1993) the chief distinctions from ICD-10 (the requirement for a 6-month course and deterioration in social functioning) remain. Moreover, the coding system for DSM-IV is still mapped to that of ICD-9. However, both sets of criteria should be used, through standardized instruments such as schedules for clinical assessment in neuropsychiatry (SCAN/PSE10) (WHO, 1994) in research and public health projects, in order to foster international comparisons as well as comparisons with locally favoured alternatives.

Testing clinical concepts

New syndromes can be derived from symptom lists by the application of statistical techniques. There is a long line of such studies, many of them initiated in the 1950s and 1960s in order to overcome the unreliability then being demonstrated in day-to-day clinical diagnosis (e.g. Kreitman, 1961; Lorr, 1966). They were successful in achieving reliability, but the usefulness of the syndromes has not been demonstrated, except in the sense that the factors often looked very similar to the diagnoses they tried to leave behind.

Kendell (1975, 1989) has addressed the problem in a more practical way. He suggests utilizing statistical methods to refine syndromes; these can then be tested against outcome and used to generate testable biological hypotheses. His own studies (Kendell & Brockington, 1980) did not demonstrate a point of statistical discontinuity between schizophrenic and affective psychoses. This must be due in part to fluctuation over time; cross-sections cannot display the full longitudinal clinical picture that emerges over time (Wing, 1988). In addition, the hierarchies that run through psychiatric classification, ensuring that disorders higher up tend to have symptoms of those lower down, must be considered. A high proportion of people with schizophrenia in the International Pilot Study of Schizophrenia (IPSS) (WHO, 1973) would have been classified by the CATEGO program as affective if symptoms discriminating for schizophrenia had been left out (Wing *et al.*, 1974).

Moreover, at least some of the affective symptoms so common in acute schizophrenia must be reactive to the stress of the primary experiences.

Kendell's third suggestion is germane to recent discussions of whether two or three syndromes, each with distinctive patterns of biological dysfunctioning, underlie part or all of the clinical picture of schizophrenia as distinct from other disorders. Recent statistical studies, one fortified by positron emission tomography (PET) results of altered perfusion at different cerebral locations, suggest that a three-factor solution is preferable to two, the third being composed of the incoherence element of the erstwhile positive syndrome (Liddle & Barnes, 1990; Mortimer *et al.*, 1990; Brown & White, 1992; Liddle *et al.*, 1992; Peralta *et al.*, 1992). There is also a suggestion that psychological aspects of depression in schizophrenia may not be correlated with the negative syndrome (Barnes *et al.*, 1989; Kibel *et al.*, 1993).

Other recent work has taken the further step of attempting to link symptoms to neuropsychological processes, which can themselves be further linked to cerebral dysfunctions (Gray *et al.*, 1991; Frith, 1992). That is the logical way for research now to proceed. It is on the cards that the relationships between symptoms, syndromes and disorders will be clarified as a result and that much polemic will be seen to have been hot air. Frith's theories are particularly interesting because he proposes three principal abnormalities that account for all the major signs and symptoms of schizophrenia and many of those of early childhood autism as well.

1 An inability to generate spontaneous (willed) acts leads to poverty of movement, speech and affect, while failure to suppress inappropriate behaviour leads to perseveration and incoherence of speech and behaviour.

2 A disorder of self-monitoring (e.g. of own thoughts and subvocal speech) leads to first-rank experiences.

3 A disorder of monitoring the intentions of others (e.g. making incorrect inferences about their intentions) can lead to delusions of reference or persecution, and what seem to others to be obscurities in speech.

The three mechanisms are all seen as special cases of a disorder of metarepresentation (Shallice, 1988). The same deficit may explain many features of early childhood autism (Frith & Frith, 1991). The theory not only claims to provide an explanation, in terms of specific cognitive processes, of the relationship between the phenomena of schizophrenia and autism, but also suggests means, using neuroimaging, of identifying the brain functions involved.

The concept of disease

Disease as entity or as deviation from normal functioning

Kendell (1987) has pointed out that none of the four types of psychosis — schizophrenic, affective, good prognosis acute and chronic paranoid — discussed above, 'has been clearly demonstrated to be a disease entity'. Does it matter? Kraepelin and Bleuler thought it did. But not even so well 'validated' a disease as leprosy or tuberculosis can be said to be an 'entity' in the sense that everyone with the vibrio or bacillus in the blood stream has the same (or any) symptoms, let alone the same course or outcome.

Cohen (1961) argued that this concept of disease, which:

> still dominates our textbook descriptions, as illustrated by the so-called classical pictures of typhoid fever, influenza, disseminated sclerosis and the rest ... is little more helpful in diagnosis than would be a composite portrait of a football team in revealing whether any one individual is a member of it.

Throughout medicine during the past 50 years, rigid disease categories have been replaced by more useful concepts that are constantly evolving in the light of the experimental evidence. As disease concepts evolve in the light of the successes and failures of hypothesis testing, it becomes more and more obvious that diseases previously thought to be 'entities' are actually linked and that the fundamental processes involve deviations or blockages in the functioning of normal homeostatic cycles. Hypertension, diabetes and coronary heart disease are obvious examples, but so, increasingly, are most well-known diseases. Defining formulae that use the same name have to fight against each other for survival. Which is more successful at any one time depends on the weight of evidence its protagonists can provide.

Such evidence includes epidemiology; the genetics, the age and sex distribution, the excess of births in the winter months and the possibility that the course and even the incidence varies both geographically and over time.

Hierarchy in psychiatric disorders

Some sense can be made of the relationships between psychiatric disorders if dimensional as well as categorical concepts are borne in mind. Both are useful so long as it is recognized that it is essential to move easily between them. The ancient hierarchies divided mental faculties into conative, cognitive and affective. If brain function is profoundly impaired, there can be no, or only negligible, function of will; movement, thought and emotion will be absent or distorted.

It is possible that each of the three faculties can be impaired independently of the others and that the conventional hierarchical system of diagnosis would have more than just practical use if based on three or four dimensions (the extra one representing motor functions). Positive and negative aspects would then be represented at every level. At the moment, in practice, diagnoses tend to be made as follows.

At the top are disorders, such as dementia, which, at least in the early stages, can be associated with any other type of problem (Burns *et al.*, 1990). For example, schizophrenic symptoms occurring in the course of Huntington's disease or temporal lobe epilepsy or mental retardation are discounted for the purpose of diagnosis.

Similarly, disorders in the autistic spectrum, if diagnosed on the developmental history, are not called schizophrenic.

In general, schizophrenic symptoms, in the absence of 'organic' disorder, generally take precedence in diagnosis over bipolar psychoses if both are present.

Affective psychoses in turn take precedence over unipolar depression and the anxiety that is so commonly associated with all the above disorders.

Symptoms such as fatigue, worry and muscular tension are regarded as non-specific.

The position of obsessional disorders is uncertain, but should probably be higher up than the affective disorders and certainly not classified with panic and anxiety (Montgomery, 1992). The hierarchy is generally non-reflexive, i.e. each disorder tends to manifest the symptoms of those lower down (Foulds, 1965; Sturt, 1981), but not those of disorders higher up. But by the same token, *all* disorders can also be seen in cross-section as well as longitudinal, manifesting a complex of symptoms, some negative and some positive, and many 'non-specific' for the 'diagnosis'. Both perspectives are legitimate for different purposes (Wing, 1978, 1991).

Other types of theory

A review of the history of concepts of schizophrenia would not be complete without reference to theories of 'not-schizophrenia', although these tend to be logically self-destructive. Most are variants of those by Goffman (1961), Laing (Laing & Esterson, 1964), Scheff (1966) and Szasz (1971), and have been dealt with elsewhere (Wing, 1978).

This is not to say that there are no other components to the aetiology of schizophrenia than those that involve purely biological elements. In fact, from the time of Kraepelin concepts of disordered attention or arousal have suggested that environmental events may influence symptoms for better or worse. Certainly, some sufferers have learned for themselves how to cope with symptoms without losing control ('going mad') and many carers have found, without help from professionals, how to provide an optimal environment (Creer & Wing, 1974; Wing, 1975). Interactive biosocial theories that suggest how environmental overstimulation and understimulation may act to improve or exacerbate the positive and negative impairments (Wing, 1978) cannot be taken seriously by those who reject any deviation from a purely biological approach. Thus, an absolute biologism is as limiting and ultimately sterile as an absolute rejection of biology.

Conclusion

This review began with 'unitary psychosis'. Has this ceased to exist because there is no code for it in ICD-10 or DSM-IV? Should those who regard basic schizophrenic phenomena as symptoms of dysfunctions in the central nervous system classify them under FO6.2 'Organic Schizophrenia-like Disorder' or F20 'Schizophrenia'? Another problem of the same order concerns the significance of the difference between G93.3 'Postviral Fatigue Syndrome' and F48, which includes 'Fatigue Syndrome'.

Being able to pose these questions does not demonstrate the futility of providing standardized definitions for international use. The examples do not inspire confidence, but the effort to provide reference criteria is essential. It does demonstrate that, whether called 'diseases' or 'disorders', we are dealing with constantly changing concepts. That is not all. The same is true of 'syndromes' and of 'symptoms'. They too are concepts that must compete with each other. The more precisely they, and the predictions that follow from them, are stated, the more easily they can be refuted if they are wrong. It may pay, in the short term, to be vague. But a greater distraction from the search after knowledge is that some protagonists, even when using an impeccably sceptical approach in their scientific work, do tend to use the terminology of 'disease entities' and seem to want to believe that the Snark or the Boojum really exists. Others react against each such provocation and waste their time and wit in polemic. Such arguments are inevitable and will continue, but looking back from our present vantage point, it is possible to discern a pattern amid the noise.

References

APA (1994) *Diagnostic and Statistical Manual of Mental Disorders*, 4th edn. American Psychiatric Association, Washington DC.

Asperger, H. (1944) Autistic psychopathy in childhood. In (1991) *Autism and Asperger syndrome*. Cambridge University Press, Cambridge. Translated and annotated by Frith, U. from Die 'autistischen psychopathen' im Kindesalter. *Archiv für Psychiatrie und Nervenkrankheiten*, 117, 76–136.

Barnes, T.R., Curson, D.A., Liddle, P.F. & Patel, M. (1989) The nature and prevalence of depression in chronic schizophrenic in-patients. *British Journal of Psychiatry*, 154, 486–491.

Bentall, R.P., Jackson, H.F. & Pilgrim, D. (1988) Abandoning the concept of schizophrenia. *British Journal of Psychology*, 27, 303–324.

Berrios, G.E. & Hauser, R. (1988) The early development of Kraepelin's ideas on classification. A conceptual history. *Psychological Medicine*, 18, 813–821.

Berze, J. (1914) Primary insufficiency of mental activity. In Cutting, J. & Shepherd, M. (eds) (1987) *The Clinical Roots of the Schizophrenia Concept*, pp. 51–58. Translated from *Die Primäre Insuffizienz der Psychischen Aktivität*. Deuticke, Leipzig.

Bleuler, E. (1911) *Dementia Praecox or the Group of Schizophrenias*. International Universities Press, New York. Translated by Zinkin, J. (1950) from Dementia Praecox oder der Gruppe der Schizophrenien. In Aschaffenburg, G. (ed.) *Handbuch der Geisteskrankheiten*. Deuticke, Leipzig.

Bleuler, E. (1919) *Das Autistisch-Indisziplinierte Denken in der Medizin und Seine Überwindung*. Springer-Verlag, Berlin.

Brown, K.W. & White, T. (1992) Syndromes of chronic schizophrenia and some clinical correlates. *British Journal of Psychiatry*, 161, 317–322.

Burns, A., Jacoby, R. & Levy, R. (1990) Psychiatric phenomena in Alzheimer's disease. *British Journal of Psychiatry*, 157, 72–94.

Cohen, H. (1961) The evolution of the concept of disease. In Lush, B. (ed.) *Concepts of Medicine*, pp. 159–169. Pergamon Press, Oxford.

Creer, C. & Wing, J.K. (1974) *Schizophrenia at Home*. Reprinted with a new preface, 1988. National Schizophrenia Fellowship, London.

Crow, T.J. (1980) Molecular pathology of schizophrenia. More than one disease process? *British Medical Journal*, 280, 66–68.

Crow, T.J. (1985) The two-syndrome concept. Origins and current status. *Schizophrenia Bulletin*, 11, 471–486.

Crow, T.J. (1987) Psychosis as a continuum and the virogene concept. *British Medical Bulletin*, 43, 754–767.

Diem, O. (1903) The simple dementing form of dementia praecox. In Cutting, J. & Shepherd, M. (eds) (1987) *The Clinical Roots of the Schizophrenia Concept*, pp. 25–34. Translated from Die einfach demente Form der Dementia Praecox. *Archiv für Psychiatrie und Nervenkrankheiten*, 37, 81–87.

Falret, J. (1854) *Leçons Cliniques de Médicine Mentale*. Ballière, Paris.

Fish, F.J. (1958) Leonhard's classification of schizophrenia.

Journal of Mental Science, **104**, 103.

Fisher, C.M. (1983) Abulia minor versus agitated behavior. *Clinical Neurosurgery*, **31**, 9–31.

Flaum, M. & Andreason, N.C. (1991) Diagnostic criteria for schizophrenia and related disorders. Options for DSM-IV. *Schizophrenia Bulletin*, **17**, 143–156.

Foulds, G.A. (1965) *Personality and Personal Illness*. Tavistock, London.

Frith, C.D. (1992) *The Cognitive Neuropsychology of Schizophrenia*. Erlbaum, Hove.

Frith, C.D. & Frith, U. (1991) Elective affinities in schizophrenia and childhood autism. In Bebbington, P.E. (ed.) *Social Psychiatry. Theory, Methodology and Practice*, pp. 65–88. Transaction, New Brunswick.

Goffman, E. (1961) Asylums. *Essays on the Social Situation of Mental Patients and Other Inmates*. Penguin, Harmondsworth.

Gray, J.A., Feldon, J., Rawlins, J.N., Hemsley, D.R. & Smith, A.D. (1991) The neuropsychology of schizophrenia. *Behavioural and Brain Sciences*, **14**, 1–84.

Griesinger, W. (1861) *Die Pathologie und Therapie der Psychischen Krankheiten*. Krabbe, Stuttgart.

Gruhle, H.W. (1929) Psychologie der Schizophrenie. In Berze, J. & Gruhle, H.W. (eds) Springer-Verlag, Berlin.

Jackson, J.H. (1869) Certain points in the study and classification of diseases of the nervous system. Reprinted in Taylor, J. (1932) *Selected Writings of John Hughlings Jackson*, Vol. 2. Hodder & Stoughton, London.

Janzarik, W. (1984) Jaspers, Kurt Schneider und die Heidelberger Psychopathologie. *Nervenarzt*, **55**, 18–24.

Janzarik, W. (1987) The concept of schizophrenia. History and problems. In Häfner, H., Gattaz, W.F. & Janzarik, W. (eds) *Search for the Causes of Schizophrenia*. Springer-Verlag, Heidelberg.

Jaspers, K. (1946) *General Psychopathology*. Manchester University Press, Manchester. Translated by Hoenig, J. & Hamilton, M. (1963) from *Allgemeine Psychopathologie*. Springer-Verlag, Heidelberg.

Kahlbaum, K. (1874) *Catatonia*. Johns Hopkins University Press, Baltimore. Translated by Levij, Y. & Priden, T. (1973) from *Die Katatonie oder das Spannungs-Irresein*. Hirschwald, Berlin.

Kanner, L. (1943) Autistic disturbances of affective contact. *Nervous Child*, **2**, 217–250.

Kendell, R.E. (1975) The concept of disease and its implications for psychiatry. *British Journal of Psychiatry*, **136**, 421–436.

Kendell, R.E. (1987) Diagnosis and classification of functional psychoses. *British Medical Bulletin*, **43**, 499–513.

Kendell, R.E. (1989) Clinical validity. *Psychological Medicine*, **19**, 45–55.

Kendell, R.E. & Brockington, I.F. (1980) The identification of disease entities and the relationship between schizophrenic and affective psychoses. *British Journal of Psychiatry*, **137**, 324–331.

Kendler, K.S. (1985) Diagnostic approaches to schizotypal personality disorder. A historical perspective. *Schizophrenia Bulletin*, **11**, 538–553.

Kibel, D.A., Laffont, I. & Liddle, P.F. (1993) The composition of the negative syndrome of chronic schizophrenia. *British Journal of Psychiatry* **162**, 744–750.

Kleist, K. (1960) Schizophrenic symptoms and cerebral pathology. *Journal of Mental Science*, **106**, 246–255.

Kraepelin, E. (1896) Dementia praecox. In Cutting, J. & Shepherd, M. (eds) (1987) *The Clinical Roots of the Schizophrenia Concept*, pp. 15–24. Cambridge University Press, Cambridge. Translated from *Lehrbuch der Psychiatrie*, 5th edn, pp. 426–441. Barth, Leipzig.

Kraepelin, E. (1920) Die Erscheinungsformen des Irreseins. *Zeitschrift für Neurologie und Psychiatrie*, **62**, 1–29.

Kreitman, N. (1961) The reliability of psychiatric diagnosis. *Journal of Mental Science*, **107**, 876–886.

Kretschmer, E. (1966) The sensitive delusion of reference. In Hirsch, S.R. & Shepherd, M. (eds) (1974) *Themes and Variations in European Psychiatry*. Wright, Bristol. Translated from *Der Sensitiver Beziehungswahn*. Springer-Verlag, Heidelberg.

Laing, R.D. & Esterson, A. (1964) *Sanity, Madness and the Family*. Tavistock, London.

Leonhard, K. (1972) Aufteilung der endogenen Psychosen in der Forschungsrichtung von Wernicke und Kleist. In: Kisker, K.P., Meyer, J.E., Müller, M. & Strömgren E. (eds) *Klinische Psychiatrie I*, 2nd edn, pp. 183–212. Springer, Heidelberg.

Lewis, A.J. (1953) Health as a social concept. *British Journal of Sociology*, **4**, 109–124.

Liddle, P.F. & Barnes, T.R. (1990) Syndromes of chronic schizophrenia. *British Journal of Psychiatry*, **157**, 558–561.

Liddle, P.F., Friston, K.J., Frith, C.D., Hirsch, S.R., Jones, T. & Frackowiak, R.S. (1992) Patterns of cerebral blood flow in schizophrenia. *British Journal of Psychiatry*, **160**, 179–186.

Lorr, M. (1966) *Explorations in Typing Psychotics*. Pergamon Press, Oxford.

McKenna, P.J., Lund, C.E., Mortimer, A.M. & Biggins, C.A. (1991) Motor, volitional and behavioural disorders in schizophrenia. 2. The 'conflict of paradigms' hypothesis. *British Journal of Psychiatry*, **158**, 328–336.

Magnan, V. (1893) *Leçons Cliniques sur les Maladies Mentales*. Battaille, Paris.

Montgomery, S. (1992) The place of obsessive compulsive disorder in the diagnostic heirarchy. *International Clinical Psychopharmacology*, **7**, 19–24.

Mortimer, A.M., Lund, C.E. & McKenna, P.J. (1990) The positive:negative dichotomy in schizophrenia. *British Journal of Psychiatry*, **157**, 41–49.

Orton, S. (1930) Some neurologic concepts applied to schizophrenia. *Archives of Neurology and Psychiatry*, **23**, 114–129.

Orton, S. (1937) *Reading, Writing and Speech Problems in Children*. Chapman and Hall, London.

Peralta, V., Leon, J. & Cuesta, M.J. (1992) Are there more than two syndromes in schizophrenia? A critique of the positive–negative dichotomy. *British Journal of Psychiatry*, **161**, 335–343.

Rogers, D. (1992) *Motor Disorder in Psychiatry. Towards a Neurological Psychiatry*. Wiley, New York.

Scheff, T.J. (1966) *Being Mentally Ill*. Aldine, Chicago.

Schneider, K. (1959) *Clinical Psychopathology*. Translated by Hamilton, M.W. Grune & Stratton, New York.

Schneider, K. (1976) *Klinische Psychopathologie*, 11th edn. Thieme, Stuttgart.

Shallice, T. (1988) *From Neuropsychology to Mental Structure*.

Cambridge University Press, Cambridge.

Sturt, E. (1981) Hierarchical patterns in the distribution of psychiatric symptoms. *Psychological Medicine*, **11**, 783–794.

Sverd, J., Montero, G. & Gurevich, N. (1993) Cases for an association between Tourette syndrome, autistic disorder and schizophrenia-like disorder. *Journal of Autism and Developmental Disorders*, **23**, 407–414.

Szasz, T. (1971) *The Manufacture of Madness*. Routledge, London.

Tantam, D. (1988) Asperger's syndrome. *Journal of Child Psychology and Psychiatry*, **29**, 245–255.

WHO (1973) *The International Pilot Study of Schizophrenia*. World Health Organization, Geneva.

WHO (1993) *The ICD-10 Classification of Mental and Behavioural Disorders. Clinical Descriptions and Diagnostic Guidelines*. World Health Organization, Geneva.

WHO (1994) *Schedules for Clinical Assessment in Neuropsychiatry (SCAN)*. World Health Organization, Geneva.

Wing, J.K. (1961) A simple and reliable subclassification of chronic schizophrenia. *Journal of Mental Science*, **107**, 862–875.

Wing, J.K. (1966) Diagnosis, epidemiology, aetiology. In Wing, J.K. (ed.) *Early Childhood Autism*. Pergamon Press, Oxford.

Wing, J.K. (ed.) (1975) *Schizophrenia From Within*. National Schizophrenia Fellowship, London.

Wing, J.K. (1976) Kanner's syndrome. A historical introduction. In Wing, L. (ed.) *Early Childhood Autism*. Pergamon Press, Oxford.

Wing, J.K. (1978) *Reasoning About Madness*. Oxford University Press, Oxford.

Wing, J.K. (1988) Comments on the long-term outcome of schizophrenia. *Schizophrenia Bulletin*, **14**, 669–672.

Wing, J.K. (1991) Social psychiatry. In Bebbington, P.E. (ed.) *Social Psychiatry. Theory, Methodology and Practice*, pp. 3–22. Transaction, New Brunswick.

Wing, J.K. & Brown, G.W. (1961) Social treatment of chronic schizophrenia. A comparative survey of three mental hospitals. *Journal of Mental Science*, **107**, 847–861.

Wing, J.K. & Brown, G.W. (1970) *Institutionalism and Schizophrenia*. Cambridge University Press, Cambridge.

Wing, J.K., Cooper, J.E. & Sartorius, N. (1974) *The Description and Classification of Psychiatric Symptoms. An Instruction Manual for the PSE and CATEGO System*. Cambridge University Press, Cambridge.

Wing, J.K., Sartorius, N. & Üstün, T.B. (In press) *Diagnosis and Clinical Measurement in Psychiatry. The SCAN System*. Cambridge University Press, Cambridge.

Wing, L. (1981) Asperger's syndrome. *Psychological Medicine*, **11**, 115–129.

Wing, L. (1982) Development of concepts, classification and relationship to mental retardation. In Wing, J.K. & Wing, L.G. (eds) *Psychoses of Uncertain Aetiology*, pp. 185–190. Cambridge University Press, Cambridge.

Wing, L. (1993) The definition and prevalence of autism. A review. *European Child and Adolescent Psychiatry*, **2**, 61–74.

Wing, L. & Gould, J. (1979) Severe impairments of social interaction and associated abnormalities in children. Epidemiology and classification. *Journal of Autism and Developmental Disorder*, **9**, 11–29.

Wolff, S. & Chick, J. (1980) Schizoid personality in childhood. A controlled follow-up study. *Psychological Medicine*, **10**, 85–100.

Chapter 2
Descriptive Psychopathology

J. CUTTING

Introduction

In schizophrenia the apparatus of the mind disintegrates, severely and pervasively. It does so, moreover, in such a fashion that an experienced clinician can distinguish the condition from all other psychiatric disorders by the pattern of what is left after the mayhem. What we encounter in an individual suffering from schizophrenia are two sets of features: (i) the absence of certain functions or aspects of the mind which should be present in a normal individual — sometimes called 'negative symptoms'; and (ii) the presence of certain phenomena which are not present in a normal individual, and which probably represent a response of the healthy part of the schizophrenic's mind to the absent functions — sometimes called 'positive symptoms'. Some schizophrenics display only the latter, some only the former, but most display a combination of both.

For practical purposes the descriptive psychopathology of schizophrenia can be treated in three sections:

1 purely positive symptoms — *hallucinations and other abnormal experiences, delusions* and *catatonia*;
2 traditional psychopathological groupings containing positive and negative symptoms — *thought disorder* and *disturbances of emotions*; and
3 what used to be referred to as *psychological deficit*, purely negative symptoms — *impaired attention, intelligence, memory, perception* and *will*.

Neither the positive symptoms (or phenomena) nor the negative symptoms (or signs, because strictly speaking they are things we observe rather than what a patient complains about) exhaust the entire gamut of a schizophrenic's subjective experience or entirely account for all the possible behaviour. The condition has such a pervasive effect on the mind that all aspects are affected, including, for example, an individual's sense of time and appreciation of space. Moreover, schizophrenics may engage in bizarre behaviour which cannot be explained in terms of the categories of negative symptoms listed above.

15

Hallucinations and other abnormal experiences

Definitions and classification

There are four categories of experience within this group of phenomena: anomalous experiences, illusions, hallucinations and pseudohallucinations.

Anomalous experiences, or distortions of a real perceptual experience, are those where a real perception of an object (i.e. the object actually perceived is really there) does not accord with its normal quality. Its colour may be different from usual, its shape may be strange, its size may be smaller or larger than realistically possible or it may be altered in a very subtle way — less or more familiar, less or more distant (or louder or softer in the auditory modality), less or more real or even less or more accentuated relative to the rest of the perceptual environment. None of these experiences is an hallucination, illusion or pseudo-hallucination (see below) because a real object is there, it is recognized as such, but it is merely registered as different from hitherto. Some of the experiences have attracted a specific label, e.g. *déjà vu* for an increase in familiarity, derealization for a loss of the sense of reality and micropsia if the perceived object looks smaller than normal.

Illusions are false perceptual experiences where an object which really exists 'out there' is completely misrecognized as an entirely different class of object, e.g. a moving curtain for a burglar or a rubber band for a snake. It is not an anomalous experience, because it is not a qualitative alteration in the perception of a correctly recognized object, but rather the complete misrecognition of something — the new 'something' looking exactly like a real example of what it would in fact look like. Illusions are mentioned here for completeness, but are not specific or indicative of schizophrenia.

A hallucination is a perception of something when in fact nothing exists in the perceptual field, a perception without an object, in short.

A pseudohallucination is variously defined in the psychopathological literature. One school of thought (Hare, 1973) considers it to be a hallucination with preserved insight. In other words,

I might perceive an elephant in front of me (when none actually exists), and at the same time be aware of the falseness of my perceptual experience, i.e. I know that no elephant is there even though I see it. Another school of thought (Jaspers, 1913) regards it as a hallucination, but one where the hallucinated object lacks the reality of a perception of the same object if it were really there — less vivid, less 'real', etc. This latter school of thought is perhaps a more philosophically correct perspective, because the distinction between a hallucination and a pseudohallucination may be more one of degree, as a careful analysis of most hallucinations (Merleau-Ponty, 1962) will reveal that the apparent object is rarely experienced as 'realistically' as the comparable real object.

Hallucinations themselves are further divided into various types, according to modality, timing with respect to sleep, their occasional precipitation by a sensory stimulus and their content (Table 2.1). There are numerous causes of hallucinations besides schizophrenia (Cutting, 1996).

Incidence and variety in schizophrenia

The incidence of all types of anomalous experiences in schizophrenia is about 50% (Cutting & Dunne, 1989), and of all types of hallucinations about 50%. Visual hallucinations occur in 15% of all subjects, auditory in 50% of all subjects and tactile in 5% of all subjects (Cutting, 1990).

The pattern of the anomalous experiences is very varied. Some examples are shown in Table 2.2. Colours and faces are often the focus of the anomalous experience, but there may be a complete alteration in the quality of the entire environment. This understandably induces a feeling of perplexity in the sufferer, and constitutes what is called delusional mood, because the experiences later solidify as beliefs about what was going on then, e.g. people looking at me in a funny way, etc. The anomalous experiences usually occur at the onset of an episode, and are often forgotten or become delusionally elaborated by the time the patient is interviewed.

The pattern of the hallucinations, on the other hand, is quite specific. The commonest halluci-

Table 2.1 Subtypes of hallucinations

Modality
Visual
Auditory
Olfactory
Gustatory
Tactile, somatic, kinaesthetic

Timing with respect to sleep
Hypnagogic: just before falling asleep
Hypnopompic: on just waking up

Precipitation by sensory stimulus
Synaesthetic: precipitation by sensation in a different
    modality from hallucination (e.g. voice after seeing
    flashing light)
Functional (or reflex): precipitation by sensation in same
    modality (e.g. voice after hearing dripping tap. NB This
    is not an illusion because the dripping tap and the voice
    are *both* heard)

Content
e.g. Musical
Autoscopic
    Of self
Lilliputian
    Smaller than realistic
Teichopsia
    Geometrical shapes, particularly of battlements,
    Characteristic of migraine

Table 2.2 Examples of anomalous experiences in
schizophrenia

Colour
'Colours meant a lot to me . . . stood out, not meant a lot,
especially traffic lights.'

'All bright colours were ones that fråghtened me most —
orange and red.'

Faces/people
'All I could see were people in a car and they looked like
ghosts. They looked different, like statues or monuments,
dead, as if cremated.'

'The right side [in his left field] of my mother's and sister's
faces went completely black. When I looked in the mirror
the right half of my own face [really the left half as it was a
mirror image] also looked black.'

Environment
'I couldn't recognize any of my surroundings — people,
places. I could recognize certain things. I could recognize
qualities of a place, of surfaces. It was the organization of
things which was different.'

'It was like being in one of my paintings [patient was an art
student]. I used to go out and see the houses with
fascination. I would stare out of the window for hours.'

nation is a voice — not just any auditory hallucination, but a voice. Moreover, this voice has
certain characteristics that make it even more
specific for the condition: it is usually heard in a
grammatical form which is different from how we
experience our own thoughts (e.g. instead of
'I wonder what I'm going to have for supper
tonight', the voice says, '*he* is wondering what to
have for supper') and the sex of the voice (male or
female) is nearly always identified, but the owner
of the voice is usually not someone who is known
to the subject. Added to all this is the fact that
schizophrenic voices diminish if there is meaningful conversation going on around, and intensify if
there is no background auditory noise or if the
background noise is devoid of meaning (Margo
et al., 1981). Moreover, schizophrenics with voices
do not differ from schizophrenics without voices
on measures of auditory acuity (Collicutt &
Hemsley, 1981) or imagery (Starker & Jolin,
1982). Typical examples of schizophrenic voices
are: 'He's getting things the wrong way' (presumably referring to how he thought about himself),
'You're not going to smoke the cigarette the way
you want to but the way we want you to.'

Schneider (1958) was so impressed with the
regular occurrence of such 'voices' in schizophrenic patients that he elevated three types to the
rank of first-rank symptoms of the condition:
1 voices speaking thoughts aloud;
2 voices arguing (two or more hallucinatory voices
discussing the person in the third person); and
3 voices commenting on the subject's actions.

Other characteristics of the 'voices' are that
they may be experienced outside the head, but
they are usually poorly localized, and some patients
do not distinguish them completely from their
thoughts, i.e. they fulfil certain criteria for a
pseudohallucination.

Finally, consider this example of ethological research: Green and Preston (1981) applied a throat microphone to one hallucinating schizophrenic, by means of which they picked up the following conversation (supporting the view that 'voices' are subvocalizations of real thoughts experienced by a subject rather than incorrect perceptual accounts of auditory stimuli in their environment). *Voice*, 'Mind your own business darling; I don't want him [referring to the experimenter] to know what I was doing.' When the experimenter asked the subject what was going on, he replied 'See that, I spoke to ask her [the owner of the voice] what she was doing, and she said, mind your own business.'

The pattern of a schizophrenic's visual hallucinations is less well established. Although infrequent, visual hallucinations do occur in a substantial minority of schizophrenics (Guttmann & Maclay, 1937; Feinberg, 1962; Cutting, 1996). They appear to be of things which do not actually exist in the real world, or of part-objects, e.g. leg on a bedroom wall, 'a big animal like an octopus', 'something like a mouse running across the floor', 'mirages of a desert', or 'rat tail coming out of own anus'.

Illusions, in general, are rare, as are pseudo-hallucinations (barring the problem of establishing the strict phenomenological status of schizophrenic 'voices'). Olfactory (Rubert *et al.*, 1961) and gustatory (De Morsier, 1938) hallucinations are also rare. Somatic hallucinations are less rare (Cutting, 1990).

Delusions

Definitions and classification

Various definitions of delusion exist (Schmidt, 1940). Possibly the three best ones are Jaspers' (1913), that of the *Diagnostic and Statistical Manual* DSM-III-R (APA, 1987) and Spitzer's (1990).

Jaspers' definition proposed three criteria: (i) it is a belief held with extraordinary conviction, with an incomparable subjective certainty; (ii) there is an imperviousness to other experiences and to compelling counterargument; and (iii) the content is impossible.

That in DSM-III-R is:

A false personal belief based on incorrect inference about external reality and firmly sustained in spite of what almost everyone else believes and in spite of what constitutes incontrovertible and obvious proof or evidence to the contrary. The belief is not one ordinarily accepted by other members of the person's culture or sub-culture (i.e. it is not an article of religious faith). When a false belief involves an extreme value judgement, it is regarded as a delusion only when the judgement is so extreme as to defy credibility.

Spitzer defines delusion as follows:

X's statement is a delusion if it concerns the world, and is not an analytic statement (i.e. a linguistic tautology), and it is held with a subjective certainty only appropriate for statements about the mind.

The main differences between these definitions are Jaspers' emphasis on the inappropriate conviction, DSM-III-R's mapping of the social context in which the delusion has to be placed, and Spitzer's restriction to a concern with the world (rather than self, body or mind). Given the complexity of the topic, all three definitions should be taken into account for their respective insights.

Delusions are currently classified according to four independent principles:

1 degree of inexplicability, e.g. primary;
2 nature of subverted mental function, e.g. delusional perception;
3 nosological significance, i.e. the extent to which the delusional state has been accorded independent status from the three major psychoses, e.g. sensitive delusion of reference; and
4 thematic content, e.g. jealousy.

These four classificatory systems are summarized in Table 2.3, along with a fifth system (Cutting, 1996) which groups the themes in a more logical way.

Incidence and variety in schizophrenia

Delusions occur at some stage of the condition in more than 90% of schizophrenics.

Concerning the various types of delusions cat-

Table 2.3 Classification of delusions

According to degree of inexplicability
Primary, pure, true
Secondary, delusion-like ideas
Overvalued idea

According to subverted mental function
Delusional perception
Delusional notion
Delusional memory
Delusional awareness
Delusional atmosphere/mood

According to degree of independent nosological status, e.g.
Paranoia
Delusional loving (de Clérambault's syndrome)
Monosymptomatic hypochondriacal psychosis

According to thematic content (traditional), e.g.
Lycanthropy (transformation into an animal)
Jealousy
Grandiosity
Influence/control

According to thematic content (logical, comprehensive,
   mutually exclusive)
Concerning the world
   Altered identity/class of things, e.g. Capgras' syndrome
   Altered quality, e.g. spouse unfaithful
   Altered chronicle of events, e.g. world going to blow up
   Altered evaluation, e.g. persecutory
   Altered self-reference, e.g. reference
   Nihilism, e.g. spouse dead
Concerning the mind
   Altered boundaries, e.g. thought broadcasting
   Altered function, e.g. cannot think
   Altered autonomy, e.g. thought insertion
Concerning the self
   Altered identity, e.g. X = Napoleon
   Altered ability, e.g. X is spiritual healer
   Altered autonomy, e.g. someone taken X over
   Altered evaluation, e.g. guilt
Concerning the body
   Altered structure, e.g. no brain
   Altered function, e.g. bowels do not work
   Altered autonomy, e.g. X's sensations are not X's

egorized in Table 2.3, some are more common than others and some have been elevated to the status of diagnostic criteria for schizophrenia.

Jaspers (1913) believed that primary delusions were pathognomonic of schizophrenia. In addition to the three properties that he believed belonged to any delusion — conviction, imperviousness to other experiences and impossibility of content — primary delusions possessed the further properties of 'ununderstandability', 'being unmediated by thought' and 'involvement of the whole personality' (Walker, 1991).

Schneider (1958) was unhappy with this general formulation because of the practical problems of establishing whether a delusion fulfilled these latter three criteria. Only in the case of delusional perception, according to Schneider, could the psychiatrist be sure that 'some abnormal significance ... were attached ... without any comprehensible rational or emotional justification'. This, according to Schneider, was because a two-stage process was involved: a normal perception and then an 'irrational and emotionally incomprehensible ... delusional course'.

As well as delusional perception, Schneider also elevated certain delusional themes to the status of first-rank symptoms — the common denominator of which is a loss of autonomy or boundaries in the spheres of body, self or mind. These are usually regarded as seven in number (Table 2.4). More recent formulations (e.g. Research Diagnostic Criteria (RDC), Carpenter *et al.*, 1973; Spitzer *et al.*, 1975; DSM-III-R) recognize the fact that deluded schizophrenics *may not have* such first-rank symptoms but manics *may have* them, and give the following categories of delusion equal diagnostic significance — bizarre, multiple or widespread (involving more than one area of life). Of the themes listed in Table 2.3, the most diagnosis-specific in schizophrenia, relative to manics and psychotic depressives (all diagnosed by non-delusional criteria), were (McGilchrist & Cutting, 1995; Cutting, 1996) altered bodily structure, altered bodily autonomy, altered boundaries of mind, altered autonomy of mind and altered identity of the world.

Catatonia

Definition and classification

Catatonia refers to a set of complex movements,

Table 2.4 Characteristic schizophrenic delusions

Delusional perception	Normal perception has private and illogical meaning
Thought withdrawal	Thoughts cease and are simultaneously experienced as removed by external force
Thought insertion	Thoughts have a quality of not being own and are ascribed to external agency
Thought broadcasting	Thoughts escape into outside world where they are experienced by others
Made feelings	Feelings do not seem to be own, but are attributable to external force
Made impulses	Drive or impulse seems to be alien and external
Made volitional acts	Actions and movements felt to be under outside control
Somatic passivity	Experience of bodily sensations imposed by external agency
Bizarre delusions	e.g. parents exist in another time and place
Multiple delusions	e.g. nurses are Japanese, mirrors reflect the wrong way, haloperidol is made from shark's pancreas
Widespread delusions	e.g. husband acted in a sexually indiscrete way at a party, earthquake happening, grandson seriously ill

Table 2.5 Catatonic phenomena

Stupor	Virtual absence of movement and speech in the presence of full consciousness
Catalepsy	Maintenance of unusual postures for long periods of time and no sense of discomfort, often accompanied by waxy flexibility (external manipulation of limb as though made of wax)
Automatism	Automatic obedience to commands, regardless of consequence
Mannerisms	Peculiar social habits, e.g. style of dress, handshake, writing or speech, at variance with social setting
Stereotypies	Repetitive movements of a single part of the body, divorced from mainstream of bodily activities
Posturing and grimacing	Peculiar positions of body (posturing) or face (grimacing) inappropriate to mainstream activity and social situation
Negativism	Behaviour which is consistently in opposition to social and apparent individual demands of a situation
Echopraxia	Automatic repetition of visually perceived actions of others

Incidence and variety in schizophrenia

According to the International Pilot Study of Schizophrenia (WHO, 1973), 7% of 811 schizophrenics exhibited one or other phenomenon. Other estimates (Morrison, 1973; Guggenheim & Barbigian, 1974) also gave a figure of between 5 and 10%. According to Abrams and Taylor (1976), mannerisms are commonest, followed, in descending order of frequency, by stereotypies, stupor, negativism, automatism and echopraxia.

Mannerisms, stereotype, negativism, catalepsy, automatism and posturing or grimacing are most specifically linked with schizophrenia. Stupor is more commonly linked with depressive psychosis or brain-stem lesions (Johnson, 1984; Barnes et al., 1986). Echopraxia is also seen in cases with frontal lobe lesions (Lhermitte et al., 1986). Abrams and Taylor (1976) claimed that all

postures and actions whose common denominator is their involuntariness (Table 2.5). Not all involuntary movements fall within the category of catatonia; tics, chorea, dyskinesia, athetosis and ballismus are involuntary but not catatonic. It is partly convention and partly complexity that allocates certain movements or postures to the category. They are a heterogeneous bunch, ranging from a peculiar way of holding the head (posturing) to the entire annihilation of free will (as in negativism).

varieties of catatonia could occur in mania, but this is not my experience.

There is evidence that catatonic phenomena have diminished in frequency since Kraepelin's turn-of-the-century estimate of 20% in his series of patients with dementia praecox. There is also evidence that they are more common in schizophrenics from developing countries (WHO, 1973).

Nowadays, there is a tendency to lump catatonic phenomena with other involuntary movements such as tics, dyskinesia and chorea, and to deny them special status in schizophrenics (Rogers, 1985).

Thought disorder

Definitions and classification

The term thought disorder covers a variety of positive *and* negative symptoms of schizophrenia, and is largely a misnomer because much of what is traditionally referred to as thought disorder is a disorder of spoken language.

The various components are set out in Table 2.6. The first distinction, identified by Schilder

Table 2.6 Components of thought disorder

Disorder of content, i.e. delusion including delusions about the autonomy of a subject's own thought processes, e.g. thought insertion

Disorder of form, i.e. formal thought disorder
Disorder of the mechanisms of thinking as characterized descriptively (intrinsic thinking disturbance, dyslogia)
  Concrete thinking
  Loosening of associations
  Overinclusion
  Illogicality
Disorder of language and speech
  Derailment, tangentiality, Knight's move thinking
  Neologisms
  Poverty of speech (alogia)
  Poverty of content of speech
  Incoherence
  Pressure of speech
  Flight of ideas
  Retarded speech, mutism

(1920), is between *disordered content* and *disordered form*. The former is synonymous with delusion. The latter comprises two categories (Andreasen, 1982a; Cutting & Murphy, 1988): (i) an intrinsic disturbance of thinking itself; and (ii) disordered language and speech.

The intrinsic disturbance of thinking includes such inferred and hypothetical descriptive notions as concrete thinking, overinclusion, illogicality and loosening of associations. *Concrete thinking* is a tendency to select one aspect of a thing or concept, usually a physical quality or a personal association, at the expense of its overall meaning. It is traditionally tested by proverb interpretation, a concrete response being one which fails to take proper account of the metaphorical nature of proverbs. *Overinclusion* is the tendency to include false or irrelevant items in a concept or category, in other words, to inappropriately widen the boundaries of a concept or category. It is sometimes assessed in the course of an object-sorting task, an overinclusive response being one which incorporates too many or inappropriate items within a category. *Illogicality* is a tendency to offer bizarre explanations for things and events, explanations which not only grossly contravene the laws of logic, but also the 'way of the world'. It is traditionally tested by inviting a subject to complete a syllogism (e.g. if all alligators are reptiles, and some reptiles are green, then are all alligators green? True or false?). *Loosening of associations* is sometimes used as a synonym for derailment (see below), in which case it refers to a disorder in the form of spoken speech. In the present context it carries the meaning of a disordered conceptual structure, as illustrated by the reply of a schizophrenic subject to one of the questions in the similarities subscale of the Wechsler Adult Intelligence Scale: in what way are an orange and a banana alike? They are Nature's produce! This is not wrong, just loose. Note that the traditional tests for these thinking disorders are not good at discriminating schizophrenics from normals, with significant numbers of the latter overlapping with the former.

Disordered language and speech is usually held to contain the following main varieties. First, there is *derailment* or tangentiality or knight's move thinking — a failure to conform to the social rules of conversation and the needs of a listener by picking up on personal or idiosyncratic aspects of a word or phrase and not sticking to the overall theme of the discourse. Next there is *neologisms*, the creation of new words, subsuming an allied phenomenon, word approximations or paraphasia, where recognized words are given a new meaning. Then there is *poverty of speech*, which is a grossly reduced output of speech, and *poverty of content of speech*, where despite an adequate fluency the number of ideas expressed is substantially reduced. *Incoherence* refers to a breakdown in the grammatical structure of what is expressed, sometimes to such an extent that the speech resembles aphasia — hence schizophasia or 'word salad'. *Pressure of speech* is a speeding-up of the flow of speech; *flight of ideas* is a combination of pressure of speech and derailment; and *retardation*, of which *mutism* is an extreme form, is self-explanatory.

Two alternative classifications are in use, one theoretical (Chaika, 1990) and one practical (Andreasen, 1979a). Chaika proposes four levels in the breakdown of language, each responsible for some of the traditional clinical varieties. Level 1, the subtlest disorder, affects the richness of expression of ideas, of which poverty of content of speech is an example. At level 2, there is an internal lack of coherence in the construction of sentences, illustrated by derailment. By level 3, the conventionally agreed shared meanings of words is dispensed with, hence neologisms. Finally, at level 4, even the conventional rules of grammar disappear, and the utterance becomes an unintelligible jumble — incoherence.

Some items of thought disorder are regarded as positive symptoms of schizophrenia, e.g. derailment and illogicality; others are regarded as negative symptoms, e.g. poverty of speech. Several schedules for the assessment of the various types exist and the most useful of these are reviewed in Cutting (1994).

Incidence and variety in schizophrenia

Andreasen's (1979a) study on the incidence of 18 varieties of thought disorder in schizophrenics

and manics still provides the best picture of its incidence and specificity in schizophrenia. Cutting and Murphy (1988) studied the incidence of four types of intrinsic thinking disturbance, and had neurotic controls, not manics.

In Andreasen's study, derailment (56%) was the commonest variety in schizophrenia, but did not significantly distinguish this group from manics, whereas poverty of content of speech (40% schizophrenics, 19% manics) did discriminate the two diagnostic groups. Pressure of speech (27% schizophrenics, 72% manics) was another significant discriminator. Neologisms (2% schizophrenics) were rare.

Cutting and Murphy found that a loosening of associations (based on impaired ability to appreciate conceptual similarities) occurred in 5% of schizophrenics, overinclusion (based on the number of category inclusions of items ranging from appropriate to inappropriate) occurred in 25% of schizophrenics, concrete thinking (rated as concreteness in proverb interpretation) occurred in none of 20 schizophrenics, and illogicality (false conclusions in syllogisms) occurred in 10% of schizophrenics. All figures refer to the proportion of subjects falling outside of two standard deviations from the control mean.

Examples of the main varieties encountered in schizophrenia are shown in Table 2.7. Four of the five examples given — loosening of associations, incoherence, poverty of content of speech and illogicality — are the only varieties of thought disorder considered to have diagnostic specificity in DSM-III-R.

Disturbance of emotion

Definitions and classification

Emotion is a general term covering *feelings* ('individual unique and radical commotions of the psyche' [Jaspers, 1913]), *affect* ('a momentary and complex emotional process of great intensity with conspicuous bodily accompaniment and sequelae' [Jaspers, 1913]) and *mood* ('states of feeling or frames of mind that come about with prolonged emotion' [Jaspers, 1913]). Philosophers such as

Table 2.7 Examples of thought disorder in schizophrenia

Derailment

'Mum loves God. She always compares me with God. I want to know if there are any eggs in my ovaries.'

'They were frightening me about wishes and when I was 20 I blew out a candle and I was frightened of my mother.'

Incoherence

'That is when God pardoned the GP at 9.30 this morning, the catching of an instant philosophically speaking into time that only occurs at both at death turkeys in the freezer.'

'To do to ask is at the behest of my parents which seems a fairly inappropriate reason to me.'

Neologisms/word approximations

'Oumana'	God's love beyond me
'Cytic'	Extrasensory perception
'I froze people out'	Made them older
'Medetary'	Smoked cannabis because it was good for him
'Criton'	Something which expresses sexual identity
'Psycasm'	Like a Lucky Strike cigarette

Poverty of content of speech

'I asked for pudding. I wanted to get a pudding. I accepted the pudding. I brought the pudding to the room. I ate the pudding. I am an affair of certain self-fermenting proteins catalysing their own growth. I am certainly not going to accept a continuous adjustment of internal to external relations.'

'I need to see the appropriatedness of today.'

Illogicality

'I went through the colour black in quite an easy task.'

'In my mind the kissing and cuddling in 1960 makes it rain in 1980.'

'I want to have a haircut because there's no oxygen on the ward.'

Table 2.8 Disturbances of emotion

Normal aspects	Main psychopathological varieties
Feeling	Loss of feeling — anhedonia Heightened feeling
Affect	Inappropriate affect Flattened, blunting of, affect
Mood	Depression Elation Anxiety
Motivation	Apathy

Feelings, affect, mood and motivation all have their psychopathological counterparts (Table 2.8), and examples from all four categories can be encountered in schizophrenia. Only one type — inappropriate affect — is generally held to be a positive symptom of schizophrenia, whereas several — blunting (or flattening) of affect, anhedonia (loss of feeling) and apathy (loss of motivation) — are regarded as negative symptoms.

Incidence and variety in schizophrenia

Anhedonia (loss of feeling) is sometimes divided into social, e.g. loss of pleasure from being with friends, and physical, e.g. loss of pleasure from seeing a beautiful sunset, being massaged, drinking, etc. It can be rated using a questionnaire (Chapman *et al.*, 1980) or at interview (Harrow *et al.*, 1977). Using the questionnaire of Chapman *et al.*, Watson *et al.* (1979) found that 45% of 312 schizophrenics fell outside the 90th percentile of alcoholic controls, although Cook and Simukonda (1981), who used the same questionnaire, found only 34% of 52 schizophrenics fell outside one standard deviation of nurses; social anhedonia accounted for most of this. Schuck *et al.* (1984) also found that physical anhedonia was no more prevalent in schizophrenics than in depressives. Harrow *et al.* (1977) found that only chronic, not acute, schizophrenics were significantly anhedonic.

Intensification of feelings is reported at the onset of schizophrenia, but there are no adequate studies

Jaspers and Wittgenstein (1980) emphasize the fact that emotion is an experience. Other philosophers (e.g. Ryle, 1949) and behaviourist psychologists (e.g. Izard & Buechler, 1980) emphasize the *motivational* aspect of emotion.

of the topic. A patient of McGhie and Chapman (1961), for example, recalled:

> You have no idea what it's like doctor. You would have to experience it yourself. When you feel yourself going into a sort of coma you get really scared. It's like waiting on a landing craft going into D-Day. You tremble and panic. It's like no other fear on earth.

Inappropriate affect or parathymia is the display of an emotion considered inappropriate to the situation. It is usually an outburst of empty giggling and occurs in about 20% of acutely ill schizophrenics (Andreasen, 1979b).

Flattening of affect or blunted affect can be observed in about 50% of acute (Andreasen, 1979b) or chronic schizophrenics (McCreadie, 1982). According to Andreasen, it is a composite rating by an observer of the following elements, in descending order of weighted significance: paucity of expressive gestures (57%), unchanging facial expression (53%), lack of vocal inflection (53%), decreased spontaneous movement (37%), poor eye contact (37%), affective non-responsivity (30%), slowed speech (17%) and increased latency of response (10%).

Depression is a non-specific accompaniment of schizophrenia. It is much more frequent in acute schizophrenia (70% — neurotic depression in *Catego* [Wing *et al.*, 1974] — Knights & Hirsch, 1981) than expected, although probably not much higher in chronic schizophrenia (clinical depression [10%] Barnes *et al.*, 1989) than in the normal population. The relationship between depression and schizophrenia is more complicated than these bare figures indicate. There is the diagnostic dilemma to consider: do you exclude patients with 'first — rank symptoms of schizophrenia' from the category of depressive psychosis even if they fulfil all other criteria for this? According to Hirsch (1982), depression and schizophrenia both arise from a 'shared pathophysiological mechanism', and depression is 'revealed' as an integral part of schizophrenia in so far as it does not become obvious until after the acute phase has subsided, although the symptoms of depression are indeed most prevalent in the acute phase if systematically rated (Knights &

Hirsch, 1981). According to Crow (1986), who revives Griesinger's (1845) unitary psychosis theory, depression and schizophrenia are only far ends of the same spectrum. According to Galdi (1983), depression is increased by the use of neuroleptics. According to McGlashan and Carpenter (1976), remitted schizophrenics experience more depression as part of a recovery of insight into what they have been through.

Elation is also a non-specific accompaniment of schizophrenia, but may complicate the diagnostic issue in the same way as depression, as discussed above.

Anxiety is particularly marked at the outset, but is pathologically absent in the chronic stages.

Apathy is the most troublesome negative symptom of all (at least for carers of the sufferer). Although regarded as the psychopathological counterpart of the motivational component of emotion, it is, in my view, better regarded as a manifestation of impaired will in the condition, and will be discussed below. Its mention here is justified because most psychologists and many psychiatrists regard motivation as an aspect of emotion.

Psychological deficit

The terms dementia praecox, deterioration, defect state and pseudodementia have all been applied to the combination of impaired attention, apparent decline in intelligence, failures in memory, perceptual impoverishment and lack of will. The individual components are also referred to as psychological deficits or negative symptoms.

Attentional impairment

There is a large body of literature demonstrating that attention, particularly maintenance of attention, is impaired in schizophrenia (e.g. Asarnow & MacCrimmon, 1978; Van den Bosch, 1982). The various components of attention — maintenance, selectivity, span, shifting of focus — are not equally affected, and the brunt is borne by maintenance, shifting, span and selectivity in that order of severity.

Intellectual decline

Numerous studies have shown a decline in formally measured intelligence from a prepsychotic state to psychosis (Rappaport & Webb, 1950) and, further, from acute to chronic psychosis (Trapp & James, 1937). The intellectual decline affects all subtests of the Wechsler Adult Intelligence Scale, but particularly the performance subtests, and particularly digit symbol and picture arrangement (Cutting, 1990). There is growing evidence, and some controversy, that schizophrenics have a particular profile of intellectual decline, relative to Alzheimer's disease (see Chapter 10).

Memory failures

Although amnesia is traditionally regarded as a symptom of organic psychosis and should not, according to this view, be prominent in a functional psychosis such as schizophrenia, there is increasing evidence that chronic schizophrenics do have a pervasive disturbance of memory. McKenna *et al.* (1990) demonstrated that the memory impairment in chronic schizophrenics was equivalent to a group of patients with definite brain injury (see Chapter 10).

Perceptual impoverishment

Schizophrenics turn away from the outside world and become preoccupied with their own subjective state (Sass, 1992), and it is difficult to assess the patency of the actual perceptual processes. There is ample evidence that their perception of the world differs qualitatively from that of a normal person (Cutting, 1990); this, in consequence, leads to an impoverishment in their appreciation of the outside world.

Lack of will

Chronic schizophrenics suffer from a profound apathy, sometimes known as abulia, and this stems from a fundamental deficiency in the mainspring of their life. Kraepelin (1913) considered this their essential psychological problem. Unfortunately, the term 'will' has fallen into disuse for most of this century and there have been no experimental studies to assess the significance of Kraepelin's views.

Clustering of phenomena/symptoms

There is no shortage of attempts to classify the above psychopathological features of schizophrenia.

Bleuler (1911) proposed a distinction between 'fundamental symptoms', those which were virtually pathognomonic, and 'accessory symptoms', those which occurred in other conditions as well. The former comprised disturbances of association and affectivity, ambivalence and autism. The latter included delusions, alterations in personality, speech and writing disorders and catatonia.

Schneider (1958) proposed a distinction between first-rank symptoms (see Table 2.4) and other symptoms, regarding the former as atheoretical diagnostic aids.

Andreasen (1982b) and Crow (1980) adapted Hughlings Jackson's formulation of positive and negative symptoms as applied to neurological disorders to schizophrenia, and this has proved, in my view, one of the most useful classifications of phenomena. Andreasen recognizes five categories of negative symptoms: affective flattening, attentional impairment, alogia (poverty of speech), avolition (apathy), and anhedonia (asociality). Hallucinations, delusions, bizarre behaviour and certain instances of thought disorder (derailment, flight of ideas, illogicality) are the positive symptoms.

Liddle (1987) identified three statistical clusters of symptoms, calling them the psychomotor poverty syndrome (poverty of speech, flattened affect and decreased spontaneous movement), the disorganization syndrome (formal thought disorder and inappropriate affect) and the reality distortion syndrome (delusions and hallucinations).

Huber *et al.* (1980) divided symptoms into 'characteristic schizophrenic deficiency' types and 'non-characteristic'. The former included what he called 'coenaesthetic symptoms', body hallucinations and the latter such complaints as 'reduced capacity for adaptation'.

All such classifications can be criticized on the grounds of either reliability or validity, and their usefulness will almost certainly be undermined or corroborated by neurobiological advances over the next decade or so.

Explanatory theories

Explanatory theories for schizophrenic phenomena abound (Cutting, 1985). It may be that all these are so closely attached to a psychological theory of the mind that subsequent generations, who eschew that particular theory, will have to grasp the schizophrenic experience afresh. The best modern account is actually given in a book that relates schizophrenia to the artistic history of the last century — *Madness and Modernism* (Sass, 1992) — emphasizing that the 'descriptive' psychopathology of schizophrenia is still a powerful source of information for all those interested in the workings of the mind in 'normals', as well as for those endeavouring to understand the nature and cause of schizophrenia.

References

Abrams, R. & Taylor, M.A. (1976) Catatonia. *Archives of General Psychiatry*, 33, 579–581.

Andreasen, N.C. (1979a) Thought, language and communication disorders. *Archives of General Psychiatry*, 36, 1315–1330.

Andreasen, N.C. (1979b) Affective flattening and the criteria for schizophrenia. *American Journal of Psychiatry*, 136, 944–947.

Andreasen, N.C. (1982a) Should the term 'thought disorder' be revised? *Comprehensive Psychiatry*, 23, 291–299.

Andreasen, N.C. (1982b) Negative symptoms in schizophrenia. *Archives of General Psychiatry*, 39, 784–788.

APA (1987) *Diagnostic and Statistical Manual of Mental Disorders*, 3rd edn. American Psychiatric Association, Washington DC.

Asarnow, R.F. & MacCrimmon, D.J. (1978) Residual performance deficit in clinically remitted schizophrenics: a marker of schizophrenia? *Journal of Abnormal Psychology*, 87, 597–608.

Barnes, M.P., Saunders, M., Walls, T.J., Saunders, I. & Kirk, C.A. (1986) The syndrome of Karl Ludwig Kahlbaum. *Journal of Neurology, Neurosurgery and Psychiatry*, 49, 991–996.

Barnes, T.R.E., Curson, D.A., Liddle, P.F. & Patel, M. (1989) The nature and prevalence of depression in chronic schizophrenic in-patients. *British Journal of Psychiatry*, 154, 486–491.

Bleuler, E. (1911) *Dementia Praecox*. International University Press, New York. Translated by Zinkin, J. (1950) from *Dementia Praecox oder die Gruppe der Schizophrenien*. Deuticke, Leipzig.

Carpenter, W.T., Strauss, J.S. & Bartko, J.J. (1973) Flexible system for the diagnosis of schizophrenia. *Science*, 182, 1275–1278.

Chaika, E. (1990) *Understanding Psychotic Speech: Beyond Freud and Chomsky*. Charles C. Thomas, Springfield.

Chapman, L.J., Chapman, J.P. & Raulin, M.L. (1980) Scales for physical and social anhedonia. *Journal of Abnormal Psychology*, 85, 374–382.

Collicutt, J.R. & Hemsley, D.R. (1981) A psychophysical investigation of auditory functioning in schizophrenia. *British Journal of Social and Clinical Psychology*, 20, 199–204.

Cook, M. & Simukonda, F. (1981) Anhedonia and schizophrenia. *British Journal of Psychiatry*, 139, 523–525.

Crow, T.J. (1980) Molecular pathology of schizophrenia: more than one disease process? *British Medical Journal*, i, 66–68.

Crow, T.J. (1986) The continuum of psychosis and its implications for the structure of the gene. *British Journal of Psychiatry*, 149, 419–429.

Cutting, J. (1985) *The Psychology of Schizophrenia*. Churchill Livingstone, Edinburgh.

Cutting, J. (1990) *The Right Cerebral Hemisphere and Psychiatric Disorders*. Oxford University Press, Oxford.

Cutting, J. (1994) The assessment of thought disorder. In Barnes, T. & Nelson, H. (eds) *Assessment of Psychosis: A Practical Handbook*. Farrand Press, London.

Cutting, J. (1996) *Two Worlds, Two Minds, Two Hemispheres: A Reinterpretation of Psychopathology*. Oxford University Press, Oxford.

Cutting, J. & Dunne, F. (1989) Subjective experience of schizophrenia. *Schizophrenia Bulletin*, 15, 217–231.

Cutting, J. & Murphy, D. (1988) Schizophrenia thought disorder. *British Journal of Psychiatry*, 152, 310–319.

De Morsier, G. (1938) Les hallucinations. *Revue d'Oto'neuro-ophthalmologie*, 16, 241–252.

Feinberg, I. (1962) A comparison of the visual hallucinations in schizophrenia with those induced by mescaline and LSD-25. In West, L.J. (ed.) *Hallucinations*, pp. 64–76. Grune & Stratton, New York.

Galdi, J. (1983) The causality of depression in schizophrenia. *British Journal of Psychiatry*, 142, 621–625.

Green, P. & Preston, M. (1981) Reinforcement of vocal correlates of auditory hallucinations by auditory feedback. *British Journal of Psychiatry*, 139, 204–208.

Griesinger, W. (1845) *Mental Pathology and Therapeutics*. New Sydenham Society, London. Translated (1867) from *Die Pathologie und Therapie der Psychischen Krankheiten*. Krabbe, Stuttgart.

Guggenheim, F.G. & Barbigian, H.M. (1974) Catatonic schizophrenia: epidemiology and clinical course. *Journal of Nervous and Mental Diseases*, 158, 291–305.

Guttmann, E. & Maclay, W.S. (1937) Clinical observations on schizophrenic drawings. *British Journal of Medical Psychology*, 16, 184–205.

Hare, E.H. (1973) A short note on pseudohallucinations. *British Journal of Psychiatry*, 122, 469–476.

Harrow, M., Grinker, R.R., Holzman, P.S. & Kayton, L.

(1977) Anhedonia and schizophrenia. *American Journal of Psychiatry*, **134**, 794–797.

Hirsch, S.R. (1982) Depression 'revealed' in schizophrenia. *British Journal of Psychiatry*, **140**, 421–424.

Huber, G., Gross, G., Schuttler, R. & Linz, M. (1980) Longitudinal studies of schizophrenic patients. *Schizophrenia Bulletin*, **6**, 592–605.

Izard, C.E. & Buechler, S. (1980) Aspects of consciousness and personality in terms of differential emotions theory. In Plutchik, R. & Kellerman, H. (eds) *Emotion; Theory, Research and Experience*, Vol. 1, pp. 165–187. Academic Press, New York.

Jaspers, K. (1913) *General Psychopathology*. Manchester University Press, Manchester. Translated by Hoenig, J. & Hamilton, M.W. (1963) from *Allgemeine Psychopathologie*. Springer Verlag, Berlin.

Johnson, J. (1984) Stupor and akinetic mutism. In Harrison, M.J.G. (ed.) *Contemporary Neurology*, pp. 96–102. Butterworths, London.

Knights, A. & Hirsch, S.R. (1981) 'Revealed' depression and drug treatment of schizophrenia. *Archives of General Psychiatry*, **38**, 806–811.

Kraepelin, E. (1913) *Psychiatrie*, 8th edn, Vol. 3, Part 2. Churchill Livingstone, Edinburgh. Translated by Barclay, R.M. (1919) as *Dementia Praecox and Paraphrenia*.

Lhermitte, F., Pillon, B. & Serdaru, M. (1986) Human autonomy and the frontal lobes. I. Imitation and utilization behaviour, a neuropsychological study of 75 patients. *Annals of Neurology*, **19**, 326–334.

Liddle, P.F. (1987) Schizophrenic syndromes, cognitive performance and neurological dysfunction. *Psychological Medicine*, **17**, 49–57.

McCreadie, R.G. (1982) The Nithsdale schizophrenia survey. I. Psychiatric and social handicaps. *British Journal of Psychiatry*, **140**, 582–586.

McGhie, A. & Chapman, J. (1961) Disorders of attention and perception in early schizophrenia. *British Journal of Medical Psychology*, **34**, 103–115.

McGilchrist, I. & Cutting, J. (1994) Bodily delusions. *British Journal of Psychiatry* (in press).

McGlashan, T.H. & Carpenter, W.T. (1976) Postpsychotic depression in schizophrenia. *Archives of General Psychiatry*, **33**, 231–239.

McKenna, P.J., Tamlyn, D., Lund, C.E., Mortimer, A.M., Hammond, S. & Baddeley, A.D. (1990) Amnesic syndrome in schizophrenia. *Psychological Medicine*, **20**, 967–972.

Margo, A., Hemsley, D.R. & Slade, P.D. (1981) The effects of varying auditory input on schizophrenic hallucinations. *British Journal of Psychiatry*, **139**, 122–127.

Merleau-Ponty, M. (1962) *Phenomenology of Perception*. Routledge & Kegal Paul, London.

Morrison, J.R. (1973) Catatonia: retarded and excited types. *Archives of General Psychiatry*, **28**, 39–41.

Rappaport, S.R. & Webb, W.B. (1950) An attempt to study intellectual deterioration by premorbid and psychotic testing. *Journal of Consulting Psychology*, **14**, 95–98.

Rogers, D. (1985) The motor disorders of severe psychiatric illness: a conflict of paradigms. *British Journal of Psychiatry*, **147**, 221–232.

Rubert, S.L., Hollender, M.H. & Mehrhof, E.G. (1961) Olfactory hallucinations. *Archives of General Psychiatry*, **5**, 313–318.

Ryle, G. (1949) *The Concept of Mind*. Penguin, Harmondsworth.

Sass, L.A. (1992) *Madness and Modernism*. Basic Books, New York.

Schilder, P. (1920) On the development of thoughts. In Rappaport, D. (ed.) *Organisation and Pathology of Thought*, pp. 497–518. Columbia University Press, New York. Translated by Rappaport, D. (1951).

Schmidt, G. (1940) A review of the German literature on delusion between 1914 and 1939. In Cutting, J. & Shepherd, M. (eds) (1987) *The Clinical Roots of the Schizophrenia Concept*, pp. 104–134. Cambridge University Press, Cambridge. Translated by Marshall, H. from Der Wahn in deutschsprachigen Schriftum der letzten 25 Jahre (1914–1939). *Zentrulblatt für die gesamte Neurologie und Psychiatrie*, **97**, 113–143.

Schneider, K. (1958) *Clinical Psychopathology*. Translated by Hamilton, M.W. (1959). Grune & Stratton, New York.

Schuck, J., Leventhal, D., Rothstein, H. & Irizarry, V. (1984) Physical anhedonia and schizophrenia. *Journal of Abnormal Psychology*, **93**, 342–344.

Spitzer, M. (1990) On defining delusions. *Comprehensive Psychiatry*, **31**, 377–397.

Spitzer, R.L., Endicott, J. & Robins, E. (1975) *Research Diagnostic Criteria*. New York State Psychiatric Institute, New York.

Starker, S. & Jolin, A. (1982) Imagery and hallucinations in schizophrenic patients. *Journal of Nervous and Mental Diseases*, **170**, 448–451.

Trapp, C.E. & James, E.B. (1937) Comparative intelligence ratings on the four types of dementia praecox. *Journal of Nervous and Mental Diseases*, **86**, 399–404.

Van den Bosch, R.J. (1982) *Attentional Correlates of Schizophrenia and Related Disorders*. Lisse, Swets & Zeitlinger,

Walker, C. (1991) Delusion: What did Jaspers really say? *British Journal of Psychiatry*, **159**, (Suppl. 14), 94–103.

Watson, C.G., Jacobs, L. & Kucala, T. (1979) A note on the pathology of anhedonia. *Journal of Clinical Psychology*, **35**, 740–743.

WHO (1973) *Report of the International Pilot Study of Schizophrenia*, Vol. 1. World Health Organization, Geneva.

Wing, J.K., Cooper, J.E. & Sartorius, N. (1974) *Measurement and Classification of Psychiatric Symptoms*. Cambridge University Press, Cambridge.

Wittgenstein, L. (1980) *Remarks on the Philosophy of Psychology*. Basil Blackwell, Oxford.

Chapter 3
Positive and Negative Symptoms

N. C. ANDREASEN, M.-A. ROY AND M. FLAUM

Introduction

The terms 'positive' and 'negative' were first applied to symptoms of brain disorders by two 19th-century English physicians, Reynolds and Jackson (Berrios, 1985). Using epilepsy as a model, Jackson hypothesized that the florid symptoms of insanity, such as delusions or hallucinations, reflected normal underlying brain processes that had been disinhibited as a result of a pathological insult to a higher level of brain functioning. 'Dissolution' of higher cortical processes resulted in negative symptoms, which were therefore conceptualized as primary. Reynolds had emphasized the distinction between positive and negative symptoms some years earlier, but without positing a hierarchical or functional relationship. While many of the pioneers of psychiatric phenomenology clearly recognized the importance of negative symptoms, they did not necessarily use these explicit terms. For example, Kraepelin wrote extensively about avolition and affective flattening as central and defining features of dementia praecox (Kraepelin et al., 1919). Bleuler included affective flattening, ambivalence and autism among his list of 'fundamental symptoms' of schizophrenia. Interest in negative symptoms waned in the 1950s and 1960s for a variety of reasons. Foremost among these was Schneider's influential contention that certain positive symptoms, which he referred to as 'first-rank symptoms', were highly specific, if not pathognomonic, of schizophrenia (Schneider, 1959).

Interest in negative symptoms re-emerged in the 1970s, as exemplified by the work of Strauss and Carpenter (1974) and Andreasen (1979a–c). Perhaps the watershed contribution came from the work of Crow who, in 1980, proposed a new typology for schizophrenia based on the positive and negative symptom dichotomy (Crow, 1980; Crow et al., 1981). The primary symptoms of the positive (or type I) subtype were hallucinations and delusions; Crow posited that the underlying pathophysiological mechanism for this subtype was a biochemical imbalance, such as an excess of dopamine D_2 receptors. Therefore, he hypothesized that the resulting clinical manifestations would be more likely to respond favourably to antipsychotic medication, to be characterized by exacerbations and remissions and to have a more favourable outcome. Conversely, the negative subtype, presenting with symptoms such as affective flattening and poverty of speech, was said to be a manifestation of an underlying structural/anatomical abnormality reflected by ventricular enlargement and cortical atrophy on computerized axial tomography (CAT) scan studies. These symptoms would therefore tend to be poorly responsive to somatic treatment, to follow a chronic course and to predict poor outcome.

Crow's original model did not specify which of the various descriptors of type I versus type II should be used in studies designed to disconfirm or verify the hypothesized dichotomy. Andreasen subsequently proposed a method that involved using standard approaches for the validation of nosological symptoms (Andreasen, 1982; Andreasen & Olson, 1982). She suggested that the hypothesis could be tested by using cross-sectional phenomenology as the initial basis for selecting experimental groups, while the other correlates of the positive and negative subtypes, as well as their longitudinal change, could be treated as experimental variables. Recognizing that most patients have a considerable overlap of positive and negative symptoms, she designated criteria for three groups rather than two: positive, mixed and negative. She also developed two detailed standardized rating scales for assessing positive and negative symptoms; these could be used to apply the proposed criteria and also to explore other aspects of the interrelationships between positive and negative symptoms and cognitive, psychosocial and neurobiological correlates of schizophrenia. As Andreasen (1985) suggested, studies should maintain a distinction between disease categories and symptom clusters. Crow's model proposed the existence of subtypes or categories, which were postulated to have differentiating correlates, while an alternative approach would speculate that the symptoms themselves were more fundamental, and that correlations to particular symptom clusters or dimensions might be noted across disease categories (Andreasen, 1985, 1986).

The concept of positive and negative symptoms, as well as the conceptual and methodological issues raised in their exploration, had a catalytic effect on studies of schizophrenia subsequently conducted during the 1980s and 1990s. The concept appears to have filled a conceptual void, and the terms have now acquired wide usage in clinical discussions of schizophrenia, as well as in research investigations. The concepts, at least at a descriptive level, have been incorporated into the diagnostic nomenclature that will be used to define schizophrenia during the 1990s, as embodied in both the *International Classification of Disease* (ICD-10) (WHO, 1992) and the fourth *Diagnostic and Statistical Manual* (DSM-IV) of the American Psychiatric Association (APA, 1993).

Psychometric issues

The increasing interest and emphasis on evaluation of positive and negative symptoms has raised a variety of psychometric issues.

Reliability

Although negative symptoms, conceptualized as 'fundamental symptoms', were given primacy in the conceptualization and diagnosis of schizophrenia by both Kraepelin *et al.* (1919) and Bleuler (1911), they were de-emphasized during the 1970s and early 1980s, largely because of a concern that they could not be rated reliably. The 1970s was an era that gave great importance to the development of standardized and structured approaches to assessment, with an emphasis on identifying objective phenomena for which good interobserver agreement and test–retest reliability could be achieved. This led to the development of standardized structured instruments such as the *Present State Examination* (PSE) (Wing, 1970) and the *Schedule for Affective Disorders and Schizophrenia* (SADS) (Endicott & Spitzer, 1978). Positive symptoms, such as delusions and hallucinations, were given prominence in these structured interviews, as well as in the diagnostic algorithms or criteria that derived from them, such as the research diagnostic criteria (RDC) (Endicott & Spitzer, 1979). The first national criterion-based diagnostic system, DSM-III, based the diagnosis of schizophrenia almost entirely upon positive symptoms.

The response to this concern about reliability led to the development of a variety of diagnostic instruments specifically designed to assess

Table 3.1 Interrater reliability of negative and positive symptoms in different cultural settings

Symptoms	Intraclass R			
	Italy	Spain	Japan	China
NEGATIVE				
Alogia				
Poverty of speech	0.632	0.870	0.604	0.801
Poverty of content of speech	0.615	0.935	0.571	0.771
Blocking	0.269	0.907	−0.014	0.825
Increased latency of response	0.803	0.939	0.591	0.824
Subjective rating		0.802	0.864	0.837
Global rating	0.694	0.945	0.628	0.989
Subscale score		0.971		
Affective flattening				
Unchanging facial expression	0.786	0.930	0.805	0.847
Decreased spontaneous movements	0.782	0.940	0.728	0.835
Paucity of expressive gestures	0.757	0.886	0.671	0.772
Poor eye contact	0.873	0.897	0.676	0.722
Affective non-responsivity	0.714	0.774	0.641	0.787
Inappropriate affect	0.774	0.805	0.294	0.034
Lack of vocal inflections	0.827	0.963	0.720	0.835
Subjective rating		0.831	0.553	0.581
Global rating	0.688	0.844	0.721	0.903
Subscale score		0.926		
Avolition-apathy				
Grooming and hygiene	0.624	0.759	0.744	0.516
Impersistence at work or school	0.715	0.734	0.752	0.732
Physical anergia	0.755	0.843	0.513	0.735
Subjective complaints		0.964	0.607	0.756
Global rating	0.747	0.860	0.749	0.817
Subscale score		0.942		
Anhedonia-asociality				
Recreational interests and activities	0.741	0.875	0.610	0.761
Sexual interest and activity	0.605	0.790	0.742	0.712
Ability to feel intimacy and closeness	0.587	0.616	0.552	0.709
Relationships with friends and peers	0.620	0.768	0.642	0.790
Subjective awareness		0.841	0.823	0.798
Global rating	0.728	0.769	0.725	0.864
Subscale score		0.810		
Attentional impairment				
Work inattentiveness	0.321	0.870	0.711	0.550
Inattentiveness during mental testing	0.854	0.937	0.987	0.925
Subjective complaints		0.857	0.462	0.672
Global rating	0.659	0.892	0.788	0.832
Subscale score		0.938		

Continued

Table 3.1 (*Continued*)

Symptoms	Intraclass R		
	Italy	Spain	China
POSITIVE			
Hallucinations			
Auditory	0.942	0.953	0.904
Voices commenting	0.944	0.876	0.862
Voices conversing	0.896	0.889	0.013
Somatic or tactile	1.000	0.827	0.451
Olfactory	0.948	0.861	0.726
Visual	0.712	0.701	0.713
Subjective rating		0.870	0.304
Global rating	0.862	0.927	0.837
Subscale score		0.895	
Delusions			
Persecutory	0.906	0.964	0.934
Delusions of jealousy	0.357	0.789	0.307
Delusions of guilt or sin	0.600	0.768	0.870
Grandiose	0.936	0.752	0.782
Religious	0.886	0.673	0.954
Somatic	0.738	0.860	0.906
Delusions of reference	0.768	0.826	0.776
Delusions of being controlled	0.889	0.869	0.914
Delusions of mind-reading	0.890	0.678	0.864
Thought broadcasting	0.664	0.698	0.879
Thought insertion	0.877	0.839	−0.160
Thought withdrawal	0.828	0.854	0.901
Subjective rating		0.954	0.232
Global rating	0.878	0.896	0.420
Subscale score		0.893	
Bizarre behaviour			
Clothing and appearance	0.796	0.775	0.920
Social and sexual	0.734	0.665	0.235
Aggressive and agitated	0.750	0.777	0.751
Repetitive or stereotyped	0.849	0.849	0.657
Subjective rating		0.884	0.745
Global rating	0.834	0.867	0.993
Subscale score		0.914	
Positive formal thought disorder			
Derailment	0.855	0.766	0.825
Tangentiality	0.693	0.599	0.727
Incoherence	0.814	0.666	0.807
Illogicality	0.492	0.836	0.159
Circumstantiality	0.525	0.560	0.423
Pressure of speech	0.761	0.617	0.363
Distractible speech	0.637	0.844	0.757
Clanging	0.441	0.564	0.858
Subjective rating	0.870		
Global rating	0.818	0.989	0.942
Subscale score		0.881	

Intraclass R, Intraclass correlation coefficient.

negative symptoms. A number of scales have now been proposed, which vary widely in their level of detail and psychometric rigour (Krawiecka *et al.*, 1977; Abrams & Taylor, 1978; Andreasen, 1979a−c; Andreasen, 1983; Lewine *et al.*, 1983; Iager *et al.*, 1985; Kay *et al.*, 1988; Alphs *et al.*, 1989; Kirkpatrick *et al.*, 1989). Among these various scales, the scale for the assessment of negative symptoms (SANS) has been the most widely used and has had the most extensive psychometric development. Interrater reliabilities from a variety of different studies are summarized in Table 3.1.

Assessment of reliability is not a simple matter, however, and clinicians and investigators should not be lulled into a false confidence that all reliability problems inherent in negative symptoms have been solved. For example, many reliability studies conducted to date have employed an inter-rater design, using either a conjoint interview or a videotaped format. This design serves to eliminate or markedly reduce the error introduced by information variance, and therefore does not account for the fact that information variance indeed exists in clinical research studies. Relatively few studies have employed a design in which ratings were based on independent interviews by multiple raters (i.e. test−retest reliability) (Andreasen *et al.*, 1992a). Most studies conducted to date have also been carried out at a single site, with much less emphasis on comparative intercentre reliability, despite the fact that the scales are often employed in multicentre studies and with raters of highly variable levels of experience or training. Nevertheless, the constancy of high-interrater reliabilities across a variety of international sites allays these concerns partially, as do the data from the DSM-IV field trials, which were a multicentre study (Flaum *et al.*, in press). A similar design has been used for a US treatment study, treatment strategies in schizophrenia, with adequate levels of reliability being achieved across the various sites. Yet another concern about reliability data arises because most reliability data reported thus far have been limited to the rating of current symptoms, in spite of the use of these rating scales to evaluate the severity of information from retrospective chart reviews or symptoms in the past (Fenton & McGlashan, 1992). Our work evaluating the reliability of retrospective recall of negative symptoms suggests that reliability is reduced when symptoms have occurred in the past (Andreasen *et al.*, 1992a).

In summary, the development of instruments designed to assess negative symptoms has been a critical first step, and it has been established that negative symptoms can be evaluated with good interrater agreement and with at least adequate test−retest reliability as well. In any given study, various steps can be taken to improve the quality of reliability, including the use of training materials, calibration with standardized videotapes, adequate attention to rater drift and calibration over time and the use of clearly defined anchors and probes.

Interrelationships between symptoms

Early efforts to identify and define 'positive' and 'negative' symptoms led inevitably to the question of how and why particular symptoms of psychopathology should be classified in one group or the other. The Jacksonian conceptualization was employed as a partial guide in some discussions (Andreasen, 1982, 1985, 1986; Andreasen & Olson, 1982), but not all (Strauss *et al.*, 1974). Jackson suggested that positive symptoms, or the 'florid' symptoms of insanity, reflected release phenomena, and would be manifested as distortions or exaggerations of functions that are normally present but have been disinhibited. Negative symptoms, on the other hand, represent a simple loss of function owing to 'dissolution'. Following this line of reasoning, early formulations categorized delusions, hallucinations, positive formal thought disorder and bizarre behaviours as 'positive symptoms', while alogia or poverty of speech, affective blunting, avolition, anhedonia and attentional impairment were designated as negative symptoms (Andreasen, 1982).

Three different approaches may be used to determine the interrelationships among symptoms. The first approach, exemplified by Jackson, involves creating a conceptual system that would explain the interrelationships. This type of conceptual system draws on cognitive and experimental psychology and postulates models about 'how the brain works'. Efforts to root the conceptualization of positive and negative symptoms in such models has been relatively rudimentary, however, largely owing to the overwhelming complexity of the human central nervous system and our equally overwhelming ignorance about the nature of normal cognitive functions. Theories about how the various symptoms of psychopathology arise from disruptions of normal functions, by whatever mechanisms, must ultimately rest on an understanding of normal human cognition. Given this inherent difficulty, a second strategy has been used in most investigations; this strategy relies heavily on statistical analyses that examine the intercorrelations between symptoms. A third strategy, also pursued to only a rudimentary degree to date, examines the interrelationships between elevations of particular symptoms or clusters of symptoms and measured brain pathologies.

The second strategy, which relies on correlational analysis, measures of internal consistency such as Cronbach's alpha and factor analysis, was initially employed by Andreasen in her original descriptions of SANS and the scale for the assessment of positive symptoms (SAPS) (Andreasen, 1982, 1983). She noted that the intercorrelations between the negative symptoms were quite high, and the internal consistency of the overall SANS was also high (0.849), while the intercorrelations between the positive symptoms were weaker, as was the internal consistency (0.397). An unrotated factor analysis reported in that study suggested a bipolar factor, which showed negative correlations between the various positive and negative symptoms; this observation was inferred at the time to suggest that positive and negative symptoms represented two separate dimensions of symptomatology. A second factor analytical study (Andreasen, 1986) indicated that multiple factors were needed, however, and subsequent analyses have indicated that the original data reported in 1982 would produce a three-factor solution if subjected to varimax rotation (Klimidis *et al.*, 1993).

During the late 1980s and early 1990s, 15 different studies of SANS and SAPS were completed, producing results that are highly convergent and suggesting that the division of positive and negative symptoms into two groups is clearly an oversimplification. Instead, these results suggest that these symptoms, at least as measured in groups of patients suffering from schizophrenia, fall into three natural dimensions. The symptoms traditionally considered to be positive subdivide into one dimension that reflects psychoticism and is comprised of delusions and hallucinations, while the second dimension represents disorganization and is comprised of disorganized/bizarre behaviour, positive formal thought disorder/disorganized speech and inappropriate affect (Bilder *et al.*, 1985; Andreasen *et al.*, 1986; Liddle, 1987). Negative symptoms remain more or less the same. The 14 studies are summarized in Table 3.2 and a sample factor analysis from one study is presented in Table 3.3 (Arndt *et al.*, 1991).

These factor analytical studies suggest that particular groups of symptoms tend to cluster or co-occur within a given patient or group of patients. That is, a patient having delusions is also likely to have hallucinations. A patient with one negative symptom is likely to have others. In any given patient, these various factors or dimensions can co-occur and overlap. Thus, dimensions do not constitute subtypes or categories and cannot be used to define 'subtypes of schizophrenia'. Rather, dimensions are continuous and additive. For example, a particular patient who has high levels of all three dimensions could be considered to have the most severe psychopathology. Not only do factors or dimensions not identify subtypes, but they also do not have any necessary relationship to mechanisms or aetiology. The identification of factors through the examination of correlational relationships simply tells the clinician or investigator that symptoms tend to co-occur or be correlated. Further studies are needed to identify what this co-occurrence means in terms of either clinical prediction or understanding the underlying neurobiology of the factor or dimension.

The third strategy for exploring the interrelationship of symptoms involves attempting to

Table 3.2 Studies of schizophrenia using factor analytical techiques

Reference	*n*	Technique	Factors	Comment
Andreasen (1982)	52	PCA	Two or three	Original PCA (unrotated) showed one large bipolar (positive and negative factor); later unpublished analysis using varimax shows three, corresponding to psychotic, disorganized and negative
Bilder *et al.* (1985)	32	PCA, varimax rotation	Three	Factor 1 combines alogia, attention, thought disorder and bizarre behaviour; factor 2, negative symptoms; factor 3, psychotic symptoms
Andreasen (1986)	117	PCA	Three, possibly four	First two factors represented negative symptoms; factor 3, delusions and hallucinations; factor 4, bizarre behaviour
Kulhara *et al.* (1986)	98	PCA	Three	Negative symptoms, psychoticism, disorganization
Moscarelli *et al.* (1987)	59	PCA	Two to three	Clear negative factor; positive factors less cohesive
Liddle (1987)	40	PCA, rotation	Three	'Psychomotor poverty, disorganization, and reality distortion'; based on only a subset of SANS/SAPS items
Lenzenweger *et al.* (1989)	302	Confirmatory FA using maximum likelihood techniques from LISREL to compare several models	Two, possibly more	Retrospective re-analysis of twin data; positive and negative factors
Schulberg *et al.* (1990)	370	PCA, varimax	Two	Clear negative factor; positive factor mainly psychoticism
Liddle and Barnes (1990)	57	PCA, varimax	Three	Psychomotor poverty, disorganization and reality distortion
Arndt *et al.* (1991)	207	PCA, varimax rotation, maximum likelihood techniques	Three	Negative symptoms, psychoticism, disorganization
Gur *et al.* (1991)	47	PCA, rotation	Three	Negative symptoms, psychotocism, disorganization
Minas *et al.* (1992)	114	Multidimensional scaling	Three	Negative symptoms, psychoticism, thought disorder; based on item analysis rather than global ratings

Continued

Table 3.2 (*Continued*)

Reference	*n*	Technique	Factors	Comment
Peralta *et al.* (1992)	115	PCA, varimax	Four	Negative symptoms, psychoticism, thought disorder, loadings on bizarre behaviour not reported
Brown & White (1992)	139	PCA, varimax	Three	Cross-sectional ratings using SANS and Manchester Scale; negative symptoms, psychoticism and inattentiveness and inappropriate affect
Miller *et al.* (1993)	90	PCA, varimax	Three	Negative symptoms, psychoticism, disorganization

PCA, principal components analysis; SANS, scale for the assessment of negative symptoms; SAPS, scale for the assessment of positive symptoms; FA, factor analysis.

Table 3.3 Varimax rotated factor loadings on positive and negative symptoms (*n* = 207)

Factor	1	2	3
Avolition	0.82	0.16	0.01
Anhedonia	0.81	−0.01	0.01
Affective flattening	0.79	0.07	0.18
Alogia	0.73	0.46	0.00
Attentional deficit	0.72	0.21	0.16
Positive thought disorder	0.07	0.86	0.12
Bizarre behaviour	0.22	0.70	−0.01
Delusions	−0.03	0.11	0.83
Hallucinations	0.22	−0.02	0.78

relate them to neurobiological measures. Studies of this type have to date been relatively rudimentary and infrequent, but have been most extensively explored by Liddle *et al.* (Liddle, 1987; Liddle *et al.*, 1989, 1992). Consonant with the conceptualization of three factors or dimensions described above, Liddle has proposed that the symptoms of schizophrenia be subdivided into three broad groups, which he refers to as psychomotor poverty, disorganization and reality distortion. He has noted these three patterns of psychopathology to have different patterns of abnormality in cerebral blood flow, as assessed by positron emission tomography (PET) (Liddle *et al.*, 1992). Andreasen *et al.* (1992b) have shown similar relationships between negative symptoms and decreased frontal blood flow using single photon emission computed tomography (SPECT), as have Lewis *et al.* (1992). Both sets of findings are consistent with the early speculation of Ingvar and Franzen (1974) that negative symptoms would be associated with hypofrontality, as well as with their observations of a relationship using measures of resting blood flow. Recently, several other attempts have shown relationships between either dimensions or specific symptoms. Barta *et al.* (1990) and Flaum *et al.* (in press) have shown a relationship between decreased size of the superior temporal gyrus and hallucinations, while Shenton *et al.* (1992) have reported a relationship between positive thought disorder and decreased hippocampal size.

In spite of all these efforts, the relationship between disorganization and the positive and negative constructs remains somewhat controversial. This is largely because it shares some features with each. Symptoms of disorganization (e.g. disorganized speech and bizarre behaviour) are often viewed as 'positive' because they are considered to be indicators of the active phase of the illness or of 'psychosis'. They often cause patients to be hospitalized acutely and lead to vigorous treatment by clinicians. For this reason, it may be best to view the psychotic and disorganized dimensions as subtypes of positive symptoms. On the other hand, some aspects of disorganization are more closely allied with negative symptoms in clinical presentation; disorganized behaviour which impairs the patient's ability to perform activities of daily living has a 'negative' quality to it, for example. During the next decade, these relationships are likely to receive further exploration, particularly in the light of the increasing number of biological measures which can be applied in order to explore differential mechanisms.

Dimensions vs. categories (syndromes)

Studies of psychopathology can emphasize either categorical or dimensional approaches. Categorical approaches divide patients into mutually exclusive subgroups, which are usually assumed to have different clinical and neurobiological correlates, as reflected in course, response to treatment and underlying neurobiology. Categorical approaches are firmly rooted in the 'disease model' that is widely used in medicine. Ultimately, categorical approaches assume that the subtypes identified will differ from one another in some type of underlying pathophysiological mechanisms or aetiology. As a first approximation, clinical presentation, as exemplified by cross-sectional symptomatology, is used as the 'entry' to identify a category; before such categories actually have an identified pathophysiology they are referred to as 'syndromes' (literally, a running together), because they constitute an identifiable clinical pattern that makes sense in the context of observed inter-relationships and making predictions about groups of patients; once a specific pathophysiology or aetiology is identified, syndromes are elevated to the status of recognized diseases. The concept of dimensions, on the other hand, is closely related to clinical psychology. While categories have traditionally arisen from disease models, dimensions often derive from the study of normal psychology; therefore, students of dimensional approaches have shown less concern about identifying brain/behaviour relationships. Dimensions

define groups of symptoms that co-occur as well, but the co-occurrence is noted through statistical techniques such as factor analysis. While the test of the robustness of a category is its ability to make clinical predictions, the test of the robustness of a dimension is normally the internal consistency of its components and its stability over time. While categories classify individuals, dimensions classify symptoms. Therefore, dimensions can overlap within a given individual and be additive.

The typology of schizophrenia proposed by Crow was inherently categorical, with subjects classified as either type I or type II. The expansion of this conceptualization by Andreasen to include a mixed type was also categorical.

Early studies suggested that the categorical classifications proposed by Crow and refined through Andreasen's criteria had some predictive validity (e.g. Andreasen & Olson, 1982, 1990), but these categories also had a variety of problems. Some problems noted by Andreasen in 1985 included the difficulty of interpreting the mixed group, the tendency of symptoms to change over time and the relative rarity of 'pure negative' and 'pure positive' patients. Some subsequent studies have shown that the classification scheme is unstable over time, with large numbers of patients reclassified during different phases of the disorder (Breier *et al.*, 1987; Marneros *et al.*, 1991b). Furthermore, the subtypes as defined by Andreasen may also have some problems with reliability, since they are heavily dependent on the selection of a cut-off point (a severity rating of 3 or greater on SANS and SAPS items) to assign patients to particular categories (Fenton & McGlashan, 1991).

As a consequence, investigators interested in psychopathology have become increasingly interested in exploring dimensional approaches to the study of disease mechanisms. This approach has been most clearly articulated by Carpenter, who has proposed the study of 'multiple domains of psychopathology' (Andreasen & Carpenter, 1993). According to this model, the dimensions that co-occur within a single patient could be due to multiple different disease processes: dimension A caused by process A, dimension B by process B and dimension C by process C. A patient who presents with only one dimension would have only one underlying disease process (e.g. frontal lobe dysfunction), while a patient manifesting multiple dimensions would have multiple underlying processes.

Primary vs. secondary negative symptoms

Crow proposed that the negative syndrome in schizophrenia was the manifestation of an underlying structural neural deficit (Crow, 1980). One of the most difficult problems in the study of negative symptoms in schizophrenia involves the recognition that negative symptoms may occur as a consequence of a wide variety of factors which may be completely unrelated to such a posited structural deficit. The most commonly implicated factors are: (i) neuroleptic side effects (e.g. akinesia); (ii) depression, which is common in schizophrenia, particularly during the residual phase (Siris, 1991); (iii) a response to positive symptoms (e.g. social avoidance secondary to paranoia); and (iv) environmental understimulation resulting from chronic institutionalization (Carpenter *et al.*, 1985). While there is consensus that it is essential to attempt to disentangle 'primary' from 'secondary' negative symptoms, there has been much debate about the best method of doing so.

Carpenter and his group have been most active in their attempts to grapple with this problem (Carpenter & Kirkpatrick, 1988). They propose that 'deficit' (or primary) negative symptoms can indeed be distinguished from secondary negative symptoms on the basis of a careful and systematic assessment of clinical signs and symptoms. They have developed a structured assessment instrument and operationalized criteria for making this distinction. According to these criteria, subjects must display prominent negative symptoms for at least 12 months in the absence of likely secondary causes. They have demonstrated adequate reliability using these instruments within their centre, and in categorizing patients as deficit versus non-deficit. They have also published a series of reports in which the validity of the deficit versus non-deficit distinction has been supported by differences in cognitive testing, magnetic resonance imaging (MRI) measures and premorbid functioning (Kirkpatrick & Buchanan, 1990).

Nevertheless, much concern remains about the practical ability for most clinical researchers to make this type of distinction with acceptable levels of reliability. This concern is supported by data from the psychotic disorders field trial for DSM-IV, in which the reliability for distinguishing between 'primary' and 'secondary' negative symptoms was consistently poor, with Kappas of <0.5 for all symptoms (Flaum, in press). This was without the benefit of an instrument designed specifically for this purpose.) The alternative approach that has been employed by other investigators involves the collection of measures of the potential causes of secondary negative symptoms, such as depression, akinesia or psychosis. Ratings of these features are then included as co-variates in analyses looking at the relationship between negative symptoms and external correlates. While this approach obviates the need for potentially unreliable judgements as to the source of a particular symptom, it can lead to cumbersome multivariate statistical procedures.

Course of positive and negative symptoms

Positive and negative symptoms are important both clinically and theoretically for a variety of reasons. For many years, clinicians have been interested in identifying from among first-episode patients those likely to have a poor prognosis from those likely to have a good prognosis in order to assist in clinical counselling. Furthermore, to the extent that symptoms are transient or persistent, they may provide some information about underlying mechanisms.

The stability of positive and negative symptoms

In his original model, Crow predicted that the negative syndrome would be stable, as it was hypothesized to reflect structural brain damage (Crow, 1980; Crow *et al.*, 1981). Studies which examined this hypothesis have generally looked at the correlation between some overall rating of positive and negative symptoms measured on two different occasions. These studies have generally shown that negative symptoms tended to be slightly more stable than positive ones (Pfohl & Winokur, 1982; Pogue-Geile & Harrow, 1985; Johnstone *et al.*, 1986; Lindenmayer *et al.*, 1986; Addington & Addington, 1991; Andreasen *et al.*, 1991). However, in spite of this relative stability of negative symptoms, there remains a significant possibility of change, even in very chronic patients (Johnstone *et al.*, 1986).

Some methodological difficulties confound the interpretation of these results. First, these studies failed to distinguish between primary (so-called deficit) and secondary negative symptoms. This distinction is critical, since the secondary negative symptoms were shown to be much less stable than the deficit ones (Carpenter & Kirkpatrick, 1988). Second, they did not take into account that the reliability level of a measure creates an upper limit for the correlation of a measure in two occasions. Thus, a substantial part of the change in the measure may reflect the unreliability of the measure rather than true variation of the intensity of the phenomenon, these changes being the consequence of the limit of the reliability of the measures. Third, the stability is likely to be influenced by the patient's state at entry into the study; in at least one study (Lindenmayer *et al.*, 1986), patients were in an acute psychosis during their baseline assessment, and thus were probably in their worst clinical state. Thus, it is expected that the stability figures which we would obtain if the original assessment was outside an acute decompensation could be very different (Lindenmayer *et al.*, 1986; Kay & Singh, 1989).

Prognostic significance of positive and negative symptoms

Early investigators attempted to establish which symptoms were more likely to predict a good versus a poor outcome in patients suffering from acute psychosis (Stephens, 1978; Vaillant, 1978).

These studies were used for an early subdivision of schizophrenia into good versus poor prognosis subtypes. To some extent, the rediscovery of the positive versus negative distinction is a re-evaluation of this early work. Based on that early framework, as well as on more recent hypotheses, negative symptoms are usually considered to be associated with a poor prognosis, while positive symptoms are associated with a better prognosis.

Studies that have looked at these issues have used either a concurrent, retrospective or prospective time frame. In order to summarize these studies, a follow-up time period proposed by McGlashan and Fenton (1992) has been used. Short-term outcome is defined as $0-2$ years after onset, medium-term as $3-6$ years after onset and long-term as 7 years or more. From study to study, the outcome is rarely consistently defined. Outcome can variously mean a remission of symptoms, an adequate level of psychosocial functioning or a failure to relapse and be rehospitalized.

Concurrent function

Studies that looked at the correlation between negative symptoms and current functioning unanimously have found that the level of negative symptoms is related to a poor level of psychosocial functioning (Johnstone *et al.*, 1979; Kolakowska *et al.*, 1985b; Keefe *et al.*, 1987; Breier *et al.*, 1991), which is somewhat tautological given that the definition of the negative syndrome includes items that could be considered part of the impairments associated with schizophrenia. However, some, but not all, studies found that a high level of positive symptoms also correlates cross-sectionally with poor functioning (Pogue-Geile & Harrow, 1984; Keefe *et al.*, 1987; Breier *et al.*, 1991).

Outcome

A general consensus exists that negative symptoms measured soon after the initial psychotic episode predict poor medium-term and long-term outcome (Pogue-Geile & Harrow, 1985; Biehl *et al.*, 1986; Breier *et al.*, 1991). The study by Pogue-Geile and Harrow (1985) suggests that the level of positive symptoms could also be predictive.

Some studies looked at the relationship between retrospectively assessed negative symptoms. They also suggest a link between negative symptoms and poor medium-term and long-term outcome (Roff & Knight, 1978; Knight *et al.*, 1979; Kolakowska *et al.*, 1985; Munk-Jorgensen & Mortensen, 1989; Fenton & McGlashan, 1992).

With regard to the prediction of short-term outcome, the situation is more confused. Indeed, most studies found that negative symptoms at the index admission (Andreasen, 1986; McCreadie *et al.*, 1989; Lieberman *et al.*, 1991) or 6 months after (Biehl *et al.*, 1986) are predictive of poor short-term outcome. Some found that patients with high ratings on both positive and negative symptoms did the worst (Pogue-Geile & Harrow, 1984). However, some studies found that negative symptoms at admission were not predictive of poor acute-phase outcomes (Lindenmayer *et al.*, 1984, 1986; Schubart *et al.*, 1986). They have even suggested that the negative ones were predictive of good short-term outcome. These investigators proposed that the negative symptoms rated in the beginning of the illness reflected depressive symptoms.

Longitudinal pattern of positive and negative symptoms

Some data show that negative symptoms predate the beginning of positive symptoms (Häfner *et al.*, 1991). Moreover, negative symptoms have been shown to be as frequent and intense in recent-onset patients as in more chronic ones (Arndt *et al.*, 1991). Four longitudinal studies have shown that the frequency and the intensity of negative symptoms did not increase with time in prospectively followed patients (Pogue-Geile & Harrow, 1985; McCreadie *et al.*, 1989; Häfner *et al.*, 1991). However, in a fifth study, the intensity of both positive and negative symptoms was found to increase (Breier *et al.*, 1991). In cross-sectional studies, the rating of negative symptoms appears uncorrelated to the length of illness (Andreasen, 1982; Rosen *et al.*, 1984; Guelfi *et al.*, 1989; Kay & Singh 1989; Andreasen *et al.*, 1990).

Neurobiological correlates

A variety of neurobiological correlates have been used to examine the validity of the positive versus negative construct. Three main areas of investigation have been especially informative: neuroimaging studies, studies of cognitive impairment and studies of response to treatment.

Neuroimaging studies

The early structural imaging literature relied heavily on the use of computerized tomography (CT) scans. This literature has been thoughtfully reviewed by Marks and Luchins (1990). While the majority ($n = 20$) of the 28 studies reviewed supported the association of negative syndrome with ventricular enlargement, five obtained no significant correlation, and three found an inverse relationship. Even if these findings generally lend support to the two-category model, the authors stressed that most studies have focused on non-specific measures, such as the ventricular brain ratio (VBR), that could not provide strong clues about the exact location of some underlying lesion. Only a few studies have used MRI to examine correlates with negative symptoms. Again, the primary correlate that has been found to be significant to date has been ventricular enlargement, although there is some suggestion that frontal involvement may also have a relationship (Andreasen, 1986; Andreasen *et al.*, 1990).

The functional imaging literature has attempted to expand the complexity of the models being used to explore brain behaviour relationships and to examine interrelationships between various brain regions and various symptom patterns. The work of Liddle *et al.* (1992) using PET is the most highly developed version of this approach. They showed that the symptoms of schizophrenic patients segregate into three syndromes, each associated with a different pattern of regional cerebral blood flow. The psychomotor poverty syndrome is associated with altered blood flow in the caudate (involving increases) and in dorsolateral frontal and superior parietal association cortex (representing decreases). The disorganization syndrome is associated with abnormalities in the cingulate gyrus and thalamus (increases in flow) and in the ventral lateral prefrontal cortex and angular gyrus (decreases in flow). The reality distortion syndrome is associated with flow changes in the left parahippocampal gyrus, left striatum (increases) and cingulate gyrus (decrease in flow). The findings are consistent with disruptions in interrelated but independent circuits that may account for differences in clinical presentation. Several other investigators have also noted that decreased frontal function may be specifically related to negative symptoms (Ingvar & Franzen, 1974; Volkow *et al.*, 1987; Andreasen *et al.*, 1992).

These neuroimaging studies point toward the importance of formulating neural models that are more complex than the one originally proposed by Crow and which will link specific types of symptoms to dysfunction in specific areas of the brain (Andreasen, 1986). Some data are available that allow the creation of such models. Thus far, neuropsychological and functional imaging studies suggest that negative symptoms could reflect a dysfunction in the prefrontal cortex. This is consistent with the similarities between patients with prominent negative symptoms and those with frontal lobe lesions in areas such as deficits in executive planning, emotional reactivity, abstract thinking, etc. (Merriam *et al.*, 1990; Liddle & Morris, 1991). Moreover, some manifestations of the negative syndrome, such as blunted affect, apathy, poverty of speech and problems with concept formation, are also shared by Parkinson's syndrome, which is underlain by a deficit in dopamine activity (Lecrubier *et al.*, 1980; Mackay, 1980; Wyatt *et al.*, 1986).

Conversely, many lines of evidence converge to suggest that positive symptoms reflect a hyperactivity of the dopamine circuits. These observations have been integrated by Weinberger (1987) into a highly heuristic model which is based on earlier work by Pycock *et al.* (1980) and Bannon and Roth (1983), whose hypotheses explain the occurrence of both syndromes at the same time by modifying the dopamine hypothesis of schizophrenia. According to Weinberger, underactivity of mesocortical dopaminergic circuits would cause negative symptoms, which would explain both its

similarities with frontal and Parkinson's syndromes. The lesion causing this defect could arise from different types of genetic or brain insults sustained *in utero*, at birth or in early childhood. Then, the normal retroactive negative feedback of the mesocortical dopaminergic tract on the mesolimbic dopaminergic tract would be released. Thus, mesolimbic activity could go unrestrained, thereby accounting for positive symptoms.

Neuropsychology and cognitive impairment

There is a remarkably consistent pattern of association of negative symptoms with various types of indicators of global cognitive deficit (Andreasen, 1982, 1990; Opler *et al.*, 1984; Cornblatt *et al.*, 1985; Gaebel *et al.*, 1987; Keilip *et al.*, 1988; Braff, 1989; Merriam *et al.*, 1990). This consistency in the association of cognitive deficits with the negative dimension is remarkable given the diversity of psychometric instruments used. Concerns may be raised, however, about an inherent circularity of the findings, which could be due to a lack of initiative, attention or effort.

The association of positive syndromes with cognitive and attentional deficits has also been examined. Results from these studies support the validity of the split of positive symptoms into two separate domains. Different measures of distractibility (Bilder *et al.*, 1985; Cornblatt *et al.*, 1985; Green & Walker, 1986; Walker & Harvey, 1986; Gaebel, 1987) and some indicators of generalized poor cognitive performance (Bilder *et al.*, 1985; Liddle & Morris, 1991) have been associated with positive formal thought disorder and other symptoms of the disorganization syndrome. The summary by Liddle *et al.* (1992) of their PET findings also provides a useful overview of the interrelationships between cognitive assessment and the three-dimensional approach.

Genetic studies

It has been proposed that negative schizophrenia would represent a more genetic subtype. In support of this hypothesis, some studies (Kay *et al.*, 1986; McGuffin & Owen, 1991), but not all

(Pearlson *et al.*, 1985; Alda *et al.*, 1991), showed that first-degree relatives of negative schizophrenics have a higher morbid risk than the relatives of positive schizophrenics. Moreover, a reanalysis of previously published studies of twins showed that negative symptoms in one twin predicts a higher concordance rate (Dworkin *et al.*, 1988).

An alternative explanation for some of these findings has been provided by McGuffin (1987; McGuffin & Owen, 1991). These investigators proposed that negative schizophrenics would present a more severe form of schizophrenia. Then, as predicted by the polygenic multifactorial model, these patients should have more affected relatives than patients with a less severe form of the disorder. However, this explanation appears difficult to reconcile with the observation that negative symptoms are often present in relatives of schizophrenics showing milder expressions of the schizophrenia spectrum, such as schizotypal or schizoid personality traits or disorders (Tsuang, 1991).

Response to treatment

Crow (1980) proposed that negative symptoms do not respond to neuroleptics. This point of view is quite prevalent, but the studies supporting this idea have methodological limitations that weaken their conclusions. Angrist *et al.* (1980) found a poor response only after changing a posteriori his definition of negative symptoms. The study by Johnstone *et al.* (1978) evaluated the neuroleptic responsivity of negative symptoms of patients rated at 0.8 on a scale going from 0 to 4. Since the patients evaluated in this study were already at the bottom of the scale, however, a floor effect was produced that made positive results difficult to obtain.

Conversely, there is a substantial bulk of literature that supports the idea that negative symptoms respond to neuroleptics (Goldberg, 1985; Meltzer *et al.*, 1986; Breier *et al.*, 1987; Van Kammen, 1987; Tandon *et al.*, 1988; Kay & Singh, 1989). Some authorities have proposed that the so-called disinhibitory neuroleptics (i.e. sulpiride, pimozide) would be more efficient in this aspect (Lecrubier *et al.*, 1980), but the evidence is rather scarce (Meltzer *et al.*, 1986). Two recent studies (reviewed in Meltzer *et al.*, 1991) suggest that clozapine might be more efficient than classic neuroleptics in reducing negative symptoms. However, those studies all involved actively psychotic patients. Thus, it is quite possible that these patients were presenting negative symptoms secondary to their psychosis and these negative symptoms would decrease as a consequence of the effect of neuroleptics on positive symptoms.

To address this issue, Boyer *et al.* (1990) have performed an open trial and a double blind placebo-controlled study of treatment of pure negative syndrome, using amisulpiride. This drug was found to be efficient in reducing the intensity of this pure negative syndrome. To our knowledge, this is the only study that has specifically targeted this type of patient.

Besides neuroleptics, other treatments, such as dopamine agonists (Levi-Minzi *et al.*, 1991), anticholinergics (Tandon *et al.*, 1988) and behavioural and psycho-education therapies (Slade & Bentall, 1989), have been advocated for negative symptoms, but very few systematic evaluations of these treatments have been performed using the positive and negative dichotomy. The development of new treatments for negative symptoms is currently a burgeoning area in psychopharmacology.

Summary and conclusions

In summary, the past decade has been a rich era for the conceptualization and study of positive and negative symptoms. These concepts have well-documented reliability and validity and have become well established in both clinical and research applications.

References

Abrams, R. & Taylor, M.A. (1978) A rating scale for emotional blunting. *American Journal of Psychiatry*, 135, 226–229.

Addington, J. & Addington, D. (1991) Positive and negative symptoms of schizophrenia: their course and relationship over time. *Schizophrenia Research*, 5(1), 51–59.

Alda, M., Zvolsky, P., Dvorakova, M. & Papezova, H. (1991) Study of chronic schizophrenics with positive and negative family histories of psychosis. *Acta Psychiatrica Scandinavica*, **83(5)**, 334–337.

Alphs, L.D., Lafferman, J.A., Ross, L., Bland, W. & Levine, J. (1989) Fenfluramine treatment of negative symptoms in older schizophrenic inpatients. *Psychopharmacology Bulletin*, **25(1)**, 149–153.

Andreasen, N.C. (1979a) Affective flattening and the criteria for schizophrenia. *American Journal of Psychiatry*, **136**, 944–947.

Andreasen, N.C. (1979b) Thought, language, and communication disorders. I. Clinical assessment, definition of terms, and evaluation of their reliability. *Archives of General Psychiatry*, **36**, 1315–1321.

Andreasen, N.C. (1979c) Thought, language, and communication disorders. II. Diagnostic significance. *Archives of General Psychiatry*, **36**, 1325–1330.

Andreasen, N.C. (1982) Negative symptoms in schizophrenia: definition and reliability. *Archives of General Psychiatry*, **39**, 784–788.

Andreasen, N.C. (1983) *The Scale for the Assessment of Negative Symptoms (SANS)*. University of Iowa, Iowa.

Andreasen, N.C. (1984) *The Scale for the Assessment of Positive Symptoms (SAPS)*. University of Iowa, Iowa.

Andreasen, N.C. (1985) Positive vs. negative schizophrenia: a critical evaluation. *Schizophrenia Bulletin*, **11**, 380–389.

Andreasen, N.C. (ed.) (1986) *Can Schizophrenia Be Localized in the Brain?* American Psychiatric Press, Washington DC.

Andreasen, N.C. (1990) Methods for assessing positive and negative symptoms. In Ban, T.A., Freedman, A.M., Godfries, C.G. *et al.* (eds) *Modern Problems of Pharmaco-psychiatry: Positive and Negative Symptoms and Syndromes*, pp. 73–88. Karger, Basel.

Andreasen, N.C. & Carpenter, W.T. (1993) Diagnosis and classification of schizophrenia. *Schizophrenia Bulletin*, **19(2)**, 199–214.

Andreasen, N.C., Ehrhardt, J.C., Swayze, V.W. *et al.* (1990) Magnetic resonance of the brain in schizophrenia: The pathophysiological significance of structural abnormalities. *Archives of General Psychiatry*, **47**, 35–44.

Andreasen, N.C., Flaum, M. & Arndt, S. (1992a) The comprehensive assessment of symptoms and history (CASH): an instrument for assessing psychopathology and diagnosis. *Archives of General Psychiatry*, **49**, 615–623.

Andreasen, N.C. & Olson, S. (1982) Negative versus positive schizophrenia: definition and validation. *Archives of General Psychiatry*, **39**, 789–794.

Andreasen, N.C., Flaum, M., Arndt, S., Alliger, R. & Swayze, V.W. (1991) Positive and negative symptoms: assessment and validity. In Morneros, A., Andreasen, N.C. & Tsuang, M. (eds) *Negative Versus Positive Schizophrenia*, pp. 28–51. Springer-Verlag, Berlin.

Andreasen, N.C., Nasrallah, H.A., Dunn, V.D. *et al.* (1986) Structural abnormalities in the frontal system in schizophrenia: a magnetic resonance imaging study. *Archives of General Psychiatry*, **43**, 136–144.

Andreasen, N.C., Rezai, K., Alliger, R. *et al.* (1992b) Hypofrontality in neuroleptic-naive and chronic schizophrenic patients: assessment with xenon-133 single-photon emission computed tomography and the Tower of London. *Archives of General Psychiatry*, **49**, 943–958.

Angrist, B., Rotrosen, J. & Gershon, S. (1980) Differential effects of amphetamine and neuroleptics on negative vs. positive symptoms in schizophrenia. *Psychopharmacology (Berlin)*, **72**, 17–19.

APA (1994) *Diagnostic and Statistical Manual of Mental Disorders (DSM-IV)*, 4th edn. American Psychiatric Association, Washington DC.

Arndt, S., Alliger, R.J. & Andreasen, N.C. (1991) The distinction of positive and negative symptoms: the failure of a two-dimensional model. *British Journal of Psychiatry*, **158**, 317–322.

Bannon, M.J. & Roth, R.H. (1983) Pharmacology of meso-cortical dopamine neurons. *Pharmacological Reviews*, **35**, 63–68.

Barta, P.E., Pearlson, G.D., Powers, R.E., Richards, S.S. & Tune, L.E. (1990) Auditory hallucinations and smaller superior temporal gyrus volume in schizophrenia. *Archives of General Psychiatry*, **147(11)**, 1457–1462.

Berrios, G.E. (1985) Positive and negative symptoms and Jackson. A conceptual history. *Archives of General Psychiatry*, **42**, 95–97.

Biehi, H., Maurer, K., Schubart, C., Krumm, B. & Jung, E. (1986) Prediction of outcome and utilization of medical services in a prospective study of first onset schizophrenics: results of a prospective 5-year follow-up study. *European Archives of Psychiatry and Neurological Science*, **236(3)**, 139–147.

Bilder, R.M., Mukherjee, S., Rieder, R.O. & Pandurangi, A.K. (1985) Symptomatic and neuropsychological components of defect states. *Schizophrenia Bulletin*, **11(3)**, 409–419.

Bleuler, E. (1911) *Dementia Praecox of the Group of Schizophrenias*. International Universities Press, New York. Translated by Zinkin, J. (1950).

Boyer, P., Lecrubier, Y. & Puech, A.J. (1990) The treatment of positive and negative symptoms: pharmacologic approaches. *Modern Problems of Pharmacopsychiatry*, **24**, 152–174.

Braff, D.L. (1989) Sensory input deficits and negative symptoms in schizophrenic patients. *American Journal of Psychiatry*, **146(8)**, 1006–1011.

Braff, D.L., Heaton, R., Kuck, J. *et al.* (1991) The generalized pattern of neuropsychological deficits in outpatients with chronic schizophrenia with heterogeneous Wisconsin Card Sorting Test results. *Archives of General Psychiatry*, **48**, 891–898.

Breier, A., Schreiber, J.L., Dyer, J. & Pickar, D. (1991) National Institute of Mental Health longitudinal study of chronic schizophrenia: prognosis and predictors of outcome. *Archives of General Psychiatry*, **48(3)**, 329–346.

Breier, A., Wolkowitz, O.M., Doran, A.R. *et al.* (1987) Neuroleptic responsivity of negative and positive symptoms in schizophrenia. *American Journal of Psychiatry*, **144(12)**, 1549–1555.

Brown, K.W. & White, T. (1992) Syndromes of chronic schizophrenia and some clinical correlates. *British Journal of Psychiatry*, **161**, 317–322.

Carpenter, W.T. & Kirkpatrick, B. (1988) The heterogeneity of the long-term course of schizophrenia. *Schizophrenia*

Bulletin, **14**, 645–659.

Carpenter, W.T., Strauss, J.S. & Bartko, J.J. (1985) On the heterogeneity of schizophrenia. In Alpert, M. (ed.) *Controversies in Schizophrenia*, pp. 25–37. Guilford Press, New York.

Cornblatt, B.A., Lenzenweger, M.F., Dworkin, R.H. & Erlenmeyer-Kimling, L. (1985) Positive and negative schizophrenic symptoms. Attention and information processing. *Schizophrenia Bulletin*, **11**, 397–407.

Crow, T.J. (1980) Molecular pathology of schizophrenia: more than one disease process? *British Medical Journal*, **280**, 66–68.

Crow, T.J., Corsellis, J.A.N., Cross, A.J. *et al.* (1981) The search for changes underlying the type II syndrome in schizophrenia. In Perris, C., Struwe, G. & Jansson, B. (eds) *Biological Psychiatry*, pp. 727–731. Elsevier, North-Holland Biomedical Press.

Dworkin, R.H., Lenzenweger, M.F., Moldin, S.O., Skillings, G.F. & Levick, S.E. (1988) A multidimensional approach to the genetics of schizophrenia. *American Journal of Psychiatry*, **145**, 1077–1083.

Endicott, J. & Spitzer, R.L. (1978) A diagnostic interview: the schedule for affective disorders and schizophrenia (SADS). *Archives of General Psychiatry*, **35**, 837–844.

Endicott, J. & Spitzer, R.L. (1979) Use of the Research Diagnostic Criteria and the Schedule for Affective Disorders and Schizophrenia to study affective disorders. *American Journal of Psychiatry*, **136**, 52–56.

Fenton, W.S. & McGlashan, T.H. (1991) Natural history of schizophrenia subtypes. II. Positive and negative symptoms and long-term course. *Archives of General Psychiatry*, **48**, 978–986.

Fenton, W.S. & McGlashan, T.H. (1992) Testing systems for assessment of negative symptoms in schizophrenia. *Archives of General Psychiatry*, **49**(3), 179–184.

Flaum, M., O'Leary, D.S., Swayze, V.W., Miller, D.D., Arndt, S.V. & Andreasen, N.C. (In press) Symptom dimensions and brain morphology in schizophrenia and related psychotic disorders. *Journal of Psychiatric Research*.

Gaebel, W., Ulrich, G. & Frick, K. (1987) Visuomotor performance of schizophrenic patients and normal controls in a picture viewing task. *Biological Psychiatry*, **22**(10), 1227–1237.

Goldberg, S.C. (1985) Negative and deficit symptoms in schizophrenia do respond to neuroleptics. *Schizophrenia Bulletin*, **11**, 453–456.

Green, M. & Walker, E. (1986) Attentional performance in positive- and negative-symptom schizophrenia. *Journal of Nervous and Mental Disease*, **174**, 208–213.

Guelfi, G.P., Faustman, W.O. & Csernansky, J.G. (1989) Independence of positive and negative symptoms in a population of schizophrenic patients. *Journal of Nervous and Mental Disease*, **177**(5), 285–290.

Gur, R.E., Mozley, D., Resnick, S.M. *et al.* (1991) Relations among clinical scales in schizophrenia. *American Journal of Psychiatry*, **148**, 472–478.

Häfner, H., Behrens, S., DeVry, J. & Gattaz, W.F. (1991) Oestradiol enhances the vulnerability threshold for schizophrenia in women by an early effect on dopaminergic neurotransmission: evidence from an epidemiological study and from animal experiments. *European Archives of Psychiatry and Clinical Neurosciences*, **241**(1), 65–68.

Iager, A.C., Kirch, D.G. & Wyatt, R.J. (1985) A negative symptom rating scale. *Psychiatry Research*, **16**, 27–36.

Ingvar, D.H. & Franzen, G. (1974) Abnormalities of cerebral blood flow distribution in patients with chronic schizophrenia. *Acta Psychiatrica Scandinavica*, **50**, 425–462.

Johnstone, E.C., Crow, T.J. Frith, C.D., Carney, M.W. & Price, J.S. (1978) Mechanism of the antipsychotic effect in the treatment of acute schizophrenia. *Lancet*, **i**, 848–851.

Johnstone, E.C., Frith, C.D., Gold, A. & Stevens, M. (1979) The outcome of severe acute shizophrenia illnesses after one year. *British Journal of Psychiatry*, **134**, 28–33.

Johnstone, E.C., Owens, D.G.C., Firth, C.D. & Crow, T.J. (1986) The relative stability of positive and negative features in chronic schizophrenia. *British Journal of Psychiatry*, **150**, 60–64.

Kay, S.R. & Singh, N.M. (1989) The positive–negative distinction in drug-free schizophrenic patients. Stability, response to neuroleptics and prognostic significance. *Archives of General Psychiatry*, **46**(8), 711–718.

Kay, S.R., Opler, L.A. & Fiszbein, A. (1986) Significance of positive and negative symptoms in chronic schizophrenia. *British Journal of Psychiatry*, **149**, 439–448.

Kay, S.R., Opler, L.A. & Lindenmayer, J.P. (1988) Reliability and validity of the positive and negative syndrome scale for schizophrenics. *Psychiatry Research* **23**, 99–110.

Keefe, R.S.E., Mohs, R.C., Losonczy, M.F. *et al.* (1987) Characteristics of very poor outcome schizophrenia. *American Journal of Psychiatry*, **144**, 889–895.

Keilp, J.G., Sweeney, J.A., Jacobsen, P. *et al.* (1988) Cognitive impairment in schizophrenia: specific relations to ventricular size and negative symptomatology. *Biological Psychiatry*, **24**, 47–55.

Kirkpatrick, B. & Buchanan, R.W. (1990) Anhedonia and the deficit syndrome of schizophrenia. *Psychiatry Research*, **31**, 25–30.

Kirkpatrick, B., Buchanan, R.W., McKenney, P.D., Alphs, L.D. & Carpenter, W.T. (1989) The schedule for the deficit syndrome: an instrument for research in schizophrenia. *Psychiatry Research*, **30**, 119–124.

Klimidis, S., Stuart, G.W., Minas, I.H., Copolov, D.L. & Singh, B.S. (1993) Positive and negative symptoms in the psychoses: re-analysis of published SAPS and SANS global ratings. *Schizophrenia Research*, **9**, 11–18.

Knight, R.A., Roff, J.D., Barrnet, J. & Moss, J.L. (1979) Concurrent and predictive validity of thought disorder and affectivity: a 22-year follow-up of acute schizophrenia. *Journal of Abnormal Psychology*, **88**(1), 1–12.

Kolakowska, T., Williams, A.O., Ardern, M. *et al.* (1985a) Schizophrenia with good and poor outcome. I. Early clinical features, response to neuroleptics and signs of organic dysfunction. *British Journal of Psychiatry*, **146**, 229–239.

Kolakowska, T., Williams, A.O., Jambor, K. & Ardern, M. (1985b) Schizophrenia with good and poor outcome. III. Neurological 'soft' signs, cognitive impairment and their clinical significance. *British Journal of Psychiatry*, **146**, 348–357.

Kraepelin, E., Barclay, R.M. & Robertson, G.M. (1919) *Dementia Praecox and Paraphrenia*. E & S Livingstone, Edinburgh.

Krawiecka, M., Goldberg, D. & Vaughan, M. (1977) A standardized psychiatric assessment for rating chronic psychiatric patients. *Acta Psychiatrica Scandinavica*, **55**, 299–308.

Kulhara, P., Kota, S.K. & Joseph, S. (1986) Positive and negative subtypes of schizophrenia: a study from India. *Acta Psychiatrica Scandinavica*, **74(4)**, 353–359.

Lecrubier, Y., Puech, A.J., Simon, P. & Widlocher, D. (1980) Schizophrenie: hyper- ou hypofonctionnement du systeme dopaminergique: une hypothese bipolaire. *Psychologie Medicale*, **12**, 2431–2441.

Lenzenweger, M.F., Dworkin, R.H. & Wethington, E. (1989) Models of positive and negative symptoms in schizophrenia: an empirical evaluation of latent structures. *Journal of Abnormal Psychology*, **98**, 62–70.

Levi-Minzi, S., Bermanzohn, P.C. & Siris, S.G. (1991) Bromocriptine for 'negative' schizophrenia. *Comprehensive Psychiatry*, **32(3)**, 210–216.

Lewine, R.R., Fogg, L. & Meltzer, H.Y. (1983) Assessment of negative and positive symptoms in schizophrenia. *Schizophrenia Bulletin*, **9**, 368–376.

Lewis, S.W., Ford, R.A., Syed, G.M., Reveley, A.M. & Toone, B.K. (1992) A controlled study of ^{99m}Tc-HMPAO single-photon emission imaging in chronic schizophrenia. *Psychological Medicine*, **22**, 27–35.

Liddle, P.F. (1987) Schizophrenic syndrome, cognitive performance and neurological dysfunction. *Psychological Medicine*, **17**, 49–57.

Liddle, P.F. & Barnes, T.R.E. (1990) Syndromes of chronic schizophrenia. *British Journal of Psychiatry*, **157**, 558–561.

Liddle, P.F. & Morris, D. (1991) Schizophrenic syndromes and frontal lobe performance. *British Journal of Psychiatry*, **158**, 340–345.

Liddle, P.F., Barnes, T.R.E., Morris, D. & Haque, S. (1989) Three symptoms in chronic schizophrenia. *British Journal of Psychiatry* (Suppl.), **7**, 119–122.

Liddle, P.F., Friston, K.J., Frith, C.D. & Frackowiak, R.S.J. (1992) Cerebral blood flow and mental processes in schizophrenia. *Journal of the Royal Society of Medicine*, **85(4)**, 224–226.

Lieberman, J.A., Saltz, B.L., Johns, C.A., Pollack, S., Borenstein, M. & Kane, J. (1991) The effects of clozapine on tardive dyskinesia. *British Journal of Psychiatry*, **158**, 503–510.

Lindenmayer, J.P., Kay, S.R. & Friedman, C. (1986) Negative and positive schizophrenic syndromes after the acute phase: a prospective follow-up. *Comprehensive Psychiatry*, **27**, 276–286.

Lindenmayer, J.P., Kay, S.R. & Opler, L. (1984) Positive and negative subtypes in acute schizophrenia. *Comprehensive Psychiatry*, **25**, 455–464.

McCreadie, R.G., Wiles, D., Grant, S. *et al.* (1989) The Scottish first episode schizophrenia study. VII. Two-year follow-up: Scottish schizophrenia research group. *Acta Psychiatrica Scandinavica*, **80(6)**, 597–602.

McGlashan, T.H. & Fenton, W.T. (1992) The positive–negative distinction in schizophrenia: review of natural history validators. *Archives of General Psychiatry*, **49**, 63–72.

McGuffin, P. (1987) The new genetics and childhood psychiatric disorder. *Journal of Child Psychology and Psychiatry and Allied Disciplines*, **28(2)**, 215–222.

McGuffin, P. & Owen, M. (1991) The molecular genetics of schizophrenia: an overview and forward view. *European Archives of Psychiatry and Clinical Neurosciences*, **240(3)**, 169–173.

Mackay, A.V.P. (1980) Positive and negative schizophrenic symptoms and the role of dopamine. *British Journal of Psychiatry*, **137**, 379–383.

Marks, R.C. & Luchins, D.J. (1990) Relationship between brain imaging findings in schizophrenia and psychopathology. In Andreasen, N.C. (ed.) Schizophrenia: Positive and Negative Symptoms and Syndromes.

Marneros, A., Deister, A. & Rohde, A. (1991a) Long-term investigation in stability of negative/positive distinction. In Marneros, A., Andreasen, N.C. & Tsuang, M. (eds) *Negative Versus Positive Schizophrenia*, Springer-Verlag, Berlin.

Marneros, A., Deister, A. & Rohde, A. (1991b) Stability of diagnoses in affective, schizoaffective and schizophrenic disorders: cross-sectional versus longitudinal diagnosis. *European Archives of Psychiatry and Clinical Neurosciences*, **241(3)**, 187–192.

Meltzer, H.Y., Sommers, A.A. & Luchins, D.J. (1986) The effect of neuroleptics and other psychotropic drugs on negative symptoms in schizophrenia. *Journal of Clinical Psychopharmacology*, **6**, 329–338.

Meltzer, H.Y., Alphs, L.D., Bastani, B., Ramirez, L.F. & Kwon, K. (1991) Clinical efficacy of clozapine in the treatment of schizophrenia. *Pharmacopsychiatry*, **24(2)**, 44–45.

Merriam, A.E., Kay, S.R., Opler, L.A., Kushner, S.F. & van Praag, H.M. (1990) Neurological signs and the positive–negative dimension in schizophrenia. *Biological Psychiatry*, **28(3)**, 181–192.

Miller, D.D., Arndt, S. & Andreasen, N.C. (1993) Alogia, attentional impairment, and inappropriate affect: their status in the dimensions of schizophrenia. *Comprehensive Psychiatry*, **34**, 221–226.

Minas, I.H., Stuart, G.W., Klimidis, S., Jackson, H.J., Singh, B.S. & Copolov, D.L. (1992) Positive and negative symptoms in the psychoses; multidimensional scaling of SAPS and SANS items. *Schizophrenia Research*, **8**, 143–156.

Moscarelli, M., Maffei, C. & Cesana, B.M. (1987) An international perspective on assessment of negative and positive symptoms in schizophrenia. *American Journal of Psychiatry*, **144**, 1595–1598.

Munk-Jorgensen, P. & Mortensen, P.B. (1989) Schizophrenia: a 13-year follow-up. Diagnostic and Psychopathological aspects. *Acta Psychiatrica Scandinavica*, **79(4)**, 391–399.

Opler, L.A., Kay, S.R., Rosado, V. & Lindenmayer, J.P. (1984) Positive and negative syndromes in chronic schizophrenic patients. *Journal of Nervous and Mental Disease*, **172**, 317–325.

Pearlson, G.D., Garbacz, D.J., Moberg, P.J., Ahn, H.S. & DePaulo, J.R. (1985) Symptomatic, familial, perinatal, and social correlates of computerized axial tomography (CAT) changes in schizophrenics and bipolars. *Journal of Nervous and Mental Disease*, **173**, 42–50.

Peralta, V., de Leon, J. & Cuesta, M.J. (1992) Are there more than two syndromes in schizophrenia: a critique of the positive-negative dichtomy. *British Journal of Psychiatry*, **161**, 335–343.

Pfohl, B. & Winokur, G. (1982) The evolution of symptoms in

institutionalized hebephrenic/catatonic schizophrenics. *British Journal of Psychiatry*, **141**, 567–572.

Pogue-Geile, M.F. & Harrow, M. (1984) Negative and positive symptoms in schizophrenia and depression: a follow-up. *Schizophrenia Bulletin*, **10(3)**, 371–387.

Pogue-Geile, M.F. & Harrow, M. (1985) Negative symptoms in schizophrenia: their longitudinal course and prognostic importance. *Schizophrenia Bulletin*, **11**, 427–439.

Pycock, C.J., Kerwin, R.W. & Carter, C.J. (1980) Effect of lesion of cortical dopamine terminals on sub-cortical dopamine receptors in rats. *Nature*, **286**, 74–77.

Roff, J.D. & Knight, R. (1978) A schizophrenia checklist: reliability without stability, concurrent without predictive validity. *Psychological Reports*, **43**, 791–794.

Rosen, W.G., Mohs, R.C., Johns, C.A. *et al.* (1984) Positive and negative symptoms in schizophrenia. *Psychiatry Research*, **13**, 277–284.

Schneider, K. (1959) *Clinical Psychopathology*. Translated by Hamilton, M.W. Grune & Stratton, New York.

Schubart, C., Krumm, B., Biehl, H. & Schwarz, R. (1986) Measurement of social disability in a shizophrenic patient group: definition assessment and outcome over two years in a cohort of schizophrenic patients of recent onset. *Social Psychiatry*, **21(1)**, 1–9.

Schulberg, D., Quinlan, D.M., Morgenstern, H. & Glazer, W. (1990) Positive and negative symptoms in chronic psychiatric outpatients: reliability, stability, and factor structure. *Psychological Assessment: A Journal of Consulting and Clinical Psychology*, **2**, 262–268.

Shenton, M.E., Kikinis, R., Jolesz, F.A. *et al.* (1992) Abnormalities of the left temporal lobe and thought disorder in schizophrenia: a quantitative magnetic resonance imaging study. *New England Journal of Medicine*, **327(9)**, 604–612.

Siris, S.G. (1991) Diagnosis of secondary depression in schizophrenia: implications for DSM-IV. *Schizophrenia Bulletin*, **17(1)**, 75–98.

Slade, P. & Bentall, R. (1989) Psychological treatments for negative symptoms. *British Journal of Psychiatry* (Suppl.), **Nov 7**, 133–135.

Stephens, J.H. (1978) Long-term prognosis and follow-up in schizophrenia. *Schizophrenia Bulletin*, **4**, 25–47.

Strauss, J.S. & Carpenter, W.T. (1974) Characteristic symptoms and outcome in schizophrenia. *Archives of General Psychiatry*, **30**, 429–434.

Strauss, J.S., Carpenter, W.T., Jr. & Bartko, J.J. (1974) Schizophrenic signs and symptoms. *Schizophrenia Bulletin*, **4**, 61–69.

Tandon, R., Greden, J.F. & Silk, K.R. (1988) Treatment of negative schizophrenic symptoms with trihexphenidyl. *Journal of Clinical Psychopharmacology*, **8(3)**, 212–215.

Tsuang, M.T. (1991) Morbidity risks of schizophrenia and affective disorders among first-degree relatives of patients with schizoaffective disorders. *British Journal of Psychiatry*, **158**, 165–170.

Vaillant, G.E. (1978) A 10-year followup of remitting schizophrenics. *Schizophrenia Bulletin*, **4**, 78–85.

Van Kammen, D.P. (1987) 5 H-T, a neurotransmitter for all seasons? *Biological Psychiatry*, **22(1)**, 1–3.

Volkow, N.D., Wolf, A.P., Van Gelder, P. *et al.* (1987) Phenomenological correlates of metabolic activity in 18 patients with chronic schizophrenia. *American Journal of Psychiatry*, **144**, 151–158.

Walker, E. & Harvey, P. (1986) Positive and negative symptoms in schizophrenia: attentional performance correlates. *Psychopathology*, **19**, 294–302.

Weinberger, D.R. (1987) Implications of normal brain development for the pathogenesis of schizophrenia. *Archives of General Psychiatry*, **44**, 660–669.

WHO (1992) *The ICD-IO Classification of Mental and Behavioral Disorders*. Geneva, World Health Organization.

Wing, J.K. (1970) A standard form of psychiatric Present State Examinations (PSE) and a method for standardizing the classification of symptoms. In Hare, E.H. & Wing, J.K. (eds) *Psychiatric Epidemiology*, Oxford University Press, Oxford.

Wyatt, R.J., Morihisa, J.M., Nakamura, R.K. & Freed, W.J. (1986) Transplanting tissue into the brain for function: use in a model of Parkinson's disease. *Research Publications Association for Research in Nervous and Mental Disease*, **64**, 199–208.

Chapter 4
Schizoaffective Disorder

M. T. TSUANG, J. J. LEVITT AND J. C. SIMPSON

Introduction

Before there was an alternative to antipsychotic medication there was little practical psychopharmacological consequence in categorizing a psychotic patient as schizophrenic or manic depressive. With the widespread introduction of lithium, manic-depressive illness became more susceptible to treatment, gained attractiveness as a diagnosis, and hence sharpened interest in the differential diagnosis of psychotic disorders. Specifically, where the boundary lies between schizophrenia and manic-depressive illness became a question of practical therapeutic importance and helped renew interest in schizoaffective disorder and other atypical psychotic conditions.

In this chapter, we will survey the widely differing views regarding the diagnosis and treatment of schizoaffective disorder in the light of recent empirical research, and refer to interesting findings from genetic, epidemiological and follow-up studies. We will begin with a selective historical review of the concept of schizoaffective disorder.

Historical overview

Controversy over the classification of those patients who share schizophrenic and affective features has existed at least since the time of Kraepelin (1919), who believed that differential diagnosis was most difficult when confronted by a 'mingling of morbid symptoms of both psychoses'. The 'acute schizoaffective psychoses', a phrase first employed by Kasanin (1933), expresses the problem succinctly. Kasanin applied this term to a group of patients characterized as having a sudden onset in a state of marked emotional turmoil, distortion of the outside world (including false sensory impressions in some) and recovery following a short-lived psychosis of a few weeks to a few months.

This type of patient, who when viewed cross-sectionally appeared schizophrenic, but who fully recovered, attracted increasing attention in the 1960s. Vaillant (1964), relying heavily on the work of Langfeldt and Kant, derived a group of prognostic features which he used to predict remission in schizophrenic patients. Stephens *et al.* (1966) generated a longer but analogous list of prognostic features, also used to predict recovery in such patients. Both these investigators were able to predict remission in approximately 80% of cases by combining various prognostic features, including affective symptoms and affective heredity (or absence of schizophrenic heredity) as predictors of remission. By labelling patients 'remitting schizophrenia', however, these authors implied their belief that mixed cases nonetheless remain schizophrenic.

Other investigators have argued that mixed cases are better thought of as variants of affective disorder. Evidence in support of this viewpoint has come primarily from studies of schizoaffective patients with a predominantly manic affective picture (e.g. see Abrams & Taylor, 1976; Pope *et al.*, 1980; Rosenthal *et al.*, 1980).

The final major three ways in which schizoaffective disorder has been viewed are: (i) that it is a heterogeneous mixture of disorders; (ii) that it is a distinct disorder separate from schizophrenia and affective illness; and (iii) that it represents an artificial categorization of clinical phenomena lying on a continuum between schizophrenia and affective disorder. Family and outcome studies (discussed below) have been the primary focus of efforts to evaluate these alternative positions. At this point, we merely note that the continuum hypothesis assumes a dimensional, as opposed to a categorical, perspective, and that although dimensional nosological approaches can have certain advantages (e.g. see Widiger & Frances, 1985), in application to psychoses there could arise conceptual (and clinical) confusion if the continuum hypothesis is taken to suggest that the psychoses can be divided into a limitless number of categories for purposes of prognosis and treatment. If, on the other hand, the heterogeneous view of schizoaffective disorder is adopted (e.g. see Levitt & Tsuang, 1988), it suggests the usefulness of the strategy of subdivivion into a few major homogeneous subtypes.

The latter approach raises the issue of how best to subtype schizoaffective disorder. For example, can schizoaffective disorder be most profitably subtyped into depressive and bipolar divisions as in the *Diagnostic and Statistical Manual* DSM-IV (APA, 1994), or should it initially be divided into schizodominant and affect-dominant types as by Tsuang *et al.* (1986), or should both approaches be used as in the Research Diagnostic Criteria (RDC)? We shall see that empirical evidence from long-term outcome studies appears to sup-

port distinctions based upon polarity, but not to the exclusion of other subtyping schemes. Unipolar and bipolar subtypes have also proved to be useful for clinical purposes, e.g. in guiding cross-sectional pharmacological treatment, but the evidence from family studies is not conclusive. It has also been pointed out that longitudinally, the course of schizoaffective disorder can often be described as polymorphous (Marneros *et al.*, 1986), which could make any dichotomy an oversimplification. Because of these complexities, this remains a very active area of schizoaffective research.

Additional interest in schizoaffective disorder has been stimulated by a recent trend to conceptualize schizophrenia in terms of negative and positive symptoms (Crow, 1980; Andreasen *et al.*, 1991), thus emphasizing the need to distinguish between the depressive component of schizoaffective disorder and the negative syndrome of schizophrenia. This distinction can be difficult cross-sectionally in view of the similarity of the two syndromes. One potential way to disentangle these two overlapping sets of symptoms is to follow patients longitudinally, as negative symptoms are thought to persist over the long term (Pfohl & Winokur, 1983; Andreasen *et al.*, 1991), whereas depressive symptoms tend to remit. An additional complication is that negative symptoms are not homogeneous and can result from such diverse causes as drug-induced akinesia, institutionalization, positive symptoms, depression (Andreasen *et al.*, 1991) or as an emotional response to psychosis itself, e.g. postpsychotic depression or demoralization.

Diagnostic criteria for schizoaffective disorder

The term 'schizoaffective disorder' has been widely used, but with considerable differences in meaning and application (Brockington & Leff, 1979). However, most definitions of schizoaffective disorder do have in common that they identify patients who concurrently share characteristic and pronounced schizophrenic and affective features, and hence do not qualify for typical diagnoses of schizophrenia or affective disorder (Levitt & Tsuang, 1990). In particular, such patients have sufficient affective symptoms to exclude an uncomplicated diagnosis of schizophrenia or, alternatively, sufficient schizophrenic features to exclude an uncomplicated diagnosis of affective disorder. It follows that one's concept of schizoaffective illness will be directly influenced by how broadly or narrowly one defines schizophrenia and affective psychosis (Kendell, 1986).

Despite Kasanin's original description of schizoaffective disorder as characterized by very sudden onset followed by recovery after a few weeks or months (Kasanin, 1933), not all subsequent definitions have emphasized the course of the illness. For example, the criteria of Welner *et al.* (1974), Abrams and Taylor (1976), Brockington *et al.* (1980a,b), and the proposed clinical criteria of Tsuang *et al.* (1986) are primarily or exclusively cross-sectional. However, in view of the complexity of schizoaffective syndromes, involving various mixtures of schizophrenic and affective features over time, it should not be surprising that there has been an increasing emphasis on the use of longitudinal features to define schizoaffective disorder.

The most widely used criteria for studies of schizoaffective disorder have been the RDC of Spitzer *et al.* (1978), which specify (but do not necessarily require) periods of time when schizophrenia-like symptoms clearly dominate the clinical picture. This concept — the persistence of psychotic symptoms in the absence of affective symptoms — is also important in RDC for distinguishing between 'mainly schizophrenic' and 'mainly affective' subtypes of schizoaffective disorder, and several major studies have demonstrated the predictive validity of this clinical feature (Brockington *et al.*, 1980a; Himmelhoch *et al.*, 1981; Coryell *et al.*, 1990a,b).

At the same time that the RDC were introduced, an influential review paper by Pope and Lipinski (1978) forcefully argued that 'schizophrenic' symptoms occur with some regularity in affective disorders, and by themselves (e.g. cross-sectionally) should not be the basis for differential diagnosis. In consequence of these several developments, there appears to have been a shift in the core concept of schizoaffective disorder from the co-occurrence of psychotic (and in particular, mood-incongruent) symptoms and affective symptoms to one that represents 'patients whose psychotic symptoms are not clearly linked to their affective episodes' (Blacker & Tsuang, 1992). In 1985, Maj and Perris proposed a set of diagnostic criteria distinguished by their emphasis on course to subclassify schizoaffective disorder. Subsequently, the DSM-III-R (APA, 1987) criteria required the persistence of delusions or hallucinations in the absence of prominent mood symptoms for at least 2 weeks; this is essentially a modified version of the RDC criteria for schizoaffective disorder, mainly schizophrenic type. This longitudinal criterion has been carried over into DSM-IV (APA, 1994) with the additional limiting requirement that this 2-week (or longer) period occur during the same period of the illness characterized by the concurrent expression of affective and schizophrenic syndromes. One effect of this requirement could be to re-emphasize somewhat the cross-sectional picture in diagnosis by, for example, not including in schizoaffective disorder a hypothetical patient who had a mixed clinical picture in one episode followed in a separate episode by 2 weeks of predominantly schizophrenic symptoms. It appears that the prognostic and nosological significance of longitudinal features will be an active area of research for some time to come.

At present, the criteria most commonly used to define schizoaffective disorder for research purposes include the RDC and the similar DSM-IV criteria. In addition, investigators have often modified these criteria (e.g. Marneros *et al.*, 1992) or proposed their own criteria (e.g. Tsuang *et al.*, 1986) as a means of studying course, family data and other potentially important defining characteristics of these patients. Doubtless there will continue to be a variety of ways used to define schizoaffective disorder, and given the controversial status of the illness this is to be preferred to settling prematurely on any one criterion set. In fact, it is perhaps best explicitly to label all current diagnostic criteria for schizoaffective disorder as provisional. To emphasize this point (which can tend to be overlooked with repeated use of the phrase 'schizoaffective disorder') it could be helpful to use alternative terms such as 'schizoaffective syndrome', 'RDC schizoaffective disorder', 'DSM-IV schizoaffective disorder', etc. in appropriate contexts.

Epidemiology

In contrast to schizophrenia, which has been the subject of innumerable epidemiological investigations, relatively little is known about the epidemiology of schizoaffective disorder, e.g. regarding incidence, prevalence, demographics, mortality and associations with socioeconomic variables and other potential risk factors. This is probably due largely to the uncertain nosological status of schizoaffective disorder, and to the resulting difficulty in reconciling across studies results that can be greatly affected by how the disorder is defined. To minimize this problem, we have emphasized in this review those studies that used objective diagnostic criteria (e.g. RDC and DSM-III-R).

Incidence

Only a few studies have examined the incidence of schizoaffective disorder. Brockington and Leff (1979) reported that patients meeting three or more definitions of schizoaffective disorder (out of eight definitions examined) comprised 4.5% of first-admission psychiatric patients in the Camberwell catchment area of London in 1973–74. 'Schizomanic' patients (manic patients with schizophrenic or paranoid symptoms) had an incidence rate of 1.7 per 100 000 population per year, which was considerably smaller than the rate of 4 per 100 000 population per year for 'schizodepressive' patients. The numbers of schizoaffective patients identified in this sample exceeded the number of manic patients, and were roughly half the number of incident schizophrenic cases, indicating that schizoaffective patients comprise a clinically significant population.

Additional evidence on this point can be obtained from a recent analysis of epidemiological catchment area study data, obtained from diagnostic interview schedule (DIS) interviews with randomly selected cases in five US communities (Tien & Eaton, 1992). These authors compared incidence rates in three non-overlapping groups of cases with delusions and hallucinations: (i) schizophrenics; (ii) cases with only delusions and hallucinations; and (iii) a 'psychotic affective syndrome' group who also had manic or depressive episodes. The latter group is similar to, but not identical with, most definitions of schizoaffective disorder because 59% of the group experienced delusions and hallucinations only when they had a mood disturbance (such cases would be classified as having a mood disorder with psychotic symptoms under DSM-IV). Despite this limitation, the study is important because it found that 1-year incidence rates for the psychotic affective group were approximately the same as for the schizophrenics, namely 1.7 per 1000 population per year vs. 2.0 per 1000 population per year for schizophrenia. Even if only 40% of the psychotic affective group would meet criteria for schizoaffective disorder, this result still exceeds by an order of magnitude the earlier estimates of Brockington and Leff (1979). In part, the difference can be attributed to the difference between a community sample and a treated sample. However, the difference between the incidence rates for schizophrenia is just as large, and not readily explained.

Prevalence

Most of the information regarding the prevalence of schizoaffective disorder has been obtained from clinical samples. An exception is Torrey's (1987) prevalence study of schizophrenia in a rural area of western Ireland. Using key informants, Torrey estimated the 6-month prevalence rate for broadly defined schizophrenia to be 12.6 per 1000 population. The actual number of cases included 21 with DSM-III schizophrenia and 11 with schizoaffective disorder; as with Brockington and Leff's (1979) incidence study, the ratio of schizophrenia to schizoaffective disorder is roughly 2:1.

Prevalence estimates of schizoaffective disorder in clinical populations have varied widely, as can be expected given the multiple factors affecting selection into treatment and duration of treatment. For example, Rosenthal *et al.* (1980) reported that 35% of the manic patients in a lithium clinic were RDC schizoaffective-manic. Müller-Oerlinghausen *et al.* (1992) found that the prevalence of schizoaffective disorder in lithium clinics varied widely from city to city: 7% (Aarhus), 15% (Berlin), 23% (Vienna) and 32% (Hamilton). Junginger *et al.* (1992) found that 14% of the delusional patients in a chronic and highly selected population of in-patients and out-patients met DSM-III-R criteria for schizoaffective disorder, compared with 60% for schizophrenia, 17% for bipolar disorder and 4% for major depression. In the Cologne study on long-term course and outcome, Marneros *et al.* (1991) applied longitudinal criteria adapted from DSM-III-R to a large sample of patients with major psychoses, and found that the number with schizoaffective disorder (28.5%) was about the same as the number with affective disorders (30%), and less than the number with schizophrenia (42%). Taken together, these studies validate current interest in schizoaffective disorder as being a clinically significant population of psychiatric patients.

A number of investigators have compared the prevalence of the manic and depressive subtypes of schizoaffective disorder. Clayton, in an influential 1982 review, concluded that the manic type is more frequent. A subsequent first-admission study by Berner and Lenz (1986) supports this conclusion in a comparison of subtypes of RDC schizoaffective disorder (12.5% schizoaffective-manic vs. 8% schizoaffective-depressed). However, a broader sample of first-admission patients in the study by Brockington and Leff (1979) showed substantially more schizodepressive patients (3.7%) than schizomanic patients (1.5%). Two recent studies of consecutive in-patient samples also indicate that the depressive subtype is more prevalent: Kitamura and Suga (1991), using RDC criteria; and Marneros *et al.* (1991), using modified DSM-III. In view of these inconsistent results, we can hypothesize that selection

factors largely determine the relative numbers of schizoaffective-manic and schizoaffective-depressed patients who are treated. More definitive findings will have to await information from future epidemiological studies of schizoaffective disorder.

Demographic factors

Given the variability in how schizoaffective disorder is defined and the evident influence of selection biases in prevalence studies, it is not surprising that studies of demographic factors, such as gender and age at onset, have produced widely varying results. Nevertheless, some general conclusions are possible.

With regard to gender, there appear to be as many or more females than males, e.g. 71% in the sample of Tsuang *et al.* (1986) and 63% in that of Marneros *et al.* (1990a). Berner and Lenz (1986) reported that the male to female ratio ranged from 0.3:1 to 1:1 depending on the definition of schizoaffective disorder employed. In their general population study, Tien and Eaton (1992) reported higher 1-year incidence rates for females with DIS psychotic affective syndrome (a heterogeneous group that probably includes schizoaffective disorder) for all age groups examined, and computed a relative risk of 6.8 for developing this syndrome in females compared with in males. Clayton (1982) hypothesized that the results also depend on polarity, e.g. approximately equal numbers of males and females in the manic subtype, compared with almost two-thirds female patients in the depressive subtype. Kitamura and Suga (1991), however, found approximately equal numbers of males and females in both schizoaffective-manic and schizoaffective-depressed subtypes.

Age at onset is one of the basic characteristics that reliably distinguishes major subgroups of patients — e.g. male vs. female schizophrenics (Goldstein *et al.*, 1989), and bipolar vs. unipolar affective disorder (Smeraldi *et al.*, 1983) — and for that reason is also of interest in schizoaffective disorder. First, age at onset appears to be a discriminating factor in comparison with other disorders. For example, in her 1982 review Clayton concluded that most studies found the average age at onset to be youngest for schizoaffective disorders compared with unipolar and bipolar disorders. Similarly, Tsuang *et al.* (1986) reported that the mean age at onset of schizoaffective disorder (29 years) was significantly younger than for manic and depressed groups defined using Washington University criteria (34 and 44 years, respectively); however, there was no difference between schizoaffective disorder and schizophrenia. Marneros *et al.* (1990a) reported that the median age at onset for schizoaffective disorder (29 years) was younger than the median age for affective disorders (35 years), and older than for schizophrenia (24 years). Berner and Lenz (1986) showed that the age at onset depends largely on the diagnostic criteria employed; for example, DSM-III identified a schizoaffective patient population that was older than the RDC schizoaffective-depressed subtype, and substantially older than the RDC schizoaffective-manic subtype of schizoaffective disorder.

Within schizoaffective disorder there might also be a substantial effect of gender on the age at onset, namely, that females tend to be older at onset of the disorder (Angst, 1986). To the extent that their DIS psychotic affective syndrome includes schizoaffective disorder, the results of Tien and Eaton (1992) also support this generalization: 1-year incidence rates for females were substantial for age groups greater than 34 years, whereas incidence rates for males declined sharply after an age of 34 years.

Information on marital status is available in a few studies (e.g. Clayton, 1982; Marneros *et al.*, 1990b), but confounding by gender makes the available results difficult to interpret or compare across studies.

Precipitating factors

One of the defining characteristics of schizoaffective disorder, as initially conceptualized by Kasanin (1933), has been the presence of precipitants such as stressors or major life events. To some extent this notion has been validated empirically. Brockington *et al.* (1980b) reported that 10 of 32 schizomanic patients had obvious recent

stress such as childbirth, surgery, head injury or the disruption of important personal relationships. Tsuang *et al.* (1986) found significantly more precipitants of any type in schizoaffective disorder (60%) compared with schizophrenia (11%), mania (27%) or depression (39%). Furthermore, schizoaffectives had significantly more psychosocial, physical and postpartum precipitants in most of the comparisons with these other diagnostic groups. In contrast, Marneros *et al.* (1990b) found equal percentages of schizoaffective and affective disorder patients with life events before onset (51%), compared with only 24% in schizophrenia. Tien and Eaton (1992) found that antecendent alcohol problems, but not daily marijuana abuse, increased the relative risk of DIS psychotic affective syndrome to 5.7.

Premorbid factors

Premorbid or predisposing factors can give useful clues to the aetiology and early course of the disorder, but unfortunately little is known about such factors in schizoaffective disorder. Marneros *et al.* (1990b) reported a significantly higher educational level in schizoaffective patients compared with that in schizophrenic patients, but no difference between schizoaffective and affective disorder patients. The same pattern was obtained for employment or vocational training. Compared with schizoaffectives, patients with schizophrenia were more often in lower social classes; this was attributed partly to the parents' social class, and partly to the schizophrenic patient's downward mobility at the time of onset. In contrast, there was no significant difference between the schizoaffective and affective disorder groups. Finally, all three diagnostic groups had similar percentages of patients from broken homes.

Mortality

Several factors combine to make premature mortality a special concern in schizoaffective disorder. Schizoaffective patients share some of the symptoms and other characteristics of schizophrenics and affective disorder patients, who have repeatedly been shown to be at increased risk of death, principally (but not exclusively) from suicides and accidents (Simpson, 1988). Buda *et al.* (1988) directly compared the mortality experience of those with DSM-III schizophrenia with a heterogeneous group that included schizoaffective disorder, schizophreniform disorder and atypical psychotic disorder; they used follow-up data beginning with index hospital stays between 1934 and 1945. Excess mortality for the atypical group in this historical sample was observed for specific causes of death including infections, neoplasms, cardiovascular disease and suicide. Furthermore, suicide occurred in excess among the other psychotics compared with shizophrenics and with the general population. Angst *et al.* (1990) compared suicides in affective disorder and schizoaffective disorder using data from Zurich, Bonn and New York, and found that the suicide risk for schizoaffective patients closely resembled that for patients with affective disorders. In particular, the risk of suicide was constant over a lifetime and did not increase or decrease with age. Marneros *et al.* (1989), in a long-term follow-up study of schizoaffective patients, reported suicide attempts over a lifetime in 43% of the unipolar subgroup and in 29% of the bipolar subgroup, usually by drug overdose. Clearly, the suicide risk in these patients is substantial and enduring.

Fortunately, there is evidence that suicide in psychiatric patients is to some extent predictable and preventable, largely in response to standard psychiatric interventions (Tsuang *et al.*, 1992). Recent evidence in support of this view was gathered by Müller-Oerlinghausen *et al.* (1992) in a study of the long-term effect of lithium treatment (average duration of treatment was 7 years) on the mortality of patients with schizoaffective and affective disorders. That study, which included clinical samples from Canada and three European countries, found that mortality was not significantly increased in lithium-treated schizoaffective patients compared with the general population, although the mortality risk in the bipolar and unipolar comparison groups was actually somewhat less than for schizoaffective disorder.

Genetic and family studies

Family studies of schizoaffective disorder have led to inconsistent results which can be attributed in part to the inherent heterogeneity of this group of patients and to the lack of uniformity in diagnosis. It is of some interest, therefore, to find three studies that used different definitions of schizoaffective disorder and yet obtained convergent results.

First, a review by Fowler (1978) summarized several studies showing schizophrenics with good prognosis to have a familial risk of affective disorder (20%) between that of unipolar depressive (16%) and manic patients (35%), and to have a familial risk of schizophrenia significantly greater (6%) than manic (<1%) or unipolar depressive patients (<1%). This was interpreted as consistent with the conclusion that good-prognosis schizophrenia had elevated risks in relatives for both affective disorder and schizophrenia, and hence was most consistent with an interpretation of heterogeneity. In contrast, Gershon *et al.* (1988) studied schizoaffective disorder as largely defined by RDC where the emphasis is more on mixing affective and schizophrenic features rather than on a good outcome. The schizoaffective, chronic subtype in this study also revealed elevated risks (compared with controls) for non-affective psychosis and affective disorder (pooling unipolar and bipolar cases). A third example of yet a different definition of schizoaffective disorder, namely cases with 'atypical psychosis' who for a variety of reasons fail to meet diagnostic criteria for schizophrenia or affective disorder, is found in a study by Tsuang (1991), where again high rates of schizophrenia and affective disorders were found in relatives of schizoaffective probands. Hence, whether good prognosis, mixing of affective and schizophrenic features, or atypicality is emphasized in the definition of schizoaffective disorder, family studies have revealed elevated rates of both schizophrenic and affective disorder in relatives of schizoaffective patients, consistent with genetic heterogeneity.

Another possibility is that schizoaffective disorder is a distinct entity. In general, however, family studies have not demonstrated an increased risk of schizoaffective disorder and no other disorders in relatives of schizoaffectives, which would be the pattern most supportive of schizoaffective disorder as a distinct entity or 'third psychosis' (Zerbin-Rüdin, 1986).

If it is true that schizoaffective disorder is heterogeneous, the next logical question is whether it can be successfully subtyped. Tsuang (1991) has demonstrated one approach to such subtyping by segregating atypical psychotic patients into those with an increased probability for schizophrenia or affective disorder, and a residual undifferentiated group. Marneros *et al.* (1989) have approached the problem longitudinally by showing that schizoaffective disorder can be divided in terms of long-term course into those with bipolar and unipolar types. Others, including Angst *et al.* (1979) and Gershon *et al.* (1988), have had difficulty subtyping schizoaffectives when using family studies as a validator.

Long-term course and outcome

Reasons for examining the long-term course of schizoaffective disorder include the importance of understanding the prognosis as the basis for clinical management and for comparisons of treatment efficacy; the possibility of identifying prognostic factors; and the use of longitudinal information to validate diagnostic concepts and to investigate diagnostic heterogeneity (e.g. by identifying homogeneous subgroups).

As a basic description of the course of the illness, we provide the following illustrative summary adapted from Samson *et al.* (1988), and subject to the limitations noted elsewhere in this chapter regarding the wide variability in the definition of schizoaffective disorder. Reported rates of recovery from schizoaffective episodes have ranged from 83% reported in a short-term follow-up study (Clayton *et al.*, 1968) to 29% at any time during a 6-month follow-up period (Coryell *et al.*, 1984). Approximately 20−30% of schizoaffective patients go on to show a deteriorating course, e.g. one typified by persistent psychosis (Holmboe & Astrup, 1957; Brockington *et al.*, 1980a,b; Gross *et al.*, 1986; Coryell *et al.*, 1990a,b; Tsuang, 1990; Grossman *et al.*, 1991).

Approximately 10% of patients show diagnostic shifts over time, becoming either more affective or more psychotic in symptom manifestation (Angst, 1986). Schizoaffective patients have been reported to spend on average about 20% of their lifetimes hospitalized or in an episode (Angst, 1986). Angst (1986) has also reported that the median number of hospitalizations over a 25-year period was between 6 and 7. Although many definitions of schizoaffective disorder allow for the sequential manifestation of psychotic and affective symptomatology, most patients show concurrent expressions of psychotic and affective symptoms (Marneros *et al.*, 1986).

To put the results of longitudinal studies of schizoaffective disorder in context, it is helpful to keep in mind that in general the long-term outcome of schizoaffective disorder is better than in schizophrenia, but worse in comparison with affective disorder (Harrow and Grossman (1984), Angst (1986) and Samson *et al.* (1988) provide extensive reviews of this topic). There is also some evidence that the long-term outcome for the manic subtype of schizoaffective disorder is similar to that for mania or bipolar disorder, whereas outcome comparisons of the depressive subtype and major depression reveal substantial differences (Brockington *et al.*, 1980a,b; Clayton, 1982). Differential outcomes of other subgroupings of schizoaffective disorder have also been investigated, with much interest focusing on the mainly affective vs. mainly schizophrenic distinction in the RDC. Earlier results indicated worse outcomes for the mainly schizophrenic subtype (Levinson & Levitt, 1987), but several recent reports have not confirmed this pattern (Coryell *et al.*, 1990a,b; Grossman *et al.*, 1991). For example, Coryell *et al.* (1990a,b) concluded that chronicity was more predictive of outcome in both depressive and manic subtypes of RDC schizoaffective disorder.

A major goal of longitudinal studies is to identify prognostic factors, particularly those variables that predict especially good or poor outcomes. The one variable that has emerged with some consistency is the persistence of psychotic symptoms in the absence of affective symptoms; this substantially increases the risk of poor outcomes such as persistent psychosis (Brockington *et al.*, 1980a; Himmelhoch *et al.*, 1981; Maj *et al.*, 1987; Coryell *et al.*, 1990a,b). Other risk factors for a negative outcome include poor premorbid personality (Coryell *et al.*, 1990a,b; del Rio Vega & Ayuso-Gutierrez, 1990), premorbid instrumental skills (McGlashan & Williams, 1990), chronicity at index assessment (Maj *et al.*, 1987; Coryell *et al.*, 1990a,b), frequency of relapses (del Rio Vega & Ayuso-Gutierrez, 1990) and the number of typically schizophrenic symptoms (McGlashan & Williams, 1990). To assist clinicians in identifying patients with an increased likelihood of having a schizophrenia-like course and outcome, Coryell *et al.* (1990a,b) developed the following 'poor-outcome prototype': a patient who has had a poor premorbid or adolescent social adjustment and inadequate social adjustment as an adult, a chronic course and, at some point, persistent psychotic features that dominated the clinical picture. This prototype appeared to be valid in both depressive and manic types of RDC schizoaffective disorder (Coryell *et al.*, 1990a,b). A focus for future research will be to validate such predictors in other patient populations, and to refine the concept of a poor-prognosis prototype in homogeneous subgroups that are identified as being nosologically important.

Treatment strategies

Studies addressing psychopharmacological treatment of schizoaffective disorder are made more difficult to generalize from because of the non-uniform way in which schizoaffective disorder has been defined in the literature. As it is our contention that schizoaffective disorder is genetically heterogeneous, subtyping is a natural next step. We have found it useful for psychopharmacological treatment purposes to divide schizoaffective disorder by polarity (e.g. bipolar vs. unipolar schizoaffective disorder) and to pay especially close attention to interepisode psychotic symptomatology (i.e. to psychotic symptoms that persist in the absence of a full affective syndrome).

When viewed cross-sectionally, schizoaffective disorder, bipolar type (or 'schizomania'), probably represents primarily a mixture of those patients

with bipolar affective disorder and others with schizophrenia in excited states (Clayton, 1982). A high index of suspicion for organic/toxic states is also important. If a certain proportion of these patients actually suffer from a form of bipolar disorder, certainly the use of antimanic agents, including neuroleptics, lithium and anticonvulsants (e.g. carbamazepine and valproate), makes sense. Such agents have been explored alone (Prien *et al.*, 1972; Abrams & Taylor, 1976; Brockington *et al.*, 1978; Pope *et al.*, 1980) and in combination (Biederman *et al.*, 1979; Okuma *et al.*, 1989a,b). Biederman *et al.* (1979), for example, found a modest benefit from the combination of lithium carbonate and haloperidol which must then be balanced against the additional risk of greater toxicity. It has been our experience that when intermorbid psychotic symptoms persist after mixed-symptom episodes subside, chronic neuroleptic therapy is more likely to be necessary. Okuma *et al.* (1989b) reported that carbamazepine in combination with neuroleptics was modestly useful in the treatment of excited states in a mixed group of schizophrenics and schizoaffectives. Potential adverse effects included increased hallucinatory behaviour and worsened psychomotor activity possibly related to the reported inducing by carbamazepine of its own metabolism and that of concomitant neuroleptics, thus lowering neuroleptic blood levels. Valproate, which is not a tricyclic structure and does not induce the metabolism of hepatically cleared agents (McElroy *et al.*, 1992), would be a possible alternative. Clozapine has recently also been proposed as an additional alternative (McElroy *et al.*, 1991) for patients with schizoaffective disorder, bipolar or depressed type.

Cross-sectional diagnoses of schizoaffective disorder, unipolar type (or 'schizodepression'), probably primarily represent a mixture of patients with psychotic affective disorder (e.g. delusional depression) and schizophrenics with depressive syndromes (Brockington *et al.*, 1980a) together with some patients with bipolar disorder and diverse other conditions (Clayton, 1982). Again, combination treatment suggests itself. The use of antidepressants from all classes in combination with neuroleptics is plausible, with tricyclics and monoamine oxidase inhibitors (MAOIs) so far being most closely examined (Siris *et al.*, 1978, 1987). It has been suggested that one source of variance in whether these patients respond to the addition of an antidepressant is whether or not patients with current florid psychotic symptoms are excluded (Kramer *et al.*, 1989). In the light of additional weight gain seen as a potential side effect of combining phenothiazines and tricyclics (Prussoff *et al.*, 1979), selective serotonin re-uptake inhibitors (which do not cause weight gain) might be an attractive alternative, although to our knowledge this alternative has so far not been studied systematically. Augmentation with lithium, analogous to that used with treatment-resistant depressions (de Montigny *et al.*, 1983), has also been suggested for the treatment of refractory psychotic depression, especially that associated with a bipolar course (Nelson & Mazure, 1986). In addition, it has been suggested by Tsuang *et al.* (1979) that electroconvulsive therapy (ECT) may reduce mortality in schizo-affective patients.

Conclusion

We have reviewed schizoaffective disorder, perhaps the most common atypical psychosis, from multiple perspectives. Our necessarily provisional view is that schizoaffective disorder is a genetically heterogeneous condition primarily composed of schizophrenia, unipolar and bipolar disorders and perhaps a residual currently undifferentiated condition. For research purposes, schizoaffective disorder can accordingly be subtyped into schizophrenic, affective and undifferentiated categories. Other subtyping schemes (e.g. chronic vs. non-chronic, and manic vs. depressive) also have potential value, and should not be prematurely excluded at this stage of investigation. For psycho-pharmacological treatment purposes, subtyping into bipolar and unipolar categories has proved to be of clinical value. Future research will be needed to resolve the continuing uncertainty regarding diagnosis, treatment and prognosis in this heterogeneous but important group of psychoses.

References

Abrams, R. & Taylor, M.A. (1976) Mania and schizo-affective disorder manic type: a comparison. *American Journal of Psychiatry*, **133**, 1145–1147.

Andreasen, N.C., Flaum, M., Arndt, S., Alliger, R. & Swayze, V.W. (1991) Positive and negative symptoms: assessment and validity. In Marneros, A., Andreasen, N.C. & Tsuang, M.T. (eds) *Negative Versus Positive Schizophrenia*, pp. 28–51. Springer-Verlag, Berlin.

Angst, J. (1986) The course of schizoaffective disorders. In Marneros, A. & Tsuang, M.T. (eds) *Schizoaffective Psychoses*, pp. 63–93. Springer-Verlag, Berlin.

Angst, J., Felder, W. & Lohmeyer, B. (1979) Are schizoaffective psychoses heterogeneous? II. Results of a genetic investigation. *Journal of Affective Disorders*, **1**, 155–165.

Angst, J., Stassen, H.H., Gross, G., Huber, G. & Stone, M.H. (1990) Suicide in affective and schizoaffective disorders. In Marneros, A. & Tsuang, M.T. (eds) *Affective and Schizoaffective Disorders*, pp. 168–185. Springer-Verlag, Berlin.

APA (1987) *Diagnostic and Statistical Manual of Mental Disorders*, 3rd edn, revised. American Psychiatric Association, Washington DC.

APA (1994) *Diagnostic and Statistical Manual of Mental Disorders*, 4th edn. American Psychiatric Association, Washington DC.

Berner, P. & Lenz, G. (1986) Definitions of schizoaffective psychosis: mutual concordance and relationship to schizophrenia and affective disorder. In Marneros, A. & Tsuang, M.T. (eds) *Schizoaffective Psychoses*, pp. 31–49. Springer-Verlag, Berlin.

Biederman, J., Lerner, Y. & Belmaker, R.H. (1979) Combination of lithium carbonate and haloperidol in schizo-affective disorder: a controlled study. *Archives of General Psychiatry*, **36**, 327–333.

Blacker, D. & Tsuang, M.T. (1992) Contested boundaries of bipolar disorder and the limits of categorical diagnosis in psychiatry. *American Journal of Psychiatry*, **149**, 1473–1483.

Brockington, I.F. & Leff, J.P. (1979) Schizo-affective psychosis: definitions and incidence. *Psychological Medicine*, **9**, 91–99.

Brockington, I.F., Kendell, R.E., Kellet, J.M., Curry, S.H. & Wainwright, S. (1978) Trials of lithium, chlorpromazine and amitriptyline in schizoaffective patients. *British Journal of Psychiatry*, **133**, 162–168.

Brockington, I.F., Kendell, R.E. & Wainwright, S. (1980a) Depressed patients with schizophrenic or paranoid symptoms. *Psychological Medicine*, **10**, 665–675.

Brockington, I.F., Wainwright, S. & Kendell, R.E. (1980b) Manic patients with schizophrenic or paranoid symptoms. *Psychological Medicine*, **10**, 73–83.

Buda, M., Tsuang, M.T. & Fleming, J.A. (1988) Causes of death in DSM-III schizophrenics and other psychotics (atypical group): a comparison with the general population. *Archives of General Psychiatry*, **45**, 283–285.

Clayton, P.J. (1982) Schizoaffective disorders. *Journal of Nervous and Mental Disease*, **170**, 646–650.

Clayton, P., Rodin, L. & Winokur, G. (1968) Family history studies. III. Schizoaffective disorder, clinical and genetic factors including a one- to two-year follow-up. *Comprehensive Psychiatry*, **9**, 31–49.

Coryell, W., Keller, M., Lavori, P. & Endicott, J. (1990a) Affective syndromes, psychotic features, and prognosis. I. Depression. *Archives of General Psychiatry*, **47**, 651–657.

Coryell, W., Keller, M., Lavori, P. & Endicott, J. (1990b) Affective syndromes, psychotic features, and prognosis. II. Mania. *Archives of General Psychiatry*, **47**, 658–662.

Coryell, W., Lavori, P., Endicott, J., Keller, M. & Van Eerdewegh, M. (1984) Outcome in schizoaffective, psychotic, and nonpsychotic depression: course during a six- to 24-month follow-up. *Archives of General Psychiatry*, **41**, 787–791.

Crow, T.J. (1980) Molecular pathology of schizophrenia: more than one disease process? *British Medical Journal*, **280**, 66–68.

Fowler, R.C. (1978) Remitting schizophrenia as a variant of affective disorder. *Schizophrenia Bulletin*, **4**, 68–77.

Gershon, E.S., DeLisi, L.E., Hamovit, J. *et al.* (1988) A controlled family study of chronic psychoses: schizophrenia and schizoaffective disorder. *Archives of General Psychiatry*, **45**, 328–336.

Goldstein, J.M., Tsuang, M.T. & Faraone, S.V. (1989) Gender and schizophrenia: implications for understanding the heterogeneity of the illness. *Psychiatry Research*, **28**, 243–253.

Gross, G., Huber, G. & Armbruster, B. (1986) Schizoaffective psychoses — long-term prognosis and symptomatology. In Marneros, A. & Tsuang, M.T. (eds) *Schizoaffective Psychoses*, pp. 188–203. Springer-Verlag, Berlin.

Grossman, L.S., Harrow, M., Goldberg, J.F. & Fichtner, C.G. (1991) Outcome of schizoaffective disorder at two long-term follow-ups: comparisons with outcome of schizophrenia and affective disorders. *American Journal of Psychiatry*, **148**, 1359–1365.

Harrow, M. & Grossman, L.S. (1984) Outcome in schizoaffective disorders: a critical review and reevaluation of the literature. *Schizophrenia Bulletin*, **10**, 87–108.

Himmelhoch, J.M., Fuchs, C.Z., May, S.J., Symons, B.J. & Neil, K.S. (1981) When a schizo-affective diagnosis has meaning. *Journal of Nervous and Mental Disease*, **169**, 277–282.

Holmboe, R. & Astrup, C. (1957) A follow-up study of 255 patients with acute schizophrenia and schizophreniform psychoses. *Acta Psychiatrica Scandinavica*, **115** (Suppl.), 9–61.

Junginger, J., Barker, S. & Coe, D. (1992) Mood theme and bizarreness of delusions in schizophrenia and mood psychosis. *Journal of Abnormal Psychology*, **101**, 287–292.

Kasanin, J. (1933) The acute schizoaffective psychoses. *American Journal of Psychiatry*, **90**, 97–126.

Kendell, R.E. (1986) The relationship of schizoaffective illnesses to schizophrenic and affective disorders. In Marneros, A. & Tsuang, M.T. (eds) *Schizoaffective Psychoses*, pp. 18–30. Springer-Verlag, Berlin.

Kitamura, T. & Suga, R. (1991) Depressive and negative symptoms in major psychiatric disorders. *Comprehensive Psychiatry*, **32**, 88–94.

Kraepelin, E. (1919) *Dementia Praecox and Paraphrenia*, facsimile 1919 edition. Krieger, Huntington.

Kramer, M.S., Vogel, W.H., DiJohnson, C. *et al.* (1989) Antidepressants in 'depressed' schizophrenic inpatients: a controlled trial. *Archives of General Psychiatry*, **46**, 922–928.

Levinson, D.F. & Levitt, M.E.M. (1987) Schizoaffective mania reconsidered. *American Journal of Psychiatry*, **144**, 415–425.

Levitt, J.J. & Tsuang, M.T. (1988) The heterogeneity of schizoaffective disorder: implications for treatment. *American Journal of Psychiatry*, **145**, 926–936.

Levitt, J.J. & Tsuang, M.T. (1990) Atypical psychoses. In Hyman, S. & Jennike, M. (eds) *Manual of Clinical Problems in Psychiatry*, pp. 45–52. Little Brown, Boston.

McElroy, S.L., Dessain, E.C., Pope H.G. Jr *et al.* (1991) Clozapine in the treatment of psychotic mood disorders, schizoaffective disorder, and schizophrenia. *Journal of Clinical Psychiatry*, **52**, 411–414.

McElroy, S.L., Keck, P.E. Jr, Pope H.G. Jr & Hudson, J.I. (1992) Valproate in the treatment of bipolar disorder: literature review and clinical guidelines. *Journal of Clinical Psychopharmacology*, **12**, 42S–52S.

McGlashan, T.H. & Williams, P.V. (1990) Predicting outcome in schizoaffective psychosis. *Archives of General Psychiatry*, **178**, 518–520.

Maj, M. & Perris, C. (1985) An approach to the diagnosis and classification of schizoaffective disorders for research purposes. *Acta Psychiatrica Scandinavica*, **72**, 405–413.

Maj, M., Starace, F. & Kemaldi, D. (1987) Prediction of outcome by historical, clinical and biological variables in schizoaffective disorder, depressed type. *Journal of Psychiatric Research*, **21**, 289–295.

Marneros, A., Deister, A. & Rohde, A. (1990a) Psychopathological and social status of patients with affective, schizophrenic and schizoaffective disorders after long-term course. *Acta Psychiatrica Scandinavica*, **82**, 352–358.

Marneros, A., Deister, A. & Rohde, A. (1990b) Sociodemographic and premorbid features of schizophrenic, schizoaffective, and affective psychoses. In Marneros, A. & Tsuang, M.T. (eds) *Affective and Schizoaffective Disorders*, pp. 130–145. Springer-Verlag, Berlin.

Marneros, A., Deister, A. & Rohde, A. (1991) Stability of diagnoses in affective, schizoaffective and schizophrenic disorders: cross-sectional versus longitudinal diägnosis. *European Archives of Psychiatry and Clinical Neuroscience*, **241**, 187–192.

Marneros, A., Deister, A. & Rohde, A. (1992) Comparison of long-term outcome of schizophrenic, affective and schizoaffective disorders. *British Journal of Psychiatry*, **161** (Suppl. 18), 44–51.

Marneros, A., Rohde, A. & Deister, A. (1989) Unipolar and bipolar schizoaffective disorders: a comparative study. II. Long-term course. *European Archives of Psychiatry and Clinical Neuroscience*, **239**, 164–170.

Marneros, A., Rohde, A., Deister, A. & Risse, A. (1986) Schizoaffective disorders: the prognostic value of the affective component. In Marneros, A. & Tsuang, M.T. (eds) *Schizoaffective Psychoses*, pp. 155–163. Springer-Verlag, Berlin.

de Montigny, C., Cournoyer, G., Morissette, R., Langlois, R. & Caille, G. (1983) Lithium carbonate addition in tricyclic antidepressant-resistant unipolar depression: correlations with neurobiologic actions of tricyclic antidepressant drugs and lithium ion on serotonin system. *Archives of General Psychiatry*, 40, 1327–1334.

Müller-Oerlinghausen, B., Ahrens, B., Grof, E. *et al.* (1992) The effect of long-term lithium treatment on the mortality of patients with manic-depressive and schizoaffective illness. *Acta Psychiatrica Scandinavica*, 86, 218–222.

Nelson, J.C. & Mazure, C.M. (1986) Lithium augmentation in psychotic depression refractory to combined drug treatment. *American Journal of Psychiatry*, 143, 363–366.

Okuma, T., Yamashita, I., Takahashi, R. *et al.* (1989a) Clinical efficacy of carbamazepine in affective, schizoaffective and schizophrenic disorders. *Pharmacopsychiatry*, 22, 47–53.

Okuma, T., Yamashita, I., Takahashi, R. *et al.* (1989b) A double-blind study of adjunctive carbamazepine versus placebo on excited states of schizophrenic and schizo-affective disorders. *Acta Psychiatrica Scandinavica*, 80, 250–259.

Pfohl, B. & Winokur, G. (1983) The micropsychopathology of hebephrenic/catatonic schizophrenia. *Journal of Nervous and Mental Disease*, 171, 296–300.

Pope, H.G. Jr & Lipinski, J. (1978) Diagnosis in schizophrenia and manic-depressive illness: a reassessment of the specificity of 'schizophrenic' symptoms in the light of current research. *Archives of General Psychiatry*, 35, 811–828.

Pope, H.G. Jr, Lipinski, J.F., Cohen, B.M. & Axelrod, D.T. (1980) Schizo-affective disorder: an invalid diagnosis? A comparison of schizo-affective disorder, schizophrenia and affective disorder. *American Journal of Psychiatry*, 137, 921–927.

Prien, R.F., Point, P., Caffey, E.M. Jr & Klett, C.J. (1972) A comparison of lithium carbonate and chlorpromazine in the treatment of excited schizoaffectives: report of the Veterans Administration and Nation Institute of Mental Health collaborative study group. *Archives of General Psychiatry*, 27, 182–189.

Prusoff, B.A., Williams, D.H., Weissman, M.M. & Astrachan, B.M. (1979) Treatment of secondary depression in schizophrenia: a double-blind, placebo-controlled trial of amitriptyline added to perphenazine. *Archives of General Psychiatry*, 36, 569–575.

del Rio Vega, J.M. & Ayuso-Gutierrez, J.L. (1990) Course of schizoaffective psychosis: a retrospective study. *Acta Psychiatrica Scandinavica*, 81, 534–537.

Rosenthal, N.E., Rosenthal, L.N., Stallone, F., Dunner, D.L. & Fieve, R.R. (1980) Toward the validation of RDC schizoaffective disorder. *Archives of General Psychiatry*, 37, 804–810.

Samson, J.A., Simpson, J.C. & Tsuang, M.T. (1988) Outcome studies of schizoaffective disorders. *Schizophrenia Bulletin*, 14, 543–554.

Simpson, J.C. (1988) Mortality studies in schizophrenia. In Tsuang, M.T. & Simpson, J.C. (eds) *Handbook of Schizophrenia*, Vol. 3; *Nosology, Epidemiology and Genetics of Schizophrenia*, pp. 245–273. Elsevier, Amsterdam.

Siris, S.G., van Kammen, D.P. & Docherty, J.P. (1978) Use of antidepressant drugs in schizophrenia. *Archives of General Psychiatry*, 35, 1368–1377.

Siris, S.G., Morgan, V., Fagerstrom, R., Rifkin, A. & Cooper, T.B. (1987) Adjunctive imipramine in the treatment of postpsychotic depression: a controlled trial. *Archives of General Psychiatry*, 42, 533–539.

Smeraldi, E., Gasperini, M., Macciardi, F., Bussoleni, C. & Morabito, A. (1983) Factors affecting the distribution of age at onset in patients with affective disorders. *Journal of Psychiatric Research*, 17, 309–317.

Spitzer, R.L., Endicott, J. & Robbins, E. (1978) *Research Diagnostic Criteria*, 3rd edn. Biometrics Research, New York State Department of Mental Hygiene, New York.

Stephens, J.H., Astrup, C. & Mangrum, J.C. (1966) Prognostic factors in recovered and deteriorated schizophrenics. *American Journal of Psychiatry*, 122, 1116–1121.

Tien, A.Y. & Eaton, W.W. (1992) Psychopathologic precursors and sociodemographic risk factors for the schizophrenia syndrome. *Archives of General Psychiatry*, 49, 37–46.

Torrey, E.F. (1987) Prevalence studies in schizophrenia. *British Journal of Psychiatry*, 150, 598–608.

Tsuang, M.T. (1990) Follow-up studies of schizoaffective disorders: a comparison with affective disorders. In Marneros, A. & Tsuang, M.T. (eds) *Affective and Schizoaffective Disorders*, pp. 123–129. Springer–Verlag, Berlin.

Tsuang, M.T. (1991) Morbidity risks of schizophrenia and affective disorders among first-degree relatives of patients with schizoaffective disorders. *British Journal of Psychiatry*, 158, 165–170.

Tsuang, M.T., Dempsey, G.M. & Fleming, J.A. (1979) Can ECT prevent premature death and suicide in 'schizoaffective' patients? *Journal of Affective Disorders*, 1, 167–171.

Tsuang, M.T., Simpson, J.C. & Fleming, J.A. (1986) Diagnostic criteria for subtyping schizoaffective disorder. In Marneros, A. & Tsuang, M.T. (eds) *Schizoaffective Psychoses*, pp. 50–62. Springer-Verlag, Berlin.

Tsuang, M.T., Simpson, J.C. & Fleming, J.A. (1992) Epidemiology of suicide. *International Review of Psychiatry*, 4, 125–138.

Vallant, G.E. (1964) Prospective perdiction of schizophrenic remission. *Archives of General Psychiatry*, 11, 509–518.

Welner, A., Croughan, J.L. & Robins, E. (1974) The group of schizoaffective and related psychoses — critique, record, follow-up, and family studies. I. A persistent enigma. *Archives of General Psychiatry*, 31, 628–631.

Widiger, T.A. & Frances, A. (1985) The DSM-III personality disorders: perspectives from psychology. *Archives of General Psychiatry*, 42, 615–623.

Zerbin-Rüdin, E. (1986) Schizoaffective and other atypical psychoses: the genetical aspect. In Marneros, A. & Tsuang, M.T. (eds) *Schizoaffective Psychoses*, pp. 225–231. Springer-Verlag, Berlin.

Chapter 5
Atypical Psychotic Disorders

C. B. PULL

Introduction

Atypical psychotic disorders designate psychotic conditions that cannot be easily classified as either schizophrenia or a mood disorder with psychotic features. They form a heterogeneous and poorly understood collection of disorders that are regarded as probably unrelated to schizophrenia and affective disorder, but on which surprisingly little empirical research has been carried out up to now. The terminology used to designate the individual disorders in this group as well as the proportion of patients that are regarded as suffering from one of these disorders varies from country to country.

Atypical psychotic disorders can conveniently be divided according to their typical duration into a group of chronic persistent delusional disorders and a group of acute and transient psychotic disorders.

Schizoaffective disorder is described in a separate chapter and will not be detailed again here.

Historical background

In the successive editions of his *Textbook of Psychiatry*, Kraepelin gradually evolved a system of classification to which all subsequent systems have paid tribute. In describing those conditions known today as functional psychoses, Kraepelin leaned heavily on clinical course and prognosis. In the sixth edition of his textbook (1899), he distinguished three classes of psychoses: manic-depressive psychoses, dementia praecox and paranoia. In the eighth edition (1909–1915), Kraepelin introduced the concept of the paraphrenias that are separated from the paranoid form of dementia praecox.

Kraepelin described dementia praecox as a

single disease progressing towards 'psychic enfeeblement' (*psychische Schwäche*) and presenting three forms: hebephrenia, catatonia and dementia paranoides. Paranoia was characterized by systematized delusions, without hallucinations, and accompanied by perfect preservation of clear and orderly thinking. Paraphrenia shared many of the characteristics of paranoia and schizophrenia. The main difference from paranoia was that in paraphrenia the delusions were accompanied by prominent hallucinations, and the main difference from schizophrenia was that paraphrenia did not progress to a dementia-like state.

Although Kraepelin's nosology was gradually to establish its position, several aspects of his classification have been either neglected or opposed, to varying degrees, depending on national schools of psychiatry. This has led to either an extension or a narrowing of the concept of dementia praecox, and consequently of schizophrenia. In Britain and in the USA, terms like paranoia and paraphrenia were rarely used in practice, and psychoses that were not organic were classified, up to a recent past, as either schizophrenic or affective (Kendell, 1993). The French, Scandinavian and German schools of psychiatry have, on the contrary, excluded from schizophrenia different types of acute and transient psychoses as well as a number of chronic delusional disorders.

Transient psychotic disorders

A considerable number of labels have been proposed to designate transient psychotic disorders which are regarded as neither schizophrenic nor affective. Although the different eponyms seem to refer to the same group of patients, systematic clinical information that would give rise to concepts that can be clearly defined and separated from each other is not yet available. The incidence of these disorders seems to be more frequent in the developing countries than in other parts of the world (Sartorius *et al.*, 1986).

Prominent concepts in this field are the *bouffées délirantes* of the French, the 'reactive' or 'psychogenic' psychoses and the 'schizophreniform' psychoses of the Scandinavian and the 'cycloid psychoses' of the German tradition, as well as a number of so-called culture-bound psychoses.

Bouffées délirantes

The concept of *bouffée délirante polymorphe des dégénérés* was introduced by Magnan and Legrain (1895), at the end of the 19th century, as part of a complex classification of the delusional states of degeneracy. The classical description of bouffée délirante, as given by Magnan's pupil Legrain (1886), rests on the following criteria: (i) sudden onset, 'like a bolt from the blue'; (ii) polymorphous delusions and hallucinations of any kind; (iii) clouded consciousness associated with emotional instability; (iv) absence of physical signs, i.e. the disorder is not due to any organic mental disorder; (v) rapid return to the premorbid level of functioning; and (vi) relapses may occur, but individual episodes are separated by symptom-free intervals.

Whereas Magnan and Legrain stated that bouffées délirantes occur without any identifiable precipitating factor, the current consensus holds that there is a variant of the disorder occasioned by psychological stressors.

Using the results of a national enquiry, the present author (Pull *et al.*, 1987) has developed explicit diagnostic inclusion and exclusion criteria for both genuine or Magnan-type as well as for stress-related bouffée délirante. The striking outcome of this enquiry is that the concept of bouffée délirante, as used by present-day French psychiatrists, has not changed in 100 years, with the exception that the theory of degeneracy is no longer used.

In the past, the disorder was diagnosed by French psychiatrists nearly three times as frequently as acute schizophrenia (Pichot & Debray, 1971). According to Pichot (1990), empirical studies currently being carried out indicate, however, that, when stringent diagnostic criteria are applied, the disorder is not commonly reported among new cases.

Psychogenic or reactive psychoses

The concept of psychogenic or reactive psychosis

has been developed in Scandinavia.

The first comprehensive survey of the concept of psychogenic psychosis is to be found in a monograph from 1916 by the Danish psychiatrist Wimmer. According to Wimmer, psychogenic psychoses are clinically independent from schizophrenia and manic-depressive psychosis, they usually develop in a predisposed individual, they are caused by psychosocial factors (which also determine the content and form of the disorder), they have a great tendency to recover and they seem never to end in deterioration.

The prognostic validity of psychogenic psychosis has been investigated by Faergeman (1963), who made a follow-up study of Wimmer's cases. Of the 113 original cases of psychogenic psychosis, 66 were confirmed by Faergeman, whereas one-third were rediagnosed as suffering from schizophrenia.

According to Strömgren (1974), 65% of psychogenic psychoses are emotional reactions, 15% are disorders of consciousness and 20% are paranoid types.

Schizophreniform psychoses

The concept of schizophreniform psychosis was described in Norway by Langfeldt in 1939. Langfeldt differentiated between two groups of psychoses usually diagnosed as schizophrenia: a group with poor prognosis, labelled 'genuine' or 'process' schizophrenia, and a group with good prognosis, labelled 'schizophreniform' psychosis.

The following factors were considered by Langfeldt to be correlated with good prognosis: a well-adjusted premorbid personality, the presence of identifiable precipitating factors, sudden onset, the presence among an otherwise schizophrenic symptomatology of a disturbance of mood, clouding of consciousness and the absence of blunted affect.

A great deal of research (Garmezy, 1968; Brockington *et al.*, 1978) has been focused on an objective separation between 'process' schizophrenia and 'schizophreniform' psychosis, but there still is no decisive evidence to prove that the two types are of a qualitatively different nature.

Cycloid psychoses

The term cycloid psychoses was coined by Leonhard (1957) to denominate endogenous psychotic syndromes characterized by a sudden onset, an admixture of symptoms belonging to the affective disorders and of symptoms belonging to schizophrenia and phasic course. Leonhard subdivided the cycloid psychoses into three forms: motility psychoses, confusional psychoses and anxiety—blissfulness psychoses.

The concept has been operationalized by Perris (1974) as follows: cycloid psychoses are psychotic episodes of sudden onset, mostly unrelated to stress, with good immediate outcome but with a high risk of recurrence, characterized by mood swings (from depression to elation) and at least two of the following: (i) various degrees of perplexity or confusion; (ii) delusions (of reference, influence or persecution) and/or hallucinations not syntonic with mood; (iii) motility disturbances (hypo- or hyperkinesia); (iv) occasional episodes of ecstasy; and (v) states of overwhelming anxiety (pananxiety).

Findings of several empirical investigations (Cutting *et al.*, 1978; Brockington *et al.*, 1982) suggest that cycloid psychoses meeting Perris' criteria represent a relatively consistent pattern of disorder with regard to onset, symptomatology, recurrence, outcome, response to treatment and family history.

Culture-specific psychoses

Disorders such as latah, amok, koro, windigo and a variety of other possibly culture-specific disorders share two principal features: (i) they are not easily accommodated by the categories in established and internationally used psychiatric classifications; and (ii) they were first described in, and subsequently closely or exclusively associated with, a particular population or cultural area.

These disorders have also been referred to as culture-bound or culture-reactive, and as ethnic or exotic psychoses. Some are rare, some may be comparatively common, and the status of most is controversial. Many researchers argue that they differ only in degree from disorders already included in existing classifications. As suggested by the tentative assignment of culture-specific disorders to categories in the *International Classification of Diseases* ICD-10 (WHO, 1993), it would appear that most of these disorders are not even related to any identified psychosis, but rather to varying personality disorders, somatoform disorders, dissociative disorders, or that they represent acute reactions to stress.

A list of culture-specific disorders and the codes suggested in ICD-10 for classifying them is given in Table 5.1.

Persistent psychotic or delusional disorders

The number and nature of persistent psychotic or delusional disorders which are regarded as neither schizophrenic nor affective varies greatly from country to country. Prominent in this field are the concepts of paranoia and paraphrenia, the *délires chroniques* of the French tradition, as well as a variety of other concepts, either included in the preceding or separated from them, such as delusional jealousy, *folie à deux*, Capgras' syndrome, erotomania, Cotard's syndrome, Kretschmer's *sensitiver Beziehungswahn* and the more recent category of schizotypal disorder.

Paranoia and paranoid disorders

In the times before Kraepelin, the term paranoia was applied to a number of quite different disorders. In the eighth edition of his textbook, Kraepelin (1909–1915) restricted the term to a group of psychoses characterized by the development of a permanent and unshakeable delusional system without hallucinations, accompanied by clear and orderly thinking, willing and acting. Kraepelin described different subtypes of paranoia, depending on the content of the delusions (persecutory, grandiose or jealous).

Since Kraepelin, the independence of paranoia from affective disorder and schizophrenia has been the object of much debate. In his 1980 literature review, Kendell concluded that the available data did not suggest that paranoia is a subtype of affective illness, and that 'the bulk of the evidence suggests that paranoia and schizophrenia are distinct syndromes'.

More recent evidence supporting the independence of paranoia from schizophrenia comes primarily from family history studies (Kendler *et al.*, 1981, 1985) and from course and outcome studies (Opjordsmoen & Retterstol, 1987; Schanda & Gariel, 1988).

The term paranoid disorders, which embraces paranoia, paraphrenia and a number of other delusional syndromes, has been the object of much controversy, in particular because the adjective 'paranoid' has had multiple different meanings over time and in different languages. In its original German meaning, it refers to all delusions relating to the subject. In the English-speaking community, it has been restricted by and large to designate persecutory delusions (Kendell, 1993). In France, the term *paranoïde* is used exclusively to differentiate a particular form of schizophrenia, i.e. paranoid schizophrenia (Pichot, 1990). In current nomenclatures, the term delusional disorder has been adopted for this group of disorders.

Paraphrenia

The concept of paraphrenia was introduced by Kraepelin in the later editions of his textbook. Kraepelin described four types of paraphrenia: systematic, expansive, confabulatory and fantastic. For Kraepelin, paraphrenias could be distinguished from dementia praecox by the absence of deterioration despite a protracted course, and from paranoia because they were accompanied by prominent auditory hallucinations.

The independence of paraphrenia from schizophrenia has been questioned early on, and although the term has been part of most classifications up to a recent past, paraphrenia has been generally subsumed under schizophrenia.

Late paraphrenia was defined by Roth (1955) as a well-organized system of paranoid delusions, with or without auditory hallucinations, existing in the setting of a well-preserved personality and

Table 5.1 Culture-bound syndromes and suggested *International Classification of Disease* ICD-10 codes

Local term	ICD-10	Suggested code
Amok	F68.8	Other specified disorders of adult personality and behaviour
Dhat, dhatu, jiryan, shen-k'uei, shen-kui	F48.8 F45.34	Other specified neurotic disorders Somatoform autonomic dysfunction of the genitourinary system
Koro, jinjin bemar, suk yeong, suo-yang	F48.8 F45.34	Other specified neurotic disorders Somatoform autonomic dysfunction of the genitourinary system
Latah	F48.8 F44.88	Other specified neurotic disorders Other specified dissociative disorders
Nerfiza, nerves nevra, nervios	F32.11 F48.0 F45.1	Moderate depressive episode with somatic syndrome Neurasthenia Undifferentiated somatoform disorder
Pa-leng, frigophobia	F40.2	Specific phobias
Pibloktoq, Arctic hysteria	F44.7 F44.88	Mixed dissociative disorders Other specified dissociative disorders
Susto, espanto	F45.1 F48.8	Undifferentiated somatoform disorder Other specified neurotic disorders
Taijin kyofusho, shinkeishitsu, anthropophobia	F40.1 F40.8	Social phobias Other phobic anxiety disorders
Ufufuyane, saka	F44.3 F44.7	Trance and possession disorders Mixed dissociative disorders
Uqamairineq	F44.88 F47.4	Other specified dissociative disorders Narcolepsy and cataplexy
Windigo	F68.8	Other specified disorders of adult personality and behaviour

affective response. Whether or not late paraphrenia should be considered a separate, though clinically not homogeneous, entity (Holden, 1987) or a late-onset form of schizophrenia (Grahame, 1984) continues to be debated up to the present (Howard *et al.*, 1993).

The chronic delusional states of French nosology

French psychiatrists traditionally separate from paranoid schizophrenia an important proportion of cases labelled délires chroniques (chronic delusional states). Chronic delusional states are subdivided into three broad categories.

1 Chronic interpretative psychosis (also known as systematized or paranoiac psychosis).
2 Chronic hallucinatory psychosis.
3 Chronic imaginative (or paraphrenic or fantastic) psychosis.

Chronic interpretative psychosis

Chronic interpretative psychosis is subdivided into intellectual and emotional delusional states, according to the content of the delusional system and to whether or not the delusions are 'polarized' around a single theme.

In intellectual delusional states, the delusions spread progressively to contaminate all areas of mental activity. The original description of the disorder was provided by Sérieux and Capgras (1909). The disorder is defined by the authors as a chronic, systematized psychosis, feeding on delusional interpretations and characterized by false reasoning originating in the misinterpretation of otherwise correctly perceived facts. The other essential features listed by Sérieux and Capgras are: (i) the complexity and coherence of the delusions; (ii) the absence of prominent hallucinations; (iii) unimpaired intellectual functioning; (iv) progressive spreading of the delusional system; and (v) chronic course. As described in current standard French textbooks, the disorder is essentially the same as that described in other nomenclatures by the term paranoia.

In emotional delusional states the delusional premise does not spread beyond the theme and person(s) involved in the original system. The disorder has been described by Sérieux and Capgras (1909) as a chronic, systematized psychosis, in which a single, relentless and patently pathological thought subdues and dominates all other mental activity. The most commonly described variants are: (i) the vindictive delusional states of litigious persons, social reformers, religious fanatics or secretive inventors; and (ii) delusional jealousy and erotomania.

Emotional delusional states have been particularly well described by de Clérambault (in a series of papers collected in 1942), according to whom these disorders are characterized by a central delusional premise: 'I am the victim of an injustice', in the case of vindictive delusional states; 'he (she) is unfaithful to me', in delusional jealousy; and 'he (she) loves me', in erotomania.

A theoretical diagram of the traditional French classification of chronic interpretative psychosis (Pichot, 1990) is presented in Table 5.2.

Chronic hallucinatory psychosis

Chronic hallucinatory psychosis was first described by Ballet in 1911 as a disorder characterized by: (i) persistent hallucinatory activity; (ii) delusions, most frequently of persecution; and (iii) clear sensorium, unimpaired speech, appropriate behaviour and intact higher intellectual functions. In addition to the preceding features, current explicit diagnostic criteria (Pull *et al.*, 1987) emphasize the absence of schizophrenic thought disorder, onset in middle or late adult life, and relatively good psychosocial adjustment.

Chronic imaginative psychosis

Chronic imaginative psychosis was originally described by Dupré and Logre in 1911. The disorder is characterized by paralogical, magical thinking, fantastic and grandiose delusions, the predominance of confabulatory delusional mechanisms and good contact with reality contrasting with the extravagance of the delusions. The diagnosis is rarely made by French psychiatrists in present days.

Delusional jealousy

Also called pathological jealousy, morbid jealousy or Othello syndrome, this disorder is characterized by an abnormal belief that one's sexual partner is unfaithful. According to Gelder *et al.* (1989), the condition is not uncommon in psychiatric practice and most full-time clinicians probably see one or two cases a year. As indicated by the results of surveys of subjects with delusional jealousy (Langfeldt, 1961; Shepherd, 1961; Mowat, 1966;

Table 5.2 Theoretical diagram of the traditional French classification of chronic delusional states. (From Pichot, 1990)

Class	Genus	Species	Variants
Chronic interpretative psychosis	Intellectual delusional states (not encapsulated)	Interpretative delusional states	
		Hypersensitive delusional states	Paranoia of spinsters and governesses Paranoia of immigrants or of culture shock
	Emotional delusional states (encapsulated)	Vindictive delusional states	Litigious paranoia Paranoia of social reformers and religious fanatics Paranoia of secretive inventors
		Sentimental delusional states	Conjugal paranoia Erotic paranoia (erotomania)

Vauhkonen, 1968; Mullen & Maack, 1985), the disorder is more frequent in men than women; the prognosis depends on a number of factors, including the nature of any underlying psychiatric disorder and the patient's premorbid personality; and there is a risk that the patient may become violent to his or her partner or supposed rival.

Folie à deux

Folie à deux was first described by Lasègue and Falret in 1877, as a disorder in which the delusions held by a sick person are induced in, or shared by, a healthy person. The disorder, which may involve more than two people, typically develops in persons who are isolated from other people. Usually, the healthy partner(s) will lose the delusional beliefs when the relationship with the primary person is interrupted. The concept of folie à deux, which is listed apart in other nomenclatures, is not considered an independent disorder in traditional French nosology, but is subsumed under the category of interpretative delusional states.

Capgras' syndrome or illusion des sosies

The *illusion des sosies* was described by Capgras and Reboul-Lachaux in 1923, as a delusional disorder in which the patient, usually a woman, is convinced that a particular person in her life, such as her husband or another person who is quite familiar and well known to her, has been replaced by a double (*sosie*), i.e. a look-alike impostor. Although originally described in France, the syndrome has received more attention in other countries (Sims & Reddie, 1976) than in France, where the concept is hardly used at all. In 1983, Berson reviewed 133 published cases of Capgras' syndrome in the English-language literature. He concluded that the syndrome appeared in both men and women over a wide age range and in a variety of illness states. In particular, the syndrome was associated with schizophrenia in more than half the cases.

Erotomania

Also called de Clérambault's syndrome outside

of France, erotomania represents one of the emotional delusional states (*délires passionnels*) described by de Clérambault. The subject, usually a woman, is unshakeably but unjustifiably convinced that another person, usually a man of higher social status or famous as a public figure, is infatuated with her. She finds 'proof' of his love for her everywhere, e.g. in casual remarks or in the way he dresses. In the beginning, the patient is quite confident that her 'lover' will eventually be able to come out of hiding, and tries to convince him with letters, phone calls or gifts. In the later stages of the disorder, the patient may become resentful, abusive, spiteful and even aggressive.

Recent reports suggest that erotomania is an aetiologically heterogeneous syndrome that may be seen in a variety of mental disorders, most commonly in schizophrenia (Sims & White, 1973; Jordan & Howe, 1980; Ellis & Mellsop, 1985). The presence of erotomania has also been noted in other conditions, including depression (Raskin & Sullivan, 1974; Staner, 1991), bipolar disorder (Remington & Book, 1984; Signer & Swinson, 1987) and organic mental disorder (Signer & Cummings, 1987).

Cotard's syndrome

Under the name *délire de négation*, Cotard (1880, 1882) described patients who complained of having lost not only their possessions and social status, but also their hearts, blood, intestines or brains. The syndrome is usually associated with a severe form of depression. It has become rarer in recent years, at least in its complete form, probably because the underlying disorder responds to pharmacotherapy before the psychopathological manifestations of the syndrome develop. Chronic forms of the syndrome may occur in organic mental disorders.

Kretschmer's sensitiver Beziehungswahn

In a monograph published in 1918, Kretschmer described a type of paranoia which developed in sensitive personalities when a precipitating event, termed key experience (*Schlüsselerlebnis*), occurred at the correct time in the person's life. According to Kretschmer, the prognosis was good. In particular, patients with the disorder did not develop schizophrenia. According to Pichot (1983), Kretschmer's description was to have a major impact on psychiatric thinking. By setting forth that a particular delusional state could be 'understood', Kretschmer 'opened the path to the dissolution of process endogeny and the establishment of the psychogenic conception of the psychoses'.

Schizotypal (personality) disorder

The term schizotypal was introduced to modern psychiatric nosology largely as the result of family studies in schizophrenia (Kety *et al.*, 1978; Kendler *et al.*, 1981). The disorder is more common among family members of individuals with schizophrenia and is believed to be part of the genetic 'spectrum' of disorders. Schizotypal disorder is characterized by eccentric behaviour and anomalies of thinking and affect which resemble those seen in schizophrenia, although no definite and characteristic schizophrenic anomalies have occurred at any stage. No single feature is invariably present. The disorder is not clearly demarcated either from simple schizophrenia or from schizoid or paranoid personality disorders. It runs a chronic course with fluctuations of intensity. There is no definite onset and the evolution and course are usually those of a personality disorder.

Atypical psychotic disorders in DSM-IV

In the fourth edition of the *Diagnostic and Statistical Manual* (DSM-IV) of the American Psychiatric Association (APA, 1994), atypical psychotic disorders (as defined here) are described under the heading 'Schizophrenia and Other Psychotic Disorders'. DSM-IV lists five major disorders in this section.
1 Delusional disorder.
2 Brief psychotic disorder.
3 Schizophreniform disorder.
4 Schizoaffective disorder.

5 Induced or shared psychotic disorder (folie à deux).

Schizotypal disorder is listed among the personality disorders.

The DSM-IV classification of atypical psychotic disorders is presented in Table 5.3.

Important changes have been made in the nomenclature and description of 'atypical' psychotic disorders, from DSM-III (APA, 1981) to DSM-III-R (APA, 1987) (Kendler *et al.*, 1989), and again from DSM-III-R to DSM-IV (APA, 1994).

Delusional disorder

According to the DSM, current evidence from demographic, family and follow-up studies suggests that delusional disorder is probably distinct from both schizophrenia and mood disorders. In the three recent editions of the classification, the essential feature of the disorder is the presence of one or more persistent delusions that are not

Table 5.3 The *Diagnostic and Statistical Manual* DSM-IV classification of non-organic atypical psychotic disorders

295.40	Schizophreniform disorder
	Specify if: without good prognostic features
	with good prognostic features
295.70	Schizoaffective disorder
	Specify type: bipolar type
	depressive type
297.1	Delusional disorder
	Specify type: erotomanic, grandiose
	jealous, persecutory
	somatic, mixed, unspecified
298.8	Brief psychotic disorder
	Specify type: with marked stressor(s)
	(brief reactive)
	without marked stressor(s)
	with postpartum onset
297.3	Shared psychotic disorder (folie à deux)
298.9	Psychotic disorder not otherwise specified

due to any other mental disorder, such as schizophrenia, schizophreniform disorder, a mood disorder, an organic factor or the direct effects of a substance. Apart from the impact of the delusion(s) or its ramifications, functioning is not markedly impaired and behaviour is not obviously odd or bizarre.

The term 'paranoid', which was used in DSM-III to designate this type of disorder, has been changed to 'delusional' disorder in DSM-III-R and DSM-IV. While the diagnosis of paranoid disorder could only be applied to people with delusions of persecution or jealousy, the inclusion criteria for delusional disorder are much broader in that they require only the presence of one or more 'non-bizarre' (i.e. non-schizophrenic) delusions, without further specification.

Two other important changes that were made in the criteria for delusional disorder in DSM-III-R have been retained in DSM-IV. First, the minimum duration of the disorder has been increased from 1 week to 1 month, and second, persistent tactile and olfactory hallucinations are no longer excluded if related to the delusional theme (whereas auditory or visual hallucinations may not be present for more than a few hours).

Delusional disorder can be subdivided according to the predominant delusional theme in erotomanic type, grandiose type, jealous type, persecutory type, somatic type, mixed type (when delusions characteristic of more than one type are present but no one theme predominates) or unspecified type.

Brief reactive psychosis and brief psychotic disorder

In DSM-III, the essential feature of brief reactive psychosis is the sudden onset of psychotic symptoms shortly after a recognizable psychosocial stressor, persisting for no more than 2 weeks, and with a full return to the premorbid level of functioning. In DSM-III-R, the maximum duration of the disorder has been increased from 2 to 4 weeks, and there is acknowledgement that the stressors may be cumulative.

In DSM-IV, brief reactive disorder is listed as a subtype of a new category labelled brief psychotic disorder. The disorder is subdivided into three subtypes: with marked stressor(s), corresponding to the definition of brief reactive psychosis; without marked stressor(s); and with postpartum onset.

Schizophreniform disorder

The essential features of this disorder are identical with those of schizophrenia, with the exception that the duration is less than 6 months (but at least 1 month). Two subtypes may be specified, according to the presence or absence of 'good prognostic features' such as rapid onset, confusion or perplexity, good premorbid functioning and absence of blunted or flat affect.

Schizoaffective disorder

The definition of schizoaffective disorder has been modified from DSM-III to DSM-III-R, and again from DSM-III-R to DSM-IV. In DSM-IV, the diagnosis is given to individuals who have had an uninterrupted period of illness during which, at some time, there was a major depressive episode or manic episode concurrent with symptoms of schizophrenia. During the same period of illness, there must have been delusions and hallucinations for at least 2 weeks in the absence of prominent mood symptoms. In addition, symptoms meeting criteria for a mood episode must be present for a substantial portion of the total duration of the illness.

Shared psychotic disorder

The DSM-IV definition of shared delusional disorder corresponds to the original description of folie à deux given by Lasègue and Falret (1877).

Schizotypal personality disorder

In DSM-III, DSM-III-R and DSM-IV, schizotypal disorder is listed among the personality disorders.

Atypical psychotic disorders in ICD-10

In ICD-10 (Sartorius *et al.*, 1993) atypical psychotic disorders (as defined here) are subdivided into five groups.
1 Persistent delusional disorders.
2 Acute and transient psychotic disorders.
3 Induced delusional disorder.
4 Schizoaffective disorder.
5 Schizotypal disorder.
The ICD-10 classification of atypical psychotic disorders is presented in Table 5.4.

Persistent delusional disorder

The group of persistent delusional disorders includes a variety of disorders in which long-standing delusions constitute the only, or the most conspicuous, clinical characteristic, and which cannot be classified as organic, schizophrenic or affective. They are probably heterogeneous and have uncertain relationships to schizophrenia. The relative importance of genetic factors, personality characteristics and life circumstances in their genesis is uncertain and probably variable.

The category is subdivided into delusional disorder, other persistent delusional disorder and unspecified persistent delusional disorder.

Delusional disorder is characterized by the development of either a single delusion or a set of related delusions other than those listed as typically schizophrenic. The delusions are highly variable in content, the commonest examples being persecutory, grandiose, hypochondriacal, jealous or erotic. They must be present for at least 3 months; they are usually persistent and sometimes lifelong. Persistent hallucinations in any modality must not be present and the general criteria of schizophrenia must not be fulfilled. Depressive symptoms may be present intermittently, provided that the delusions persist at times when there is no disturbance of mood. The following subtypes may be specified: persecutory, litigious, self-referential, grandiose, hypochondriacal or somatic, jealous and erotomanic.

The diagnostic criteria for research that are

Table 5.4 The *International Classification of Diseases* ICD-10 classification of non-organic atypical psychotic disorders

F21   Schizotypal disorder

F22   Persistent delusional disorders
    F22.0 Delusional disorder
           The following types may be specified if desired: persecutory, litiginous, self-referential, grandiose, hypochondriacal, jealous, erotomanic
    F22.8 Other persistent delusional disorders
    F22.9 Persistent delusional disorder, unspecified

F23   Acute and transient psychotic disorders
    F23.0 Acute polymorphic psychotic disorder without symptoms of schizophrenia
    F23.1 Acute polymorphic psychotic disorder with symptoms of schizophrenia
    F23.2 Acute schizophrenia-like psychotic disorder
    F23.3 Other acute predominantly delusional psychotic disorder
    F23.8 Other acute and transient psychotic disorders
    F23.9 Acute and transient psychotic disorders, unspecified

    A fifth character may be used to identify the presence or absence of associated acute stress:
    F23.×0 Without associated acute stress
    F23.×1 With associated acute stress

F24   Induced delusional disorder

F25   Schizoaffective disorders
    F25.0 Schizoaffective disorder, manic type
    F25.1 Schizoaffective disorder, depressed type
    F25.2 Schizoaffective disorder, mixed type
    F25.8 Other schizoaffective disorders
    F25.9 Schizoaffective disorder, unspecified

F28   Other non-organic psychotic disorders

F29   Unspecified non-organic psychosis

Table 5.5 Delusional disorder: *International Classification of Diseases* ICD-10 diagnostic criteria for research

A   A delusion or set of related delusions, other than those listed as typically schizophrenic (i.e. other than completely impossible or culturally inappropriate), must be present. The commonest examples are persecutory, grandiose, hypochondriacal, jealous or erotic delusions

B   The delusion(s) in the first criterion must be present for at least 3 months

C   The general criteria for schizophrenia are not fulfilled

D   There must be no persistent hallucinations in any modality (but there may be transitory or occasional auditory hallucinations that are not in the third person or giving a running commentary)

E   Depressive symptoms (or even a depressive episode) may be present intermittently, provided that the delusions persist at times when there is no disturbance of mood

F   Most commonly used exclusion criteria. There must be no evidence of primary or secondary organic mental disorder, or of a psychotic disorder due to psychoactive substance use

Specification for possible subtypes. The following types may be specified if desired: persecutory, litiginous, self-referential, grandiose, hypochondriacal (somatic), jealous, erotomanic

posed in ICD-10 for delusional disorder are presented in Table 5.5.

The category 'other persistent delusional disorders' should be used to classify disorders in which delusions are accompanied by persistent hallucinatory voices or by schizophrenic symptoms that are insufficient to meet criteria for schizophrenia.

Acute and transient psychotic disorders

ICD-10 explicitly recognizes that systematic clinical information that should provide definite guidance on the classification of acute and transient psychotic disorders is not yet available, and the limited data and clinical tradition that must therefore be used instead do not give rise to concepts that can be clearly defined and separated from each other.

The general diagnostic criteria for research

that are proposed in ICD-10 for the group of acute and transient psychotic disorders are presented in Table 5.6.

To classify the disorders in this group, ICD-10 uses a diagnostic sequence that reflects the order of priority given to selected key features. Acute and transient psychotic disorders are subdivided according to whether the onset is acute (within a period of 2 weeks or less) or abrupt (within 48 h or less), whether the typical syndrome is polymorphic or typical of schizophrenia, and whether or not it is associated with acute stress. None of the disorders in the group meets criteria for manic or depressive episodes, although emotional changes may be prominent from time to time. The disorders are also defined by the absence of organic causation and should not be diagnosed in the presence of obvious intoxication by a psychoactive substance.

The syndrome called 'polymorphic' is defined as a rapidly changing and variable state in which hallucinations, delusions, perceptual disturbances, and emotional turmoil with intense feelings of happiness and ecstasy or anxiety and irritability are obvious but markedly variable, changing from day to day or even from hour to hour.

The most appropriate duration of acute and transient psychotic disorders is specified with regard to the duration of symptoms required for a diagnosis of schizophrenia and persistent delusional disorders. In ICD-10, the diagnosis of schizophrenia depends upon the presence of typical schizophrenic symptoms that persist for at least 1 month. When schizophrenic symptoms are consistently present during an acute psychotic disorder, the diagnosis should be changed to schizophrenia if the schizophrenic symptoms persist for more than 1 month. For patients with psychotic, but non-schizophrenic, symptoms that persist beyond 1 month, there is no need to change the diagnosis until the duration requirement of delusional disorder is reached (3 months).

Table 5.6 Acute and transient psychotic disorders: *International Classification of Diseases* ICD-10 diagnostic criteria for research

G1 There is acute onset of delusions, hallucinations, incomprehensible or incoherent speech, or any combination of these. The interval between the first appearance of any psychotic symptoms and the presentation of the fully developed disorder should not exceed 2 weeks

G2 If transient states of perplexity, misidentification or impairment of attention and concentration are present, they do not fulfil the criteria for organically caused clouding of consciousness

G3 The disorder does not meet the symptomatic criteria for manic episode, depressive episode or recurrent depressive disorder

G4 There is insufficient evidence of recent psychoactive substance use to fulfil the criteria for intoxication, harmful use, dependence or withdrawal states. The continued moderate and largely unchanged use of alcohol or drugs in amounts or with the frequency to which the individual is accustomed does not necessarily rule out the use of this category; this must be decided by clinical judgement and the requirements of the research project in question

G5 Most commonly used exclusion clause. There must be no organic mental disorder or serious metabolic disturbances affecting the central nervous system (this does not include childbirth)

A fifth character should be used to specify whether the acute onset of the disorder is associated with acute stress (occurring 2 weeks or less before evidence of first psychotic symptoms)

For research purposes it is recommended that change of the disorder from a non-psychotic to a clearly psychotic state is further specified as *either* abrupt (onset within 48 h) *or* acute (onset in more than 48 h but less than 2 weeks)

Induced delusional disorder

The ICD-10 definition of induced delusional disorder corresponds to the original description by Lasègue and Falret (1877).

Schizoaffective disorders

According to ICD-10, schizoaffective disorders

Table 5.7 Schizotypal disorder: *International Classification of Diseases* ICD-10 diagnostic criteria for research

---

A The subject must have manifested at least four of the following over a period of at least 2 years, either continuously or repeatedly:
   1 inappropriate or constricted affect, with the individual appearing cold and aloof
   2 behaviour or appearance that is odd, eccentric or peculiar
   3 poor rapport with others and a tendency to social withdrawal
   4 odd beliefs or magical thinking, influencing behaviour and inconsistent with subcultural norms
   5 suspiciousness or paranoid ideas
   6 ruminations without inner resistance, often with dysmorphophobic, sexual or aggressive contents
   7 unusual perceptual experiences, including somatosensory (bodily) or other illusions, depersonalization or derealization
   8 vague, circumstantial, metaphoric, overelaborate or often stereotyped thinking, manifested by odd speech or in other ways, without gross incoherence
   9 occasional transient quasi-psychotic episodes with intense illusions, auditory or other hallucinations and delusion-like ideas, usually occurring without external provocation

B The subject must never have met the criteria for schizophrenia

---

are episodic disorders in which both affective and schizophrenic symptoms are prominent within the same episode of illness, and concurrently for at least part of the episode. The diagnosis rests upon an approximate equilibrium between the number, severity and duration of schizophrenic and affective symptoms. The disorder is subdivided into manic, depressive and mixed types. Two further subtypes may be specified according to the longitudinal development of the disorder, i.e. to whether or not schizophrenic symptoms persist beyond the duration of affective symptoms.

Schizotypal disorder

In ICD-10, schizotypal disorder is listed together with schizophrenia and delusional disorders. The diagnostic criteria for research that are proposed

in ICD-10 for schizotypal disorder are presented in Table 5.7.

Comment

Atypical psychotic disorders represent a heterogeneous and poorly understood group of disorders. The nomenclature of these disorders is as uncertain as their nosological status. Little empirical evidence is available up to now, and the limited data and clinical tradition that are used instead to define these disorders have generated concepts that remain controversial. There seems to be considerable international consensus, however, as to which of these disorders should be classified, at least provisionally, apart from schizophrenia and the mood disorders. It is hoped that the specified atypical psychotic disorders that have been included in recent classification systems will lead to widespread critical appraisal of their usefulness and to increasingly rigorous empirical investigations into their true clinical value.

References

APA (1981) *Diagnostic and Statistical Manual of Mental Disorder*, 3rd edn. (DSM-III). American Psychiatric Association, Washington DC.

APA (1987) *Diagnostic and Statistical Manual of Mental Disorder*, 3rd edn. revised (DSM-III-R). American Psychiatric Association, Washington DC.

APA (1994) *Diagnostic and Statistical Manual of Mental Disorder*, 4th edn. (DSM-IV). American Psychiatric Association, Washington DC.

Ballet, G. (1911) La psychose hallucinatoire chronique. *Encéphale*, **11**, 401–411.

Berson, R.J. (1983) Capgras' syndrome. *American Journal of Psychiatry*, **140**, 969–978.

Brockington, I.F., Kendell, R.E. & Leff, J.P. (1978) Definitions of schizophrenia: concordance and prediction of outcome. *Psychological Medicine*, **8**, 387–398.

Brockington, I.F., Perris, C., Kendell, R.E., Hillier, V.E. & Wainwright, S. (1982) The course and outcome of cycloid psychosis. *Psychological Medicine*, **12**, 97–105.

Capgras, J. & Reboul-Lachaux, J. (1923) L'illusion des 'sosies' dans un délire systématisé chronique. *Annales Médico-Psychologiques*, **81**, 186–193.

de Clérambault, G. (1942) *Oeuvre Psychiatrique*. Presses Universitaires de France, Paris.

Cotard, J. (1880) Du délire hypochondriaque dans une forme grave de la mélancolie anxieuse. *Annales Médico-Psychologiques*, **38**, 168–174.

Cotard, J. (1882) Du délire des négations. *Archives de Neurologie*, **11**, 152−170 and **12**, 282−296.

Cutting, J.C., Clarke, A.W. & Mann, A.H. (1978) Cycloid psychosis: an investigation of the diagnostic concept. *Psychological Medicine*, **8**, 637−648.

Dupré, E. & Logre, L. (1911) Les délires d'imagination. Mythomanie délirante. *Encéphale*, **10**, 209−232.

Ellis, P. & Mellsop, G. (1985) De Clérambault's syndrome-A nosological entity? *British Journal of Psychiatry*, **146**, 90−95.

Faergeman, P.M. (1963) *Psychogenic Psychoses. A Description and Follow-up of Psychoses Following Psychological Stress*. Butterworths, London.

Garmezy, N. (1968) Process and reactive schizophrenia: some conceptions and issues. In Katz, M.M., Cole, J.O. & Barton, W.E. (eds) *The Role and Methodology of Classification in Psychiatry and Psychopathology*, pp. 419−430. United States Government Printing Office, Washington.

Gelder, M., Gath, D. & Mayou, R. (1989) Paranoid symptoms and paranoid syndromes. In *Oxford Textbook of Psychiatry*, 2nd edn., pp. 324−344. Oxford University Press, Oxford.

Grahame, P.S. (1984) Schizophrenia in old age (late paraphrenia). *British Journal of Psychiatry*, **145**, 493−495.

Holden, N.L. (1987) Late paraphrenia or the paraphrenias? A descriptive study with a 10-year follow-up. *British Journal of Psychiatry*, **150**, 635−639.

Howard, R., Castle, D., Wessely, S. & Murray, R. (1993) A comparative study of 470 cases of early-onset and late-onset schizophrenia. *British Journal of Psychiatry*, **163**, 352−357.

Jordan, H.W. & Howe, G. (1980) De Clérambault syndrome (erotomania): a review and case presentation. *Journal of the National Medical Association*, **72**, 979−985.

Kendell, R.E. (1993) Paranoid disorders. In Kendell, R.E. & Zealley, A.K. (eds) *Companion to Psychiatric Studies*, pp. 459−471. Churchill Livingstone, Edinburgh.

Kendler, S.K. (1980) The nosologic validity of paranoia (simple delusional disorder). A review. *Archives of General Psychiatry*, **37**, 699−706.

Kendler, S.K., Gruenberg, A.M. & Strauss, J.S. (1981) An independent analysis of the Copenhagen sample of the Danish Adoption Study of schizophrenia. *Archives of General Psychiatry*, **38**, 985−987.

Kendler, S.K., Masterson, C.C. & Davis, K.L. (1985) Psychiatric illness in first-degree relatives of patients with paranoid psychosis, schizophrenia and medical illness. *British Journal of Psychiatry*, **147**, 524−531.

Kendler, S.K., Spitzer, R.L. & Williams, J.B.W. (1989) Psychotic disorders in DSM-III-R. *American Journal of Psychiatry*, **146**, 953−962.

Kety, S.S., Rosenthal, D., Wender, P.H., Schulsinger, F. & Jacobson, B. (1978) The biologic and adoptive families of adopted individuals who became schizophrenic: prevalence of mental illness and other characteristics. In Wynne, L.D. (ed.) *The Nature of Schizophrenia*. John Wiley & Sons, New York.

Kraepelin, E. (1899) *Psychiatrie. Ein Lehrbuch für Studierende und Aerzte*, 6th edn. Barth, Leipzig.

Kraepelin, E. (1909−1915) *Psychiatrie. Ein Lehrbuch für Studierende und Aerzte*, 8th edn. Barth, Leipzig.

Kretschmer, E. (1918) *Der sensitive Beziehungswahn*. Springer-Verlag, Berlin.

Langfeldt, G. (1939) *The Schizophreniform States*. Munsksgaard, Copenhagen (1939) and Oxford University Press, Oxford.

Langfeldt, G. (1961) The erotic jealousy syndrome. A clinical study. *Acta Psychiatrica Scandinavica*, Suppl. **151**.

Lasègue, C. & Falret, J. (1877) La folie à deux ou folie communiquée. *Annales Médico-Psychologiques*, **18**, 321.

Legrain, M. (1886) *Du Délire Chez les Dégénérés*. Deshaye et Lecrosnier, Paris.

Leonhard, K. (1957) *Aufteilung der Endogenen Psychosen*, 1st edn. Akademie Verlag, Berlin.

Magnan, V. & Legrain, M. (1895) *Les Dégénérés (Etat Mental et Syndromes Episodiques)*. Rueff et Cie, Paris.

Mowat, R.R. (1966) *Morbid Jealousy and Murder*. Tavistock, London.

Mullen, P.E. & Maack, L.H. (1985) Jealousy, pathological jealousy and aggression. In Farington, D.P. & Gunn, J. (eds) *Aggression and Dangerousness*. Wiley, Chicester.

Opjordsmoen, S. & Retterstol, N. (1987) Hypochondriacal delusions in paranoid psychoses: course and outcome compared with other types of delusions. *Psychopathology*, **20**, 272−284.

Perris, C. (1974) A study of cycloid psychoses. *Acta Psychiatrica Scandinavica*, Suppl. **253**, 77 pp.

Pichot, P. (1983) *A Century of Psychiatry*. Editions Roger Dacosta, Paris.

Pichot, P. (1990) The diagnosis and classification of mental disorders in the French-speaking countries: background, current values and comparison with other classifications. In Sartorius, N., Jablensky, A., Regier, D.A. *et al.* (eds) *Sources and Traditions of Classification in Psychiatry*, pp. 7−58. Hofgrete & Huber, Toronto.

Pichot, P. & Debray, H. (1971) *Hospitalisation Psychiatrique. Statistique Descriptive*. Sandoz Editions, Paris.

Pull, C.B., Pull, M.C. & Pichot, P. (1987) Des critères empiriques français pour les psychoses. III. Algorithmes et arbre de décision. *Encéphale*, **XIII**, 59−66.

Raskin, D.E. & Sullivan, K.E. (1974) Erotomania. American Journal of Psychiatry, **131**, 1033−1035.

Remington, G. & Book, H. (1984) Case report of de Clérambault syndrome, bipolar affective disorder, and response to lithium. *American Journal of Psychiatry*, **141**, 1285−1287.

Roth, M. (1955) The natural history of mental disorder in old age. *Journal of Mental Science*, **101**, 281−301.

Sartorius, N. *et al.* (1986) Early manifestations and first contact incidence of schizophrenia in different cultures. A preliminary report on the initial evaluation phase of the WHO Collaborative Study on Determinants of Outcome of Severe Mental Disorders. *Psychological Medicine*, **16**, 909−928.

Sartorius, N. *et al.* (1993) Progress toward achieving a common language in psychiatry. Results from the field trial of the Clinical Guidelines accompanying the WHO Classification of Mental and Behavioural Disorders in ICD-10. *Archives of General Psychiatry*, **50**, 115−124.

Schanda, H. & Gabriel, E. (1988) Position of affective symptomatology in the course of delusional psychoses. *Psycho-*

pathology, **21**, 1−11.

Sérieux, P. & Capgras, J. (1909) *Les Folies Raisonnantes. Le Délire d'Interprétation*. Felix Arcan, Paris.

Shepherd, M. (1961) Morbid jealousy: some clinical and social aspects of a psychiatric symptom. *Journal of Mental Science*, **107**, 687−753.

Signer, S.F. & Cummings, J.L. (1987) De Clérambault's syndrome in organic affective disorder. Two cases. *British Journal of Psychiatry*, **151**, 404−407.

Signer, S.F. & Swinson, R.P. (1987) Two cases of erotomania (de Clérambault's syndrome) in bipolar affective disorder. *British Journal of Psychiatry*, **151**, 853−855.

Sims, A. & Reddie, M. (1976) The de Clérambault and Capgras history. *British Journal of Psychiatry*, **129**, 95−96.

Sims, A. & White, A. (1973) Coexistence of Capgras and de Clérambault's syndromes: a case history. *British Journal of Psychiatry*, **123**, 635−637.

Staner, L. (1991) Sleep, dexamethasone suppression test, and response to somatic therapies in an atypical affective state presenting as erotomania: a case report. *European Psychiatry*, **6**, 269−271.

Strömgren, E. (1974) Psychogenic psychoses. In Hirsch, S.R. & Shepherd, M. (eds) *Themes and Variations in European Psychiatry*, pp. 97−117. Wright & Sons, Bristol.

Vauhkonen, K. (1968) On the pathogenesis of morbid jealousy. *Acta Psychiatrica Scandinavica*, Suppl. **202**, 1−261.

Wimmer, A. (1916) Psykogene sindssygdomsformer. In *Sct. Hans Mental Hospital 1816−1916, Jubilee Publication*, pp. 85−216. Gad, Copenhagen.

WHO (1992) *The ICD-10 Classification of Mental and Behavioural Disorders. Clinical Descriptions and Diagnostic Guidelines*. World Health Organization, Geneva.

WHO (1993) *The ICD-10 Classification of Mental and Behavioural Disorders. Diagnostic Criteria for Research*. World Health Organization, Geneva.

Chapter 6
Late-Life Schizophrenia

D. V. JESTE, P. L. GILBERT, A. KODSI, S. C. HEATON,
D. D. SEWELL AND J. P. LACRO

Introduction

Patients with late-life schizophrenia include those with late-onset schizophrenia (LOS; i.e. with onset of schizophrenia after age 45 years) as well as those with early-onset schizophrenia (EOS) who are now over the age of 45 years. Late-life schizophrenia is a relatively unstudied (especially in the USA), yet increasingly important, entity. During the next 30 years, the proportion of persons in the general population over the age of 45 years is expected to increase by about one-third (National Institute on Aging, 1987). Hence, there will be a greater number of new cases of LOS, along with a higher number of EOS patients living into and beyond middle age. Understanding the pathophysiology of LOS as well as the course of EOS in older age is important for developing a comprehensive theory of schizophrenia.

Most of the early work on LOS and on the long-term course of EOS was carried out in Europe. Investigators such as Bleuler, Roth, Kay, Post and others have made major contributions to this area. It is only in the last 15 years or so that interest in late-life schizophrenia in the USA has become noticeable.

One serious problem for research in LOS has been that of terminology and definitions. Labels such as LOS, paraphrenia, late paraphrenia and paranoia have been used without clear distinctions (Harris & Jeste, 1988). Kraepelin (1909) utilized the term 'paraphrenia' in reference to certain chronic patients who exhibited hallucinations and paranoid delusions in middle age without any loss of volition, coherence or reality testing outside the realm of their delusions. Subsequent investigators used this label with varying connotations. Neither the *Diagnostic and Statistical Manual* DSM-IV nor the *International Classification of Disease* ICD-10 will include a diagnosis of 'paraphrenia'. It is to be hoped that in future research, issues of diagnostic validity and reliability will be given due consideration.

In this chapter we will discuss the characteristics of late-life schizophrenia, giving special attention to the differences between the LOS population and the older EOS population. Also, we will focus on more recent research in this area.

Demographics

The reported prevalence of schizophrenia in the

Chapter 6

elderly varies from 0.1 to 1.0% (Gurland & Cross, 1982). A conservative estimate of the ratio of EOS to LOS among older schizophrenic patients is 9:1. Based on a literature review, Harris and Jeste (1988) noted that 23% of all schizophrenic in-patients reportedly had onset of their illness after age 40. There seemed to be a progressive decline in the number of patients with onset in older age. Recently, however, Castle and Murray (1993) found in an analysis of a London-based sample of patients with non-affective functional psychoses, that there were three peaks of onset: the highest one in the 16- to 25-year age group, a slight one in the 46- to 55-year group and a more emphatic one in those over 65.

While schizophrenia in later life is similar in a number of ways to that in earlier life, there are also differences between patients with EOS who have carried the illness into later life and patients who have recently manifested LOS. One of the most striking demographic differences between EOS and LOS is in gender distribution. Unlike the schizophrenic population with onset in early life in whom we find a relatively high proportion of men, in LOS there is a higher ratio of women to men.

Clinical studies

Clinical investigations of LOS face some serious logistical difficulties.

1 DSM-III (1980) criteria precluded a clinical diagnosis of schizophrenia if the onset of psychosis occurred after age 45. Jeste *et al.* (1988), using DSM-III-R criteria for an operational definition of LOS, were able to diagnose LOS in 15 patients who had previously been diagnosed, using DSM-III criteria, as having atypical psychosis or paranoid disorder.

2 Since the onset of symptoms of schizophrenia is often protracted, insidious and subtle, it is difficult to demarcate the exact age of onset in many patients, especially older patients. Age-associated memory problems, as well as a lack of insight make it difficult for elderly patients to recall previous medical histories. Premorbid schizoid or paranoid personality traits may further

cloud onset data. Social patterns may enable older adults to conceal more successfully their early symptoms from the observation of others than is usually possible for children and young adults.

3 Symptoms of LOS may be intermixed with, or impinged upon by, symptoms of other medical and psychiatric conditions. Longitudinal studies are difficult since financial, social and geriatric medical issues all interfere with long-term psychiatric evaluation or care.

4 The schizophrenic syndrome is not a homogeneous entity, but a concatenation of several different subtypes or a spectrum of multifactorial origin (Faraone & Tsuang, 1985; Kendler *et al.*, 1985). The symptomatology of schizophrenia exhibits substantial variation, suggesting the possibility of aetiological and pathogenetic heterogeneity. Only detailed assessments of relevant clinical and biological variables can provide the data needed to define EOS and LOS either as distinct homogeneous subtypes or as variants along the schizophrenic spectrum.

Symptoms

In general, patients with EOS and LOS are similar in terms of positive symptoms such as hallucinations and delusions. With advancing age, however, EOS patients tend to show a reduction of positive symptoms (Winokur *et al.*, 1987) when compared with younger EOS patients. In a multicentre study of LOS, Jeste *et al.* (1988) found that delusions, particularly of persecution, and auditory hallucinations were prominent in patients with LOS. The authors observed that LOS typically resembled the paranoid subtype of EOS. Other subtypes of schizophrenia, including catatonic and disorganized types, were very rare in old age. Castle and Murray (1993) reported that persecutory delusions and auditory hallucinations were more common in LOS than in EOS, while the reverse was true for formal thought disorder, passivity phenomenon, thought interference, paucity of thought/speech and restricted affect.

Studies of deficit syndrome and negative symptoms in older schizophrenic patients should be of clinical as well as theoretical interest. In an investigation of 46 schizophrenic patients over the age of 45 years, Harris *et al.* (1991) found that 17 patients (37%) met the criteria for deficit syndrome as described by Carpenter *et al.* (1988). This prevalence was 2.5 times greater than the 15% prevalence of deficit syndrome reported by Carpenter *et al.* in a group of young schizophrenic adults. Harris *et al.* (1991) also found a trend for the older patients with deficit syndrome to have greater impairment on the Halstead–Reitan neuropsychological test battery. The higher frequency of deficit syndrome in older patients may be attributable to ageing or to a longer duration of illness.

In a subsequent study of the same group of subjects using the scale for the assessment of negative symptoms (SANS; Andreasen *et al.*, 1982), Harris *et al.* (1993) proposed a three-factor model of negative symptoms in older schizophrenic patients: core symptoms, defect symptoms and incidental symptoms. The core symptoms (alogia and anhedonia-asociality) were present to a similar extent in the LOS and EOS groups. The defect symptoms (affective blunting and avolition-apathy) were more severe in the EOS patients than in the LOS group. The incidental symptom (attentional impairment) was of similar severity in the schizophrenic (LOS and EOS) and normal comparison subjects, possibly suggesting a significant improvement in this symptom in the schizophrenic patients as a result of neuroleptic treatment. We have described an illustrative case history of a patient with LOS in the Appendix.

Premorbid personality features

Schizoid and paranoid premorbid personality traits tend to be common in LOS. Pearlson and Rabins (1988) noted that patients who developed LOS had been described by their families as having been aloof, suspicious and eccentric with odd beliefs. Despite these abnormal characteristics, patients with LOS were more likely to have been employed, married and had children than were patients with EOS. In EOS, the illness (at least the prodromal phase) frequently begins during the teenage years, prior to marriage or entry into the workplace, and may interfere with, or even preclude, these activities which help to further develop social skills. While LOS patients tend to have better premorbid functioning than EOS patients, the premorbid adjustment of LOS patients is usually worse than that of normal controls. These deficits may be related to the higher percentage of schizoid or paranoid premorbid personality traits that can be found in the LOS population compared with normal subjects.

Physical comorbidity

In terms of overall survival, Allebeck (1989) commented upon the higher mortality rate of schizophrenic patients compared with that of the general population, related to both natural causes and unnatural ones such as suicide and violence. Given that physical comorbidity increases with age, one may expect a high prevalence of medical illnesses among older schizophrenic patients. In a recent study of elderly psychiatric patients, however, Gierz and Jeste (1993) found that schizophrenic patients actually had a lower total number of physical ailments than did patients with other diagnoses, including anxiety and mood disorder. This finding was confirmed by Lacro and Jeste (1994) in a different patient population. The authors studied 78 patients with schizophrenia, 41 with major depression and 62 with Alzheimer's disease; all the patients were over age 45, and had a mean age of 68 years. The patients with schizophrenia had the lowest number of physical illnesses, the difference in physical comorbidity between schizophrenic and depressed groups being statistically significant. These results may reflect biological differences or may be due to differences in psychiatric treatment or the use of healthcare resources. An alternative explanation is that the lower physical comorbidity in older schizophrenic patients may represent a survivor or healthier cohort of patients.

Sensory deficits

Kay and Roth (1955, 1961) were among the first investigators to report an association between sensory impairment (deafness or blindness) and late-onset paranoid psychosis. Pearlson and Rabins (1988) supported such a relationship between visual and hearing impairment and the onset of both EOS and LOS, with a more pronounced association with LOS. In addition, these authors postulated that almost any type of sensory impairment might lead to the development of schizophrenia in certain predisposed individuals.

Prager and Jeste (1993) reviewed the literature published over the past 40 years and found 27 studies of sensory (visual or auditory) impairment in psychotic patients. Twenty-two of the studies assessed sensory loss among patients with late-life psychosis, and five studies examined psychopathology in subjects with sensory impairment. The authors then conducted a case-control study involving a comparison of schizophrenic patients (EOS and LOS) with mood-disorder patients and normal control subjects in terms of visual and auditory impairment. The results showed that all the psychiatric groups were similar to normal controls on uncorrected vision or hearing, but were significantly more impaired on corrected (i.e. with eyeglasses or hearing aids) sensory function. From this study, Prager and Jeste (1993) suggested that the association between sensory impairment and late-life psychosis may be, at least in part, a result of insufficient correction of sensory deficits in older schizophrenic patients compared with normal controls. This could reflect a difficulty for these patients to access optimal healthcare, especially for the treatment of sensory impairment.

Brain imaging

Ventricular enlargement has been reported in numerous studies of younger schizophrenic patients (Johnstone *et al.*, 1976; Weinberger *et al.*, 1979; Gur & Pearlson, 1993). Rabins *et al.* (1987) found that ventricular size was larger in LOS patents compared with an age-matched normal cohort, but smaller than that of an age-matched group of patients with probable Alzheimer's disease who had psychotic symptoms. Krull *et al.* (1991) also reported a trend for an increased ventricle:brain ratio with magnetic resonance

imaging (MRI) of LOS patients compared with normal controls. The ventricles of LOS patients were, however, smaller than those of patients with Alzheimer's disease. In another study of patients with LOS ($n = 11$) or Alzheimer's disease ($n = 12$) and age- and gender-matched normal controls ($n = 18$), Lesser *et al.* (1993) found significant increases in third ventricular volume, lateral ventricular size and total percentage cerebrospinal fluid (CSF) in patients with Alzheimer's disease, while only the third ventricular volume was significantly increased in those with LOS compared with the controls. In a comparison of EOS and LOS patients on visual analogue measures of atrophy, Pearlson *et al.* (1993) reported a similar degree of atrophy in these two patient groups. In a rare longitudinal investigation, Hymas *et al.* (1989) observed that the ventricle:brain ratio was not associated with clinical course or outcome.

A number of investigators have reported large areas of white matter hyperintensities and vascular lesions in patients with late-life psychoses compared with age-matched normal comparison subjects (Miller & Lesser, 1988; Breitner *et al.*, 1990; Coffey *et al.*, 1990; Flint *et al.*, 1991; Miller *et al.*, 1991; Lesser *et al.*, 1992). Several of these studies, however, included mixed diagnostic groups.

Using single photon emission computed tomography (SPECT), Lesser *et al.* (1993) noted that 83% of their late-life psychotic subjects and 27% of normals had temporal or frontal areas of hyperfusion. We too have observed lower global cortical uptake (particularly in the left posterior frontal region and bilateral inferior temporal regions) in late-life schizophrenic patients ($n = 11$) than in normal comparison subjects ($n = 11$) (Dupont *et al.*, in press). While the uptake was slightly lower in LOS patients compared with EOS patients, there was no overall correlation between cortical uptake and age of onset or duration of schizophrenia, current neuroleptic dose, severity of psychopathology, or global cognitive impairment. Finally, one study using positron emission tomography (PET) reported elevated B_{max} values for D_2 receptors in 13 neuroleptic-naive LOS patients compared with age- and gender-matched normal controls (Pearlson *et al.*, 1993).

Neuropsychological impairment

Two contrasting views of the progression of neuropsychological impairment in schizophrenia have been reported. On the one hand, cognitive deficits are thought to follow a course analogous to, and suggestive of, a progressive dementia (Davidson *et al.*, 1991). On the other hand, cognitive deficits are viewed as being relatively stable, and thus more consistent with the notion of a static encephalopathy (Goldberg *et al.*, 1993). After the onset of clinical symptoms, the patient remains in a cognitively stable, but impaired, condition for many years.

Heaton *et al.* (1993) evaluated neuropsychological performance in 38 normal comparison subjects, 83 early-onset schizophrenia younger (EOS-Y) patients, 22 subjects with LOS, 35 age-comparable patients with early-onset schizophrenia (early-onset schizophrenia old, EOS-O) and 42 patients with Alzheimer's disease. All the subjects received an expanded Halstead–Reitan neuropsychological test battery. Raw scores on the neuropsychological tests were converted to age-, education- and gender-corrected T-scores (Heaton, 1992). Next, 'deficit scores' were computed to summarize the entire test battery into eight cognitive ability areas. All the schizophrenia groups were worse than the normal comparison group on deficit scores for all the ability areas except memory. The LOS, EOS-O and EOS-Y groups were similar to one another in all the cognitive ability areas. Age of onset and duration of schizophrenia illnesses did not have a major impact on the associated neuropsychological impairment. Furthermore, the authors reported that the patterns of neuropsychological deficits were different when patients with schizophrenia and Alzheimer's disease were compared. Schizophrenic patients were impaired in their ability to learn new information, but were normal with respect to recalling such information after a delay. This finding was similar to that reported by Gold *et al.* (1992). Patients with Alzheimer's disease performed worse than the normal subjects on all the deficit scores, including memory; they had greater learning and memory impairments than

had the schizophrenia groups. Finally, neuropsychological discriminative functions rarely misclassified a schizophrenia subject (LOS or EOS) as having Alzheimer's disease.

According to the neurodevelopmental model (Weinberger, 1987), the brain lesions putatively related to the pathogenesis of schizophrenia are of developmental origin and are not progressive or degenerative in nature. Furthermore, long-term treatment with neuroleptics and other environmental factors are not major contributors to cognitive deficits and brain abnormalities associated with schizophrenia.

Our studies suggest that the neurodevelopmental model also applies to LOS. Differences in severity and specific locations or the nature of these 'lesions' may account for a delay in the onset of schizophrenia. Additionally, the peak in dopaminergic activity related to the schizophrenic breakdown, as per the neurodevelopmental theory (Weinberger *et al.*, 1987), may be delayed until later in life in patients with LOS. Wong *et al.* (1984) suggest that the later age of onset and a better prognosis for schizophrenia in women may relate to a later peak and delayed regression of dopaminergic activity.

Course

While Kraepelin's definition of dementia praecox included a poor prognosis, the current view of the natural history of schizophrenia is less pessimistic and suggests a more variable outcome in both LOS and EOS. McGlashan (1988) reported that nearly one-third of EOS patients had remission or marked improvement with age. Ciompi (1980) suggested that advancing age might mitigate the intensity of schizophrenic illness and that the so-called residual states might be the most commonly seen manifestations of schizophrenia in old age.

Finally, although there have been no consistent predictors of outcome in schizophrenia, Ciompi (1980) suggested that a better premorbid personality and advancing age were potential indicators of a more positive outcome for schizophrenia.

Diagnosis

Comparison of DSM-III-R and DSM-IV criteria

The criteria for diagnosis of schizophrenia according to the *DSM-IV Draft Criteria* (APA, 1993) are similar to those in the DSM-III-R (APA, 1987), except for a few novel features. One important modification for schizophrenia in general is the addition of negative symptoms to symptom list A, 'Characteristic Symptoms', in the *DSM-IV Draft Criteria* (APA, 1993). The negative-symptom category includes the symptom 'flat affect' listed in the DSM-III-R (APA, 1987), and adds 'alogia' and 'avolition' to the examples of negative symptoms. One significant modification found in DSM-IV (APA, 1993) is that there is no longer any specification in terms of the age of onset of schizophrenia. Thus, no distinction is made between early-onset and late-onset (after age 45) schizophrenia in the *DSM-IV Draft Criteria*.

In the DSM-II (APA, 1968) the diagnosis of schizophrenia had no restriction in terms of age of onset. This was revised in the DSM-III (APA, 1980) such that a diagnosis of schizophrenia required an onset before age 45. In the DSM-III-R (APA, 1987), the age of onset restriction was removed and LOS was specified to indicate onset of schizophrenia after age 45. The proposed DSM-IV would revert back to the criteria in the DSM-II, which made no mention of age of onset in the diagnosis of schizophrenia.

Differential diagnosis

The differential diagnosis of schizophrenia in late life must begin with the elimination of any organic aetiology for psychosis, as a vast number of medical and neurological illnesses have symptoms that can mimic those of schizophrenia (Kaplan & Sadock, 1988). Especially in the elderly, dementia and other organic mental syndromes with psychotic features must be distinguished from schizophrenia by the history and clinical examination. A diagnosis of dementia rather than schizophrenia is suggested by a prominent disturbance of memory, language, personality and judgement as well as a presumed underlying organic aetiology. Delirium is manifested by disorientation, alteration in level of consciousness and fleeting hallucinatory experiences, whereas the acute or subacute phase of schizophrenia is associated with more organized, prominent hallucinations and delusions and a generally clear sensorium.

Next, the mood disorders with psychotic features, including major depression and bipolar disorder, must be excluded. In contrast to the prominence of affective signs and symptoms in the mood disorders, the diagnosis of schizophrenia is made when the total duration of all mood symptoms has been brief relative to the primary psychotic symptoms.

Schizoaffective disorder, either the depressive or the bipolar type, may be differentiated from schizophrenia by the occurrence of a full major depressive or manic episode coexistent with the characteristic psychotic symptoms of the active phase of schizophrenia. Thus, in shizoaffective disorder, the duration of all episodes of mood disorder has not been brief relative to the total duration of psychosis.

Delusional disorder is distinguished from schizophrenia by the presence of non-bizarre delusions of at least 1 month's duration; behaviour which is not obviously odd or bizarre, apart from that which is based on the delusional system; and an absence of prominent auditory or visual hallucinations.

Certain personality disorders, notably schizotypal personality disorder, may resemble schizophrenia but do not usually include frank psychotic symptoms. If present, the psychotic symptoms are of a transient and incomplete quality.

Finally, a number of miscellaneous psychoses, including brief reactive psychosis, schizophreniform disorder, induced psychotic disorder and psychotic disorder not otherwise specified, must be considered when establishing a diagnosis of schizophrenia.

Treatment of late-life schizophrenia with neuroleptics

Neuroleptics are commonly prescribed to the elderly population. They constitute the most effective treatment for LOS as well as EOS. Supportive psychosocial therapy is, however, an important adjunct.

The use of neuroleptics, as well as other medications, in the elderly is complicated by the altered pharmacokinetics and pharmacodynamics with ageing. The elderly are more sensitive to both the beneficial and the adverse effects of medications. One particularly troublesome side effect associated with the use of neuroleptics is tardive dyskinesia. Newer 'atypical' neuroleptics, such as clozapine, remoxipride and risperidone, may prove to be useful alternatives in the treatment of the elderly population.

Below, we discuss in greater detail the pharmacology of neuroleptics in older schizophrenic patients.

Pharmacokinetic considerations in the elderly

Pharmacokinetics is defined as the study of the movement of drugs through the body, specifically with reference to the absorption, distribution, metabolism and elimination of the substance (Maletta *et al.*, 1991). The physiological alterations associated with the ageing process have an impact on the pharmacokinetics of various substances.

Absorption

Although there is an increase in gastric pH and a decrease in gastric emptying, splanchnic blood flow and gastrointestinal motility associated with increasing age, very few drugs exhibit a delayed rate or extent of absorption. The bioavailability of most drugs is also unaltered in the elderly (Williams & Lowenthal, 1992).

Distribution

The ageing process is associated with a decrease in total body water, extracellular water and lean body mass with an increase in adipose tissue. As a result, lipid-soluble medications such as neuroleptics exhibit an increased volume of distribution and therefore a prolonged action (Williams & Lowenthal, 1992). Serum albumin concentrations are also decreased in the elderly and this leads to an increase in the unbound concentration, or pharmacologically active portion, of drugs. This increase in the unbound concentration of medications is the equivalent of an increase in the dosage, and may often lead to adverse effects. The approximate decrease of 15–25% in serum albumin in patients over the age of 60 may be related to a decrease in liver function as well as to poor dietary intake of proteins (Cherry & Morton, 1989).

Metabolism

The extent of metabolism of drugs by the liver is variable among the elderly. The liver is the primary site of conversion of drugs to more water-soluble substances to enhance their elimination through the kidneys. The elderly exhibit a decrease in hepatic mass and hepatic blood flow. In addition, there is an age-related decrease in the number of oxidative enzymes. Taken together, these alterations in the functioning of the liver often lead to an increased bioavailability and serum concentration of medications, which in turn may increase the risk of toxicity (Cherry & Morton, 1989). Cohen and Sommer found the serum concentrations of thioridazine and its metabolites to be 1.5–2 times higher in eight elderly patients compared with the level in eight younger patients after a single 25-mg dose (Cohen & Sommer, 1988).

Excretion

The elimination of drugs from the body, like other pharmacokinetic parameters, is altered during the ageing process. After the age of 40, there is a 6–10% decrease in the glomerular filtration rate and renal blood flow every 10 years such that a 70-year-old person exhibits a 40–50% decrease in renal function (Williams & Lowenthal, 1992). As a result, medications that are renally eliminated may have an increased plasma concentration and possibly a higher risk of causing adverse effects in the elderly.

Pharmacodynamic considerations in the elderly

Pharmacodynamics is defined as the study of the effect of a drug on the target site, or as the physiological or psychological response to a drug (Williams & Lowenthal, 1992). At the same serum concentration as in younger patients, the elderly population has been found to respond differently to medications. Relating specifically to neuroleptics, akathisia, parkinsonism and tardive dyskinesia have been found to be more prevalent with increasing age (Rosen *et al.*, 1990). The elderly are also at an increased risk of developing delirium secondary to the use of a neuroleptic with anticholinergic properties. Elderly patients receiving neuroleptics, especially low-potency agents, should also be closely monitored for orthostatic hypotension. In general, higher potency neuroleptics which have a lower incidence of orthostatic hypotension and anticholinergic side effects may be a safer choice in the elderly with abnormal blood pressure, urinary retention, glaucoma, etc. (Rosen *et al.*, 1990).

Therapeutics of neuroleptics in late-life schizophrenia

In contrast to the large amount of literature on the efficacy of neuroleptics in young schizophrenic adults, there have been only a few double-blind placebo-controlled studies in middle-aged and elderly schizophrenic patients (Jeste *et al.*, 1993). In one such investigation, Honigfeld *et al.* (1965) compared acetophenazine, trifluoperazine and placebo among 308 schizophrenic men over the age of 50 (mean age 66 years). This 24-week double-blind study found both the neuroleptics to be superior to placebo in controlling the symptoms

of psychosis. Other studies have not shown an obvious difference among different types of neuroleptics in terms of their antipsychotic efficacy in older patients. When non-compliance is a problem, depot neuroleptics may be preferable (Raskind *et al.*, 1979). The dosages of neuroleptics appropriate for older patients are usually much lower (even one-third or less) than those used in younger adults (Salzman, 1990). In a cross-sectional study of the correlates of neuroleptic dose in 64 middle-aged and elderly schizophrenic patients, Jeste *et al.* (1993) found an inverse correlation between age and daily dose of neuroleptics expressed in milligram chlorpromazine equivalents. A later age of onset of schizophrenia was associated with lower dosages, possibly indicating a better prognosis or greater therapeutic response in that patient population. Finally, there was a suggestion that cognitively impaired patients needed higher doses of neuroleptics.

Tardive dyskinesia

Neuroleptic-induced tardive dyskinesia appears to be more prevalent among elderly patients. Patients over 40 years old are 3 times as likely to develop neuroleptic-induced tardive dyskinesia as patients less than 40 years (Jeste & Wyatt, 1982). In a recent report, Jeste *et al.* found a 26% cumulative incidence of tardive dyskinesia by the end of a 1-year study in 236 patients all over 45 years old (Jeste *et al.*, 1993). These results are consistent with other reports of neuroleptic-induced tardive dyskinesia in the elderly (Yassa *et al.*, 1992). Saltz *et al.* (1991) reported a 31% incidence of tardive dyskinesia in 163 elderly patients after 43 weeks of cumulative treatment with neuroleptics. This study identified several risk factors for the development of neuroleptic-induced tardive dyskinesia: (i) non-organic psychiatric diagnoses (affective disorders); (ii) a history of treatment with electroconvulsive therapy; and (iii) a history of parkinsonian side effects during the first 4 weeks of neuroleptic therapy. The incidence of neuroleptic-induced tardive dyskinesia was not found to be significantly associated with the daily neuroleptic dosage.

Tardive dyskinesia has been found to be somewhat more common in women (26.6%) than in men (21.6%) (Yassa & Jeste, 1992). Yassa *et al.* (1987) noted that smoking was associated with an increased prevalence of tardive dyskinesia. Other potential risk factors for the disorder include diabetes mellitus and organic mental syndromes (Ganzini *et al.*, 1991).

Neuroleptic withdrawal

Owing to the increased incidence of neuroleptic-induced tardive dyskinesia among the elderly, neuroleptic withdrawal is often initiated in this population. Furthermore, approximately one-third of elderly schizophrenic patients exhibit remission or a marked improvement in symptoms (McGlashan, 1988) and may, therefore, no longer require treatment with neuroleptics. Jeste *et al.* (1993) recently reviewed six double-blind, controlled studies of neuroleptic withdrawal in patients over 45 years old. The mean rate of relapse in the neuroleptic-withdrawn groups was 39.9% compared with 11.4% in the neuroleptic-maintained groups. Jeste *et al.* also conducted a 3-week study of neuroleptic withdrawal in 20 chronic schizophrenic patients. None of these patients met the criteria for relapse by the end of the study. While neuroleptic withdrawal may be clinically indicated in chronic schizophrenic patients, this population should be closely monitored for early signs of relapse.

Atypical neuroleptics

Unlike traditional neuroleptics, the newer 'atypical' neuroleptics are associated with lower extrapyramidal side effects. These agents, such as clozapine, remoxipride and risperidone, may be useful in the treatment of the elderly psychiatric population, although relatively little information is available on their use in late-life schizophrenia.

Clozapine

Clozapine is a dibenzodiazepine antipsychotic agent which exhibits relatively potent cholinergic, serotonergic, histaminergic and adrenergic activity (Kane *et al.*, 1988). Unlike typical neuroleptics,

clozapine is a weak antagonist of the dopamine D_2 receptor, while it exhibits a higher affinity for the dopamine D_1 receptor. It has been suggested that clozapine selectively blocks dopamine receptors in the mesolimbic and mesocortical dopamine pathways, areas associated with the efficacy of neuroleptics. Clozapine is not, however, thought to have an effect on the nigrostriatal dopamine neurones, which have been linked to the development of extrapyramidal side effects. In addition, clozapine's blockade of the serotonin 2 receptor may contribute to its lack of extrapyramidal symtoms (EPS) and efficacy against the negative symptoms of schizophrenia (Gerlach, 1991). The most frequent side effects noted in patients receiving clozapine are sedation (34%), weight gain (34%), hypersalivation (23%), gastro-intestinal symptoms (17%), hypotension (11%), tachycardia (7%), seizures (4%) and leuko-penia or agranulocytosis (1%) (Baldessarini & Frankenburg, 1991). There are few reports of the use of clozapine in the elderly, except for the treatment of drug-induced psychosis in patients with Parkinson's disease (Scholz & Dichgans, 1985; Ostergaard & Dupont, 1988; Wolters *et al.*, 1990; Wolk & Douglas, 1992). The patients in these reports ranged in age from 57 to 80 years and were treated with clozapine in dosages ranging from 25 to 250 mg/day. Several patients receiving the higher dosages of clozapine experienced sedation, anticholinergic delirium and orthostatic hypotension.

Bajulaiye and Addonizio (1992) reported the use of clozapine in the treatment of psychosis in an 82-year-old woman with tardive dyskinesia. Clozapine was initiated at 25 mg/day and increased over a 5-week period to 125 mg/day. After 3 weeks, the patient's tardive dyskinesia abated and her psychosis improved. The patient did not experience any adverse effects.

Remoxipride

Remoxipride is a novel neuroleptic of the benzamide class. Like clozapine, remoxipride exhibits preferential activity in the mesolimbic brain areas and therefore is associated with a low incidence of EPS. As a result, remoxipride may be another treatment alternative in the elderly population (Widerlov *et al.*, 1991). Remoxipride at dosages of 150—600 mg/day has been shown to have anti-psychotic activity equal to that of haloperidol administered at 5—45 mg/day. Remoxipride appears to be slightly better than haloperidol in the treatment of negative symptoms of schizo-phrenia (Lewander *et al.*, 1990). Widerlov *et al.* (1991) evaluated the pharmacokinetics of remoxi-pride in eight elderly patients with tardive dys-kinesia (mean age of 66 years). The investigators found that the pharmacokinetics of remoxipride were comparable with those in middle-aged schizophrenic patients. Compared with healthy volunteers, however, there was a 30% increase in maximal blood concentration (C_{max}) and area under curve (AUC) values. Other studies have found in elderly patients increased C_{max} and AUC values of remoxipride ranging from 50 to 80% of that seen in younger subjects (Andersson *et al.*, 1985; Movin *et al.*, 1990).

Risperidone

Risperidone is a benzisoxazole derivative exhibi-ting combined dopamine D_2 and serotonin 2 receptor blockade. Like clozapine and remoxi-pride, risperidone has been suggested to offer benefit in the treatment of the negative symptoms of schizophrenia, with a low incidence of EPS (Gerlach, 1991). There is little or no information relating to the use of risperidone in the elderly. Heykants *et al.* (1993) evaluated the pharmaco-kinetics of a single 1-mg oral dose of risperidone in young and elderly patients, and patients with liver disease and renal insufficiency. The renal clearance of risperidone was found to be related to creatinine. In the elderly and in the renally impaired patients, there was an increase in the elimination half-life of the drug. Based on these findings, a dosage reduction of risperidone is recommended in the elderly and in the renally impaired patient.

Summary

There is excellent evidence that schizophrenia can manifest for the first time after age 45, although such LOS is much less common than EOS. It seems most likely that the basic patho-genesis of LOS may be broadly similar to that of EOS, with some differences being responsible for the late onset of the disorder. The long-term course of EOS suggests a lack of progressive deterioration in cognitive function in such patients, thus differentiating them from patients with Alzheimer's disease and similar dementias. Both these findings support the hypothesis of a static encephalopathy during the developmental period in schizophrenic patients, irrespective of the age of onset, and a lack of progressive cognitive decline in later stages of the illness. Nonetheless, further research is needed to understand better the factors that protect the LOS patients from developing symptoms earlier in life, the factors that are associ-ated with precipitation of the disorder during middle age or thereafter and the factors that may be responsible for the somewhat heterogeneous course of the psychotic symptoms in EOS.

Appendix: illustrative case history

Mr L. was a retired 61-year-old single man with a college degree in business management. He dated the beginning of his psychiatric problems at age 59, a few months after he had sold his house, owing to financial difficulties, and moved in with his sister and niece. Mr L. began to express concern about Mormons setting him up and fol-lowing him. He also reported that he had in his nose an electronic bug which was broadcasting his thoughts on a CB radio. He started hearing voices. Initially, the voices were incoherent and barely audible to Mr L. However, over the next 6 months, the voices grew in volume and clarity, finally becoming very loud, clear and persistent. The voices talked to one another and to him, saying 'Let's shoot him in the head. How heavy is he? Can we fit his body into the trunk?'. The voices were loudest when he lay in his bed at night and he was afraid to fall asleep for fear that he might be shot in the head by the voices. He therefore reportedly slept only approximately 2 h/night. During this period, Mr L. also complained that he heard prowlers at night. One day he came into the house with two loaded guns and later dialled the police to inform them that he was going to shoot two prowlers outside. The police impounded his guns and brought him to the hospital. The police reported that Mr L. had threatened to shoot his sister and niece. Mr L. explained that he had not wanted to shoot his sister and niece, but was simply trying to defend them because the voices were telling him that they were going to kill him.

Mr L. and his sister both denied that he had a history of alcohol or other substance abuse. He did not meet DSM-III-R criteria for a mood disorder and denied suicidal or homicidal ideation (except for a desire to shoot the threatening voices). Mr L. had no history of head injury, stroke or unconsciousness.

His past psychiatric history was not significant. There were no psychiatric hospitalizations, counselling, medications or other treatment reported prior to the described hospitalization.

There was no family history of a psychiatric illness except for some documentation that Mr L.'s mother had been hospitalized for 2−3 months after his birth for possible postpartum psychosis or depression, and apparently had some bizarre behaviour for some years prior to her death at age 60.

Personal history. Mr L. was the third of four children. He was a healthy child and did well in school and college. After obtaining a BA in business management, he served 2 years in the army as a clerk and then was given an honourable discharge. From age 28−45, Mr L. worked as the manager of the accounting department at a hospital. He had several close friends that he would see a couple of times a week, reported extensive dating history but was never married and had no children. When the management at the hospital he was working for changed, Mr L. went to work as an accountant in an advertising firm. There, Mr L. did not find his work so rewarding and eventually quit (or might have been made to leave for unclear reasons) after 2 years, around age 52. Soon after quitting his job Mr L.

won a relatively large amount of money in horse racing. He lived off the winnings and invested in some property over the next few years. At age 59, most of his savings had been spent and he was forced to sell his house to raise money.

Medical history. His medical history was significant for mild essential hypertension and late-onset diabetes mellitus.

Mental status examination. At the time of his hospitalization, he showed reasonable appearance, normal speech and normal orientation and memory. Mr L.'s judgement and insight were, however, poor. His mood was dysphoric and his affect was somewhat flat. Mr L. presented an elaborate paranoid delusional system with ongoing feelings of being harassed, talked about, monitored by various electronic devices and under the threat of his life. He reported thought insertion, and that people were trying to control his thinking but he would not allow it.

Neurological and other physical examinations. These were within normal limits. Of note, he was diagnosed with moderate sleep apnoea after participating in a sleep study. Routine laboratory tests were all within normal limits. His Mini Mental State Examination score was 29/30.

Neuropsychological testing. Mr L. was given an extensive neuropsychological test battery. It showed moderate impairment in strength and fine motor control, and mild impairment in attention, speed of information processing and learning, but no deficit in memory.

MRI. This showed moderate central and mild cortical volume loss, and multiple areas of focal hyperintensities in the deep white matter of the cerebral hemispheres.

Illness course. Following hospitalization, Mr L. was diagnosed as having late-onset paranoid schizophrenia, and was started on 10 mg haloperidol, 1 mg benztropine and supportive therapy. Mr L. reported that within a few days of beginning to take haloperidol, he started to feel better. The voices as well as the paranoia diminished somewhat. Mr L. was discharged after 14 days, returned to his sister's house and continued to see a psychiatrist and take haloperidol at a reduced dose of 5 mg/day. Over the next year, he remained relatively stable and his haloperidol dose was further lowered. He then decided on his own to discontinue the medication, but 6 months later had a relapse of symptoms. He believed that his sister was trying to steal money from him, began to hear the threatening voices again and thought his food was being poisoned. He moved out of his sister's house and lived in motels for several days before he went to see his psychiatrist, who suggested he be readmitted into the hospital, which he did voluntarily. At this time, Mr L. was started on 6 mg haloperidol. As with his first hospitalization, Mr L. was stabilized on haloperidol within days. He was released from the hospital 5 days later and was maintained on 6 mg haloperidol for the next year. Neuropsychological testing repeated 2 years after the baseline tests showed no decline in memory or other cognitive function.

References

Allebeck, P. (1989) Schizophrenia: a life-shortening disease. *Schizophrenia Bulletin*, **15**, 81–89.

Andersson, U., Nilsson, M.I., Häggström, J.E. & Widerlov, E. (1985) Antidyskinetic action and pharmacokinetics of remoxipride, a substituted benzamide, in elderly patients with tardive dyskinesia. In Burrows, G., Burrows, G.D., Norman, T.R. & Dennerstein, L. (eds) *Clinical and Pharmacological Studies in Psychiatric Disorders*, pp. 381–388. Libbey, London.

Andreasen, N., Nasrallah, H.A., Dunn, V. & Olsen, S. (1982) Negative versus positive schizophrenia. *Archives of General Psychiatry*, **39**, 789–794.

APA (1968) *Diagnostic and Statistical Manual of Mental Disorders*, 2nd edn. American Psychiatric Association, Washington DC.

APA (1980) *Diagnostic and Statistical Manual of Mental Disorders*, 3rd edn. American Psychiatric Association, Washington DC.

APA (1987) *Diagnostic and Statistical Manual of Mental Disorders*, 3rd edn, revised. American Psychiatric Association, Washington DC.

APA (1993) *DSM-IV Draft Criteria: 3–1–93*. American Psychiatric Association, Washington DC.

Bajulaiye, R. & Addonizio, G. (1992) Clozapine in the treatment of psychosis in an 82-year-old woman with tardive dyskinesia. *Journal of Clinical Psychopharmacology*, **12**, 364–365.

Baldessarini, R.J. & Frankenburg, F.R. (1991) Clozapine: a novel antipsychotic agent. *New England Journal of Medicine*, **324(11)**, 746–754.

Breitner, J., Husain, M., Figiel, G., Krishnan, K. & Boyko, O. (1990) Cerebral white matter disease in late-onset psychosis. *Biological Psychiatry*, **28**, 266–274.

Carpenter, W.T. Jr, Heinrichs, D.W. & Wagman, A.M.I. (1988) Deficit and nondeficit forms of schizophrenia: the concept. *American Journal of Psychiatry*, **145**, 578–583.

Castle, D.J. & Murray, R.M. (1993) The epidemiology of late-onset schizophrenia. *Schizophrenia Bulletin*, **19(4)**, 691–700.

Cherry, K.E. & Morton, M.R. (1989) Drug sensitivity in older adults: the role of physiologic and pharmacokinetic factors. *International Journal of Aging and Human Development*, **28(3)**, 159–174.

Ciompi, L. (1980) Catamnestic long-term study on the course of life and aging of schizophrenics. *Schizophrenia Bulletin*, **6**, 606–618.

Coffey, C.E., Figiel, G.S., Djang, W.T. & Weiner, R.D. (1990) Subcortical hyperintensity on magnetic resonance imaging: a comparison of normal and depressed elderly subjects. *American Journal of Psychiatry*, **47**, 187–189.

Cohen, B.M. & Sommer, B.R. (1988) Metabolism of thioridazine in the elderly. *Journal of Clinical Psychopharmacology*, **8**, 336–339.

Davidson, M., Powchik, V., Haroutunian, V. *et al.* (1991) Dementia-like symptoms in elderly schizophrenic patients. *American College of Neuropsychopharmacology*, **Dec**, 67 (Abstract).

Dupont, R.M., Lehr, P., Lamoureaux, G., Halpern, S., Harris, M.J. & Jeste, D.V. (1993) Preliminary report: cerebral blood flow abnormalities in late-life schizophrenia. *Psychiatry Research*, (in press).

Faraone, S.V. & Tsuang, M.T. (1985) Quantitative models of the genetic transmission of schizophrenia. *Psychological Bulletin*, **98**, 41–66.

Flint, A.J., Rifat, S.I. & Eastwood, M.R. (1991) Late-onset paranoia: distinct from paraphrenia? *International Journal of Geriatric Psychiatry*, **6**, 103–109.

Ganzini, L., Heintz, R.T., Hoffman, W.F. & Casey, D.E. (1991) The prevalence of tardive dyskinesia in neuroleptic-treated diabetics: a controlled study. *Archives of General Psychiatry*, **48**, 259–263.

Gerlach, J. (1991) New antipsychotics: classification, efficacy, and adverse effects. *Schizophrenia Bulletin*, **17**, 289–309.

Gierz, M. & Jeste, D.V. (1993) Physical comorbidity in elderly schizophrenic and depressed groups. *American Journal of Geriatric Psychiatry*, **1**, 165–170.

Gold, J.M., Randolph, C., Carpenter, C.J., Goldberg, T.E. & Weinberger, D.R. (1992) Forms of memory failure in schizophrenia. *Journal of Abnormal Psychology*, **101(3)**, 487–494.

Goldberg, T.E., Hyde, T.M., Kleinman, J.E. & Weinberger, D.R. (1993) The course of schizophrenia: neuropsychological evidence for a static encephalopathy. *Schizophrenia Bulletin*, **19**, 797–804.

Gur, R.E. & Pearlson, G.D. (1993) Neuroimaging in schizophrenia research. *Schizophrenia Bulletin*, **19**, 337–353.

Gurland, B.J. & Cross, P.S. (1982) Epidemiology of psychopathology in old age: some implications for clinical services. *Psychiatric Clinics of North America*, **5**, 11–26.

Harris, M.J. & Jeste, D.V. (1988) Late-onset schizophrenia: an overview. *Schizophrenia Bulletin*, **14**, 39–55.

Harris, M.J., Jeste, D.V., Krull, A.J., Montague, J. & Heaton, R.K. (1991) Deficit syndrome in older schizophrenic patients. *Psychiatry Research*, **39**, 285–292.

Harris, M.J., McAdams, L.A. & Heaton, S. (1994) Negative symptoms in late-life schizophrenia. *American Journal of Geriatric Psychiatry*, **2**, 9–20.

Heaton, R.K. (1992) *Comprehensive Norms for an Expanded Halstead–Reitan Battery: A Supplement for the Wechsler Adult Intelligence Scale*, revised. Psychological Assessment Resources Inc, Odessa.

Heaton, R., Paulsen, J., McAdams, L.A. *et al.* (1994) Neuropsychological deficits in schizophrenia: relationship to age, chronicity and dementia. *Archives of General Psychiatry*, **51**, 469–476.

Heykants, J., Snoeck, E., Van Peer, A., Sack, M., Horton, M. & Meibach, R. (1993) Risperidone pharmacokinetics: effect of age, renal and liver impairment. *9th World Congress of Psychiatry*, **June**, 741 (Abstract).

Honigfeld, G., Rosebaum, M.P., Blumenthal, I.J., Lambert, H.L. & Roberts, A.J. (1965) Behavioral improvement in the older schizophrenic patient: drug and social therapies. *Journal of the American Geriatric Society*, **13**, 57–71.

Hymas, N., Naguib, M. & Levy, R. (1989) Late paraphrenia – a follow-up study. *International Journal of Geriatric Psychiatry*, **4**, 23–29.

Jeste, D.V. & Wyatt, R.J. (1982) *Understanding and Treating Tardive Dyskinesia*. Guilford Press, New York.

Jeste, D.V., Harris, M.J., Pearlson, G.D. *et al.* (1988) Late-onset schizophrenia: studying clinical validity. *Psychiatric Clinics of North America*, **11**, 1–14.

Jeste, D.V., Lacro, J.P., Gilbert, P.L., Kline, J. & Kline, N. (1993) Treatment of late-life schizophrenia with neuroleptics. *Schizophrenia Bulletin*, **19**, 817–830.

Johnstone, E.V., Crow, T.J., Frith, C.D., Husband, J. & Kreel, L. (1976) Cerebral ventricular size and cognitive impairment in chronic schizophrenia. *Lancet*, **2**, 924–926.

Kane, J.M., Honigfeld, G., Singer, J., Meltzer, H. & Clozaril Study Group (1988) Clozapine for the treatment resistant schizophrenic: a double-blind comparison vs. chlopromazine/benztropine. *Archives of General Psychiatry*, **45**, 789–796.

Kaplan, H.I. & Sadock, B.J. (1988) *Synopsis of Psychiatry*. Williams & Wilkins, Baltimore.

Kay, D.W.K. & Roth, M. (1955) Physical accompaniments of mental disorder in old age. *Lancet*, **269**, 740–745.

Kay, D.W.K. & Roth, M. (1961) Environmental and hereditary factors in the schizophrenias of old age ('late paraphrenia') and their bearing on the general problem of causation in schizophrenia. *Journal of Mental Science*, **107**, 649–686.

Kendler, K.S., Gruenberg, A.M. & Tsuang, M.T. (1985) Subtype stability in schizophrenia. *American Journal of Psychiatry*, **142**, 827–832.

Kraepelin, E. (1909) *Psychiatrie. Ein Lehrbuch für Studierende und Aerzte*. Barth, Leipzig.

Krull, A.J., Press, G., Dupont, R., Harris, M.J. & Jeste, D.V. (1991) Brain imaging in late-onset schizophrenia and related psychoses. *International Journal of Geriatric Psychiatry*, **6**, 651–658.

Lacro, J.P. & Jeste, D.V. (1994) Physical comorbidity and polypharmacy in older psychiatric patients. *Biological Psychiatry*, **36**, 146–152.

Lesser, I.M., Jeste, D.V., Boone, K.B. *et al.* (1992) Late-onset psychotic disorder, not otherwise specified: clinical and neuroimaging findings. *Biological Psychiatry*, **31**, 419–423.

Lesser, I.M., Miller, B.L., Swartz, J.R., Boone, K.B., Mehringer, C.M. & Mena, I. (1993) Brain imaging in late-life schizophrenia and related psychosis. *Schizophrenia Bulletin*, **19**, 773–782.

Lewander, T., Weterbergh, S.E. & Morrison, D. (1990) Clinical profile of remoxipride – a combined analysis of a comparative double-blind multicentre trial programme. *Acta Psychiatrica Scandinavica*, **82(358)**, 92–98.

McGlashan, T.H. (1988) A selective review of recent North American long-term followup studies of schizophrenia. *Schizophrenia Bulletin*, **14**, 515–542.

Maletta, G., Mattox, K.M. & Dysken, M. (1991) Guidelines for prescribing psychoactive drugs in the elderly: part 1. *Geriatrics*, **46(9)**, 40–47.

Miller, B.L. & Lesser, I.M. (1988) Late-life psychosis and modern neuroimaging. In Jeste, D.V. & Zisook, S. (eds) *The Psychiatric Clinics of North America: Psychosis and Depression in the Elderly*, pp. 33–46. WB Saunders, Philadelphia.

Miller, B.L., Lesser, I.M., Boone, K.B., Hill, E., Mehringer, C.M. & Wong, K. (1991) Brain lesions and cognitive function in late-life psychosis. *British Journal of Psychiatry*, **158**, 76–82.

Movin, G., Gustafson, L., Franzen, G. *et al.* (1990) Pharmacokinetics of remoxipride in elderly psychotic patients. *Acta Psychiatrica Scandinavica*, **358**, 176–180.

National Institute on Aging (1987) *Personnel for Health Needs of the Elderly Through the Year 2020*. US Dept of Health and Human Services, Bethesda.

Ostergaard, K. & Dupont, E. (1988) Clozapine treatment of drug-induced psychotic symptoms in late stages of Parkinson's disease. *Acta Neurologica Scandinavica*, **78**, 349–350.

Pearlson, G. & Rabins, P. (1988) The late-onset psychoses: possible risk factors. In Jeste, D.V. & Zisook, S. (eds) *The Psychiatric Clinics of North America: Psychosis and Depression in the Elderly*, pp. 15–32. WB Saunders, Philadelphia.

Pearlson, G.D., Tune, L.E., Wong, D.F. *et al.* (1993) Quantitative D2 dopamine receptor PET and structural MRI changes in late-onset schizophrenia: a preliminary report. *Schizophrenia Bulletin*, **19**, 783–795.

Prager, S. & Jeste, D.V. (1993) Sensory impairment in late-life schizophrenia. *Schizophrenia Bulletin*, **19**, 755–772.

Rabins, P., Pearlson, G., Jayaram, G., Steele, C. & Tune, L. (1987) Elevated VBR in late-onset schizophrenia. *American Journal of Psychiatry*, **144**, 1216–1218.

Raskind, M., Alvarez, C. & Herlin, S. (1979) Fluphenazine enthanthate in the outpatient treatment of late paraphrenia. *Journal of American Geriatric Society*, **27**, 459–463.

Rosen, J., Bohon, S. & Gershon, S. (1990) Antipsychotics in the elderly. *Acta Psychiatrica Scandinavica*, **82** (Suppl. **358**), 170–175.

Saltz, B.L., Woerner, M.G., Kane, J.M. *et al.* (1991) Prospective study of tardive dyskinesia incidence in the elderly. *Journal of American Medical Association*, **266**, 2402–2406.

Salzman, C. (1990) Principles of psychopharmacology. In Bienenfeld, D. (ed.) *Verwoerdt's Clinical Geropsychiatry*, pp. 235–249. Williams & Wilkins, Baltimore.

Scholz, E. & Dichgans, J. (1985) Treatment of drug-induced exogenous psychosis in Parkinsonism with clozapine and fluperlapine. *European Archives of Psychiatry and Neurological Sciences*, **235**, 60–64.

Weinberger, D.R. (1987) Implications of normal brain development for the pathogenesis of schizophrenia. *Archives of General Psychiatry*, **44**, 660–669.

Weinberger, D.R., Jeste, D.V., Wyatt, R.J. & Teychenne, P.F. (1987) Cerebral atrophy in elderly schizophrenic patients: effects of aging and of long-term institutionalization and neuroleptic therapy. In Miller, N.E. & Cohen, G.D. (eds) *Schizophrenia and Aging: Schizophrenia, Paranoid and Schizophreniform Disorders in Later Life*, pp. 109–118. Guilford Press, New York.

Weinberger, D., Torrey, E., Neophytides, A. & Wyatt, R. (1979) Lateral cerebral ventricular enlargement in chronic schizophrenia. *Archives of General Psychiatry*, **36**, 735–739.

Widerlov, E., Andersson, U., Von Bahr, C. & Maj-Inger, N. (1991) Pharmacokinetics and effects on prolactin of remoxi-pride in patients with tardive dyskinesia. *Psychopharmacology*, **103**, 46–49.

Williams, L. & Lowenthal, D.T. (1992) Drug therapy in the elderly. *Southern Medical Journal*, **85(2)**, 127–131.

Winokur, G., Pfohl, B. & Tsuang, M. (1987) A 40-year follow-up of hebephrenic-catatonic schizophrenia. In Miller, N. & Cohen, G. (eds) *Schizophrenia and Aging*, pp. 52–60. Guilford Press, New York, NY.

Wolk, S.I. & Douglas, C.J. (1992) Clozapine treatment of psychosis in Parkinson's disease: a report of 5 consecutive cases. *Journal of Clinical Psychiatry*, **53**, 373–376.

Wolters, E.C., Hurwitz, T.A., Mak, E. *et al.* (1990) Clozapine in the treatment of parkinsonian patients with dopamino-mimetic psychosis. *Neurology*, **40**, 832–840.

Wong, D.F., Wagner, H.N. Jr, Dannals, R.F. *et al.* (1984) Effects of age on dopamine and serotonin receptors measured by positron emission tomography in the living human brain. *Science*, **226**, 1393–1396.

Yassa, R. & Jeste, D.V. (1992) Gender differences in tardive dyskinesia: a critical review of the literature. *Schizophrenia Bulletin*, **18(4)**, 701–715.

Yassa, R., Lal, S., Korpassy, A. & Ally, J. (1987) Nicotine exposure and tardive dyskinesia. *Biological Psychiatry*, **22**, 67–72.

Yassa, R., Nastase, C., Dupont, D. & Thibeau, M. (1992) Tardive dyskinesia in elderly psychiatric patients: a 5-year study. *American Journal of Psychiatry*, **149(9)**, 1206–1211.

Chapter 7
The Schizophrenia Spectrum Personality Disorders

L. J. SIEVER, A. J. BERGMAN AND R. S. E. KEEFE

The schizophrenia spectrum

While it has long been appreciated that the schizophrenic disorders comprise a 'schizophrenia spectrum' from severe chronic psychotic forms of schizophrenia to the milder schizophrenia-related personality disorders, the study of schizophrenia spectrum disorders has been revitalized in the context of new genetic and biological studies into the aetiology, pathophysiology and treatment of schizophrenia. European phenomenologically orientated psychiatrists such as Bleuler and Kahn were among the first to observe that there may be gradations of schizophrenia-related disorders, with relatives of schizophrenic patients displaying milder psychotic-like symptoms and asociality that were similar in character, if not in severity, to those observed in chronic schizophrenic patients (Siever & Gunderson, 1983; Kendler, 1985). These milder, schizophrenia-related disorders were designated as 'schizoid' by Bleuler and others to acknowledge the relationship of their symptomatology to schizophrenia, although the individuals lacked overt psychotic symptoms. While the term schizoid became more broadly applied to individuals who tended to be isolated or had an active fantasy life, a picture that may be consistent with a variety of disorders including affective disorders, other terms such as borderline schizophrenia or schizotype (Rado, 1962) replaced the term schizoid and were developed to identify more specifically a disorder genetically and clinically related to schizophrenia.

This diagnostic concept was revitalized when the diagnosis schizotypal personality disorder, a relatively new diagnosis in psychiatric nomenclature, was introduced in the *Diagnostic and Statistical Manual* DSM-III (APA, 1980). The criteria for schizotypal personality disorder were based on the clinical profiles of probands and relatives in the adoptive studies of Kety, Rosenthal and Wender (Kety *et al.*, 1975) with diagnoses of 'borderline schizophrenia' or 'latent schizophrenia'. The inclusion of schizotypal personality disorder provided a more easily targeted construct for clinical investigation of the schizophrenia spectrum. In this context, a series of studies pertaining to the phenomenology, genetics, biology, outcome and treatment response suggested that schizotypal personality disorder was indeed closely related to chronic schizophrenia in all these domains. Newer, more sophisticated studies have gone further in suggesting that schizotypal and other schizophrenia-related personality disorders may allow an opportunity to disentangle and clarify the multifactorial convergent genetic and biological processes underlying schizophrenia. In this chapter, we highlight the results of many of these studies in the context of developing notions of the schizophrenia spectrum.

Phenomenology

DSM-III-R and DSM-IV diagnostic criteria for schizotypal personality disorder consist of attenuated psychotic-like symptoms such as ideas of reference and cognitive/perceptual distortions, as well as deficit-like symptoms of constricted affect and social isolation and related criteria reflecting eccentric appearance and speech. The ideas of reference of schizotypal personality disorder, while not held with the conviction characteristic of the chronic schizophrenic, are often persistent and disturbing to the patient. Schizotypal individuals may feel that others are staring at them or talking about them when they enter a bus or attend a social occasion. They often entertain unusual beliefs that are outside the social norms of their culture, sometimes in a superstitious or religious context and other times in an idiosyncratic fashion. For example, they may manifest 'magical thinking' such as the belief that one's thoughts anticipate tragic events like accidental deaths. Illusions and other perceptual experiences are common, particularly in situations where information is ambiguous, such as in a darkened room, or in an altered state, such as drowsiness or fatigue. Schizotypal individuals may be socially isolated and have few friends in whom they confide and to whom they feel close in an enduring way. Their affect may be constricted, and they may be difficult to engage interpersonally; rapport with others may be severely lacking. At other times, they may smile inappropritely and react emotionally in a way that appears dysynchronous from their speech context. They tend to be suspicious and guarded, attributing negative or persecutory intents to others. Their behaviour and appearance may be odd with idiosyncratic movements, expressions, mannerisms and style of dress. Their speech may also be unusual and may be concrete and impoverished or extraordinarily elaborate with frequent nonsequiturs.

The diagnostic criteria for paranoid personality disorder emphasize suspicious and mistrustful traits; distortions in cognition and perception may not be present. Thus, persons with this disorder have an expectancy of malevolent intent and behaviour on the part of others. They constantly question the loyalty of friends and close colleagues and see hidden, threatening meanings that tend to justify their preconceptions. Because of their fear of the ill will of others, they are reluctant to confide in them and are often volatile in response to perceived slights.

Finally, schizoid personality disorder is grounded in the core traits of asociality and lack of enjoyment of interpersonal engagement. The schizoid person, like the schizotypal individual, may have no close friends or confidants, although people with schizoid personality disorder do not necessarily have the cognitive/perceptual distortions that are criteria for schizotypal personality disorder. The schizoid individual appears to prefer being alone and does not evidence desire for, or pleasure from, close relationships, whether friendly or intimate. Such individuals often appear indifferent to criticism and praise, and share with the schizotypal individual an aloof, detached, constricted appearance.

These three disorders are highly overlapping in clinical samples (Siever *et al.*, 1991). Schizoid personality is least common in the clinical setting, perhaps because these individuals are stably isolated and thus do not experience the dysphoria, disruption of relationships and work function, and more eccentric appearance associated with the cognitive peculiarities of schizotypal and paranoid personality disorders. Paranoid and schizotypal personality disorders are highly overlapping in most clinical studies (Siever *et al.*, 1991), which is not surprising given the overlap between the criteria. However, it is not clear whether there is perhaps a group of individuals with paranoid personality disorder distinct from individuals meeting criteria for schizotypal personality disorder, who may be more closely related to delusional disorder or, in some cases, to the histrionic and dramatic spectrum of personality disorders.

The generally high comorbidity of these disorders and close relationship of their criteria raise a question of whether they are defining distinct disorders or are actually gradations of severity along the schizophrenia spectrum. According to the latter conception, schizoid personality disorder would represent one end of the continuum, at the other end of which is schizophrenia, with schizotypal personality disorder between the two. Obviously, as one moves towards the more schizoid end of the spectrum, the relationship to schizophrenia is less strong and specific. However, from an aetiological point of view, heterogeneity might be found throughout the spectrum, since a variety of pathophysiological processes may lead to a final outcome of chronic schizophrenia.

There is also an overlap between schizophrenia spectrum personality disorders and borderline and avoidant personality disorders. The overlap with borderline personality disorder has been diminished as criteria for each have become refined; also, the diagnosis of schizotypal personality disorder requires five rather than four criteria in DSM-III-R. An attempt to differentiate the psychotic-like symptoms of borderline personality disorder as transient and often dissociative, in contrast to those of schizotypal personality disorder, which are more persistent and pervasive, has been incorporated into the criteria for DSM-IV and will hopefully further clarify this diagnostic distinction. Conceptually, avoidant personality disordered individuals yearn for social relationships but require an unusually strong degree of acceptance before engaging in them because of their anxiety, while schizoid and schizotypal individuals do not actively want or seek these relationships. In practice, however, these distinctions are difficult to make. Schizotypal and schizoid individuals may acknowledge a wistfulness for relationships and experience the limitations of their isolation. Furthermore, avoidant individuals may at times appear aloof and distant, and on neuropsychological testing even show cognitive impairment (Hollander *et al.*, 1992) that may not be clearly distinct in character from the neuropsychological abnormalities observed in the schizophrenia spectrum disorders.

Some of the symptoms characterizing these personality disorders have also been studied in non-clinical samples, who may be at the furthest end of the schizophrenia spectrum continuum. This line of research has focused on applying psychometric procedures to a normal population in order to detect individuals with an increased liability for schizophrenia. This psychometric high-risk strategy, which is used to identify hypothetically psychosis-prone individuals, is based on Meehl's conception of 'schizotaxia' reflecting an underlying schizophrenic genotype (Meehl, 1962). Meehl hypothesized that individuals with schizotaxia who possess the genetic predisposition for schizophrenia but do not manifest the disorder will usually display some evidence of deviant psychological functioning, labelled 'schizotypy'. Meehl described a set of signs and symptoms that he believed were evident in those non-psychotic, schizotypic individuals (Meehl, 1964).

Since Meehl's original description of schizotypic individuals, many self-report instruments have been developed to measure schizotypy in primarily non-clinical populations (e.g. Chapman *et al.*, 1976, 1978; Eckblad & Chapman, 1983; Claridge & Broks, 1984; Venables, 1990; Raine, 1991). When used as a high-risk methodology, this approach is a useful complement to the traditional genetic high-risk strategy because it should result in a more representative sample of future schizophrenics, given that only about 5–10% of schizophrenics have a schizophrenic parent (Chapman & Chapman, 1985). Venables *et al.* (1990) also pointed out that this high-risk methodology has the advantage of targeting adult subjects instead of children so that the period of follow-up is economically shortened. Furthermore, the benefits of studying non-clinical populations include accessibility to larger numbers of subjects, elimination of potential confounds such as medication and institutionalization, and additional insight into the boundaries of the disorder.

The plethora of self-report scales differ in a number of ways, including item construction, conceptual bias and theoretical assumptions. Despite the wide range of techniques and conceptual frameworks evident in the various schizo-typy scales, there are a number of findings that are relevant for the study of schizophrenia and schizophrenia spectrum personality disorders. When compared with schizophrenic patients, there is consistent evidence that non-clinical samples identified through these self-report inventories show similar (although less severe) deficits in a number of areas, such as neuropsychological, cognitive and psychophysiological functioning (e.g. Simons *et al.*, 1982; Barlogh & Merritt, 1985; Simons & Katkin, 1985; Rosenbaum *et al.*, 1988; Spaulding *et al.*, 1989; Lenzenweger *et al.*, 1991). These findings support the hypothesis that mild expression of schizotypy is genetically and clinically related to schizophrenia.

Another relevant contribution of the psycho-metric high-risk paradigm has been a number of studies investigating the factor structure underlying schizotypy. Despite the fact that these studies differed in terms of the specific scales used, some compatible findings have emerged. The most consistent factor to emerge from these studies seems to measure 'positive' schizotypy, consisting of psychotic-like cognitive and perceptual experiences (Muntaner *et al.*, 1988; Bentall *et al.*, 1989; Hewitt & Claridge, 1989; Raine & Allbutt, 1989; Venables, 1990; Kendler & Hewitt, 1992). Another factor comprises items reflecting 'negative' or deficit-like characteristics (Muntaner *et al.*, 1988; Bentall *et al.*, 1989; Kendler & Hewitt, 1992). Some studies also find a third factor, which can be described as cognitive disorganization (Bentall *et al.*, 1989), while others report a third factor of non-conformity (Muntaner *et al.*, 1988; Bentall *et al.*, 1989; Raine & Allbutt, 1989; Kendler & Hewitt, 1992). These factors, which were based on data primarily gathered from non-clinical populations, may parallel the positive, negative and thought-disordered factors frequently found in studies of schizophrenia. Furthermore, in a study of twins, Kendler *et al.* (1991) found two independent dimensions (i.e. positive and negative) of both clinically rated and self-rated schizotypy. The findings indicated that both positive and negative dimensions of both clinically rated and self-rated schizotypy were correlated

more highly in monozygotic twins than in dizygotic twins. A later paper focused solely on self-report scales of schizotypy and found three distinct factors (positive trait schizotypy, non-conformity and social schizotypy), all of which were influenced by genetic factors (Kendler & Hewitt, 1992). These results suggest that genetic factors are important in all these areas of schizotypy.

While much of the research investigating the aetiology, pathophysiology and treatment of schizophrenia involves studies with schizophrenic patients, the concept of a schizophrenia spectrum has stimulated interest in studying both clinical and non-clinical schizotypic subjects. The results of studies utilizing self-report psychometric inventories of schizotypy confirm the importance and relevance of this research for the study of schizophrenia and schizophrenia spectrum personality disorders. In particular, it seems that the positive and negative factors of schizotypy may provide an important area to explore, as it has been suggested that positive and negative symptoms along the schizophrenia spectrum may be associated with distinct pathophysiologies (Siever, 1991; Siever *et al.*, 1993b).

Spectrum personality disorders in premorbid clinical profiles of schizophrenic patients

Interest in the premorbid personality of schizophrenic patients is well established in the psychiatric literature. Both Kraepelin (1919) and Bleuler (1950) observed that a proportion of schizophrenic patients displayed abnormal behaviour long before the onset of adult psychosis. Kretschmer's (1921) description of schizoid personality included solitariness, cold affect and eccentricity. Other descriptions have often included suspiciousness, rigidity and unusual speech (Foerster *et al.*, 1991a). Given the recent interest in viewing schizophrenia spectrum personality disorders as milder, schizophrenia-related disorders, the study of premorbid personality characteristics in schizophrenia may help clarify the relationship between schizophrenia spectrum personality disorders and schizophrenia.

A variety of methodologies have been used to investigate the characteristics of adult psychiatric patients before the onset of an illness. These include follow-back studies of adult schizophrenic patients looking at school records (Watt, 1978) or child guidance centre records (Ambelas, 1992), follow-up studies of children who have attended child guidance clinics (Robins, 1966) and prospective high-risk studies following children who are presumably at high risk for schizophrenia, usually based on the genetic risk (Parnas & Jorgensen, 1989). The majority of these studies did not involve the assessment of schizophrenia spectrum personality disorders as premorbid features of schizophrenia. However, some recent retrospective and high-risk studies have used assessments of personality features based on both patient report and interviews with relatives (Squires-Wheeler *et al.*, 1988; Foerster *et al.*, 1991a,b; Peralta *et al.*, 1991).

Many of the early retrospective and follow-back studies found that preschizophrenic boys were shy and withdrawn (Bower *et al.*, 1960; Warnken & Seiss, 1965; Barthell & Holmes, 1968). One investigation of the school records of male and female schizophrenic patients indicated that preschizophrenic males were described as emotionally unstable and disagreeable beginning in grade seven which corresponds to early adolescence (Watt, 1978). Preschizophrenic females, on the other hand, were described as emotionally unstable and introverted. A more recent study utilized information in the case notes of adult schizophrenic patients (male only) who had attended a child guidance centre as children (Ambelas, 1992). The findings indicated that the diagnoses of these boys tended to consist of mixed emotional and conduct disorders. In terms of follow-up studies, most have found that preschizophrenic boys were both aggressive and withdrawn (Michael *et al.*, 1957; O'Neal & Robins, 1958). However, those who were predominantly withdrawn seemed to have the poorest adult outcome (Ricks & Berry, 1970; Roff *et al.*, 1976).

A more efficient way of prospectively following preschizophrenic individuals is to identify children who are at increased genetic risk for developing schizophrenia as adults. All the studies that have compared high-risk children with normal controls have found significant behavioural differences. Some investigators have found high-risk children to be more emotionally unstable (Glish *et al.*, 1982), while others have reported that high-risk children who later developed schizophrenia were characterized by poor affective control and cognitive disturbances (Parnas *et al.*, 1982). There is also evidence that those high-risk subjects who develop predominantly negative-symptom schizophrenia will present with different premorbid behaviours than those subjects who develop predominantly positive-symptom schizophrenia (Cannon *et al.*, 1990). This study reported that premorbid teacher ratings of predominantly negative-symptom schizophrenic patients consisted of more negative-type premorbid behaviours (i.e. passivity, lack of spontaneity, social unresponsiveness and isolation), while the predominantly positive schizophrenic patients were rated with more positive-type premorbid behaviours (i.e. overactivity, irritability, distractibility and aggression).

While the above studies clearly indicate that preschizophrenic and high-risk children are deviant compared with normal controls, some questions remain about the specificity of behavioural deviance to schizophrenia and whether these behaviours can be identified as schizophrenia spectrum personality disorders or traits. Some studies that have compared the behaviour of high-risk children with that of a psychiatric control group have found few, if any, behavioural differences (El-Guebaly *et al.*, 1978; Weintraub & Neale, 1984). Squires-Wheeler *et al.* (1988, 1989, 1992) have investigated the rate of schizotypal personality traits in the subjects of the New York high-risk project. They report that the rates of schizotypal personality traits do not differ between the offspring of schizophrenic parents and the offspring of affective disorder parents (Squires-Wheeler *et al.*, 1988, 1989). More recently, they have reported that, with longitudinal assessments, a subgroup of the offspring of affective disorder parents may be distinguished who exhibit transformation of schizotypal features to depression and/or anxiety (Squires-Wheeler *et al.*, 1992). Taken together, these results do not provide conclusive evidence as to the specificity of schizotypal personality traits to schizophrenia in high-risk populations.

In contrast, there is some support for the specificity of schizotypal traits in the premorbid personalities of schizophrenic patients versus patients with affective psychosis (Foerster *et al.*, 1991b). It is clear that before the onset of illness a significant proportion of schizophrenic adults exhibit deviant characteristics including schizoid and schizotypal traits (Fish, 1986; Hogg *et al.*, 1990; Foerster *et al.*, 1991b; Peralta *et al.*, 1991). Furthermore, some investigators have found that premorbid personality traits are associated with specific dimensions of schizophrenic symptomatology (Jorgensen & Parnas, 1990). For instance, there is evidence to support a relationship between premorbid schizoid personality disorder and negative symptoms in schizophrenic patients (Jorgensen & Parnas, 1990; Peralta *et al.*, 1991). These results are consistent with one hypothesis that the 'primary' genetic susceptibility to schizophrenia is manifested as deficit-like or negative traits (Siever, 1991; Siever *et al.*, 1993b).

While findings of premorbid schizoid and schizotypal personality traits in schizophrenic patients lend support to the notion of a schizophrenia spectrum, it must also be noted that not all schizophrenic patients evidence abnormal personality traits before the onset of schizophrenia. In fact, one study found that a normal personality was the most frequent premorbid characterization of the schizophrenic sample (44%; Peralta *et al.*, 1991). Another report indicated that 42% of the sample had no premorbid diagnosis based on the schedule for interviewing DSM-III personality disorders (SIDP), although when the Million Multiaxial Clinical Inventory (MCMI-I) was used, 70% of the same sample had at least one personality disorder diagnosis (Hogg *et al.*, 1990). Once again, the heterogeneous nature of schizophrenia seems apparent.

In conclusion, it seems likely that a subgroup of schizophrenic patients can be characterized by premorbid personality disorders that are clearly related to schizophrenia. However, the relationship between abnormal personality traits and later schizophrenia is not clear. It may be that the presence of schizophrenia spectrum personality disorders is indicative of a higher morbidity for the development of schizophrenia, or that these personality disorders are part of the extended phenotype of schizophrenia. Furthermore, it is not clear whether a schizophrenia spectrum personality disorder is a necessary transitional stage before the development of schizophrenia, which would indicate that all schizophrenic patients have a premorbid personality disturbance. Research investigating schizophrenia spectrum personality disorders in a variety of populations, including the premorbid personalities of schizophrenic patients, non-affected relatives of schizophrenic patients and clinically referred personality disordered patients, may help to answer some of the questions regarding the role of early personality disturbances in the development of schizophrenia.

Biology

Neuroanatomical imaging

One of the first observations of alteration of brain structure in schizophrenic patients was an increase in the size of the ventricle:brain ratio (VBR). This finding has remained one of the most consistent abnormalities in schizophrenia research (Shelton & Weinberger, 1986). Both increased VBR and evidence of cortical atrophy on computerized axial tomography (CAT) scans have been associated with the deficit-like symptoms of schizophrenia, impairment of cognitive functions, decreased dopaminergic activity and poor outcome in schizophrenic patients (Shelton & Weinberger, 1986). More recent studies using magnetic resonance imaging (MRI) have demonstrated decreases in the size of the temporal lobes and perihippocampal structures (Suddath *et al.*, 1989).

Imaging of neuroanatomical structures has only just begun to be applied to other patients in the schizophrenia spectrum. Adolescents with spectrum disorders have been reported to have increases in VBR compared with the ratio in controls (Schulz *et al.*, 1983). Two studies of schizotypal patients from clinical populations have suggested increases in VBR in the schizotypal patients compared with other personality disorder patients and/or normal controls (Cazzulo *et al.*, 1991; Siever, 1991; Siever *et al.*, 1993b,c). In the latter study, increases were found in lateral VBR (particularly the left lateral VBR) in the schizotypal patients compared with the patients with other personality disorders (Siever, 1991; Siever *et al.*, 1993b,c). Abnormal left to right asymmetry, as reflected by an increased left, compared with right, frontal horn has been found to distinguish schizophrenics with severe social deterioration from other schizophrenics (Keefe *et al.*, 1987; Frecska *et al.*, 1991). This measure also discriminates schizotypal patients from the other personality disorder control group and is highly correlated with schizotypal symptoms (Siever *et al.*, 1993c). Furthermore, increases in frontal horn size were associated with increased errors on neuropsychological tests that are sensitive to frontal dysfunction; these include the Wisconsin card sort test (WCST) and Trails B (Siever, 1991; De Vegvar *et al.*, 1993; Siever *et al.*, 1993b).

Studies of relatives of schizophrenic patients also suggest the possibility of increased ventricular size (particularly in frontal horn areas) associated with defects in tests of frontal function and deficit-like symptoms of asociality (Silverman *et al.*, 1992). One study of siblings of schizophrenic patients initially showed increases, but in a larger sample showed no differences from normal (Olson *et al.*, 1993). A third study assessing relatives of schizophrenic patients used the genetic 'high-risk' strategy, evaluating the offspring of schizophrenic patients. The offspring were evaluated as to whether they had neither, one or both parents in the schizophrenia spectrum (e.g. one schizophrenic and one schizotypal) as well as birth defects. Increases in the genetic risk for schizophrenia, as indicated by the number of parents with schizophrenia spectrum disorders, were associated with increased VBR values, with particular prominence of the cortical sulci in temporal and other cortical areas. In contrast, birth complications were more associated with increases in ventricular size. Offspring with schizotypal diagnoses, who had fewer perinatal complications than the chronic schizophrenic patients, demonstrated a ventricular size that did not differ from normal (and was actually decreased in the initial series), while sulcal enlargement was common to both schizotypal and schizophrenic offspring (Schulsinger *et al.*, 1984; Cannon *et al.*, 1990, 1993). These results are compatible with the model that perinatal complications may interact with a genetic susceptibility to schizophrenia spectrum disorders, resulting in a clinical phenotype of schizophrenia as well as the CAT finding of enlarged ventricles. The genetic susceptibility alone would be associated with sulcal enlargement and reduced cortical size, but not necessarily with ventricular enlargement. These considerations could explain why ventricular enlargement may be more likely to manifest in clinical samples than in genetic 'high-risk' samples.

Neuropsychological profile

Numerous studies implicate cognitive/neuropsychological dysfunction in schizophrenic patients. These involve deficits in abstraction, executive function, verbal memory and problem solving (see Gray *et al.* (1991) for a recent review). In contrast, some functions such as perceptual skills may be relatively spared. While no specific regional brain impairment can be implicated from these findings in general, they suggest dysfunction in temporal and frontal cortical circuits.

One hypothesis that has stimulated a great deal of research in schizophrenia is that schizophrenia may be particularly associated with impairment in the dorsolateral prefrontal cortex (Weinberger, 1987). Tests sensitive to prefrontal dysfunction, such as the WCST, are performed relatively poorly by schizophrenic patients. Furthermore, imaging studies of blood flow during the undertaking of these tasks suggest that schizophrenic patients show diminished activation of this region during the WCST. Since the WCST evaluates executive function, particularly the capacity to both maintain and appropriately shift cognitive set in relation to verbal feedback, which is believed to be mediated in part by the frontal cortex, the impairment of schizophrenics on this and similar tasks may suggest dysfunction of the frontal lobes in schizophrenia. Schizophrenic patients with deficit symptoms may perform particularly poorly on tests of frontal function (Andreasen *et al.*, 1992).

Several studies raise the possibility that neuropsychological impairment may be observed in schizotypal personality disorder patients as well as schizophrenic patients. Abnormalities of WCST performance have been identified in both clinical samples (DeVegvar *et al.*, 1993) and in volunteers selected by virtue of their schizotypal characteristics (Lyons *et al.*, 1991; Raine *et al.*, 1992). In the clinical study, schizotypal personality disorder patients, patients with other personality disorders and normal controls were administered a variety of neuropsychological tasks including the WCST, a test of verbal fluency sensitive to frontal dysfunction and Trails B, which is also sensitive to frontal dysfunction (Reitan, 1958; Picton *et al.*, 1986). In addition, tests of more generalized cortical function (Wechsler Adult Intelligence Scale-Revised vocabulary and block design) were administered. In general, the schizotypal personality disorder patients performed intermediately between the controls and other personality disorder patients on the one hand, and schizophrenic patients on the other hand. During the WCST, the schizotypal personality disorder patients made significantly more perseverative errors and completed a lower number of categories than did patients with other personality disorders and/or normal controls. The schizotypal personality disorder patients took longer to complete the Trails B test than did comparison groups, but they were not significantly different from either comparison group on the WAIS-R or verbal fluency. In general, these data suggest that tests sensitive to prefrontal function may be particularly impaired in patients with schizotypal personality disorder. Studies of the relatives of schizophrenic patients who may display schizotypal psychopathology suggest that these individuals may perform worse than controls on measures of set alternation and verbal fluency (Keefe *et al.*, 1994) as well as abstraction and verbal memory. A full battery of neuropsychological and cognitive tests on these patients have not been completed to identify a specific profile of functional and possible neuroanatomical abnormalities. The data collected to date, however, suggest that, as in schizophrenic patients, functions mediated in part by the frontal cortex may be impaired.

If defects in the dopaminergic function in the cortex are contributing to or associated with deficits in frontally related cognitive function, agents that would enhance dopaminergic function might be expected to improve performance. Indeed, D_1 receptors may play a crucial role in modulating working memory performance, which can be impaired by dopaminergic blockade of these receptors (Sawaguchi & Goldman-Rakic, 1991). D_2 agonists, such as bromocryptine, also may improve working memory (Luciana *et al.*, 1992). To evaluate this possibility, a pilot study of amphetamine effects on neuropsychological performance was initiated in our laboratory. Preliminary results suggest that schizotypal personality disorder patients almost uniformly improve their neuropsychological performance on the WCST; the most impaired performers improve to the greatest degree. Plasma homovanillic acid (HVA) concentrations tend to be reduced after amphetamine administration; this is consistent with the reuptake blockade and releasing effects of amphetamine, suggesting that increased dopamine was available for synaptic transmission (Wainberg *et al.*, 1993). Interestingly, an increase in psychotic-like symptoms was not seen in these patients. These very preliminary results are consistent with studies of schizophrenic patients suggesting that prefrontal activation on the WCST is correlated with dopaminergic function as measured by concentrations of cerebrospinal fluid (CSF) HVA (Weinberger, 1987). They further hint at the possibility that enhancement of dopaminergic function may be effective in improving cognitive performance in schizotypal patients. While studies of amphetamine administration in schizophrenic patients with regard to neurocognitive testing and frontal function have not yielded to conclusive results (Daniel *et al.*, 1991), the schizotypal patient with presumably more potentially intact cortical processing capacity may be a more fruitful target of research into the interaction of dopamine and cognition in schizophrenia-related disorders.

Finally, while functional imaging studies have only recently been applied to schizotypal patients, our preliminary results of studies using single photon emission computed tomography (SPECT) imaging suggest inefficient processing in schizotypal patients, such that these patients relatively overactivate both frontal cortex and other cortical areas compared with normal controls (Siever *et al.*, unpublished data). Increased activation of an inefficient frontal cortex, as well as compensatory activation of other cortical areas not normally utilized in this task, may help to partially normalize the schizotypal patient's performance in comparison with that of the schizophrenic patient. In contrast, schizophrenic patients may avoid use of the highly functionally impaired frontal cortex in favour of other regions, resulting in frontal hypoactivation. Although speculative, these possibilities invite further investigation.

Attentional/psychophysiological tasks

Schizophrenic patients show impairment on a variety of tests that demand sustained attention and information processing. While these tasks encompass a range of cognitive/attentional functions, they seem to involve high-order cortical processing, particularly by frontal and temporal association areas.

Perhaps one of the most robust and consistent findings of impairment in the psychophysiological task is that of eye movement impairment in schizophrenic patients. In this group of patients the quality of smooth pursuit eye movement is significantly poorer than in normal controls, and includes disruptions of smooth pursuit by saccadic eye movements ('catch-up' saccades serve to compensate for slow velocity or 'low-gain' pursuit; 'anticipatory' saccades move the eye ahead of the target in anticipation of its arrival). Low-velocity pursuit or reduced gain is also characteristic of schizophrenic patients. Approximately two-thirds to three-quarters of schizophrenic patients show

smooth pursuit eye movement impairment (see the review by Clementz and Sweeney (1990)). While eye movement impairment is not entirely specific to schizophrenia and may also be observed in psychotic affective disorders, particularly bipolar disorder, eye movement impairment is present in approximately half the relatives of schizophrenics, while it is present in only a very small proportion of relatives of bipolar patients (Holzman *et al.*, 1984). Furthermore, eye movement impairment in affective disorder patients may differ in character (Iacono *et al.*, 1981; Amador *et al.*, 1991) and may be more state dependent (Iacono *et al.*, 1981) than in schizophrenic patients.

Because of its prevalence in relatives of schizophrenic patients, eye movement impairment may reflect a genetically determined 'latent trait' that may less frequently manifest itself as chronic schizophrenia (Matthysse *et al.*, 1986). Since schizotypal personality disorder also appears to be genetically related to schizophrenia, it is logical to hypothesize that schizotypal personality disorder and eye tracking impairment may be associated. Indeed, such an association has been demonstrated in relatives of schizophrenic patients (Clementz *et al.*, 1990; Grove *et al.*, 1992), volunteers selected by virtue of their low tracking accuracy (Siever *et al.*, 1984, 1989), volunteers selected by scoring high on the Chapman physical anhedonia scale (Simons *et al.*, 1982), and patients with schizotypal personality disorder (Siever *et al.*, 1990; Moskowitz *et al.*, 1992). In the clinical sample, qualitative ratings were increased in the schizotypal patients compared with the controls, and low-quality tracking was negatively correlated with the number of deficit-like symptoms, but not with the number of psychotic-like symptoms (Siever, 1991; Moskowitz *et al.*, 1992; Siever *et al.*, 1993b). Similarly, in relatives of schizophrenic patients poor-quality tracking has been associated with high scores on the social anhedonia subscale of the Chapman psychosis — proneness scale (Clementz *et al.*, 1992).

Another test of attentional performance, the continuous performance task (CPT), has also been shown to be impaired in schizotypal individuals as well as in schizophrenic patients. The CPT is a test of sustained attention that requires the subject to respond by pressing a button when a 'target' sequence occurs among a series of presented stimuli. Offspring of schizophrenic patients, schizotypal volunteers and schizotypal patients may demonstrate CPT abnormalities (Siever et al., 1991).

Measurements of evoked potentials, widely found to be abnormal in schizophrenic patients, may also be disturbed in patients with schizotypal personality disorder. Amplitude reduction of P_{300} and N_{200} has been reported to be reduced in volunteers scoring high on the Chapman anhedonia scales (Simons et al., 1982). In two studies, a reduced P_{300} amplitude was noted in schizotypal personality disorder patients (Blackwood et al., 1986; Kutcher et al., 1989), but in these same studies was also found in individuals with borderline personality disorder. In another study of clinically selected schizotypal patients, the P_{300} amplitude was intermediate between schizophrenic and normal controls, but, in contrast to the amplitude of P_{300} in the schizophrenic patients compared with that in the controls, the P_{300} amplitude in the schizotypal patients did not significantly differ from that of adequate controls. Furthermore, P_{300} amplitudes did not correlate with deficit-like symptoms, although N_{200} amplitudes did tend to correlate with the deficit-like symptoms of schizotypal personality disorder, and did correlate negatively with ventricular size in these studies (Siever, 1991; Siever et al., 1993b). Thus, while a reduced P_{300} amplitude may not be a robust and specific correlate of schizotypal personality disorder, it is similar to the other psychophysiological tests in that the pattern of abnormalities is not as severe as in schizophrenic patients, yet is worse than in controls.

Neurochemistry

Dopamine and its metabolites

The dopamine hypothesis, driven by the efficacy of neuroleptic medications in improving the symptoms of schizophrenia, has often yielded dis-

appointing results in defining the pathophysiology of schizophrenia. However, a variety of evidence from postmortem, metabolite and imaging studies suggests the possibility of dopaminergic abnormalities in schizophrenia (Davis et al., 1991). Among medication-free schizophrenic patients, plasma homovanillic acid (HVA) concentrations correlate with symptom severity. Clinical improvement with neuroleptic treatment is associated with higher baseline plasma HVA concentrations and lower concentrations following treatment (Pickar et al., 1984; Davis et al., 1985, 1991). The most recent version of the dopamine hypothesis in schizophrenia posits differences in dopaminergic function among brain regions, with hypodopaminergic in cortical areas and hyperdopaminergia in subcortical areas. Deafferentation of limbic dopamine systems associated with higher cortical impairment may result in disinhibition of limbic dopamine systems with increased receptor responsiveness and release of dopamine (Davis et al., 1991). These complex relationships of differential regional dopaminergic dysfunction in schizophrenic patients may obscure potential relationships between dopamine and symptoms in other milder disorders along the schizophrenia spectrum.

The study of schizotypal personality disorder provides a unique opportunity to understand the pathophysiology of the dopamine system in relation to schizophrenia-related psychopathology. Given the efficacy of neuroleptics in reducing psychotic symptoms by virtue of their dopamine antagonist properties and the psychotogenic effects of stimulant medications which increase dopamine concentrations in the synapse, it has been hypothesized that plasma HVA and CSF HVA concentrations would correlate with the positive or psychotic-like symptoms of schizotypal personality disorder. Indeed, this possibility was supported by the clinical improvement documented in response to the administration of neuroleptic medications (Goldberg et al., 1986; Hymowitz et al., 1986). Plasma HVA concentrations have in fact been found to be significantly higher in schizotypal personality disorder patients compared with normal controls and other personality disorder comparison groups, but do not seem to be related to any of the usual confounding variables endemic to schizophrenia studies, such as neuroleptic treatment, institutionalization, etc. (Siever *et al.*, 1991). Plasma HVA concentrations are significantly positively correlated with the psychotic-like symptoms of schizotypal personality disorder but not with other deficit-related symptoms of schizotypal personality disorder. Similarly, CSF HVA concentrations have been found to be elevated in schizotypal personality disorder patients compared with patients with other personality disorders; they again correlate with psychotic-like schizotypal personality disorder symptoms but not deficit-like symptoms. When the effect of the psychotic-like symptoms on plasma HVA was used as a covariate in these analyses, the difference between groups was no longer present (Siever *et al.*, 1993a). These results raised the possibility that the psychotic-like symptoms may be associated with hyperfunction of the dopamine system.

In contrast, in the relatives of schizophrenic patients with schizotypal personality disorder, who are primarily characterized by negative or deficit-like symptoms (Lenzenweger & Dworkin, 1984; Lyons *et al.*, 1992), concentrations of plasma HVA were in fact lower than those observed in non-schizotypal relatives of schizophrenic patients or controls (Amin *et al.*, 1993). These differences remained when the effects of plasma 3-methoxy-4-hydroxyphenylglycol (MHPG) were covaried from the analyses to factor out effects of increased peripheral noradrenergic metabolism that may contribute to plasma HVA concentrations. These results suggest that the plasma HVA concentrations did perhaps reflect reductions in central dopaminergic metabolism in these patients. The reductions in HVA correlated with the degree of deficit-like symptoms and with neuropsychological measures sensitive to frontal dysfunction (Keefe *et al.*, 1991), although they also correlated negatively with the degree of psychotic-like symptoms. Thus, in the relatives, reductions in plasma HVA seem to be related to deficit-like symptoms, but also to account for the mild psychotic-like symptoms in these individuals. These results

are compatible with the hypotheses that the schizotypal relatives, who are genetically related to schizophrenic patients, may have reduced dopaminergic terminals in cortical areas, while increases in dopaminergic activity, seen primarily in clinically selected schizotypal patients, may be more associated with the psychotic-like symptoms of this disorder (Siever, 1991; Siever *et al.*, 1993b).

Catecholamine-related enzymes

Both monoamine and plasma amine oxidase have been studied in schizotypal subjects, selected on the basis of schizotypal traits from a volunteer population, as well as in schizotypal relatives of schizophrenic patients (Baron & Levitt, 1980; Baron *et al.*, 1980). As the amine oxidases metabolize dopamine, reduced concentrations of these enzymes might contribute to increased functional dopamine activity.

Responses to dopaminergic challenge

Schizophrenic patients have been shown to have a variety of responses to amphetamine, which may worsen their psychotic symptoms, although in some cases may improve their deficit symptoms (Van Kammen *et al.*, 1983). Patients meeting criteria for both borderline and schizotypal personality disorder demonstrated a worsening of psychotic-like symptoms and anxiety after an amphetamine infusion (Schulz *et al.*, 1988). From the preliminary results of an amphetamine study with schizotypal patients, the schizotypal personality disorder patients showed responses that suggest an improvement in neurocognitive performance, although there was no marked worsening of psychotic-like symptoms (Wainberg *et al.*, 1993).

Treatment

Studies of the treatment of schizotypal personality disorder have been influenced by the biological and phenomenological similarities between schizophrenia and schizotypal personality disorder. Thus, these treatment studies have focused primarily on neuroleptic medications. Low-dose thiothixene significantly reduced the symptoms of ideas of reference, illusions and social isolation compared with placebo in patients with schizotypal personality disorder and patients with borderline personality disorder (Goldberg *et al.*, 1986). Patients with more severe symptoms were especially responsive to thiothixene vs. placebo. A 2-week low-dose haloperidol treatment resulted in significant decreases in ideas of reference, odd communication and social isolation in 17 patients with schizotypal personality disorder (Hymowitz *et al.*, 1986). One of the difficulties in treating schizotypal personality disorder patients with neuroleptic medications is that the medication side effects may overwhelm the treatment benefits. As a result of this poor cost: benefit ratio, 50% of patients refused to participate in the full treatment regimen of these 6-week (Hymowitz *et al.*, 1986) or 12-week (Goldberg *et al.*, 1986) neuroleptic trials. Thus, while low-dose dopamine blockade may have a mild symptom-reducing effect in some patients, particularly in those with more severe baseline symptoms, treatment non-compliance may reduce the effectiveness of currently available neuroleptic medications. It is conceivable that treatment-responsive schizotypal patients, like schizophrenic parents, may have higher plasma HVA concentrations, a possibility that invites investigation. A more sophisticated understanding of the relationship between symptoms, neuro-anatomical abnormalities, cognitive deficits and HVA levels in plasma and CSF may contribute to the identification of patients with schizotypal personality disorder who may best benefit from low-dose neuroleptic treatment.

Although patients with schizotypal personality disorder are often likely to seek treatment owing to depressive symptoms that result from the social, cognitive and emotional disturbances associated with schizotypy, few studies have assessed the effect of antidepressant medications on the symptoms. In earlier years, the monoamine oxidase inhibitors, tricyclics and lithium have reportedly improved symptoms in pseudoneurotic schizophrenia, a forerunner of the schizotypal diagnosis (Klein, 1972; Rifkin *et al.*, 1972). More recently, patients meeting the criteria for schizotypal and/ or borderline personality disorders responded to a non-blind, 12-week trial of fluoxetine with reductions in self-injury and in scores on the Hopkins symptom checklist (Markovitz *et al.*, 1991). In a non-blind trial of amoxapine, patients with schizotypal personality disorder showed improvements, while patients with borderline personality disorder did not (Jensen & Andersen, 1989). However, it was concluded that the efficacy of amoxapine in the former group was due to its neuroleptic activity.

One potential untested pharmacological model for reducing the symptoms of schizotypal personality disorder is, paradoxically, the activation of dopamine function. As reflected by their poor performance on tests, such as the WCST, requiring frontal functions, some patients with schizotypal personality disorder may have the reduced cognitive functions found in schizophrenia, yet they do not manifest psychotic symptoms. Treatment of these patients with dopamine-enhancing agents may improve cognition without exacerbating psychosis. As mentioned previously, a preliminary study at our centre has indicated that schizotypal personality disorder patients with poor performance on the WCST demonstrated an improvement in performance following amphetamine administration. To date, no patients have demonstrated an exacerbation of psychotic or psychotic-like symptoms following amphetamine administration. This strategy is in the beginning stages of development and additional work will be required to establish its efficacy.

The effect of psychotherapy on schizotypal personality disorder has not been extensively studied. One recent study reported the effects of a day-hospital therapeutic community treatment (psychodynamic orientation) for patients with personality disorders (Karterud *et al.*, 1992). The results indicated that patients with schizotypal personality disorder did not show significant improvements, unlike patients with other personality disorders, including borderline personality disorder. It has been suggested that exploratory psychotherapeutic approaches have the potential effect of facilitating decompensation, but more structured approaches, including reality testing, interpersonal boundary reinforcement, and psychoeducation, may help patients with schizotypal personality disorder (Stone, 1992). Models for the psychoeducational treatment of schizophrenia, if extended to patients with schizotypal personality disorder, suggest that patients and their family members should be encouraged to allow the patients to remove themselves from stressful situations, particularly situations that may require the activation of attention and information processing that is beyond the patient's capacities (MacFarlane, 1990). Schizotypal personality disorder patients with working memory deficits may be particularly vulnerable to symptom exacerbation in stressful situations such as lively group interaction, as these patients may be unable to follow the pace of the interpersonal communication; this leads to social anxiety, cognitive aberrations and odd styles of communication.

Outcome

As for schizophrenia, the long-term outcome of schizotypal personality disorder is variable. Owing to the severity of their deficit-like symptoms, many schizotypal patients are presumed to have poor social outcomes, but these presumptions are biased by the same ascertainment flaw as studies of the long-term outcome of schizophrenia: only patients who remain dependent upon treatment remain in the study under investigation (Harding *et al.*, 1992). Few studies have investigated this issue empirically. Patients with schizotypal personality disorder have been shown to have a long-term outcome that is more similar to that of chronic schizophrenia than to that of borderline personality disorder, another severe personality disorder (McGlashan, 1986). One study that compared the outcome of personality disordered patients found that, at follow-up, schizotypal patients had the poorest ratings on global functioning level, social activity and social adjustment (Mehlum *et al.*, 1991). Other findings have indicated that patients who meet criteria for both schizotypal and borderline personality disorders are more similar to patients with borderline personality disorder than to 'pure' schizotypal patients. While the capacity of these 'mixed'

patients for more intimate relationships seemed poorer than that of the pure borderline patients, their social relationships and functioning were less isolative than those of patients with pure schizotypal personality disorder (McGlashan, 1983, 1986), suggesting that borderline symptoms may play a protective role in the long-term outcome of the schizotypal individual, possibly by reducing the impact of severe social isolation.

It is not clear what percentage of patients diagnosed as having schizotypal personality disorder actually are in a protracted prodrome of an eventual schizophrenia. Estimates from a follow-up study of a young adult population with schizotypal personality disorder suggest that about 25% developed schizophrenia (Schulz & Soloff, 1987). In the Chestnut Lodge follow-up study, 17% of the schizotypal personality disorder sample received a later diagnosis of schizophrenia (Fenton & McGlashan, 1989). Other samples, however, have shown a much lower prevalence (Siever *et al.*, 1991). Predictors of the later onset of schizophrenia in schizotypal patients have been reported to include symptoms of paranoid ideation, social isolation and magical thinking (Fenton & McGlashan, 1989). Even when schizotypal patients do not develop schizophrenia, however, many studies have reported outcomes that are similar to DSM-III diagnosed schizophrenic patients (Plakun *et al.*, 1985; McGlashan 1986; Modestin *et al.*, 1989).

While schizoid and paranoid personality disorders may be considered within the schizophrenia spectrum, the outcome of these disorders needs further study. One investigation involved 'schizoid' children who, as adults, showed the features of DSM-III schizotypal personality disorder (Wolff *et al.*, 1991). The six core features used for a diagnosis of schizoid were: solitariness; impaired empathy; rigidity; the single-minded pursuit of special interests; increased sensitivity; and unusual styles of communication. It is clear that additional longitudinal studies are required to evaluate the overlap between these disorders and their relationship to schizophrenia.

Conclusions

The symptoms of schizophrenia spectrum disorders are similar to the symptoms of schizophrenia, with the important exception that patients with spectrum disorders are rarely psychotic. Although intensive research into the spectrum disorders is only just beginning, several tentative conclusions can be made regarding the biological, genetic and psychological similarities between schizophrenia spectrum disorders and schizophrenia.

The symptoms of schizotypal personality disorder appear to be heritable and genetically related to schizophrenia. The negative or deficit-like symptoms of schizotypal personality disorder, such as restricted affect and social isolation, may be more genetically mediated than the positive or psychotic-like symptoms, such as magical thinking and perceptual aberrations. However, there is considerable overlap between schizotypal symptoms and symptoms of personality disorders outside the schizophrenia spectrum, and further study is required to refine the boundaries of schizotypal personality disorder as an expression of a schizophrenia-related phenotype. Future pharmacological treatment studies should focus on the identification of patients with profiles of symptoms, cognitive deficits and biology that more closely match patients with schizophrenia, as these patients may benefit more from neuroleptic treatment than patients without these profiles.

Patients with schizotypal personality disorder symptoms demonstrate psychophysiological and cognitive deficits that are similar to, but milder than, those found in schizophrenic patients. Although no single deficit is found in all schizotypal patients, normal performance on many of the tests that are impaired in these patients require adequate functioning of the 'working memory'. A rationale for the development of schizotypal symptoms as a result of working memory deficits has already been proposed by the authors (Keefe *et al.*, in press). One important question that needs to be addressed is whether the improvement of working memory functions is associated with symptom reduction in patients with schizotypal personality disorder. Since there are few data available regarding the pharmacological treatment of working memory deficits, tentative arguments can be made in favour of treatment with either dopamine augmentation or blockade. Research to address these questions is currently under way in our laboratory.

The neurochemistry and pharmacological treatment of schizotypal personality disorder requires further investigation. Our laboratory has found that schizotypal personality disorder symptoms are associated with HVA levels in plasma and CSF. Psychotic-like symptoms are correlated with higher HVA levels, while neuropsychological deficits and deficit-like symptoms are correlated with lower HVA levels. These data, coupled with findings of modest responses to low-dose neuroleptics in schizotypal personality disorder patients, suggest that schizotypal symptoms in some patients may be mediated by dopaminergic abnormalities that are responsive to dopamine blockade. However, about 50% of schizotypal personality disorder patients refuse to continue treatment with neuroleptic medication because of the side effects. These important initial studies need to be supplemented with data addressing the issues of non-compliance. In addition, the effect of antidepressant medications or dopamine augmentation treatment on patients with schizotypal personality disorder has not been assessed fully enough to warrant definitive conclusions.

Enhancement of catecholaminergic function by antidepressants or dopamine precursors or direct activation of frontal D_1 receptors by D_1 agonists could prove useful in ameliorating the negative or deficit-like symptoms of the schizophrenia spectrum disorders. The study of schizotypal personality disorder represents an unusual opportunity to dissect out and clarify the multifactorial pathophysiological processes involved in the schizophrenic disorders. In chronic schizophrenia, frontal cortical abnormalities associated with hypodopaminergia and deficit symptoms have been hypothesized to result in deafferentation and up-regulation of subcortical dopamine systems associated with psychotic symptoms (Weinberger, 1987; Davis *et al.*, 1991). Schizotypal patients with prominent deficit-like or negative symptoms, as seen in the relatives of schizophrenic patients, exhibit evidence of cortical structure/function abnormalities, but may be less sensitive, or better buffered, than schizophrenic patients to cortical/subcortical disconnection with consequent subcortical dopamine up-regulation and associated psychotic symptoms. Schizotypal personality disorder patients with prominent psychotic-like symptoms may have subcortical dopaminergic hyperactivity without necessarily having cortical processing deficits (Siever *et al.*, 1993b). While there is no evidence for discrete subtypes of the schizophrenia spectrum, an investigation of the dimensions of deficit-like and psychotic-like syndromes in schizotypal personality disorder may help clarify the role of cortical/subcortical dysfunction in the schizophrenic disorders. As regional imaging techniques of both metabolism and dopaminergic activity are refined, the study of schizotypal personality disorder patients may provide important data for the elucidation of the pathophysiology of the schizophrenia spectrum. Ultimately, such studies can help clarify the boundaries of the schizophrenia spectrum and determine why some individuals on the spectrum are more susceptible to psychosis than others; this would have important preventative implications.

References

Amador, X.F., Sackeim, H.A., Mukherjee, S. *et al.* (1991) Specificity of smooth pursuit eye movement and visual fixation abnormalities in schizophrenia. *Schizophrenia Research*, **5**, 135–144.

Ambelas, A. (1992) Preschizophrenics: adding to the evidence, sharpening the focus. *British Journal of Psychiatry*, **160**, 401–404.

Amin, F., Silverman, J.M., Dumont, L. *et al.* (1993) Plasma HVA in non-psychotic first-degree relatives of schizophrenic probands. *American Psychiatric Association 146th Annual Meeting*, NR221.

Andreasen, N.C., Karim, R., Alliger, R. *et al.* (1992) Hypofrontality in neuroleptic-naive patients and chronic schizophrenic patients: a SPECT study. *Archives of General Psychiatry*, **49**, 943–959.

Andreasen, N.C., Olson, S.A., Dennet, J.W. & Smith, M.R. (1982) Ventricular enlargement in schizophrenia: relationship to positive and negative symptoms. *American Journal of Psychiatry*, **139**, 297–302.

APA (1980) *Diagnostic and Statistical Manual of Mental Disorders*, 3rd edn. American Psychiatric Association, Washington DC.

Barlogh, D.W. & Merritt, R.D. (1985) Susceptibility to type A backward pattern masking among hypothetically psychosis prone college students. *Journal of Abnormal Psychology*, **94**, 377–383.

Baron, M. & Levitt, M. (1980) Platelet monoamine oxidase activity: relation to genetic load of schizophrenia. *Psychiatry Research*, **3**, 69–74.

Baron, M., Levitt, M. & Perlman, R. (1980) Low platelet monoamine oxidase activity: a possible biochemical correlate of borderline schizophrenia. *Psychiatry Research*, **3**, 329–335.

Barthell, C. & Holmes, D. (1968) High school yearbooks: a non-reactive measure of social isolation in graduates who later became schizoprhenic. *Journal of Abnormal Psychology*, **78**, 313–316.

Bentall, R.P., Claridge, G.S. & Slade, P.D. (1989) The multidimensional nature of schizotypal traits: a factor analytic study with normal subjects. *British Journal of Clinical Psychology*, **28**, 363–375.

Blackwood, D.H.R., St Clair, D.M. & Kutcher, S.P. (1986) P300 event-related potential abnormalities in borderline personality disorder. *Biological Psychiatry*, **21**, 557–560.

Bleuler, E. (1950) *Dementia Praecox or the Group of Schizophrenias*. International Universities Press, New York.

Bower, E.M., Schellhammer, T.A. & Daily, J.A. (1960) School characteristics of male adolescents who later become schizophrenic. *American Journal of Orthopsychiatry*, **30**, 712–729.

Cannon, T.D., Mednick, S.A. & Parnas, J. (1990) Antecedents of predominantly negative- and predominantly positive-symptom schizophrenia in a high risk population. *Archives of General Psychiatry*, **47**, 622–632.

Cannon, T.D., Mednick, S.A., Parnas, J., Schuksinger, F., Praestholm, J. & Vestergaad, A. (1993) Developmental brain abnormalities in the offspring of schizophrenic mothers. *Archives of General Psychiatry*, **50**, 551–564.

Cazzulo, Vita, A., Giobbio, G.M., Dieci, M. & Sacchetti, E. (1991) Cerebral structural abnormalities in schizophreniform disorder and in schizophrenia spectrum personality disorders. In Tamminga, C.A. & Schulz, S.C. (eds) *Advances in Neuropsychiatry and Psychopharmacology*, Vol. 1. *Schizophrenia Research*.

Chapman, L.J. & Chapman, J.P. (1985) Psychosis proneness. In Alpert, M. (ed.) *Controversies in Schizophrenia: Changes and Constancies*, pp. 157–174. Guilford Press, New York.

Chapman, L.J., Chapman, J.P. & Raulin, M.L. (1976) Scales for physical and social anhedonia. *Journal of Abnormal Psychology*, **85**, 374–382.

Chapman, L.J., Chapman, J.P. & Raulin, M.L. (1978) Body-image aberration in schizophrenia. *Journal of Abnormal Psychology*, **87**, 399–407.

Claridge, G. & Broks, P. (1984) Schizotypy and hemisphere function. I. Theoretical considerations and the measurement of schizotypy. *Personality and Individual Differences*, **5**, 633–648.

Clementz, B.A. & Sweeney, J.A. (1990) Is eye movement

dysfunction a biological marker for schizophrenia? A methodological review. *Psychological Bulletin*, **108**, 77–92.

Clementz, B.A., Grove, W.M., Iacono, W.G. & Sweeney, J. (1992) Smooth pursuit eye movement dysfunction and liability for schizophrenia: implications for genetic modelling. *Journal of Abnormal Psychology*, **101**, 117–129.

Clementz, B.A., Sweeney, J.A., Hirt, M. & Haas, G. (1990) Pursuit gain and saccadic intrusions in first-degree relatives of probands with schizophrenia. *Journal of Abnormal Psychology*, **99**, 327–335.

Daniel, E.G., Weinberger, D.R., Goldberg, T.E. *et al.* (1991) The effect of amphetamine on regional cerebral blood flow during cognitive activation in schizophrenia. *Journal of Neuroscience*, **11**, 1907–1917.

Davis, K.L., Davidson, M., Mohs, R.C. *et al.* (1985) Plasma homovanillic acid concentration and the severity of schizophrenic illness. *Science*, **227**, 1601–1602.

Davis, K.L., Kahn, R.S., Ko, G. & Davidson, M. (1991) Dopamine and schizophrenia: a reconceptualization. *American Journal of Psychiatry*, **148**, 1474–1486.

DeVegvar, M.L., Keefe, R.S.E., Moskowitz, J. *et al.* (1993) Frontal lobe dysfunction and schizotypal personality disorder. *American Psychiatric Association 146th Annual Meeting*, San Francisco.

Eckblad, M. & Chapman, L.J. (1983) Magical ideation as an indicator of schizotypy. *Journal of Consulting and Clinical Psychology*, **51**, 215–225.

El-Guebaly, N., Offord, D.R., Sullivan, K.T. & Lynch, G.W. (1978) Psychosocial adjustment of the offspring of psychiatric inpatients: the effect of alcoholic, depressive, and schizophrenic parentage. *Canadian Psychiatric Association Journal*, **23**, 281–289.

Fenton, T.S. & McGlashan, T.H. (1989) Risk of schizophrenia in character disordered patients. *American Journal of Psychiatry*, **146**, 1280–1284.

Fish, B. (1986) Antecedents of an acute schizophrenic break. *Journal of the American Academy of Child Psychiatry*, **25**, 595–600.

Foerster, A., Lewis, S., Owen, M. & Murray, R. (1991a) Premorbid adjustment and personality in psychosis: effects of sex and diagnosis. *British Journal of Psychiatry*, **158**, 171–176.

Foerster, A., Lewis, S., Owen, M. & Murray, R. (1991b) Low birth weight and a family history of schizophrenia predict poor premorbid functioning in psychosis. *Schizophrenia Research*, **5**, 13–20.

Freskca, E., Keefe, R.S.E., Apter, S., Davidson, M., Mohs, R.C. & Davis, K.L. (1991) Clinical study of Kraepelinian schizophrenia. *American Psychiatric Association 144th Annual Meeting*, p. 50, NR8. New Orleans, Louisiana.

Glish, M.A., Erlenmeyer-Kimling, L. & Watt, N.F. (1982) Parental assessment of the social and emotional adaptation of children at high risk for schizophrenia. In Lahey, B. & Kazdin, A. (eds) *Advances in Child Clinical Psychology*. Wiley, New York.

Goldberg, S.C., Schulz, C., Schulz, M., Resnick, R.J., Hamer, R.M. & Friedal, R.O. (1986) Borderline and schizotypal personality disorders treated with low-dose thiothixene vs. placebo. *Archives of General Psychiatry*, **43**, 680–686.

Gray, J.A., Feldon, J., Rawlins, J.N.P., Hemsley, D.R. & Smith, A.D. (1991) The neuropsychology of schizophrenia. *Behavioral and Brain Sciences*, **14**, 1–84.

Grove, W.M., Clementz, B.A., Iacono, W.G. & Katsanis, J. (1992) Smooth pursuit ocular motor function in schizophrenia; evidence for a major gene. *American Journal of Psychiatry*, **149**, 1362–1368.

Harding, C.M., Zubin, J. & Strauss, J.S. (1992) Chronicity in schizophrenia: revisited. *British Journal of Psychiatry*, **161** (Suppl. 28), 27–37.

Hewitt, J.K. & Claridge, G.S. (1989) The factor structure of schizotypy in a normal population. *Personality and Individual Differences*, **10**, 323–329.

Hogg, B., Jackson, H.J., Rudd, R.P. & Edwards, J. (1990) Diagnosing personality disorders in recent-onset schizophrenia. *Journal of Nervous and Mental Disease*, **178**, 194–199.

Hollander, E., Stein, D.J., DeCaria, C.M., Klein, D.F. & Liebowitz, M.R. (1992) Neuropsychiatry and 5-HT function in OCD and social phobia. *American College of Neuropsychopharmacology, 31st Annual Meeting*. San Juan. (Abstract).

Holzman, P.S., Solomon, C.M., Levin, S. & Waternaux, C.S. (1984) Pursuit eye movement dysfunctions in schizophrenia; family evidence for specificity. *Archives of General Psychiatry*, **41**, 136–139.

Hymowitz, P., Frances, A., Jacobsberg, L.B., Sickles, M. & Hoyt, R. (1986) Neuroleptic treatment of schizotypal personality disorders. *Comprehensive Psychiatry*, **27**, 267–271.

Iacono, W.G., Tuasow, V.B. & Johnson, R.A. (1981) Dissociation of smooth pursuit and saccadic eye tracking in remitted schizophrenics. *Archives of General Psychiatry*, **38**, 991–996.

Jensen, H.Z. & Andersen, J. (1989) An open non-comparative study of amoxapine in borderline disorders. *Acta Psychiatrica Scandinavica*, **79**, 89–93.

Jorgensen, A. & Parnas, J. (1990) The Copenhagen high risk study: premorbid and clinical dimensions of maternal schizophrenia. *Journal of Nervous and Mental Disease*, **178(6)**, 370–376.

Karterud, S., Vaglum, S., Friis, S., Irion, T., Johns, S. & Vaglum, P. (1992) Day hospital therapeutic community treatment for patients with personality disorders: an empirical evaluation of the containment function. *Journal of Nervous and Mental Disease*, **180(4)**, 238–243.

Keefe, R.S.E., Mohs, R.C., Losonczy, M.F. *et al.* (1987) Characteristics of very poor outcome schizophrenia. *American Journal of Psychiatry*, **144**, 889–895.

Keefe, R.S.E., Siever, L. & Davis, K. The neurobiology of schizotypal personality disorder. *Journal of Clinical Neuropharmacology*, (in press).

Keefe, R.S.E., Silverman, J.M., Lees, S.E. *et al.* (1994) Performance of nonpsychotic relatives of schizophrenic patients on cognitive tests. *Psychiatry Research*, **53**, 1–12.

Keefe, R.S.E., Silverman, J.M., Moskowitz, J. *et al.* (1991) Eye tracking and CPT in the relatives of schizophrenic probands: independence of deficits and association with schizotypal traits. *Society of Biological Psychiatry 46th Annual Convention*, **29**, 95A. New Orleans, Louisiana.

Kendler, K. (1985) Diagnostic approaches to schizotypal

personality disorder: a historical perspective. *Schizophrenia Bulletin*, **11**(4), 538−553.

Kendler, K.S. & Hewitt, J.K. (1992) The structure of self-report schizotypy in twins. *Journal of Personality Disorders*, **6**, 1−17.

Kendler, K.S., Ochs, A.L., Gorman, A.M. *et al.* (1991) The structure of schizotypy: a pilot multitrait twin study. *Psychiatry Research*, **36**, 19−36.

Kety, S.S., Rosenthal, D., Wender, P.H. *et al.* (1975) Mental illness in the biological and adoptive families of adopted individuals who have become schizophrenic: preliminary report based on psychiatric interviews. In Fieve, R.R., Rosentahal, D. & Brill, H. (eds) *Genetic Research in Psychiatry*, pp. 147−165. John Hopkins University Press, Baltimore.

Klein, D.F. (1972) *Psychiatric Case Studies: Treatment, Drugs, and Outcome*. Williams & Wilkins, Baltimore.

Kraepelin, E. (1919) *Dementia Praecox and Paraphrenia*. Livingstone, Edinburgh.

Kretschmer, E. (1921) *Physique and Character*. Kegan Paul, London. Translated 1936.

Kutcher, S.P., Blackwood, D.H.R., Gaskell, D.F., Muir, W.J. & St Clair, D.M. (1989) Auditory P300 does not differentiate borderline personality disorder from schizotypal personality disorder. *Biological Psychiatry*, **26**, 766−774.

Lenzenweger, M.A. & Dworkin, R.H. (1984) Symptoms and the genetics of schizophrenia: implications for diagnosis. *American Journal of Psychiatry*, **141**, 1541−1546.

Lenzenweger, M.F., Cornblatt, B.A. & Putnick, M. (1991) Schizotypy and sustained attention. *Journal of Abnormal Psychology*, **100**, 84−89.

Luciana, M., Depue, R.A., Arbisi, P. & Leon, A. (1992) Facilitation of working memory in humans by a D_2 dopamine receptor agonist. *Journal of Cognitive Neuroscience*, **4**, 58−68.

Lyons, M.J. Merla, M.E., Young, L. & Kremen, W.S. (1991) Impaired neuropsychological functioning in symptomatic volunteers with schizotypy: preliminary findings. *Biological Psychiatry*, **30**, 424−426.

Lyons, M., Tsuang, M., Faraone, S. & Kremen, W. (1992) Characteristics of schizotypal subjects related to schizophrenia versus affective probands: symptomatology, co-morbidity, and familial psychopathology. *Society of Biological Psychiatry 47th Annual Meeting*, **31**, 68A. Washington, DC.

MacFarlane, W.F. (1990) Psychoeducational treatment of schizophrenia. In Herz, M.L., Keith, S.J. & Docherty, J.P. (eds) *Handbook of Schizophrenia*, Vol. 4. Elsevier, New York.

McGlashan, T.H. (1983) The borderline syndrome. II. Is it a variant of schizophrenia or affective disorder? *Archives of General Psychiatry*, **40**, 1319−1323.

McGlashan, T.H. (1986) Schizotypal personality disorder, Chestnut Lodge follow-up study. VI. Long-term follow-up perspective. *Archives of General Psychiatry*, **43**, 329−334.

Markovitz, P.J., Calabrese, J.R., Schulz, S.C. & Meltzer, H.Y. (1991) Fluoxetine in the treatment of borderline and schizotypal personality disorders. *American Journal of Psychiatry*, **148**, 1064−1067.

Matthysse, S., Holtzman, P.S. & Lange, K. (1986) The genetic transmission of schizophrenia: application of Mendelian latent structure analysis to eye tracking dysfunctions in schizophrenia and affective disorder. *Journal of Psychiatric Research*, **20**, 57−67.

Meehl, P.E. (1962) Schizotaxia, schizotypy, schizophrenia. *American Psychologist*, **17**, 827−839.

Meehl, P.E. (1964) *Manual for Use with Checklist of Schizotypic Signs*. Unpublished manuscript, University of Minnesota, Minneapolis.

Mehlum, L., Friis, S., Irion, T. *et al.* (1991) Personality disorders 2−5 years after treatment: a perspective follow-up study. *Acta Psychiatrica Scandinavica*, **84**, 72−77.

Michael, C.M., Morris, D.P. & Soroker, E. (1957) Follow-up studies of shy, withdrawn children. II. Relative incidence of schizophrenia. *American Journal of Orthopsychiatry*, **27**, 331−337.

Modestin, J., Foglia, A. & Toffler, G. (1989) Comparative study of schizotypal and schizophrenia patients. *Psychopathology*, **22**, 1−13.

Moskowitz, J., Lees, S., Friedman, L., Keefe, R., Mohs, R. & Siever, L.J. (1992) The relationship between eye tracking impairment and deficit symptoms. *Society of Biological Psychiatry 47th Annual Meeting*, **31**, 149A. Washington, DC.

Muntaner, C., Garcia-Sevilla, L., Alberto, A. & Torrubia, R. (1988) Personality dimensions, schizotypal and borderline personality traits and psychosis proneness. *Personality and Individual Differences*, **9**, 257−268.

Olson, S.C., Nasrallah, H.A. & Lynn, M.B. (1993) Brain morphology in schizophrenics and their siblings. *American Psychiatric Association 146th Annual Meeting*, p. 126, NR263. San Francisco, CA.

O'Neal, P. & Robins, L.N. (1958) Childhood patterns predictive of adult schizophrenia: a 30-year follow-up study. *American Journal of Psychiatry*, **115**, 385−391.

Parnas, J. & Jorgensen, A. (1989) Pre-morbid psychopathology in schizophrenia spectrum. *British Journal of Psychiatry*, **155**, 623−627.

Parnas, J., Schulsinger, F., Schulsinger, H., Mednick, S.A. & Teasdale, T.W. (1982) Behavioral precursors of schizophrenia spectrum. *Archives of General Psychiatry*, **39**, 658−664.

Peralta, V., Cuesta, M.J. & de Leon, J. (1991) Premorbid personality and positive and negative symptoms in schizophrenia. *Acta Psychiatrica Scandanavica*, **84**, 336−339.

Pickar, D., Labarca, R., Linnoila, M. *et al.* (1984) Neuroleptic-induced decrease in plasma homovanillic acid and antipsychotic activity in schizophrenic patients. *Science*, **225**, 954−956.

Picton, T.W., Stuss, D.T. & Marshall, K.C. (1986) Attention and the brain. In Friedman, S.L., Klivington, K.S. & Peterson, R.W. (eds) *The Brain, Cognition, and Education*, pp. 19−79. Academic Press, New York.

Plakun, E.M., Burkhardt, P.E. & Muller, J.P. (1985) 14-year follow-up of borderline and schizotypal personality disorders. *Comprehensive Psychiatry*, **26**, 448−455.

Rado, S. (1962) Theory and therapy: the theory of schizotypal organization and its application to the treatment of decompensated schizotypal behavior. In Rado, S. (ed.) *Psychoanalysis of Behavior*, Vol. 2, pp. 127−140. Grune &

Stratton, New York.

Raine, A. (1991) The SPQ: a scale for the assessment of schizotypal personality based on DSM-III-R criteria. *Schizophrenia Bulletin*, **17**, 555−564.

Raine, A. & Allbutt, J. (1989) Factors of schizoid personality. *British Journal of Clinical Psychology*, **28**, 31−40.

Raine, A., Sheard, C., Reynolds, G.P. & Lencz, T. (1992) Pre-frontal structural and functional deficits associated with individual differences in schizotypal personality. *Schizophrenia Research*, **7**, 237−247.

Reitan, R.M. (1958) Validity of the trail-making test as an indicator of organic brain damage. *Perception and Motor Skills*, **8**, 271−276.

Ricks, D.F. & Berry, J.C. (1970) Family and symptom patterns that precede schizophrenia. In Roff, M. & Ricks, D.F. (eds) *Life History Research in Psychopathology*, Vol. 1. University of Minnesota Press, Minneapolis.

Rifkin, A., Quitkin, F. & Carrillo, C. (1972) Lithium carbonate in emotionally unstable character disorder. *Archives of General Psychiatry*, **27**, 519−523.

Robins, L.N. (1966) *Deviant Children Grown Up*. Williams & Wilkins, Baltimore.

Roff, J.D., Knight, R. & Wertheim, E. (1976) Disturbed preschizophrenics: childhood symptoms in relation to adult outcome. *Journal of Nervous and Mental Disease*, **162**, 274−281.

Rosenbaum, G., Shore, D.L. & Chapin, K. (1988) Attention deficit in schizophrenia and schizotypy: marker versus symptom variables. *Journal of Abnormal Psychology*, **97**, 41−47.

Sawaguchi, T. & Goldman-Rakic, P.S. (1991) D_1 dopamine receptors in prefrontal cortex: involvement in working memory. *Science*, **251**, 947−950.

Schulsinger, F., Parnas, J., Peterson, E. *et al.* (1984) Cerebral ventricular size in the offspring of schizophrenic mothers. *Archives of General Psychiatry*, **41**, 602−606.

Schulz, P.M. & Soloff, P.H. (1987) Still borderline after all these years. *140th Annual Meeting of the American Psychiatric Association*. Chicago, Illinois.

Schulz, S.C., Cornelius, J., Schulz, P.M. & Soloff, P.H. (1988) The amphetamine challenge test in patients with borderline disorder. *American Journal of Psychiatry*, **145**, 809−814.

Schulz, S.C., Koller, M.M., Kishore, P.R., Hamer, R.M., Gehl, J.J. & Friedel, R.O. (1983) Ventricular enlargement in teenage patients with schizophrenia spectrum disorder. *American Journal of Psychiatry*, **140**, 1592−1595.

Shelton, R.C. & Weinberger, D.R. (1986) X-ray computerized tomography studies in schizophrenia: a review and synthesis. In Nasrallah, H.A. & Weinberger, D.R. (eds) *The Neurology of Schizophrenia*, pp. 207−250. Elsevier, New York.

Siever, L.J. (1991) The biology of the boundaries of schizophrenia. In Tamminga, C.A. & Schulz, S.C. (eds) *Advances in Neuropsychiatry and Psychopharmacology*, Vol. 1, *Schizophrenia Research*, pp. 181−191. Raven Press, New York.

Siever, L.J. & Gunderson, J.G. (1983) The search for a schizotypal personality: historical origins and current status. *Comprehensive Psychiatry*, **24**, 199−212.

Siever, L.J., Kalus, O.F. & Keefe, R.S.E. (1993b) The boundaries of schizophrenia. *Psychiatric Clinics of North America*, **16**(2), 217−244.

Siever, L.J., Coursey, R.D., Alterman, I.S., Buchsbaum, M.S. & Murphy, D.L. (1984) Impaired smooth-pursuit eye movement: vulnerability marker for schizotypal personality disorder in a normal volunteer population. *American Journal of Psychiatry*, **141**, 1560−1566.

Siever, L.J., Rotter, M., Trestman, R., Coccaro, E., Losonczy, M. & Davis, K. (1993c) Lateral ventricle enlargement in schizotypal personality disorder. *American Psychiatric Association 146th Annual Meeting*, p. 126, NR263. San Francisco, CA.

Siever, L.J., Amin, F., Coccaro, E.F. *et al.* (1991) Plasma homovanillic acid in schizotypal personality disorder patients and controls. *American Journal of Psychiatry*, **148**, 1246−1248.

Siever, L.J., Amin, F., Coccaro, E.F. *et al.* (1993a) Cerebrospinal fluid homovanillic acid in schizotypal personality disorder. *American Journal of Psychiatry*, **150**, 149−151.

Siever, L.J., Coursey, R.D., Alterman, I.S. *et al.* (1989) Clinical, psychophysiologic, and neurologic characteristics of volunteers with impaired smooth pursuit eye movements. *Biological Psychiatry*, **26**, 35−51.

Siever, L.J., Keefe, R., Bernstein, D.P. *et al.* (1990) Eye tracking impairment in clinically identified schizotypal personality disorder patients. *American Journal of Psychiatry*, **147**, 740−745.

Silverman, J.M., Keefe, R.S.E., Losonczy, M.F. *et al.* (1992) Schizotypal and neuro-imaging factors in relatives of schizophrenic probands. *Society of Biological Psychiatry 47th Annual Meeting*, **31**, 70A. Washington, DC.

Simons, R.F. & Katkin, W. (1985) Smooth pursuit eye movements in subjects reporting physical anhedonia and perceptual aberrations. *Psychiatry Research*, **14**, 275−289.

Simons, R.F., MacMillan, F.W. & Ireland, F.B. (1982) Reaction time crossover in preselected schizotypic subjects. *Journal of Abnormal Psychology*, **6**, 414−419.

Spaulding, W., Garbin, C.P. & Dras, S.R. (1989) Cognitive abnormalities in schizophrenic patients and schizotypal college students. *Journal of Nervous and Mental Disease*, **177**, 717−728.

Squires-Wheeler, E., Skodol, A.E., Bassett, A. & Erlenmeyer-Kimling, L. (1989) DSM-III-R schizotypal personality traits in offspring of schizophrenic disorder, affective disorder, and normal control parents. *Journal of Psychiatric Research*, **23**, 229−239.

Squires-Wheeler, E., Skodol, A.E. & Erlenmeyer-Kimling, L. (1992) The assessment of schizotypal features over two points in time. *Schizophrenia Research*, **6**, 75−85.

Squires-Wheeler, E., Skodol, A.E., Friedman, D. & Erlenmeyer-Kimling, L. (1988) The specificity of DSM-III schizotypal personality traits. *Psychological Medicine*, **18**, 757−765.

Stone, M. (1992) Treatment of severe personality disorder. In Tasman, A. & Riba, M. (eds) *Annual Review of Psychiatry Press*, pp. 98−115. American Psychiatric Association, Washington DC.

Suddath, R.L., Casanova, M.F., Goldberg, T.E., Daniel, D.G., Kelsoe, J.R. Jr & Weinberger, D.R. (1989) Temporal lobe pathology in schizophrenia: a quantitative magnetic resonance imaging study. *American Journal of Psychiatry*, **146**, 464–472.

Van Kammen, D.P., Mann, L.S., Sternberg, D.E. *et al.* (1983) Dopamine beta-hydroxylase activity and homovanillic acid in spinal fluid in schizophrenics with brain atrophy. *Science*, **220**, 974–976.

Venables, P.H. (1990) The measurement of schizotypy in Mauritius. *Personality and Individual Differences*, **11**, 965–971.

Venables, P.H., Wilkins, S., Mitchell, D.A., Raine, A. & Bailes, K. (1990) A scale for the measurement of schizotypy. *Personality and Individual Differences*, **11**, 481–495.

Wainberg, M.L., Trestman, R.L., Keefe, R.S., Cornblatt, B., DeVegvar, M. & Siever, L.J. (1993) CPT in schizotypal personality disorder. *American Psychiatric Association 146th Annual Meeting*, p. 186, NR501. San Francisco, C.A.

Warnken, R.G. & Seiss, T.F. (1965) The use of the cumulative record in the prediction of behavior. *Personnel and Guidance Journal*, **31**, 231–237.

Watt, N.F. (1978) Patterns of childhood social development in adult schizophrenics. *Archives of General Psychiatry*, **35**, 160–165.

Weinberger, D.R. (1987) Implications of normal brain development for the pathogenesis of schizophrenia. *Archives of General Psychiatry*, **44**, 660–670.

Weintraub, S. & Neale, J.M. (1984) Social behavior of children at risk for schizophrenia. In Watt, N.F., Anthony, E.J., Wynne, L.C. & Rolf, J.E. (eds) *Children at Risk for Schizophrenia: A Longitudinal Perspective*, pp. 279–285. Cambridge University Press, New York.

Wolff, S., Tonshend, R., McGuire, R.J. & Weeks, D.J. (1991) Schizoid personality in childhood and adult life. II. Adult adjustment and continuity with schizotypal personality disorder. *British Journal of Psychiatry*, **159**, 620–629.

Chapter 8
Course and Outcome of Schizophrenia

H.-J. MÖLLER AND D. VON ZERSSEN

Introduction

There is an abundance of older and more recent literature concerning the course of schizophrenia. Starting with E. Bleuler's and Kraepelin's descriptions of this disorder in 1911 and 1913, respectively, questions regarding its course have remained in the centre of psychiatric research. Studies on this subject have played a particularly important role not only in establishing the nosological uniqueness of schizophrenia, by demonstrating the existence of a specific course pattern, but also in revealing the significance of social, biographical and symptomatological characteristics and of therapeutic and other influences on the course of the disorder.

Methodological problems in outcome research

Although numerous studies dealing with the course of schizophrenia exist, and many of these studies show significant results in specific areas, it has not been possible to derive a well-rounded, comprehensive view of the course of schizophrenic disorders from the available data. There are many reasons for this state of affairs (WHO, 1979; Kringlen, 1980): varying methods of patient selection owing to the lack of standardized patient characteristics and diagnostic classification, varying consideration of modifying factors, varying lengths of follow-up and different follow-up strategies.

The diagnosis of schizophrenia

A major problem affecting all past and present schizophrenia outcome research is presented by unevenly applied and/or unclearly defined diagnostic criteria (Schwarz *et al.*, 1980; Landmark, 1982; WPA, 1983). For example, while M. Bleuler (1972) and Huber *et al.* (1979) employ a relatively broad concept of schizophrenia similar to the one used in the eighth version of the *International Classification of Disease* (ICD-8), other authors, especially in Scandinavia, have tended to employ stricter definitions which exclude conditions such as brief schizophreniform episodes and reactive schizophreniform states (Langfeldt, 1937, 1956; Achté, 1961; Vaillant, 1962; Astrup & Noreik, 1966; Leonhard, 1966; see also Chapters 1 & 2, this volume). The idea behind the latter approach is that only those schizophrenic conditions not classified as brief or reactive demonstrate the

106

characteristic unfavourable course of schizophrenia as described by Kraepelin. With Bleuler and Huber, the diagnosis of schizophrenia is based primarily on cross-sectional findings and there is no implication that the course of the disorder must be unfavourable, while the last-mentioned authors combine the cross-sectional findings and the course description in order to establish the diagnosis. Following this line, the *Diagnostic and Statistical Manual* DSM-III-R criteria allow the diagnosis of schizophrenia only if symptoms have persisted for at least 6 months or if total remission has not taken place (APA, 1987). The resulting selection of patients with prognostically unfavourable characteristics and/or incipient chronicity ultimately leads via circular reasoning to the confirmation of the unfavourable course of schizophrenic illness by means of outcome studies (Möller *et al.*, 1989). The problems inherent in such an approach and their effect on outcome research have been pointed out in particular by Bleuler *et al.* (1976) and Huber *et al.* (1979).

As to psychopathological symptoms, Bleuler (1972), in assigning the diagnosis of schizophrenia, proceeds from 'fundamental symptoms' defined by E. Bleuler in 1911 (thought disorder, affective impairment, impaired social relations and impaired expression), giving these priority over 'accessory symptoms' (delusions, hallucinations and catatonia), while Huber *et al.* (1979), following Schneider, give greater diagnostic weight to abnormal experiences, i.e. to first-rank and (to a lesser extent) second-rank symptoms, than to the Schneiderian expressive symptoms, which correspond to Bleuler's 'fundamental symptoms' (Schneider, 1987; see also Chapter 2).

Elsewhere, particularly in North America, a broader concept of schizophrenia was used for many years to label as schizophrenic cases which in Europe would have been diagnosed as mania, severe neurosis or simply an adolescent adjustment disorder characterized by strong ambivalence and antisocial behaviour (Mombour, 1975). Apart from these relatively clear differences in diagnostic conceptions, there are many less obvious examples of imprecise definitions of the concept of 'schizophrenia'.

As has been shown by a number of studies, varying and imprecise definitions of diagnostic concepts have constituted the main reason for the interinstitutional and the intra- and international lack of reliability with regard to the diagnosis of schizophrenia (Cooper *et al.*, 1972; Kendell, 1975; Cranach & Strauss, 1978; Möller & von Zerssen, 1980). This lack of reliability has been a major problem in schizophrenia research, as it leads to different methods of patient selection, thereby seriously restricting the comparability of results from different studies. Since the definitions put forth by ICD-8 and ICD-9 did not result in a satisfactory solution to this problem, in recent years operational definitions and algorithms, based on combinations of Kraepelinian, Bleulerian and Schneiderian concepts as well as those of Langfeldt, have been developed to achieve greater consensus across centres internationally and form a more reliable reference point for therapy and outcome studies. Among these newer classificatory systems are the criteria of Feighner *et al.* (1972), which in modified form have been incorporated into the research diagnostic criteria (RDC; Spitzer *et al.*, 1977), and DSM-III (APA, 1980) and its revised version, DSM-III-R (APA, 1987). A further possibility of obtaining a less ambiguous diagnosis with regard to schizophrenia is offered by structured interviews for clinical assessment and the application of defined algorithms to the data by means of computer programs, thus reducing the subjective leeway available in assigning symptom combinations to specific nosological groups. Current examples of such methods are the *Present State Examination* (PSE)/CATEGO program (Wing *et al.*, 1974) or the *Structured Clinical Interview for DSM-III-R (SCID)* (Spitzer *et al.*, 1987). Further details regarding assessment methods are dealt with in the following section.

Assessment and description of findings

Along with the above-mentioned variability and imprecision of nosological classifications, there are other sources of unreliability in diagnoses which are due to differences in the assessment (recognition) and description of psychiatric phenomena (Kendell, 1975; Mombour, 1975; Möller *et al.*, 1978; von Zerssen & Möller, 1980). The lack of reliability occurs with the identification and description of symptoms as well as errors in the nosological classification of individual cases, but also not infrequently involves unsound documentation of the initial findings, which usually serve as the basis for comparison in the evaluation of subsequent findings in the course of the disorder. Therefore, the reliable description of these initial findings is of the utmost importance for the study of the course of the disorder. In particular, the 'free interview' and 'freehand' formulations of psychopathology still customary in many or most clinical settings proves to be inadequate for long-term follow-up studies of schizophrenia. The inadequacies of the initial database reduce the significance of better and more differentiated symptom descriptions in the follow-ups, since comparable baseline data are absent. The lack of standardization in the recording of findings not only leads to qualifications and constraints in the conclusions of follow-up studies, but also limits comparison with the results of other studies.

Structured and semi-structured interviews developed over the past 30 years have successfully addressed the principle of standardization (von Zerssen, 1979; Möller, 1989). A very strictly defined method of information gathering, such as the structured PSE (Wing *et al.*, 1972), offers perhaps the best chance of high interrater reliability; this advantage is, however, offset by the limited practicality of such instruments. It is for this reason that instruments which are less restrictive with respect to the method of information gathering are more widely used, for example standardized rating scales like the brief psychiatric rating scale (BPRS) (Overall & Gorham, 1962) or the in-patient multidimensional psychiatric scale (IMPS) (Lorr & Klett, 1967). These scales cover the whole spectrum of psychopathology but are less specific and do not rate specific recognized psychiatric symptoms and signs. The problem with the relatively short BPRS is that it rates a group of symptoms confounding traditional symptoms and syndromes under behaviourally recognized concepts. In the last

decade, special focus has been placed on the differentiation of positive and negative symptoms, resulting in rating scales for this specific purpose (see also Chapters 2 and 3, this volume). All these scales are completed on the basis of a relatively free interview but have nonetheless been shown to be sufficiently reliable between interviewers. In the statistical analyses of such scales, the individual items are customarily assigned to factors (syndromes) via multivariate procedures. This method has the advantages of reducing the data mass and possessing greater reliability when compared with the individual-item analysis (Möller & von Zerssen, 1982, 1983). The more differentiated assessment of psychopathology offered by such multidimensional scales is, with regard to precision and the amount of information obtained, generally preferable to the use of the time-saving, but otherwise imprecise, global rating scales.

The development of instruments for the assessment of the impairment in social functioning of schizophrenics has not reached a similar level of precision. The long-lasting neglect of a standardized assessment of social adaptation in follow-up research may stem from the implicit assumption that the presence of a clearcut symptomatology is closely tied to impairment in social functioning, an assumption which in this strict form has not been substantiated by recent findings in psychotherapy research (Seidenstücker & Baumann, 1978) or in the follow-up studies of schizophrenics (Brown *et al.*, 1966; Strauss & Carpenter, 1972). It is perhaps for this reason that more recent outcome-research work has been striving towards a more standardized description of social functioning using methods capable of achieving a degree of precision comparable with that of the psychopathology rating scales (Schubart *et al.*, 1986a; Möller *et al.*, 1988; Marneros *et al.*, 1991). In evaluating social functioning, one has to consider the greatest possible number of variables in the most differentiating way possible. This evaluation must not be restricted to the area of occupation, but must include other areas of social functioning such as social contacts, leisure-time activities, etc. Although a number of observer and self-rating scales for the evaluation of social functioning have already been developed (Weissman & Sholomskas, 1981), a standard set has yet to emerge by consensus among researchers in this field. An important problem for most instruments available for evaluating social functioning is the absence of adequate reference data from clinical or non-clinical populations. However, the social interview schedule (SIS) has more reference data than most scales (Clare & Cairns, 1978; Faltermaier *et al.*, 1987). For a global assessment of psychopathological symptoms and social adjustment, the global assessment scale (GAS; Spitzer *et al.*, 1976) has been widely used during the last decade. The disability assessment schedule (DAS), developed by a WHO research group (WHO, 1988), should also be mentioned in this context.

Outcome criteria

The results of outcome studies vary depending on the weight given to the symptomatological or social-adaptive perspective and the criteria used to assess outcome and remission.

The improvement criteria used by Bleuler (1972) and by Ciompi and Müller (1976) are formulated in a manner that the course of illness on the whole must appear favourable for the afflicted individuals. In a long-term follow-up study, Bleuler classifies cases which remained stable for 5 years into the following categories: complete remission, mild illness, moderate illness and severe illness. Complete remission was based on the social criterion that 'the former patient was fully employable and could maintain his/her previous place in society, in particular within the family as parent or housewife'. Further requirements are that the individual is no longer identified by his or her family as mentally ill and that in subsequent psychiatric examinations no psychotic symptoms are present. Such individuals, previously considered schizophrenic, are still considered to be 'cured' even if an exhaustive psychiatric examination showed residual delusions, lack of insight in the episodes of illness, odd behaviour or constricted interests and social

activity (Bleuler, 1972). Mild illness is defined as follows:

> A mild 'end state' is assumed to be present in those patients who despite the existence of clear schizophrenic symptoms speak in an ordered fashion, at least as regards topics which do not relate to their delusional and hallucinatory experiences. Their appearance is generally unremarkable and their illness will not become immediately apparent if one's contact with them remains superficial. They perform useful work and they live either off the hospital grounds or in open wards. Correspondingly, in this group there are many schizophrenics whose delusions or hallucinations are more in the background and whose personalities have not disintegrated — in short, older outsiders who have turned away from the mainstream of life, who hardly show normal interests, and who perform some sort of monotonous work or live out their lives following some eccentric idea (Bleuler, 1972).

Criteria of this sort are the opposite of more stringent standards such as those defined by Achté (1967), according to whom a patient is classified as 'fully cured' if no psychotic symptoms are present and no personality change has occurred and if the individual is employed at the level of premorbid functioning. A patient is judged to be improved if no symptoms are apparent and if the level of current employment corresponds to, or is slightly below, the level of premorbid functioning, but a complete remission is considered doubtful or slight deficits cannot be completely ruled out. Other authors apply different mixtures of cross-sectional and longitudinal criteria considering psychopathological and/or social adjustment (Prudo & Blum, 1987; Sartorius *et al.*, 1987). It is obvious from the consideration of such divergent global evaluation criteria that valid comparisons of research results are almost impossible. Unfortunately, these studies have not employed a standardized global scale that summarizes the psychopathological state and the state of social adaptation like the GAS (Spitzer *et al.*, 1976), which has only subsequently become available.

Other investigators have restricted themselves to determining only rates of recidivism and rehospitalization in outcome studies, thereby avoiding reliance on 'soft' data relating to symptomatology and social functioning (Shepherd, 1957; Niskanen & Achté 1972; May *et al.*, 1976). The frequency and length of hospitalization are not direct illness-dependent measures because they are influenced by factors such as environmental tolerance, admission practices of psychiatrists and the presence or absence of alternatives to the hospital, such as community care, etc. This dependence on factors not directly related to the illness makes such improvement criteria as the sole basis for evaluation questionable.

Other methodological problems

The methodological problems discussed above are usually associated with economic and technical constraints. Studies using samples of schizophrenic patients from a single hospital offer fewer organizational problems than does the epidemiologically more representative survey of all schizophrenic patients in a particular region, but only the latter can provide a sound basis for generalization which might be applicable to other populations. Such studies are rare because they can only be carried out where there have been clinically organized catchment areas (Schwarz *et al.*, 1980; Watt *et al.*, 1983). Follow-up studies with a restricted set of instruments are easier and less strenuous for the patient and can be carried out with less financial expense than more complicated studies possessing a comprehensive battery of instruments. Retrospective studies can be carried out more quickly than prospective studies. Studies in which information is collected solely from hospital charts or is solicited from patients and/or their relatives by telephone or by a mailed questionnaire is less complicated than the direct follow-up examination of patients. The assessment of only present findings during the outcome interview is simpler than the additional gathering of data from the entire follow-up period, so that usually the former is preferred, albeit along with the gathering of rudimentary data relating to the course of

illness, such as the frequency and duration of rehospitalization. In most cases, the studies involve mixed samples consisting of first-episode and relapses as well as chronic cases. The follow-up of pure samples of first-episode patients would allow clear conclusions to be drawn with respect to the course of the illness, but such collectives are usually difficult to recruit.

Intervening variables which influence the outcome

A further problem is the consideration of those factors which can influence the course of illness. Especially in retrospective studies, these factors can rarely be sufficiently taken into account for practical reasons, but in prospective studies at least some of them will be neglected as well, for the same reasons.

Thus, depending on the respective financial and recruitment potential of outcome studies, restrictions in the protocol will be present which will ultimately lead to restrictions in the conclusions drawn.

Results of outcome research

The results of outcome research in schizophrenia can be classified according to various emphases: the patient's condition at follow-up, typology of course, influencing factors, predictors or the comparison with the course of other psychiatric disorders.

The patient's condition at the time of follow-up

While earlier studies concerning the course of schizophrenia described rather unfavourable outcomes (Gerloff, 1936), later investigations in this area have, on the whole, given a much more favourable picture of this disorder (Stephens, 1970). This view can be interpreted as being largely a reflection of the therapeutic advances achieved over the years. The outcome studies of Bleuler (1972) and Huber *et al.* (1979) represent important summaries of the course of schizophrenia in patients over a period of 20−30 years. Both studies follow a retrospective design and describe the state of the patients at follow-up in terms of descriptive psychopathology without using standardized procedures in the sense of modern psychometrics. The diagnosis of schizophrenia was a clinical one, based on the clinical constructs described by Bleuler (study of Bleuler) or Schneider (study of Huber *et al.*), without using defined operationalization criteria in the modern sense.

Bleuler (1972) published the following results regarding the retrospective long-term follow-up of 208 schizophrenic patients he had treated personally and who had been in-patients in the Burghölzli Psychiatric Hospital in Zurich in 1942: approximately 60% of the patients from the original sample achieved 'end states' that were stable over 5 years; of these patients, 20% were considered to be in complete remission, 33% mildly ill, 24% moderately ill and 24% severely ill. Bleuler emphasizes that among those patients with 'non-stabilized' courses of illness, there was a large number of patients with high relapse rates whose illness demonstrated a phasic course, including periods of full remission, so that over the whole group of patients the results are even more favourable. At the time of follow-up (22 years after discharge from the hospital), 43% of all patients were employed either at or below their premorbid occupational level. These results were confirmed by Bleuler's observations of four other patient samples at different follow-up points. Altogether, Bleuler observed the long-term course of schizophrenia in 650 patients; he concludes:

> If one views the long-term remissions, the remissions which are interrupted only by brief psychotic episodes, and the mild chronic 'end states' as characteristics of benign schizophrenia, the moderate and severe 'end states' as characteristics of malignant schizophrenia, then one can derive the rule that about two-thirds to three-fourths of schizophrenics will have a benign course and only about one-third or less a malignant course (Bleuler, 1972).

In presenting Bleuler's optimistic view, one should not forget that the concept of 'mild chronic final state' can, as mentioned above, include relatively severe psychopathological findings and hospitalizations of long duration because the classification depends first and foremost on the patient's state of functioning in society.

In their follow-up assessment of the psychopathology of schizophrenic patients, Huber *et al.* (1979) utilized a different classification system, one that is difficult to compare with Bleuler's. Their survey encompassed approximately 500 schizophrenics who had been treated as in-patients in the University of Bonn Psychiatric Hospital between 1945 and 1959. Complete remission was reported for 22% of the patients, 'uncharacteristic residual symptoms' for 43% and 'characteristic residual symptoms' for 35%. They attempted to translate these findings into M. Bleuler's classificatory system (Bleuler *et al.*, 1976; Huber *et al.*, 1979) and reported on patients who had achieved a stable condition over at least 5 years (73% of the total sample). They found that 26% had a complete remission, while 31% had mild, 29% moderate and 14% severe 'end states'. At the time of follow-up, 56% of the patients were fully able to work: 39% at the premorbid level and 17% at a lower level. A further 19% were classified as capable of working to a limited degree, 17% as incapable of working in their learned trades and 8% as completely incapable of working. While the 'social remissions' (i.e. fully able to earn a living) in the Bonn sample were somewhat more frequent than in the Zurich sample, there were no essential differences between the two groups with respect to psychopathology.

In the Bonn study, very subtle psychopathological differentiations were employed in the attempt to delineate 15 types of schizophrenic residual states, of which only the main groups, the 'uncharacteristic' and 'characteristic', will be discussed here. The uncharacteristic remission types are defined as residual states in which the patients' cross-sectional findings would not suffice to diagnose schizophrenia. Among such states are 'minimal residual states' and 'pure deficits' for which the loss of potential is typical, as are structural alterations as exemplified by schizophrenic 'eccentrics' and 'originals'. The characteristic remission types are, apart from the 'chronic pure pychoses', marked by the loss of potential or suffering personality alteration in combination with productive schizophrenic symptoms. Even on the basis of a purely cross-sectional assessment, such patients will be diagnosed as schizophrenic. Huber *et al.* emphasize the importance of this psychopathological differentiation by pointing out that uncharacteristic residual states have a higher 'social remission rate' than do the characteristic ones.

There is not sufficient space to describe here other important long-term studies, like those of Tsuang *et al.* (1979), Harding *et al.* (1987) and Marneros *et al.* (1991).

Many other studies have reported results after shorter follow-up periods (Table 8.1). It is probably not meaningful to discuss in detail these studies (see Möller & von Zerssen, 1986). Some of them (e.g. Holmboe & Astrup, 1957; Brown *et al.*, 1966; Henisz, 1966; Achté, 1967; Affleck *et al.*, 1976; Bland *et al.* 1976; Ciompi & Müller, 1976; Lo & Lo, 1977) describe a relatively favourable course of illness; others (e.g. Johanson, 1958; Astrup & Noreik, 1966) depict a considerably less favourable course and outcome. It is generally difficult to judge which factors are responsible for the differences in these two sets of studies. Part of the differences are surely due to varying diagnostic concepts and different improvement criteria. Conspicuously, the two last-cited articles are from Scandinavia, where they separate diagnoses 'schizophreniform psychosis' and 'reactive psychosis', which have a favourable course

Table 8.1 Studies in which the mean length of follow-up is at least 10 years and in which it is possible to grade stated outcome in terms of recovered, improved or not improved. (From Johnstone, 1991)

Reference[*]	No. of cases	Mean length of follow-up (years)	Recovered (%)	Improved (%)	Not improved (%)
Mayer-Gross (1932)	294	16	30	8	62
Rennie (1939)	222	20	27	13	60
Muller (1951)	194	17	16	17	67
Errera (1957)	54	16	26	26	48
Holmboe and Astrup (1957)	225	12	29	29	42
Eitinger *et al.* (1958)	154	11	12	22	66
Ey (1958)	120	15	45	20	35
Johansen (1958)	98	14	2	35	63
Astrup *et al.* (1963)	435	12	15	17	68
Faergeman (1963)	85	17	52	22	26
Retterstøl (1966)	126	16	41	16	43
Vaillant and Funkenstein (1966)	61	11	26	10	64
Achté (1967)	76	15	35	15	50
Noreik *et al.* (1967)	219	22	16	38	46
Beck (1968)	84	30	7	10	83
Stephens (1970)	143	12	24	46	30
Shimazono (1974)	110	13.5	29	37	35
Huber *et al.* (1975)	502	22	22	43	35
Roff (1975)	125	22	43	39	18
Tsuang and Winokur (1975)	139	35	10	35	47
Bland *et al.* (1976)	88	11	51	25	17
Ciompi (1980)	269	37	20	42	38

[*] References given in Johnstone (1991).

(Retterstøl, 1978, 1983), from the diagnosis of schizophrenia with an unfavourable course. In his review of outcome studies with a follow-up period of at least 5 years, Stephens (1970) comes to the conclusion that, when using a narrow definition of schizophrenia, 60% of all patients are unimproved after 5 years, while the proportion of unimproved schizophreniform psychoses is only about 20%.

Many modern studies on schizophrenia have used modern standardized rating proceedings and some of them included different scales for the measurement of psychopathology and social adaptation. In the 5-year follow-up of the Washington group within the International Pilot Study of Schizophrenia (IPSS), 60% of the patients showed a very good or good outcome as measured by a global score encompassing symptomatology and social functioning (Hawk *et al.*, 1975). In the 5-year follow-up of the London group within the IPSS, 49% of the patients had a good symptomatological outcome, and 42% had a good social outcome according to a composite measure of social functioning (Prudo & Blum, 1987).

It is not necessary to report similar outcome results of other recent follow-up studies: Watt *et al.* (1983), Möller *et al.* (1986), Schubart *et al.* (1986b), Sartorius *et al.* (1987), Leff *et al.* (1991) and the Scottish Schizophrenia Research Group (1992). Generalizing the results found in these more recent studies, which give the findings of patients during the course of their treatment, the conclusion can be drawn that, at the time of the follow-up examination, about 50% of the patients demonstrated an unfavourable condition with respect to psychopathology and social functioning. Approximately 50% required one or more readmissions during the follow-up period. However, chronic hospitalization was much less frequent than reported in earlier studies, and long-term hospitalization has become rare.

Studies following shorter follow-up examinations do not show more favourable outcomes than those covering longer time spans. This fact could be due to the more stringent improvement criteria used in shorter term studies. On the other hand, it could be due to the phenomenon observed by Bleuler *et al.* (1976) that schizophrenics as a group show no tendency to deteriorate after the first 5 years. Thus, the results of Bleuler's long-term finding and more recent shorter term studies do not support the hypothesis that schizophrenics continue to deteriorate over a longer term of say 20 years.

There have been few follow-up studies which assess the change of psychopathology progressively over time, for example Möller *et al.* (1981) at admission, discharge and at 5-year follow-up, and Biehl *et al.* (1988) at 6-month intervals during a follow-up period of 5 years. Such data give a more detailed insight into the development of psychopathological symptoms during clinical treatment than do the usual two-point measurements. They demonstrate that treatment with neuroleptics at index hospitalization leads to a reduction of productive symptoms in a high proportion of patients, a considerable proportion of patients achieve an unsatisfactory result with an increase of schizophrenic symptoms in the intervening period (Möller *et al.* 1986). However, Biehl *et al.* (1988) concluded that the increase of symptoms over the 5-year period is due more to negative and non-specific symptoms than to positive symptoms.

With neuroleptic treatment the majority of schizophrenics are spared long-term hospitalization and are able to live in society, but this does not mean that they are symptom free or socially well functioning. The frequent presence of considerably disturbed social functioning has been documented in several of the more recent follow-up studies (Strauss & Carpenter, 1972; WHO, 1979; Möller & von Zerssen, 1986; Schubart *et al.*, 1986b; Sartorius *et al.*, 1987; Leff *et al.*, 1991). Thus, the apparently favourable picture which arises through the application of relatively unrefined improvement criteria in several long-term follow-up studies has to be balanced against the less favourable outcomes found in more recent shorter term studies that have employed more stringent outcome criteria through the use of a more discriminating assessment of social functioning which takes account of such parameters as occupational performance, social contacts, leisure activities, etc. (see Chapter 13 for an epidemiological perspective).

The effect of therapeutic and other mediating factors

Whether the course of schizophrenia has improved since the introduction of neuroleptic medication has various interpretations (Hogarty, 1977), but most opinions support an important positive effect of neuroleptic treatment. In the pre-neuroleptic era, it could be assumed that only perhaps 20–25% of patients receiving the diagnosis of schizophrenia would achieve 'social remission' (Bleuler, 1941). As the literature discussed above shows, this number has doubled in recent years.

However, this change in the long-term prognosis of schizophrenia cannot be attributed to neuroleptic therapy alone. There are indications that the course of schizophrenia improved following the introduction of insulin-shock, coma and electroconvulsive treatments in the 1930s. In 1972, Bleuler concluded that with the improvement in therapeutic possibilities 'catastrophic schizophrenias' (marked by an acute initial phase with a rapid transition to a severe chronic state: Mauz, 1930) would no longer occur and that severe psychoses in general had become less frequent. In Bleuler's opinion, however, the proportion of patients with long-term remissions would not alter.

There are many findings that in catamnestic studies, which focus on patients admitted after the introduction of neuroleptics, the duration of hospital stay is shorter than in studies before. Apparently, there was also a marked reduction in the number of psychiatric beds required after the introduction of neuroleptics. However, many of the epidemiological studies indicate that the decrease in the number of psychiatric beds required, which at least in the 1950s, 1960s and 1970s was perhaps a stable indicator of the severity of illness and the degree to which it caused dependency, began before the introduction of neuroleptic medication, and was possibly related to changes in the milieu of psychiatric hospitals and to social-psychiatric efforts. Therefore, the shorter stay in hospital and the reduction in number of psychiatric beds cannot be explained

simply by the introduction of neuroleptic treatment. It can only be supposed that the neuroleptic treatment contributed to this effect.

Huber *et al.* (1979) concluded from a comparison of the follow-up of patients from earlier and more recent first hospitalizations that there was a significantly more favourable long-term development in the course of patients hospitalized after 1951, reflecting the benefit of early in-patient treatment with neuroleptic medication. For patients who were not treated at the beginning of their illness, full remissions were significantly rarer and 'characteristic residual states' were more frequent than in the total sample. Huber *et al.* interpreted their results to conclude that long-term treatment with medication leads to a 'pharmacogenic syndrome shift' which, within the subgroup of the characteristic residual states, consists in a symptomatological shift from the typical 'schizophrenic deficit psychosis' to more favourable 'mixed residual states'.

Achté (1967) compared two samples of schizophrenic patients, one with the first hospitalization in 1950 and the other with the first hospitalization in 1960 after the introduction of neuroleptics. Among these patients, 65% of the earlier hospitalized and 76% of the more recently hospitalized could be classified as 'socially cured'. In a comparison of the patients with unfavourable prognoses who were diagnosed according to Langfeldt's (1937) more stringent criteria of schizophrenia, the improvement in prognosis since the introduction of neuroleptics was more obvious: only 31% of the patients from the 1950 sample achieved social remission, while 51% of the patients from the 1960 group did so.

Using modern methods of multivariate statistics, An der Heiden *et al.* (An der Heiden & Krumm, 1985; An der Heiden *et al.*, 1989) demonstrated that out-patient long-term treatment by psychiatrists is able to improve the prognosis of schizophrenic patients. Under the aspect that this treatment includes neuroleptic medication as an essential part, this result also provides some evidence for the efficacy of neuroleptic treatment under natural treatment conditions.

Naturalistic follow-up studies are not the best

way to demonstrate the efficacy of specific therapies, but prospective randomized controlled
studies are inevitably short term. Nevertheless,
they provide conclusive evidence that the acute
treatment with neuroleptic medication as well as
maintenance treatment (Fig. 8.1) with neuroleptics
has a significantly better outcome than treatment
without medication, with on average a 50% lower
rate of relapse (Davis *et al.*, 1980; Johnstone *et al.*,
1986), and that psychosocial interventions of different kinds add only marginal benefits to the
rate of relapse (Hogarty, 1977; Mosher &
Keith, 1979).

However, it has to be questioned whether this
general statement concerning psychosocial interventions needs to be modified after some groups
demonstrated efficacy, at least for some methods
of family therapy, e.g. family therapy based on the
high-expressed emotion concept (Hogarty *et al.*,
1986). There is also no question that social-
psychiatric activities, especially rehabilitation, are
of great importance for long-term outcome in
schizophrenia. However, the scientific evaluation
in this field is complicated by severe methodological problems.

Another factor of great interest arises from the
results of the 5-year follow-up of the IPSS. This
showed that the outcome of schizophrenia in
developing countries was better than in developed
countries (Sartorius *et al.*, 1987). Leff (1987) has
suggested that higher exposure of families in
developed countries to a greater degree of negative
and intense 'expressed emotion', which is less
prevalent in the situation of the extended family
with community support found in less-developed
countries, accounts for the worse prognosis in
developed countries.

A positive influence of extended families,
originally supposed to be a crucial factor, would,
however, not be confirmed in a comparison of
data from the Columbian centre of the IPS
and an independent German follow-up study.
Furthermore, the 5- to 10-year outcome was not
generally better in the Columbian than in the
German sample, but rather more heterogeneous
with more positive and more negative and less
intermediate outcomes (von Zerssen *et al.*, 1990).
This difference may in part be due to a lack
of aftercare with neuroleptic medication in the
Columbian patients.

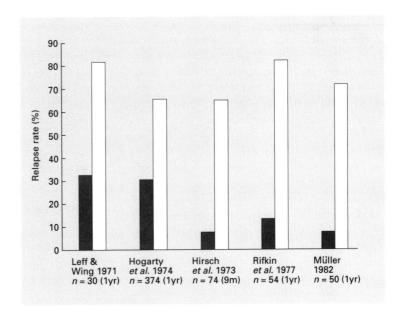

Fig. 8.1 Relapse-preventing
therapy with oral neuroleptics.
(From Möller, 1990.)
■ Neuroleptic; □ placebo.

Typology of the course of schizophrenia

Several authors have attempted to delineate a course typology for schizophrenia on the basis of their results. In these typologies, aspects of the onset of illness (acute, gradual) are tied to characteristics of the course (phasic, episodic, chronic) and the condition at follow-up (remission, personality alteration, psychosis). Bleuler's typology (1972) is perhaps most well known. In Fig. 8.2, the percentage frequencies stated are derived from two of Bleuler's long-term follow-up studies. This typology has not been established in practice, possibly because of the difficulties inherent in attempting to reliably assign a case to such complex course types. In their study on interrater reliability, Ciompi and Müller (1976) determined that despite extensive training there was only 30% agreement among raters in assigning patients to Bleuler's typology. The disagreement was high for all aspects of the course of illness: onset, type of course and end state. Satisfactory concordance rates in the area of 70% were reached only when the three characteristics were judged separately. Ciompi and Müller found an acute onset of illness in 43% and a chronic onset in 44% of patients. For the type of course, 43% of patients showed a linear course and 50% an undulatory course. At the time of follow-up, 27% of the patients were reportedly in complete remission ('cured'), and 22% had achieved a mild, 24% a moderately severe and 18% a severe 'end state'. It can be concluded that typologies of the course of schizophrenia are difficult to employ and do not allow for a sufficient degree of reliability among researchers.

For these reasons, a typology of the post-hospital course of mental disorders was developed on the basis of a retrospective global rating of psychopathology in quarterly intervals over a follow-up period of 5–8 years. One approach used a clustering of quantitative characteristics of time courses to group the individual courses; another consisted of a diagnostically blind, visual analysis of 'chronograms' (plots of data against time). The results were similar but somewhat easier to interpret with respect to the visual typing

procedure. Here, besides complete enduring remissions, relatively constant courses at different levels of severity and several rather variable courses emerged. The latter comprised chronic symptomatology with more or less pronounced changes without a long-standing trend and courses with a trend towards remission or with a trend towards deterioration and, finally, clearcut episodic courses. The latter courses prevailed in affective and schizoaffective psychoses; constant courses and courses with only slight or moderate variability predominated in neurotic and personality disorders; and more or less variable courses with or without an obvious trend were most prevalent in schizophrenic psychoses. This also applied to courses with a trend towards remission (von Zerssen, 1990).

Most investigators who attempt a typology of the clinical course would apply relatively simple categorizations relating to course and condition at follow-up. For example, in their 5-year outcome study, Watt *et al.* (1983) applied the following classification.

1 Single episode, no lasting impairment: 16%.
2 Several episodes, no or minimal impairment: 32%.
3 Repeated episodes, lasting impairment at a constant level, no complete remission: 9%.
4 Repeated episodes, increasingly severe residual symptoms, no complete remission: 43%.

These percentages are related to the whole group of 121 patients. If only patients with first manifestations of their illness at index time are included, the results appear more favourable. This is important because the clinicians' impression of prognosis is based partly on the patients seen, but such an impression will be biased by a disproportion of patients who have more frequent and enduring symptoms.

Prediction of the course of illness

A large number of studies reflect attempts to find predictors of the long-term course of schizophrenia. The problem of prediction has thereby often been tied to efforts to differentiate between 'typical' or 'process' schizophrenia, having an

Linear courses

1 Acute course to severe end states
   (to schizophrenic dementia)
   A 5 – 18%
   B   1% ± 0.69
   C   0

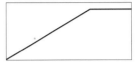

2 Chronic course to severe end states
   (to schizophrenic dementia)
   A 10 – 20%
   B   12% ± 2.27
   C   8% ± 2.44

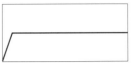

3 Acute course to moderate or mild
   end states (to defect state)
   A hardly over 5%
   B   2% ± 0.97
   C   4% ± 1.75

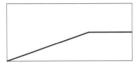

4 Chronic course to moderate or mild
   end states (to defect state)
   A 5 – 10%
   B   23% ± 2.94
   C   20% ± 3.61

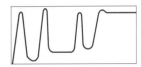

Undulatory courses

5 Undulatory course to severe end
   states (to schizophrenic dementia)
   A hardly over 5%
   B   9% ± 1.99
   C   3% ± 1.53

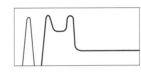

6 Undulatory course to moderate or
   mild end states (to defect states)
   A 30 – 40%
   B   27% ± 3.1
   C   22% ± 3.73

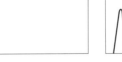 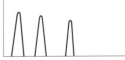

7 Undulatory course ending in
   complete remission
   A 25 – 35%
   B   22% ± 2.89
   C   39% ± 4.39

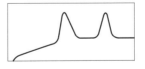 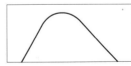

Atypical courses
   A about 5%
   B   4% ± 1.37
   C   4% ± 1.76

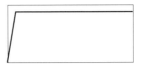

Fig. 8.2 Frequencies of the different course types in Bleuler's investigations of 1941 and 1972. (From Bleuler, 1972.) A, findings in the investigation of 1941; B, findings of all patients in the investigation of 1972. From these results prognostic conclusions can be drawn for all schizophrenics at hospital admission; C, findings in first admission patients and their siblings in the investigation of 1972. From these results prognostic conclusions can be drawn for patients with an onsetting schizophrenia provided that the disorder is that severe that the patient has to be hospitalized for at least once in his life.

unfavourable course, and schizophreniform psychosis, reactive schizophrenia, schizoaffective psychosis and atypical psychosis, all of which purportedly have a more favourable course. It was with this distinction in mind that Langfeldt (1937), on the basis of a 10-year follow-up of schizophrenic patients, developed criteria which were supposed to be helpful in predicting a favourable or an unfavourable course (Langfeldt, 1956). Accordingly, predictors of a favourable course would be specific symptoms such as manic or depressive affective symptoms, but also characteristics of the onset of illness, such as rapidity of onset and the presence or absence of psychogenic factors. Kant (1940, 1941a,b) presented the results of his outcome studies in a similar manner. Some studies appear to confirm the prognostic value of Langfeldt's criteria (Vaillant, 1962; Stephens & Astrup, 1965; Achté, 1967). In contrast, Welner and Strömgren (1958), using the same criteria, could not make useful prognoses with regard to favourable and unfavourable courses of schizophrenic illness; Strauss and Carpenter (1974), applying only the symptomatological criteria for the course of process schizophrenia, were likewise unable to support Langfeldt's work.

This leads us to consider attempts to predict the course of schizophrenia solely on the basis of psychopathological symptoms or syndromes, or of the diagnostic subtypes closely correlated with psychopathology. Achté (1967) found that patients presenting with hebephrenic symptoms or diagnosed as 'simple' schizophrenia (schizophrenia simplex) demonstrated the most unfavourable course, while patients with catatonic symptoms and, even more so, those diagnosed as schizophreniform psychoses showed the most favourable course. Huber *et al.* (1979) came to essentially the same conclusions: catatonic and 'cenesthetic-depressive' syndromes, especially in women, indicate a favourable course; a paranoid syndrome at onset and paranoid-hallucinatory syndromes in general indicate a less favourable course. The evaluation of the data from the 2-year outcome investigation carried out within the framework of the IPSS (WHO, 1979) showed that catatonic schizophrenia, schizoaffective psychoses and acute schizophrenic episodes usually take a favourable course, while the course for hebephrenic, paranoid and simple schizophrenia is unfavourable. Conversely, Tsuang and Winokur (1974) found a more favourable course for hebephrenic compared with paranoid schizophrenia. However, these authors also described a particularly favourable long-term course for schizoaffective psychoses; in this case, the course of illness approximated that of bipolar disorders (Tsuang *et al.*, 1979; see also Chapter 4, this volume).

These results seem to allow the conclusion that some specific characteristics of cross-sectional psychopathology have prognostic significance with regard to the long-term course and the outcome of schizophrenic illness; yet there are contradictory findings. Hargreaves *et al.* (1977), in their 2-year follow-up study, found no significant influence of the various subtypes of schizophrenia on prognosis. The Washington study group of the IPSS, using data from the 5-year outcome investigation, was unable to make adequate prognostic predictions on the basis of Langfeldtian criteria and Schneiderian first-rank symptoms or according to the subtypes paranoid/non-paranoid schizophrenia, schizoaffective psychosis/schizophrenia, schizophrenic episodes and borderline cases/schizophrenia (Gunderson *et al.*, 1975; Hawk *et al.*, 1975; Strauss & Carpenter, 1977). It is possible that these negative results are influenced by the fact that the samples were smaller and the duration of follow-up shorter than in the other studies cited above.

It appears that the use of standardized rating procedures for the assessment of the psychopathological state at admission or at index period does not increase the prognostic power with respect to global outcome at follow-up. The published findings with respect to the prognostic value of certain symptoms or syndromes vary considerably. Negative symptoms seem to have a stronger prognostic power than positive symptoms. The analysis of psychopathological findings recorded at admission, discharge and follow-up demonstrates that the patient's symptoms at discharge are especially relevant because they correlate in a more or less syndrome-specific way with the corresponding psychopathological picture at follow-up (Möller *et al.*, 1982). Dimensions of psychopathology which can be self-rated also have prognostic significance (Möller *et al.*, 1982; Martin, 1991). In the effort to predict the course of illness, a number of characteristics other than psychopathological ones have been studied (Table 8.2).

It has to be considered that predictors are often related to certain outcome criteria and they might not be confirmed as predictors when they are analysed in relation to other outcome criteria (Strauss & Carpenter, 1977; Möller *et al.*, 1982; Pietzcker & Gaebel, 1983). In addition to this, often predictors reported in the literature cannot be replicated. In general, they explain only a small percentage of variance. Psychopathological predictors are weaker in their predictive power than the clinical history and social adaptation. Notwithstanding, the favourable prognostic significance of good social contacts, less frequent work absenteeism and shorter hospital stays in the period prior to the index investigation has been confirmed by several groups (Mintz *et al.*, 1976; Pokorny *et al.*, 1976; Goldberg *et al.*, 1977; Strauss & Carpenter, 1977; Möller *et al.*, 1986; Carpenter & Strauss, 1991). Other authors have emphasized the prognostic value of the psychopathological findings at the time of discharge from hospital (Renton *et al.*, 1963; Affleck *et al.*, 1976; Mintz *et al.*, 1976; Wittenborn *et al.*, 1977; Möller *et al.*, 1986) (Table 8.3).

Individual predictors can usually explain only a small proportion of the outcome variance. This proportion can be considerably increased by pooling several prognostically relevant factors. Of the prognosis scales described in the literature, the most successful ones are those which involve combinations of traits from different areas (previous history, psychopathology and social functioning). But even relatively simple scales for assessing premorbid functioning are relatively powerful. The best results in this regard have been achieved by the Strauss–Carpenter scale and the Stephens scale (Möller *et al.*, 1982, 1984) (Table 8.4).

Newer approaches to formulating a prognosis

for schizophrenic illness employ multivariate analysis of known or newly derived predictors in order to identify combinations of traits which explain a higher proportion of the variance of outcome criteria (Strauss & Carpenter, 1977; WHO, 1979; Möller *et al.*, 1986). A problem with such approaches is that the predictor patterns identified by applying multivariate techniques to small samples can be replicated by other groups only to a limited extent, since multivariate statistics fit predictor patterns optimally into the special characteristics of the data set at hand. They are a *post hoc* statement of what correlated best with what in the particular data set, rather than a true set of prospectively stated predictors, confirmed in a follow-up study.

Comparison with the course of other functional psychoses

There are only relatively few studies which address the discrimination of the course of schizophrenia from that of other psychiatric illnesses. These studies come to basically the same conclusions. Astrup and Noreik (1966) found that the course of schizophrenia was unfavourable compared with that of affective disorders, as measured by symptomatology and social integration at the time of follow-up. Similar findings have been described by Shepherd (1957) and Norris (1959), who used length and frequency of rehospitalization as the assessment criteria. This has been confirmed by recent research (Tsuang *et al.*, 1979; WHO, 1979; Möller *et al.*, 1988, 1989; Grossman *et al.*, 1991; Marneros *et al.*, 1991).

Two of these studies are worth mentioning in detail. Tsuang and Fleming (1987) reported on about 700 patients with schizophrenia, affective disorders and surgical controls followed up for 30–40 years. There was a clear and significant difference between schizophrenic and affective psychoses with respect to occupational and psychiatric outcome 30–40 years after index admission. Among schizophrenics 20% had a good psychiatric outcome compared with 50% of patients with mania and 61% with depression, and 83% of controls. The schizophrenia group

Table 8.2 Summary of hypotheses on predictors of course and outcome in schizophrenia derived from previous studies. (From WHO, 1979)

Variables	Good prognosis	Poor prognosis
Sociodemographic		
Age at onset	Above 20–25	Below 20
Sex	Inconclusive evidence	Inconclusive evidence
Socioeconomic status	Average, high	Low
Occupational record	Stable	Irregular
Level of education	Uncertain	Uncertain
Urban/rural residence	Uncertain	Uncertain
Belonging to minority group	No	Yes
Other adverse social factors	Absent	Present
Past history and personality		
Family history of mental illness	Affective	Schizophrenic
Previous personality	Syntonic, affective	Schizoid
Somatotype	Pyknic	Asthenic, leptosome
Behaviour disorder in past	Uncertain	Uncertain
Intelligence level	Not subnormal	Subnormal
Psychosexual adjustment	At least one lasting heterosexual relationship	No lasting heterosexual relationship
Past physical illnesses	Uncertain	Uncertain
Past psychotic illness	Affective	Schizophrenic
Past neurotic illnesses	Obsessional	Uncertain
Precipitating factors	Present	Absent
Type of onset	Acute, sudden	Insidious
Rate of progression of symptoms	Rapid, florid	Slow, barren
Length of episode prior to assessment	Months or less	Years
Presenting psychopathology		
Psychological intelligibility of symptoms	Present	Absent
State of consciousness, sensorium	Clouding, confusion	Clear
Affective symptoms	Depression, elation, fear	Absent
Affective blunting or incongruity	Absent	Present
Neurotic symptoms	Obsessional, hysterical, anxiety	Absent
Catatonic symptoms	Excitement, agitation	Stupor in absence of affective features
Speech, thinking	Flight of ideas, incoherence	Poverty of speech
Depersonalization and derealization (in Langfeldt's sense)	Absent	Present
Thought insertion, broadcast, hearing, spoken aloud, etc.	Uncertain	Uncertain
Hallucinations	Visual	Bodily, esp. sexual, haptic, olfactory

Continued

Table 8.2 (*Continued*)

Variables	Good prognosis	Poor prognosis
'Characteristic' hallucinations (voices discussing patient, etc.)	Uncertain	Uncertain
Predelusional experiences	Delusional mood, misidentification	Uncertain
Ideas of reference	Uncertain	Uncertain
Delusions	Guilt, grandeur, fantastic, hypochondriacal	Body change, sex change, influence, passivity, persecution
Systematization of delusions	Absent	Present
Early signs of autism	Absent	Present

Table 8.3 Predictors for the general 'level of functioning' (global assessment scale (GAS) score). (From Möller & von Zerssen, 1986)

Prognosis	Predictors of GAS	Explained variance	
		≤10%	11−20%
(−)	Higher socioeconomic status of parents	×	
(−)	Premorbid working dysfunction	×	
(+)	More advanced age at first manifestation	×	
(+)	More advanced age at first hospitalization	×	
(+)	Precipitating factors before first manifestation	×	
(−)	Duration of psychiatric hospitalization (5 years before index admission)	×	
(−)	Duration of occupational disintegration (5 years before index admission)		×
(+)	Lasting heterosexual relationship	×	
(−)	Impairment of working ability (1 year before index admission)		×
(−)	Personality change (1 year before index admission)		×
(−)	Diagnosis of schizophrenia	×	
(−)	Poor psychopathological state at discharge		×
(−)	IMPS superfactor of organic syndrome at discharge	×	
(−)	IMPS superfactor of depressive-apathetic syndrome at discharge	×	
(+)	Ratio of amelioration of the IMPS superfactor of psychotic excitement	×	
(−)	Self-rating factor of paranoid tendencies at discharge		×
(+)	Ratio of amelioration of the self-rating factor of paranoid tendencies		×

(+), Good prognosis; (−), poor prognosis; IMPS, in-patient multidimensional psychiatric scale.

Table 8.4 Product−moment correlations of prognostic scales with the outcome criteria. Munich follow-up study on schizophrenia: samples I and II (replication sample). (From Möller *et al.*, 1986, 1988)

Prognostic Scale	Impairment of 'level of functioning' (GAS)		Paranoid-hallucinatory syndrome (IMPS)		Depressive-apathetic syndrome (IMPS)		Duration of occupational disintegration		Duration of psychiatric hospitalization	
	I	II	I	II	I	II	I	II	I	II
Gittelman−Klein (*n* = 55−70/35−37)	•				••	••			••	••
Goldstein (*n* = 55−61/32−35)					••				•	
Phillips (*n* = 75−78/42−46)	•	•••			••	•••	•	••	•••	••
Vaillant (*n* = 72−76/42−46)	••	••			•	••	••		••	••
Stephens (*n* = 72−76/42−46)	•••	•••	•	••	•	••	••	••	•••	••
Strauss−Carpenter (*n* = 67−77/39−43)	••	••	••		••	••	•	••	•••	•••

Explained variance: •, ≤10%; ••, 11−20%; •••, 21−30%. GAS, global assessment scale; IMPS, in-patient multidimensional psychiatric scale.

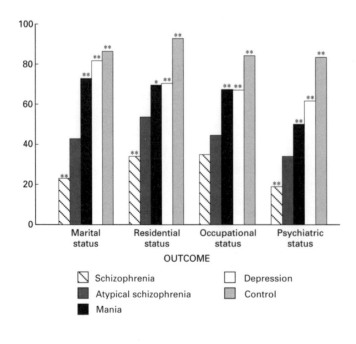

Fig. 8.3 Comparison of good outcomes in atypical schizophrenia with those in schizophrenia, mania, depression and a matched control group. (From Tsuang & Fleming, 1987.) *p < 0.05; **p < 0.01.

has the largest percentage of poor ratings at 45%, compared with 29% in mania, 22% in depression and 4% in the control group. Among schizophrenic patients 35% had a good occupational status compared with 67% of patients with mania, 67% with depression and 84% of controls. Overall, almost 60% of the schizophrenics received a poor rating, compared with 24% for mania, 17% for depression and 2% for the control group (Fig. 8.3).

Similarly, the study by Marneros *et al.* (1991) of 335 patients over 25 years found a difference in outcome between schizophrenia, schizoaffective psychoses and affective psychoses. Depending on the variable studied, a favourable prognosis was found in between 7 and 41% of schizophrenics (7% for psychological deficits and 41% for preservation of full autonomy), in 50−78% for schizoaffective disorders and in 65−93% for affective disorders. Very poor adjustment according to the DAS (WHO, 1988) was found in 27% of the schizophrenics but in only 9% of the schizoaffective patients and in 2% of those with affective disorders. Severe and very severe disturbances of functioning, as measured by the GAS (scores under 50), were found in 70% of the schizophrenics, 21% of the schizoaffective patients and only 4% of those with affective disorders.

In some of these studies, attention was given to the special position of schizoaffective psychoses. In terms of outcome they were mostly placed closer to the affective psychoses than to the schizophrenic psychoses (Marneros *et al.*, 1991).

Conclusion

The review demonstrates that even under the conditions of modern treatment possibilities, schizophrenia is still a severe disease with a relatively poor outcome in about 50% of patients. Compared with other functional psychoses, schizophrenia still has the poorest outcome. The differentiation between schizophrenia and schizoaffective disorder seems meaningful under the aspect that the outcome of schizoaffective psychoses is on average more favourable than the

outcome of schizophrenia, showing some similarities with the outcome of affective psychoses. In comparison with the time before the introduction of neuroleptics, the outcome of schizophrenia is nowadays more favourable, especially with respect to the duration of hospitalization and also with respect to psychopathological states. But it remains open whether this development can be definitely attributed to the introduction of neuroleptics or whether it might also be caused by changes in psychosocial strategies. Severe methodological differences in long-term studies, especially the retrospective long-term studies and the more recent prospective studies, make it impossible to give a final answer to this question. Apart from this special problem, there is no doubt that neuroleptic medication is very efficacious in reducing acute symptoms of schizophrenia and in preventing relapses of schizophrenia. In spite of all the efforts which have been made to establish predictors, the results in this field are controversial, and as far as predictors have been replicated they mostly explain only a low percentage of outcome variance. In particular, psychopathological predictors described in some of the classical long-term studies are, in the light of modern studies, not of such great importance. It would appear that other variables, such as characteristics of the history of the illness and the history of social adaptation, are of greater importance. Of greatest prognostic power are combinations of several predictors in prognosis scales. However, even on such a basis the prognostic capacity is limited and allows only a group differentiation but not a single-case prediction.

References

Achté, K.A. (1961) Der verlauf der schizophrenien und der schizophreniformen psychosen. *Acta Psychiatrica Scandinavica*, **36** (Suppl. 155), 1−273.

Achté, K.A. (1967) On prognosis and rehabilitation in schizophrenic and paranoid psychoses. *Acta Psychiatrica Scandinavica*, **43** (Suppl. 196), 1−217.

Affleck, J.W., Burns, J. & Forrest, A.D. (1976) Long-term follow-up of schizophrenic patients in Edinburgh. *Acta Psychiatrica Scandinavica*, **53**, 227−237.

An der Heiden, W. & Krumm, B. (1985) Does outpatient treatment reduce hospital stay in schizophrenics? *European*

Archives of Psychiatry and Neurological Sciences, **235**, 26−31.

An der Heiden, W., Krumm, B. & Häfner, H. (1989) *Die Wirksamkeit ambulanter psychiatrischer Versorgung. Ein Modell zur Evaluation extramuraler Dienste.* Springer, Berlin.

APA (1980) *Diagnostic and Statistical Manual of Mental Disorders*, 3rd edn. American Psychiatric Association, Washington DC.

APA (1987) *Diagnostic and Statistical Manual of Mental Disorders*, 3rd revised edn. DSM-III-R. American Psychiatric Association, Washington DC.

Astrup, C. & Noreik, K. (1966) *Functional Psychoses. Diagnostic and Prognostic Models.* Charles C. Thomas, Springfield.

Biehl, H., Maurer, K., Jung, E., Krüger, G. & Bauer-Schubart, C. (1988) Reported symptoms in schizophrenic patients within five years of the onset of illness. A report from the prospective Rhine Neckar cohort study. In Dencker, S.J. & Kulhanek, F. (eds) *Treatment Resistance in Schizophrenia*, pp. 108−118. Vieweg, Braunschweig.

Bland, R.C., Parker, J.H. & Orn, H. (1976) Prognosis in schizophrenia. A ten-year follow-up of first admissions. *Archives of General Psychiatry*, **33**, 949−954.

Bleuler, E. (1911) Dementia praecox oder Gruppe der Schizophrenien. In Aschaffenburg, G. (ed.) *Handbuch der Psychiatrie.* spez. Teil, 4. Abt. Deuticke, Leipzig.

Bleuler, M. (1941) *Krankheitsverlauf, Persönlichkeit und Verwandtschaft Schizophrener und ihre gegenseitigen Beziehungen.* Thieme, Leipzig.

Bleuler, M. (1972) *Die schizophrenen Geistesstörungen im Lichte langjähriger Kranken- und Familiengeschichten.* Thieme, Stuttgart.

Bleuler, M., Huber, G., Gross, G. & Schüttler, R. (1976) Der langfristige Verlauf schizophrener Psychosen. Gemeinsame Ergebnisse zweier Untersuchungen. *Nervenarzt*, **47**, 477−481.

Brown, G.W., Bone, M., Dalison, B. & Wing, J.K. (1966) *Schizophrenia and Social Care.* Oxford University Press, Oxford.

Carpenter, W.T. & Strauss, J.S. (1991) The prediction of outcome in schizophrenia. IV. Eleven-year follow-up of the Washington IPSS cohort. *Journal of Nervous and Mental Disease*, **179**, 517−525.

Ciompi, L. & Müller, C. (1976) *Lebensweg und Alter der Schizophrenen. Eine katamnestische Langzeitstudie bis ins Senium.* Springer, Berlin.

Clare, A.W. & Cairns, V.E. (1978) Design, development and use of a standardized interview to assess social maladjustment and dysfunction in community studies. *Psychological Medicine*, **8**, 589−604.

Cooper, J.E., Kendell, R.E., Gurland, B.J., Sharpe, L., Copeland, J.R.M. & Simon, R. (1972) *Psychiatric Diagnoses in New York and London.* Oxford University Press, Oxford.

Cranach, M. von & Strauss, A. (1978) Die internationale Vergleichbarkeit psychiatrischer Diagnosen. In Häfner, H. (ed.) *Psychiatrische Epidemiologie*, pp. 209−220. Springer, Berlin.

Davis, J.M., Schaffer, C.B., Killian, G.A., Kinnard, C. & Chan, C. (1980) Important issues in the drug treatment of schizophrenia. *Schizophrenia Bulletin*, **6**, 70−87.

Faltermaier, T., Hecht, H. & Wittchen, H.U. (1987) *Die Social Interview Schedule.* (German modified version) Roderer, Regensburg.

Feighner, J.P., Robins, B., Guze, R., Woodruff, R.A. & Winokur, B. (1972) Diagnostic criteria for use in psychiatric research. *Archives of General Psychiatry*, **26**, 57−63.

Gerloff, W. (1936) Über Verlauf und Prognose der Schizophrenie. *Archiv für Psychiatrie und Nervenkrank Leiten*, **106**, 585−597.

Goldberg, S.C., Schooler, N.R., Hogarty, G.E. & Roper, M. (1977) Prediction of relapse in schizophrenic outpatients treated by drug and sociotherapy. *Archives of General Psychiatry*, **34**, 171−184.

Grossman, L.S., Harrow, M., Goldberg, J.F. & Fichtner, C.G. (1991) Outcome of schizoaffective disorder at two long-term follow-ups: comparisons with outcome of schizophrenia and affective disorders. *American Journal of Psychiatry*, **148**, 1359−1365.

Gunderson, J.G., Carpenter, W.T. & Strauss, J.S. (1975) Borderline and schizophrenic patients: a comparative study. *American Journal of Psychiatry*, **132**, 1257−1264.

Harding, C.M., Brooks, G.W., Ashikaga, T., Strauss, J.S. & Breier, A. (1987) The Vermont longitudinal study of persons with severe mental illness. I. Methodology, study sample and overall status 32 years later. *American Journal of Psychiatry*, **144**, 718−726.

Hargreaves, W.A., Glick, I.D., Drues, J., Showstack, J.A. & Feigenbaum, E. (1977) Short vs. long hospitalization. VI. Two-year follow-up results for schizophrenics. *Archives of General Psychiatry*, **34**, 305−311.

Hawk, A.B., Carpenter, T.W. & Strauss, J.S. (1975) Diagnostic criteria and five-year outcome in schizophrenia: a report from the International Pilot Study of Schizophrenia. *Archives of General Psychiatry*, **32**, 343−347.

Henisz, J.A. (1966) A follow-up study of schizophrenic patients. *Comprehensive Psychiatry*, **12**, 524−528.

Hirsch, S.R., Gaind, R., Rohde, P., Stevens, B. & Wing, J.K. (1973) Outpatient maintenance treatment of chronic schizophrenics with fluphenazine decanoate injections: a double-blind placebo trial. *British Medical Journal*, **1**, 633−637.

Hogarty, G.E. (1977) Treatment and the course of schizophrenia. *Schizophrenia Bulletin*, **3**, 587−599.

Hogarty, G.E., Goldberg, S., Schooler, N. & Ulrich, R. (1974) Drug and sociotherapy in the aftercare of schizophrenic patients. II. Two-year relapse rates. *Archives of General Psychiatry*, **31**, 603−608.

Hogarty, G.E., Anderson, C.M., Reiss, D.J. *et al.* (1986) Family psychoeducation, social skills training, and maintenance chemotherapy in the aftercare treatment of schizophrenia. I. One-year effects of a controlled study on relapse and expressed emotion. *Archives of General Psychiatry*, **43**, 633−642.

Holmboe, R. & Astrup, C. (1957) A follow-up study of 255 patients with acute schizophrenia and schizophreniform psychoses. *Acta Psychiatrica Scandinavica*, **32** (Suppl. 115), 1−61.

Huber, G., Gross, G. & Schüttler, R. (1979) *Schizophrenie. Eine verlaufs- und sozialpsychiatrische Langzeitstudie.* Springer, Berlin.

Johanson, E. (1958) A study of schizophrenia in the male. *Acta*

Psychiatrica Scandinavica, **33** (Suppl. 125), 1–132.

Johnstone, E.C. (1991) What is crucial for the long-term outcome of schizophrenia? In Häfner, H. & Gattaz, W.F. (eds) *Search for the Causes of Schizophrenia*, Vol. II, pp. 67–76. Springer, Berlin.

Johnstone, E.C., Crow, T.J., Johnson, A.L. & Macmillan, J.F. (1986) The Northwick Park study of first episodes of schizophrenia. I. Presentation of the illness and problems relating to admission. *British Journal of Psychiatry*, **148**, 115–120.

Kant, O. (1940) Types and analyses of the clinical pictures of recovered schizophrenics. *Psychiatric Quarterly*, **14**, 676–700.

Kant, O. (1941a) Study of a group of recovered schizophrenic patients. *Psychiatric Quarterly*, **15**, 262–283.

Kant, O. (1941b) A comparative study of recovered and deteriorated schizophrenic patients. *Journal of Nervous and Mental Disease*, **93**, 616–624.

Kendell, R.E. (1975) *The Role of Diagnosis in Psychiatry*. Blackwell Scientific Publications, Oxford.

Kraepelin, E. (1913) *Psychiatrie*. Barth, Leipzig.

Kringlen, E. (1980) Principles and methods in psychiatric follow-up studies. In Schimmelpenning, G.W. (ed.) *Psychiatrische Verlaufsforschung. Methoden und Ergebnisse*, pp. 19–32. Huber, Bern.

Landmark, J. (1982) A manual for the assessment of schizophrenia. *Acta Psychiatrica Scandinavica*, **65** (Suppl. 298), 1–88.

Langfeldt, G. (1937) The prognosis in schizophrenia and the factors influencing the course of disease. *Acta Psychiatrica Scandinavica*, (Suppl. 13), 1–228.

Langfeldt, G. (1956) The prognosis of schizophrenia. *Acta Psychiatrica Scandinavica*, (Suppl. 110), 1–66.

Leff, J. (1987) A model of schizophrenic vulnerability to environmental factors. In Häfner, H., Gattaz, W.F. & Janzarik, W. (eds) *Search for the Causes of Schizophrenia*, Vol. I, pp. 317–330. Springer, Berlin.

Leff, J. & Wing, J.K. (1971) Trials of maintenance therapy in schizophrenia. *British Medical Journal*, **III**, 599–604.

Leff, J., Sartorius, N., Jablensky, A. *et al.* (1991) The International Pilot Study of Schizophrenia: five-year follow-up findings. In Häfner, H. & Gattaz, W.F. (eds) *Search for the Causes of Schizophrenia*, Vol. II, pp. 57–66. Springer-Verlag, Berlin.

Leonhard, K. (1966) *Aufteilung der endogenen Psychosen*. Akademie Verlag, Berlin.

Lo, W. & Lo, T. (1977) A ten-year follow-up study of Chinese schizophrenics in Hong Kong. *British Journal of Psychiatry*, **131**, 63–66.

Lorr, M. & Klett, C.J. (1967) *Manual for the Inpatient Multidimensional Psychiatric Scale* (revised). Consulting Psychologists Press, Palo Alto.

Marneros, A., Deister, A. & Rohde, A. (1991) *Affektive, schizoaffektive und schizophrene Psychosen. Eine vergleichende Langzeitstudie*. Springer, Berlin.

Martin, M. (1991) *Verlauf der Schizophrenie im Jugendalter unter Rehabilitationsbedingungen*. Enke, Stuttgart.

Mauz, F. (1930) *Die Prognostik der endogenen Psychosen*. Thieme, Leipzig.

May, P.R.A., Tuma, A.H. & Dixon, W.J. (1976) Schizophrenia — A follow-up study of results of treatment. *Archives of General Psychiatry*, **33**, 474–478.

Mintz, J., O'Brien, C.P. & Luborsky, L. (1976) Predicting the outcome of psychotherapy for schizophrenics. *Archives of General Psychiatry*, **33**, 1183–1187.

Möller, H.J. (1989) Standardisierte psychiatrische Befunderhebung. In Kisker, K.P., Lauter, H., Meyer, J.-E., Müller, C. & Strömgren, E. (eds) *Psychiatrie der Gegenwart*, 3rd edn, Vol. 9, pp. 13–45. Springer, Berlin.

Möller, H.J. (1990) Neuroleptische Langzeittherapie schizophrener Erkrankungen. In Heinrich, K. (ed.) *Leitlinien neuroleptischer Therapie*, pp. 97–115. Springer, Berlin.

Möller, H.J. & von Zerssen, D. (1980) Probleme und Verbesserungsmöglichkeiten der psychiatrischen Diagnostik. In Biefang, S. (ed.) *Evaluationsforschung in der Psychiatrie. Fragestellungen und Methoden*, pp. 167–207. Enke, Stuttgart.

Möller, H.J. & von Zerssen, D. (1982) Psychopathometrische Verfahren. I. Allgemeiner Teil. *Nervenarzt*, **53**, 493–503.

Möller, H.J. & von Zerssen, D. (1983) Psychopathometrische Verfahren. II. Standardisierte Beurteilungsverfahren. *Nervenarzt*, **54**, 1–16.

Möller, H.J. & von Zerssen, D. (1986) *Der Verlauf schizophrener Psychosen unter den gegenwärtigen Behandlungsbedingungen*. Springer, Berlin.

Möller, H.J., Pirée, S. & von Zerssen, D. (1978) Psychiatrische Klassifikation. *Nervenarzt*, **49**, 445–455.

Möller, H.J., Scharl, W. & von Zerssen, D. (1984) Strauss–Carpenter–Skala: Überprüfung ihres prognostischen Wertes für das 5-Jahres-'outcome' schizophrener Patienten. *European Archives of Psychiatry and Neurological Sciences*, **234**, 112–117.

Möller, H.J., Schmid-Bode, W. & von Zerssen, D. (1986) Prediction of long-term outcome in schizophrenia by prognostic scales. *Schizophrenia Bulletin*, **12**, 225–234.

Möller, H.J., von Zerssen, D., Werner-Eilert, K. & Wüschner-Stockheim, M. (1982) Outcome in schizophrenic and similar paranoid psychoses. *Schizophrenia Bulletin*, **8**, 99–108.

Möller, H.J., von Zerssen, D., Wüschner-Stockheim, M. & Werner-Eilert, K. (1981) Die prognostische Bedeutung psychopathometrischer Aufnahme- und Entlassungsbefunddaten schizophrener Patienten. *Archiv für Psychiatrie und Nervenkrank Leiten*, **231**, 13–34.

Möller, H.J., Schmid-Bode, W., Cording-Tömmel, C., Wittchen, H.U., Zaudig, M. & von Zerssen, D. (1988) Psychopathological and social outcome in schizophrenia versus affective/schizoaffective psychoses and prediction of poor outcome in schizophrenia: results from a 5–8 years follow-up. *Acta Psychiatrica Scandinavica*, **77**, 379–389.

Möller, H.J., Hohe-Schramm, M., Cording-Tömmel, C. *et al.* (1989) The classification of functional psychoses and its implications for prognosis. *British Journal of Psychiatry*, **154**, 467–472.

Mombour, W. (1975) Klassifikation, Patientenstatistik, Register. In Kisker, K.P., Meyer, J.E., Müller, C. & Strömgren, E. (eds) *Psychiatrie der Gegenwart*, 2nd edn, Vol. 3, pp. 81–118. Springer, Berlin.

Mosher, L.R. & Keith, S.J. (1979) Research on the psychosocial treatment of schizophrenics: a summary report. *American Journal of Psychiatry*, **136**, 623–631.

Müller, P. (ed.) (1982) Die Patienten und das Ergebnis der Rezidivprophylaxe. In *Zur Rezidivprophylaxe schizophrener Psychosen*, pp. 15–23. Enke, Stuttgart.

Niskanen, P. & Achté, K. (1972) *The Course and Prognosis of Schizophrenic Psychoses in Helsinki. A Comparative Study of First Admissions in 1950, 1960 and 1965*. Monographs from the Psychiatric Clinic of the Helsinki University Central Hospital, No. 4.

Norris, V. (1959) *Mental Illness in London*. Maudsley Monographs No. 6. Chapman and Hall, London.

Overall, J.E. & Gorham, D.R. (1962) The brief psychiatric rating scale. *Psychological Reports*, **10**, 799–812.

Pietzcker, A. & Gaebel, W. (1983) Prediction of 'natural' course, relapse and prophylactic response in schizophrenic patients. *Pharmacopsychiatry*, **16**, 206–211.

Pokorny, A.D., Thornby, J., Kaplan, H.W. & Ball, D. (1976) Prediction of chronicity in psychiatric patients. *Archives of General Psychiatry*, **33**, 932–937.

Prudo, R. & Blum, H.M. (1987) Five-year outcome and prognosis in schizophrenia: a report from the London Field Research Centre of the International Pilot Study of Schizophrenia. *British Journal of Psychiatry*, **150**, 345–354.

Renton, C.A., Affleck, J.W., Carstairs, G.M. & Forrest, A.D. (1963) A follow-up of schizophrenic patients in Edinburgh. *Acta Psychiatrica Scandinavica*, **39**, 548–581.

Retterstøl, N. (1978) The Scandinavian concept of reactive psychosis, schizophreniform psychosis and schizophrenia. *Psychiatric Clinics*, **11**, 180–187.

Retterstøl, N. (1983) Course of paranoid psychoses in relation to diagnostic grouping. *Psychiatric Clinics*, **16**, 198–206.

Rifkin, A., Quitkin, F., Rabiner, C.J. & Klein, D.F. (1977) Fluphenazine decanoate, fluphenazine hydrochloride given orally, and placebo in remitted schizophrenics. Relapse rate after one year. *Archives of General Psychiatry*, **34**, 43–47.

Sartorius, N., Jablensky, A., Ernberg, G., Leff, J., Korten A. & Gulbinat, W. (1987) Course of schizophrenia in different countries: some results of a WHO international comparative 5-year follow-up study. In Häfner, H., Gattaz, W.F. & Janzarik, W. (eds) *Search for the Causes of Schizophrenia*, Vol. I, pp. 107–113. Springer, Berlin.

Schneider, K. (1987) *Klinische Psychopathologie*, 13th edn. Thieme, Stuttgart.

Schubart, C., Krumm, B., Biehl, H. & Schwarz, R. (1986a) Measurement of social disability in a schizophrenic patient group. Definition, assessment and outcome over 2 years in a cohort of schizophrenic patients of recent onset. *Social Psychiatry*, **21**, 1–9.

Schubart, C., Schwarz, R., Krumm, B. & Biehl, H. (1986b) *Schizophrenie und soziale Anpassung. Eine prospektive Längsschnittuntersuchung*. Springer, Berlin.

Schwarz, R., Biehl, H., Krumm, B. & Schubart, C. (1980) Case-finding and characteristics of schizophrenic patients of recent onset in Mannheim. A report from the WHO collaborative study on the assessment of disability associated with schizophrenic disorders. *Acta Psychiatrica Scandinavica*, **62** (Suppl. 285), 212–219.

Scottish Schizophrenia Research Group (1992) The Scottish

first episode schizophrenia study. VIII. Five-year follow-up: clinical and psychosocial findings. *British Journal of Psychiatry*, **161**, 496–500.

Seidenstücker, G. & Baumann, U. (1978) Multimethodale Diagnostik. In Baumann, U., Berbalk, H. & Seidenstücker, G. (eds) *Klinische Psychologie. Trends in Forschung und Praxis*, I, pp. 134–183. Huber, Bern.

Shepherd, M. (1957) *A Study of the Major Psychoses in an English Country*. Chapman and Hall, London.

Spitzer, J., Endicott, R.L. & Fleiss, L. (1976) The global assessment scale. A procedure for measuring overall severity of psychiatric disturbances. *Archives of General Psychiatry*, **33**, 766–771.

Spitzer, J., Endicott, J.E. & Robins, E. (1977) *Research Diagnostic Criteria (RDC) for a Selected Group of Functional Disorders*, 3rd edn. New York State Psychiatric Institute, New York.

Spitzer, R.L., Williams, J.B.W. & Gibbon, M. (1987) *Structured Clinical Interview for DSM-III-R. Interview and Manual*. New York State Psychiatric Institute, New York.

Stephens, J.H. (1970) Long-term course and prognosis in schizophrenia. *Seminars in Psychiatry*, **2**, 464–485.

Stephens, J.H. & Astrup, C. (1965) Treatment outcome in 'process' and 'non-process' schizophrenics treated by 'A' and 'B' types of therapists. *Journal of Nervous and Mental Disease*, **140**, 440–465.

Strauss, J.S. & Carpenter, W.T. (1972) The prediction of outcome in schizophrenia. I. Characteristics of outcome. *Archives of General Psychiatry*, **27**, 739–746.

Strauss, J.S. & Carpenter, W.T. (1974) Characteristic symptoms and outcome in schizophrenia. *Archives of General Psychiatry*, **30**, 429–434.

Strauss, J.S. & Carpenter, W.T. (1977) The prediction of outcome in schizophrenia. III. Five-year outcome and its predictors. *Archives of General Psychiatry*, **34**, 159–163.

Tsuang, M.T. & Fleming, J.A. (1987) Long-term outcome of schizophrenia and other psychoses. In Häfner, H., Gattaz, W.F. & Janzarik, W. (eds) *Search for the Causes of Schizophrenia*, Vol. I, pp. 88–97. Springer, Berlin.

Tsuang, M.T. & Winokur, G. (1974) Criteria for subtyping schizophrenia. Clinical differentiation of hebephrenic and paranoid schizophrenia. *Archives of General Psychiatry*, **31**, 43–47.

Tsuang, M.T., Woolson, R.F. & Fleming, J.A. (1979) Long-term outcome of major psychoses. I. Schizophrenia and affective disorders compared with psychiatrically symptom-free surgical conditions. *Archives of General Psychiatry*, **36**, 1295–1301.

Vaillant, G. (1962) The prediction of recovery in schizophrenia. *Journal of Nervous and Mental Disease*, **135**, 534–543.

Watt, D.C., Katz, K. & Shepherd, M. (1983) The natural history of schizophrenia: a 5-year prospective follow-up of a representative sample of schizophrenics by means of a standardized clinical and social assessment. *Psychological Medicine*, **13**, 663–670.

Weissman, M.M. & Sholomskas, J.K. (1981) The assessment of social adjustment: an update. *Archives of General Psychiatry*, **38**, 1250–1258.

Welner, J. & Strömgren, E. (1958) Clinical and genetic studies on benign schizophreniform psychoses based on follow-up. *Acta Psychiatrica Scandinavica*, **33**, 377–399.

WHO (1979) *Schizophrenia. An International Follow-up Study.* Wiley, Chichester.

WHO (1988) *WHO Psychiatric Disability Assessment Schedule (WHO/DAS).* World Health Organization, Geneva.

Wing, J.K., Cooper, J.E. & Sartorius, N. (1972) *Instruction Manual for the Present State Examination and CATEGO.* Institute of Psychiatry, London.

Wing, J.K., Cooper, J.E. & Sartorius, N. (1974) *The Measurement and Classification of Psychiatric Symptoms.* Cambridge University Press, Cambridge.

Wittenborn, J.R., McDonald, D.C. & Maurer, H.S. (1977) Persisting symptoms in schizophrenia predicted by background factors. *Archives of General Psychiatry*, **34**, 1059–1061.

WPA (1983) *Diagnostic Criteria for Schizophrenic and Affective Psychoses.* World Psychiatric Association, Washington.

von Zerssen, D. (1979) Klinisch-psychiatrische Selbstbeurteilungsfragebögen. In Baumann, U., Berbalk, H. & Seidenstücker, G. (eds) *Klinische Psychologie. Trends in Forschung und Praxis*, Vol. II, pp. 130–159. Huber, Bern.

von Zerssen, D. (1990) Langzeitverläufe funktioneller psychischer Störungen: Veränderung versus Konstanz. In Baumann, U., Fähndrich, E., Stieglitz, R.-D. & Woggon, B. (eds) *Veränderungsmessung in Psychiatrie und Klinischer Psychologie*, pp. 46–76. Profil, Munich.

von Zerssen, D. & Möller, H.J. (1980) Psychopathometrische Verfahren in der psychiatrischen Therapieforschung. In Biefang, S. (ed.) *Evaluationsforschung in der Psychiatrie: Fragestellungen und Methoden*, pp. 129–166. Enke, Stuttgart.

von Zerssen, D., León, C.A., Möller, H.J., Wittchen, H.U., Pfister, H. & Sartorius, N. (1990) Care strategies for schizophrenic patients in a transcultural comparison. *Comprehensive Psychiatry*, **31**, 398–408.

Chapter 9
Depression and Schizophrenia

S. G. SIRIS

Introduction

Much psychiatric wisdom has been generated on the basis of Kraepelin's astute separation of what we now know as mood disorders from what we now know as schizophrenia. Nevertheless, the fact has remained, and been noted for many years, that a goodly proportion of patients with schizophrenia, no matter how defined, suffer from 'depression-like' symptomatology during the longitudinal course of their disorder.

Historically, Bleuler noted early on that symptoms of depression often occur during the course of schizophrenia (Bleuler, 1950). Subsequently, the concept of depression in schizophrenia became largely steeped in psychoanalytically influenced writings. Mayer–Gross discussed depression in schizophrenia as being a denial of the future or a reaction of despair to the psychotic experience (McGlashan & Carpenter, 1976b). Others found themes of loss to be central to the dynamics of depressed schizophrenic patients (Semrad, 1966; Roth, 1970; Miller & Sonnenberg, 1973). Semrad (1966) also considered that the depression of these patients represented important progress out of a more pathological narcissistic regressed state

which more immediately followed the florid psychosis, although he also considered this state to be influenced by pain and/or the despair of an 'empty ego'. Both Semrad and Eissler (1951) were of the opinion that the occurrence of depression in schizophrenia represented a moment of psychotherapeutic opportunity, with the possibility of insight and mastery which would attend the less primitive defensive state that was then manifest. In this regard, depression was interpreted as having positive prognostic significance.

Later, however, more data-based research was collected which documented the course, frequency and intensity of depression in schizophrenia (Bowers & Astrachan, 1967; McGlashan & Carpenter, 1976a; Siris, 1991). As the definitions of both depression and schizophrenia became more operationalized over time, and when medication treatment of the subjects involved in the studies became more highly controlled, investigations began to indicate that the outcomes are often less favourable in those schizophrenic patients who manifest depression during the longitudinal course of their disoders. Such depressions were noted to be associated with

128

higher risks of relapse or rehospitalization (Mandel *et al.*, 1982; Roy *et al.*, 1983; Johnson, 1988; Birchwood *et al.*, 1993), as well as with an increased rate of suicide (Roy *et al.*, 1983; Drake & Cotton, 1986; Caldwell & Gottesman, 1990).

Various descriptors have been applied over the years to states of depression occurring in the course of schizophrenia, and nosological agreement has been difficult to achieve. Although the designation is controversial and may even be misleading, a full depressive syndrome presenting in the longitudinal course of schizophrenia has often come to be called postpsychotic depression. Indeed, despite the problems with its name, postpsychotic depression has been listed as a diagnosis in the *International Classification of Disease* ICD-10 (WHO, 1988), and is also included in the appendix of the *Diagnostic and Statistical Manual* DSM-IV (APA, 1994). Previously, although postpsychotic depression *per se* had not been discussed in either ICD or DSM manuals, 'depression superimposed on residual schizophrenia' was included as a diagnostic category in the research diagnostic criteria (RDC) (Spitzer *et al.*, 1978).

Whatever its designation, depressive-like symptomatology clearly plays a role in the devastating long-term character of schizophrenia. The subjective state involved leads to great personal suffering for the patients afflicted and for their families. No doubt the mood state also contributes to the associated loss of social and vocational capacity which these individuals experience; this is exacerbated by their reduction in energy level, absence of self-confidence and impaired concentration.

Many explanations and discussions have been advanced in attempts to describe and/or explain depression in schizophrenia, and address aspects of its appropriate treatment. Yet, truly firm conclusions have not so far been drawn in a number of areas. Probably this is because the presenting condition is heterogeneous. Therefore, after this chapter has discussed the topic of incidence and prevalence, it will go on to address a working differential diagnosis of 'depression' in schizophrenia. Then the validation of the construct, approaches to treatment and further implications

of the concept of such an associated syndrome in the course of schizophrenia will be discussed.

Incidence and prevalence of depression in schizophrenia

Close to 30 studies have been published and reviewed concerning the occurrence of depression-like symptomatology over the longitudinal course of schizophrenia (Siris, 1991). These vary substantially in a number of characteristics, including the definition employed for schizophrenia, the definition of depression, the duration observed, the treatment situation of the patients and in-patient vs. out-patient status. What is remarkable is that no matter what the definitions or conditions, all the studies found at least some meaningful rate of depression in the course of schizophrenia.

The rate of depression described in all these studies varied from a low of 7%, in a cross-sectional assessment study of chronically hospitalized DSM-III schizophrenic patients, which nevertheless emphasized postpsychotic depression's distinct nature from 'negative' symptoms (Hirsch *et al.*, 1989), to a high of 65% in a study which followed 'Feighner-criteria' schizophrenic patients for whom an effort had been made to exclude neuroleptic-induced akinesia, with ratings at least every 3 months, for 3 years after they had been free of acute psychotic symptoms (Johnson, 1988). The modal rate for all these various investigations was 25%, a rate which has consistently seemed to be a benchmark in such reports (Winokur, 1972; McGlashan & Carpenter, 1976b; Johnson, 1981a; Mandel *et al.*, 1982; Siris, 1991). Table 9.1 describes the studies that have reported incidence or prevalence figures for episodes of depression in the course of schizophrenia as defined by recent common criteria such as DSM-III, RDC, ICD, *Present State Examination* (PSE), International Pilot Study of Schizophrenia (IPSS), New Haven Schizophrenia Index, Feighner, CATEGO or Schneiderian first rank. The very diversity of diagnostic criteria for schizophrenia and depression, and the variety of patient settings and means of observation sup-

Table 9.1 Studies reporting the incidence or prevalence of secondary depression in cases of schizophrenia diagnosed by popular criteria. (After Siris, 1991)

Study (*n*)	Definition of psychosis	Definition of postpsychotic interval	Definition of depression	Percentage depressed	Comment
McGlashan and Carpenter (1976a) (*n* = 30)	IPSS: more than 90% chance of schizophrenia	Cross-sectional assessment at discharge and at 1-year follow-up	Depression as per PSE	43 (at discharge) 50 (cummulative as per 1-year follow-up)	Depression dimension of PSE had a bimodal distribution
Weissman *et al.* (1977) (*n* = 50)	Out-patients with New Haven Schizophrenia Index diagnosis of schizophrenia	Point prevalence	Raskin scale score of 7 or more	28	No differences in demography of depressed group
Van Putten and May (1978) (*n* = 94)	Newly admitted patients with Feighner criteria for schizophrenia	Length of acute hospital stay	Increase in BPRS depression scale rating	38	57% for patients with akinesia 22% for patients without akinesia
Knights *et al.* (1979) (*n* = 37)	CATEGO criteria: 87% = unequivocal schizophrenia	6 months or until relapse while on depot neuroleptic	PSE-based depression rating scale	54	43% had onset or increase in depression ratings during interval
Roy (1980) (*n* = 100)	DSM-III chronic paranoid schizophrenia	Chart review for mean of 6 years	DSM-III for major depressive disorder, secondary type	30	Depressed mood as assessed by PSE: 9% depressed at follow-up
Johnson (1981a)	Schizophrenia diagnosis based on Schneiderian first-rank symptoms		Lowered mood state lasting at least 1 week		The risk of an episode of depression was 3 times the risk of an episode of psychosis for patients maintained on depot neuroleptic
Cohort A (*n* = 41)		Cohort A: 2 months prospective prevalence study	Cohort A: HAM-D rating scale score and/or BDI score = 15 or more	Cohort A: 24	
Cohort B (*n* = 100)	Out-patients free of acute symptoms for at least 3 months	Cohort B: cross-sectional prevalence	Cohort B: nurses' rating and self-rating	Cohort B: 26	
Cohort C (*n* = 30)	Patients maintained on depot neuroleptic	Chort C: 2-year follow-up	Cohort C: HAM-D and/ or BDI = 15 or more	Cohort C: 50 (excluding episodes associated with psychotic relapse)	

Continued

Table 9.1 (*Continued*)

Study (n)	Definition of psychosis	Definition of postpsychotic interval	Definition of depression	Percentage depressed	Comment
Siris *et al.* (1981) (n = 50)	Acutely admitted in-patients diagnosed by RDC	Duration of hospitalization after resolution of flagrant psychotic symptoms	RDC for major or minor depression by chart review of symptoms	6 (major depression) 22 (minor depression)	34% appeared depressed to staff 40% manifested subjective sadness
Roy (1981) (n = 100)	DSM-III for schizophrenia	Chart review: 4–10 years	Treated for depression by antidepressants or ECT	39	More early parental loss among patients with depression
Möller and von Zerssen (1982) (n = 81)	In-patients with schizophrenia (77%) *or* paranoid psychosis (23%) by ICD criteria	Point prevalence at hospital discharge	Three consecutive actual mood scores at or above 21	23	17% developed new episodes of depression
Guze *et al.* (1983) and Martin *et al.* (1985) (n = 44)	Feighner criteria for schizophrenia	Retrospective survey at 6–12 years follow-up	Feighner criteria for depression	57	Criteria were not exactly those of Feighner, but were extremely close
Summers *et al.* (1983) Cohort A (n = 161)	RDC for schizophrenia Cohort A: chronic	Cohort A: at admission to aftercare	Cohort A: SCL-90 scales	Cohort A: as a group schizophrenics more depressed than normals	Acute and chronic patients found to have comparable depression symptoms after hospitalization
Cohort B: (n = 72)	Cohort B: acute	Cohort B: past month assessment (average 2.13 years post discharge)	Cohort B: two composite depression scales from KAS	Cohort B: 37% poor, 68% poor *or* equivocal	
Watt and Shepherd (1983) (as reported in Roy, 1986) (n = 121)	Chronic schizophrenia (PSE criteria)	PSE at admission and 1 month, 1 year and 5 years after discharge	PSE assessment of depression syndrome	40 at 1 month and 1 year ('severe' in 25% of these); 19 at 5 years	Prospective epidemiological study

Continued on p.132

Table 9.1 (*Continued*)

Study (*n*)	Definition of psychosis	Definition of postpsychotic interval	Definition of depression	Percentage depressed	Comment
Munro *et al.* (1984) (*n* = 100)	Out-patients with DSM-III for schizophrenia	Clinic cross-sectional prevalence	Carroll rating scale	41	10% severe depression; 18% moderate depression; 13% mild depression
Leff *et al.* (1988) (*n* = 31)	Newly admitted patients with PSE/CATEGO definition of schizophrenia	Until discharged or until 6 months	Depressed mood as assessed by PSE	45	Patients were not on neuroleptics Correlation between improvement in depressive symptoms and in psychosis suggested depression was an 'integral part' of these cases
Johnson (1988) (*n* = 80)	Feighner criteria for schizophrenia Presence of Schneiderian first-rank symptoms	Period began when patients were free of all acute symptoms Period A: 0−12 months Period B: 12−36 months (ratings at least every 3 months)	Altered mood state lasting at least 7 days with HAM-D and BDI each more than 15 Meet DSM-III for depression	13−30 for period A 65 for period B	Akinesia excluded by physical examination for parkinsonism Risk of psychotic relapse was significantly higher for patients depressed in second or third years than for patients depressed in first year or not depressed
Hirsch *et al.* (1989)	DSM-III for schizophrenia *Also*				Depressive symptoms are less common in chronic schizophrenic in-patients than would be predicted if they were a manifestation of negative symptoms or neuroleptic-induced parkinsonism Depressed patients had more auditory hallucinations in cohort B
Cohort A (*n* = 46)	Cohort A: thought by nurses to be depressed	Cohorts A and B: cross-sectional assessment	Cohort A: HAM-D and BDI	Cohort A: 7	
Cohort B (*n* = 196) (also Barnes *et al.*, 1989)	Cohort B: long-stay in-patients		Cohort B: item number 23 ('depression') of PSE	Cohort B: 13	

Continued

Table 9.1 (*Continued*)

Study (n)	Definition of psychosis	Definition of postpsychotic interval	Definition of depression	Percentage depressed	Comment
Cohort C (n = 44)	Cohort C: out-patients with no florid symptoms in previous 6 months	Cohort C: repeated bimonthly assessments for 1 year while randomly assigned to depot neuroleptic or placebo	Cohort C: depression item = 2 or more on Manchester scale	Cohort C: 73 of psychotic relapses were preceded prodromal symptoms which included depression	
Bandelow *et al.* (1991) (n = 364)	ICD-9 and RDC for schizophrenia	Point prevalence 3 months after discharge and stabilization on neuroleptic medication for an acute psychotic episde	BPRS anxious– depression scale ≥10	19.5	Two other scales for depression rated between 26.6 and 42.8% of patients as depressed, depending on cut-off scores; 35.7% of patients were rated as depressed when a milder BPRS cut-off was employed
Brier *et al.* (1991) (n = 58)	RDC diagnosis of schizophrenia (n = 42) or schizoaffective disorder (mostly schizophrenic) (n = 16, of whom 12 were depressed type)	Average follow-up period = 6 ± 3 years	Episode of major depression as diagnosed by RDC	24	38% of the sample had made at least one suicide attempt
Birchwood *et al.* (1993) (n = 49)	CATEGO class 's' for schizophrenia	Randomly selected from urban out-patient 'depot' treatment clinic	Score of at least 15 on BDI	29	Patients with lesser sense of control concerning their illness were more likely to manifest depression

Continued on p. 134

Table 9.1 (*Continued*)

Study (*n*)	Definition of psychosis	Definition of postpsychotic interval	Definition of depression	Percentage depressed	Comment
Harrow *et al.* (1994) (*n* = 54)	RDC diagnosis of schizophrenia	Prevalence during 1 year preceding follow-up interview, which was an average of 4.5 years after hospital discharge for index psychotic episode	Presence of a full depressive syndrome by RDC	37	Patients receiving neuroleptics were more likely to have depression (*P* < 0.01) or experience anhedonia (*P* < 0.001) Depression finding remains when psychosis was controlled for

IPSS, International Pilot Study of Schizophrenia; PSE, *Present State Examination*; BPRS, brief psychiatric rating scale; DSM, *Diagnostic and Statistical Manual*; HAM-D, Hamilton depression (scale); BDI, Beck depression inventory; RDC, research diagnostic criteria; ECT, electroconvulsive therapy; ICD, *International Classification of Disease*; SCL, symptom check list; KAS, Katz adjustment scales.

port the broad 'generalizability' of the concept that some form or forms of phenotypic depression occur in the longitudinal course of a substantial proportion of patients with schizophrenia.

Differential diagnosis of depression in schizophrenia

Organic factors

There are many potential origins of depression, or a phenocopy of depression, in schizophrenia. The first of these is represented by organic causes of a depressive syndrome (Bartels & Drake, 1989). These can arise from medical conditions, such as anaemias, carcinomas, endocrinopathies, metabolic abnormalities, infectious diseases or neurological disorders; from the use of commonly prescribed medications, such as sedative hypnotics, beta blockers, various other antihypertensive medications, sulphonamides or indomethacin; or from the discontinuation of certain other prescribed medications such as corticosteriods or stimulants. Substances of abuse can also be involved in the creation of depressed states, either through their acute or chronic use, or through discontinuation. Alcohol can predispose to a depression-like state through either acute or chronic use; the chronic use of cannabis can lead to an anergic state which shares many features with depression; and the withdrawal state from cocaine involves well-described depressive phenomenology. Withdrawal from commonly used legal substances, such as caffeine or nicotine (both often used to excess by schizophrenic patients), can also lead to dysphoric states which can be confused with depression.

Neuroleptic-induced dysphoria

One pertinent question concerns the issue of whether or not neuroleptic medications themselves can predispose to a depressed state among schizophrenic patients. On a theoretical level, this issue arises because neuroleptic medications block dopamine receptors, and dopamine receptors are known to be involved in brain pathways which mediate 'reward' (Wise, 1982; Harrow *et al.*,

1994). Therefore, if a neuroleptic interfered with the experience of reward or pleasure, the resultant experience of relative anhedonia could become a phenocopy of a depressed state. Indeed, one well-designed recent study comparing anhedonia in schizophrenic patients who either were or were not taking neuroleptics found significantly more anhedonia as well as depression in those who were taking neuroleptics (Harrow *et al.*, 1994); and several early reports implicated neuroleptics as an aetiological agent for depression among schizophrenic patients (DeAlarcon & Carney, 1969; Floru *et al.*, 1975; Galdi *et al.*, 1981; Johnson, 1981b; Galdi, 1983). Most recent evidence, however, has tended to refute the notion that appropriately administered neuroleptic medication causes a full depressive state to emerge in schizophrenic patients (Knights & Hirsch, 1981; Möller & von Zerssen, 1986; Siris, 1991).

This negative evidence comes from three directions. First, the evaluation of psychotic schizophrenic patients throughout the course of treatment for their acute episodes has revealed that, in fact, the greatest level of depressive symptomatology exists at the height of the psychosis, and tends to resolve, though often at a slower rate than the psychosis, when the psychosis is treated with a neuroleptic (Knights & Hirsch, 1981; Möller & von Zerseen, 1982; Strian *et al.*, 1982; Szymanski *et al.*, 1983; Leff *et al.*, 1988; Hirsch *et al.*, 1989; Green *et al.*, 1990). These observations oppose the notion that depression is caused by neuroleptics by demonstrating that depressive symptomatology was present before the neuroleptic was administered and actually decreases as the patient receives treatment with these compounds. Second, when patients being treated with neuroleptics were compared with patients not being treated with neuroleptics, the patients treated with neuroleptics were not found to be more depressed (Hirsch *et al.*, 1973; Wistedt & Palmstierna, 1983; Hogarty & Munetz, 1984; Hirsch *et al.*, 1989). Third, when schizophrenic patients with and without depression were compared with each other, the depressed group was not found to be receiving higher doses of neuroleptic drugs, or to have higher neuroleptic blood levels (Roy *et al.*, 1983; Roy, 1984; Berrios & Bulbena, 1987; Siris *et al.*, 1988a; Barnes *et al.*, 1989; Bandelow *et al.*, 1991). This group-data refutation of the hypothesis that neuroleptic drugs can cause depression is not entirely conclusive, especially in the presence of one well-designed positive study (Harrow *et al.*, 1994), and certainly does not rule out the possibility that in individual cases this might not be a factor.

Akinesia and akathisia

Antipsychotic drugs may clearly be a factor in the production of a depression-like state when depressive-like features occur in association with the extrapyramidal neuroleptic side effects of akinesia and akathisia. Neuroleptic-induced akinesia, a syndrome of reduced spontaneity as well as reduced generalized motor activity, can at times produce a rather exact phenocopy of depression, even when muscle stiffness or cogwheeling are not present (Rifkin *et al.*, 1975, 1978; Van Putten & May, 1978; Martin *et al.*, 1985; Bermanzohn & Siris, 1992). This phenocopy includes blue mood as well as reduced energy, pessimism and anhedonia, and is principally differentiated from depression by its responsiveness to antiparkinsonian medication, which is usually not thought to be a treatment for other forms of depression. Akinesia may be particularly problematic in terms of its diagnosis when it occurs in an insidious and subtle form, or in the absence of large muscle extrapyramidal signs, such as shuffling gait or reduced arm swing. Unfortunately, most studies of depression in the course of schizophrenia make scant effort to rule out neuroleptic-induced akinesia as a confounding factor.

Neuroleptic-induced akathisia is another extrapyramidal side effect which is easy to diagnose in its blatant form, owing to prominent motor restlessness, but equally easy to misdiagnose in its subtle form where the patient may be more dysphoric than outwardly restless (Van Putten, 1975; Siris, 1985). Such patients may still be prone, however, to more subtle behavioural excesses such as overtalkativeness or wandering into other people's territory. This dysphoric form of akathisia can be easily mistaken for agitated depression. Indeed, the dysphoria of akathisia may be intense, and both suicidal ideation and suicidal behaviour have been associated with this state (Shear *et al.*, 1983; Drake & Ehrlich, 1985).

Negative symptoms

The negative symptoms of schizophrenia, like akinesia, can also present in a way which resembles depression in a number of substantial respects (Crow, 1980; Andreasen & Olsen, 1982; Carpenter *et al.*, 1985; Siris *et al.*, 1988b; Bermanzohn & Siris, 1992), although clear distinctions may also be evident (Barnes *et al.*, 1989; Lindenmayer *et al.*, 1991; Norman & Malla, 1991; Kuck *et al.*, 1992). Features such as anhedonia and anergia may indeed be common between these two states (Bermanzohn & Siris, 1992). However Barnes *et al.* (1989) found very little overlap between the diagnosis of the negative symptoms of schizophrenia and the diagnosis of depression in chronic in-patients. Thus, in many cases, with careful attention, these syndromes need not be confused. The clinical feature most likely to set these two conditions apart is blue mood, which is generally present in depression. Negative symptoms, on the other hand, are usually marked by blunted affect. Since one prominent hypothesis concerning the pathogenesis of negative symptoms involves it representing a hypo-dopaminergic state (Davis *et al.*, 1991), it is conceivable that neuroleptic medications at too high a dose may exacerbate this condition, thereby contributing to the reputation of neuroleptic agents as being 'depressogenic'.

Disappointment reactions

Schizophrenic patients often have a considerable amount to be disappointed about in the ways in which their lives are progressing, and they may certainly manifest their psychological reaction to this. Acute disappointment reactions may occur in reaction to any events which go awry in an individual's life. Operationally, this is most easily distinguished by the presence of an immediate stressful event, and the fact that the reaction is transient — seldom lasting more than 1–2 weeks. More difficult to distinguish from depression may be the chronic variety of disappointment reaction known as the demoralization syndrome (Frank, 1973; Klein, 1974). In this situation, patients become chronically discouraged and dispirited on the basis of repeated failures or the sense that important life goals have become impossible to achieve. Of interest in this regard is the observation that schizophrenic patients who feel less of a sense of control concerning their illness are more prone to experience depression (Birchwood *et al.*, 1993). From an aetiological point of view, demoralization reactions may be particularly worthy of diagnosis, because they may represent a clinical state more amenable than others to psychosocial treatments and supports.

Prodrome of psychotic relapse

Depression has been described as a common symptom that schizophrenic patients may manifest during the process of decompensation into a new episode of psychosis (Docherty *et al.*, 1978; Herz & Melville, 1980; Herz, 1985; Johnson, 1988; Hirsch *et al.*, 1989; Green *et al.*, 1990). In these cases the dysphoric state is often accompanied by social withdrawal, anxiety and/or other stigmata such as hypervigilance suggestive of early manifestations of psychosis, but the differential diagnosis may be difficult. Because of this possibility, the lowering of neuroleptic dosage is not necessarily advisable among schizophrenic patients in whom depressive-like symptomatology is newly emergent. Rather, increased monitoring may be the indicated intervention. Initiation of antidepressant medications under this circumstance may have contributed to the early impression, not subsequently validated, that antidepressant medications could be psychotogenic in schizophrenic patients even when neuroleptic medications are maintained (Siris *et al.*, 1978).

Schizoaffective disorder

Another interplay between the syndrome of

depression and the phenotypic psychosis of schizophrenia, which belongs in the differential diagnosis of secondary depression in schizophrenia, occurs in schizoaffective disorder. In this instance, the full depressive syndrome coincides with the florid psychotic syndrome in ways which have been defined variously according to different diagnostic schemes (Levitt & Tsuang, 1988; Coryell *et al.*, 1990; Taylor, 1992). Since the definition of the requisite level of psychotic symptomatology coexisting with depression will differ according to the diagnostic system employed, the technical boundary between schizoaffective disorder and secondary depression in residually psychotic schizophrenic patients will vary. Conceptually, though, the pertinent issue is that a full depression syndrome coincides with the appropriate manifestations of psychosis during at least part of an episode of schizoaffective depression. A fuller exposition of schizoaffective disorder carries us beyond the boundaries of this chapter (Siris, 1993; Siris & Lavin, in press; see also Chapter 4, this volume). Schizoaffective disorder additionally enters into the differential diagnosis of postpsychotic depression in schizophrenia, of course, in that episodes of secondary depression can also occur in the course of schizoaffective disorder.

Validation of postpsychotic depression

Prognosis

The literature concerning the prognostic implications of depressive symptomatology in schizophrenia is complicated by the issue of whether the depressive symptoms coincide with the timing of the psychosis or occur apart from it (Siris, 1991). Although depressive symptoms coinciding with the psychosis carry favourable prognostic implications (McGlashan & Carpenter, 1976b), such symptoms occurring in intervals during which the patient is not psychotic have been found to predict oppositely (Bartels & Drake, 1988; Becker, 1988). Specifically, those patients who manifest secondary depressions in schizophrenia have been noted to be more likely to experience psychotic relapse, even when 'prodromal' depressive symp-

tomatology has been accounted for (Falloon *et al.*, 1978; Mandel *et al.*, 1982). Consistent with this unfavourable implication is the observation that postpsychotic depression in schizophrenia is also associated with other negative predictors of outcome, such as poor premorbid adjustment and insidious onset of the first or index psychotic episodes (Möller & von Zerssen, 1986).

Suicide

The most blatantly disastrous outcome in schizophrenia is suicide, an event which tragically is not rare and has been estimated to be the way in which approximately 10% of schizophrenic lives end (Miles, 1977; Caldwell & Gottesman, 1990). A greater number of schizophrenic suicides (Roy, 1982; Drake & Cotton, 1986) and suicide attempters (Roy, 1986; Prasad & Kumar, 1988) have been found to have past or recent histories of depressive symptomatology, especially its psychological aspects such as hopelessness (Drake & Cotton, 1986). Suicidal ideation has also been found to be associated with depression in schizophrenia (Barnes *et al.*, 1989).

Life events

More undesirable events, more exit events and more life events altogether have been observed in those schizophrenic patients who manifest secondary depressions (Roy, 1981). In addition, schizophrenic patients with secondary depressions have been found to have histories of more early parental loss (Roy, 1980, 1981; Roy *et al.*, 1983).

Biological measures

Inconsistent results have been reported in the several studies which have examined the results of the dexamethasone suppression test (DST) in schizophrenic patients with secondary depressions (Siris, 1991). One confounding variable in these investigations may have been the failure to control for the effects of antiparkinsonian or other anticholinergic medications on dexamethasone suppression. Only one study has been reported concerning the thyrotropin releasing hormone (TRH) test in postpsychotic depressed patients (Siris, 1991). Although that study showed rates of blunted response comparable with that of patients with primary depression, it contained no control group of non-depressed schizophrenic patients. Another study awaiting replication is the finding of higher levels of platelet monoamine oxidase (MAO) activity in patients with schizophrenia-related depression (Schildkraut *et al.*, 1980).

Genetic studies

Schizophrenic patients who have first-degree relatives with unipolar depression have been found to have a significantly higher likelihood of developing a depression syndrome following the resolution of a psychotic episode (Kendler & Hays, 1983). On the other hand, two relatively small studies ($n = 44$ and $n = 70$) failed to find significant differences in rates of primary affectively disordered relatives between schizophrenic patients with and without depression (Berrios & Bulbena, 1987; Guze *et al.*, 1983). Finally, one unique study found a relationship between neuroleptic-induced depressive symptomatology and those schizophrenic patients who had depressed relatives (Galdi *et al.*, 1981).

Treatment implications

The existence of a syndrome of depression in schizophrenia raises several important implications for treatment. A newly emergent syndrome of depression in a patient with schizophrenia is certainly cause for an increased level of observation and support. Such a condition may represent an early stage in the process of decompensation into a new episode of psychosis. If such proves to be the case, increased structure, decreased stress and augmentation or change of antipsychotic medication may be called for. Intercepting and treating new episodes of psychosis quickly may substantially curtail both psychiatric and social morbidity. To do so, therefore, is a valuable objective in the longitudinal treatment of individuals with schizophrenia.

Alternatively, emergence of a new episode of depression in schizophrenia may represent a transient disappointment reaction. Such an event represents a life stressor. Again, in this case, patients will not be harmed and are likely to benefit from support, although there may be no need to adjust medications. By definition, such episodes are transient and will resolve with the passage of time, generally within a week or two.

When a new state of depression in schizophrenia persists or becomes chronic, reduction of the dose of neuroleptic medication should be considered. Although evidence leans away from the view that neuroleptics cause an otherwise characteristic depressed illness in schizophrenic patients, neuroleptic agents may play a role in generating syndromes which mimic depression. These include akinesia, akathisia and perhaps even the 'negative symptoms' state. Therefore, when treating non-acute episodes of depression in schizophrenia, an effort should be made to decrease the neuroleptic dose to the lowest level consistent with maintaining remission from flagrant psychotic symptomatology. Indeed, the minimization of neuroleptic dosage in this manner is generally advocated for the long-term maintenance of patients with schizophrenia as a means of reducing side effects and optimizing psychosocial functioning (Kane *et al.*, 1983; Marder *et al.*, 1987).

Antidepressant medications

After the possibilities of impending psychotic relapse and transient disappointment reaction have been accounted for, and an effort has been made to rule out neuroleptic-induced akinesia or akathisia through appropriate adjustments of medication, the efficacy of treatment with antidepressant medication must be considered. Studies addressing this question have had mixed results, but are generally regarded as favourable (Plasky, 1991; Siris, 1991). Table 9.2 reviews the double-blind, placebo-controlled studies that have been reported concerning the addition of an adjunctive antidepressant medication in cases of secondary depression in schizophrenia. Most of the negative reports have design issues which make their interpretation difficult; these issues include brief duration of treatment (4 weeks), low antidepressant dose (maprotiline as low as 50 mg/day), antidepressant dose which may be too high for some patients (nortriptyline 150 mg/day, especially in the presence of a concomitant neuroleptic which could reduce metabolism) or antidepressant medication being given to patients on one neuroleptic while placebo is given to patients receiving a different neuroleptic. The studies in Table 9.2 which are positive have fewer limitations of design, although even the most favourable results (Siris *et al.*, 1987) demonstrated 'much improved' responses in fewer than half (42%) of the patients treated with adjunctive antidepressant. In addition, most of the studies in Table 9.2 did not make an attempt to rule out the syndrome of akinesia in their design, so the results have to be interpreted in that light. The final study listed in Table 9.2 (Kramer *et al.*, 1989) differs from the others in that it involved patients who were floridly psychotic at the time of the trial (acutely admitted patients with schizoaffective depression). That these patients did not benefit from the addition of an antidepressant to their neuroleptic regimen may relate to their being flagrantly psychotic at the time of the trial (Siris, 1991). Also, in general, out-patients in the studies in Table 9.2 did better with an adjunct antidepressant than did in-patients (Fisher exact test, $P = 0.048$).

Only one study has been reported of maintenance adjunctive antidepressant, compared double-blindly to adjunctive placebo, in neuroleptic-treated schizophrenic or schizoaffective patients with postpsychotic depressions. That study strongly favoured the adjunctive antidepressant both in terms of preventing relapse into depression and in terms of reducing the chance of relapse into psychosis (Siris *et al.*, 1994).

MAO inhibitor antidepressants have not been adequately studied in schizophrenic patients with depression. Of possible relevance, however, is a double-blind adjunctive tranylcypromine study which found this MAO inhibitor to be of benefit for schizophrenic patients with negative symptoms

(Bucci, 1987). Preliminary results have suggested that selegiline, an MAO-B inhibitor, may have value as an adjunctive treatment for negative symptoms (Bodkin *et al.*, 1992; Perenyi *et al.*, 1992), but interpretation of these results is complicated by the fact that selegiline has antiparkinsonian properties (Parkinson Study Group, 1993) and the effects observed may therefore represent treatment of akinesia. Small double-blind studies have also indicated that an adjunctive serotonin reuptake-inhibiting (Silver & Nassar, 1992) or tricyclic (Siris *et al.*, 1991) antidepressant may be of use to some schizophrenic patients with negative symptoms, and an open trial has suggested that adjunctive fluoxetine may be of benefit for negative symptoms (Goff *et al.*, 1990). These results have yet to be confirmed.

Lithium

Most of the studies involving the use of lithium in schizophrenia have involved the acute treatment of psychotic exacerbations, rather than its use in the maintenance phase of treatment (Christison *et al.*, 1991; Plasky, 1991), and the most frequently cited predictors of favourable response are excitement, overactivity and euphoria, rather than depression. Nevertheless, depressive symptomatology has also been identified as a positive prognosticator of adjunctive lithium response in schizophrenia (Lerner *et al.*, 1988), along with previous affective episodes, family history of affective disorder and an overall episodic course (Atre-Vaidya & Taylor, 1989). Therefore, it is reasonable to attempt a trial of adjunctive lithium in patients with postpsychotic depression who have been otherwise non-responsive, although the efficacy of this has not been established in the literature. It is also rational to try lithium in addition to an adjunctive antidepressant for schizophrenic patients whose depression does not respond, although a specific documentation for this approach does not exist. Support for the use and safety of lithium in patients who have both affective and psychotic characteristics derives from the fact that it may be useful in patients with the

Table 9.2 Double-blind studies of antidepressants in depressed schizophrenic patients. (After Siris, 1991)

Study (*n*)	Patients	Neuroleptic	Antidepressant	Duration	Result
Singh *et al.* (1978) (*n* = 60)	Schizophrenia by Feighner criteria Chronic patients with symptoms of depression HAM-D rating scale score of 18 or more In-patients	Previous phenothiazine continued	Trazodone (300 mg/day) or placebo	6 weeks	Trazadone favoured by HAM-D and CGI scale changes No significant differences in BPRS
Prussoff *et al.* (1979) (*n* = 35)	Schizophrenia by New Haven Index criteria A score of at least 7 on the Raskin depression rating scale Out-patients	Perphenazine (16−48 mg/day)	Amitriptyline (100−200 mg/day) or placebo	1,2,4 or 6 months	With amitriptyline: some decrease in depression ratings some increase in thought disorder and agitation ratings improvement in social well-being overall impression: mildly positive
Waehrens and Gerlach (1980) (*n* = 17; cross-over design)	'Schizophrenia' (no criteria given) Chronic and 'emotionally withdrawn' 'Long-term' in-patients	Continuation of previous neuroleptics	Maprotiline (50−200 mg/day) or placebo	8 weeks	No benefit found from addition of maprotiline
Johnson (1981a) (*n* = 50)	Schizophrenia by Feighner or Schneiderian symptoms Beck depression inventory score 15 or more for episode of 'acute' depression All 'chronic' patients (unstated whether in-patients or out-patients)	Fluphenazine decanoate or flupenthixol decanoate (doses not specified)	Nortriptyline (150 mg/day) or placebo	5 weeks	No statistically significant benefit to depression from adding nortriptyline, although 40% placebo response rate would make such a finding difficult to detect Increased side effects with nortriptyline
Kurland and Nagaraju (1981) (*n* = 22)	Schizophrenia (no criteria given) HAM-D score of 18 or more Patients treated with antiparkinsonian medications were specifically excluded In-patients	Chlorpromazine (75−300 mg/day or) haloperidol (6−15 mg/day)	Viloxazine to 300 mg/day maximum in final week only, or placebo	4 weeks	No differences between groups Majority of patients in both groups improved

Continued

Table 9.2 (*Continued*)

Study (*n*)	Patients	Neuroleptic	Antidepressant	Duration	Result
Becker (1983) (*n* = 52)	Schizophrenia by RDC RDC for major depressive syndrome (superimposed on schizophrenia) In-patients	Chlorpromazine (100–1200 mg/day) or thiothixene (5–60 mg/day)	Imipramine (150–250 mg/day) for patients on chlorpromazine, or placebo for patients on thiothixene	4 weeks (after 2 weeks drug free)	Both treatments effective compared with baseline on BPRS and HAM-D but neither treatment statistically superior to the other More sedative and autonomic side effects with chlorpromazine–imipramine combination
Siris *et al.* (1987) (*n* = 33)	Schizophrenia or schizoaffective disorder by RDC (non-psychotic or residually psychotic) RDC for major or minor depression Depression unresponsive to benztropine (2 mg p.o. TID) Out-patients	Fluphenazine decanoate — clinically adjusted stable weekly dose	Imipramine (150–200 mg/day) or placebo	6 weeks	Imipramine group superior on global measure (CGI) and depression scales No difference between groups in psychosis or side effects
Dufresne *et al.* (1988) (*n* = 38)	Schizophrenia by DSM-III Superimposed atypical affective disorder (equivalent to DSM-III major depression) In-patients	Thiothixene — clinically adjusted stable dose	Bupropion (150–750 mg/day) flexible dose, or placebo	4 weeks	Both groups improved, but placebo group improved more Majority of bupropion-treated patients dropped out
Kramer *et al.* (1989) (*n* = 58)	Initial DSM-III diagnosis of schizophrenia RDC for schizoaffective disorder (mainly schizophrenic), depressive subtype HAM-D score >17 Treated with benztropine (2–8 mg/day) In-patients, actively psychotic	Haloperidol (0.4 mg/kg per day p.o.)	Amitriptyline (3.5 mg/kg per day), desipramine 3.5 mg/kg per day), or placebo	4 weeks	Addition of neither amitriptyline nor desipramine showed significant therapeutic advantage Patients treated with antidepressant tended to score worse at the end on BPRS hallucinatory behaviour and thinking disturbance

Continued on p. 142

Table 9.2 (*Continued*)

Study (*n*)	Patients	Neuroleptic	Antidepressant	Duration	Result
Siris *et al.* (1989; 1994) (*n* = 24)	Schizophrenia or schizoaffective disorder by RDC (non-psychotic or residually psychotic) RDC for major depression History of favourable response to adjunctive imipramine (150–300 mg/day) Out-patients	Fluphenazine decanoate — clinically adjusted stable dose	Open continuation treatment with imipramine (100–300 mg/day) for 6 months Then, *either* maintained on imipramine *or* tapered to placebo double-blind for 1 year maintenance trial	18 months	Significantly more relapse into depression in group tapered to placebo No exacerbation of psychosis while on adjunctive imipramine, and significantly more exacerbation of psychosis in group tapered to placebo

HAM-D, Hamilton depression; CGI, clinical global impression; BPRS, brief psychiatric rating scale; RDC, research diagnostic criteria; DSM, *Diagnostic and Statistical Manual.*

closely related symptomatology of schizoaffective disorder (Siris, 1993).

Psychosocial interventions

Although psychosocial interventions have not been specifically studied in a controlled fashion in schizophrenic patients with depression, it is clear that appropriate psychosocial approaches can be valuable in the long-term management of schizophrenia (Hogarty *et al.*, 1986). Such interventions include skill building, psychoeducation, stress reduction, problem solving and family work aimed at reducing expressed emotion. Appropriate structure and support, along with treatments aimed at building self-esteem and realistic components of hope, may also be quite useful (see Chapters 30 and 31). Schizophrenic patients with depressions would appear to be particularly likely to benefit from such interventions because of their otherwise compromised status and fragility.

Conclusion

Depressive syndromes occur frequently during the longitudinal course of schizophrenia. They are associated with considerable morbidity, and a number of alternatives must be considered in their differential diagnosis. They also carry important prognostic and treatment implications, and their proper understanding may also have heuristic relevance.

References

Andreasen, N.C. & Olsen, S. (1982) Negative symptoms in schizophrenia: definition and reliability. *Archives of General Psychiatry*, **39**, 789–794.

APA (1994) *Diagnostic and Statistical Manual of Mental Disorders*, 4th edn, pp. 711–712. American Psychiatric Association, Washington DC.

Atre-Vaidya, N. & Taylor, M.A. (1989) Effectiveness of lithium and schizophrenia: do we really have an answer? *Journal of Clinical Psychiatry*, **50**, 170–173.

Bandelow, B., Muller, P., Gaebel, W. *et al.* (1991) Depressive syndromes in schizophrenic patients after discharge from hospital. *European Archives of Psychiatry and Clinical Neuroscience*, **240**, 113–120.

Barnes, T.R., Curson, D.A., Liddle, P.F. & Patel, M. (1989) The nature and prevalence of depression in chronic schizophrenic in-patients. *British Journal of Psychiatry*, **154**, 486–491.

Bartels, S.J. & Drake, R.E. (1988) Depressive symptoms in schizophrenia: comprehensive differential diagnosis. *Comprehensive Psychiatry*, **29**, 467–483.

Bartels, S.J. & Drake, R.E. (1989) Depression in schizophrenia: current guidelines to treatment. *Psychiatric Quarterly*, **60**, 337–357.

Becker, R.E. (1983) Implications of the efficacy of thiothixene and a chlorpromazine–imipramine combination for depression in schizophrenia. *American Journal of Psychiatry*, **140**, 208–211.

Becker, R.E. (1988) Depression in schizophrenia. *Hospital and Community Psychiatry*, **39**, 1269–1275.

Bermanzohn, P.C. & Siris, S.G. (1992) Akinesia: a syndrome common to parkinsonism, retarded depression, and negative symptoms. *Comprehensive Psychiatry*, **33**, 221–232.

Berrios, G.E. & Bulbena, A. (1987) Post psychotic depression: the Fulbourn cohort. *Acta Psychiatrica Scandinavica*, **76**, 89–93.

Birchwood, M., Mason, R., Macmillan, F. & Healy, J. (1993) Depression, demoralization and control over psychotic illness: a comparison of depressed and non-depressed patients with a chronic psychosis. *Psychological Medicine*, **23**, 387–395.

Bleuler, E. (1950) *Dementia Praecox or the Group of Schizophrenias*. International Universities Press, New York.

Bodkin, A., Cannon, S., Cohen, B., Alpert, J., Zornberg, G. & Cole, J. (1992) Selegiline treatment of negative symptoms of schizophrenia and schizoaffective disorder. Presented at the *31st Annual Meeting of the American College of Neuropsychopharmacology, San Juan, December 1992.*

Bowers, M.D. & Astrachan, B.M. (1967) Depression in acute schizophrenic psychosis. *American Journal of Psychiatry*, **123**, 976–979.

Brier, A., Schreiber, J.L., Dyer, J. & Pickar, D. (1991) National Institute of Mental Health longitudinal study of chronic schizophrenia: prognosis and predictors of outcome. *Archives of General Psychiatry*, **48**, 239–246.

Bucci, L. (1987) The negative symptoms of schizophrenia and the monamine oxidase inhibitors. *Psychopharmacology*, **91**, 104–108.

Caldwell, C.B. & Gottesman, I.I. (1990) Schizophrenics kill themselves too: a review of risk factors for suicide. *Schizophrenia Bulletin*, **16**, 571–589.

Carpenter, W.T. Jr, Heinrichs, D.W. & Alphs, L.D. (1985) Treatment of negative symptoms. *Schizophrenia Bulletin*, **11**, 440–452.

Christison, G.W., Kirch, D.G. & Wyatt, R.J. (1991) When symptoms persist: choosing among alternative somatic treatments for schizophrenia. *Schizophrenia Bulletin*, **17**, 217–240.

Coryell, W., Keller, M., Lavori, P. & Endicott, J. (1990) Affective syndromes, psychotic features, and prognosis. I. Depression. *Archives of General Psychiatry*, **47**, 651–657.

Crow, T.J. (1980) Molecular pathology of schizophrenia: more than one disease process? *British Medical Journal*, **280**, 66–68.

Davis, K.L., Kahn, R.S., Ko, G. & Davidson, M. (1991) Dopamine in schizophrenia: a review and reconceptualization. *American Journal of Psychiatry*, **148**, 1474–1486.

DeAlarcon, R. & Carney, M.W.P. (1969) Severe depressive mood changes following slow-release intramuscular fluphenazine injection. *British Medical Journal*, **3**, 564–567.

Docherty, J.P., van Kammen, D.P., Siris, S.G. & Marder, S.R. (1978) Stages of onset of schizophrenic psychosis. *American Journal of Psychiatry*, **135**, 420–426.

Drake, R.E. & Cotton, P.G. (1986) Depression, hopelessness and suicide in chronic schizophrenia. *British Journal of Psychiatry*, **148**, 554–559.

Drake, R.E. & Ehrlich, J. (1985) Suicide attempts associated with akathisia. *American Journal of Psychiatry*, **142**, 499–501.

Dufresne, R.L., Kass, D.J. & Becker, R.E. (1988) Bupropion and thiothixene versus placebo and thiothixene in the treatment of depression in schizophrenia. *Drug Development Research*, **12**, 259–266.

Eissler, K.R. (1951) Remarks on the psycho-analysis of schizophrenia. *International Journal of Psychoanalysis*, **32**, 139–156.

Falloon, I., Watt, D.C. & Shepherd, M. (1978) A comparative controlled trial of pimozide and fluphenazine decanoate in the continuation therapy of schizophrenia. *Psychological Medicine*, **8**, 59–70.

Floru, L., Heinrich, K. & Wittek, F. (1975) The problem of postpsychotic schizophrenic depressions and their pharmacological induction. *International Pharmacopsychiatry*, **10**, 230–239.

Frank, J.D. (1973) *Persuasion and Healing*. Johns Hopkins University Press, Baltimore.

Galdi, J. (1983) The causality of depression in schizophrenia. *British Journal of Psychiatry*, **142**, 621–625.

Galdi, J., Rieder, R.O., Silber, D. & Bonato, R.R. (1981) Genetic factors in the response to neuroleptics in schizophrenia: a pharmacogenetic study. *Psychological Medicine*, **11**, 713–728.

Goff, D.C., Brotman, A.W., Waites, M. & McCormicks, S. (1990) Trial of fluoxetine added to neuroleptics for treatment-resistant schizophrenic patients. *American Journal of Psychiatry*, **147**, 492–494.

Green, M.F., Nuechterlein, K.H., Ventura, J. & Mintz, J. (1990) The temporal relationship between depressive and psychotic symptoms in recent-onset schizophrenia. *American Journal of Psychiatry*, **147**, 179–182.

Guze, S.B., Cloninger, C.R., Martin, R.L. & Clayton, P.J. (1983) A follow-up and family study of schizophrenia. *Archives of General Psychiatry*, **40**, 1273–1276.

Harrow, M., Yonan, C.A., Sands, J.R. & Marengo, J. (1994) Depression in schizophrenia: are neuroleptics, akinesia, or ankedonia involved? *Schizophrenia Bulletin*, **20**, 327–338.

Herz, M. (1985) Prodromal symptoms and prevention of relapse in schizophrenia. *Journal of Clinical Psychiatry*, **46**(11), 22–25.

Herz, M. & Melville, C. (1980) Relapse in schizophrenia. *American Journal of Psychiatry*, **137**, 801–805.

Hirsch, S.R. & Jolley, A.G. (1989) The dysphoric syndrome in schizophrenia and its implications for relapse. *British Journal of Psychiatry*, **155** (Suppl. 5), 46–50.

Hirsch, S.R., Gaind, R., Rohde, P.D., Stevens, B.C. & Wing, J.T. (1973) Outpatient maintenance of chronic schizophrenic patients with long-acting fluphenazine: double-blind placebo trial. *British Medical Journal*, **1**, 633–637.

Hirsch, S.R., Jolley, A.G., Barnes, T.R.E. *et al.* (1989) Dysphoric and depressive symptoms in chronic schizophrenia. *Schizophrenia Research*, **2**, 259–264.

Hogarty, G.E. & Munetz, M.R. (1984) Pharmacogenic depression among outpatient schizophrenic patients: a failure to substantiate. *Journal of Clinical Psychopharmacology*,

4, 17–24.

Hogarty, G.E., Anderson, C.M., Reiss, D.J. *et al.* (1986) Family psychoeducational, social skills training, and maintenance chemotherapy in the aftercare treatment of schizophrenia. I. One-year effects of a controlled study on relapse and expressed emotion. *Archives of General Psychiatry*, **43**, 633–642.

Johnson, D.A.W. (1981a) Studies of depressive symptoms in schizophrenia. *British Journal of Psychiatry*, **139**, 89–101.

Johnson, D.A.W. (1981b) Depressions in schizophrenia: some observations on prevalence, etiology, and treatment. *Acta Psychiatrica Scandinavica*, **63** (Suppl. 291), 137–144.

Johnson, D.A.W. (1988) The significance of depression in the prediction of relapse in chronic schizophrenia. *British Journal of Psychiatry*, **152**, 320–323.

Kane, J.M., Rifkin, A., Woerner, M. *et al.* (1983) Low-dose neuroleptic treatment of outpatient schizophrenics. I. Preliminary results for relapse rates. *Archives of General Psychiatry*, **40**, 893–896.

Kendler, K.S. & Hays, P. (1983) Schizophrenia subdivided by the family history of affective disorder: a comparison of symptomatology and cause of illness. *Archives of General Psychiatry*, **40**, 951–955.

Klein, D.F. (1974) Endomorphic depression: a conceptual and terminological revision. *Archives of General Psychiatry*, **31**, 447–454.

Knights, A. & Hirsch, S.R. (1981) 'Revealed' depression and drug treatment for schizophrenia. *Archives of General Psychiatry*, **38**, 806–811.

Knights, A., Okasha, M.S., Salih, M.A. & Hirsch, S.R. (1979) Depressive and extrapyramidal symptoms and clinical effects: a trial of fluphenazine versus flupenthixol in maintenance of schizophrenic out-patients. *British Journal of Psychiatry*, **135**, 515–523.

Kramer, M.S., Vogel, W.H., DiJohnson, C. *et al.* (1989) Antidepressants in 'depressed' schizophrenic inpatients: a controlled trial. *Archives of General Psychiatry*, **46**, 922–928.

Kuck, J., Zisook, S., Moranville, J.T., Heaton, R.K. & Braff, D.L. (1992) Negative symptomatology in schizophrenic outpatients. *Journal of Nervous and Mental Disease*, **180**, 510–515.

Kurland, A.A. & Nagaraju, A. (1981) Viloxazine and the depressed schizophrenic — methodological issues. *Journal of Clinical Pharmacology*, **21**, 37–41.

Leff, J., Tress, K. & Edwards, B. (1988) The clinical course of depressive symptoms in schizophrenia. *Schizophrenia Research*, **1**, 25–30.

Lerner, Y., Mintzer, Y. & Schestatzky, M. (1988) Lithium combined with haloperidol in schizophrenic patients. *British Journal of Psychiatry*, **153**, 359–362.

Levitt, J.J. & Tsuang, M.T. (1988) The heterogeneity of schizoaffective disorder: implications for treatment. *American Journal of Psychiatry*, **145**, 926–936.

Lindenmayer, J.-P., Grochowski, S. & Kay, S.R. (1991) Schizophrenic patients with depression: psychopathological profiles and relationship with negative symptoms. *Comprehensive Psychiatry*, **32**, 528–533.

McGlashan, T.H. & Carpenter, W.T. Jr (1976a) An investigation of the post psychotic depressive syndrome. *American Journal of Psychiatry*, **133**, 14–19.

McGlashan, T.H. & Carpenter, W.T. Jr (1976b) Postpsychotic depression in schizophrenia. *Archives of General Psychiatry*, **33**, 231–239.

Mandel, M.R., Severe, J.B., Schooler, N.R., Gelenberg, A.J. & Mieske, M. (1982) Development and prediction of postpsychotic depression in neuroleptic-treated schizophrenics. *Archives of General Psychiatry*, **39**, 197–203.

Marder, S.R., Van Putten, T., Mintz, J., Lebell, M., McKenzie, J. & May, P.R.A. (1987) Low- and conventional-dose maintenance therapy with fluphenazine decanoate: two-year outcome. *Archives of General Psychiatry*, **44**, 518–521.

Martin, R.L., Cloninger, R.C., Guze, S.B. & Clayton, P.J. (1985) Frequency and differential diagnosis of depressive syndromes in schizophrenia. *Journal of Clinical Psychiatry*, **46(11)**, 9–13.

Miles, C. (1977) Conditions predisposing to suicide: a review. *Journal of Nervous and Mental Disease*, **164**, 221–246.

Miller, J.B. & Sonnenberg, S.M. (1973) Depression following psychotic episodes: a response to the challenge of change? *Journal of the American Academy of Psychoanalysis*, **1**, 253–270.

Möller, H.J. & von Zerssen, D. (1982) Depressive states occurring during the neuroleptic treatment of schizophrenia. *Schizophrenia Bulletin*, **8**, 109–117.

Möller, H.J. & von Zerssen, D. (1986) Depression in schizophrenia. In Burrows, G.D., Norman, T.R. & Rubinstein, G. (eds) *Handbook of Studies on Schizophrenia*, Part 1, pp. 183–191. Elsevier, Amsterdam.

Munro, J.G., Hardiker, T.M. & Leonard, D.P. (1984) The dexamethasone suppression test in residual schizophrenia with depression. *American Journal of Psychiatry*, **141**, 250–252.

Norman, R.M.G. & Malla, A.K. (1991) Dysphoric mood and symptomatology in schizophrenia. *Psychological Medicine*, **21**, 897–903.

Parkinson Study Group (1993) Effects of tocopherol and deprenyl on the progression of disability in early Parkinson's disease. *New England Journal of Medicine*, **328**, 176–183.

Perenyi, A., Goswami, U., Frecska, E. & Arato, M. (1992) L-Deprenyl in treating negative symptoms of schizophrenia. *Psychiatry Research*, **42**, 189–191.

Plasky, P. (1991) Antidepressant usage in schizophrenia. *Schizophrenia Bulletin*, **17**, 649–657.

Prasad, A.J. & Kumar, N. (1988) Suicidal behavior in hospitalized schizophrenics. *Suicide and Life-Threatening Behavior*, **18**, 265–269.

Prusoff, B.A., Williams, D.H., Weissman, M.M. & Astrachan, B.M. (1979) Treatment of secondary depression in schizophrenia. *Archives of General Psychiatry*, **36**, 569–575.

Rifkin, A., Quitkin, F. & Klein, D.F. (1975) Akinesia: a poorly recognized drug-induced extrapyramidal behavioral disorder. *Archives of General Psychiatry*, **32**, 672–674.

Rifkin, A., Quitkin, F., Kane, J., Struve, F. & Klein, D.F. (1978) Are prophylactic antiparkinsonian drugs necessary? A controlled study of procyclidine withdrawal. *Archives of General Psychiatry*, **35**, 483–489.

Roth, S. (1970) The seemingly ubiquitous depression following acute schizophrenic episodes, a neglected area of clinical discussion. *American Journal of Psychiatry*, **127**, 51–58.

Roy, A. (1980) Depression in chronic paranoid schizophrenia.

British Journal of Psychiatry, **137**, 138–139.

Roy, A. (1981) Depression in the course of chronic undifferentiated schizophrenia. *Archives of General Psychiatry*, **38**, 296–297.

Roy, A. (1982) Suicide in chronic schizophrenia. *British Journal of Psychiatry*, **141**, 171–177.

Roy, A. (1984) Do neuroleptics cause depression? *Biological Psychiatry*, **19**, 777–781.

Roy, A. (1986) Depression, attempted suicide, and suicide in patients with chronic schizophrenia. *Psychiatric Clinics of North America*, **9**, 193–206.

Roy, A., Thompson, R. & Kennedy, S. (1983) Depression in chronic schizophrenia. *British Journal of Psychiatry*, **142**, 465–470.

Schildkraut, J.J., Orsulak, P.J., Schatzberg, A.F. & Herzog, J.M. (1980) Platelet monoamine oxidase activity in subgroups of schizophrenic disorders. *Schizophrenia Bulletin*, **6**, 220–225.

Semrad, E.V. (1966) Long-term therapy of schizophrenia: formulation of the clinical approach. In Usdin, G. (ed.) *Psychoneuroses and Schizophrenia*, pp. 155–173. J.B. Lippincott, Philadelphia.

Shear, K., Frances, A. & Weiden, P. (1983) Suicide associated with akathisia and depot fluphenazine treatment. *Journal of Clinical Psychopharmacology*, **3**, 235–236.

Silver, H. & Nassar, A. (1992) Fluvoxamine improves negative symptoms in treated chronic schizophrenia: an add-on double-blind, placebo-controlled study. *Biological Psychiatry*, **31**, 698–704.

Singh, A.N., Saxena, B. & Nelson, H.L. (1978) A controlled clinical study of trazodone in chronic schizophrenic patients with pronounced depressive symptomatology. *Current Therapeutics Research*, **23**, 485–501.

Siris, S.G. (1985) Akathisia and 'acting-out'. *Journal of Clinical Psychiatry*, **46**, 395–397.

Siris, S.G. (1991) Diagnosis of secondary depression in schizophrenia: implications for DSM-IV. *Schizophrenia Bulletin*, **17**, 75–98.

Siris, S.G. (1993) The treatment of schizoaffective disorder. In Dunner, D.L. (ed.) *Current Psychiatric Therapy*, pp. 160–165. WB Saunders, Philadelphia.

Siris, S.G. & Lavin, M.R. Schizoaffective disorder, schizophreniform disorder, and acute psychotic disorder. In Kaplan, H.I. & Sadock, B.J. (eds) *Comprehensive Textbook of Psychiatry*, Vol. VI. Williams & Wilkins, Baltimore, (in press).

Siris, S.G., Harmon, G.K. & Endicott, J. (1981) Postpsychotic depressive symptoms in hospitalized schizophrenic patients. *Archives of General Psychiatry*, **38**, 1122–1123.

Siris, S.G., van Kammen, D.P. & Docherty, J.P. (1978) The use of antidepressant medication in schizophrenia: a review of the literature. *Archives of General Psychiatry*, **35**, 1368–1377.

Siris, S.G., Bermanzohn, P.C., Mason, S.E. & Shuwall, M.A. (1994) Maintenance imipramine for secondary depression in schizophrenia: a controlled trial. *Archives of General Psychiatry*, **51**, 109–115.

Siris, S.G., Morgan, V., Fagerstrom, R., Rifkin, A. & Cooper, T.B. (1987) Adjunctive imipramine in the treatment of postpsychotic depression: a controlled trial. *Archives of General Psychiatry*, **44**, 533–539.

Siris, S.G., Strahan, A., Mandeli, J., Cooper, T.B. & Casey, E. (1988a) Fluphenazine decanoate dose and severity of depression in patients with post-psychotic depression. *Schizophrenia Research*, **1**, 31–35.

Siris, S.G., Adan, F., Cohen, M., Mandeli, J., Aronson, A. & Casey, E. (1988b) Post-psychotic depression and negative symptoms: an investigation of syndromal overlap. *American Journal of Psychiatry*, **145**, 1532–1537.

Siris, S.G., Bermanzohn, P.C., Gonzalez, A., Mason, S.E., White, C.V. & Shuwall, M.A. (1991) The use of antidepressants for negative symptoms in a subset of schizophrenic patients. *Psychopharmacology Bulletin*, **27**, 331–335.

Siris, S.G., Cutler, J., Owen, K., Mason, S., Gingrich, S. & Lang, M.P. (1989) Adjunctive imipramine maintenance in schizophrenic patients with remitted postpsychotic depressions. *American Journal of Psychiatry*, **146**, 1495–1497.

Spitzer, R.L., Endicott, J. & Robins, E. (1978) Research diagnostic criteria: rationale and reliability. *Archives of General Psychiatry*, **35**, 773–782.

Strian, F., Heger, R. & Klicpera, C. (1982) The time structure of depressive mood in schizophrenic patients. *Acta Psychiatrica Scandinavica*, **65**, 66–73.

Summers, F., Harrow, M. & Westermeyer, J. (1983) Neurotic symptoms in the postacute phase of schizophrenia. *Journal of Nervous and Mental Disease*, **171**, 216–221.

Szymanski, H.V., Simon, J.C. & Gutterman, N. (1983) Recovery from schizophrenic psychosis. *American Journal of Psychiatry*, **140**, 335–338.

Taylor, M.A. (1992) Are schizophrenia and affective disorder related? A selective literature review. *American Journal of Psychiatry*, **149**, 22–32.

Van Putten, T. (1975) The many faces of akathisia. *Comprehensive Psychiatry*, **16**, 43–47.

Van Putten, T. & May, P.R.A. (1978) 'Akinetic depression' in schizophrenia. *Archives of General Psychiatry*, **35**, 1101–1107.

Waehrens, J. & Gerlach, J. (1980) Antidepressant drugs in anergic schizophrenia: a double-blind cross-over study with maprotiline and placebo. *Acta Psychiatrica Scandinavica*, **61**, 438–444.

Weissman, M.M., Pottenger, M., Kleber, H., Ruben, H.L., Williams, D. & Thompson, W.D. (1977) Symptom patterns in primary and secondary depression: a comparison of primary depressives with depressed opiate addicts, alcoholics, and schizophrenics. *Archives of General Psychiatry*, **34**, 854–862.

WHO (1988) *International Classification of Disease (ICD-10): Clinical Descriptions and Diagnostic Guidelines*. World Health Organization, Geneva, Switzerland. (Draft of Field Trials.)

Winokur, G. (1972) Family history studies. VIII. Secondary depression is alive and well, and . . . . *Diseases of the Nervous System*, **33**, 94–99.

Wise, R.A. (1982) Neuroleptics and operant behavior: the anhedonia hypothesis. *Behavioral and Brain Sciences*, **5**, 39–87.

Wistedt, B. & Palmstierna, T. (1983) Depressive symptoms in chronic schizophrenic patients after withdrawal of long-acting neuroleptics. *Journal of Clinical Psychiatry*, **44**, 369–371.

Chapter 10
Neurocognitive Deficits in Schizophrenia

T. E. GOLDBERG AND J. M. GOLD

Introduction

Abnormalities in attentional, associative and volitional cognitive processes have been considered central features of schizophrenia since the original clinical descriptions of Kraepelin (1919) and Bleuler (1950). The application of formal psychological assessment techniques in hundreds of studies in dozens of independent laboratories over the past 70 years has more than amply documented that such abnormalities are common occurrences in patients with the disorder. For example, about 40 years ago, Rappaport *et al.* (1945/46) published *Diagnostic Psychological Testing*, an influential two-volume set reporting findings from the application of a broad test battery to a wide variety of psychiatric patients. In describing deteriorated chronic schizophrenic patients, they noted that such patients have their greatest impairments in 'judgement, attention, concentration, planning ability and anticipation'. They further commented on the memory difficulties, inadequate concept formation and general intellectual inefficiency of patients with schizophrenia. Although interpreted within a psychodynamic framework and prior to the narrowing of the diagnostic conceptualization of schizophrenia and introduction of modern pharmacotherapy, the empirical observations made in the early 1940s are remarkably consistent with current findings. Indeed, we would suggest that the vast body of data on cognitive functioning in schizophrenia has been remarkably stable over many years. What has changed is the significance attributed to these results.

A most dramatic change occurred in the late 1970s. Three different review papers examined the ability of neuropsychological tests to distinguish the performance of 'functional' and 'organic' patients (Goldstein, 1978; Heaton *et al.*, 1978; Malec, 1978). All three concluded that such tests were quite successful except with patients with chronic schizophrenia, for whom classification hit rates approached chance. With the initial publications of *in vivo* evidence of ventricular enlargement in schizophrenia, as revealed by computerized tomography (CT) (Johnstone *et al.*, 1976; Weinberger *et al.*, 1979), a new era of neuropsychological study of schizophrenia began: there was a growing realization that patients with schizophrenia performed in the range typically seen in brain-damaged populations because schizophrenia involved a primary structural abnormality of the brain.

In the last 10 years, the routine use of clinical neuropsychological assessment and experimental neuropsychological paradigms has offered a new look to accounts of schizophrenia. Recent studies have thrown light on several of the more problematic facets of the disorder. In particular, they have made important contributions to understanding the frequency and severity of neurocognitive impairment in schizophrenia, the specificity of profiles of cognitive impairment to schizophrenia, the course of cognitive impairment and the prognostic importance of deficits. Careful reading of the studies also raises three conceptual issues of paramount importance.

1 Are the deficits reliable given the clinical variability of the disorder within and across patients?

2 Are the deficits generalized or differential in their severity?

3 Are the deficits restricted to various subgroups?

In the remainder of this chapter, we will address these issues with the aim of providing a coherent and up-to-date view of the cognitive impairments that may well burden schizophrenic patients as they attempt to succeed in the variegated transactions of everyday life.

Symptoms and cognition

In understanding schizophrenia, an important issue relevant for clinicians and researchers alike is the relationship between symptomatology and cognitive impairment. In clinical settings, it has often been assumed that the neurocognitive deficits in schizophrenia are due to the distracting impact of hallucinations, distortions and anxiety caused by paranoid delusions, motivational problems and lack of persistence. That is, it has been argued that deficits are dependent upon non-task-specific epiphenomena that might be psychological. This argument would seem to undercut any claim that neuropsychological performance provides an avenue into the brain—behaviour relations in schizophrenia.

The literature examining the impact of antipsychotic medications on cognitive performance provides a body of data relevant to the issue of symptom—cognition relations. Although the bulk of this literature is 20–30 years old and suffers from significant methodological flaws, it provides some grounds for examining whether the cognitive deficits of schizophrenia are primarily secondarily to the symptomatic state. If this were the case,

then one would expect successful pharmacological treatment to enhance cognitive performance. However, several recent reviews have come to a different conclusion: antipsychotic treatment offers relatively limited cognitive benefit [for reviews see Medalia *et al.* (1988) and Spohn and Strauss (1989)]. Certain attentional functions tend to improve, and measures of abstraction which demand a verbal response tend to show positive changes with treatment. However, most cognitive measures are surprisingly stable in the face of changes in medication status and, presumably, clinical state. The positive changes that are observed, while significant, typically fall short of bringing patients to normal levels. Indeed, it has been our observation that the most dramatic positive change occurs in the ability of some patients to co-operate with an evaluation when medicated. Thus, the cognitive impairment in schizophrenia appears to have significant stable, trait-like features with some functions having additional clinical 'state'-related variation.

Treatment with antipsychotic and anticholinergic medications may also have adverse effects on some cognitive functions. Such negative effects have been most frequently observed in studies of acute treatment; more chronic treatment rarely produces clear cognitive 'costs'. There is some evidence that complex motor functions may be impaired by treatment with antipsychotic medications and that memory functions may be impaired by either anticholinergic effects of antiparkinsonian medications or the anticholinergic activity inherent in many neuroleptics. However, effects have not been large across studies. In short, there is little evidence that the cognitive impairments in schizophrenia either result from or can be substantially improved by treatment with conventional neuroleptic medications.

We have also examined this issue by attempting to dissociate symptoms and cognition in a study involving the neuroleptic medication clozapine (Goldberg *et al.*, 1993b). Clozapine was chosen not because it is a so-called atypical neuroleptic with pharmacological effects on many neurotransmitter systems, but because it is known to produce large symptomatic changes in a notoriously treatment-resistant group, namely chronic schizophrenic patients, and because it does not induce parkinsonian side effects. The design of this study was straightforward. First, patients has symptoms rated on the brief psychiatric rating scale (BPRS) and neurocognitive function assessed by a standard screening battery while they were receiving a variety of 'typical' neuroleptic medications. Then, the patients were given clozapine. They were retested, on average, about 15 months later (still receiving clozapine). Symptoms improved dramatically: BPRS scores were reduced by approximately 40%. However, in this sample of 15 patients, neurocognitive scores did not improve. Moreover, we found no difference in cognitive change scores between the group that improved the most symptomatically and the group that improved the least (based upon the median split of BPRS change scores). These results suggest that cognitive impairment is not simply a function of symptomatology. We are not arguing that symptoms have no role in the cognitive impairment in schizophrenia; clearly, they cannot help cognitive performance. Rather, we are adumbrating the view that there is much variance in schizophrenic cognition that is not explained by symptoms.

We (Goldberg *et al.* 1993a) have also compared symptom—cognition relationships in a large group of patients with schizophrenia and with affective disorder. A statistical technique involving redundancy analysis was used, which yields a measure of the strength and directionality of an association between two sets of variables. It was found that for the schizophrenia group, BPRS factor scores accounted for about 5% of the variance in cognitive measures including intelligence quotient (IQ), memory, set shifting and visual spatial performance. Moreover, it appeared that cognitive failure may, in fact, have had an impact on symptomatology, i.e. cognitive measures accounted for 10% of the variance in BPRS scores. In unipolar and bipolar affective groups, the amount of variance in cognition for which symptoms accounted was much greater, ranging from 20% to 30%. Redundancy analyses also suggested that, in contradistinction to the schizophrenic group, the effect of

cognition on symptoms in the affectively disordered groups was small. The results in the affective disorders group are consistent with a large body of literature that suggests that cognitive functioning in depressed patients varies at least partially as a function of symptom severity (Weingartner, 1986).

Another clinically germane question is whether poor performance can be attributed to a lack of motivation or co-operation. We attempted to explore this aspect of the nature of impairment on the Wisconsin Card Sorting Test (WCST) by providing incremental instructions about categorization and set shifting to patients, followed by intensive card-by-card teaching in an effort to ensure that patients established and maintained an optimal test-taking set (Goldberg *et al.*, 1987). Incremental information did not improve the performance of these patients, but card-by-card teaching normalized their performance. Their willingness to attend to intensive teaching suggested that patients were capable of being co-operative, attentive and motivated. However, when the card-by-card teaching was stopped and normal testing procedures were reimplemented, patients' performance returned to baseline. This suggested that 'psychological' factors were not the primary explanation for the patients' difficulties. We believe that this study indicated that patients truly could not do the test rather than would not do it. We were neither the first nor the last group to examine this issue (Stuss *et al.*, 1983; Schneider & Asarnow, 1987; Levin *et al.*, 1989). Published studies by four other groups have suggested that the effects of instructions and/or reinforcements could improve WCST performance in patients with schizophrenia (Bellack *et al.*, 1990; Summerfelt *et al.*, 1991; Tompkins *et al.*, 1991; Green *et al.*, 1992). However, none of these groups were able to normalize patients' performance. Indeed, similar results have been found in patients with well-documented neurological conditions, including amnesia and dementia (Richardson, 1992). The results of these studies do not argue that the conditions are somehow less real, or unrelated to neural dysfunction, but rather illustrate that motivation, encouragement and test-taking strategies may improve the function of even compromised neural systems, perhaps by increasing arousal, diminishing neural 'noise', modulating reward systems or aiding in the recruitment of neural systems not usually involved in the task. However, the results also indicate that in schizophrenia, the relevant neural systems function in a deficient manner (Goldberg & Weinberger, 1994).

Differential deficits?

One of the goals of neuropsychological and cognitive research in schizophrenia is to identify abnormalities in particular cognitive processes that are linked to specific brain regions or systems. The search for such a 'fundamental' deficit or deficits faces a basic methodological challenge. As noted by Chapman and Chapman (1973), patients with schizophrenia tend to perform more poorly than normal controls on a wide variety of tasks: they demonstrate a 'generalized' deficit whose origin remains undetermined. Such a deficit might conceivably reflect the experience of institutionalization, failures in co-operation or diffuse brain dysfunction. Of greater theoretical interest, however, is the existence of 'differential' deficits, i.e. deficits more severe than might be anticipated on the basis of the generalized deficit. Such differential deficits could provide evidence of regionally specific neurocognitive impairment. Current clinical assessment test batteries are not capable of rigorously supporting inferences of differential deficit. To demonstrate differential deficit adequately, tasks should be matched on the basis of difficulty level and reliability, so that ceiling effects or measurement error do not skew the results. Very few matched tasks have been developed (Calev, 1984) and these tasks have not been incorporated into standard clinical assessment batteries.

Another aspect of task matching which is frequently overlooked involves the dispersion of scores. Some tests are constructed such that it is difficult to score more than two standard deviations below the normal control mean, while on many other tests it is possible to score many standard deviations below normal (Randolph *et al.*, 1993). Therefore, one could conclude incorrectly that performance on the latter group is worse than on the former group of tests. It should be recognized, however, that when a difference is found between groups, that difference is valid in terms of its existence. On the other hand, claims that one impaired performance is necessarily more deficient than another impaired performance, or that a normal performance is 'truly' normal, are not valid if tasks are not matched. In sum, the interpretation of neuropsychological findings remains largely a matter of clinical judgement, a process which has clear limitations for supporting more specific inferences about areas of maximal dysfunction in a population with widespread cognitive difficulties.

There are no easy solutions to these problems of measurement. One statistical approach involves comparing the residuals from a regression line that is derived from two variables of interest (Chapman & Chapman, 1989). First, a regression equation is determined in the normal or control group and its residuals are calculated. Then, this equation is applied to the experimental sample, and the residuals of the actual and predicted values are compared. In patients with verified neurological disorders, an approach that has been fruitful in identifying differential deficit patterns involves a search for double dissociations (Teuber, 1955; Shallice, 1988). In this method, two patient groups are compared on two tests. If one group outperforms the other on the first test, but is itself outperformed on the second, then one infers that the groups have a differential profile of performance. This latter approach, underutilized in previous schizophrenia research, has recently been used by Gold *et al.* (1994) in a study of temporal lobe epilepsy and schizophrenia, and by Goldberg *et al.* (1990a) in a study of Huntington's disease and schizophrenia. In the former, patients with schizophrenia had worse attentional, but better semantic, functioning than did patients with left temporal lobe epilepsy. In the latter, patients with schizophrenia had reduced prefrontal and increased parietal cerebral blood flow in comparison with patients with Huntington's disease. While the double-dissociation approach is not immune to psychometric artefacts, i.e. one test is 'harder' than the other, it appears to have a distinct advantage over studies comparing patients and normal controls.

Core neurocognitive deficits

It has been possible to establish the cognitive geography of much of the brain despite the difficult methodological issues involved in establishing differential deficits. This is because the clinical interpretation of test data can often point to multiple studies that converge on a set of frequent, severe and selective deficits. In our view, patients with schizophrenia typically demonstrate abnormalities in attention, memory and executive function which stand out against a background of diffuse impairment. Although this view cannot, at present, be proven, the apparent impairments in these cognitive functions are of interest in relation to other neurobiological findings in the illness, such as structural abnormalities of the temporal lobe, functional hypometabolism of the prefrontal cortex and abnormalities in catecholamine function.

Attention

Even the casual observer may often be struck by deficits in the capacity of patients to cull information from their environment. Simply put, patients do not seem to focus attention and to concentrate. Moreover, they sometimes appear to be preoccupied with internal stimuli, or are easily distracted by external stimuli. Such observations, both historical and clinical, have been amply supported by numerous studies of sustained and selective attention. One of the early experimental studies of attention, devised by Shakow (1979), found that patients with schizophrenia demonstrate slowed reaction time and, moreover, cannot improve their performance in a reaction time paradigm even when intervals between warning and stimulus are both predictable and long. Thus, the patients appeared to be unable to sustain attention, compromising their readiness to respond across longer time intervals. In other set

of attentional paradigms, schizophrenic patients had deficits maintaining vigilance during a continuous performance test involving specific combinations of stimuli (Mirsky, 1988). Patients typically failed to respond to target stimuli and also responded inappropriately to lures, thereby making both omission and commission errors.

Other paradigms have regularly demonstrated that patients with schizophrenia have difficulty with focused attention. For instance, in a span of apprehension tests (Asarnow *et al.*, 1991), schizophrenic patients had difficulty in accurately and selectively stating whether a target was present in a briefly presented array. Other tests of inhibition to distractors (Oltmanns & Neale, 1975) have also revealed deficits. It is worth noting that even the basic 'freedom from distractibility' factor on the WAIS-R is compromised in schizophrenic patients (Gold *et al.*, 1994). This attentional deficit in schizophrenia may be found across many different paradigms.

It is clear that attention is not a unitary construct, but it is unclear whether there is a particular dimension that is maximally impaired in schizophrenia. Posner and Petersen (1990) developed an elegant model of the components of spatial attention. An initial examination of this model in schizophrenia was potentially promising: Posner *et al.* reported that schizophrenic patients displayed an asymmetrical slowing in response to stimuli that appeared in the right visual field after so-called invalid cues for a response (Posner *et al.*, 1988). However, attempts to replicate this study have not met with success (Gold *et al.*, 1992).

It is also important to consider the extent to which attention is modularized. That is, attentional impairments may or may not disrupt many other cognitive functions. One might assume that poor attention would prevent many types of information from being processed fully. However, correlational studies have generally suggested that attentional dysfunction explains only a small portion of the variance in many cognitive functions (Kenny & Meltzer, 1991). Perhaps this should not come as a complete surprise, as patients with well-documented attentional deficit disorders often display many areas of intact cognitive function (Barkley *et al.*, 1990). It remains to be seen whether this is due to the properties of the distributed neural system underlying attention (Mesulam, 1983), or whether it simply reflects some dissociation between the ecology of the testing situation and real life.

Memory

Memory function in schizophrenia was one of the first cognitive abilities to be studied (Hull, 1917). The results, however, have been difficult to characterize. Patients with schizophrenia generally remember stories, verbal paired associates and visual designs more poorly than do normal subjects. Moreover, differences between normal controls and patients may be large (Saykin *et al.*, 1991; Gold *et al.*, 1994). The rate of learning may also differ between normal subjects and schizophrenic patients (Goldberg *et al.*, 1989). In tests of recognition memory in which retrieval strategies are minimized, patients sometimes have been found to be impaired and sometimes have been found to be relatively intact (Bauman & Murray, 1968; Calev, 1984; Goldberg *et al.*, 1989; Gold *et al.*, 1992). Deficits have been attributed not only to consolidation impairments, but to inefficient encoding (Traupmann, 1980), poor use of retrieval strategies in effortful recall (Goldberg *et al.*, 1989) and rapid forgetting (Sengel & Lovalla, 1983; McKenna *et al.*, 1990).

Some of the difficulty in characterizing schizophrenic memory functioning may be due to methodological factors. First, poorly matched control groups might obscure real between-group differences. Second, many studies have not distinguished among 'stages' or 'types' of memory. There is now much evidence to suggest that memory is not unitary, but rather can be dissociated into various subtypes. These include explicit memory, in which there is conscious recollection of material, implicit memory, in which there is evidence of learning but without conscious awareness and procedural memory, in which a motor skill is learned by performing it. Third, many studies have not carefully examined the role

of possible confounds in memory testing, namely symptoms and medication, including anticholinergics (see above).

Three recent studies have attempted to address these methodological concerns. In the first, Gold *et al.* (1992) compared the performance of schizophrenic patients and a normal group matched on measures of semantic memory, namely visual confrontation naming, word knowledge and reading (a measure of premorbid intellect). Tasks of free recall, recognition and frequency estimation were administered and the patients demonstrated impairments despite differences in attentional demands and so-called automaticity of the tasks. Second, Goldberg *et al.* (1993c) used a paradigm which examined monozygotic twins discordant for schizophrenia. It controlled for differences in genome, and minimized differences in early education, socioeconomic status and family emotional climate. They found that the affected twins performed significantly worse than the unaffected group on measures of story recall, paired associate learning and visual recall of designs. Recognition memory appeared to be relatively preserved in the affected twins. The groups did not differ on a measure of procedural memory that involved procedural learning on a rotary pursuit test. In addition, it was found that anticholinergic medication did not significantly contribute to the results.

In the third study, which examined implicit memory using a stem-completion paradigm, Randolph *et al.* (1993a) found that while patients exhibited impaired implicit memory performance on a standard version of the stem-completion task, a manipulation that increased the semantic encoding of the word appeared to normalize performance on the task. This manipulation had no effect on normal controls, suggesting that the patients may have approached the task in an unusual fashion. However, a recent study by Schwartz *et al.* (1993) reported that schizophrenic patients displayed impaired explicit memory in paired associate learning coupled to normal implicit memory performance for degraded word identification and category production tasks (i.e. fluency for semantic categories). Thus, the status of implicit memory in schizophrenia remains unclear.

In summary, schizophrenic patients demonstrate marked deficits in episodic memory measures. That is, patients have difficulty retrieving episodes of experience within distinct spatio-temporal contexts. Procedural learning that involves motor skills may be relatively intact (with the emphasis on 'relatively'). The situation for item-specific implicit memory is unclear, given the contrary findings to date.

Executive functions

Clinicians have frequently observed that schizophrenic patients have difficulty generating and implementing plans. Patients also appear to have difficulty solving problems whose solutions are not readily apparent, or when they must rely upon novel recombinations of existing knowledge. From the neuropsychological standpoint, such deficits are often considered to be 'executive' in nature, in the sense that they involve use of information rather than fundamental processing of the information. Formal tests of analogues of these abilities have usually revealed deficits in patients. For instance, Fey (1951) demonstrated that schizophrenic patients have performance deficits on the WCST of abstraction, set shifting and response to feedback. More recent studies (Stuss *et al.*, 1983; Braff *et al.*, 1991) have also showed that chronic schizophrenic patients performed poorly on the WCST. Not only do patients have difficulty abstracting a concept, but they often perseverate to incorrect responses even when provided with regular feedback to the contrary. Not surprisingly, many schizophrenic patients also demonstrate deficits on a difficult test of concept formation and rule learning, namely the category test from the Halstead−Reitan battery (Goldstein, 1990).

What might be the foundation for such deficits? Recently, interest has increased in cognitive operations presumed to be involved in a supervisory attentional or working memory system that could control information flow on tasks like the WCST or category test. Importantly, it has been premised that when the system is dysfunctional, it might

result in two seemingly contradictory behaviours: (i) distractibility, because all environmental stimuli appear to be equally relevant and thus produce 'capture' errors; and (ii) perseveration, in that new strategies might not be brought 'on-line' after responses that had once been correct were now no longer so (Shallice, 1988).

A number of studies provide evidence that working memory (here defined as the capacity to maintain information over short delays while that information is being transformed or co-ordinated with other ongoing mental operations in the service of a response) is compromised in schizophrenia. Cohen and Servan-Schreiber (1992) found that patients with schizophrenia had differential difficulty in using contextual phrases to comprehend a sentence when these phrases were temporally remote from ambiguous words, i.e. the phrases had to be held 'in mind' longer. Park and Holzman (1992) reported deficits in an oculomotor version of a delayed response task sensitive to prefrontal lesions in non-human primates and in a novel haptic task. Gold *et al.* (submitted) reported that patients had difficulty learning a delayed alternation task and continued to have difficulty even after instruction.

Studies of auditory tasks reveal similar deficits in working memory. Gold *et al.* (1994) found that schizophrenic patients performed more poorly than patients with temporal lobe epilepsy on the digit span and arithmetic subtests of the Wechsler Adult Intelligence Scale − Revised (WAIS-R). There are multiple reports of poor performance by patients with schizophrenia on variants of the Brown−Peterson task. This task (which appears to require a combination of short- and long-term memory) involves remembering a short list of words over a brief delay (e.g. 12 s) during which interpolated activities draw off 'processing resources' and/or prevent rehearsal. Fleming *et al.* (in press) found that the recall of schizophrenic patients was sensitive to other processing demands performed during the retention interval. Even simple counting resulted in a performance decrement, suggesting that patients were not able to rehearse when asked simultaneously to remember and perform even a simple task. This finding suggests a very basic defect in the ability to allocate attentional resources and is theoretically consistent with an impaired central executive of working memory.

Intact cognitive functions?

It is a truism that schizophrenic patients do more poorly than normal subjects on almost every test. However, some areas of function appeared to be relatively more intact than others. For instance, the verbal (language) subtests of the WAIS-R that involve expressive vocabulary, expression of knowledge of commonplace information and abstraction of similarities between words are all relatively well preserved (Gold *et al.*, 1994). In addition, language factors comprised of a variety of measures that included comprehension and naming also appear to be relatively uncompromised (Saykin *et al.*, 1991). While Andreasen and Grove (1979) suggested that schizophrenic language, when marked by derailments, fragmentation and neologisms, was similar to that of patients with receptive aphasia, this has not been empirically discerned, as Daniels *et al.* (1988) found the language of schizophrenic patients to be similar to that of patients with right hemisphere lesions. In particular, the comprehension and naming in schizophrenic patients is not markedly impaired and the errors that they make on formal tests, including the Token Test of auditory understanding of syntax and semantics, are not similar to those of aphasic patients (Barr *et al.*, 1989).

The view that language is relatively unimpaired is subject to several qualifications, however. For example, Tamlyn *et al.* (1992) found that patients had deficits in their remote knowledge or semantic system and made remarkable errors on tests of simple 'real-world' comprehension (but see above, Gold *et al.*, 1994). There has also been speculation that the semantic system may have a role in the disorganization sometimes found in the expressive language of schizophrenic patients (i.e. thought disorder). In this regard, studies that have assessed the ease with which target words might be activated by semantically related words (called 'primes') have rather often indicated that schizophrenic patients display excessive priming effects, in that their reaction-time scores decline more than do those of normal controls. Such excessive activation might plausibly be a critical factor in producing disorganized speech. This interface between cognition and symptomatology will probably receive much experimental attention in the near future (Frith, 1993).

Another domain that may not be markedly impaired in schizophrenia involves visual spatial processing. Patients with schizophrenia usually perform within normal limits on tests that assess the ability to analyse the relationship between the location of objects in space (Kolb & Whishaw, 1983). Thus, patients do relatively well in performing tasks that involve block design construction, right/left orientation on a road-map test and judgement of the orientation of angled lines (Goldberg *et al.*, 1990b). Data on so-called object recognition visual tests are somewhat more equivocal (Goldberg *et al.*, 1993a). Further examination of these two visual systems appears to be warranted.

In light of the attentional impairments found in schizophrenia, it is noteworthy that patients do not appear to perform differentially worse on certain measures of complex attentional function. For example, the Stroop test is considered a classic measure of selective attention in that the subject must name the colour of ink used to print a word identifying an opposing colour. Thus, the automatic reading response must be inhibited. Although patients perform abnormally in this condition, they are also unusually slow at simple word reading and colour naming, and it is not at all clear that the additional selective attention demand amplifies the patient control differences (Goldberg *et al.*, 1990b). Similarly, performance on Trail Making test B, a test which demands rapid, sequenced shifts of attention between letter and number stimuli, does not appear to be more impaired than performance on trailmaking test A, which requires the sequencing of number stimuli alone (Goldberg *et al.*, 1990b). In both the Stroop and Trail Making tests, it appears likely that deficits in more basic processing account for much of the variance in the more complex condition.

Neuroanatomical implications

The neuropsychological profile delineated above, in which prominent attentional, memory and executive function deficits are observed in the context of milder impairments in some aspects of language and some types of visual spatial processing, implicates specific brain regions. As noted by Kolb and Whishaw (1983) and by Taylor and Abrams (1984), such a pattern suggests frontal–medial temporal dysfunction. Posterior areas may be relatively spared. More direct correlative evidence, as opposed to inferential evidence, has also been found. Thus, Goldberg *et al.* (1994) studied monozygotic twins discordant for schizophrenia in an attempt to ascertain precisely the degree to which cognitive, neurophysiological and neuroanatomical measures deviate from their genetically and environmentally determined potential level. The method involved correlating the difference scores between the unaffected member and affected member of a twin pair for each measurement. Significant associations between the left hippocampus and verbal memory for stories (when IQ was partialled) and prefrontal cerebral blood flow with perseveration on the WCST were found. Moreover, Weinberger *et al.* (1992) found a very high correlation between the two biological measures, prefrontal cerebral blood flow and anterior hippocampal volume, suggesting that the connectivity between these two regions may be important in understanding both the cognitive and the symptomatological manifestations of schizophrenia.

Efforts to correlate ventricular or brain size with cognitive impairment have met with mixed results (Goldberg *et al.*, 1994). It may be that the diminutions in size or ability typically found in schizophrenia are not of sufficient magnitude to produce a range necessary to finding more robust associations. If this is the case, then it might be necessary to combine chronic in-patient samples, out-patient samples and so-called spectrum samples (that presumably vary along a severity dimension) to increase the range of abnormalities present.

Frequency of neurocognitive impairment and subtyping

Using binary cut-offs, the frequency of neuropsychological impairment in schizophrenia is often between 40 and 60% on individual tests known to demonstrate deficits in brain-damaged patients (Goldberg *et al.*, 1988b). However, a recent study using a paradigm involving monozygotic twins discordant for schizophrenia suggests that the frequency of impairment may be considerably higher. We (Goldberg *et al.*, 1990b) found that affected twins consistently performed worse than their unaffected cotwins on many of the tests in a neuropsychological battery. For instance, 'hit rates' (i.e. instances in which the affected twin performed worse than the unaffected cotwin) for the Wechsler Memory Scale, WCST and full-scale IQ were 95, 85 and 80%, respectively. Especially important was the fact that even when the affected twin was ostensibly performing within the normal range, the cotwin performed at a still higher level.

Prior to this study, it was difficult to know whether patients who appear to be performing normally on a given test may not have suffered any substantial decline. These data suggest that it may be crucial to know not only the patients' current level of performance, but also how far they have fallen relative to their potential genetic and environmental endowment. These data also suggest that the intercession of disease appears either to prevent the affected twin from reaching his or her potential or, more likely, to reduce performance on many of the cognitive tasks. In short, results from the study of discordant twins indicate that neuropsychological dysfunction appears to be an extremely frequent, if not fundamental, feature of schizophrenia.

These results also have certain implications for subtype analysis. For instance, a number of studies have suggested that patients with predominantly negative symptoms have more severe cognitive impairments than those with predominantly positive symptoms. The study of twins indicated that cognitive impairment is present in nearly all patients, irrespective of symptom profile, although the precise severity of cognitive impairment may vary. The study also indicated that cognitive impairment was present in both paranoid and undifferentiated diagnoses. Rather than a bimodal distribution, these data argue for a normal, or perhaps slightly skewed, distribution of cognitive scores shifted to the left of the normal distribution.

It has also been argued that female patients have a milder course than males, respond more completely to neuroleptics and may have a different pathogenesis (Goldstein and Tsuang, 1990; Castle & Murray, 1991). If females with schizophrenia comprise a valid subgroup, differences in neuropsychological performance between females and males might be expected. We (Goldberg *et al.*, in press) examined four independent samples of schizophrenic patients. One sample was comprised of consecutive admissions to a private psychiatric hospital, another was comprised of the aforementioned discordant twins and two others were comprised of chronic patients at a research hospital. In over 100 comparisons on different neurocognitive tests, no sex differences favouring females were found. These data argue that from a neuropsychological standpoint, subtyping patients on the basis of their sex is not informative.

Neuroanatomical and neurophysiological data may also support arguments for homogeneity rather than heterogeneity. In studying discordant twins, Suddath *et al.* (1990) found that ventricular enlargement and hippocampal volumetric reduction were present in nearly all affected individuals as compared with their well cotwins. That is, a subgroup of patients with uncompromised morphologies was not present. Similarly, Berman *et al.* (1993) found that all affected twins had lower prefrontal regional cerebral blood flow while being administered the WCST than did their unaffected cotwins. Again, no evidence for subgroups was found. In another study, Daniel *et al.* (1991) examined the distribution of over 1000 ventricular brain ratio values culled from the literature on CT for evidence of bimodality. Such a distribution might have indicated the presence of one subgroup of patients with very large ventricles and a second subgroup with ventricles well within the normal range. Using a mixture distribution technique that involved curve-fitting procedures, the results were negative. That is, no subgroup of patients with exceptionally large ventricular brain ratios was found. What was perhaps most striking about the data was the paucity of cases in which schizophrenic patients had very small ventricles. This set of results provided further evidence that all patients in the distribution had suffered some degree of insult and thus showed increased cerebrospinal fluid (CSF) spaces.

Comparative studies

The identification of a characteristic neurocognitive profile of schizophrenia relative to other disorders provides useful information concerning the fundamental validity of the accumulated neurocognitive findings. Differences in overall global impairment (i.e. level) may have important implications for everyday functioning. Differences in profile of impairment (i.e. shape) may help sharpen the discussion of anatomical implications of deficits and identify useful measures for high-risk or linkage studies. Furthermore, these comparative differential deficits could provide targets for rehabilitative and pharmacological treatment efforts.

The comparison of schizophrenic patients and patients with mood disorders offers some insight into the clinical importance of neuropsychological functioning, given the fact that the outcome of schizophrenia is generally far worse in terms of social and vocational functioning than that observed in mood disorders. If the disability of schizoprenic patients reflects neuropsychological impairment, then one would expect formal testing to distinguish the diagnostic groups. The results of a recent study (Goldberg *et al.*, 1993a) support this view. A schizophrenic group performed significantly below affective groups (unipolar and bipolar) on tests of attention and psychomotor speed, verbal and visual memory, and problem solving and abstraction. Values of IQ were also low in the schizophrenic group and appeared to have deteriorated from a normal premorbid level. Moreover, when the analysis was restricted to patients with IQ scores of 90 or more, the patients with schizophrenia still performed more poorly than did the mood disorder group on the WCST and visual memory, suggesting that inadequacy of global cognitive competence was not the sole source of the between-group difference. On the other hand, patients with schizophrenia did not differ from patients with schizoaffective disorder on this neuropsychological screening battery (Goldberg, unpublished data). This result is consistent with other data that schizoaffective disorder is more similar to schizophrenia than to affective disorder.

A number of investigators have suggested that schizophrenia might be considered a form of subcortical dementia (Pantelis *et al.*, 1992). We (Goldberg *et al.*, 1990a) directly compared patients with schizophrenia with those with Huntington's disease, the archetypal 'subcortical dementia' (Cummings & Benson, 1984) in which there is marked atrophy of the caudate. In this study, we matched performance of the groups on the WCST; both groups also had equivalent full-scale IQs. However, the patients with Huntington's disease demonstrated somewhat better language and attentional abilities, while demonstrating considerably worse visual spatial abilities. This difference between the groups could not be attributed to differences in executive function because, as noted, they were matched on perseverative tendencies. We found double dissociation in cerebral blood flow, measured while the patients performed the WCST. Patients with schizophrenia had relatively low frontal and relatively high parietal activity, while patients with Huntington's disease exhibited the reverse pattern. These data suggest not only that schizophrenia is dissimilar to Huntington's disease, but also that a final common cognitive impairment in executive function may be associated with two markedly dissimilar pathophysiological states.

In light of recent evidence of structural abnormalities in the mesial temporal lobe of those with schizophrenia, the neuropsychological comparison of patients with schizophrenia and patients with temporal lobe epilepsy (TLE) may offer some insight into the role of lateralized temporal lobe dysfunction in the genesis of schizophrenic impairment. We (Gold *et al.*, 1994) studied patients with left and right temporal lobe epilepsy with clearly lateralized seizure foci who had medication-resistant disorders and whose chronic seizures generally began in early or middle childhood. In short, these epilepsy groups represent the severe end of the epileptic spectrum. We found striking differences in group performance patterns. The patients with schizophrenia demonstrated superior word reading and verbal semantic memory relative to the TLE groups, with marked and consistent differences observed in comparison with the left TLE patients. The patients with schizophrenia demonstrated significant attentional, motor and problem-solving deficits relative to both right and left TLE groups. We argued that this pattern of findings suggests that in schizophrenia there is a loss of function, whereas in epilepsy the acquisition of academic and linguistic skill is compromised. The contrasts in memory function have varied across memory measures. The schizophrenic group demonstrated worse visual memory than either TLE group on the visual memory index of the Wechsler Memory Scale — Revised. On this test the immediate recall of verbal materials was highly similar in the left TLE and schizophrenic groups, but the groups clearly differed on measures of delayed recall where the left TLE group was particularly impaired. Somewhat different results were obtained using the California Verbal Learning Test, a test of list learning. Here, the schizophrenic and right TLE groups both performed somewhat better than the left TLE group, although it should be noted that all three groups performed well below normal controls. Thus, our examination of memory performance has not yet yielded clear-cut results. However, the relationship between memory and other cognitive functions appears to be quite different between these disorders. In TLE, particularly left TLE, memory is selectively impaired relative to attention. In schizophrenia, both functions are equally impaired. Thus, it is the pattern of findings rather than absolute performance level that appears to be most useful in distinguishing the cognitive deficits of these disorders.

Course

The course of schizophrenia has often been considered similar to that of progressive dementia in that there is relentless social and presumably cognitive decline (Miller, 1989). There are, however, a great many neuropsychological studies that do not support this view (Heaton & Drexler, 1987).

A broad literature can be drawn upon to support a different account which emphasizes features in the course consistent with the notion of 'static encephalopathy'. For instance, prior to the emergence of symptoms patients had relatively normal IQs and performed relatively well in school (although not necessarily at the level of their peers or siblings) despite findings of subtle attenuations in various aspects of memory, abstraction and set shifting, and attention (Offord & Cross, 1971; Cornblatt & Erlenmeyer-Kimling, 1985; Nuechterlein, 1985; Pogue-Geile, 1989; Asarnow *et al.*, 1991; Walker & Lewine, 1990; Goldberg *et al.*, in press). Within the first few years of their clinical illness, patients typically performed poorly on a wide range of tests that include those assessing memory, executive functions and attentional abilities (Goldberg *et al.*, 1988a; Bilder *et al.*, in press). In this period, variability in repeated assessment might also occur, as patients' scores may even improve slightly (Sweeney *et al.*, 1991). Longitudinal studies of armed forces personnel, prior to the onset of illness and during its active phase, are consistent with results that suggest relatively abrupt declines in functioning. Thus, on armed forces classification tests patients performed similarly to their controls in the premorbid period and then displayed significant decrements of nearly 0.5 standard deviations after the onset of illness (Lubin *et al.*, 1962; Schwartzman & Douglas, 1962).

Crucially, deterioration does not appear to occur during the (more) chronic phase of the illness. For instance, over intervals of 8 years, the performance of patients did not decline on tests such as the WAIS and the Porteus maze test (Smith, 1964; Klonoff *et al.*, 1970).

Another approach to the issue of dementia in schizophrenia involves the use of a well-validated cross-sectional cohort comparison design. We (Hyde *et al.*, 1994) studied successive cohorts of patients in their third, fourth, fifth, sixth and seventh decades of life. Patients were administered a battery of tests known to be sensitive to progressive dementia (Mini-Mental State Examination, Dementia Rating Scale, list learning and Boston Naming). While the methodology has obvious shortcomings, notably increased variability because comparisons are made between age groups rather than within subjects, the study design nonetheless allowed for comparisons over an extremely wide age range and duration of illness while minimizing attrition effects. In addition, the groups were matched on premorbid intellectual ability by use of reading recognition, a putative measure of premorbid intellect. Patients were carefully screened to exclude those with confounding systemic and neurological conditions that might also lead to impairment on neuropsychological testing. We found no significant differences between age cohorts on verbal list learning, semantic fluency, the Mini-Mental State examination and the dementia rating scale. A cohort effect was found for naming, but it correlated with age rather than with duration of illness. We therefore concluded that the course of cognitive function in schizophrenia appeared to be consistent with a static encephalopathy rather than with a progressive dementing disorder. Goldstein and Zubin (1990) also found that on tests from a neuropsychological battery younger schizophrenic patients did not differ from older patients above and beyond the effects of ageing. Also, the length of institutionalization did not have a significant effect on neuropsychological results. This study is important because of its large sample size and extensive assessment procedures (i.e. the Halstead–Reitan battery). These results are also consistent with Kraepelin's original observation: 'As a rule, if no essential improvement intervenes in at most two or three years after the appearance of the more striking morbid phenomena, a state of weak mindedness will be developed, which usually changes only slowly and insignificantly'. Shakow also noted that despite individual variations in course 'the most frequent type is that which resembles temporally the process of oblivescence, a considerable drop at first with the tapering off through a slowed period to a stable level' (Shakow, 1946).

These neuropsychological observations are also consistent with neuroimaging and neuropathological studies. For instance, 'first-episode' patients who underwent serial magnetic resonance imaging (MRI) or CT scanning over a period as long as 9 years did not appear to exhibit progressive changes (Abi-Dargham *et al.*, 1991). Also, longitudinal CT studies of chronic patients have generally not revealed changes (Illowsky *et al.*, 1988). In a number of neuropathological studies, gliosis, considered to be a marker of an active degenerative process, has rarely been observed (Bruton *et al.*, 1990). On the contrary, the most common abnormalities have involved ventricular enlargement, reductions in grey matter volume or cytoarchitectonic irregularities. All these abnormalities may be consistent with a non-progressive neurodevelopmental lesion (for further discussion of prognostic factors see Chapter 8).

Concurrent and predictive validity of neuropsychological impairment

Neurocognitive deficits may be a rate-limiting factor in the rehabilitation of patients with schizophrenia. For instance, in our study of clozapine (Goldberg *et al.*, 1993b), we observed that while patients' symptoms improved markedly over the 15-month study period, the patients still required supervised living arrangements and could not work in high-level competitive situations. Because their neuropsychological profile remained impaired and unchanged, neurocognitive deficits might have accounted for some of the continuing disabilities. Strong concurrent relations between the global level of functioning and specific neurocognitive test scores have been found (Goldberg *et al.*, 1990b, 1993c). On cognitive measures that included memory for stories from the Wechsler memory scale, verbal fluency, WCST and IQ, intratwin pair differences were strongly and significantly associated with differences in social and vocational functioning as measured by the global

assessment scale (GAS). Breier *et al.* (1991) also found that the WCST was a powerful predictor of the current level of functioning. In addition, in monozygotic twins concordant for schizophrenia, a group in whom symptomatology was similar, as was the experience of having a chronic illness, differences in a set of cognitive measures (trails, IQ, WCST and memory quotient) accounted for over 95% of the variance in intrapair differences in GAS scores (Goldberg *et al.*, in press).

Neuropsychological impairment also may contribute to long-term outcome in schizophrenia. For instance, Perlick *et al.* (1992) found that a composite measure of neuropsychological functioning was more effective than symptomatology, premorbid status or age of onset in discriminating between patients who remained continually hospitalized and those who were able to live in the community. In particular, measures of motor co-ordination, perseveration memory and attention distinguished between patient groups. Moreover, symptoms, especially of the florid, psychotic type, may not have a strong relationship with economic self-support in the long term (Jonnson & Nyman, 1991). Kolakowska *et al.* (1985) studied patients for up to 20 years following the onset of illness and found that cognitive impairment was one of the variables associated with unfavourable outcome. This is not to downplay the role of symptoms, which certainly play a role in outcome (Pogue-Geile, 1989), nor family functioning which can sometimes emerge as an important predictor of outcome (McGlashan, 1986). The data do suggest, however, that these are not the whole story (see also Chapter 30).

Summary

A number of conclusions can be drawn from the foregoing discussion. First, schizophrenic patients exhibit prominent impairments in attention, memory and executive functions. This profile of impairment implicates frontal−medial temporal cerebral regions. Second, these deficits are not restricted to a group of 'outliers', but can be discerned to varying degrees throughout the population of patients. Third, these deficits may be independent of clinical state to a surprising degree. Fourth, they reflect deterioration from some higher level of functioning and then stabilization, as consistent with a static encephalopathy. Finally, because these deficits may account for some of the social and vocational morbidity associated with schizophrenia, they probably should be considered targets for various remediation modalities, including cognitive training and nootropics.

References

Abi-Dargham, A., Jaskiw, G., Suddath, R. & Weinberger, D.R. (1991) Evidence against progression of *in vivo* anatomical abnormalities in schizophrenia. *Schizophrenia Research*, **5**, 210.

Andreasen, N.C. & Grove, W. (1979) The relationship between schizophrenic language, manic language, and aphasia. In Gruzelier, J. & Flor-Henry, P. (eds) *Hemisphere Asymmetries of Function in Psychopathology*. Elsevier/North-Holland Biomedical Press, pp. 373–390.

Asarnow, R.F., Granholm, E. & Sherman, T. (1991) Span of apprehension in schizophrenia. In Steinhauer, S.R., Gruzelier, J.H. & Zubin, J. (eds) *Handbook of Schizophrenia, Vol. 5, Neuropsychology, Psychophysiology and Information Processing*. Elsevier, New York, pp. 335–370.

Barkley, R.A., DuPaul, G.J. & McMurray, M.B. (1990) Comprehensive evaluation of attention deficit disorder with and without hyperactivity as defined by research criteria. *Journal of Consulting and Clinical Psychology*, **58**, 775–789.

Barr, W.B., Bilder, R.M., Goldberg, E.H. & Kaplan, E. (1989) The neuropsychology of schizophrenic speech. *Journal of Communication Disorders*, **22**, 327–349.

Bauman, E. & Murray, D.J. (1968) Recognition versus recall in schizophrenia. *Canadian Journal of Psychology*, **22**, 18–25.

Bellack, A.S., Mueser, K.T., Morrison, R.L., Tierney, A. & Podell, K. (1990) Remediation of cognitive deficits in schizophrenia. *American Journal of Psychiatry*, **147**, 1650–1655.

Berman, K.F., Torrey, E.F. & Weinberger, D.R. (1993) rCBF in monozygotic twins discordant for schizophrenia. *Archives of General Psychiatry*, **49**, 927–934.

Bilder, R.M., Lipschutz-Broch, L., Reiter, G., Geisler, S., Mayerhoff, D. & Lieberman, J.A. (1994) Intellectual deficits in first episode and chronic schizophrenia: evidence for progressive deterioration? *Schizophrenia Bulletin*, (in press).

Bleuler, E. (1950) *Dementia Praecox or the Group of Schizophrenia*. International Universities Press, New York.

Braff, D.L., Heaton, R., Kuck, J. *et al.* (1991) The generalized pattern of neuropsychological deficits in outpatients with chronic schizophrenia with heterogeneous Wisconsin Card Sorting Test results. *Archives of General Psychiatry*, **48**, 891–898.

Breier, A., Schreiber, J.L., Dyer, J. & Pickar, D. (1991) National Institute of Mental Health longitudinal study of schizophrenia: prognosis and predictors of outcome. *Archives of General Psychiatry*, **49**, 239–246.

Bruton, C.J., Crow, T.J., Frith, C.D., Johnstone, E.C., Owens, D.G.C. & Roberts, G.W. (1990) Schizophrenia and the brain: a prospective clinico-neuropathological study. *Psychological Medicine*, **20**, 285–304.

Calev, A. (1984) Recall and recognition in mildly disturbed schizophrenics: the use of matched tasks. *Psychological Medicine*, **14**, 425–429.

Castle, D.J. & Murray, R.M. (1991) The neurodevelopmental basis of sex differences in schizophrenia. *Psychological Medicine*, **21**, 565–575.

Chapman, L.J. & Chapman, J.P. (1973) Problems in the measurement of cognitive deficit. *Psychological Bulletin*, **79**, 380–385.

Chapman, L.J. & Chapman, J.P. (1989) Strategies for resolving the heterogeneity of schizophrenics and their relatives using cognitive measures. *Journal of Abnormal Psychology*, **98**, 357–366.

Cohen, J.D. & Servan-Schreiber, D. (1992) Context, cortex and dopamine: a connectionis approach to behavior and biology in schizophrenia. *Psychological Review*, **99**, 45–77.

Cornblatt, R.A. & Erlenmeyer-Kimling, L. (1985) Global attentional deviance as a marker of risk for schizophrenia: specificity and predictive validity. *Journal of Abnormal Psychology*, **96**, 470–486.

Cummings, J.L. & Benson, F. (1984) Subcortical dementia: review of an emerging concept. *Archives of Neurology*, **41**, 874–879.

Daniel, D.G., Goldberg, T.E., Gibbon, R. & Weinberger, D.R. (1991) Lack of a bimodal distribution of ventricular size in schizophrenia: a Gaussian mixture analysis of 1056 cases and controls. *Biological Psychiatry*, **30**, 887–903.

Daniels, E.K., Shenton, M.E., Hozlman, P.S. *et al.* (1988) Patterns of thought disorder associated with right cortical damage, schizophrenia, and mania. *American Journal of Psychiatry*, **145**, 944–949.

Fey, E.T. (1951) The performance of young schizophrenics and young normals on the Wisconsin Card Sorting Test. *Journal of Consulting Psychology*, **15**, 311–319.

Fleming, K., Goldberg, T.E., Gold, J.M. & Weinberger, D.R. (In press). Brown Peterson performance in patients with schizophrenia. *Psychiatry Research*.

Frith, C. (1993) *The Cognitive Neuropsychology of Schizophrenia*. Erlbaum, Hove.

Gold, J.M., Hermann, B.P., Wyler, A., Randolph, C., Goldberg, T.E. & Weinberger, D.R. (1994) Schizophrenia and temporal lobe epilepsy: a neuropsychological study. *Archives of General Psychiatry*, **51**, 265–272.

Gold, J.M., Randolph, C., Carpenter, C.J., Goldberg, T.E. & Weinberger, D.R. (1992) Forms of memory failure in schizophrenia. *Journal of Abnormal Psychology*, **101**, 487–494.

Gold, J.M., Berman, K.F., Randolph, C., Goldberg, T.E. & Weinberger, D.R. (Submitted) PET validation and clinical application of a novel prefrontal task: delayed response alternation.

Goldberg, T.E. & Weinberger, D.R. (1994) Schizophrenia, training paradigms, and the Wisconsin Card Sorting Test redux. *Schizophrenia Research*, **11**, 291–296.

Goldberg, T.E., Berman, K.F., Mohr, E. & Weinberger, D.R. (1990a) Regional cerebral blood flow and cognitive function in Huntington's disease and schizophrenia. *Archives of Neurology*, **47**, 418–422.

Goldberg, T.E., Gold, J.M., Greenberg, R. *et al.* (1993a) Contrasts between patients with affective disorder and patients with schizophrenia on a neuropsychological screening battery. *American Journal of Psychiatry*, **150**, 1355–1362.

Goldberg, T.E., Greenberg, R., Griffin, S. (1993b) The impact of clozapine on cognition and psychistric symptoms in patients with schizophrenia. *British Journal of Psychiatry*, **162**, 43–48.

Goldberg, T.E., Karson, C.N., Leleszi, P.J. & Weinberger, D.R. (1988a) Intellectual impairment in adolescent psychosis. A controlled psychometric study. *Schizophrenia Research*, **1**, 261–266.

Goldberg, T.E., Kelsoe, J.R., Weinberger, D.R., Pliskin, N.H., Kirwin, P.D. & Berman, K.F. (1988b) Performance of schizophrenic patients on putative neuropsychological tests of frontal lobe function. *International Journal of Neuroscience*, **42**, 51–58.

Goldberg, T.E., Ragland, D.R., Gold, J., Bigelow, L.B., Torrey, E.F. & Weinberger, D.R. (1990b) Neuropsychological assessment of monozygotic twins discordant for schizophrenia. *Archives of General Psychiatry*, **47**, 1066–1072.

Goldberg, T.E., Torrey, E.F., Berman, K.B. & Weinberger, D.R. (1994) Relations between neuropsychological performance and brain morphological and physiological measures in monozygotic twins discordant for schizophrenia: use of an intrapair difference method. *Psychiatry Research: Neuroimaging*, **55**, 51–61.

Goldberg, T.E., Torrey, E.F., Gold, J.M. *et al.* Risk of neuropsychological impairment in monozygotic twins discordant and concordant for schizophrenia. *Schizophrenia Research* (in press).

Goldberg, T.E., Torrey, E.F., Gold, J.M., Ragland, J.D., Bigelow, L.B. & Weinberger, D.R. (1993c) Learning and memory in monozygotic twins discordant for schizophrenia. *Psychological Medicine*, **23**, 71–85.

Goldberg, T.E., Weinberger, D.R., Berman, K.F., Pliskin, N.H. & Podd, M.G. (1987) Further evidence for dementia of the prefrontal type in schizophrenia? A controlled study of teaching the Wisconsin Card Sorting Test. *Archives of General Psychiatry*, **44**, 1008–1014.

Goldberg, T.E., Weinberger, D.R., Pliskin, N.H., Berman, K.B. & Podd, M.H. (1989) Recall memory deficit in schizophrenia. *Schizophrenia Research*, **2**, 251–257.

Goldstein, G. (1978) Cognitive and perceptual differences between schizophrenics and organics. *Schizophrenia Bulletin*, **4**, 160–185.

Goldstein, G. (1990) Neuropsychological heterogeneity in schizophrenia: a consideration of abstraction and problem-solving abilities. *Archives of Clinical Neuropsychology*, **5**, 251–264.

Goldstein, G. & Zubin, J. (1990) Neuropsychological differences between young and old schizophrenics with and without associated neurological dysfunction. *Schizophrenia Research*, **3**, 117–126.

Goldstein, J.M. & Tsuang, M.T. (1990) Gender and schizophrenia: an introduction and synthesis of findings. *Schizophrenia Bulletin*, **16**, 179–183.

Green, M.F., Satz, P., Ganzell, S. & Vaclav, J.F. (1992) Wisconsin Card Sorting Test performance in schizophrenia: remediation of a stubborn deficit. *American Journal of Psychiatry*, **149**, 62–67.

Heaton, R.K. & Drexler, M. (1987) Clinical neuropsychological findings in schizophrenia and aging. In Miller, N.E. & Cohen, G.D. (eds) *Schizophrenia and Aging: Schizophrenia, Paranoia and Schizophreniform*, pp. 145–161. Guilford Press, New York.

Heaton, R.K., Baade, L.E. & Johnson, K.L. (1978) Neuropsychological test results associated with psychiatric disorders in adults. *Psychological Bulletin*, **85**, 141–162.

Hull, C.L. (1917) The formation and retention of associations among the insane. *American Journal of Psychology*, **28**, 419–435.

Hyde, T.M., Nawroz, S., Goldberg, T.E. *et al.* (1994) Is there cognitive decline in schizophrenia? A cross-sectional study. *British Journal of Psychiatry*, **164**, 494–500.

Illowsky, B.P., Juliano, D.M., Bigelow, L.B. & Weinberger, D.R. (1988) Stability of CT scan findings in schizophrenia: results of an eight-year follow-up study. *Journal of Neurology, Neurosurgery and Psychiatry*, **51**, 209–213.

Johnstone, E.C., Crow, T.J., Frith, C.D., Husband, J. & Kreel, L. (1976) Cerebral ventricular size and cognitive impairment in chronic schizophrenia. *Lancet*, **II**, 924–926.

Jonsson, H. & Nyman, A.K. (1991) Predicting long-term outcome in schizophrenia. *Acta Psychiatrica Scandinavica*, **83**, 342–346.

Kenny, J.T. & Meltzer, H.Y. (1991) Attention and higher cortical functions in schizophrenia. *Journal of Neuropsychiatry*, **3**, 269–275.

Klonoff, H., Hutton, G.H. & Fibiger, C.H. (1970) Neuropsychological patterns in chronic schizophrenia. *Journal of Nervous and Mental Disease*, **150**, 291–300.

Kolakowska, T., Williams, A.O., Ardern, M. *et al.* (1985) Schizophrenia with good and poor outcome. I. Early clinical features, response to neuroleptics and signs of organic dysfunction. *British Journal of Psychiatry*, **146**, 229–246.

Kolb, B. & Whishaw, I.Q. (1983) Performance of schizophrenic patients on tests sensitive to left or right frontal temporal, and parietal function in neurologic patients. *Journal of Nervous and Mental Disease*, **171**, 435–443.

Kraepelin, E. (1919) *Dementia Praecox and Paraphrenia*, Robertson, G.M. (ed.) Translated by Barclay, R.M. & Krieger, R.E. (1971) Huntington, New York.

Levin, S., Yurgelun-Todd, D. & Craft, S. (1989) Contributions of clinical neuropsychology to the study of schizophrenia. *Journal of Abnormal Psychology*, **98**, 341–356.

Lubin, A., Gieseking, G.F. & Williams, H.L. (1962) Direct measurement of cognitive deficit in schizophrenia. *Journal of Consulting Psychology*, **26**, 139–143.

McGlashan, T.H. (1986) The prediction of outcome in chronic schizophrenia. *Archives of General Psychiatry*, **43**, 167–176.

McKenna, P.J., Tamlyn, D., Lund, C.E., Mortimer, A.M., Hammond, S. & Baddeley, A.D. (1990) Amnesic syndrome in schizophrenia. *Psychological Medicine*, **20**, 967–972.

Malec, J. (1978) Neuropsychological assessment of schizophrenia versus brain damage: a review. *Journal of Nervous and Mental Disease*, **166**, 507–516.

Medalia, A., Gold, J.M. & Merriam, A. (1988) The effects of neuroleptics on neuropsychological test results of schizoprenics. *Archives of Clinical Neuropsychology*, **3**, 249–271.

Mesulam, M.M. (1983) The functional anatomy and hemisphere specialization for directed attention. *Trends in Neuroscience*, 384–387.

Miller, R. (1989) Schizophrenia as a progressive disorder: relations to EEG, CT, neuropathological and other evidence. *Progress in Neurobiology*, **33**, 17–44.

Mirsky, A.F. (1988) Research on schizophrenia in the NIMH Laboratory of Psychology and Psychopathology, 1954–1987. Schizophrenia Bulletin, **14**, 151–156.

Nuechterlein, K.H. (1985) Converging evidence for vigilance deficit as a vulnerability indicator for schizophrenic disorders. In Alpert, M. (ed.) *Controversies in Schizophrenia*, pp. 175–198. Guilford Press, New York.

Offord, D.R. & Cross, L.A. (1971) Adult schizophrenia with scholastic failure and low IQ in childhood. A preliminary report. *Archives of General Psychiatry*, **24**, 431–436.

Oltmanns, T.F. & Neale, J.M. (1975) Schizophrenic performance when distractors are present: attentional deficit or differential task difficulty? *Journal of Abnormal Psychology*, **84**, 204–209.

Pantelis, C., Barnes, T.R.E. & Nelson, H.E. (1992) Is the concept of frontal-subcortical dementia relevant to schizophrenia? *British Journal of Psychiatry*, **160**, 442–460.

Park, S. & Holzman, P.S. (1992) Schizophrenics show spatial working memory deficits. *Archives of General Psychiatry*, **49**, 975–982.

Perlick, D., Mattis, S., Stasny, P. & Teresi, J. (1992) Neuropsychological discriminators of long-term inpatient or outpatient status in chronic schizophrenia. *Journal of Neuropsychiatry and Clinical Neurosciences*, **4**, 428–434.

Pogue-Geile, M.F. (1989) The prognostic significance of negative symptoms in schizophrenia. *British Journal of Psychiatry*, **155**, 123–127.

Posner, M.I. (1990) The attention system of the human brain. In Cowan, W.M., Shooter, E.M., Stevens, C.F. & Thompson, R.F. (eds) *Annual Review of Neuroscience*. Annual Review Inc., California, pp. 25–42.

Posner, M.I., Early, T.S., Reiman, E., Pardo, P.J. & Dhawan, M. (1988) Asymmetries in hemispheric control of attention in schizophrenia. *Archives of General Psychiatry*, **45**, 814–821.

Randolph, C., Gold, J.M., Carpenter, C.J., Goldberg, T.E. & Weinberger, D.R. (1993a) Implicit memory in patients with schizophrenia and normal controls: effects of task demands and susceptibility to priming. *Journal of Clinical and Experimental Neuropsychology*, **15**, 853–866.

Randolph, C., Goldberg, T.E. & Weinberger, D.R. (1993b) The neuropsychology of schizophrenia. In Heilman, K.M. & Valenstein, E. (eds) *Clinical Neuropsychology*, 3rd edn. Oxford, New York pp. 499–522.

Rappaport, D., Gill, M. & Schafer, R. (1945/46) *Diagnostic Psychological Testing*. Year Book Publishers, Chicago.

Richardson, J.T.E. (1992) Imagery, mnemonics and memory remediation. *Neurology*, **42**, 283–286.

Saykin, J.A., Gur, R.C., Gur, R.E. *et al.* (1991) Neuropsychological function in schizophrenia: selective impairment in memory and learning. *Archives of General Psychiatry*, **48**, 618–624.

Schneider, S.G. & Asarnow, R.F. (1987) A comparison of cognitive/neuropsychological impairments of nonretarded autistic and schizophrenic children. *Journal of Abnormal Child Psychology*, **15**, 29–46.

Schwartz, B.L., Rosse, R.L. & Deutsch, S.I. (1993) Limits of the processing view in accounting for dissociations among memory measures in a clinical population. *Memory and Cognition*, **21**, 63–72.

Schwartzman, A.E. & Douglas, V.I. (1962) Intellectual loss in schizophrenia, part II. *Canadian Journal of Psychology*, **16**, 161–168.

Sengel, R.A. & Lovalla, W.R. (1983) Effects of cueing on immediate and recent memory in schizophrenics. *Journal of Nervous and Mental Disease*, **171**, 426–430.

Shakow, D. (1946) The nature of deterioration in schizophrenic conditions. *Nervous and Mental Disease Monographs*, 70.

Shakow, D. (1979) *Adaptation in Schizophrenia: the Theory of Segmental Set*. John Wiley & Sons, New York.

Shallice, T. (1988) *From Neuropsychology to Mental Structure*. Cambridge University Press, Cambridge.

Smith, A. (1964) Mental deterioration in chronic schizophrenia. *Journal of Nervous and Mental Disease*, **39**, 479–487.

Spohn, H.E. & Strauss, M.E. (1989) Relation of neuroleptic and anticholinergic medication to cognitive function in schizophrenia. *Journal of Abnormal Psychology*, **98**, 367–380.

Stuss, D.T., Benson, D.F., Kaplan, E.F. *et al.* (1983) The involvement of orbitofrontal cerebrum in cognitive tasks. *Neuropsychologia*, **21**, 235–248.

Suddath, R.L., Christison, G.W., Torrey, E.F., Casanova, M.F. & Weinberger, D.R. (1990) Anatomical abnormalities in the brains of monozygotic twins discordant for schizophrenia. *New England Journal of Medicine*, **22**, 789–794.

Summerfelt, A.T., Alphs, L.D., Wagman, A.M.I., Funderburk, F.R., Hierholzer, R.M. & Strauss, M.E. (1991) Reduction of perseverative errors in patients with schizophrenia using monetary feedback. *Journal of Abnormal Psychology*, **100**, 613–616.

Sweeney, J.A., Haas, G.L., Keilp, J.G. & Long, M. (1991) Evaluation of the stability of neuropsychological functioning after acute episode of schizophrenia: one-year followup study. *Psychiatry Research*, **38**, 63–76.

Tamlyn, D., McKenna, P.J., Mortimer, A.M., Lund, C.E., Hammond, S. & Baddeley, A.D. (1992) Memory impairment in schizophrenia: its extent, affiliations and neuropsychological character. *Psychological Medicine*, **22**, 101–115.

Taylor, M.A. & Abrams, R. (1984) Cognitive dysfunction in schizophrenia. *American Journal of Psychiatry*, **141**, 196–201.

Teuber, H.L. (1955) Physiological psychology. *Annual Review of Psychology*, **9**, 267–298.

Tompkins, L., Goldman, R.S. & Axelrod, B.N. (1991) Modifiability of neuropsychological dysfunction in schizophrenia (abstract). *Journal of Experimental and Clinical Neuropsychology*, **14**, 57.

Traupmann, K.L. (1980) Encoding processes and memory for categorically related word by schizophrenic patients. *Journal of Abnormal Psychology*, **89**, 704–716.

Walker, E. & Lewine, R.J. (1990) Prediction of adult-onset schizophrenia from childhood home movies of the patients. *American Journal of Psychiatry*, **147**, 1052–1056.

Weinberger, D.R., Berman, K.F., Suddath, R. & Torrey, E.F. (1992) Evidence for dysfunction of a prefrontal-limbic network in schizophrenia: an MRI and rCBF study of discordant monozygotic twins. *American Journal of Psychiatry*, **149**, 890–897.

Weinberger, D.R., Torrey, E.F., Neophytides, A.N. & Wyatt, R.J. (1979) Lateral cerebral ventricular enlargement in chronic schizophrenia. *Archives of General Psychiatry*, **36**, 735–739.

Weingartner, H. (1986) Automatic and effort-demanding cognitive processes in depression. In Poon, L.W., Crook, T., David, K.L. & Eisdorefer, C. (eds) *Handbook for Clinical Memory Assessment of Older Adults*, pp. 218–225. American Psychological Association, Hyattsville.

Chapter 11
Schizophrenia and the Risk of Violence

P. J. TAYLOR

Historical introduction to the concept of violence and the mentally ill

In reading the history of nations . . . we find that whole communities suddenly fix their minds upon one object, and go mad in its pursuit; that millions of people become simultaneously impressed with one delusion, and run after it . . . . We see one nation suddenly seized, . . . another as suddenly becoming crazed . . . and neither of them recovering its senses until it has shed rivers of blood and sowed a harvest of groans and tears, to be reaped by its posterity . . . .

Charles Mackay (1869) thus introduced his monograph on extraordinary popular delusions. He leaves the reader in no doubt that, although unsubstantiated beliefs are far from invariably indicative of disease, they not uncommonly lead to violence even in supposedly healthy populations.

Lay and psychiatrist observers alike have remarked on links between violence and beliefs founded in mental pathology, the latter commonly, but not invariably, schizophrenia. In spite of this, general psychiatry and psychology texts are striking for their omission of analysis of the impact of delusions on action. Buchanan (1993) attributes

this in part to the powerful influence of the behaviourists on psychological theory, but it is likely that the fluctuating attitudes of wider society have also taken their toll on understanding. Although a wide range of actions occur in relation to beliefs, violent or potentially dangerous actions (like fire setting) tend to be the ones most readily observed. These evoke fear, and banishment of such patients from mainstream services and society, to the detriment of developments in their assessment, treatment and safety. An opposite form of denial that was gaining ground — to the effect that people with schizophrenia and other mental illnesses are at no special risk of violence — is equally unlikely to be conducive to helping patients or promoting safety.

Among the few expert commentators is Lewis (1941): 'Patients often do not act in accordance with their delusional beliefs', although he goes on to suggest that if these beliefs become more persistent 'a patient will then act on his beliefs violently or in terror'. Jaspers (1946) does suggest something of the range and progression of actions: '*Persecuted paranoiacs* not only write to the papers, compose pamphlets, write to the Public Prosecutor, but take their own steps to murder.' Neither Lewis nor Jaspers, however, had much to add to the wisdom of their early 19th century colleagues.

Where curiosity driven simply by uncomplicated clinical presentations may have resulted in only modest progress in thinking about links between mental disorder and violence, concepts of fairness and justice prompted lawyers to demand an understanding of such associations, perhaps especially where psychosis was apparent. In the early 19th-century two principal approaches were established which still influence practice — each affecting different geographical areas. In much of Europe the Napoleonic code prevailed, resulting in unified concepts of 'responsibility' and 'irresponsibility', the dimension covering both the capacity to understand and the capacity to control behaviour. The other, English approach provided the basis for legal developments and consequent concepts of interaction between disease and behaviour for Australia, Canada and the USA as well as a range of countries with very different cultures, but influenced by temporary colonization. The issues that arise are as important to good clinical practice as to 'justice' when violence and psychosis do occur together. The case of Hadfield, in 1800, was a key landmark in this respect.

James Hadfield was a man who shot at King George III. Erskine, who was Hadfield's advocate, asserted: 'I must convince you, not only that the unhappy prisoner was a lunatic, within my own definition of lunacy, but that the act in question was the immediate unqualified offspring of the disease' (West & Walk, 1977). This statement contains three important principles, which still hold good. The first is that legal definitions of mental disorder do not necessarily coincide with medical ones, and the second is that to establish an association between mental disorder and a violent act the mental disorder must have been present *at the time of the act*. The third point is that it is generally important both in a defence to a crime (as opposed to mere mitigation at sentencing) and in good clinical management of any such case to draw out more than mere coincidence of disorder and violence. Erskine succeeded in carrying his arguments, but had three great advantages in his client. Hadfield had been of previous

impeccable record; he was patently deluded, and there were manifest organic brain deficits resulting from his war injury to which his symptoms could be attributed. At the time it was also important that he had not actually killed his victim.

The case in 1840 of Oxford, also tried for treason but for an attempt on Queen Victoria's life, followed a similar pattern. It is to McNaughton though, or rather the House of Lords' ruling that followed the outcry in 1843 when he was acquitted of murder, that many nations still owe their current concepts of legal insanity. West and Walk's book (1977) includes a transcript of the State Trials Report of the McNaughton case, in which the psychiatric evidence is set out in full. Dr Monro was one of the expert psychiatric witnesses and his evidence, including his description of McNaughton's account of events, is included:

> In reply to the questions put to him, the prisoner said he was persecuted by a system or crew at Glasgow, Edinburgh, Liverpool, London, and Boulogne. That this crew preceded or followed him wherever he went; that he had no peace of mind, and he was sure it would kill him; that physicians could be of no service to him, for if he took a ton of drugs it would be of no service to him . . . .
> . . . they had followed him to Boulogne on two occasions; they would never allow him to learn French, and wanted to murder him . . . . He mentioned having applied to Mr A Johnston, M.P. for Kilmarnock, for protection; Mr Johnston had told him that he [the prisoner] was labouring under a delusion, but that he was sure he was not . . .; that on one or two occasions something pernicious had been put into his food; . . . the person at whom he fired at Charing Cross to be one of the crew . . . . He observed that when he saw this person . . . every feeling of suffering which he had endured for months and years rose up at once in his mind, and that he conceived that he should obtain peace by killing him.

Psychiatrists of the late 20th century have evidently lost some of the confidence of their predecessors, or the courts some of their confidence in psychiatrists. At the more recent English trial of Peter Sutcliffe, who was charged with 13 serial murders, and several attempted murders, the defence advanced was of diminished responsibility under the Homicide Act 1957, notionally based on less stringent criteria than insanity but requiring similar issues to be addressed. All five psychiatrists called between defence and prosecution were agreed on the supportive psychiatric evidence, but they had difficulty establishing in court the validity of their claims. Monro had no such problems. He was asked: 'Do you think that your knowledge of insanity enables you to judge between the conduct of a man who feigns a delusion and one who feels it?'

'I do, certainly' said Monro, 'I am quite satisfied that they [the delusions] were real. I have not a shadow of a doubt on the point.'

The general public similarly had no difficulty in accepting the madness of McNaughton, but could not accept that that should result in a spirit of understanding or in the 'special verdict'. Queen Victoria added her own personal protest. Fear of insane violence was fanned by fears that 'the authorities' might no longer impose controls. The resulting public outcry may, in part, have coloured the dire observer account of insanity and violence in *Jane Eyre* (Bronte, 1847), almost certainly reflective of attitudes at the time.

> In a room without a window . . . in the deep shade, at the farther end of the room, a figure ran backwards and forwards. What it was, whether beast or human being, one could not, at first sight tell; it grovelled, seemingly, on all fours; it snatched and growled like some strange wild animal; but it was covered with clothing, and a quantity of dark, grizzled hair, wild as a mane, hid its head and face. The maniac bellowed; . . . the lunatic sprang and grappled his throat viciously, and laid her teeth to his cheek . . . .

Over 100 years later, in a different social climate, another writer (Rhys, 1966) provided a very different perspective on Mrs Rochester, this fictional character first described in *Jane Eyre*, who finally killed herself in setting fire to the house.

Grace Poole [the nurse, caretaker] said, 'So you don't remember that you attacked this gentleman with a knife?'

'I remember now that . . . he [her brother] looked and spoke to me as though I were a stranger. What do you do when something happens to you like that? Why are you laughing at me? Have you hidden my red dress too? If I had been wearing that he'd have known me . . . . But I held the dress in my hand wondering if they had done the last and worst thing. If they had *changed* it when I wasn't looking . . . and it wasn't my dress at all . . . . I let the dress fall on the floor, and looked from the fire to the dress and from the dress to the fire . . . it was as if the fire had spread across the room. It was beautiful and it reminded me of something I must do . . . .

There is some hope that such an apparently less hostile, more perceptive, and empathic attitude to people who have a mental disorder, even to those who are also violent, is reflective of something more widespread. It certainly opens the prospect of interventions which are simultaneously more humane, safe and therapeutic. Monahan (1992) offered a brief history of public perceptions of the dangers of madness. In spite of continuing media presentations emphasizing links between violence and mental illness, he noted some possible evolution in attitudes between a poll conducted for the California Department of Mental Health in the early 1980s (Field Institute, 1984), in which nearly two-thirds of the sample agreed with the proposition 'the person who is diagnosed as schizophrenic is more likely to commit a violent crime than a normal person', and a later, USA-wide poll (DYG Corporation, 1990) in which only one-quarter of the sample agreed with such a sentiment, while nearly half concurred with the view 'the mentally ill are far less of a danger than most people believe'. Unfortunately, the wording of the questions and the samples studied differ sufficiently that these comparisons must be regarded as indicative, not conclusive. Link *et al.* (1987) showed that people at the extremes of such perceptions behaved very differently. Those who believed people with a mental disorder to be violence prone were rejecting, those who did not believe in a connection were accepting of the reintegration of people with a mental disorder into the community. Given that the more accepting attitude is not only the more humane and appropriate but also probably the safer, it is more important than ever to safeguard shifts in public attitude by being accurate in the judgement of real risk and in the implementation of interventions that can limit the risk. Among people with schizophrenia in particular, the risk of violence is almost invariably due to the illness (Taylor, 1985; and below) and thus can generally be managed. Often it is not managed, and the person with schizophrenia has to bear the brunt of that burden as well as the symptoms of the illness.

The frequency of association between schizophrenia and violence

Epidemiology is a potentially useful tool in this field. It can offer the basis for effective calculation of the level of service provision necessary for people who have schizophrenia and are violent, but also it may provide fundamental evidence in support or refutation of a real relationship between illness and violent acts. Unfortunately, however, at least one of two major criticisms can be levelled at most of such work: that either or both of the key variables were inadequately defined; or that the nature of the sampling was too specific to allow any general conclusions. Monahan and Steadman (1983) illustrated particularly clearly the importance of identifying true disorder rates and true violence or crime rates rather than simply those formally recognized by mental health or criminal justice systems respectively, and went on to show that no study to that date had achieved both goals simultaneously. Wessely and Taylor (1991) explored other sources of bias, drawing out too the extent to which different disciplinary approaches — from criminology and from clinical practice — have contributed.

Presentational descriptions of schizophrenia no longer give overwhelming problems. Although some classification systems are more inclusive

than others, and for none of them is it absolutely clear that true diagnostic entities are being pinpointed, at least there are a number of reliable systems for such descriptions which have some clinical meaning, and implications for treatment. Researchers or clinicians in one part of the world will know what their colleagues in another country mean by particular designations and can themselves go out and identify similar cases. There is much greater difficulty with violence. Unlike schizophrenia, violence is not always regarded as abnormal or undesirable. Controlled violence may well be fundamental to the making and maintenance of societies (Gunn, 1991). Then, humans, unlike other animals, no longer have to be in direct contact with each other in order to inflict the most terrible harm. Issues of primary motivation, balanced risk or coincidental consequence also come into play. Is the national leader who declares war but strikes no blows him/herself committing a violent act, which should be so rated in any study? What about the ordering of cost-cutting activities, or their implementation, if these contribute to the death or maiming of people in industry, or in a transport disaster? The catalogue is endless. Although the violence that is of most concern to society is that violence which it does not sanction, and for that when destruction is merely a byproduct of some other activity, its disapprobation seems slight, it is important to note in considering any relationship between schizophrenia and violence that in the substantial areas of sanctioned or coincidental 'industrial' violence, people with schizophrenia make very little contribution. Once the illness has emerged, it would be extremely rare for such individuals to be retained in a national army, to be recruited by professional criminals or to be in such a position of responsibility in industry or public service that they could inflict significant damage. It is probably even less common for people with schizophrenia to drive motor vehicles, thereby reducing their contribution to 'accidental violence'. Reference to the likely significant under-representation of people with schizophrenia among perpetrators of these sorts of violence is almost never made.

Schizophrenia and homicide

There are some good reasons for focusing on unlawful homicide when estimating the frequency of association between violence and schizophrenia. Homicide is the most serious and finite of crimes, and thus is thought to be minimally susceptible to the problems of under-reporting, underdetection and attrition through the criminal justice system. These are all problems that are widely acknowledged for other violence, which, however, may in turn be better detected, although not necessarily better reported, than non-violent crime [e.g. for Britain, Hough & Mayhew (1983); for the USA, Reiss & Roth (1993)]. Nevertheless, there are reasons for interpreting homicide figures with caution too. It is not necessarily an offence from which generalizations about other violence can be made; it is not, for example, generally a recidivist offence. Furthermore, one substantial group of unlawful homicides is rarely included in national figures, namely death by dangerous driving. Above all, in seeking to calculate links between homicide and schizophrenia it is clear from studies reviewing international statistics that apparent relationships are influenced powerfully by the overall national homicide rates (Schipkowensky, 1973; Coid, 1983; Reiss & Roth, 1993). Crudely, in jurisdictions with high national rates of unlawful homicide, the contribution of schizophrenia and other mental disorders is relatively small, with the converse occurring for countries with low national rates. To some extent this is reassuring; given that rates of schizophrenia are relatively constant internationally, it would be difficult to explain widely different homicide rates if these were accounted for principally by people with schizophrenia, or indeed other mental disorders.

Many studies exploring mental abnormality and homicide have been conducted on samples of individuals selected for likely mental abnormality, for example samples of patients admitted to hospitals or specialist units for pretrial reports. These serve principally to show the importance of a diagnosis of schizophrenia in a psychiatrically selected sample of homicides, and will not be considered further. With one exception, the only

studies to be highlighted will be those in the decade from 1980, which marks the advent of international attempts to obtain consistency and reliability in diagnosis.

Petursson and Gudjonsson (1981) had by far the most complete sample of homicide offenders — all unlawful killers in Iceland between 1900 and 1979. The drawback to the study is that such a small, stable island population is in itself unusual, and so, for once, even a complete sample may not be representative of anything other than itself. Nevertheless, the diagnostic breakdown is of interest. Seven of the 47 offenders identified (15%) had a diagnosis of schizophrenia; in fact, this varies only slightly from the rest of western Europe. Gottlieb *et al.* (1987) studied all homicides in Copenhagen, Denmark, over a period of 25 years. Among men, 20% were said to have a psychosis, although the proportion of women was much higher (44%). Lindqvist (1989) evaluated all such offenders in north Sweden and Stockholm, and among 16 women and 106 men found that 8% of the sample had schizophrenia, and a further 4% a schizophreniform psychosis.

For 4 months of 1 year (1979–80), the present author studied all men charged with homicide (except by dangerous driving) among one-third of the population of England and Wales (Taylor & Gunn, 1984); all such men were then first remanded to Brixton Prison, including teenagers and those subsequently bailed. Sixty-one were identified, yielding a yearly rate of about 180 for the population in the then catchment area of Brixton, or an estimate of 540 for all of England and Wales. Figures in 1979 for offences initially recorded as homicide were between 520 and 555 men; thus, the Brixton sample was close to the expected size. Whether an area that included Greater London was wholly representative of the country is harder to say. Of the 61 men, five had undoubted schizophrena; these constituted 8% of the group charged, or 11% of the convicted group. In Camberwell, an area of London typical of those from which most of the offenders were drawn, the inception rate for schizophrenia was 0.1% (i.e. the rate of presentations and representations to medical services in 1 year of people with schizophrenia, and probably therefore the most comparable rate in a largely non-offender population); the annual prevalence was 0.4% and the life expectancy around 1% so, by comparison with any of these figures, men with schizophrenia were heavily overpresented in the homicide sample.

The most comparable research carried out in the USA was probably that by Wilcox (1985). He studied all people who had committed homicide, other than death by dangerous driving, in Contra Costa County, California, over roughly the same time period (1978–80) as the Brixton study was carried out. As described above, when making international comparisons it is important to take account of the local base rate for homicides. For this study, the figures were explicit. The mean number of homicides per 100 000 population in that part of California for the 3 years of the study was 6, closer to the British figures of 1–2 per 100 000 than the USA national average of over 10 per 100 000. Again, the numbers were small, but comparable. Of the 71 people convicted, seven (10%) had schizophrenia.

The 'exceptional' study is that of homicidal people in former West Germany during the 10 years between 1955 and 1964 (Hafner & Boker, 1973). Although substantially earlier than the others, it is of particular importance for two reasons. The first is its sheer size, but the second is the acknowledgement of a very important point — that at extremes of violence it is often very much a matter of chance whether the victim dies or not. The 'lucky' offender, for example, picks a poor weapon, lacks strength or strikes a rib instead of slipping the knife through an intercostal space, while the 'unlucky' one strikes a victim with an exceptionally thin skull, or for whom the ambulance is delayed. Hafner and Boker's sample therefore included people who had made serious homicide attempts as well as actually having killed. Among 2996 men who thus assaulted others, 232 (7.7%) had schizophrenia. The corresponding proportion for the much smaller group of women was 6.4%.

There is thus no room for doubt that people with schizophrenia are consistently, even similarly, over-represented in samples of people who have

unlawfully killed and, given the high clear-up rates of this crime, it seems unlikely that this could be accounted for simply on the grounds that people with schizophrenia are more susceptible to detection. *Significant* though these figures may be, their *importance* must be kept in perspective. Their importance is undeniable in the context of individual prevention considerations, but it remains true that only a tiny minority of unlawful homicides are committed by people with schizophrenia. Hafner and Boker also expressed the position from the perspective of a person with schizophrenia. The risk of committing a homicidal attack, they calculated, is about 0.05% — over 100 times less than the risk of suicide.

Non-fatal violence and schizophrenia

The two most important cross-sectional studies of relationships between violence and schizophrenia are both from the USA. The first was part of the epidemiologic catchment area (ECA) project. For about 10 000 respondents, representative of the populations of three of the sites (Baltimore, Raleigh-Durham and Los Angeles), Swanson *et al.* (1990) pooled data on violence, collected as part of the diagnostic interview schedule (DIS) ratings. Full details of the sampling are given in Eaton *et al.* (1984) and Holzer *et al.* (1985). The overall prevalence of at least one self-reported incident of actual assault in the 12 months prior to the interview was 3.7% (368 of the 10 059 respondents). People without a psychiatric diagnosis were least likely to report violence, and did so at a rate of 2.05%. The diagnosis of schizophrenia was associated with a risk 4 times as high, but if the schizophrenia were complicated by other psychiatric disorders, then the risk was much higher still — up to 30% of people also using drugs or alcohol reported violence. There have been attempts to explain away these differences with the argument that the rates of assault among the healthy seemed spuriously low, and the survey was a better measure of candour or disinhibition in telling the tale among those with schizophrenia than of the reality of violence. For 1988, however the US Bureau of Justice Statistics (1990) estimated from community sampling an overall rate of report of victimization of nearly 3% among people aged 12 years and over. The addition of child victims would perhaps make the figure very close indeed to the Swanson figure of 3.7% of self-reported violence. The other issue, perhaps of more importance, is that the study was of a true community sample, and thus may have excluded significant numbers of the very people of interest because they were in institutions, namely the violent or those with schizophrenia. This, however, would have biased the study against support of the hypothesis that there is a relationship between mental disorder and violence, but the association showed through nonetheless.

Link *et al.* (1992) drew their samples both directly from the community and from psychiatric in- and out-patient groups in the Washington Heights section of New York City, but excluded people in prisons or other correctional institutions. Their argument in support of this decision was that, on checking the 1980 New York State census data, they found that only 0.6% of the target population were institutionalized. Again, however, they were not measuring variables unrelated to admission to such institutions, and they may have introduced an uneven bias in that they did choose to adjust the samples for the loading of one key set of variables, namely those related to psychiatric disorder, but not for the other, namely those related to more serious crime, including violence. In other respects though, the study is exemplary; it demonstrated that non-responders were unlikely to differ from responders, covered both subject interview and independent data, and allowed for some key community context variables, such as ethnic heterogeneity or residential mobility. Patients in any category were significantly more likely to show at least two of the key violence indicators than community residents who had never been treated. Psychosis, not explicitly broken down by diagnosis but likely to have been mostly schizophrenia, significantly predicted hitting, fighting and weapon use over and above any general psychiatric disorder factor.

For all forms of violence, therefore, it appears that people with schizophrenia may be more likely than their healthy community peers to commit violent acts, but again the relative risk must be qualified. In the substantial sample employed by Swanson *et al.* (1990), people with schizophrenia still accounted for only 3% of the total violence. Link *et al.* (1992) were even more pointed:

> If higher rates of violence/illegal behaviour are a 'rational' justification for the exclusion of mental patients and former patients one might just as well advocate exclusion of men or high school graduates in preference for women or college graduates!

Schizophrenia as the foundation of a career of violence

If a cross-sectional picture of populations is suggestive of a more than chance association between schizophrenia and offending, how much more powerful are the longitudinal studies. Aside from a few German studies carried out earlier this century and based on small numbers of cases (e.g. Wilmanns, 1940), research consistently shows that people who are violent and have schizophrenia tend to present later than those with one of the problems in isolation. Hafner and Boker (1973) noted that in their homicidal sample just eight of the 284 people with schizophrenia had committed the crime in the first month of illness; 84% had been ill for over a year and 55% for more than 5 years. Walker and McCabe (1973) commented on the particular absence of first admissions for schizophrenia among their sample of less serious offenders compared with non-offender patients. In a much later sample (Johnstone *et al.*, 1986), selected for schizophrenia but not for violence, at first admission the rate of life-threatening violence seemed to challenge this point on timing. By the early 1980s, however, with changes in admission policies, the first admission *per se* was probably relatively immaterial. It did not necessarily imply recent pathology. Re-examination of these data showed that behaviour threatening to the life of others, manifested by as many as 20% of patients, was significantly more common the longer people had been ill (Humphreys *et al.*, 1992). Over half had been ill for over a year by the time of the incident, and presentation was not uncommonly deferred after that.

In the overview sample of 1241 Brixton pretrial male prisoners, men with schizophrenia were more or less intermediately distributed for age between the non-psychotic remandees to the prison and men with schizophrenia in the general population of Camberwell (Taylor & Parrott, 1988). The most convincing evidence of the impact of schizophrenia, however, came from the smaller, interviewed sample of 90 men with schizophrenia, 31 men with other psychoses and 82 men without psychosis. The psychotic men seemed reliable in recollecting the time of onset of their illness. There was little discrepancy between their recall for this landmark and the contemporaneously recorded time. The onset of illness by no means always coincided with the first admission. Although there was a highly significant correlation between the events ($r = 0.9$), in 25% of cases the illness onset predated first admission by anything from 1 to 15 years. In no case did admission precede onset.

Within the sample of 203 men interviewed, those with psychosis were, on average, older than those without. The age ranges were similar — 20–69 years for the psychotic men and 16–62 years for the non-psychotic men — but the means were significantly different and reflected the greater clustering of the psychotic men towards the older age bands. More importantly, there was a significant difference in age of the onset of violence. This was a pinpointing of timing fraught with difficulty, in that there can be few males who graduate to adulthood without some sort of violent outburst, if only in playground fights, and yet it was important to capture all significant violence and not just that which had come to the attention of the courts. The men, in fact, seemed to have little difficulty in locating the onset of their violence careers. Some act of aggression had, they said, been remarked on by someone, or even simply impinged on their own awareness as worthy of note. There was nothing to contradict their accounts and often something to support them in contemporaneous medical, social or criminal records — and one or more of these existed for all

but two of the men. Ratings were made on the basis of balancing all possible information from all sources. As far as possible, only those outbursts which seemed slightly beyond the ordinary were recorded. The men with psychosis were significantly older than those without psychosis at the time of their first offensive behaviour involving any kind of violence — including threats and damage to property — with the means being 30.7 and 26.8 years, respectively. The means and ratio differed very little at the time of first injury inflicted on another person — 31 and 27 years, respectively.

In striking contrast to indicators of general delinquency, a career of violence was most likely to have started after the onset of schizophrenia or other psychosis. A general criminal career was just as likely to have started before the onset of schizophrenia as after it, but among the men with schizophrenia who had ever been violent, 79% had first acted in a way that could have been construed as strikingly aggressive after the onset of their illness. For the 75 men with schizophrenia for whom data regarding the age of onset of symptoms were available, one had verified symptoms at the age of 5 (albeit not developing to full-blown schizophrenia until much later) and one was as old as 55 years, but the mean age of onset was 23 with two-thirds of the men being between 17 and 27 years. The relationship between symptom onset and first violence was even more striking when first activity resulting in actual injury was considered. In nearly 90% of cases this followed the onset of the illness. In only one case did it long predate the apparent onset, and it would indeed be surprising if it were never the case that a man who had previously been violent developed schizophrenia. The other thing that was apparent and important was that first assaults were being noted up to 30 years after the onset of illness (see also Taylor, 1993). The most usual patten, however, was for violence to emerge between 5 and 10 years after the first documentation of symptoms.

Four other studies have confirmed the importance of the illness through the examination of comparative illness and violence careers, and each leads to a similar conclusion about the impact. In Sweden, Lindqvist and Allebeck (1990) followed a sample of over 600 discharged patients with schizophrenia for 15 years, although they were wholly dependant on records. In this context they felt unable to pinpoint the onset of illness, but noted that official criminal violence was 4 times more common among men with schizophrenia than among men without, and was sustained to much older ages in the schizophrenic group. The much smaller group of women with schizophrenia showed a much higher rate of all criminal offences than occurred among the general population, and not just of violent offending. Hodgins (1992) followed a different Swedish sample of discharged patients drawn from a birth cohort of over 7000 men and 7000 women. For those with 'major mental disorder', a term equating with psychosis and commonly meaning a research diagnosis of schizophrenia, follow-up was conducted from records, this time for over 30 years. Hodgins made the interesting observation that there were two peaks of first offending as measured by criminal records for the men with major mental illness. One peak was between the ages of 15 and 18 years and the second, smaller peak between 21 and 30 years. Only the later peak was evident for the women. In a personal communication, Hodgins has confirmed that the peaks represent rather different patterns of crime for the men; the earlier peak generally represents the onset of usually trivial, non-violent offending, and the later peak the more serious, usually violent offending. By the later peak, the psychotic illness was well established. For the women, whose onset of schizophrenia tended to be later than for men, all offending was delayed, as in the Lindqvist and Allebeck series.

A study by Wessely *et al.* (1994) is of particular importance because it is of a substantial community sample of those ever contacting a psychiatric service and not of people selected for offending or for schizophrenia. All people with possible schizophrenia, together with the next adjacent case with a mental disorder other than schizophrenia, were extracted from the Camberwell register and rated for diagnosis and criminality from hospital and official criminal records. There were 491 cases and 383 'controls', approximately evenly distributed between men and women; the nature of the controls meant that it was possible to separate out, at least in part, the specific impact of schizophrenia over and above that of any mental disorder. For women, the rate of all criminal convictions was increased (rate ratio 3.3), but for men it was increased for violent offending only (3.8 for violent offending), a finding entirely consistent with the Swedish studies. The risk of first conviction of any kind was increased by unemployment, ethnic group, substance abuse and low social class, but schizophrenia accounted for small, but significant, additional variance. There were also distinctive timings in the criminal careers of people with schizophrenia. Even when adjusted for time at risk — here meaning time at liberty in the community, as the most appropriate time when counting registered criminal offences — the criminal careers of people with schizophrenia began later and apparently finished sooner than did those of the controls. Thus, relative to their psychiatrically disordered but non-schizophrenic peers, the violent offending of the men with schizophrenia was not only more frequent but also packed into a shorter time; this was true for all classes of offence among the women.

A further important perspective in career studies has been provided by Coid *et al.* (1993). Their sample was of twins with a functional psychosis seen at the Bethlem and Maudsley hospital between 1948 and 1988. Two hundred and eighty probands and 238 cotwins were traced; these consented and provided enough clinical information by interview or questionnaire to supplement data on the National Health Service Register to be included in the study. Official criminal records were obtained. It was found that 35% of the probands (98) and less than 10% (21) of the cotwins had schizophrenia; a bare majority of the probands had an affective psychosis and the rest had schizophrenia, organic or atypical psychosis. The number of women in the criminal sample was small (10), but the effect of diagnosis was similar for men and women. Among the men, those with schizophrenia were significantly more often convicted than were men with an affective psychosis, and also significantly more often convicted of violent offences. The offending of men with schizophrenia started at a significantly younger age than that of those with an affective psychosis, but offending among men with psychosis was very significantly and importantly ($r = 0.66$) correlated with the onset of illness, post dating the first psychiatric contact in nearly 60% of cases. Subsequent reanalysis has confirmed that 16 of the 18 men convicted of a violent offence and both such women were first violent after the onset of the illness (B. Coid, personal communication).

Risk and schizophrenia

Some pointers in assessment

Both cross-sectional and longitudinal studies show that, although many of the factors which appear to predispose to criminal or violent careers in healthy or non-psychotic people also foreshadow such careers among people with schizophrenia, the schizophrenia has some direct bearing. Risk assessment among people with schizophrenia must, therefore, take account of the general and the specific.

The key to limiting harm to and by a person with schizophrenia is for the clinician to discard the all-or-nothing concept of dangerousness and accept the multiplicity and variety of risks that may arise, their multifactorial basis and the mixed intervention strategies that may thus be necessary to influence the risks. The judgement of risk is best viewed as a continuum, with predictors, counteractions and monitoring taking place within recognized limits of confidence, time scale and circumstances. Slovic and Monahan (submitted) have indeed shown that while the probability of harm is likely to be rated on a continuum by intelligent lay judges (mostly university students) recruited for a study rating clinical vignettes, the transition to a dangerousness judgement produced a step function. The 'probability of harm' statements could be transposed fairly easily to a binary dangerousness statement, but the loss of data in so doing is considerable — principally in reliable and valid understanding of the transition value between the two sorts of statements, and where in

excess of that transition the probability of harm lies (or the converse). It is also the case that a dangerousness statement cannot readily be transposed back and, unless the categorical decision on dangerousness is imposed only very late in the process of risk assessment, serious misjudgements in management of the patient could follow. Happily for third parties, but less so for the patient, misjudgements usually lie in the overprediction of violence. One of the best systems, for example, tested on over 300 adult male general psychiatric patients, not all with schizophrenia, correctly classified 85% of the sample. Of those predicted to be non-violent, 94% were non-violent, although this still left 18 men who were apparently unexpectedly violent. Of those predicted to be violent, 59% were violent, leaving just over 40% falsely predicted (Klassen & O'Connor, 1988).

In spite of many years of pessimism about predicting the risk of violence or other dangerous behaviour, this study presaged further good evidence that clinical effort is worthwhile, if still in need of considerable improvement. In the USA (Pittsburgh), Lidz *et al.* (1993) recruited 357 patients, whom clinicians had assessed as likely to be violent, from a consecutive sample of nearly 2500 people attending a psychiatric emergency department, and 357 controls matched on sex, race, age and admission status but for whom violence had not elicited concern. In such a sample, random predictions of violence by clinicians would have a sensitivity (rate of true positives) and specificity (rate of true negatives) of 50%. In fact, the clinicians' predictions overall were significantly better than this — 60 and 58%, respectively. Neither race nor age influenced the results, but the apparent effectiveness in predicting violence held for the men only. Violence was seriously underpredicted among the women. The crucial question, however, was how far a clinical prediction added any advantage to actuarial predictors based on characteristics generally recognized to increase risk, for example an established history of previous violence. Certainly, the sensitivity of a prediction appeared better using the history as a predictor (69%), but the specificity was considerably weaker (48%). The patient pairs were split into two groups — history present ($n = 171$ pairs) and history absent ($n = 186$ pairs) — to test further the role of violence history in prediction. Clinician accuracy was significantly better than chance in both groups, with no significant differences between them in sensitivity or specificity. Thus, even in a heterogeneously mentally disordered population, over half of whom fell into one of the 'softer' diagnostic classes, such as personality disorder, clinical predictions do have something to add to actuarial predictions. The author hypothesizes that if the diagnostic groups were to be treated separately, prediction would be significantly better for the group with schizophrenia than for most of the others. Some of the data below would tend to support that.

The first task in a clinical situation is to draw up a list of risks as they seem to apply to a particular patient, without any attempt to weight them. These may range from specific aspects of mental state, through activities like wandering, failure to eat properly, increased smoking or refusal of treatment, to more obviously aggressive or violent acts like suicidal activities, accosting strangers and violent thinking, planning or actions. A system that serves quite well for developing a practical shortlist that can serve as the focus of concern is offered by Steadman *et al.* (1993). Three questions can be used to interrogate the longer list.

1 What is the seriousness of the risk?
2 What is the imminence of the risk?
3 What is the probability of the risk becoming actual?

Judgement of seriousness is in part obvious and in part based on extensive knowledge of the individual. A clear threat to kill someone, or a known propensity to set fire to petrol stations, for example, in the face of a claim of urges to do so would count as serious by any reckoning. The rejection of all food cooked by the hospital canteen might at first sound to be an eminently reasonable decision but, linked to a belief that the cook has specifically poisonous intent and must be stopped in his or her activities *and* with finality, the food rejection takes on a different order of seriousness. Critical belief systems can only be inferred from a complex process of inquiry and previous knowledge. Persistent, professional curiosity about patients is essential.

Imminence of risk merely adds urgency to the assessment and need for intervention. To follow on from the previous example, an expressed intention to eliminate the cook at once must bring concern into sharper focus than an intention, expressed in January, to be watchful until the next Christmas dinner when the taste of the pudding may give the final, incontrovertible proof to the patient of a need to act. The clinician will need to maintain watchfulness too, but while the former situation might call for immediate, even enforced, admission to hospital with specific treatment, the latter might allow for time to negotiate solutions with the patient.

The probability of a risk being converted into reality is a slightly different calculation again. By no means are all threats enacted, and if the risk is for an activity or withdrawal of activity of low seriousness, it may be regarded as a risk worth taking, even if the probability of its becoming real is high. Even in the USA, however, where the 'dangerousness standard' has been adopted as the key to involuntary mental hospital admission, there remains concern about other matters which under English legislation might broadly fit conceptually with 'the interests of his/her own health' (e.g. APA, 1983). Slovic and Monahan (1995) showed that 'young adults' (described above) rated between one-quarter and one-third of cases that were *not* judged as dangerous to others as candidates for involuntary hospitalization. The presence of delusional beliefs or prior admissions was among the criteria for 'not dangerous, but coercible'.

The likelihood of an event taking place rarely depends on one factor alone, but usually on a balance between characteristics of the patient, characteristics of potential victims and features of the environment. For the person with schizophrenia, perhaps the characteristics of the patient, which are largely determined by the illness, become disproportionately important, and most of the remainder of this chapter will be concerned with those, although factors external to the patient cannot be ignored. Ultimately, safety will depend on the quality of fit between the patient's characteristics and circumstances. A crucial question after a serious threat, or an actual occurrence of violence is always whether the balance in the tripartite relationship between the patient, victim or potential victims and environment has changed sufficiently to restore safety. For example, where there is one named victim who fully appreciates the risks and is prepared to take evasive action, or is able to negotiate safety, the clinician may be able to allow the patient a much greater choice in physical freedom or treatment than where, say, a mother who has been attacked on several occasions steadfastly refuses to believe that her child is really capable of harming her, or where the potential targets for violence are vague and unknown, such as people with blue eyes. There is almost no such thing as a safe environment, but factors like the ready availability of alcohol or potential weapons, and the patient's capacity for capitalizing on these must be particularly influential. The evidence is mixed for the importance of alcohol in the violence of people with psychosis. In the author's series of remand prisoners, among whom much of the violence was serious, use of alcohol at the time of the offence was unusual among psychotic men who were violent (Taylor, 1993), and in this they differed significantly from their non-psychotic peers. This echoed findings in some hospital admission studies (e.g. Tardiff & Sweillam, 1980). However, other prison studies in the USA have suggested a strong relationship between violent offending and the use of alcohol around the time of the offence, even among men with psychosis (e.g. Abram & Teplin, 1991). In the community, the ECA study suggested that use of alcohol or other drugs increased the risk of violence by people with schizophrenia as well as by any other group (Swanson *et al.*, 1990). There can certainly, therefore, be no complacency about the possible impact of alcohol on people with schizophrenia, but it may not be quite as much a matter of concern as among the mentally healthy.

Risk factors within the patient

Each patient has some characteristics which are fixed or relatively fixed, some past experiences with answering reactions that may be crucial and some characteristics which are primarily, if not exclusively, features of the acquired illness. Of characteristics in the first category, it has been thought that gender influences the propensity for violence as much, and in the same direction, within sick as within healthy groups. One exception long recognized is that of homicidal violence in the context of affective psychosis, in which category women outnumber men by at least 3:1, a reversal of the usual ratio (Hafner & Boker, 1973). The work of Lidz *et al.* (1993), however, calls old ideas into question. Although in both the USA (Tardiff, 1983) and England (Fottrell, 1980) it has been shown that in the *in-patient* setting women seemed more likely than men to be assaultive, Lidz *et al.* showed that in an emergency room sample, afterwards followed for 6 months, the level of violent incidents was also higher among women (49%) than among men (42%). The prediction of violence among women, however, was very poor (22%) and certainly no better than chance. Among people with a mental disorder, and given the predominance of schizophrenia in in-patient samples perhaps particularly among people with schizophrenia, women may be much closer to men in posing a similar risk of harm to others than has been previously supposed. Their relative absence from prison and security hospital samples may reflect better an underestimate of risk than their true needs. Advancing age is perhaps less of a safeguard in sick groups, particularly among people with schizophrenia. Nevertheless, although for the population of people with schizophrenia the decline in risk of violence may be later and less complete than in the healthy, overall it does occur. Relatively little work has been carried out to date on whether such characteristics as impulsivity, often enduring, are much influenced by the onset of psychosis, and even whether they are much influenced by the delivery of specific treatments.

The power of historical events other than acts

of violence by the patient is only just being recognized fully. There is nothing that can be done about traumatic experiences in childhood or as an adult, but it is likely that, even among people with schizophrenia, their impact could be better addressed than it has been. There is certainly need. In the Brixton series, substantial, but roughly equal, proportions of the psychotic and non-psychotic men had been without a mother (33%) or father (over 40%) for a substantial period of their childhood. By definition, this was for 1 year or more before the age of 16, but most of those who had lost parents by death or separation had lost them by the age of 5. By the same token, up to one-quarter of the men had spent at least a year in institutional care. Those men, however, who were driven to the index crime, usually a seriously violent crime, by their delusions stood out as different from all the other men. They were significantly more likely to have retained their mother throughout childhood. At first sight it seemed puzzling that an apparent indicator of greater stability during development should be associated with later serious problems, but in these cases the mother was often ill and her presence was generally undiluted by any other influences. Serious emotional traumas in childhood may predispose to antisocial behaviours (e.g. Widom, 1991), but there is some evidence that the traumas experienced by at least a subgroup of psychotic men may be special and need addressing as such.

One example of a distorted maternal relationship which was extreme, because the man finally killed his mother, but not otherwise atypical, was of a man who was the last born of her children. When he was 2 years old his much older siblings drove the father from the house after a violent quarrel, and then also left. The subject's relationship with his mother was then exclusive. The first recognition of illness in him came after she had presented to her doctor with malnutrition, claiming that she could not eat because she had to give all her food to her ailing son. He, in turn, construed her physical frailties as his own, although physically he was entirely healthy. The first warning of impending disaster came after he smashed his beloved record player — it came to him that the

world had stopped and he had no choice. The second warning came when, after a home visit, his mother was noticed to have a very bruised face. She emphatically denied any assault from her son and gave the kind of flamboyant account of her injury that is not uncommon in family abuse. She insisted that a wardrobe had fallen downstairs and had happened to strike her a glancing blow on the cheek. She was keeping her son away from all other human contact at the time, in bed in pyjamas, because she recognized him as ill. On the night his mother died, the man called the police to the house; they found his new record player was smashed and his only other loved object — his mother — had been killed. In this case the man believed too much that was not true, the victim not enough that was (i.e. the real risk at the time from her son) and the environment of isolation reinforced his desperation and any limited remaining contact with reality, while supplying all the weaponry that he needed.

Assessment of delusions

Of all the positive symptoms of schizophrenia and attendant neurotic symptoms, only delusions stand out as directly and significantly relevant to serious violent offending. They are the most widely experienced symptoms of schizophrenia (e.g. Lucas *et al.*, 1962; Taylor *et al.*, 1982), but there is, nevertheless, more than a chance association with violence. Several lines of evidence all point in this same direction (Taylor *et al.*, 1993a). They include the demonstration that seriously violent offenders with schizophrenia are more likely to be delusional than are their non-violent schizophrenic peers (Hafner & Boker, 1973). It is of interest to note that there is also historical evidence linking delusions and violence. Wilkins (1993) studied the records of over 1000 children and teenagers admitted to the Bethlem Royal Hospital during the 19th century. Delusions were significantly more common among boys than girls. The unexpectedly high overall rate (65%) for this age group, compared with present-day expectations, related more closely with the exceptionally high rate of dangerousness (49%) or suicidal

(28%) ratings than with any other factor considered as a possible basis for an explanatory hypothesis. Another piece of evidence for the risk posed by delusions is that paranoid schizophrenia — the form with the most predominantly delusional presentation — is more often shown to be significantly associated with violence (e.g. Hafner & Boker, 1973; Rofman *et al.*, 1980) than are other forms (e.g. schizo-affective schizophrenia: Shader *et al.*, 1977), even when allowance is made for the relative frequency of occurrence of the paranoid subtype. Furthermore, G. Robertson and this author found, in a second Brixton series, some evidence for a gradient in likelihood of violence, with the highest occurrence among men with a relatively pure delusional form of schizophrenia, through a mixed type of presentation, to a form in which delusions had no prominence at all and violence was rare (Taylor *et al.*, 1993a). Delusions have also been shown to be significantly more likely to be cited by sufferers as motivation for seriously violent offending compared with more rational motives which were more likely to be associated with more trivial offending among psychotic men (Taylor, 1985). Among the first series of Brixton pretrial men it was also shown that some characteristics of delusions appeared to be particularly likely to be associated with delusional drive and, in turn, violent acting. They included the level of conviction with which the beliefs were held, which was intense among the delusionally driven, and the content of the belief. Contrary to expectation, delusions of persecution were not particularly associated with delusional drive. This is not to say that they were anything but frequently present, but they were equally likely to be present among the men without delusional drive. The delusions that seemed particularly likely to predispose to action in this series were the related cluster of delusions of passivity, paranormal and religious influence. Link and Stueve (1994) have subsequently shown a similar effect with respect to violent actions including hitting, fighting and using a weapon. The sample studied has been briefly described above (Link *et al.*, 1992). They found a strong dose—response curve between threat/control override symptoms (mind domi-

nated by forces beyond the individual's control, thought insertion and people wishing to cause the individual harm) and each class of violent act. The lower the rating for threat/control symptoms, the lower the rate of occurrence of a violent act. The threat/control symptoms remained prominent and significant through models testing the relative impact of patient non-patient status, other psychotic symptoms and when controls for other potential determinants of violent behaviour were included.

Hallucinations were rarely cited as motives for offending in the first pretrial Brixton series (Taylor, 1985), and men who experienced auditory hallucinations were equally distributed between the delusionally and non-delusionally driven groups. The literature is consistent in refuting the importance of auditory hallucinations in relation to serious violence (e.g. Hafner & Boker, 1973), although the situation may possibly be different for hallucinations of taste or smell when they occur in conjunction with delusions of being poisoned (e.g. Mowat, 1966; Mawson, 1985). In hospital samples, perhaps particularly during early phases of admission, and in association with more trivial violence, auditory hallucinations may play a more important role where the diagnosis of schizophrenia predominates (e.g. Depp, 1983; Werner *et al.*, 1984; Hellerstein *et al.*, 1987; Junginger, 1990) or in more heterogeneous samples (e.g. Janofsky *et al.*, 1988; Lowestein *et al.*, 1990). McNiel (1994) noted that, overall, where significant positive associations have been shown between hallucinations and violence, this has been in the context of other psychotic symptoms. Command hallucinations have invariably provoked the most interest. It is particularly striking in the Hellerstein study that although neither self-directed nor other-directed violence was more commonly recorded among hallucinating patients overall or in the subgroup with command hallucinations, the hallucinating patients were significantly more likely to have been placed in seclusion or under special nursing than those without. Goodwin *et al.* (1971) reported that none of their series of 117 hallucinating patients, 42 with command hallucinations, had admitted to destructive or antisocial acts. Our own work (Reed *et al.*, in press) suggests a very similar pattern. Of 83 deluded patients consecutively admitted to one of two hospitals, nearly half (37) had auditory hallucinations; among these, three-quarters described command hallucinations in the 28 days before the study. Two-thirds (15 individuals) of the command group reported acting on the command, but although the commands included instructions to kill not one harmed self or others as a result during the 28-day study period.

The Maudsley assessment of delusions schedule (MADS) gives the possibility for rating delusions along nine dimensions, and can also be used to rate hallucinations along similar dimensions if it seems clinically relevant to do so (Taylor *et al.*, 1994). Patients are asked to select a belief which is most important to them; most deluded patients can do so without any further prompting. They are then asked to describe the belief and its effects in their own words. A semi-structured interview follows which allows the belief to be rated on dimensions that include conviction, belief maintenance factors, affective impact of the belief, positive actions and negative behaviours that follow from it, idiosyncrasy of the belief, the degree to which it is preoccupying, its level of systematization and the degree of insight that patients have. The type of content is also noted. All these attributes can be measured reliably on this scale, and each appears to be independent of the other. The schedule was evaluated with 83 general psychiatry in-patients (Taylor *et al.*, 1994), and the opportunity taken to observe those features most associated with acting on a belief. The first important finding was that acting on a belief is very common. Of the men and women in this general psychiatric patient sample, all known to be deluded, about 70% with schizophrenia, 60% said that within the 28 days prior to the interview they had acted on their principal belief at least once (Wessely *et al.*, 1993). Only nine patients (11%) had acted violently, but again it must be stressed that this was during only one 28-day period.

For further analysis patients were divided into a group of 'actors on delusions', which included all those who had taken violent or other positive or repeated action (27% of the sample), and a group of 'non-actors', comprising those who had either not acted at all or acted in a negative way. A negative action usually meant something like stopping watching television or stopping speaking with certain people, and was the sort of 'action' that had generally gone unnoticed by observers such as relatives, hostel and hospital workers, whose views on the patients' actions were also rated, but rated blind to the patients' account. There was more congruence between observers and patients on the positive or violent acting. Two dimensions were particularly associated with such delusional acting. One was belief maintenance and the other affective consequence of the belief (Buchanan *et al.*, 1993).

With respect to belief maintenance, significantly more actors than non-actors were able to cite having noted so-called evidence for their belief sometime during their illness, significance being even more striking for the period of the week prior to interview. Furthermore, significantly more actors than non-actors claimed to have been looking for evidence. A pointer of some surprise was that, when challenged strongly about a belief, significantly more actors than non-actors appeared to change their level of conviction and incorporate the challenge into their belief, modifying it slightly at least for a day or two, and often showing less conviction. On the one hand, this would fit with the 'open mindedness' of apparent evidence seeking, but on the other hand it was in contradiction to the data in the Brixton pretrial series that indicated that strength and unshakeability of conviction correlated positively with delusional motivation and action. The difference in the quality of the actions between the two series may be important. Perhaps serious violence does follow almost exclusively from full conviction, and less serious violence or other forms of 'testing action' from less commitment, but this is an area for further elucidation. The other dimension that was so important was the affective impact of the belief. Actors were significantly more likely than non-actors to appear to have been made to feel angry, sad or frightened by their belief.

The relationship between a violent offender with schizophrenia and the victim

One of the qualities that is often cited as important in the psychiatric evaluation of a potentially violent patient is the capacity for empathy with the victim. A lack of it is traditionally associated with notions of psychopathic disorder. Something very akin to this problem may arise, however, among people with schizophrenia.

A striking feature in the evaluation of the offender—victim interaction in the Brixton pretrial series was that although the men with psychosis were only slightly less likely to have known their victim than those without psychosis, the men with psychosis were significantly less likely to admit to any feelings for their victim (Taylor, 1993). Only one man with psychosis, and five without it, admitted to disliking their victim, but while over half of the non-psychotic men admitted to liking their victim, this was true for well under a third of the men with psychosis. Of the 29 psychotic men insisting on indifference 22 had schizophrenia. Indirectly supporting this finding was evidence that the personal assaults by the non-psychotic men had more often occurred during a period of real interaction with the victim. Aggressive behaviour on the part of the victim, for example, was significantly more often cited by the non-psychotic men as a factor in their violence, and indeed independent evidence tended to support a significantly higher rate of provocation of some kind from the victim, than was the case for the men with psychosis. Alcohol use by the victim as well as the offender at or around the time of the offence was also more commonly evident in the context of non-psychotic assaults, again suggesting more social interaction at the time.

It therefore seems likely to be the case that among people with schizophrenia or affective psychosis, the ones that should give cause for particular concern are those who have prominent beliefs which are important to them, for which they believe they have evidence and have already acted to seek it, and which greatly frighten them or otherwise make them unhappy, and all in the context of their claiming relative indifference towards their potential victim and perhaps not even knowing the victim particularly well. Passivity, religious or paranormal delusions may hold particular potential danger, while, although the case is less clear statistically for delusions of persecution being risky, some subgroups, such as those with delusions of poisoning, should always be taken seriously.

Treatment issues

It seems shocking, but it is true, that people who are psychotic and become seriously violent rarely present to services for the first time with their violence, and even if they do they have generally been ill for a long time (Humphreys *et al.*, 1992). In the first Brixton Prison series, over 90% of the psychotic men had been previously known to psychiatric services, and almost as many had had in-patient treatment. Few, however, were receiving treatment by the time of their offence — just a quarter claimed to be taking specific antipsychotic medication. The records of the definitely delusionally driven subgroup, most of whom were seriously violent, were searched particularly thoroughly for their treatment histories. Just two were receiving full treatment at the time of their offence. One, who had killed, had been desperately trying to get treatment in the 3 days before the killing, as had his family on his behalf, but the hospital services had been doubtful about the genuineness of his madness. This is not atypical. Hafner and Boker (1973) showed that in their series of people with schizophrenia who had killed or nearly killed, almost all had been receiving treatment, although few were still in treatment at the time of the crime. Very few had defaulted. Almost all had been discharged with the full agreement, if not active encouragement, of the treating staff. Albeit in a less terrible context, Johnstone *et al.* (1984) confirmed that in an English follow-up study of people with schizophrenia, most had failed to sustain the interest of psychiatric or social services, or even their general practitioner. Of those traced, alive and in the community in the UK, only nine patients refused to take part in the study, but still only half of the original group was available for interview. Among the sample 27% had no contact with any services, 14% saw *only* a community nurse and 24% saw *only* their general practitioner. Fifty-four people from the sample of 66 had not seen a psychiatrist in the 12 months before the study and yet over 50% were undoubtedly psychotic. The greatest levels of distress reported by patients or their relatives were found among those receiving no medical or social attention and, although one or two of this group seemed healthy, the more aggressive or violent behaviour also tended to be in this no-treatment group. At least in Europe, general psychiatry thus has much more potential not only for improving the health of people with schizophrenia but also for preventing consequent violence.

Pressure in England for compulsory community treatment orders has been reported in the national press, and reached a peak in 1993 because of a number of cases where dangerous behaviour had occurred in the context of untreated illness in the community. Ironically, at least one of these patients was already under such an order (a probation order with condition of treatment), which, while it does not allow the *enforcement* of treatment in the community, can usually ensure treatment through the structure it offers. If this is not sufficient, it allows the probation officer, prompted by the psychiatrist if necessary, to return to court to ask for more appropriate provisions, which may include compulsory treatment in hospital. Both for civil patients and offender patients the Mental Health Act 1983 makes provision for guardianship, which again offers social workers and psychiatrists almost all the powers that they should need to ensure that a patient complies with safe living conditions and treatment while in the community. Neither provision is much used. They bind the services into a legal requirement to ensure resources for the patient as well as the patient into certain obligations. Is it too cynical to suggest that this is why the provisions are so little used? Legislators should be aware that a compulsory requirement on a patient to take medication in the community, quite apart from the difficulties of enforcing this (e.g. Leong, 1987) as an isolated requirement, will not in itself prevent relapse and risky behaviour. Appropriate accommodation, occupation, relaxation, support and supervision for the patient will be essential, not to mention professional support for, and liaison with, any family and those friends still in contact. Experience of community compulsory treatment is already extensive in some parts of the world, including the USA (e.g. Miller, 1992) and Australia (Bottomley, 1987).

It can only be emphasized again that the making of laws is relatively easy — the hard part is interpreting and using them in the best interests of all those that have to be served by them. Mulvey *et al.* (1987) provide an excellently balanced view of such dilemmas in this small area.

Schizophrenia is not commonly a disease which goes into complete remission, and even more rarely one in which such remission is sustained. Symptoms and circumstances change and develop. In general psychiatric practice, treatment, supervision and support must not only be offered in the first place, but also sustained. That becomes proportionally more important when there is a threat of violence to others, or a clear history of actual violence or other dangerous behaviour like firesetting. It is not always easy for psychiatrists and their colleagues to keep confronting what can sometimes seem like their failures, as patients persist in their symptoms and sometimes their antisocial activities too, but it is proportionately harder for patients, and indeed their families, to cope. Indeed, partly because it is not invariably fully successful in relieving their symptoms or it produces unpleasant side effects, patients are often erratic in their commitment to treatment. At times, patients may further be explicit in their preference for damaging alternatives, including alcohol and illicit drugs. It is often this, combined with only intermittent treatment compliance, that enables treaters, supervisors and patients to collude in the abandonment of treatment, even by going through a relabelling process, which denies the schizophrenia and emphasizes only the personality disorder or substance abuse. For these patients community care is certainly not a cheap alternative to hospital care, but for many community care can be successful if it is comprehensive, and it may be helpful to add the structure and reinforcement offered by one of the legislative procedures which most jurisdictions now offer.

For patients who really cannot survive in the community, most western jurisdictions also provide for compulsory detention in hospital, and compulsory treatment as an additional and separate issue once a patient has been compulsorily admitted, providing there is evidence that the patient will either not comply voluntarily with admission to hospital, if offered, or, if admitted, remain voluntarily. In the UK it is very clear in the mental health acts that the first criterion for civil commitment of a patient is 'the interests of his/her own health', and in North America, while there has been a swing towards dependence on 'dangerousness' criteria, still it is risk to the patient that predominates in reasons for such admission. In 1982, for example, Monahan *et al.* found that in California 70% of patients civilly committed were perceived by the committing psychiatrist to be dangerous to themselves, 29% dangerous to others and 43% 'gravely disabled'; one-third of the patients satisfied two or more criteria. More recently, also in California, Segal *et al.* (1988) found that 60% of patients were admitted as dangerous to self, 49% as dangerous to others and 32% as gravely disabled. There is generally some provision too for people who have committed a criminal offence to be detained in hospital under an order from the courts instead of receiving a sentence. In England and Wales it is the case that the majority — about two-thirds of patients, mostly men — who are so detained in purpose-built secure forensic psychiatry facilities have schizophrenia or a similar illness. Such mental disorder also raises questions in the courts of specific pretrial issues, including fitness to plead to the indictment, defences at the trial and matters of mitigation if it comes to sentencing. For a more detailed exposition of the law in relation to the adult mentally disordered offender in the UK, see Gunn *et al.* (1993) and for a comparative international perspective see Harding (1993) in the same volume.

For most people who have schizophrenia and are also violent, the principles of assessment and treatment differ very little from the principles for those with schizophrenia alone; a comprehensive picture of the patient, including assimilation of all previous records, clear informant accounts of the qualities of personal relationships and enquiry about any violence, is particularly important. Attention to the environment for treatment and to staffing levels may have to be consistently higher for the person with both sets of problems. The safe and effective use of physical security, occasionally including seclusion, calls for specialist skills which must be learned. It is probably more commonly the case where violence complicates the illness that medication may have to be used as part of emergency management of a patient, and that consistently higher than average doses of neuroleptic medications may be required to gain even partial control of the symptoms of illness and associated behaviour. Whether or not extremes of hospital care or specific treatments become necessary, accurate *contemporaneous* notes of events, management and treatment plans are essential. This may be as important to protecting the interests of the clinician or health authority as to satisfactory treatment of the patient (see Monahan, 1993). Although much of the evidence is based on case accounts rather than systematic study, the risk of violence may in itself have to be a consideration in the choice of medication. Some relatively energizing medications, for example sulpiride in higher doses, may increase the risk of violence in those with a history of repeated assault, whatever its impact on symptoms. The consequences of abrupt withdrawal from clozapine, a medication of undoubted hope for some long-incarcerated violent patients with schizophrenia, may be proportionally more serious than for the non-violent patient because there is anecdotal evidence for a risk of rebound into serious violence in conjunction with rebound psychosis. For a more extensive review of the treatment issues that are more particular to individuals who are violent as well as having schizophrenia (and other mentally disordered offenders), see Taylor *et al.* (1993b).

Once people with schizophrenia have crossed the divide into serious violence, provided that they respond to treatment in hospital they seem to do quite well. A number of studies which have followed offender patients who have been discharged from hospitals, including high-security hospitals, suggest that serious offender patients with schizophrenia, and indeed the very few additional ones with other psychoses, rarely reoffend once they return to the community, and indeed generally do better in these terms than non-psychotic patients who have been discharged (e.g. Acres, 1975; Black, 1982; Gibbens & Robertson, 1983a,b; Tennent & Way, 1984, in England; and Steadman & Cocozza, 1974, in the USA). Unfortunately, the studies to date have paid little attention to the context of rehospitalization or reoffending, although Acres noted that the relatively unplanned discharges following from a Mental Health Review Tribunal ruling were less likely to be successful. Gibbens and Robertson (1983a,b) and, in a subsequent series, Robertson (1987) drew attention to the relatively high mortality that this group has in common with other mentally disordered offenders; up to 50% of cases die from suicide, accident or other violent death.

It ought to be an attainable goal that secondary prevention of serious violence by people with schizophrenia or other psychosis could be almost complete. A further achievable aim would be the primary prevention of violence, at least to the level that there is no significant disadvantage for people with schizophrenia over those in the general population with respect to violent behaviour. These targets will, however, require services that are sufficiently attractive to make people present early, and that offer not only short-term, intensive responses when they do present, but also sustained, committed multidisciplinary work at all levels of in- and out-patient provision.

Acknowledgements

Grateful thanks are owed to Nengi Charles and Karen Elliott for their work preparing the manuscript. The chapter has emerged not only from literature review and much personal research, supported variously by the MRC of the UK and the MacArthur Foundation of the USA, but also from extensive, constructive challenge from colleagues in the Department of Forensic Psychiatry at the Institute of Psychiatry, London, UK and at the many conferences where elements of the work have been presented. Particular personal thanks in this respect are due to Professors John Gunn of the Institute of Psychiatry and John Monahan of the University of Virginia, Charlottesville, USA.

References

Abram, K.M. & Teplin, L.A. (1991) Co-occurring disorders among mentally ill jail detainees. *American Psychologist*, **46**, 1036–1045.

Acres, D.I. (1975) The after-care of special hospital patients. Appendix 3 to the *Report of the Committee on Mentally Abnormal Offenders*, Home Office, DHSS, Cmnd 6244. HMSO, London.

APA (1983) Guideline for legislation on the hospitalization of adults. *American Journal of Psychiatry*, **140**, 672–679.

Black, D.A. (1982) A 5-year follow-up study of male patients discharged from Broadmoor Hospital. In Gunn, J. & Farrington, D.P. (eds) *Abnormal Offenders, Delinquency and the Criminal Justice System*, pp. 307–332. Wiley, Chichester.

Bottomley, S. (1987) Mental health and law reform and psychiatric deinstitutionalization: the issues in New South Wales. *International Journal of Law and Psychiatry*, **10**, 369–381.

Bronte, C. (1847) *Jane Eyre*. Penguin Books, Harmandsworth.

Buchanan, A. (1993) Acting on delusion: a review. *Psychological Medicine*, **23**, 123–134.

Buchanan, A., Reed, A., Wessely, S. *et al.* (1993) Acting on delusions. II. The phenomenological correlates of acting on delusions. *British Journal of Psychiatry*, **163**, 77–83.

Bureau of Justice Statistics (1990) *Criminal Victimization in the United States, 1988*. A National Crime Survey Report. NCJ – 122024.

Coid, B., Lewis, S.W. & Reveley, A.M. (1993) A twin study of psychosis and criminality. *British Journal of Psychiatry*, **162**, 87–92.

Coid, J. (1983) The epidemiology of abnormal homicide and murder followed by suicide. *Psychological Medicine*, **13**, 855–860.

Depp, F.C. (1983) Assaults in a public mental hospital. In Lion, J.R. & Reid, W.H. (eds) *Assaults within Psychiatric Facilities*, pp. 21–45. Grune & Stratton, New York.

DYG Corporation (1990) *Public Attitudes Toward People with Chronic Mental Illness*. DYG Corporation, New York.

Eaton, W.W., Holzer, C.E. & Von Korff, M. *et al.* (1984) The design of the epidemiological catchment area surveys. *Archives of General Psychiatry*, **41**, 942–948.

Field Institute (1984) *In Pursuit of Wellness: A Survey of Californian Adults*, Vol. 4. Californian Department of Mental Health, Sacramento.

Fottrell, E. (1980) A study of violent behaviour among patients in psychiatric hospitals. *British Journal of Psychiatry.* **136**, 216–221.

Gibbens, T.C.N. & Robertson, G. (1983a) A survey of the criminal careers of hospital order patients. *British Journal of Psychiatry*, **143**, 362–369.

Gibbens, T.C.N. & Robertson, G. (1983b) A survey of the criminal careers of restriction order patients. *British Journal of Psychiatry*, **143**, 370–375.

Goodwin, D., Anderson, W.P. & Rosenthal, R. (1971) Clinical significance of hallucinations in psychiatric disorders. *Archives of General Psychiatry*, **24**, 76–80.

Gottlieb, P., Gabrielsen, G. & Kramp, P. (1987) Psychotic homicides in Copenhagen from 1959 to 1983. *Acta Psychiatrica Scandinavica*, **76**, 285–292.

Gunn, J. (1991) Human violence: a biological perspective. *Criminal Behaviour and Mental Health*, **1**, 34–54.

Gunn, J., Briscoe, D., Carson, D. *et al.* (1993) The law, adult mental disorder, and the psychiatrist in England and Wales, with commentary from the rest of the UK and Eire. In Gunn, J. & Taylor, P.J. (eds) *Forensic Psychiatry: Clinical, Legal and Ethical Issues*, pp. 21–117. Butterworth-Heinemann, Oxford.

Hafner, H. & Boker, W. (1973) *Crimes of Violence by Mentally Abnormal Offenders*. Translated by Marshall, H. (1982). Cambridge University Press, Cambridge.

Harding, T. (1993) A comparative survey of medico-legal systems. In Gunn, J. & Taylor, P.J. (eds) *Forensic Psychiatry: Clinical, Legal and Ethical Issues*, pp. 118–166. Butterworth-Heinemann, Oxford.

Hellerstein, D., Frosch, W. & Koeningsberg, H.W. (1987) The clinical significance of command hallucinations. *American Journal of Psychiatry*, **144**, 219–221.

Hodgins, S. (1992) Mental disorder, intellectual deficiency and crime. *Archives of General Psychiatry*, **49**, 476–483.

Holzer, C.E., Spitznagel, E., Jordan, K.B., Timbers, D.M., Kessler, L.G. & Anthony, J.C. (1985) Sampling the household population. In Eaton, W.W. & Kessler, L.G. (eds) *Epidemiological Field Methods in Psychiatry*, Academic Press, New York.

Hough, M. & Mayhew, P. (1983) *The British Crime Survey: First Report*. A Home Office Research and Planning Unit Report 76. HMSO, London.

Humphreys, M.S., Johnstone, E.C., MacMillan, J.F. & Taylor, P.J. (1992) Dangerous behaviour preceding first admissions for schizophrenia. *British Journal of Psychiatry*, **161**, 501–505.

Janofsky, J.S., Spears, S. & Neubauer, D.N. (1988) Psychiatrists accuracy in predicting violent behavior on an inpatient unit. *Hospital and Community Psychiatry*, **39**, 1090–1094.

Jaspers, K. (1946) *General Psychopathology*. Manchester University Press, Manchester. Translated by Hoenig, J. & Hamilton, M.W. (1963) from *Allgemeinè Psychopathologie*.

Johnstone, E.C., Crow, T.J., Johnson, A.I. & MacMillan, J.F. (1986) The Northwick Park study of first episodes of schizophrenia. 1. Presentation of the illness and problems relating to admission. *British Journal of Psychiatry*, **148**, 115–120.

Johnstone, E.C., Owens, D.G.C., Gold, A., Crow, T.J. & MacMillan, J.F. (1984) Schizophrenic patients discharged

from hospital — a follow-up study. *British Journal of Psychiatry*, **145**, 586–590.

Junginger, J. (1990) Predicting compliance with command hallucinations. *American Journal of Psychiatry*, **147**, 245–247.

Klassen, D. & O'Connor, W. (1988) A prospective study of predictors of violence in adult male mental patients. *Law and Human Behaviour*, **12**, 143–158.

Leong, G.B. (1987) Outpatient civil commitment. *American Journal of Psychiatry*, **144**, 694–695.

Lewis, A.J. (1941) Psychological medicine. In Price, F.W. (ed.) *A Textbook of the Practice of Medicine*, 6th edn, pp. 1804–1893. Oxford University Press, Oxford.

Lidz, C.W., Mulvey, E.P. & Gardner, W. (1993) The accuracy of predictions of violence to others. *Journal of the American Medical Association*, **269**, 1007–1011.

Lindqvist, P. (1989) *Violence Against a Person. The Role of Mental Disorder and Abuse*, New Series No. 254. Umea University Medical Dissertations, Umea.

Lindqvist, P. & Allebeck, P. (1990) Schizophrenia and crime. A longitudinal follow-up of 644 schizophrenics in Stockholm. *British Journal of Psychiatry*, **157**, 345–350.

Link, B.G. & Stueve, A. (1994) Psychiatric symptoms and the indent/illegal behaviour of mental patients compared to community controls. In Monahan, J. & Steadman, H. (eds) *Violence and Mental Disorder: Developments in Risk Assessment*, pp. 137–159. University of Chicago Press, Chicago.

Link, B.G., Andrews, H. & Cullen, F.T. (1992) The violent and illegal behaviour of mental patients reconsidered. *American Sociological Review*, **57**, 275–292.

Link, B., Cullen, F., Frank, J. & Wozniak, J. (1987) The social rejection of former mental patients: understanding why labels matter. *American Journal of Sociology*, **92**, 1461–1500.

Lowestein, M., Binder, R.L. & McNeil, D.E. (1990) The relationship between admission symptoms and hospital assaults. *Hospital and Community Psychiatry*, **41**, 311–313.

Lucas, C., Sainsbury, P. & Collins, J. (1962) A social and clinical study of delusions in schizophrenia. *Journal of Mental Science*, **108**, 747–758.

Mackay, C. (1869) *Memoirs of Extraordinary Popular Delusions and the Madness of Crowds*. Routledge, London.

McNiel, D.E. (1994) Hallucinations and violence. In Monahan, J. & Steadman, H. (eds) *Violence and Mental Disorder: Developments in Risk Assessment*, pp. 183–202. University of Chicago Press, Chicago.

Mawson, D. (1985) Delusions of poisoning. *Medicine, Science and the Law*, **25**, 279–287.

Miller, R.D. (1992) Involuntary civil commitment to outpatient treatment: an update. *Hospital and Community Psychiatry*, **43**, 79–80.

Monahan, J. (1992) Mental disorder and violent behaviour. *American Psychologist*, **47**, 511–521.

Monahan, J. (1993) Limiting therapist exposure to Tarasoff liability. *American Psychologist*, **48**, 242–250.

Monahan, J. & Steadman, H.J. (1983) Crime and mental disorder: an epidemiological approach. In Tonry, M. & Morris, N. (eds) *Crime and Justice: An Annual Review of Research*, Vol. 4, pp. 145–189. University of Chicago Press, Chicago.

Monahan, J., Ruggiero, M. & Fredlander, H. (1982) The

Stone–Roth model of civil commitment and the California dangerousness standard: an operational comparison. *Archives of General Psychiatry*, **39**, 1267–1271.

Mowat, R.R. (1966) *Morbid Jealousy and Murder*. Tavistock, London.

Mulvey, E.P., Geller, J.L. & Roth, L.H. (1987) The promise and peril of involuntary outpatient civil commitment. *American Psychologist*, **42**, 571–584.

Petursson, H. & Gudjonsson, G.H. (1981) Psychiatric aspects of homicide. *Acta Psychiatrica Scandinavica*, **64**, 363–372.

Reed, A., Buchanan, A., Wessely, S., Garety, P., Dunn, G. & Taylor, P.J.T. Do schizophrenia patients resist or respond to command hallucinations? *Schizophrenia Bulletin* (in press).

Reiss, A.J. & Roth, J.A. (eds) (1993) *Understanding and Preventing Violence*. National Academy Press, Washington DC.

Rhys, J. (1966) *Wide Sargasso Sea*. Penguin Books, Harmandsworth.

Robertson, G. (1987) Mentally abnormal offenders: manner of death. *British Medical Journal*, **295**, 632–634.

Rofman, E.S., Askinazi, C. & Fant, E. (1980) The prediction of dangerous behaviour in emergency civil commitment. *American Journal of Psychiatry*, **137**, 1061–1064.

Schipkowensky, N. (1973) Epidemiological aspects of homicide. In Arieti, E. (ed.) *World Biennial of Psychiatry and Psychotherapy*, Vol. 2, pp. 192–215. Basic Books, New York.

Segal, S., Watson, M., Goldfinger, S. & Averbuck, D. (1988) Civil commitment in the psychiatric emergency room. II. Mental disorder indication and three dangerousness criteria. *Archives of General Psychiatry*, **45**, 753–758.

Shader, R.I., Jackson, A.H., Houmatz, J.S. & Appelbaum, P.S. (1977) Patterns of violent behaviour among schizophrenic inpatients. *Diseases of the Nervous System*, **38**, 13–16.

Slovic, P. & Monahan, J. (1955) Probability, danger and coercion. *Law and Human Behavior*, **19**, 49–64.

Steadman, H.J. & Cocozza, J. (1974) *Careers of the Criminally Insane*. Lexington Books, Lexington.

Steadman, H.J., Monahan, J., Robbins, P.C. *et al.* (1993) From dangerousness to risk assessment: implications for appropriate research strategies. In Hodgins, S. (ed.) *Mental Disorder and Crime*, pp. 39–62. Sage, Newbury Park.

Swanson, J.W., Holzer, C.E., Ganju, V.K. & Jono, R.T. (1990) Violence and psychiatric disorder in the community: evidence from the Epidemiologic Catchment Area surveys. *Hospital and Community Psychiatry*, **41**, 761–770.

Tardiff, K. (1983) A survey of assault by chronic patients in a state hospital system. In Lion, J.R. & Reid, W.H. (eds) *Assault within Psychiatric Facilities*, pp. 3–19. Grune & Stratton, New York.

Tardiff, K. & Sweillam, A. (1980) Assault, suicide and mental illness. *Archives of General Psychiatry*, **37**, 164–169.

Taylor, P.J. (1985) Motives for offending among violent and psychotic men. *British Journal of Psychiatry*, **147**, 491–498.

Taylor, P.J. (1993) Schizophrenia and crime: distinctive patterns in association. In Hodgins, S. (ed.) *Mental Disorder*

and Crime, pp. 63–85. Sage, Newbury Park.

Taylor, P.J. & Gunn, J.C. (1984) Violence and psychosis. 1. Risk of violence among psychotic men. *British Medical Journal*, **288**, 1945–1949.

Taylor, P.J. & Parrott, J.M. (1988) Elderly offenders. *British Journal of Psychiatry*, **152**, 340–346.

Taylor, P.J., Dalton, R. & Fleminger, J.J. (1982) Handedness and schizophrenic symptoms. *British Journal of Medical Psychology*, **55**, 287–291.

Taylor, P.J., Mullen, P. & Wessely, S. (1993a) Psychosis, violence and crime. In Gunn, J. & Taylor, P.J. (eds) *Forensic Psychiatry: Clinical, Legal and Ethical Issues*, pp. 329–372. Butterworth-Heinemann, Oxford.

Taylor, P.J., Gunn, J., Browne, F., Gudjonsson, G., Rix, G. & Sohn, L. (1993b) Principles of treatment for the mentally disordered offender. In Gunn, J. & Taylor, P.J. (eds) *Forensic Psychiatry: Clinical, Legal and Ethical Issues*, pp. 646–690. Butterworth-Heinemann, Oxford.

Taylor, P.J., Garety, P., Buchanan, A. *et al.* (1994) Delusions and violence. In Monahan, J. & Steadman, H. (eds) *Violence and Mental Disorder*, pp. 161–182. Chicago University Press, Chicago.

Tennent, G. & Way, C. (1984) The English special hospitals — 12–17 year follow-up study: a comparison of violent and non-violent re-offenders and non-offenders. *Medicine, Science and the Law*, **24**, 81–91.

Walker, N. & McCabe, S. (1973) *Crime and Insanity in England*, Vol. 2, *New Solutions and New Problems*. Edinburgh University Press, Edinburgh.

Werner, P.D., Rose, T.L., Tesavage, J.A. & Seeman, K. (1984) Psychiatrists' judgements of dangerousness in patients on an acute care unit. *American Journal of Psychiatry*, **141**, 263–266.

Wessely, S. & Taylor, P.J. (1991) Madness and crime: criminology versus psychiatry. *Criminal Behaviour and Mental Health*, **1**, 193–228.

Wessely, S., Buchanan, A., Reed, A. *et al.* (1993) Acting on delusions. I. Prevalence. *British Journal of Psychiatry*, **163**, 69–76.

Wessely, S.C., Castle, D., Douglas, A.J. & Taylor, P.J. (1994) The criminal careers of incident cases of schizophrenia. *Psychological Medicine*, **24**, 483–502.

West, D.J. & Walk, A. (eds) (1977) *Daniel McNaughton. His Trial and the Aftermath*. Gaskell Books, Ashford.

Widom, C.S. (1991) Avoidance of criminality in abused and neglected children. *Psychiatry*, **54**, 162–174.

Wilcox, D.E. (1985) The relationship of mental illness to homicide. *American Journal of Forensic Psychiatry*, **6**, 3–15.

Wilkins, R. (1993) Delusions in children and teenagers admitted to Bethlem Royal Hospital in the 19th century. *British Journal of Psychiatry*, **162**, 487–492.

Wilmanns, K. (1940) Uber Morde in Prodromalstadium der Schizophrenie. *Zeitschrift für die gesamte Neurologie*, **170**, 583–662.

PART 2
BIOLOGICAL ASPECTS

Chapter 12
Risk Factors for Schizophrenia: from Conception to Birth

J. McGRATH AND R. MURRAY

Introduction

The neurodevelopmental hypothesis of schizo-phrenia can be traced back to the first part of the century (S.W. Lewis, 1989), and the various strands of evidence that support it have been described elsewhere (Weinberger, 1987; Murray *et al.*, 1988; Lyon *et al.*, 1989). In short, the hypothesis states that a substantial group of patients who receive the diagnosis of schizophrenia in adult life, have experienced a disturbance of the orderly develop-ment of the brain decades before the symptomatic phase of the illness. The neurodevelopmental model therefore directs attention to risk factors that may have impacted on the developing brain during prenatal and perinatal life.

The sturdiest of the known risk factors for schizophrenia is, of course, the presence of an affected relative. The evidence for a genetic contribution to schizophrenia is addressed in Chapter 14, but it is worth noting that Jones and Murray (1991) suggest that this could operate through variation in one or more of the genes involved in the control of early brain development. The aim of this chapter, however, is to review non-genetic risk factors operating between conception and birth that have been linked to schizophrenia.

Definitions

A *teratogen* is a 'factor extrinsic to the developing organism that acts in the interval between concep-tion and birth to injure the progeny or provoke abnormal development' (Kline *et al.*, 1989). This term is sometimes narrowly linked to the effect of drugs on the developing fetus, but, more correctly, includes a range of external insults.

The term *prenatal* describes the period from conception to birth. Birth may be at term or premature. The term *perinatal* describes the time around the period of birth, that is before, during and after birth; the limits of this period are somewhat arbitrary.

Summary terms such as *pregnancy and birth complications* (PBCs) or *obstetric complications* (OCs) have often been employed in psychiatric research. These include a host of factors from antepartum haemorrhage, birth asphyxia to twin-ning and breech birth. Various methods to score such complications have been devised (McNeil & Kaij, 1978; Parnas *et al.*, 1982; Lewis *et al.*, 1989b; McNeil *et al.*, 1993b).

Pregnancy and birth complications and schizophrenia

There is considerable evidence that PBCs are

Table 12.1 The association between pregnancy and birth complications (PBCs) and schizophrenia

Reference	Samples	Source of PBC information	Conclusions
Pollack *et al.* (1966)	$n = 33$ Sz $n = 33$ well sibs	Maternal recall	Non-significant trend for more PBCs in the Sz group
Lane and Albee (1966)	$n = 52$ Sz $n = 115$ well sibs	Birth records	The Sz group had significantly lower birth weight and higher rates of prematurity
Woerner *et al.* (1971)	$n = 34$ Sz $n = 42$ well sibs	Birth records	Non-significant trend for lower birth weight in the Sz group
Woerner *et al.* (1973)	$n = 46$ Sz $n = 37$ well sibs $n = 17$ affected sibs	Maternal recall and birth records	The Sz group had more PBCs than did well siblings
McNeil and Kaij (1978)	$n = 54$ process Sz $n = 46$ Sz-like psychoses $n = 100$ controls	Birth records	Process Sz group had more PBCs
Jacobsen and Kinney (1980)	$n = 63$ Sz $n = 63$ controls	Birth records	The Sz group had significantly more PBCs
Parnas *et al.* (1982)	$n = 12$ Sz $n = 25$ schizotypal $n = 55$ controls All subjects had mothers with Sz	Birth records	The Sz group had more PBCs, the schizotypal group had least PBCs
Lewis and Murray (1987)	$n = 955$ psychiatric patients	Case note review (mostly maternal recall)	Patients with Sz had more PBCs than did other psychiatric patients
Schwarzkopf *et al.* (1989)	$n = 15$ Sz $n = 6$ schizoaffective $n = 10$ bipolar affective disorder	Maternal recall	The Sz and schizoaffective groups had significantly more perinatal complications than did the bipolar group
Eagles *et al.* (1990)	$n = 27$ Sz $n = 27$ well sibs	Birth records	The Sz group had significantly more PBCs than did the well siblings
Done *et al.* (1991)	$n = 57$ Sz $n = 32$ affective disorder $n = 16\,980$ full cohort	Birth records	The Sz group did *not* have an excess of PBCs; however, the affective psychoses group had decreased length of gestation and increased rates of vitamin K administration at birth
Foerster *et al.* (1991)	$n = 45$ Sz $n = 28$ affective disorders	Maternal recall	The Sz group had significantly more PBCs than did the affective group
O'Callaghan *et al.* (1992b)	$n = 65$ Sz $n = 65$ controls	Birth records	Case control study: found that the Sz group, especially males, have an excess of PBCs, and that this group have a younger age of onset than patients without PBCs

Continued

Table 12.1 (*Continued*)

Reference	Samples	Source of PBC information	Conclusions
McCreadie *et al.* (1992)	$n = 54$ Sz $n = 114$ sibs (4 of whom had Sz)	Maternal interview	No difference found in levels of PBCs between the groups. In the Sz cases, there was no link between PBCs and absent family history, but did find link between PBCs and drug-induced parkinsonism
Buka *et al.* (1993)	$n = 7$ Sz $n = 1$ schizophreniform $n = 1068$ full cohort	Birth records	Prospective birth cohort with subject recontacted at age $18-27$ years. Preterm subjects had more cognitive impairment. Subjects with chronic fetal hypoxia were twice as likely to develop a psychotic disorder, but this did not reach significance because of the small number of cases
Verdoux and Bourgeois (1993)	$n = 23$ Sz $n = 23$ bipolar affective disorder $n = 23$ controls	Maternal recall	The Sz group had significantly more PBCs than did the bipolars and the well siblings

Sz, schizophrenia.

detrimental to the health of the developing fetus and, in particular, its neurodevelopment (Low *et al.*, 1985; Taylor *et al.*, 1985; Paneth & Pinto-Martin, 1991). It seems obvious, therefore, to examine the possible role of PBCs in increasing the risk of later schizophrenia, and a number of such studies have been carried out. The available data have been presented in detail in scholarly reviews by McNeil (McNeil & Kaij, 1978; McNeil, 1991), but the main studies are summarized in Table 12.1. Several of these have relied upon maternal recall to search for a link between PBCs and schizophrenia (e.g. Pollack *et al.*, 1966; Schwarzkopf *et al.*, 1989; Foerster *et al.*, 1991; Verdoux & Bourgeois, 1993) but there has, of course, been concern about the reliability of maternal recall. This has been addressed by a recent study (O'Callaghan *et al.*, 1990) which goes some way to showing that maternal recollection can provide reasonably accurate information about PBCs. In addition, birth certificates and midwives' reports have also been used (e.g. Lane & Albee, 1966; Woerner *et al.*, 1973; McNeil & Kaij, 1978; Jacobsen & Kinney, 1980; Parnas *et al.*, 1982; Eagles *et al.*, 1990; O'Callaghan *et al.*, 1992b) to provide more robust data.

The majority of studies, using various sources of data and various scoring methods, have supported an association between the presence of PBCs and an increased risk of schizophrenia. The PBCs implicated have included low birth weight (Lane & Albee, 1966), prematurity and 'small for dates' status (McNeil & Kaij, 1978), pre-eclampsia (McNeil & Kaij, 1978), prolonged labour (McNeil & Kaij, 1978; Jacobsen & Kinney, 1980), hypoxia (McNeil & Kaij, 1978; Buka *et al.*, 1993) and fetal distress (O'Callaghan *et al.*, 1992b).

However, not all studies have been positive (e.g. McCreadie *et al.*, 1992) and the links between pregnancy and birth complications and schizophrenia in adult life have not been universally accepted. Indeed, a recent study by Done *et al.* (1991) claims that there is no association between PBCs and schizophrenia. This group used record linkage between a large birth cohort (the British perinatal mortality sample, $n = 16\,980$) and the Mental Health Inquiry concerning psychiatric hospital admissions. The authors calculated a summary score of PBCs and compared the mean of this score for the 57 members of the cohort who appeared in the Mental Health Inquiry with the diagnosis of schizophrenia, with the mean score for the entire cohort. There was no significant difference between these groups. Curiously, a significantly higher summary score was found for the affective psychosis group ($n = 32$); in particular, the affective psychosis group had a shorter gestation (mean difference 7.3 days) and higher rate of vitamin K administration at birth (19% of cases vs. 5% of controls).

The study of Done *et al.* (1991) can be criticized on the grounds of: (i) an idiosyncratic definition of PBCs; (ii) the low rates of detection of schizophrenia; and (iii) the inadequacies of the diagnostic process. However, its negative findings should not be lightly dismissed, particularly since a second prospective study (Buka *et al.*, 1993) has also failed to find an association between PBCs in general and adult schizophrenia. This second group noted that chronic fetal hypoxia appeared to double the risk of psychosis, but this did not reach statistical significance because of the small number of cases identified. However, because members of the cohort were interviewed at a mean age of 23, only a fraction of the subset who would eventually develop psychosis could have been identified.

What are we to make of these apparent contradictions? First, even the most enthusiastic proponent of the link between PBCs and schizophrenia must agree that considerable caveats are required concerning the specificity and predictive power of PBCs. Most fetuses exposed to the broad range of PBCs do not develop schizophrenia, and most patients with schizophrenia have not had overt PBCs. Goodman (1988) concludes that PBCs (as currently detected) increase an individual's lifetime risk of schizophrenia from about 0.6 to only about 1.5%.

Of course, it is likely that only some PBCs, perhaps low birth weight or chronic hypoxia, have a risk-increasing effect, and even these are only indirect indicators of likely hazards to the developing brain. In addition, any increased risk may be for a subtype of schizophrenia rather than the whole spectrum of conditions. Thus, a number of studies suggest that PBCs are particularly associated with schizophrenia of severe rather than mild type (McNeil & Kaij, 1978), male sex

(O'Callaghan *et al.*, 1992b) and early onset (O'Callaghan *et al.*, 1992b). Rifkin *et al.* (1994) found that low birth weight was associated in male (but not female) schizophrenics with cognitive and social impairment in childhood, and cognitive defects and negative symptoms in adult life. These findings are reminiscent of the evidence that PBCs predict increased risk of cognitive impairment in the general population (e.g. Buka *et al.*, 1993).

Thus, one possible explanation for the disparity between the findings of clinical studies which implicate a causal role for PBCs, and cohort studies such as that of Done *et al.* (1991) concerns the different types of schizophrenics sampled. The clinical studies tend to include more severe and chronic cases than does the cohort methodology.

Another suggestion has been that PBCs are only of aetiological importance in those individuals who already carry some genetic predisposition to schizophrenia (Mednick *et al.*, 1987). Against this are a range of studies that found that PBCs were more common among those schizophrenics without a family history of the illness (McNeil & Kaij, 1978; Lewis & Murray, 1981). The direction of causality is also open to question. Last century, Freud noted that the links between cerebral palsy and birth complications may be the result of pre-existing abnormalities of brain development causing the birth complications (Freud, 1897). It has been shown that a pre-existing neural defect can be the cause of PBCs (Nelson & Ellenberg, 1986), and it is possible that the postulated neurodevelopmental abnormality underlying schizophrenia is directly or indirectly the cause of PBCs. McNeil (1987) argues against this being the case for schizophrenia.

More recently, McNeil *et al.* (1993a) have examined the more specific variable of head size at birth, as measured by midwives; this was significantly smaller in a series of preschizophrenics as compared with a comparable group of normal controls. The smaller head size of the schizophrenics was not accounted for by their greater frequency of prematurity, and indeed the head size of the schizophrenics was disproportionately small in relation to their total body length.

Structural neuroimaging and PBCs

There are, of course, now more sophisticated ways of assessing brain structure than extrapolating from a midwife's tape measure. Evidence from computerized tomography (CT) played a pivotal role in the resurgence of the neurodevelopmental model of schizophrenia (Murray *et al.*, 1985, 1988; Lewis, 1989, 1990), and evidence from structural neuroimaging has been used in an attempt to establish the pathogenic mechanism linking PBCs to adult schizophrenia.

It is widely accepted that patients with schizophrenia have larger cerebral ventricles than do normal controls (Lewis, 1990; Raz & Raz, 1990). There has been controversy for a number of years over the issue of whether cases of schizophrenia with an affected relative (familial) are less likely to show ventricular enlargement than non-familial or 'sporadic' cases in whom non-genetic factors are presumed to play a more important role. A meta-analysis of all the relevant studies and two large independent studies has now demonstrated that indeed male sporadic patients have larger lateral ventricles than do male familial patients, but this relationship does not hold for female schizophrenics (Vita, personal communication; P.B. Jones *et al.*, 1993). These findings remind one that a number of studies have reported more structural abnormality in the brains of male than female schizophrenics (e.g. Williams *et al.*, 1985; Andreasen *et al.*, 1990; Falkai *et al.*, 1993; Lewine *et al.*, 1993). This and the fact that PBCs have been more closely associated with male than female schizophrenia has encouraged researchers (e.g. Murray *et al.*, 1985; Owen *et al.*, 1988) to consider whether PBCs might be responsible for the increased ventricular size. This view appeared to gain support from the evidence from perinatal medicine of a link between PBCs (e.g. prematurity) and enlarged ventricles in the general population of neonates (DeVries *et al.*, 1985). Table 12.2 collates the studies that have attempted to relate findings on neuroimaging of schizophrenics to PBCs.

A review of the salient studies reveals an inconsistent picture. Nine of the studies support an association between the presence of PBCs and either enlarged ventricles or wider sulci and fissures (Roberts, 1980; Reveley *et al.*, 1984; Schulsinger *et al.*, 1984; Pearlson *et al.*, 1985; Silverton *et al.*, 1985; DeLisi *et al.*, 1986; Turner *et al.*, 1986; Owen *et al.*, 1988; Cannon *et al.*, 1989). These studies included differing designs and a range of CT measures, and included high-risk offspring of schizophrenics and twins. Eight studies, using CT and magnetic resonance imaging (MRI), either found no relationship or an inverse relationship between the variables of interest (DeLisi *et al.*, 1988; Nimgaonkar *et al.*, 1988; Johnstone *et al.*, 1989; Kaiya *et al.*, 1989; Reddy *et al.*, 1990; Nasrallah *et al.*, 1991; Harvey *et al.*, 1993; Jones *et al.*, 1994).

Thus, this attractive hypothesis has not been adequately supported by empirical evidence and yet it has not been convincingly rejected by the majority of studies. Research therefore continues, using the greater resolution of MRI to address the issue of whether PBCs, or more particularly some PBCs, may be associated with more discrete cerebral abnormalities.

Separate from the studies examining quantitative aspects of brain morphology, a number of reports have cited an increased frequency of gross neurodevelopmental abnormalities on CT or MRI scanning of schizophrenic individuals. These include aqueduct stenosis (Reveley & Reveley, 1983), agenesis of the corpus callosum (S. Lewis *et al.*, 1989a) and cavum septum pellucidum (Lewis & Mezey, 1985). Indeed, recently Degreef *et al.* (1992) claim to have found the latter abnormality in 21% of the schizophrenics in whom they carried out MRI scans and in 61% of schizophrenics examined at post mortem. Such abnormalities are probably not of pathogenic significance in themselves but are simply markers of neurodevelopmental disturbance.

What pathogenic mechanisms might link PBCs and schizophrenia? Over 20 years ago, Mednick (1970) proposed that hypoxia associated with PBCs could damage the developing hippocampus, increasing the risk of the fetus later developing schizophrenia. Despite considerable advances having been made in developmental neurobiology

Table 12.2 The relationship between pregnancy and birth complications (PBCs) and structural brain imaging

Reference	Samples	Measure	Conclusions
Roberts (1980)	$n = 341$ general psychiatric patients	CT	Excess of 'early traumatic events' in those with abnormal scans
Reveley et al. (1984)	$n = 21$ MZ Sz $n = 18$ MZ controls	CT ventricular volume	Twin study; larger ventricles in those with PBCs from both groups
Pearlson et al. (1985)	$n = 19$ Sz $n = 27$ bipolar affective disorder $n = 19$ controls	CT VBR lateral ventricle	Trend towards higher VBR in the four Sz patients with PBC compared with those Sz without PBC ($P = 0.06$)
Pearlson et al. (1989)	$n = 50$ Sz $n = 87$ controls	CT VBR lateral ventricle and brain area	Abnormal delivery predicted VBR in multiple regression
Turner et al. (1986)	$n = 30$ Sz $n = 26$ controls	CT VBR lateral ventricle	VBR correlated positively with 'early physical trauma'
DeLisi et al. (1986)	$n = 26$ Sz $n = 10$ well siblings of Sz	CT VBR frontal horn and lateral ventricle	Link between PBCs and increased frontal horn VBR supported
Schulsinger et al. (1984) Silverton et al. (1985) Cannon et al. (1989)	$n = 35$ (subsets) offspring of Sz mothers	CT Various measures	VBR correlated negatively with length and weight at birth and positively with prematurity. Periventricular damage was associated with PBCs
Lewis and Murray (1987)	$n = 236$ psychiatric patients	CT	CT scan reported as abnormal by radiologist in 62% of those with define or probable PBCs and in 13% of those with no PBCs
Owen et al. (1988)	$n = 61$ Sz	CT lateral ventricle Sulci and fissure width	PBCs associated with a combination of increased VBR and widening of the cortical sulci and fissures
Nimgaonkar et al. (1988)	$n = 48$ Sz divided into familial and non-familial	CT Various measures	No associations demonstrated between PBCs and CT scan measures
Nasrallah et al. (1991)	$n = 30$ Sz $n = 11$ controls	MRI measures of mid-sagittal cerebellar vermal lobule size	Hypothesis that PBC would be associated with smaller cerebella was not confirmed. Those with PBC tended to have larger cerebella (non-significant increase)
DeLisi et al. (1988)	$n = 123$ Sz $n = 148$ well siblings of Sz Drawn from 53 families	MRI Several measures of limbic system	No difference in size of limbic system between those with PBCs and those without. No data on VBR reported
Johnstone et al. (1989)	$n = 172$ psychiatric patients (including 101 Sz in-patients)	CT Various measures	No significant relationships found between CT measures and birth trauma

Continued

Table 12.2 (*Continued*)

Reference	Samples	Measure	Conclusions
Kaiya *et al.* (1989)	$n = 80$ Sz $n = 45$ controls	VBR lateral ventricle VBR third ventricle Measures of sulci and fissure width	VBR lateral ventricles increased in those Sz without PBCs. No information on PBCs in the control group
Reddy *et al.* (1990)	$n = 44$ Sz	CT Various measures	No association between PBCs and CT findings
Harvey *et al.* (1993)	$n = 60$ Sz $n = 36$ controls	MRI Various measures	No association between PBCs and MRI measures
Jones *et al.* (1994)	$n = 121$ Sz $n = 41$ schizoaffective $n = 67$ controls	CT Lateral and third ventricle volume	In Sz, a history of PBCs was associated with smaller ventricles, but in schizoaffective, PBCs were associated with larger ventricles

MZ, monozygotic twin; Sz, schizophrenia; CT, computerized tomography; VBR, ventricular brain ratio; MRI, magnetic resonance imaging.

over the last two decades, our knowledge base still remains relatively limited.

A common denominator of many PBCs is their ability to produce fetal hypoxia. As with all lesions of the developing brain, the long-term sequelae of hypoxia depend not only on the extent of the damage (the 'dose') but also on the timing of the event. For example, prior to the last few weeks of gestation, the cerebral vasculature is fragile and more sensitive to perturbations of oxygenation. Haemorrhages and secondary ischaemia at this stage may result in periventricular leukomalacia, a potential antecedent of ventricular enlargement (Leichty *et al.*, 1983). Hypoxia later in gestation can result in more damage to the cortex, especially the hippocampus and subiculum, as well as the more familiar pattern of 'watershed' infarcts seen in adults (S.W. Lewis *et al.*, 1989). Recent findings concerning neurochemical abnormalities of the temporal lobes of patients with schizophrenia have been incorporated into the neurodevelopmental hypothesis (Kerwin & Murray, 1992). These authors propose that the deleterious effect of

hypoxia on excitatory amino acid receptors could lead to a disturbance in the important tropic role that these neurotransmitters play in brain development.

In brief, PBCs may impact on the complex temporal and spatial cascade of brain development via a multitude of mechanisms including cell proliferation, cell migration, cell differentiation, synaptic connectivity and cell death. Evidence has been presented linking schizophrenia to evidence of deviations at several of these stages (Goodman, 1989; Jones & Murray, 1991).

Minor physical anomalies

Minor physical anomalies (MPAs) comprise a range of subtle alterations in the development of various organs. They include such abnormalities as variations in the shape and proportions of the fingers and hands, or of the mouth, but variations of dermatoglyphics (finger and hand prints) can also be included under this broad heading. These signs are of interest because they may serve as

Table 12.3 Minor physical anomalies (MPAs) and schizophrenia

Reference	Samples	Method	Comment
Gualtieri *et al.* (1982)	$n = 64$ Sz $n = 127$ other psychiatric $n = 171$ controls	Subset of Waldrop scale	Highest scores found in the Sz group. Significantly higher scores in Sz compared with controls. High scores also in hyperkinetic and autistic children
Guy *et al.* (1983)	$n = 40$ Sz (males only)	Waldrop scale	Sz had higher rates of MPAs than did unpublished norms. No associations between MPAs and cognitive functioning or premorbid level of functioning
Green *et al.* (1989)	$n = 67$ Sz $n = 88$ controls	Waldrop scale	Sz had significantly more abnormalities, especially mouth abnormalities. Younger age of onset for the high-MPA group. No association with tests of vigilance, attention and orientation
O'Callaghan *et al.* (1991b)	$n = 41$ Sz	Waldrop scale	Higher levels of MPAs were associated with positive family history, male sex, poor score on trail B test and presence of PBCs. No association with age of onset
McNeil *et al.* (1992)	$n = 84$ offspring of women with non-organic psychosis $n = 100$ offspring of controls	Ekelund system	No statistical difference between groups; suggests that the higher rates of MPAs in Sz are due more to PBCs than to genes
Alexander *et al.* (1992)	$n = 61$ Sz $n = 11$ bipolars $n = 20$ mentally retarded $n = 15$ controls	Waldrop scale	No differences between the Sz, bipolar or control groups. Within the Sz group, high MPAs linked to poor premorbid performance, but not to age of onset, PBCs family history or CT findings
Cantor-Graae *et al.* (1994)	10 MZ twins concordant for Sz 22 MZ twins discordant for Sz 6 MZ twins, well controls	Waldrop scale	Early pregnancy complications associated with higher levels of MPAs overall. Trend level increased MPAs in ill discordant cotwin
C.A.H. Jones *et al.* (1993)	$n = 60$ Sz	Waldrop scale Structured clinical examination (SCE) for MPAs	No gender differences noted on either scale. The SCE may be more sensitive than the Waldrop scale in adult psychiatric patients
Lane *et al.* (1993)	$n = 58$ Sz $n = 18$ well controls	Waldrop scale	Patients had more MPAs than did controls. Comment on a new scale for MPAs
Markow and Wandler (1986)	$n = 81$ Sz $n = 49$ affective disorders $n = 14$ schizoaffective $n = 69$ well controls	Finger dermal ridge count and pattern asymmetry	Sz group displayed greater asymmetry than did controls. Those with more asymmetry had an earlier age of onset and more severe course of the illness

Continued

Table 12.3 (*Continued*)

Reference	Samples	Method	Comment
Cannon *et al.* (1992)	$n = 45$ Sz $n = 43$ well controls	Hand and finger print features	Increased secondary creases over the fingers and palmar area in the Sz group
Bracha *et al.* (1991)	23 MZ twins discordant for Sz	Various measures of hand morphology	Affected cotwin had significantly more hand anomalies compared with the well twin. No significant difference between right- and left-hand levels of anomalies
Bracha *et al.* (1992)	23 MZ twins discordant for Sz 7 MZ twins, normal controls	Finger dermal ridge count compared within pairs	The Sz twins had significantly greater ridge count differences than did the well twins. Evidence supports a second trimester insult
Mellor (1992)	$n = 482$ Sz	Four measure of dermatoglyphic asymmetry	Sz group had significantly higher levels of asymmetry on all four measures. No gender differences noted
Markow and Gottesman (1989)	16 MZ twins concordant for Sz 6 DZ twins concordant for Sz 3 MZ twins discordant for Sz 16 DZ twins discordant for Sz	Finger dermal ridge count and pattern asymmetry	Greater fluctuating asymmetry in concordant pairs than in discordant pairs; supports polygenic transmission and prenatal epigenetic vulnerability in Sz
Fañanás *et al.* (1989)	$n = 139$ Sz $n = 72$ well controls	Finger and hand dermal ridge count	Patients had lower ridge counts than did controls, especially those patients without a positive family history of Sz
Trent *et al.* (1993)	$n = 20$ Sz $n = 81$ well controls	Finger pattern asymmetry	More dermatoglyphic asymmetry in patients than in controls
Fañanás *et al.* (1991)	$n = 139$ Sz $n = 916$ controls	Palmar flexion creases	Different frequencies of patterns found in patients without positive family history compared with controls

Sz, schizophrenia; PBC, pregnancy and birth complication; MZ, monozygotic; DZ, dizygotic; CT, computerized tomography.

persistent markers or 'fossilized' evidence of a teratogenic influence on development. Alternatively, they may derive from the faults within the genetic code, and in the context of schizophrenia serve as overt epiphenomena of this genetic vulnerability. Most probably, they result from a variable interaction of genetic and epigenetic factors. Interest in MPAs in psychosis is not new. Last century, Clouston reported that palatal abnormalities (steep, narrow-roofed palates) were more common in those patients he regarded as having 'adolescent insanity', a type of psychosis that he noted had a strong familial tendency (Clouston, 1891).

Table 12.3 lists the key findings related to MPAs and selected recent studies of dermatoglyphic features. Overall, it appears that a subgroup of patients with schizophrenia do have increased levels of MPAs (broadly defined) compared with controls; 13 studies report evidence supporting an association (Gualtieri *et al.*, 1982; Guy *et al.*, 1983; Markow & Wandler,

1986; Fañanás *et al.*, 1989, 1991; Green *et al.*, 1989; Markow & Gottesman, 1989; Bracha *et al.*, 1991, 1992; Cannon *et al.*, 1992; Mellor, 1992; Lane *et al.*, 1993; Trent *et al.*, 1993) and one group reject an association (Alexander *et al.*, 1992). McNeil *et al.* (1992) have examined rates of MPAs in the offspring of women with psychoses but no differences in rates of MPAs were found between this high-risk group and the offspring of matched controls. In the light of Clouston's findings last century (1891), it is of interest to note that two groups have recently commented particularly on the higher rates of palatal abnormalities in schizophrenia (Green *et al.*, 1989; O'Callaghan *et al.*, 1991b).

What type of patients have MPAs? Males had a statistically significant higher rate of MPAs in the study by O'Callaghan *et al.*, (1991b), but no difference was detected by Green *et al.* (1989) or C.A.H. Jones *et al.* (1993). There is a similar lack of consensus between the studies that examined the issue of age at onset. Green *et al.* (1989) reported an association between the presence of MPAs and an earlier age of onset in a group of patients with schizophrenia, a finding congruent with an association between a dermatoglyphic measure of asymmetry and an early age of onset (Markow & Wandler, 1986). However, Guy *et al.* (1983) and O'Callaghan *et al.* (1991b) could find no association between these variables (the former study included males only).

An association between a positive family history of schizophrenia and the presence of MPAs was found by O'Callaghan *et al.* (1991b), but this same group also reported an association between MPAs and PBCs; the latter association was restricted to patients whose mothers had had bleeding early in pregnancy. The differences in the dermatoglyphic patterns of discordant twins are more suggestive of teratogenic factors operating in the second trimester (Bracha *et al.*, 1992).

Three studies provide information on the association between MPAs and cognitive function in schizophrenia. Guy *et al.* (1983) assessed Wechsler Adult Intelligence Scale (WAIS) vocabulary and a summary score derived from two memory-related tasks and the trailmaking test.

Neither score was correlated with rates of MPAs. More refined psychometric measures of vigilance, selective attention and orientation were employed by Green *et al.* (1989); however, once again no association between these measures and MPAs was found. A positive association was reported by O'Callaghan *et al.* (1991b), using the trailmaking task. Schizophrenic patients with high MPA scores were significantly slower on part B of the test, a measure of motor speed and cognitive flexibility.

Several groups have commented on the need for more sensitive and valid scales for the assessment of MPAs in adult psychiatric patients (C.A.H. Jones *et al.*, 1993; Lane *et al.*, 1993). The frequently used Waldrop scale (Waldrop *et al.*, 1968), originally developed for children with neurodevelopmental disorders, has items that rely on the rater's subjective assessment, and lacks information on the laterality of the MPAs. Techniques based on quantitative anthropometric techniques (line and angle measurements) may have improved psychometric properties, but may be more difficult to administer. In light of the interest in fluctuating asymmetry (Markow, 1992), information on laterality should be recorded.

It is important to reflect once again on the issue of specificity. As with PBCs, increased rates of MPAs are found in a range of other neurodevelopmental disorders such as mental retardation (Alexander *et al.*, 1992) and cerebral palsy (Illingworth, 1979; Coorssen *et al.*, 1992).

In summary, the excess of MPAs provides tantalizing but tangential evidence about the earliest phases of the pathogenesis of a subgroup of patients with schizophrenia. The role of genes and/or teratogens in the production of MPAs may shed light on the their parallel role in the orderly development of the brain.

The search for candidate teratogens

One of the most consistently replicated epidemiological features of schizophrenia is the slight excess of winter−spring births (Bradbury & Miller, 1985). Equally commonly found, but somehow attracting less attention, is a diminution in the number of schizophrenics born in late summer and autumn. M.S. Lewis (1989) argued that this 'season of birth' effect was an artefact of 'age incidence', but his arguments have been frequently refuted (e.g. Torrey & Bowler, 1990). Various theories have been put forward to explain this stubborn association; the most widely accepted theories postulate teratogenic agents that fluctuate over the seasons. It seems sensible to search for candidate teratogens within the framework provided by this finding. Seasonal variations in temperature, diet, PBCs and exposure to infective agents have been examined, with the last the most promising explanation.

Indeed, prenatal exposure to influenza as a candidate teratogen has been the focus of much research in recent years (Table 12.4). In particular, several studies have suggested that fetuses exposed during the second trimester to the 1957 A2 influenza pandemic have an increased risk of schizophrenia (Mednick *et al.*, 1988, 1990; O'Callaghan *et al.*, 1991c; Fahy *et al.*, 1992; Kunugi *et al.*, 1992; Welham *et al.*, 1993). Furthermore, this link with second-trimester influenza exposure held true when the relationship between influenza epidemics and schizophrenic births was assessed over several decades in both Denmark and England (Barr *et al.*, 1990; Sham *et al.*, 1992; Takei *et al.*, 1994). The finding has not always been replicated, and two studies report no association between the variables of interest (Crow *et al.*, 1991; Torrey *et al.*, 1992). Initially, Kendell and Kemp (1989) reported no effect of the 1957 Asian flu on schizophrenic births in Scotland, but in a subsequent more thorough analysis they not only reversed their earlier conclusion concerning Scotland, but also replicated the multi-epidemic study of Sham *et al.* (1992) for England (Adams *et al.*, 1993).

Thus, the balance of the reported studies is that exposure to influenza epidemics about the second trimester of gestation does increase the later risk of schizophrenia. This hypothesis is compatible with neuropathological evidence which suggests that the nature of the cytoarchitectonic abnormalities found in schizophrenia suggests that they have their origins about the fifth or sixth month of fetal life (e.g. Jakob & Beckman, 1986). The

weakness of these studies is that the association is at the population rather than individual level, and that the link within individuals between maternal infection with influenza and later schizophrenia has yet to be proven. Assuming, however, that there is such a link, then what could the mechanism be?

Conrad and Scheibel (1987) have suggested that neuraminidase, which is an important pathogenic component of the jacket of the influenza virus, may impair neuronal—glial adhesion, and in this way interfere with the migration of neurones into the hippocampal region. However, there is no evidence that the influenza virus commonly crosses the placenta so 'humoral' hypotheses have been proposed.

Such theories implicate not the infection itself, but rather the mother's immune response to the virus, and relies on evidence that inoculation of rabbits with certain strains of influenza results in production of an antibody that cross-reacts with a neuronal protein (Laing *et al.*, 1989). Wright *et al.* (1993a) suggest, therefore, that certain mothers produce an anti-influenza antibody which crosses the immature blood—brain barrier of the fetus, and becomes an autoantibody to the developing fetal cortex. This hypothesis gains some indirect support from a preliminary report that mothers of schizophrenics, where there appears to be maternal transmission of disease, show an excess of the histocompatibility antigen (HLA) type B44 (Wright *et al.*, 1993b); many autoimmunal diseases are known to be HLA related. Autoimmune diseases are also more common in women, and so far studies that have shown the 'schizophrenic' effect of influenza epidemics have consistently found this effect to be more demonstrable for female than male schizophrenics (see Takei *et al.*, 1994).

Nevertheless, it remains to be seen whether prenatal influenza has a specific effect. Other viruses acting prenatally have been suggested as candidate teratogens, including poliovirus (Eagles, 1992) and the mumps virus (King *et al.*, 1985). However, the two studies that have applied the same methodology that was used to demonstrate the influenza—schizophrenia link (Barr *et al.*, submitted; O'Callaghan *et al.*, 1993) have failed to

Table 12.4 Schizophrenia and influenza epidemics

Reference	Location	Epidemic(s)	Base sample size	Comments regarding association between exposure and increased risk of schizophrenia
Watson *et al.* (1984)	Minnesota, USA	1916−58	3246	Associations found with diphtheria, pneumonia and influenza
Torrey *et al.* (1988)	10 USA states	1920−55	2519	Associations found with measles, polio, varicella-zoster, but only trend-level association with influenza
Mednick *et al.* (1988, 1990)	Helsinki, Finland	1957	1781 (subset)	Second-trimester exposure associated with increased risk of being admitted to a psychiatric hospital with the diagnosis of schizophrenia
Kendell and Kemp (1989)	Edinburgh Scotland	1957 1919−20	2371 13540	Edinburgh data showed an association with sixth-month exposure for the 1957 data which was not found for Scotland as a whole. No association found with 1919−20 epidemic
Torrey *et al.* (1992)	10 USA states	1957	43814	No associations found
O'Callaghan *et al.* (1991c)	England and Wales	1957	1670 (subset)	Associations between exposure during the fifth month, especially for females
Crow *et al.* (1991)	UK	1957	30724	No associations found using record linkage with a large birth cohort
Kunugi *et al.* (1992)	Japan	1957	836 (subset)	Associations with exposure during second trimester
Fahy *et al.* (1992)	Afro-Caribbeans in England	1957	1722	Associations between exposure during second trimester found in Afro-Caribbean patients
McGrath *et al.* (1994)	Queensland, Australia	1954 1957 1959	7858	Associations between exposure during second trimester after the 1954 (mainly males) and the 1957 (mainly females) epidemics. No associations found after the 1959 epidemic
Sham *et al.* (1992)	England and Wales	1939−60	14830	Association between exposure during third and seventh months
Barr *et al.* (1990)	Denmark	1911−50	7239	Association found for exposure during sixth month of gestation
Morris *et al.* (1993)	Ireland	1921−71	2846	Association found for exposure in late third trimester

Continued

Table 12.4 (*Continued*)

Reference	Location	Epidemic(s)	Base sample size	Comments regarding association between exposure and increased risk of schizophrenia
Adam *et al.* (1993)	Denmark	1911–65	18 723	1957 data demonstrate second-trimester association for all three countries. General association between epidemics and schizophrenia only found in the English data (lag of 2 and 3 months)
	Scotland	1932–60	16 960	
	England	1921–60	22 021	
Takei *et al.* (1994)	England and Wales	1938–65	3827	Association with second-trimester exposure

find plausible associations with other infectious diseases.

Maternal malnutrition has also recently been implicated as a risk factor for schizophrenia in one study (Susser & Lin, 1992). The large number of candidate epidemiological variables impacting during early life makes the task of linking early living conditions and schizophrenia daunting. Nevertheless, there is evidence that early environmental factors may be important in a range of adult diseases such as cardiovascular disease, respiratory disease and diabetes mellitus (Barker *et al.*, 1992). With respect to schizophrenia, several groups have suggested that being raised in an urban region exposes individuals to more risk factors compared with those raised in a rural region (David *et al.*, 1992; O'Callaghan *et al.*, 1992a; Takei *et al.*, 1992). A range of candidate teratogens, including infection, toxins and diet, could be postulated to account for this effect.

Prenatal exposure to alcohol as a risk factor for schizophrenia has been suggested (Lohr & Bracha, 1989), with recent animal work linking exposure to alcohol and altered hippocampal development in rats (Tanaka *et al.*, 1991). Unlikely as it may seem, prenatal exposure to neurotoxins from mould has also been proposed as a risk factor for schizophrenia (Schoental, 1985), as there is evidence of the teratogenic effect of certain mycotoxins on the developing brain (Kuiper-Goodman & Scott, 1989). The links between heavy metal poisoning and neuro-

developmental disorders are also well documented (Fryers, 1991).

Lessons from other neurodevelopmental disorders

Stepping back from the literature on prenatal and perinatal risk factors for schizophrenia, the overall pattern of results leaves the objective reviewer feeling dissatisfied. So many studies have yielded inconsistent findings, and those findings that do seem to be more replicable appear to have very limited predictive power. The fact that the underlying hypothesis, the neurodevelopmental model, remains firmly held is testament to either the strength of the paradigm or the delusional-like intensity with which researchers cling to their cherished hypotheses. Before rejecting the neurodevelopmental hypothesis, it may be prudent to briefly review another major neurodevelopmental disorder, cerebral palsy.

Cerebral palsy, like dementia praecox, was first accurately delineated in the late 19th century. As is the case with schizophrenia, cerebral palsy is a heterogeneous group of conditions with shifting nosological boundaries (Ingram, 1984), but within the core group are patients with a syndrome of recognizable motor abnormalities. The rates of cerebral palsy have generally fallen in western countries over the last 50 years, levelling off to a prevalence at school age of 2.0 per 1000 live births. There is an excess of male over female cases and there is higher concordance in mono-zygotic twin pairs than in dizygotic twin pairs. Only a small percentage of cases have a positive family history of cerebral palsy, and most cases are thought to be the result of prenatal factors (Stanley, 1984). The reader will immediately appreciate that many features are common to both schizophrenia and cerebral palsy. For example, recent schizophrenia research has focused on the possible declining incidence (Der *et al.*, 1990), the greater incidence of severe cases in males (Castle & Murray, 1991; Castle *et al.*, 1993) and the relative importance of genetic vs. prenatal factors.

The search for candidate teratogens in cerebral palsy is therefore instructive for schizophrenia research. Just as the search for links between PBCs and clinical variables in patients with schizophrenia (age of onset, sex, CT changes, etc.) has been undertaken, so too in cerebral palsy (Hagberg & Hagberg, 1984). One of the most comprehensive investigations, the Collaborative Perinatal Project, followed up 54 000 pregnancies (Nelson & Ellenberg, 1986). When all the predictors were combined they appeared to explain only 37% of the cases of cerebral palsy. Clearly, there are other factors that influence brain development in cerebral palsy apart from overt PBCs and family history.

Such findings help us focus on research impediments salient to schizophrenia. In particular, it is clear that the detectable variables included as PBCs are only a small subset of all teratogens. It seems likely that many teratogens that impact on the orderly development of the brain are silent, and are not, at present, open to measurement. This point has been made with respect to cerebral palsy by Niswander and Kiely: 'Our means for evaluating fetal health during the pregnancy are so crude as to be meaningless in most cases' (1991).

We know too little about the range of factors that can impact on the orderly development of the brain, and our current methods of assessing neurodevelopment are crude in the extreme. Indeed, it is obvious that more cross-fertilization should take place between researchers involved in different neurodevelopmental disorders such as schizophrenia, mental retardation, learning disorders and cerebral palsy. In particular, any prospective longitudinal studies of candidate teratogens should encompass a wide spectrum of neurodevelopmental disorders rather than just schizophrenia.

Conclusions

Susser (1991) has pointed out that an association between a variable and a disease can be weighed up with respect to strength and specificity, consistency (replicability and survivability), predictive performance and coherence (theoretical or general biological coherence). With respect to schizophrenia, the neurodevelopmental model has considerable coherence, with supporting evidence coming from a range of sources including those concerning minor physical anomalies, childhood premorbid deficits and neuropathological findings. The paradigm suggests a number of testable hypotheses, including the prediction that prenatal and perinatal hazards should increase the risk of schizophrenia developing in adult life. Numerous variables have been proposed as candidate teratogens but none of these rate well on specificity or predictive performance. Many studies implicate PBCs in the aetiology of schizophrenia but there are also well-designed negative studies and the risk-increasing effect for PBCs in general is likely to be modest. Rather than an effect for PBCs on schizophrenia in general, it is more likely that certain types of PBCs could be linked to features of schizophrenia (e.g. early age of onset, negative symptoms, male predominance). Because of the strong consistency of the season of birth findings, candidate teratogens that display seasonal variation deserve closer inspection. With the available data, prenatal hypoxia, low birth weight and prenatal exposure to influenza appear to be candidate teratogens that warrant further scrutiny.

The state of knowledge concerning the prenatal risk factors for cerebral palsy reminds us that the problem lies not in the neurodevelopmental model but in our current ignorance of the factors that influence neurodevelopment and, as a consequence, our inability to measure them. The issue for the reader is whether to dwell on the feebleness or otherwise of the findings, or to ponder on how we can refine our measures and ask better questions. The authors believe that the latter will be the more productive path in the long term, as the research focus slowly advances from the generation of testable hypotheses to the stage at which we will be able to use the knowledge we have gained to introduce rational attempts at the primary prevention of schizophrenia.

One particular question which deserves attention is whether the teratogens that impair neurodevelopment result in lesions which directly cause psychotic symptoms several decades later. This view suggests that the nature of the lesion is such that its interaction with some unknown brain maturational facilitating factor inevitably produces schizophrenia. The alternative to this deterministic model is one that postulates an early lesion which induces a more general neurodevelopmental impairment. This impairment could lead to childhood deficits in cognition and behaviour that interact iteratively with a broader range of variables (biological, psychological and social) which are also known to directly or indirectly influence neurodevelopment. Depending on the 'fit' between the child and the environment, the child could go on to develop one of several neurodevelopmental/psychiatric syndromes (e.g. schizophrenia). In other words, the factors that impact between conception and birth may be neither necessary nor sufficient 'causes' of schizophrenia, but in some cases be key, initiating events in a complex, multidetermined cascade of risk factors.

References

Adams, W., Kendell, R.E., Hare, E.H. & Munk-Jorgensen, P. (1993) Epidemiological evidence that maternal influenza contributes to the aetiology of schizophrenia: an analysis of Scottish, English and Danish data. *British Journal of Psychiatry*, **163**, 522–534.

Alexander, R.C., Reddy, R. & Mukherjee, S. (1992) Minor physical anomalies in schizophrenia. *Biological Psychiatry*, **31**, 209.

Andreasen, N.C., Erhardt, J.C., Swayze, V.W. *et al.* (1990) Magnetic resonance imaging of the brain in schizophrenia. The pathophysiologic significance of structural abnormalities. *Archives of General Psychiatry*, **47**, 35–44.

Barker, D.J.P. (1992) *Fetal and Infant Origins of Adult Disease*. British Medical Journal, London.

Barr, C.E., Mednick, S.A. & Munk-Jorgensen, P. (1990) Exposure to influenza epidemics during gestation and adult schizophrenia: a 40-year study. *Archives of General Psychiatry*, **47**, 869–874.

Barr, C.E., Mednick, S.A. & Munk-Jorgensen, P. (1990) Prenatal infection and schizophrenia in the offspring: a survey of 25 diseases. (Submitted)

Bracha, H.S., Torrey, E.F., Bigelow, L.B., Lohr, J.B. & Linnington, B.B. (1991) Subtle signs of prenatal maldevelopment of the hand ectoderm in schizophrenia: a preliminary monozygotic twin study. *Biological Psychiatry*, **30**, 719–725.

Bracha, H.S., Torrey, E.F., Gottesman, I.I., Bigelow, L.B. & Cunniff, C. (1992) Second-trimester markers of fetal size in schizophrenia: a study of monozygotic twins. *American Journal of Psychiatry*, **149**, 1355–1361.

Bradbury, T.N. & Miller, G.A. (1985) Season of birth in schizophrenia: a review of evidence, methodology, and etiology. *Psychological Bulletin*, **98**, 569–594.

Buka, S.L., Tsuang, M.T. & Lipsitt, L.P. (1993) Pregnancy/delivery complications and psychiatric diagnosis: a prospective study. *Archives of General Psychiatry*, **50**, 151–156.

Cannon, M., Byrne, M., Cotter, D., Sham, P., Larkin, C. & O'Callaghan, E. (1992) Abnormal creases in the handprints of schizophrenic patients. *Schizophrenia Research*, **6**, 105.

Cannon, T.D., Mednick, S.A. & Parnas, J. (1989) Genetic and perinatal determinants of structural brain deficits in schizophrenia. *Archives of General Psychiatry*, **46**, 883–889.

Cantor-Graae, E., McNeil, T.F., Torrey, E.F. *et al.* (1994) Links between pregnancy and birth complications and minor physical anomalies in monozygotic twins discordant for schizophrenia. *American Journal of Psychiatry*, **151**, 1188–1193.

Castle, D.J. & Murray, R.M. (1991) The neurodevelopmental basis of sex differences in schizophrenia. *Psychological Medicine*, **21**, 565–575.

Castle, D.J., Scott, K., Wessely, S. & Murray, R.M. (1993) Does social deprivation during gestation and early life predispose to later schizophrenia? *Social Psychiatry and Psychiatric Epidemiology*, **28**, 1–4.

Clouston, T.S. (1891) *The Neuroses of Development; Being the Morison Lectures for 1890*. Oliver & Boyd, Edinburgh.

Conrad, A.J. & Scheibel, A.B. (1987) Schizophrenia and the hippocampus: the embryological hypothesis extended. *Schizophrenia Bulletin*, **13**, 577–587.

Coorssen, E.A., Msall, M.E. & Duffy, L.C. (1992) Multiple minor malformations as a marker for prenatal etiology of cerebral palsy. *Developmental Medicine and Child Neurology*, **33**, 730–736.

Crow, T.J., Done, D.J. & Johnstone, E.C. (1991) Schizophrenia and influenza. *Lancet*, **338**, 116–117.

David, A.S., Lewis, G.H., Allebeck, P. & Andreasson, S. (1992) Urban–rural differences in place of upbringing and later schizophrenia. *Schizophrenia Research*, **6**, 101.

Degreef, G., Bogarts, B., Falkai, P. *et al.* (1992) Increased prevalence of the cavum septum pellucidum in MRI scans and postmortem brains of schizophrenic patients. *Schizophrenia Research*, **6**, 145.

DeLisi, L.E., Dauphinais, I.D. & Gershon, E.S. (1988) Perinatal complications and reduced size of brain limbic structures in familial schizophrenia. *Schizophrenia Bulletin*, **14**, 185–191.

DeLisi, L.E., Goldin, L.R., Hamovit, J.R., Maxwell, E., Kurtz, D. & Gershon, E.S. (1986) A family study of the association of increased ventricular size with schizophrenia. *Archives of General Psychiatry*, **43**, 148–153.

Der, G., Gupta, S. Murray, R.M. (1990) Is schizophrenia disappearing? *Lancet*, **335**, 513–516.

DeVries, L.S., Dubowitz, L.M.S., Dubowitz, V. *et al.* (1985) Predictive value of cranial ultrasound in the newborn baby: a reappraisal. *Lancet*, **i**, 137–140.

Done, D.J., Johnstone, E.C., Frith, C.D., Golding, J., Shepherd, P.M. & Crow, T.J. (1991) Complications of pregnancy and delivery in relation to psychosis in adult life: data from the British perinatal mortality survey sample. *British Medical Journal*, **302**, 1576–1580.

Eagles, J.M. (1992) Are polioviruses a cause of schizophrenia. *British Journal of Psychiatry*, **160**, 598–600.

Eagles, J.M., Gibson, I., Bremner, M.H., Clunie, F., Ebmeier, K.P. & Smith, N.C. (1990) Obstetric complications in DSM-III schizophrenics and their siblings. *Lancet*, **335**, 1139–1141.

Fahy, T.A., Jones, P.B. & Sham, P.C. (1992) Schizophrenia in Afro-Carribeans in the UK following prenatal exposure to the 1957 A2 influenza epidemic. *Schizophrenia Research*, **6**, 98–99.

Falkai, P., Bogerts, B., Greve, B. *et al.* (1993) Loss of sylvian fissure asymmetry in schizophrenia: a quantitative post mortem study. *Schizophrenia Research*, **7**, 23–32.

Fañanás, L., Marti-Tusquets, J. & Bertranpetit, J. (1989) Seasonality of birth in schizophrenia: an insufficient stratification of control population? *Social Psychiatry and Psychiatric Epidemiology*, **24**, 266–270.

Fañanás, L., Moral, P. & Bertranpetit, J. (1991) Palmar flexion creases in schizophrenia. *International Journal of Anthropology*, **6**, 239–242.

Foerster, A., Lewis, S., Owen, M. & Murray, R. (1991) Low birth weight and a family history of schizophrenia predict poor premorbid functioning in psychosis. *Schizophrenia Research*, **5**, 13–20.

Freud, S. (1897) *Infantile Cerebral Paralysis*. University of Miami Press, Coral Cables. Translated by Russin, L.A. from *Die Infantile Cerebrallähmung*.

Fryers, T. (1991) Pre- and perinatal factors in the etiology of mental retardation. In Kiely, M. (ed.) *Reproductive and Perinatal Epidemiology*, pp. 171–204. CRC Press, Boca Raton.

Goodman, R. (1988) Are complications of pregnancy and birth causes of schizophrenia? *Developmental Medicine and Child Neurology*, **30**, 391–395.

Goodman, R. (1989) Neuronal misconnections and psychiatric disorder. Is there a link? *British Journal of Psychiatry*, **154**, 292–299.

Green, M.F., Satz, P., Gaier, D.J., Ganzell, S. & Kharabi, F. (1989) Minor physical anomalies in schizophrenia. *Schizophrenia Bulletin*, **15**, 91–99.

Gualtieri, C.T., Adams, A., Shen, C.D. & Loiselle, D. (1982) Minor physical anomalies in alcoholic and schizophrenic adults and hyperactive and autistic children. *American Journal of Psychiatry*, **139**, 640–643.

Guy, J.D., Majorski, L.V., Wallace, C.J. & Guy, M.P. (1983) The incidence of minor physical anomalies in adult male schizophrenics. *Schizophrenia Bulletin*, **9**, 571–582.

Hagberg, B. & Hagberg, G. (1984) Prenatal and perinatal risk factors in a survey of 681 Swedish cases. In: Stanley, F. & Alberman, E. (eds) *The Epidemiology of the Cerebral Palsies*, pp. 116–134. London: Spastics International Medical Publications.

Harvey, I., de Boulay, G., Wicks, D., Lewis, S.W., Murray, R.M. & Ron, M. (1993) Reduction in cortical volume in schizophrenia on magnetic resonance imaging. *Psychological Medicine*, **23**, 591–604.

Illingworth, R.S. (1979) Why blame the obstetrician? *British Medical Journal*, **1**, 797–801.

Ingram, T.T.S. (1984) A historical review of the definition and classification of the cerebral palsies. In Stanley, F. & Alberman, E. (eds) *The Epidemiology of the Cerebral Palsies*, pp. 1–11. Spastics International Medical Publications, London.

Jacobsen, B. & Kinney, D.K. (1980) Perinatal complications in adopted and non-adopted schizophrenics and their controls: preliminary results. *Acta Psychiatrica Scandinavica*, **285**, (Suppl.), 337–351.

Jakob, H. & Beckman, H. (1986) Prenatal development disturbances in the limbic allocortex in schizophrenia. *Journal of Neural Transmission*, **65**, 303–326.

Johnstone, E.C., Owens, D.G.C., Bydder, G.M., Colter, N., Crow, T.J. & Frith, C.D. (1989) The spectrum of structural brain changes in schizophrenia: age of onset as a predictor of cognitive and clinical impairments and their cerebral correlates. *Psychological Medicine*, **19**, 91–103.

Jones, C.A.H., Bassett, A.S., McGillivray, B.D. *et al.* (1993) Physical anomalies in schizophrenia. *Schizophrenia Research*, **9**, 118

Jones, P. & Murray, R.M. (1991) The genetics of schizophrenia is the genetics of neurodevelopment. *British Journal of Psychiatry*, **158**, 615–623.

Jones, P.B., Harvey, I., Lewis, S.W. *et al.* (1994) Cerebral ventricle dimensions as risk factors for schizophrenia and affective psychoses: an epidemiological approach to analysis. *Psychological Medicine* (in press).

Kaiya, H., Uematsu, M., Ofuji, M. *et al.* (1989) Computerised tomography in schizophrenia: familial versus non-familial forms of illness. *British Journal of Psychiatry*, **155**, 444–450.

Kendell, R.E. & Kemp, I.W. (1989) Maternal influenza in the etiology of schizophrenia. *Archives of General Psychiatry*, **46**, 878–882.

Kerwin, R.W. & Murray, R.M. (1992) A developmental perspective on the pathology and neurochemistry of the temporal lobe in schizophrenia. *Schizophrenia Research*, **7**, 1–12.

King, D.J., Cooper, S.J., Earle, J.A.P. *et al.* (1985) A survey of serum antibodies to eight common viruses in psychiatric patients. *British Journal of Psychiatry*, **147**, 137–144.

Kline, J., Stein, Z. & Susser, M. (1989) *Conception to Birth. Epidemiology of Prenatal Development.* Oxford University Press, Oxford.

Kuiper-Goodman, T. & Scott, P.M. (1989) Risk assessment of the mycotoxin ochratoxin A. *Biomedicine and Environmental Science*, **2**, 179–248.

Kunugi, H., Nanko, S. & Takei, N. (1992) Influenza and schizophrenia in Japan. *British Journal of Psychiatry*, **161**, 274–275.

Laing, P., Knight, J.G., Hill, J.M. *et al.* (1989) Influenza viruses induce autoantibodies to a brain-specific 37-KDa protein in rabbits. *Proceedings of the National Academy of Science*, **86**, 1998–2002.

Lane, A., Cassidy, B., Sheppard, N. *et al.* (1993) Dysmorphogenesis in schizophrenia and its quantitative assessment. *Schizophrenia Research*, **9**, 135–136.

Lane, E.A. & Albee, G.W. (1966) Comparative birth weight of schizophrenics and their siblings. *Journal of Psychology*, **64**, 277–231.

Leichty, E.A., Gilmore, R.L., Bryson, C.Q. & Bull, J. (1983) Outcome of high-risk neonates with ventriculomegaly. *Developmental Medicine and Child Neurology*, **25**, 162–168.

Lewine, R.J., Hudgins, P., Brown, F., Caudle, J. & Risch, S.C. (1993) Gender differences in qualitative brain morphology findings in schizophrenia. *Schizophrenia Research*, **9**, 202.

Lewis, M.S. (1989) Age incidence and schizophrenia. I. The season of birth controversy. *Schizophrenia Bulletin*, **15**, 59–73.

Lewis, S.W. (1989) Congenital risk factors for schizophrenia. *Psychological Medicine*, **19**, 5–13.

Lewis, S.W. (1990) Computerised tomography in schizophrenia 15 years on. *British Journal of Psychiatry*, **157** (Suppl. 9), 16–24.

Lewis, S.W. & Mezey, G.C. (1985) Clinical correlates of septum pellucidum cavities. *Psychological Medicine*, **15**, 43.

Lewis, S.W. & Murray, R.M. (1987) Obstetric complications, neurodevelopmental deviance, and risk of schizophrenia. *Journal of Psychiatric Research*, **21**, 413–421.

Lewis, S.W., Reveley, M.A., David, A.S. & Ron, M.A. (1989a) Agenesis of the corpus callosum and schizophrenia: a case report. *Psychological Medicine*, **18**, 341–347.

Lewis, S.W., Owen, M.J. & Murray, R.M. (1989b) Obstetric complications and schizophrenia: methodology and mechanisms. In Schulz, S.C. & Tamminga, C.A. (eds) *Schizophrenia: Scientific Progress*, pp. 56–68. Oxford University Press, Oxford.

Lohr, J.B. & Bracha, H.S. (1989) Can schizophrenia be related to prenatal exposure to alcohol? Some speculations. *Schizophrenia Bulletin*, **15**, 595–603.

Low, J.A., Galbraith, R.S., Muir, D.W., Broekhoven, L.H., Wilkinson, J.W. & Karchmar, E.J. (1985) The contribution of fetal-newborn complications to motor and cognitive deficits. *Developmental Medicine and Child Neurology*, **27**, 578–587.

Lyon, M., Barr, C.E., Cannon, T.D., Mednick, S.A. & Shore, D. (1989) Fetal neurodevelopment and schizophrenia. *Schizophrenia Bulletin*, **15**, 149–161.

McCreadie, R.G., Hall, D.J., Berry, I.J., Robertson, L.J.,

Ewing, J.I. & Geals, M.F. (1992) The Nithdale schizophrenia surveys. X. Obstetric complications, family history and abnormal movements. *British Journal of Psychiatry*, **161**, 799–805.

McGrath, J.J., Pemberton, M., Welham, J.L. & Murray, R.M. (1994) Schizophrenia and the influenza epidemics of 1954, 1957 and 1959: a southern hemisphere study. *Schizophrenia Research*, (in press).

McNeil, T.F. (1987) Perinatal influences in the development of schizophrenia. In Helmchem, H. & Henn, F.A. (eds) *Biological Perspectives of Schizophrenia*, pp. 125–138. Wiley, Chichester.

McNeil, T.F. (1991) Obstetric complications in schizophrenic parents. *Schizophrenia Research*, **5**, 89–101.

McNeil, T.F. & Kaij, L. (1978) Obstetric factors in the development of schizophrenia: complications in the births of preschizophrenics and in reproductions by schizophrenic parents. In Wynne, L.C., Cromwell, R.L. & Matthysse, S. (eds) *The Nature of Schizophrenia: New Approaches to Research and Treatment*, pp. 401–429. Wiley, New York.

McNeil, T.F., Blennow, G. & Lunberg, L. (1992) Congenital malformations and structural developmental anomalies in groups at high risk for psychosis. *American Journal of Psychiatry*, **149**, 57–61.

McNeil, T.F., Cantor-Graae, E., Nordström, L.G. & Rosenlund, T. (1993a) Head circumference in 'preschizophrenic' and control neonates. *British Journal of Psychiatry*, **162**, 517–523.

McNeil, T.F., Cantor-Graae, E. & Sjostrom, K. (1993b) A new comprehensive scale for measuring obstetric complications histories of schizophrenics: content analysis and empirical test on schizophrenic samples. *Schizophrenia Research*, **9**, 136.

Markow, T.A. (1992) Genetics and developmental stability: an integrative conjecture on aetiology and neurobiology of schizophrenia. *Psychological Medicine*, **22**, 295–305.

Markow, T.A. & Gottesman, I.I. (1989) Fluctuating dermatoglyphic asymmetry in psychotic twins. *Psychiatry Research*, **29**, 37–43.

Markow, T.A. & Wandler, K. (1986) Fluctuating dermatoglyphic asymmetry and the genetics of liability to schizophrenia. *Psychiatry Research*, **19**, 323–328.

Mednick, S.A. (1970) Breakdown in individuals at high risk for schizophrenia: possible predispositional perinatal factors. *Mental Hygiene*, **54**, 50–63.

Mednick, S.A., Machón, R.A. & Huttnen, M.O. (1990) An update on the Helsinki influenza project. *Archives of General Psychiatry*, **47**, 292.

Mednick, S.A., Machón, R.A., Huttunen, M.O. & Bonett, D. (1988) Adult schizophrenia following prenatal exposure to an influenza epidemic. *Archives of General Psychiatry*, **45**, 189–192.

Mednick, S.A., Parnas, J. & Schulsinger, F. (1987) The Copenhagen high-risk project, 1962–86. *Schizophrenia Bulletin*, **13**, 485–495.

Mellor, C.S. (1992) Dermatoglyphic evidence of fluctuating asymmetry in schizophrenia. *British Journal of Psychiatry*, **160**, 467–472.

Morris, M., Cotter, D., Takei, N. *et al.* (1993) An association between schizophrenic births and influenza deaths in Ireland in the years 1921–1971. *Schizophrenia Research*, **9**, 137.

Murray, R.M., Lewis, S.W., Owen, M.J. & Foerster, A. (1988) The neurodevelopmental origins of dementia praecox. In Bebbington, P. & McGuffin, P. (eds) *Schizophrenia: The Major Issues*, pp. 90–106. Heinemann, London.

Murray, R.M., Lewis, S.W. & Reveley, A.M. (1985) Towards an aetiological classification of schizophrenia. *Lancet*, **i**, 1023–1026.

Nasrallah, H.A., Schwarzkopf, S.B., Olson, S.C. & Coffman, J.A. (1991) Perinatal brain injury and cerebellar vermal lobules I–X in schizophrenia. *Biological Psychiatry*, **29**, 567–574.

Nelson, K.B. & Ellenberg, J.H. (1986) Antecedents of cerebral palsy: Multivariate analysis of risk. *New England Journal of Medicine*, **315**, 81–86.

Nimgaonkar, V., Wessely, S. & Murray, R. (1988) Prevalence of familiality, obstetric complications, and structural brain damage in schizophrenic patients. *British Journal of Psychiatry*, **153**, 191–197.

Niswander, K.R. & Kiely, M. (1991) Intrapartum asphyxia and cerebral palsy. In Kiely, M. (ed.) *Reproductive and Perinatal Epidemiology*, pp. 357–368. CRC Press, Boca Raton.

O'Callaghan, E., Larkin, C. & Waddington, J.L. (1990) Obstetric complications in schizophrenia and the validity of maternal recall. *Psychological Medicine*, **20**, 89–94.

O'Callaghan, E., Gibson, T., Colohan, H.A. *et al.* (1991a) Season of birth in schizophrenia: evidence for confinement of an excess of winter births to patients without a family history of mental disorder. *British Journal of Psychiatry*, **158**, 764–769.

O'Callaghan, E., Larkin, C., Kinsella, A. & Waddington, J.L. (1991b) Familial, obstetric, and other clinical correlates of minor physical anomalies in schizophrenia. *American Journal of Psychiatry*, **148**, 479–483.

O'Callaghan, E., Sham, P., Takei, N., Glover, G. & Murray, R.M. (1991c) Schizophrenia after prenatal exposure to 1957 A2 influenza epidemic. *Lancet* **337**, 1248–1250.

O'Callaghan, E., Gibson, T., Colohan, H.A. *et al.* (1992) Risk of schizophrenia in adults born after obstetric complications and their association with early onset of illness: a controlled study. *British Medical Journal*, **305**, 1256–1259.

O'Callaghan, E., Sham, P.C., Takei, N. *et al.* (1993) Schizophrenic births in England and Wales and their relationship to infectious diseases. *Schizophrenia Research*, **9**, 138.

Owen, M.J., Lewis, S.W. & Murray, R.M. (1988) Obstetric complications and schizophrenia: a computed tomographic study. *Psychological Medicine*, **18**, 331–339.

Paneth, N. & Pinto-Martin, J. (1991) The epidemiology of germinal matrix/intraventricular hemorrhage. In Kiely, M. (ed.) *Reproductive and Perinatal Epidemiology*, pp. 371–399. CRC Press, Boca Raton.

Parnas, J., Schulsinger, F., Teasdale, T.W., Schulsinger, H., Feldman, P.M. & Mednick, S.A. (1982) Perinatal complications and clinical outcome within the schizophrenia spectrum. *British Journal of Psychiatry*, **140**, 416–420.

Pearlson, G.D., Garbacz, D.J., Moberg, P.J., Ahn, H.S. & DePaulo, J.R. (1985) Symptomatic, familial, perinatal, and social correlates of computerized axial tomography (CAT) changes in schizophrenics and bipolars. *Journal of Nervous and Mental Disease*, **173**, 42–50.

Pearlson, G.D., Kim, W.S., Kubos, K.L. *et al.* (1989) Ventricle-brain ratio, computed tomographic density, and brain area in 50 schizophrenics. *Archives of General Psychiatry*, **46**, 690–697.

Pollack, M., Woerner, M.G., Goodman, W. & Greenberg, I.M. (1966) Childhood developmental patterns of hospitalized adult schizophrenic and nonschizophrenic patients and their siblings. *American Journal of Orthopsychiatry*, **36**, 510.

Raz, S. & Raz, N. (1990) Structural brain abnormalities in the major psychoses: a quantitative review of the evidence from computerized imaging. *Psychological Bulletin*, **108**, 93–108.

Reddy, R., Mukherjee, S., Schnur, D.B., Chin, J. & Degreef, G. (1990) History of obstetric complications, family history, and CT scan findings in schizophrenic patients. *Schizophrenia Research*, **3**, 311–314.

Reveley, A.M. & Reveley, M.A. (1983) Aqueduct stenosis and schizophrenia. *Journal of Nervous and Mental Disease*, **46**, 18.

Reveley, A.M., Reveley, M.A. & Murray, R.M. (1984) Cerebral ventricular enlargement in non-genetic schizophrenia: a controlled twin study. *British Journal of Psychiatry*, **144**, 89–93.

Rifkin, L., Lewis, S.W., Jones, P.B., Toone, B.K. & Murray, R.M. (1994) Low birth weight and schizophrenia. *Schizophrenia Research*, **11**, 94.

Roberts, J. (1980) *The Use of the CT Scanner in Psychiatry*. MPhil Thesis, University of London.

Schoental, R. (1985) Fusarial mycotoxins and behaviour: possible implications for psychiatric disorder. *British Journal of Psychiatry*, **146**, 115–119.

Schulsinger, F., Parnas, J., Petersen, E.T. *et al.* (1984) Cerebral ventricular size in the offspring of schizophrenic mothers. A preliminary study. *Archives of General Psychiatry*, **41**, 602–606.

Schwarzkopf, S.B., Nasrallah, H.A., Olson, S.C., Coffman, J.A. & McLaughlin, J.A. (1989) Perinatal complications and genetic loading in schizophrenia: preliminary findings. *Psychiatry Research*, **27**, 233–239.

Sham, P.C., O'Callaghan, E., Takei, N., Murray, G.K., Hare, E. & Murray, R.M. (1992) Schizophrenia following prenatal exposure to influenza epidemics between 1939 and 1960. *British Journal of Psychiatry*, **160**, 461–466.

Silverton, L., Finello, K.M., Mednick, S.A. & Schulsinger, F. (1985) Low birth weight and ventricular enlargement in a high-risk sample. *Journal of Abnormal Psychology*, **94**, 405–409.

Stanley, F. (1984) Prenatal risk factors in the study of cerebral palsy. In Stanley F. & Alberman, E. (eds) *The Epidemiology of the Cerebral Palsies*, pp. 87–97. Spastics International Medical Publications, London.

Susser, E.S. & Lin, S.P. (1992) Schizophrenia after prenatal exposure to the Dutch hunger winter of 1944–1945. *Archives of General Psychiatry*, **49**, 938–988.

Susser, M. (1991) What is a cause and how do we know one? A grammar for pragmatic epidemiology. *American Journal of Epidemiology*, **133**, 635–648.

Takei, N., O'Callaghan, E., Sham, P., Glover, G. & Murray,

R.M. (1992) Winter birth excess in schizophrenia: its relationship to place of birth. *Schizophrenia Research*, **6**, 102.

Takei, N., Sham, P., O'Callaghan, E., Glover, G. & Murray, R.M. (1994) Prenatal influenza and schizophrenia: is the effect confined to females? *American Journal of Psychiatry*, **151**, 117–119.

Tanaka, H., Nasu, F. & Inomata, K. (1991) Fetal alcohol effects: decreased synaptic formations in the field CA3 of fetal hippocampus. *International Journal of Developmental Neuroscience*, **9**, 509–517.

Taylor, D.J., Howie, P.W., Davidson, D. & Drillien, C.M. (1985) Do pregnancy complications contribute to neuro-developmental disability? *Lancet*, **i**, 713–716.

Torrey, E. & Bowler, A.E. (1990) The seasonality of schizophrenic births: a reply to Marc S. Lewis. *Schizophrenia Bulletin*, **16**, 1–3.

Torrey, E.F., Rawlings, R. & Waldman, I.N. (1988) Schizophrenic births and viral diseases in two states. *Schizophrenia Research*, **1**, 73–77.

Torrey, E.F., Bowler, A.E. & Rawlings, R. (1992) Schizophrenia and the 1957 influenza epidemic. *Schizophrenia Research*, **6**, 100.

Trent, M.E., Kruger, S., Perkins, D.O. & Gelernter, J. (1993) Dermatological asymmetry in schizophrenia. *Schizophrenia Research*, **9**, 141.

Turner, S.W., Toone, B.K. & Brett-Jones, J.R. (1986) Computerised tomographic scan changes in early schizophrenia — preliminary findings. *Psychological Medicine*, **16**, 219–225.

Verdoux, H. & Bourgeois, M. (1993) A comparative study of obstetric history in schizophrenics, bipolar patients and normal subjects. *Schizophrenia Research*, **9**, 67–69.

Waldrop, M.F., Pedersen, F.A. & Bell, R.Q. (1968) Minor physical anomalies and behavior in preschool children. *Child Development*, **39**, 391–400.

Watson, C.G., Kucala, T., Tilleskjor, C. & Jacobs, L. (1984) Schizophrenic birth seasonality in relation to the incidence of infectious diseases and temperature extremes. *Archives of General Psychiatry*, **41**. 85–90.

Weinberger, D.R. (1987) Implications of normal brain development for the pathogenesis of schizophrenia. *Archives of General Psychiatry*, **44**, 660–669.

Williams, A.O., Reveley, M.A., Kalakowska, T., Ardern, M. & Mandelbrote, B.M. (1985) Schizophrenia with good and poor outcome. II. Cerebral ventricular size and its clinical significance. *British Journal of Psychiatry*, **146**, 239–246.

Woerner, M.G., Pollack, M. & Klein, D.F. (1971) Birth weight and length in schizophrenics, personality disorders, and their siblings. *British Journal of Psychiatry*, **118**, 461–464.

Woerner, M.G., Pollack, M. & Klein, D.F. (1973) Pregnancy and birth complications in psychiatric patients: a comparison of schizophrenic and personality disorder patients with their siblings. *Acta Psychiatrica Scandinavica*, **49**, 712–721.

Wright, P., Gill, M. & Murray, R.M. (1993a) Schizophrenia: genetics and the maternal immune response to viral infection. *American Journal of Medical Genetics (Neuropsychiatric Genetics)*, **48**, 40–46.

Wright, P., Murray, R.M., Donaldson, P.T. & Underhill, J.A. (1993b) Do maternal HLA antigens predispose to schizophrenia? *Lancet*, **342**, 117–118.

Chapter 13
Schizophrenia:
the Epidemiological Horizon

A. JABLENSKY

Introduction

Establishing the epidemiological identity of a disease, i.e. its frequency in specified populations and groups (clinical and non-clinical), spatial distribution, temporal variation and associations with other conditions and risk factors, is an essential step towards unravelling its causes and a prerequisite for its ultimate prevention and control. In a number of instances the epidemiological mapping of a syndrome has delineated patterns suggestive of possible causation and enabled a better focusing of subsequent clinical and laboratory research. Classic examples illustrating the successes of the epidemiological method are pellagra, rubella encephalopathy, fetal alcohol syndrome and kuru.

Attempts to apply this approach to the study of schizophrenia have not met with comparable success in spite of the fact that epidemiological investigations into all major aspects of the schizophrenic disorders have been conducted for nearly a century. A principal source of uncertainty is the nature of the disease concept of schizophrenia itself. The defining attributes of schizophrenia are primarily inferential and depend critically on self-reported subjective experiences; the underlying structural and functional pathology is still hypothetical and there is no objective diagnostic test that could provide a concurrent validity criterion for the clinical diagnostic concept. As pointed out by Jaspers (1963), the disease concept of schizophrenia is 'an idea in Kant's sense', i.e. a guiding methodological principle helping to organize knowledge, but it should not be mistaken for a piece of empirical reality.

In the absence of firm conceptual grounding, the epidemiological study of schizophrenia assumes the features of a bootstrapping operation seeking anchorage points in the surface manifestations of the disorder. This is not to say that the epidemiological study of schizophrenia is predicated on the eventual discovery of a reliable diagnostic test or a disease marker. Advancing the understanding of the neurobiology of a complex disorder with ill-defined boundaries requires a sound descriptive database and an epidemiological horizon for the proper questions to be asked when planning or interpreting genetic, neuropathological and neurophysiological research. No less important is the demand for epidemiological techniques and baseline data that would aid the clinician in day-to-day diagnostic decision-making and enable the evaluation of treatments and services. In reviewing the existing epidemiological knowledge about schizophrenia, it is therefore essential to identify findings which are replicable and likely to be valid, despite the vast variation in concepts and research methods that still befogs the field.

Earlier reviews of the epidemiology of schizophrenia (e.g. Gruenberg, 1974; Wing, 1975; Eaton, 1985; Wyatt *et al.*, 1988) have tended either to present a bird's-eye view of the entire subject, or to focus on selected aspects. The present chapter aims to survey a broad range of topics which add up to a composite epidemiological picture of a complex disease. Special attention is given to findings reported in the last few years and to the epidemiological implications of recent clinical and biological research.

Sources of variation in the epidemiology of schizophrenia related to the method of investigation

The measurement of the prevalence, incidence and morbid risk of schizophrenia as a framework and prerequisite for research into risk factors and possible causes, and for refinements of taxonomy, depends critically on: (i) the capacity for identifying in a given population all possibly affected persons (or the great majority of them); and (ii) the availability of a diagnostic assessment system which would validly select 'true' cases corresponding to established clinical concepts. The first prerequisite refers to the sensitivity of the case-finding method (which should minimize the probability of both simple misses and false-negative exclusions), while the second has to do with the specificity of disease category allocation needed to minimize the rate of false-positive diagnoses.

Case finding

Existing case-finding designs fall into three groups:
1 case detection among clinical populations (persons in contact with a relevant, usually psychiatric, service);
2 door-to-door field surveys (including census investigations of entire communities and sample surveys); and
3 birth cohort studies.

Cases in treatment contact

At any time, psychiatric hospital or out-patient populations contain varying, but usually substantial, percentages of persons with the diagnosis of schizophrenia. This provides a relatively easy access to cases for epidemiological investigation. However, the probability of being in treatment depends on nosocomial factors such as the availability of services, their location and structure and the rate of their utilization by different population groups which may not be correlated with the burden of morbidity. As a rule, patients admitted to hospital are not a representative sample of all the individuals with a given disorder, and the distributions of age and sex, marital state, socioeconomic status, ethnicity and severity of illness in hospital-admission samples tend to differ from those describing the larger pool of people in the community exhibiting the disorder of interest. The nature and extent of the selection bias characterizing treated populations may vary widely from one setting to another (e.g. in a developing country compared with a developed country) and between different points in time.

Under exceptional circumstances of stable social conditions, adequate service provision and lack of major changes in legislation, admission policies and treatment philosophy, the presumption that the great majority of people with schizophrenic disorders eventually become admitted to hospital (Odegaard, 1952) may be justified. However, such conditions hardly obtain anywhere at present and, in addition, the general trend in mental health care is away from hospital treatment. It has been shown, for example, that an increasing number of schizophrenic patients are being managed on an out-patient basis without admission to hospital (over 50% of first-episode schizophrenics in Nottingham, UK, are not admitted within 3 months of their first contact with a primary care facility — Harrison *et al.*, 1991). Therefore, epidemiological case finding for schizophrenia which is restricted to the hospital setting, and particularly the estimation of incidence on the basis on first admissions, should be regarded as methodologically flawed.

The deficiencies of case finding through the hospitals can be overcome by using the psychiatric case registers, where such exist. Registers usually cover a wider spectrum of morbidity by collating data from multiple sources, including the ambulatory services. The cumulative nature of the register, the coverage of a defined population and the capacity for record linkage to other registers and databases make it a highly effective tool of epidemiological research.

However, the advantages of the case register do not offset the problem that an unknown number of schizophrenic individuals may never contact the psychiatric services. The proportion of patients with schizophrenic symptoms who never present has been estimated to be of the order of 17% in the USA (Link & Dohrenwend, 1980). According to a survey of a random sample of the population aged over 60 in Moscow (Gavrilova, 1979), a lifetime diagnosis of schizophrenia could be made in 0.5% of the subjects who had never consulted a psychiatrist, i.e. in a proportion comparable with that of the treated prevalence of schizophrenia (the majority of these cases were women). On the other hand, there is no convincing evidence that schizophrenic patients who do not contact the psychiatric services are being treated by non-psychiatric physicians. In both Denmark (Munk-Jorgensen & Mortensen, 1992) and the UK (Bamrah *et al.*, 1991), the number of such patients managed by general practitioners is thought to be negligible. Generally, no standard estimate of the 'hidden' schizophrenic morbidity seems to be possible. The presence of such morbidity, however, is a factor that should be taken into account in epidemiological studies of schizophrenia. Its size is likely to be on the increase for diverse reasons, including the spread of alternative life styles, 'counter-culture' groups and the marginalization of the destitute and homeless.

Door-to-door surveys

The field survey is the method which to date has produced the most robust epidemiological data on schizophrenia. Its earliest version, the so-called genealogical random sample test (*genealogischer Stichprobentest*), was introduced in Germany by Rüdin (1916). It consisted of an inquiry about cases of psychoses among the first-degree relatives of accessible 'probands' hospitalized for physical disease, based on the assumption that the frequency of psychoses in their families would correspond to that in the general population.

A later version of the method was the door-to-door census type of survey, used by Brugger (1931, 1933) in his investigations of the prevalence of psychoses in Thuringia and Bavaria. The method was applied most successfully by the Scandinavian investigators in the 1930–60s

(Strömgren, 1938; Sjogren, 1948; Bremer, 1951; Essen-Möller *et al.*, 1956; Hagnell, 1966; Bojholm & Strömgren, 1989). In the majority of the Scandinavian studies a single investigator, or a small group of researchers, either interviewed and diagnosed every member of a well-defined, usually small, community, or traced and assessed every person known to key informants to be possibly psychotic. Several of these studies were prospective and the same population was re-examined after an interal of 10 or more years. New cases were identified along with the ascertainment of the outcome of those formerly detected. The main difficulty in interpreting data from this type of study is the uncertain representativeness of the small population investigated and the possibility that the community might be atypical.

A viable substitute for the census is the sample survey, in which statistically representative population samples are interviewed to establish the presence of current disorders (point prevalence) or disorders that have occurred at any time in the past (lifetime prevalence). An example of a sample survey is the National Institute of Mental Health (NIMH) epidemiological catchment area (ECA) study in which some 20 000 persons at five research sites in the USA were interviewed using a structured diagnostic instrument (Robins & Regier, 1991).

Birth cohorts

Ideally, the birth-cohort study should be the method of choice for determining incidence and morbid risk because its results produce a morbidity and mortality life table. The method was first applied to the major psychoses by Klemperer (1933), who took a random sample of 1000 individuals born in Germany in 1881−90 and attempted to trace them as adults in their fourth decade of life. However, he succeeded in tracing only 44% and in interviewing 271 probands or key informants, an effect of the high cohort attrition levels which are encountered in mobile populations. Nevertheless, there are examples of remarkable success when the method is applied to stable captive populations such as island inhabi-

tants. Thus, Fremming (1947) in Denmark, and Helgason (1964) and Helgason and Magnusson (1989) in Iceland were able to trace 92 and 99.4%, respectively, of the members of birth cohorts and to collect data for the estimation of morbid risk for schizophrenia; these are of particular importance as reference values.

Diagnosis *

Diagnostic concepts, classifications and assessment instruments play a critical role in the epidemiology of schizophrenia since: (i) a certain proportion of the variation in the results of individual studies is due to variation in diagnostic concepts and practices; (ii) the diagnostic classification of cases may not be comparable across studies that have been carried out at different locations and at different points in time; and (iii) in any particular study the diagnosis of schizophrenia may either include or exclude conditions of uncertain nosological status, such as acute schizophreniform episodes, schizoaffective disorders of 'spectrum' disorders. In addition, the questions how and by whom the diagnosis is made is an important qualifier of the reported results.

Diagnosis-related biases usually are difficult to disentangle in reviewing past epidemiological research. Until the late 1960s the diagnostic rules used in epidemiological research were seldom explicitly stated and the description of the assessment techniques often lacked sufficient detail to enable an independent evaluation. As demonstrated by the US−UK diagnostic study (Cooper *et al.*, 1972), concepts of schizophrenia used by psychiatrists trained in different medical cultures could differ to an extent that might invalidate direct comparisons of symptomatology and morbidity data. The WHO International Pilot Study of Schizophrenia (IPSS − WHO, 1973, 1979) examined diagnostic variation across nine cultures by applying a standard reference classification (CATEGO − Wing *et al.*, 1974) to the clinical diagnoses made by psychiatrists in field research centres. The picture that transpired was reassuring in so far as in the majority of settings psychiatrists were found to be using similar diagnostic concepts of schizophrenia which generally corresponded to the descriptive definitions of the Kraepelin–Bleuler tradition. There were two notable exceptions represented by psychiatrists in the USA and in the former USSR.

In the USA, a broader definition of schizophrenia, which included cases that elsewhere might be diagnosed as mania or atypical affective psychosis, was current prior to the introduction of the St Louis diagnostic criteria (Feighner *et al.*, 1972) and the adoption of the Diagnostic and Statistical Manual DSM-III in the 1980s. In Russia, a similarly broad diagnostic concept of schizophrenia incorporated some of the personality disorders and other non-psychotic illnesses. The existence of such divergent definitions should be taken into account, especially when interpreting epidemiological data from the relevant time periods in these two countries.

In most other settings, the core of the diagnostic concept of schizophrenia does not seem to have undergone major changes over time. A reanalysis of Kraepelin's original case material from 1908 (Jablensky *et al.*, 1993) demonstrated that clinical data on dementia praecox and manic-depressive psychosis collected early this century can be coded and analysed using present-day Present State Examination (PSE)–CATEGO syndromes, and that the agreement between the 1908 diagnosis of dementia praecox and the CATEGO classification of the same cases is 88.6%. It should be remembered, however, that although the core of the schizophrenia concept remained constant, its periphery has become more diffuse by incorporating such variously defined syndromological entities as schizoaffective disorder, pseudoneurotic schizophrenia, schizophreniform psychosis and acute schizophrenic episodes.

Since 1980, the comparability of epidemiological data on schizophrenia over time has been affected by the introduction of operational diagnostic criteria such as research diagnostic criteria (RDC) and DSM-III. Brockington *et al.* (1978) applied 10 different definitions of schizophrenia to the same clinical material and obtained an 11-fold difference in the frequency of the disorder depending on the criteria chosen. Similarly, Stephens *et al.* (1982), using nine diagnostic

systems, established that only 7% of the cases were diagnosed as schizophrenic by all systems. The DSM-III requirement of 6 months prior duration of symptoms and the upper age limit of 45 years for a first diagnosis of schizophrenia excludes from incidence estimates as many as two-thirds of the cases which meet the less rigorous *International Classification of Disease* ICD-9 glossary definition of the disorder. This is evident from at least two recent studies (see Table 13.3) in which first-admission rates have been calculated for alternative diagnostic classifications of the cases.

While restrictive diagnostic criteria, such as DSM-III and DSM-III-R, select more homogeneous patient groups and reduce the rate of false-positive diagnoses in clinical and biological research, their place in epidemiological research is not unequivocal. Applying RDC as inclusion/exclusion categories at the case-finding stage of field surveys is likely to result in falsely rejecting an unspecified number of potentially eligible cases which at the time of initial assessment fail to satisfy the full set of criteria. Depending on the objectives and design of the study, it might be desirable to apply such criteria at a later stage when more extensive clinical assessment and/or follow-up data are available, in order to evaluate the extent to which epidemiologically identified cases are similar to, or different from, clinical samples of schizophrenic patients. As a general rule, erring on the over-inclusive side is preferable to over-restrictiveness in a two-stage design, since false-positive cases could easily be eliminated from the analysis. In contrast, falsely rejected cases are unlikely to be retrieved.

At present, there is no agreed, standard set of screening criteria for case finding for schizophrenia in field research, and no generally accepted screening instrument. Based on a reanalysis of ECA data, Eaton *et al.* (1991) have suggested that a combination of DSM-III criterion A and 16 diagnostic interview schedule (DIS) items might identify two-thirds of the psychotic cases in a community survey; the addition of a question on past psychiatric hospitalization would increase the hit rate to nearly 90%. However, such a screening device has not yet been tested.

Investigators

Epidemiological studies of schizophrenia vary with regard to how and by whom potential cases are identified, examined and diagnosed. Many of the European studies up to the 1960s were carried out by a single investigator (usually a psychiatrist) or a very small group of researchers. This had the advantage of diagnostic consistency, although systematic bias could not be excluded. Single-investigator studies are the exception in recent research, where multicentre designs or large samples, as well as economic factors, preclude such a strategy. Lay interviewers or professionals other than psychiatrists are increasingly involved in case finding and interviewing, and psychiatrists intervene only at the point of diagnostic decision-making, or not at all. The effects of interviewer variation (e.g. professional vs. lay) have been studied only partially (Robins, 1989) but the data of the NIMH ECA project (Robins & Regier, 1991) suggest that the probability of response error (any kind of error in the information volunteered by the respondent) may be considerable with lay interviewers, even if a highly structured interviewing schedule is employed.

Instruments

Instruments used in epidemiological research in psychotic disorders differ with regard to their purpose and scope, sources of data, setting of application, output format and user. At a basic conceptual level, the most widely used current diagnostic instruments fall into two categories.

The first category comprises fully structured instruments such as the NIMH DIS (Robins *et al.*, 1981) and the related WHO−ADAMHA (Alcohol, Drug Abuse, and Mental Health Administration) composite international diagnostic interview (CIDI − Robins *et al.*, 1988); these have been written to match specifically and exclusively the diagnostic criteria of DSM-III-R and ICD-10. Such instruments are designed for use by non-psychiatric interviewers and clinical judgement plays no part in their administration and scoring.

The second category includes semi-structured interview schedules, such as the PSE (Wing *et al.*, 1974) and the Schedules for Clinical Assessment in Neuropsychiatry (SCAN − Wing *et al.*, 1990), which have been developed to cover a broad range of psychopathology using professional clinical judgement, and to elicit primary data that can be processed by alternative diagnostic algorithms (including ICD-10, DSM-III-R and DSM-IV).

Each type of instrument has both advantages and disadvantages. The DIS/CIDI type can be used by lay interviewers with brief (2-week) training and achieves a high level of interrater reliability. It is capable of generating standard diagnoses in a single-stage survey design. However, the range of psychopathology covered is restricted to the diagnostic system with which it is interlocked. Its clinical validity in terms of sensitivity and specificity in diagnosing schizophrenia is open to question (see pp. 214−215).

The PSE type of interview allows a great amount of descriptive information to be collected and this can be processed and interpreted in alternative ways; both the reliability and the validity of the PSE are to a large extent a function of the training and skills of the interviewer. However, a proper diagnosis requires collateral information (for which additional modules are available in the SCAN system) and this may be feasible only in a clinical setting.

Measures of morbidity

Different aspects of morbidity are captured by the indices of prevalence, incidence and morbid risk (disease expectancy), depending on the number and type of cases included in the numerator and the time period covered (see next section). However, common problems arise in relation to the definition of the denominator, i.e. the population base from which the affected subjects derive.

The total population size (all age groups) as a denominator may have some meaning when service needs are being estimated but it is not a proper base for measuring disease occurrence, since the probabilities of onset are unevenly distributed over the life span. The denominator, therefore, should reflect the pooled risk of developing schizophrenia within a given population and exclude those groups for which the risk practically equals zero. Three different methods can be used to achieve this, depending on the design of the study.

First, age correction should be applied and it is usual to set the lower limit for schizophrenia risk at 15 years. There is less consistency in selecting an upper limit. It is as often set at age 44 as at 54, but there is no prima-facie reason why it should not be higher. Weinberg's abridged method of estimating the person-years of exposure (Bezugsiffer, BZ) to the risk of disease (Weinberg, 1925; Reid, 1960) may be applied. Second, especially in determining lifetime incidence (morbid risk) in cohort studies, both the numerator and the denominator need to be adjusted for the mortality experience of the population in question by: (i) weighting each affected person in the numerator for average life expectancy at the age of ascertainment (or at the age at death for patients who had died prior to survey); and (ii) adjusting the denominator for persons who had died unaffected prior to the survey. Third, to enable comparisons of rates, the denominator data may need to be recalculated to a standard population.

Although epidemiological techniques are available for such data analysis operations, they are not always applied in schizophrenia research, either because of unavailability of adequate population data, or because of the time-consuming data processing involved. A lack of proper standardization of the measures of morbidity may seriously jeopardize comparisons between studies, and introduces additional uncontrolled variation affecting the figures reported in the literature.

Prevalence, incidence and morbid risk (disease expectancy)

Few epidemiological studies of schizophrenia carried out to date satisfy all the methodological requirements linked to the sources of variation outlined above. For this reason the descriptive epidemiology of schizophrenia should still be regarded as provisional, even though the global picture obtained by surveying multiple data sources does suggest certain patterns and tentative conclusions.

Prevalence

Prevalence is defined as the number of cases (per 1000 persons at risk) present in a population at a given time or over a defined period. Point prevalence refers to the cases which are active (i.e. symptomatic) on a given date, or within a brief interval with the census date as a midpoint. Since asymptomatic cases, e.g. complete remissions, will be missed in a point prevalence survey, it is useful to supplement the assessment of the present mental state with an inquiry about past episodes of the disorder being investigated. This will result in a lifetime prevalence index, or proportion of survivors affected (PSA). In disorders tending towards a chronic course, such as schizophrenia, the values of point and lifetime prevalence will be closer to each other than in remitting illnesses.

Period prevalence, i.e. the number of cases per 1000 population which are active during a specified period (e.g. 6 months or 1 year), is of doubtful usefulness since it confounds point prevalence with incidence.

An overview of selected prevalence studies of schizophrenia, spanning a period of 60 years, is presented in Table 13.1. The studies differ in their methodology but have in common a high intensity of case finding (many of them were census investigations). Several among them are repeat surveys in which the original population was reinvestigated following an interval of 10 or more years (the resulting consecutive prevalence figures are indicated by →).

The majority of the studies listed in Table 13.1 have produced prevalence figures in the range 1.4−4.6 per 1000 population at risk. Considering the variation in case definition and ascertainment, and the differences in the denominator − e.g. the population at risk in Brugger's studies included ages 10 and over, while in the majority of studies a lower limit of 15 years was adopted (18 in the ECA studies) − this appears to be a narrow range. However, prevalence figures that are similar could easily mask wide differences in the incidence rates

Table 13.1 Selected studies of the prevalence of schizophrenia

Reference	Country	Population	Method	Prevalence per 1000
Brugger (1931)	Germany	Area in Turingia ($n = 37\,561$); age 10+	Census	2.4
Strömgren (1938); Bojholm and Strömgren (1989)	Denmark	Island population ($n = 50\,000$)	Repeat census	$3.9 \rightarrow 3.3$
Lemkau *et al.* (1943)	USA	Household sample	Census	2.9
Sjogren (1948)	Sweden	Island population ($n = 25\,000$)	Census	4.6
Böök (1953); Böök *et al.* (1978)	Sweden	Area in northern Sweden (genetic isolate); ($n = 9000$); age 15–50	Census	$9.5 \rightarrow 17.0$
Essen-Möller *et al.* (1956); Hagnell (1966)	Sweden	Community in southern Sweden ($n = 2550$)	Repeat census	$6.7 \rightarrow 4.5$
Rin and Lin (1962); Lin *et al.* (1989)	Taiwan	Population sample ($n = 19\,931$)	Repeat census: 1946–48, 1961–63	$2.1 \rightarrow 1.4$
Bash and Bash-Liechti (1969)	Iran	Rural ($n = 11\,585$)	Census	2.1
Crocetti *et al.* (1971)	Croatia	Sample of 9201 households	Census	5.9
Dube and Kumar (1972)	India	Four areas of Agra ($n = 29\,468$)	Census	2.6
Temkov *et al.* (1975)	Bulgaria	Urban area ($n = 140\,000$)	Census	2.8
Nielsen (1976)	Denmark	Total population of island of Samso	Census	2.7
Rotstein (1977)	Former USSR	Population sample ($n = 35\,590$)	Census	3.8
Keith *et al.* (1991)	USA	Aggregated data across five epidemiological catchment area sites	Sample survey	15.0 (lifetime); 7.0 (point)

between populations with different mortality experiences, age structure and migration rates, such as, for example, rural Iran (2.1 per 1000) and the Danish island of Samsø (2.7 per 1000). Crude prevalence figures are difficult to interpret in the absence of detailed demographic data, and it would be misleading to assume that the modal prevalence rate, which is within the 1.4–4.6 per

1000 range, reflects the true rate of occurrence of schizophrenia in the different populations.

There are outliers which deviate from the central tendency. In a birth-cohort study, Klemperer (1933) reported a rate of 10 per 1000. However, since only 440 of his 1000-member birth cohort were traced and 271 interviewed, this is probably a biased estimate. Several of the other high rates are correct and reflect the unusual features of the populations concerned.

Böök's data (Böök, 1953; Böök *et al.*, 1978) refer to a geographical and genetic isolate beyond the polar circle in northern Sweden. The high prevalence and morbid risk figures may result from a high consanguinity rate and a founder effect traceable to two Finnish ancestors who migrated into the area at the end of the 18th century. The density of cases of psychosis within individual pedigrees has attracted genetic researchers, but some doubt persists as to the diagnostic classification of the disorders observed in these families. While Böök *et al.* (1953) considered the majority of the cases to be catatonic or undifferentiated schizophrenia, a re-examination by Perris (1974) led to the conjecture that many of them were cycloid psychoses, i.e. illnesses more closely related to the affective disorders than to schizophrenia.

The high prevalence rate of schizophrenia in Croatia (Crocetti *et al.*, 1971) is restricted to a circumscribed area comprising the Istrian peninsula and several adjacent communities. The finding has been confirmed by several sample surveys employing slightly different methods. No consistent risk factors have been identified (the same population also exhibits high rates of hypertension and psoriasis). Since the area has been characterized by an above-average level of out-migration during the 19th and early 20th centuries, negative selection has been hypothesized, but no unequivocal evidence for this has been presented.

Another extreme is the finding of a near absence of schizophrenia and a relatively high rate of depression among the Hutterites in South Dakota, a Protestant sect whose members live in close-knit communities virtually sheltered from the outside world (Eaton & Weil, 1955). Endogamy has

been a common practice among the Hutterites since the 17th century and the number of outsiders joining the sect is small. The unusual findings have provoked some fascinating theories about the role of social pressure and cohesion in genetic selection: negative selection for schizoid individuals who do not fit into the collective life style of the community and positive selection for individuals with accentuated affective traits. The finding, however, has not been replicated in other Hutterite communities (Murphy, 1980) and remains an epidemiological curiosity rather than a solid fact.

The two surveys in Taiwan (Rin & Lin, 1962; Lin *et al.*, 1989) were separated by an interval of 15 years (1946−48 and 1961−63), during which time major changes had taken place in the structure of Taiwanese society. However, against a background of a general increase in total mental morbidity (from 9.4 to 17.2 per 1000), the prevalence of schizophrenia decreased from 2.1 to 1.4 per 1000. In both surveys, the native (aboriginal) Taiwanese had significantly lower rates than the mainland Chinese who had migrated to Taiwan after World War II, and the decrease in prevalence was most marked in the lower social class (in which aboriginal people were overrepresented). The authors suggest that excess mortality among low-class schizophrenic patients may be responsible for the drop in overall prevalence (24% of the schizophrenic patients alive in 1946−48 died within 5 years and 49% died within 15 years).

The results of the NIMH ECA study are a special case. In both the early publication reporting data from three of the ECA sites (Robins *et al.*, 1984) and the final report of the study (Keith *et al.*, 1991) based on all five areas, the lifetime prevalence rates for DSM-III schizophrenia are extremely high: 10−19 per 1000 according to the 1984 paper, and 15 per 1000 according to the 1991 report. A 1-year period prevalence of 10 per 1000 and a 1-month point prevalence of 7 per 1000 are also quoted in the 1991 report. There are age- and sex-related inconsistencies among the study areas (e.g. a 13-fold difference in the rates for age group 18−24 across the sites, and a higher prevalence in females in two of the sites). Black people had a higher rate (21 per 1000 lifetime and 16 per 1000 1-year) and Hispanic people a lower rate (8 per 1000 lifetime and 4 per 1000 1-year) than white people. There was a fivefold social class differential (higher rates in the lower socioeconomic groups) which, when taken into account, explained the high prevalence rate among black people but did not explain the low Hispanic rate. In addition, the survey found that 3.3% of the persons in the household sample had experienced at some time at least one DSM-III criterion A schizophrenic symptom, such as bizarre delusions and auditory hallucinations, and that 3.7% had such symptoms at the point of interview.

These results are hard to interpret. Since the lower age limit for the sample and for the standardized population figures in the denominator was 18 years, and not 15 years as in other studies, part of the explanation for the high rates may be in the reduced population denominator. In addition, an early version of the DIS was used in the area which produced the highest rates (Robins *et al.*, 1984). Although the DIS has been shown to result in many false-negative assessments of delusions and hallucinations (Eaton *et al.*, 1991), it seems more likely that at some of the ECA sites the DIS, administered by lay interviewers after 2-week training, elicited mainly false-positive psychotic symptoms. The ECA data on schizophrenia should therefore be treated with caution.

The prevalence of schizophrenia may be sensitive to small-area variation. Rates varying between 0.0 and 14.3 per 1000, as well as some non-random clustering of cases, have been found in 36 electoral divisions in a rural area of Ireland with a total population of 25 178 (Youssef *et al.*, 1991). Such findings are common in low-prevalence chronic disorders and their significance with regard to specific risk factors has yet to be established.

Incidence

The incidence rate (annual number of new cases in a defined population per 1000 individuals at risk) is of greater interest than the prevalence of schizophrenia since it represents with less distor-

tion the so-called force of morbidity (the probability of disease occurrence at a point in time) in a given population. The estimation of incidence depends critically on the capacity to pinpoint disease onset or inception, and a knowledge of the age and sex distribution of onsets is a prerequisite for the application of tests for the effects of potential risk factors.

There is no agreed definition of inception in schizophrenia and the idea of onset as a point event raises some fundamental difficulties: (i) the socially visible onset (the appearance of conspicuous behavioural abnormalities leading to consultation, admission or other action) rarely coincides with the true onset of the diagnostic symptoms of the disorder; (ii) the onset of the diagnostic (psychotic) symptoms is in many cases preceded by a prodromal phase of subclinical abnormalities of varying duration; and (iii) precursors of the symptoms and signs of schizophrenia may appear very early in life (as suggested by the prospective high-risk studies of children born to schizophrenic women).

While, for the time being, (iii) cannot conceivably provide a reference point for dating onset (precursors can be recognized as such only retrospectively), any point or segment on the continuum extending back from the social onset through the appearance of psychotic symptoms and into the prodromal phase might be arbitrarily selected as the beginning of a schizophrenic illness. As this continuum may extend over 2–6 years (Häfner *et al.*, 1993), the choice of different onset points will result in widely differing incidence estimates.

Since the timing of the true onset of any cerebral dysfunction or biochemical lesion underlying schizophrenia is impossible to determine, a strategy which as a minimum would ensure consistency is to define the onset as the point in time when the disorder becomes diagnosable according to specified criteria.

Unfortunately, a convention of this kind has not been observed in incidence studies. Part of the reasons may be that the ascertainment of the earliest appearance of diagnosable schizophrenic disorder requires reliable information which is difficult to obtain. In the majority of studies, the easily dateable event of the first hospital admission has been used as a proxy index of onset on the assumption that it provides the required consistency. However, this assumption is difficult to support in view of the wide variation that exists between individuals, across settings and over time, in the lag between symptomatic onset and first admission. Therefore, comparisons of first admission rates (the so-called administrative incidence) are unlikely to be valid approximations to comparisons of the true incidence rates.

A better approximation is offered by the rate of first contacts, i.e. the points at which any psychiatric or general medical service is contacted by symptomatic individuals for the first time. The majority of first contacts are ambulatory and often precede admission to hospital by many months; in a number of instances hospitalization may not take place at all. Such out-patient contacts are ascertainable through the psychiatric case registers. In the WHO studies (described below) a modification of this approach was used and included first contacts with a variety of services, including non-medical ones.

Table 13.2, which presents the essential features of 11 incidence studies of schizophrenia, should be read with this proviso in mind. Leaving out the rates based on the RDC or DSM-III definition of schizophrenia, the first admission and first contact rates range from 0.17 to 0.54 per 1000 population per year, i.e. they show a threefold difference. There is a remarkable similarity among the Scandinavian rates (0.20–0.27 per 1000), probably owing to the nearly complete enumeration of the cases, fairly uniform diagnostic practices and accurate denominator data. It is likely that the high Dublin rate was based on a different administrative definition of a first admission (first admission to the services in a particular area but not necessarily first admission in a lifetime). The low Moscow rates (Lieberman, 1974), appearing as not consistent with the broad Russian concept of schizophrenia, may be explained by the method of estimating incidence in this particular study; this involved a retrospective dating of onsets in a prevalence sample of patients.

The lowest rates in Table 13.2 refer to non-European populations: Hindu and Moslem Indians in Mauritius (0.14 and 0.09 per 1000) and Chinese and aborigines in Taiwan (0.17 per 1000). Since the Mauritian data are first admission rates, they may have been influenced by a nosocomial hospitalization threshold (this does not apply to the Taiwan data, which were collected in a survey).

The two recent studies employing a polydiagnostic (ICD, RDC and DSM-III) classification of the cases illustrate the impact of the restrictive diagnostic criteria which, compared with ICD-9, result in at least a threefold decrease of the incidence rate for the same population.

To date, the only study which has generated comparative incidence data for different populations using contemporaneous case finding and identical research techniques in 12 catchment areas is the WHO 10-country investigation (Sartorius *et al.*, 1986; Jablensky *et al.*, 1992). Incidence counts in the WHO study were based on first-in-lifetime contacts with any 'helping agency' in the area (including traditional healers in the developing countries), monitored prospectively over a 2-year period. Potential cases and key informants were interviewed in detail using standardized instruments, and the timing of the onset of psychotic symptoms diagnostic of schizophrenia was ascertained for the majority of patients (1022 out of 1379). For 86% of the 1022 patients, the first appearance of diagnostic symptoms of schizophrenia was within the year preceding the first contact and therefore the first-contact incidence rate was accepted as a close approximation to the onset rate.

Two kinds of case definition, differing in the degree of specificity, were used to determine the incidence rates in the WHO study: a broad clinical definition comprising ICD-9 schizophrenia and paranoid psychoses, and a restrictive research definition including only cases classified as 'nuclear' schizophrenia with first-rank symptoms (S+) by the CATEGO computer program (Wing *et al.*, 1974). The rates for eight catchment areas are shown in Table 13.3.

The differences between the rates for broadly

Table 13.2 Selected studies of the incidence of schizophrenia

Reference	Country	Population	Method	Rate per 1000
Ödegaard (1946a)	Norway	Total population	All FAs 1926−35 ($n = 14\,231$)	0.24
Adelstein *et al.* (1968)	UK	Salford population (150 000)	FA	0.35 (M) 0.20 (F)
Walsh (1969)	Ireland	Dublin population (720 000)	FA	0.57 (M) 0.46 (F)
Häfner and Reimann (1970)	Germany	Mannheim population (330 000)	Register	0.54
Raman and Murphy (1972)	Mauritius	Population (257 000)	All FAs 1956	0.24 (A) 0.14 (IH) 0.09 (IM)
Lieberman (1974)	Former USSR	Moscow area population (248 000)	Follow-back	0.20 (M) 0.19 (F)
Nielsen (1976) Helgason (1977)	Denmark Iceland	Island of Samsø Total population	FA All FAs 1966−67 ($n = 2388$)	0.20 0.27
Lin *et al.* (1989)	Taiwan	Three communities ($n = 39\,024$)	Household survey	0.17
Castle *et al.* (1991)	UK	Camberwell	Register	0.25 (ICD) 0.17 (RDC) 0.08 (DSM)
Nicole *et al.* (1992)	Canada	Quebec area population (338 300)	FA	0.31 (ICD) 0.09 (DSM)

FA, first admission; M, male; F, female; A, Africans; IH, Indian Hindus; IM, Indian Moslems; ICD, *International Classification of Disease*; RDC, research diagnostic criteria; DSM, *Diagnostic and Statistical Manual*.

defined schizophrenia are highly significant ($P < 0.001$, two-tailed test); those for the 'nuclear' schizophrenia syndrome are not significant. It should be pointed out that no consistent differences were found between cases meeting the broad criteria only and cases classified as S+ with regard to either the course and outcome of the disorder or the type of onset (acute or insidious).

Therefore, the similar incidence rates for 'nuclear' schizophrenia across the study areas do not imply that the schizophrenic illnesses occurring in the different populations are of similar severity and/ or chronicity. Nor is there any reason to assume that the S+ patients are 'truer' schizophrenics than the broadly defined cases. The main point about the WHO data is not so much the lack of

Table 13.3 Incidence rates per 1000 in eight areas in the WHO 10-country study. (From Jablensky *et al.*, 1992)

Area	'Broad' diagnosis (ICD-9 or CATEGO S,P,O)			'Narrow' diagnosis (CATEGO S+)		
	M	F	M + F	M	F	M + F
AAR	0.18	0.13	0.18	0.09	0.05	0.07
CHA-R	0.37	0.48	0.26	0.13	0.09	0.11
CHA-U	0.34	0.35	0.35	0.08	0.11	0.09
DUB	0.23	0.21	0.22	0.10	0.08	0.09
HON	0.18	0.14	0.16	0.10	0.08	0.09
MOS	0.25	0.31	0.28	0.10	0.14	0.12
NAG	0.23	0.12	0.21	0.11	0.09	0.10
NOT	0.28	0.15	0.24	0.17	0.12	0.14
P	0.001	0.0001		NS	NS	

AAR, Åarhus (Denmark); CHA-R, Chandigarh (India), rural area; CHA-U, Chandigarh (India), urban area; DUB, Dublin (Ireland); HON, Honolulu, Hawaii (USA); MOS, Moscow (Russia); NAG, Nagasaki (Japan); NOT, Nottingham (United Kingdom); ICD, *International Classification of Disease*; S, schizophrenia; P, paranoid psychosis; O, other psychosis; S+, nuclear schizophrenia; M, male; F, female; NS, not significant.

statistically significant differences in the S+ rates as the demonstration of a relatively narrow band of variation (0.16–0.42 per 1000) in the incidence of ICD-9 schizophrenia when standard case and onset definitions, research instruments and case-finding techniques are used in different populations (i.e. when several of the methodological difficulties outlined above have been at least partially resolved).

Morbid risk (disease expectancy)

This is the probability (usually expressed as a percentage) that an individual born into a particular population or group will develop the disease if he/she survives through the entire period of risk for that disease. In the instance of schizophrenia, the period of risk is defined as either 15–44 years or 15–54 years. If the age- and sex-specific incidence rates are known, disease expectancy is estimated directly by a summation of the rates across the ages within the period of risk (under the assumption that the age-specific incidence rates are constant over time). Indirectly, disease expectancy can be estimated from census data

by the so-called abridged method of Weinberg (1925):

$$P = \frac{A}{B - (B_o + \frac{1}{2}B_m)}$$

where P is disease expectancy (%), A the number of cases, B the total population surveyed, B_o persons who have not yet entered the risk period and B_m persons within the risk period. A modification of Weinberg's method has been proposed (Stromgren, 1935; Bojholm & Strömgren, 1989) and this weights the numerator for the excess mortality observed among schizophrenic patients.

Whether estimated directly from age-specific incidence data or indirectly from census data, disease expectancy provides more reliable comparisons between rates of occurrence of schizophrenia in different populations than the prevalence or incidence rates. Notwithstanding the different methods of data collection and risk estimation, the figures indicate a fair degree of consistency across populations and over time. Excluding the northern Swedish isolate, the maximum of the risk ratio (highest to lowest morbid risk) is about 5.0; for the WHO study it is 2.9 (ICD-9 schizophrenia) and 2.0 (CATEGO S+). As most studies have produced morbid risk estimates in the range 0.50–1.60, the often quoted 'rule of thumb' estimate of the morbid risk for schizophrenia at around 1% seems to be consistent with the evidence.

The question whether significant differences exist among populations in the 'true' rate of occurrence of schizophrenia (Torrey, 1987) has no simple answer. Depending on the size of the populations or samples surveyed, statistically significant differences are bound to occur; whether such differences are epidemiologically salient is a different matter. In view of the large number of potentially confounding factors which may affect in different and subtle ways the incidence and morbid risk estimates produced by individual studies, such figures should not be quoted as absolutes but interpreted in the context of the methods applied and the general knowledge about the populations concerned. For example, it would hardly make sense to interpret the sevenfold difference in estimated population incidence of DIS/DSM-III schizophrenia between two of the ECA study sites (Tien & Eaton, 1992) as evidence of the existence of large variation in the incidence of schizophrenia in the USA.

Ideally, a meta-analysis involving a standardized recalculation of the rates from many previous studies should generate a distribution allowing one to estimate with some probability the extent to which populations differ. In the absence of ultimate proof, the weight of the current evidence does not suggest the existence of major population differences in the incidence and disease expectancy of schizophrenia, such as are known to occur in common multifactorial diseases, e.g. diabetes or ischaemic heart disease. In so far as pockets of high incidence as well as small area variations in the incidence rate exist, they seem to be local exceptions rather than the general rule in the epidemiology of schizophrenia.

Secular trends in the incidence and prevalence of schizophrenia

The rarity of descriptions of identifiable schizo-phrenia in the medical literature before the 18th century has led to speculations that the condition did not exist (Torrey, 1980) or was rare (Hare, 1983) until the Industrial Revolution. The earliest references to psychotic states matching the description of the schizophrenic syndrome can be found in Pinel (1803) and Haslam (1809). An examination of the 19th-century asylum statistics (Jablensky, 1986) indeed suggests that 'mono-maniac insanity', 'delusional insanity' and 'ordinary dementia' (i.e. the labels likely to contain schizo-phrenics in pre-Kraepelinian psychiatry) comprised between 5.3 and 18.9% of all institutionalized patients. The records of the Munich University Psychiatric Clinic, under the direction of Kraepelin in 1908, indicate that in the course of a year dementia praecox accounted for only 9.1% of the first admissions among men and for 7.3% among women (Jablensky *et al.*, 1993).

While no strong evidence has been supplied to support the claim that schizophrenia is of recent origin (this would be extremely unlikely considering its genetics and comparable rates of occurrence in diverse populations), it is possible that substantial increases in the number of people diagnosed as schizophrenic took place late in the 19th century and during the 20th century. Whether the increase was real (resulting from a decreasing mortality, rising incidence, or both) or spurious (increased likelihood of the diagnosis, social pressures lowering the threshold for institutionalizing the mentally ill) remains an open question. The similarity of the incidence rates in the developing countries and in industrialized societies today argues against schizophrenia being a 'disease of civilization' (Torrey, 1980). There is no clear relationship between the level of socioeconomic development and the incidence rate of schizophrenia, although some case studies of small traditional communities (e.g. the Achinese in Sumatra or the Tallensi in Ghana — Murphy, 1982) do suggest shifts in prevalence following major socioeconomic upheaval.

The question whether long-term trends can be detected in the incidence of schizophrenia has attracted renewed interest following the publication of several reports since 1985 (Table 13.4);

Table 13.4 Temporal trends in the administrative incidence of schizophrenia (per 1000)

Reference	Country	Period	Source of data	Change
Eagles and Whalley (1985)	Scotland	1969−78	DHSS	0.20 → 0.12
Munk-Jorgensen (1986)	Denmark	1970−84	Register (national)	0.31 → 0.16
Joyce (1987)	New Zealand	1974−84	National Health Statistics Centre	0.20−0.09
Eagles et al. (1988)	Scotland	1969−84	Register (Aberdeen)	0.13 → 0.06
Der et al. (1990)	England and Wales	1970−78	DHSS	0.15 → 0.09
Castle et al. (1991)	England	1965−84	Register (Camberwell)	0.20 → 0.25
Bamrah et al. (1991)	England	1974−84	Register (Salford)	0.17 → 0.19
Harrison et al. (1991)	England	1975−87	Register	0.11 → 0.10

DHSS, Department of Health and Social Services (UK).

these indicate a 40% or more reduction in the first admissions with a diagnosis of schizophrenia in Denmark, the UK and New Zealand over the last three decades. In fact, a decline in the hospitalization rate for schizophrenia had been described earlier by Weeke and Strömgren (1978), who noted that the national census of hospitalized schizophrenics in Denmark had dropped from 6200 in 1957 to 4500 in 1972, the reduction being most pronounced in women aged 35−54.

The recent data can be summed up as follows.
1 A trend of diminishing administrative incidence rates (both first hospital admissions and first contacts with a psychiatric case register) has indeed been demonstrated, but the data provided by the different studies are inconsistent as regards the age- and sex-specific rate reduction.
2 The trend has been identified in large aggregated databases for the populations of Denmark, Scotland, England and Wales but has not been consistently reproduced on local or regional case register data (two case registers have identified a downward trend: Eagles et al., 1988; de Alarcon et al., 1992; another two have shown increases: Bamrah et al., 1991; Castle et al., 1991; and one has reported no change: Harrison et al., 1991).
3 The studies in which research diagnoses (RDC, DSM-III or CATEGO) were made after a case review (Bamrah et al., 1991; Castle et al., 1991) have shown no decline in rates.
4 In the same areas and for the same period there have been concomitant declines in the total number of beds, all first admissions and the first admissions for affective psychoses and neurotic and personality disorders.
5 In several of the areas increases have been reported in the excess mortality of schizophrenic patients (Munk-Jorgensen & Mortensen, 1992), in the diagnoses of paranoid and reactive psychoses or borderline states on first admission (Munk-Jorgensen, 1986; Der et al., 1990; Harrison et al., 1991) and in the delay between first ambulatory contact and first hospital admission (Harrison et al., 1991).

Although a genuine trend of diminishing rates of schizophrenia cannot be excluded, the combined effects of several factors are capable of explaining the observed changes: variations in the definitions of first admission or first contact, changes in diagnostic practices over time, changes in the treatment modalities and settings, increases in the mortality of schizophrenic patients and changes in the age composition of the populations concerned. An increasing reluctance to make a diagnosis of schizophrenia on first admission has been noted among Danish psychiatrists (Munk-Jorgensen, 1986), and the same may be true of the diagnostic practice in other countries. The reported size of the compensatory increase of other first-admission diagnoses is sufficient to account for the drop in schizophrenia diagnoses. In addition, the time lag in the diagnosis of schizophrenia, which in many instances is made months or years after the first contact of the patient with the services, may artificially depress the first-admission rates for the last years of the observation period and thus enhance the overall trend. The imminent disappearance of schizophrenia is therefore a provocative but yet unproven hypothesis.

Associations with other diseases (comorbidity)

Comorbidity in schizophrenia encompasses: (i) relatively common physical diseases occurring among schizophrenic patients at a frequency different from chance expectation; (ii) co-occurrence of schizophrenia and certain rare conditions or abnormalities; and (iii) other psychiatric or behavioural disorders in individuals with a main diagnosis of schizophrenia.

Physical disease is common among schizophrenic patients but is rarely diagnosed. Between 46 and 80% of the schizophrenic in-patients and between 20 and 43% of the schizophrenic out-patients have been found in different surveys to suffer from concurrent medical illnesses. In 46% of the patients a physical illness was thought to aggravate the mental state, and in 7% it was life threatening (Adler & Griffith, 1991). In addition to the increased susceptibility to infection, and especially pulmonary tuberculosis prior to hospitalization (Baldwin, 1979), schizophrenic patients have a higher than expected rate of arteriosclerotic disease and myocardial infarction (Saugstad & Ödegaard, 1979).

Negative comorbidity, i.e. a lower than expected rate of occurrence of a specified disease in schizophrenic patients, has to date been demonstrated for rheumatoid arthritis (Österberg, 1978). Schizophrenic patients have proportionally lower cancer mortality than the general population, but the significance of this finding has been discounted on the grounds of the excess suicide and accident mortality which reduces the number of schizophrenic subjects entering the peak risk period for malignancies. However, in a WHO record linkage study based on the Danish national psychiatric and cancer case registers, the relative risk of malignancies of all sites, but particularly lung cancer, was significantly and consistently reduced in male schizophrenic patients, and a similar though less consistent, trend was found in female schizophrenic patients (Dupont *et al.*, 1986; Gulbinat *et al.*, 1992). There is no obvious explanation for this finding but some protective effect of long-term neuroleptic medication is suggested by the data (Mortensen, 1987).

Minor physical anomalies, including a high-steepled palate, malformed ears, epicanthus, single palmar crease, finger and toe abnormalities, etc. are found significantly more frequently in schizophrenic patients than in control subjects (Green *et al.*, 1989) and may be related to atypical fetal development during the first gestational trimester.

Co-occurrence of schizophrenia and rare genetic or idiopathic disorders has been reported for: basal ganglia calcification (Francis & Freeman, 1984); aqueductus Sylvii stenosis (Reveley & Reveley, 1983; Roberts *et al.*, 1983); corpus callosum agenesis (Lewis *et al.*, 1988); septal cysts (Lewis & Mezey, 1985); acute intermittent porphyria (Propping, 1983); coeliac disease (Dohan, 1966); and Marfan syndrome (Sirota *et al.*, 1990). If exceeding chance co-occurrence, such associations may be suggestive of a pathogenetic or genetic link between the two conditions; alternatively, they may represent either phenocopies or 'genocopies' (Gottesman *et al.*, 1987) of schizophrenia. In both instances they should be of considerable research interest.

Substance abuse is by far the most common behavioural comorbidity problem among schizophrenic patients (Schneier & Siris, 1987; Drake & Wallach, 1989). It may involve alcohol, stimulants, benzodiazepines, hallucinogens, antiparkinsonian drugs, caffeine and tobacco (Lohr & Flynn, 1992). In the WHO 10-country study, a history of alcohol use in the year preceding the first contact was given for a total of 57% of the male patients, and in three of the study areas drug abuse (mainly with marijuana and cocaine) was reported by 24–41% of the patients. Cannabis use can exacerbate the symptoms of schizophrenia (Treffert, 1978; Mathers & Ghodse, 1992) and was found in the WHO study to be a predictor of poor 2-year outcome in schizophrenia of recent onset (Jablensky *et al.*, 1992).

Mortality and fertility

The excess mortality of schizophrenic patients is a well-documented phenomenon. The data of the Norwegian psychiatric case register (Saugstad & Ödegaard, 1979) indicate that while the total mortality of hospitalized psychiatric patients decreased significantly between 1926–41 and 1950–74, the relative mortality of patients with a diagnosis of schizophrenia remained unchanged at 21 per 1000 for males and 15 per 1000 for females (age-standardized annual rate), i.e. at a level more than twice as high as that of the general population. Very similar results have been reported from the Oxford record linkage study (Herrman *et al.*, 1983).

More recent data from Denmark (Munk-Jorgensen & Mortensen, 1992) suggest an alarming trend of increasing mortality in successive cohorts of first-admission patients with schizophrenia. The 5-year cumulated standard mortality ratio (SMR) has increased from 5.30 (males) and 2.27 (females) in 1971–73 to 7.79 (males) and 4.52 (females) in 1980–82. Particularly striking is the SMR of 16.4 for male schizophrenics in the

first year after the diagnosis has been made.

At present, the most common cause of death among schizophrenic patients is suicide. It accounted for the majority of deaths in the Danish data. In the WHO IPSS (Leff *et al.*, 1992) suicide was the cause in 19 of the 52 deaths among the 807 patients followed up over 5 years; of the 19 patients who committed suicide 14 had a diagnosis of schizophrenia. High cumulated SMRs for suicide of 6.4 (males) and 3.3 (females) have been reported by Tsuang (1978) but the basis for his estimates was a much longer follow-up period of 40 years. The suicide-related SMRs of 1.42 (males) and 2.83 (females) established in the follow-up of 532 schizophrenic patients in the UK (Anderson *et al.*, 1991) were also based on a longer period (3–13 years). The Danish data, being based on 5-year cumulated SMRs, point to a higher and still increasing rate of early schizophrenic suicide. If replicated in other countries, such findings may be the signal of a new wave of mortality associated with the drastic changes in the management of schizophrenia in the post-institutional era.

In a review of published studies, Caldwell and Gottesman (1990) point to several risk factors which appear to be specific to schizophrenic suicide: being young and male, experiencing chronic disabling illness with multiple relapses and remissions, realistic awareness of the deteriorating course of the condition, excessive treatment dependence and loss of faith in treatment. Positive symptoms are better predictors of suicide risk in schizophrenia than are negative symptoms (Fenton & McGlashan, 1991b).

The low fertility of both men and women diagnosed as schizophrenic has been extensively documented by Essen-Möller (1935) and Larson and Nyman (1973) in Sweden and by Ödegaard (1980) in Norway. The average number of children fathered by schizophrenic men was 0.9 in Sweden, and the average number of live births over the entire reproductive period of women treated for schizophrenia in Norway during 1936–75 was 1.8, compared with 2.2 for the general female population. Similar results (1.5 live births in schizophrenic women compared with 2.0 in the general population of women) have been reported by Shmaonova *et al.* (1976) in Moscow. A slight upward trend in the fertility of schizophrenic women in more recent decades has been noted by both Ödegaard and Shmaonova *et al.* and it is likely that this trend is continuing. It should be noted that little is known about the fertility of schizophrenic men.

Several studies (Lindelius, 1970; Buck *et al.*, 1975; Rimmer & Jacobsen, 1976; Erlenmeyer-Kimling, 1978) have examined the fertility of siblings of schizophrenic probands and found no significant difference in comparison with a control sample or the general population. No evidence has been produced to date of any reproductive advantage for the non-psychotic biological first-degree relatives of schizophrenic patients that would offset the low fertility and high mortality associated with the disease. However, a reproductive advantage supporting the transmission of schizophrenia in the population remains a possibility if extended pedigrees are considered, and it would be premature to discard the hypothesis of a balanced polymorphism in schizophrenia (Huxley *et al.*, 1964)

Course and outcome of schizophrenia and their prediction

Systematic investigation of the course and outcome of schizophrenia was initiated by Kraepelin, who believed that in the absence of demonstrable brain pathology and identifiable causes, careful observation of the natural history of clinical syndromes could establish the validity of the disease entities he had delineated. Later, Kraepelin revised his claim that the prognosis of dementia praecox was invariably poor and noted that 'permanent cures' had occurred in about 15% of cases (Kraepelin, 1919). Subsequent longitudinal studies have highlighted the striking variability of the course of schizophrenia, which seems to be the most salient characteristic of its natural history.

In reviewing research into the natural course of schizophrenia, Ram *et al.* (1992) grouped studies into: (i) statistical reports on admissions and discharges; (ii) long-term follow-back studies (in which cases identified retrospectively from admission records were traced and reassessed); and (iii) prospective investigations (in which patients were enlisted at an early stage of the disorder and followed up for a varying length of time). Each design is vulnerable to bias: admission and discharge statistics usually comprise patients at different stages of disease progression; follow-back studies rely on prevalence samples in which chronic cases tend to be overrepresented; and prospective studies, though superior to other designs, often exlude those patients who have diagnoses other than schizophrenia at the start of the observation but are subsequently rediagnosed as schizophrenic. The lack of operational definitions, and measurement variation affecting such key variables as psychotic eposide, relapse, remission, improvement, end state, etc. hamper the interpretation of data. In particular, the failure to evaluate symptoms of disease, impairments of function and social disabilities independently from one another may blur important distinctions between different aspects of outcome. Nevertheless, the sum of the evidence emerging from the different types of investigation is more consistent than could be expected and points in the same general direction (see also Chapter 8).

The natural history of schizophrenia prior to the introduction of neuroleptic treatment

One of the earliest follow-up studies (Rosanoff, 1914) reported that within 5 years of first admission to a New York state hospital in 1908–13, 13.6% of the 169 patients under observation had died, 23.1% had been discharged and 58.6% remained in hospital. Very similar results were reported by Rupp and Fletcher (1940) for patients admitted in 1929–39. The high mortality of the patients was mainly accounted for by pulmonary tuberculosis (48% of all deaths).

Jonsson and Jonsson (1992) examined the lifetime records of 70 Swedish patients first admitted in 1925, and rediagnosed them in accordance with DSM-III. None of these patients had received neuroleptics. The final outcome was rated as good in 33% (but no patient was considered to be completely recovered), 'profoundly deteriorated' in 43% and intermediate in 24%. Ciompi and Muller (1976) interviewed 289 surviving patients in Switzerland first admitted between 1900 and 1962 (median follow-up length 36.9 years) and found that 49% had either remitted or exhibited mild residual abnormalities which did not interfere with their living in the community; on the other hand, 44% were severely disabled and still in hospital.

Observations on 208 patients, first admitted in 1942–43 and followed up intensively for 22 years or until death, have been published by M. Bleuler (1972). Another 23-year follow-up study of 504 patients admitted in 1945–59 has been completed by Huber *et al.* (1980). A joint paper (Bleuler *et al.*, 1976) summarizes the findings on which both studies agree. These are worth retaining as an important record of the preneuroleptic prognosis of schizophrenia (although some of the patients were medicated at later stages of the follow-up):

lasting recovery ('complete cure') in 20–26%;

severe chronic states in 14–24%;

no further deterioration after the fifth year since onset and development of a clinically stable state in 50–75% of the patients;

remitting course characterized by multiple episodes and full remissions in 22%;

catastrophic course (rapid onset of chronic deterioration) in 4%; and

20-year suicide rate in 14–22%.

At least four studies on the outcome of schizophrenia in the preneuroleptic era provide evidence that the hospital prognosis was improving prior to the introduction of the phenothiazines. Israel and Johnson (1956) showed that the 10-year discharge rates were increasing from 54.9 to 72.5% for each consecutive cohort of patients first admitted in 1913–22, 1923–32, 1933–42 and 1943–52. By tabulating the discharges of schizophrenic patients first admitted in 1936–42, 1945–52 and 1955–59, Ödegaard (1964) demonstrated that the greatest improvement in the discharge rates occurred in the period 1936–50. Achte and Apo (1967) found no clear differences in the discharge rates and outcomes of first admissions in the

preneuroleptic period 1950–52 and the post-neuroleptic period 1957–59. A similar trend had been described by Shepherd (1957).

Insulin coma treatment, introduced in the late 1930s, is unlikely to have contributed substantially to the shortening of the hospital stay. Harris *et al.* (1956) found no relation between the 5-year outcome of 126 patients admitted in 1945–48 and the number of comas, insulin dosage or weight changes occurring during the treatment these patients received. The improving discharge rate of schizophrenia seems to be related to the progressive changes in attitudes and hospital regime which occurred in a number of institutions on both sides of the Atlantic in the 1930s and 1940s, as well as to the revival of the labour market following the Great Depression (Ödegaard, 1964). This conclusion is strengthened by the evidence that low levels of institutionalism for schizophrenic patients was related to the availability of in-patient rehabilitation and aftercare (Wing & Brown, 1970). Neuroleptic treatment was introduced at a time when the average length of hospital treatment of schizophrenia was already declining under the influence of environmental factors, and this fact may have attenuated its impact.

Recent course and outcome studies

Longitudinal research in the past two decades has added data which tend to corroborate rather than challenge the pattern of outcomes outlined by the earlier studies.

The reported rates of improvement without relapse are in the range between 21 (Bland & Orn, 1978) and 30% (Scottish Schizophrenia Research Group, 1992); poor outcome in terms of continuous psychotic symptoms and/or increasing social disability is between 24 (Salokangas, 1983) and 43% (Shepherd *et al.*, 1989).

There is a relationship of some consistency between the length of the follow-up and the proportions of patients who are reported as recovered, remitting or deteriorating, with a general trend towards higher improvement rates in long-term studies. To illustrate this, the proportion of good outcomes increased from 10% at the 2.5-year follow-up to 17% at 5 years (Carone *et al.*, 1991); it was nearly 60% at the end of the 32-year follow-up reported by Harding *et al.* (1987a,b). The same trend was observed in the WHO studies described below.

The three prospective WHO investigations, the IPSS (WHO 1973, 1979; Leff *et al.*, 1992), the 10-country study on determinants of outcome (Jablensky *et al.*, 1992) and the study on assessment of psychiatric disability (Jablensky *et al.*, 1980; Schubart *et al.*, 1986), provide a cross-cultural database for the evaluation of the course and outcome of schizophrenia which comprises extensive initial and follow-up information on a total of 2736 patients diagnosed as schizophrenic according to strictly comparable criteria. The standardized assessment methods and instruments used in the three studies were quite similar, so that comparisons across the study populations are possible. Illustrative results of the WHO 10-country study (pooled data on patients in all the research sites) are presented in Table 13.5. The WHO findings lead to five general conclusions

(other aspects of the results are reviewed in the section on cultural differences, see pp. 230–32.

1 The striking variability of the course and outcome of schizophrenia has been cross-culturally confirmed. There is a continuum of outcomes ranging from stable clinical and social recovery after a single psychotic episode to chronic unremitting psychosis and severe impairment, in patients who had similar clinical and daignostic characteristics at the initial assessment. The intensive follow-up and the low cohort attrition rate resulted in the ascertainment of a higher proportion of good outcomes (over 30% in the WHO studies) than in the case of less intensive surveys in which a disproportionately large number of recovering patients may be lost to follow-up.

2 The probabilities of both relapses and remissions tend to increase over time: while at 2-year follow-up 11% of the patients had experienced two or more psychotic episodes followed by complete remission and another 18% had two or more episodes followed by residual symptoms and impairments, the corresponding proportions at 5-year follow-up were 15 and 33%.

Table 13.5 Two-year course and outcome of 1070 schizophrenic patients followed up in the WHO 10-country study: percentage time psychotic, in complete remission, in hospital and on antipsychotic medication. (From Jablensky *et al.*, 1992)

	Percentage time of the follow-up					
	0	1–5	6–15	16–45	46–75	76–100
Psychotic						
Men	–	20.3	32.1	21.0	7.9	18.7
Women	–	18.9	36.4	22.0	5.4	17.3
Remission						
Men	44.2	0.3	3.4	10.0	13.8	28.2
Women	40.7	1.2	1.0	9.8	17.8	29.5
In hospital						
Men	30.3	21.0	28.5	15.1	3.3	1.8
Women	34.6	19.8	25.2	17.3	2.7	0.4
On medication						
Men	4.1	7.0	13.1	16.8	19.9	39.2
Women	6.1	7.4	12.7	20.4	14.9	38.6

3 Regardless of the increasing relapse rate, the proportion of cumulated follow-up time during which patients experience psychotic symptoms, as a percentage of the total follow-up time, tends to remain stable or to decrease. At the end of the 5-year follow-up period, 57% of the patients had cumulated less than 9 months of active psychotic episodes, and only 22% had been psychotic for 45−60 months.

4 The levels of social impairment established at 2 years changed very little during the 5-year follow-up. Overall, most of the clinical and social adjustment changes occurring between the 2-year follow-up and the 5-year follow-up are in the direction of improvement rather than deterioration.

5 Compared with the IPSS 2-year follow-up , the corresponding data from the WHO 10-country study indicate a better course and outcome. Part of the explanation may be linked to a cohort effect (a 10-year interval between the starting dates of the two studies), but a more likely reason is the prospective case-finding design of the second study, in which patients were identified as they made first contact with a service. At that point the majority of the subjects were in an early post-onset stage of the disorder.

Staging the course of schizophrenia

At present, it does not seem possible to define with any precision discrete stages in the progression of schizophrenic illnesses using combined clinical and pathological criteria, as in cancer or cardiovascular disease. Nevertheless, a 'softer' form of staging is worth attempting as a testable working hypothesis in longitudinal research, since there is on the whole a good agreement between the results of different studies on the global aspects of the course of schizophrenia.

On the basis of a long-term follow-up, Ciompi (1984) distinguished between a premorbid phase (from birth to the onset of psychosis), a phase of acute or positive schizophrenic symptomatology and a residual phase. Breier *et al.* (1991) proposed another phasic model comprising three stages.

1 An early deteriorating phase (the first 5−10 years).

2 A middle (stabilization) phase.

3 A gradual improvement phase.

This model tentatively links the succession of phases to the decrement in brain dopamine receptors associated with normal ageing. Whatever the hypothetical pathophysiological base of the process, a descriptive three-stage scheme agrees well with the empirical evidence and could be a useful focus for establishing baseline data on individual risks and prognosis.

Stability of the clinical syndromes over time

Longitudinal studies suggest that the symptomatology of schizophrenia 'breeds true' in the sense that relatively few patients are eventually reclassified into other disease categories following a firm initial diagnosis of a schizophrenic illness. In the 2-year follow-up of the IPSS (WHO, 1979), 75% of the patients with an initial diagnosis of schizophrenia who experienced relapses of any type had schizophrenic symptoms only, and another 3% had both schizophrenic and other types of episodes. On 5-year follow-up these proportions were 59 and 17%, respectively, i.e. there was an increase in the number of patients who in the course of time developed other symptoms (mainly affective) in addition to their persisting or episodic schizophrenic symptoms.

First-rank symptoms (and the corresponding CATEGO class S+ of 'nuclear' schizophrenia) tend to recur in subsequent psychotic episodes. For patients with first-rank symptoms on initial examination the relative risk of experiencing such symptoms in any late stage of the disorder is 2.7, compared with patients with no first-rank symptoms on initial examination (Jablensky *et al.*, 1992).

The most common non-schizophrenic syndrome developing in the course of schizophrenia is depression. In the course of 2 years, 17% of the IPSS patients with a diagnosis of schizophrenia who remitted and then relapsed had clearcut depressive episodes (Sheldrick *et al.*, 1977). This proportion remained almost unchanged at 15% at the end of the 5-year follow-up (Leff *et al.*, 1992). Similarly, the frequency of major depressive episodes was 24% during the 2−12 years of follow-up in the NIMH study (Breier *et al.*, 1991). In contrast, subsequent schizophrenic illnesses develop in only 9.7% of the patients with an initial diagnosis of major depression (WHO, 1978).

These data suggest that depression is not an accidental event in the course of schizophrenia but part of its clinical spectrum. Based on such data, the diagnostic rubric of post-schizophrenic depression has been added to the classification of schizophrenia in ICD-10.

Prognosis of schizophrenia subtypes

According to Kraepelin (1904) and Bleuler (1911), the classic subtypes of schizophrenia were well distinguished by their prognosis: invariably poor in hebephrenia and the simple type, less uniform in catatonia and the paranoid form and relatively favourable in the cyclic or periodic forms. There is little epidemiological evidence to support or reject this clinical view because of a surprising scarcity of well-designed longitudinal studies of schizophrenia subtypes.

Recently, consistent differences between paranoid, hebephrenic and undifferentiated schizophrenia (diagnosed according to DSM-III) have been reported by Fenton and McGlashan (1991a,b) for 187 patients followed up for an average of 19 years. Paranoid schizophrenia tended to be of a later and more acute onset than the other two subtypes, to have a remittent course, and to be associated with less disability. In contrast, hebephrenia had an insidious onset and poor long-term prognosis, while undifferentiated schizophrenia occupied an intermediate position.

In the IPSS (WHO, 1979), four alternative groupings of the ICD-9 subtypes were tested by a discriminant function for differences with regard to a composite of six course and outcome measures. Clear discrimination was achieved between simple and hebephrenic schizophrenia on the one hand and the schizoaffective subtype on the other hand. However, the comparison of simple and hebephrenic schizophrenia with paranoid schizophrenia suggested a considerable degree of overlap between the two groups.

Better levels of outcome discrimination have been claimed for groups of patients diagnosed according to the criteria of Leonhard (1957). Stephens and Astrup (1963) reported on 5–13 years of follow-up of 178 patients admitted during 1944–54 with a diagnosis of schizophrenia and rediagnosed retrospectively by the authors as systematic schizophrenia, atypical (unsystematic) schizophrenia, cycloid psychosis or reactive psychosis. The first two rubrics were labelled as 'process', and the latter two as 'non-process' schizophrenia. While 10% of the process schizophrenics were found on a blind outcome assessment to be 'recovered', 41% 'improved' and 49% 'unimproved', the corresponding proportions for the non-process group were 38, 59 and 3%.

The question whether good-prognosis, remitting schizophrenia of an acute onset is a subtype that may have a different symptom profile from the chronic, deteriorating schizophrenic illnesses was addressed in the WHO 10-country study (Jablensky *et al.*, 1992). A comparison between 274 patients with an initial ICD-9 diagnosis of acute schizophrenic episode and 752 patients with diagnoses of other schizophrenia subtypes demonstrated that the acute cases tended to be younger and to show a lower male:female ratio than the rest of the schizophrenic patients. However, the two groups did not differ with respect to symptom profiles on initial assessment, which argues against acute schizophrenia being a discrete syndrome.

Similar conclusions were reached by Vaillant (1978), who reassessed 51 schizophrenic patients remitting after an acute episode in a 4–16-year follow-up. The 20 patients who relapsed in the course of the follow-up and the 31 patients who sustained a remission both tended to have more affective features, a non-schizoid premorbid personality, and more often to be married than a group of 128 non-remitting schizophrenics in the same hospital. However, these were differences of degree rather than of kind, and did not warrant a relabelling of the remitting schizophrenics as a discrete disease entity.

The course and outcome data on schizoaffective disorders do not resolve all the issues relating to their classification but seem to support their current placement within the broad category of schizophrenia. A retrospective and prospective study of 150 schizoaffective patients and 95 bipolar affective patients (Angst *et al.*, 1980) established general similarities between the two groups, but the schizoaffective cases were less likely to achieve a full remission and more likely to develop a residual state (in 57% compared with 24% for the bipolar group). An intermediate outcome between that of schizophrenia and bipolar affective disorder is a common finding (Tsuang & Dempsey, 1979; Maj, 1985; Marneros *et al.*, 1992).

Predictors of course and outcome

The variables which have been identified as predictors of course and outcome in schizophrenia fall into six classes: (i) sociodemographic and family background characteristics; (ii) characteristics of the premorbid personality and preindex functioning; (iii) history of past psychotic episodes and treatments; (iv) characteristics of the onset; (v) characteristics of the initial clinical state; and (vi) mixed findings related to brain morphology, treatment response and habit behaviour. A synopsis of predictors is presented in Table 13.6.

Many of the predictors listed in Table 13.6 have been established independently by different investigators and there is reasonable agreement on the general direction of their effects. However, the methods employed differ in the degree of statistical discrimination (e.g. the capacity to measure the independent contribution of individual predictors) and in the definition and operationalization of both the independent (the predictors) and the dependent variables (the specific aspects of course and outcome).

The explanatory power of the predictors (in terms of outcome variance explained by a set of variables) is likely to vary depending on the setting, sample size, homogeneity of patient groups, number of predictors and dependent variables and measurement error, but generally tends to be low. For example, the set of five best predictors in the IPPS (WHO, 1979) explained 30% of the 2-year outcome variance using step-wise multiple regression analysis. This suggests that background and premorbid characteristics of the individual, as well as the variables describing the early manifestations of disease, are not particularly strong determinants of the outcome of schizophrenic illnesses; emerging events or mid-course changes in the predictor variables may have an equal, or greater, impact on the ultimate outcome. Certain variables have been shown to gain in predictive power if they are assessed during the middle course; in particular, this seems to be the case with the negative symptoms which are better predictors if ascertained 2 or more years after the onset (Biehl *et al.*, 1987; Fenton & McGlashan, 1991b), or when the patients have received adequate treatment (Breier *et al.*, 1991). On the other hand, the prognostic power of predictors such as a high index of expressed emotion (Leff *et al.*, 1990) and the mode of onset (Ciompi, 1984) may become attenuated in the course of time.

Generally, several variables — male sex, single marital status, premorbid social withdrawal, insidious onset and preindex chronicity — emerge as robust predictors of a poor outcome in the short to medium term (2–5 years), while female sex, being married, having social contacts outside the home and acute onset predict a relatively good outcome (Angermeyer *et al.*, 1990; Childers & Harding, 1990; Jablensky *et al.*, 1992). In the short term, the best predictor of relapse is antipsychotic drug withdrawal (Dencker *et al.*, 1986), notwithstanding the predictive validity of stressful life events (Brown & Birley, 1968; Bebbington *et al.*, 1993) and a high-expressed emotion (EE) index (Vaughn *et al.*, 1984).

With the exception of the negative symptoms (when assessed under the conditions referred to above), the initial clinical symptoms of schizophrenia have less predictive power than do the variables listed above.

Recent entries in the list of predictors of poor outcome are: brain imaging findings of cortical atrophy on first admission (Vita *et al.*, 1991) and habitual use of cannabis prior to the first contact (Jablensky *et al.*, 1992). Predictors of good outcome are: good initial response to neuroleptics

Table 13.6 Synopsis of predictors of course and outcome in schizophrenia

Poor outcome	Good outcome
Sociodemographic and family	
*Single, divorced, separated	*Married
Male sex	Female sex
High EE (short term)	Low EE
	Affective disorder in relatives
Premorbid personality and adjustment	
Schizoid personality	*Extrovert or cyclothymic personality
Poor psychosexual adjustment	*Good work, social and sexual adjustment
*Social isolation	Social contacts outside the family
Adjustment problems in adolescence	Precipitating stress or life events pre-onset
Past episodes and treatment	
*Longer duration of preindex illness	*Shorter duration of preindex illness
Mode of onset	
*Insidious	*Acute, associated with excitement, elation, perplexity, anxiety or depression
Initial clinical state	
*Negative symptoms on first admission	Affective features confusion, clouding
Affective blunting	
Primary delusions	Secondary delusions
Bizarre delusions	
Somatic delusions	
Voices from body	
Conversing with voices	
Hearing own thoughts	
Haptic and tactile hallucinations	Soft neurological signs
Social withdrawal	
Other variables	
Abnormal MRI	Good initial response to neuroleptics
Cortical atrophy on CT	
Street drug use (cannabis)	Response to placebo

*, 'Robust' predictors (replicated across multiple studies); EE, expressed emotion; MRI, magnetic resonance imaging; CT, computerized tomography.

(Breier *et al.*, 1991) and a positive response to placebo (Johnstone *et al.*, 1990).

Cultural differences in the course and outcome of schizophrenia

To date, not a single population or culture has been demonstrated to be free of schizophrenia. Although the issue of the real size and importance of the observed differences in incidence and prevalence across populations has not been fully resolved, it is unlikely that sharp contrasts between cultures will be revealed in the overall frequency of the disorder and there is little to support the view that culture plays a primary causative role in schizophrenia.

However, schizophrenia is a complex disorder and most of its characteristic symptoms unfold in layers of the subjective psyche related to the self concept and in behaviours linked to social communication. Seen from this perspective, culture, as the 'ideas, values, habits, and other patterns of behaviour which a human group consciously or unconsciously transmits from one generation to another' (Murphy, 1982), permeates the manifestations of schizophrenia at all levels: the organization of the self, the content and meaning of perceptual and ideational anomalies, the communication of meaning through language and non-verbal behaviour and the response of the social environment to the behavioural expression of schizophrenic phenomena.

A number of clinical studies have highlighted differences in the clinical presentation of schizophrenia in non-industrialized societies when compared with Western settings: a higher frequency of acute excitement, confusion, catatonic features, lability of affect, magic–mystic ideation and anxiety (Lambo, 1965; Pfeiffer, 1976; Wulff, 1976). Physical comorbidity may on occasions be responsible for part of the atypical presentation of the syndrome but the causes of such cross-cultural differences remain essentially unknown.

Systematic studies employing standardized methods of assessment have, on the other hand, underscored more the similarities than the differences in the clinical symptoms of schizophrenia in different cultures (WHO, 1979; Jablensky *et al.*, 1992). Thus, the PSE symptom profiles of patients in developing countries and in developed countries are similar (Fig. 13.1), although some symptoms (e.g. visual hallucinations) tend to be more frequent among patients in developing countries, while others (e.g. primary delusions) are more often diagnosed in patients in the developed countries.

The area in which cultural differences are most accentuated and consistent is that of the course and outcome of schizophrenia. A higher rate of symptomatic recovery (59%) at 5- to 12-year follow-up has been reported in Mauritius as compared with a London rate of 34% (Murphy & Raman, 1971). In Sri Lanka, Waxler (1979) found on a 5-year follow-up that 40% of a cohort of first-admission patients had experienced no further illness episodes and 45% showed no social deterioration.

Extensive evidence that the course and outcome of schizophrenia are more favourable in developing countries than developed countries has been provided by the WHO studies. In both the IPSS (WHO, 1979; Leff *et al.*, 1992) and the 10-country study (Jablensky *et al.*, 1992), a higher proportion of schizophrenic patients in Colombia, India and Nigeria showed recovery or significant improvement than patients with similar initial symptomatology in the developed countries. Data comparing the outcome at 2-year follow-up in these two types of setting are shown in Table 13.7.

The possibility that the observed differences could be explained by a different composition of patient samples, e.g. by a higher percentage of acute schizophreniform illnesses of good prognosis among Third World patients, is practically ruled out by the fact that better outcome in developing countries applies to patients with all types of onset, including the insidious type which generally predicts unfavourable course of the disorder.

The sociocultural setting, i.e. a developing country or a developed country, was the best predictor of 2-year and 5-year outcome in the two WHO studies. Exactly what underlying factors may be responsible for these marked cultural differences in the prognosis of schizophrenia

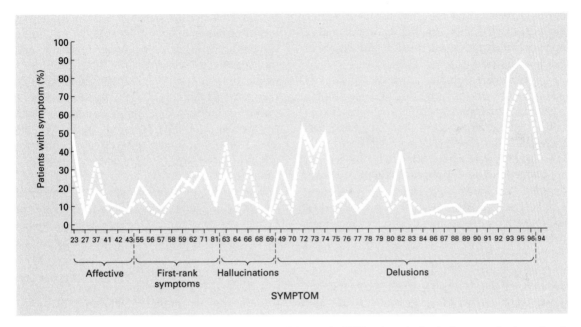

Fig. 13.1 Symptom profiles (44 *Present State Examination* (PSE) items) of 551 patients in developing countries (– – –) and 737 patients in developed countries (———), all meeting 'broad'. (From Jablensky *et al.*, 1992.)

Table 13.7 Two-year pattern of course (percentage of patients) by type of onset and setting (WHO 10-country study)

Setting	Onset	Pattern of course (percentage of patients)		
		Mild	Intermediate	Severe
Developed countries	Acute	52.1	25.1	22.6
	Subacute	41.3	23.9	34.7
	Insidious	29.8	17.5	52.6
	All types	38.9	21.1	39.8
Developing countries	Acute	62.0	21.0	16.9
	Subacute	58.7	23.8	17.4
	Insidious	40.2	16.3	43.4
	All types	55.7	20.2	24.0

remains an unresolved issue. Short-term differences in the relapse rate might be related to the finding that families with high EE scores were rarer in the Indian subsample than in the European centres (Wig *et al.*, 1987). However, the IPSS follow-up demonstrated that in the developing countries the outcome was also better for diagnostic categories other than schizophrenia categories, such as paranoid psychoses and affective disorders. The impact of culture on course and outcome therefore seems to be of a more general nature and may result from the additive effects of beliefs and expectations about mental illness, strong social support networks and a non-stigmatizing sick role in the early stages of psychotic illness.

An interesting question is whether the better outcome of schizophrenia in the developing countries is 'transportable' following migration to other settings. Preliminary data on immigrants treated for first episodes of schizophrenia in the UK suggest that while Asian patients have a considerably lower relapse and readmission rate than British-born whites, Afro-Caribbeans show a higher rate (Birchwood *et al.*, 1992). The marked social and family structure differences which exist between the Asian and Afro-Caribbean immigrant communities suggest that the likelihood of a favourable pattern of course in a new setting depends on the degree to which the immigrant group retains its traditional cultural values and intragroup cohesion.

Associated and risk factors

Several classes of variables have been investigated for clues to the aetiology of schizophrenia, using case-control comparisons: demographic descriptors such as age and gender, patterns of occurrence of the disease in families, premorbid antecedents of the disorder and exposures to specified psychosocial or non-psychosocial factors. The finding of an association may lead to the identification of risk factors increasing the probability of occurrence of the disorder (without necessarily being causally connected). Since the ultimate proof of a causal link is the experiment, the closest approximation to experimental evidence of causality should be the identification of a risk factor modifiable through an intervention that ultimately leads to a reduction of incidence or improvement of outcome.

Gender

Gender has been shown consistently to be significantly related to major aspects of schizophrenia in at least three ways.

First, the mean age at onset is lower in men

than in women. This difference in the timing of onset is claimed to be: (i) robust to the diagnostic system used; (ii) cross-culturally invariant; and (iii) specific to schizophrenia. The recent evidence from a study of 392 first admissions in Germany (Häfner *et al.*, 1991b), from a comparison of German and Danish case register data (Häfner *et al.*, 1991c) and from analysis of two WHO studies in a total of 17 different countries (Hambrecht *et al.*, 1992a,b) is concordant and supports this conclusion.

The timing of points which mark sequential phases of the onset was a special objective of Häfner *et al.* (1991b), and the corresponding mean ages estimated in this study provide a useful reference:

earliest sign of mental disorder — age 24.3 in males and 27.5 in females;
earliest psychotic symptom of schizophrenia — age 26.5 in males and 30.6 in females; and
first admission — age 28.5 in males and 32.4 in females.

There is agreement between the German data and the findings of the WHO 10-country study in which the mean age at onset (pooled data from all research sites) was 25.3 for men and 28.9 for women.

Second, men and women developing schizophrenia show different age–incidence curves. Onsets in men peak steeply in the age group 20–24; thereafter, the rate of inception remains more or less constant at a lower level. In women, a less prominent peak in the age group 20–24 is followed by another increase in incidence in age groups older than 35.

The question whether the total lifetime risks for men and women are about the same, or different, has not been answered definitively. Earlier investigations have reported higher incidence rates for men; today, this is usually the case when the DSM-III definition of schizophrenia is used. A sampling bias apparently is responsible for such differences, considering that the upper age limit for the DSM-III diagnosis is 45 years, that the onset of the disorder is later in women and that schizophrenic women tend to be under-represented in epidemiological samples (Hambrecht *et al.*

1992c). Both the WHO 10-country study and the German study referred to above find approximately equal cumulated risks for the two sexes up to age 54 (Jablensky *et al.*, 1992) or age 59 (Häfner *et al.*, 1993). This is at variance with other studies reporting either a higher lifetime risk (up to age 60) in men (Böök *et al.*, 1978; Hagnell, 1989), or a higher lifetime risk in women (Bojholm & Strömgren, 1989; Helgason & Magnusson, 1989). The latter should be of particular interest since the cohorts of subjects at risk in these two studies were followed up to a very old age (81+ and 85+, respectively). Therefore, the possibility cannot be excluded that the cumulated risk in females is actually higher than in men but this may only be detectable if the follow-up is extended to a very advanced age and both late-onset schizophrenia and late paraphrenia are included.

Third, male–female differences have been described in relation to the premorbid history (better premorbid functioning in women), the occurrence of brain abnormalities (more frequent in men), course (a higher percentage of remitting illness episodes and shorter hospital stays for women) and outcome (higher survival rate in the community, less disability among women) of schizophrenia (WHO, 1979; Lewis, S.W. 1989; Angermeyer *et al.*, 1990; Childers & Harding, 1990; Jablensky *et al.*, 1992). However, notwithstanding claims to the contrary (Castle & Murray, 1991), there is no unequivocal evidence of consistent sex differences in the symptom profiles of schizophrenia (Jablensky *et al.*, 1992), and in particular in the frequency of positive and negative symptoms (Häfner *et al.*, 1993).

While a less disabling course in women could be explained by the later onset and the more sheltered female role in most cultures, the consistent sex difference in the timing of onset, which is specific to schizophrenia, does not seem to be reducible to behavioural factors. A modulating, neuroleptic-like effect of oestradiol on central dopaminergic neurotransmission (Seeman & Lang, 1990; Häfner *et al.*, 1991a), a protective effect of the earlier central nervous system maturation in females (Saugstad, 1989) and a genetic basis (DeLisi, 1992) have all been invoked as

possible factors. A genetic mechanism would be consistent with the view that the age at onset in chronic, heritable disorders is under genetic control. There is some evidence that within sibships concordant for schizophrenia the ages at onset are significantly intercorrelated and the gender difference in the age at onset disappears (DeLisi *et al.*, 1987). Hypothetically, this could arise if, in addition to a general liability to schizophrenia, a specific sex-linked 'protective' gene exists which tends to delay the onset of manifest disorder. Such a gene would be prevented from expression by the random inactivation of the X chromosome in 50% of the females but in none of the males in sibship. The age at onset would then be correlated for all males and for 50% of the females; the effect of the actually delayed onset in the remaining (protected) 50% of the females might be too small to reach significance within a single sibship or in a small number of sibships, but should be detectable across sibships and in large samples.

Age

There is adequate evidence that the risk of inception of schizophrenia extends beyond the arbitrary limit of 45 years set by the DSM-III definition, and also beyond the equally arbitrary age of 54 or 59 which has been adopted in many epidemiological studies. The clinical characteristics of the late forms of schizophrenia have recently been reviewed by Harris and Jeste (1988) and by Castle and Howard (1992). The relevant features include: a predominance of paranoid delusions; evidence of paranoid or schizoid premorbid traits; hallucinations in multiple sensory modalities; a low incidence of formal thought disorder; an increased frequency of hearing loss (up to 25% of the patients) and ocular pathology; a tendency towards chronicity; and poor response to neuroleptics. The familial risk for schizophrenia is lower than in the younger age groups and there is an increased probability of organic cerebral lesions and of a higher ventricle: brain ratio (VBR).

A major effect of the inclusion of late-onset schizophrenia (onset after age 40) and late paraphrenia (onset after age 60) would be the change in the sex ratio in prevalence and first-admission studies (the male:female ratio becomes 1:1.9 after age 40 and 1.4 or even 1.6 after age 60 — Bleuler, 1972; Huber *et al.*, 1979). Although the presenting features of late-onset schizophrenia may in some ways appear as contrasting in respect of schizophrenia of early onset, the current evidence does not provide much support for the idea that schizophrenia is a 'conflation' of two separate disorders, one arising mainly in young males and the other in older females (Castle & Murray, 1991). No real 'point of rarity' can be demonstrated between the symptomatology of late-onset schizophrenia and schizophrenia of an early onset. Rather, each successive developmental stage, including ageing, seems to imprint the presenting clinical symptomatology, resulting in a predominance of nonspecific psychotic symptoms in the age group 15–24, of delusions of reference and affective symptoms in ages 25–34, and of persecutory delusions and negative symptoms in ages 35–59 (Häfner *et al.*, 1993). Still, the nature of late-onset schizophrenia is far from being fully understood and the issue clearly calls for fresh research.

Ethnicity

The possible association between ethnicity and the risk for schizophrenia has recently been brought to attention by reports of exceptionally high (up to 10-fold) first-admission and first-contact rates for schizophrenia in Afro-Caribbeans born in the UK (Harrison *et al.*, 1988; Harvey *et al.*, 1990; Wessely *et al.*, 1991). By and large, diagnostic bias and misclassification have been ruled out as an explanation. If substantiated, such data would provide the first evidence for a population group defined by ethnic origin which differs sharply from all other studied populations with regard to the risk for schizophrenia. The potential interest in such data is strengthened by the finding by Fahy *et al.* (1992) of an excess of births in March 1958 for first-generation Afro-Caribbean patients, which the authors link to the hypothesis of a causal role of the influenza pandemic in autumn 1957 (see Non-psychosocial environ-

mental factors, p. 24). Other suggested explanations include: a lower admission threshold for Afro-Caribbeans; behavioural toxic factors, such as cannabis use, which may precipitate psychosis in predisposed individuals; and a higher neonatal survival rate of low birth weight infants, which is thought to be characteristic of Afro-Caribbeans and could be a risk factor for schizophrenia (Eagles, 1991).

However, the present evidence does not permit a conclusion as to whether a true elevation of schizophrenia risk has been established because of the lack of reliable figures on the size and age structure of the Afro-Caribbean population in the UK (Wessely *et al.*, 1991). If the reported risk elevation is real and not an artefact of a population denominator error, it is more likely to be the result of additive effects of several of the above factors, rather than the operation of a single factor.

Familial and genetic risks

The significant contribution of genetic factors to the aetiology of schizophrenia must be accepted as established. As pointed out by Shields (1977), 'no environmental indicator predicts a raised risk of schizophrenia in small or moderate-sized samples of persons not already known to be genetically related to a schizophrenic'. Heritability estimates range from 66 to 93% and the contribution of all non-genetic factors including cultural transmission is at best around 24% (McGue *et al.*, 1983). However, the nature of the genetic basis of the disorder remains elusive and the question whether such basis is: (i) necessary but not sufficient (i.e. always present but requiring an additional, non-genetic trigger for its expression); (ii) both necessary and sufficient; or (iii) sufficient to cause the disease in a proportion of the cases but not necessary in all cases of schizophrenia, cannot be answered at present.

Genetic linkage studies using high-resolution markers and association studies using cloned candidate genes have so far produced negative or inconclusive results (Owen, 1992) and some of the methodological aspects and underlying assumptions of current research practices have been queried (Weeks *et al.*, 1990). For example, although family segregation studies are not a prerequisite for linkage analysis, they provide information that augments the power of linkage analysis. Family segregation analysis depends on knowledge obtained from family studies. Deficiencies and errors in the epidemiological database may therefore become a bottleneck for genetic research. The major issues of the genetic epidemiology of schizophrenia have been reviewed by Gottesman and Shields (1982) and Gottesman *et al.* (1987).

The estimation of familial risk may be complicated by dilemmas for which epidemiological data are required in order to be resolved. Thus, diagnostic variation predictably affects the risk estimates. Complications arise not only, and not so much, from differences in the degree of inclusiveness of the diagnosis of schizophrenia ('broad' or 'high-yield' vs. 'narrow' or 'low-yield' definitions) but also from the non-hierarchical relationships between alternative diagnostic systems (e.g. a 'narrow' DSM-III diagnosis cannot be said to be 'nested' within the broader ICD-9 concept). In other words, alternative diagnostic systems identify different, only partially overlapping groups of patients. To remedy this, an inclusion/exclusion diagnostic hierarchy has been proposed by a recent workshop on genetic linkage studies (Weeks *et al.*, 1990); in this the DSM-III-R diagnoses of chronic schizophrenia, schizoaffective disorder, paranoid psychosis and other non-affective psychosis and schizotypal personality disorder are arranged along an axis of increasing inclusiveness. However, this scheme leaves the acute remitting schizophrenias (constituting some 15–25% of the total schizophrenia morbidity) and schizophreniform psychosis entirely out of consideration as either inclusions or exclusions, and thus fails to address an important issue in schizophrenia research.

Allowing for diagnostic variation, the risk estimates generated by the different studies appear nonetheless to be similar. They suggest a general pattern of descending risk as the proportions of shared genes between any two individuals decrease. However, such estimates may have to be amended and refined in the light of data indicating

gender differences in the risk for first-degree relatives. Thus, Goldstein *et al.* (1992) found a 5.2% lifetime risk in the relatives (both male and female) of female schizophrenics but only 2.2% in the relatives of male schizophrenics. Furthermore, the present lack of family risk data for non-European populations (i.e. for 75% of the world's population) makes the generalizability of the current estimates uncertain.

The evidence from family studies suggests that both a degree of homotypia and extensive nosological overlap characterize the psychiatric morbidity in families of schizophrenic probands. The complexity of risk segregation in families identified by a schizophrenic proband is illustrated by a study of 269 probands and 1577 first-degree relatives (Scharfetter & Nüsperli, 1980) in which the highest risk for schizophrenia (any subtype) was found in the relatives of probands with schizoaffective psychoses (13.5%) and catatonic schizophrenia (12.8%). The risk for affective disorder (unipolar or bipolar) was also increased: 9.6% in the relatives of schizoaffectives and 4.1% in the relatives of catatonics. However, the most common schizophrenia subtypes in the relatives of schizoaffective probands were catatonia and hebephrenia, and not schizoaffective psychosis. Hebephrenic schizophrenia in this study tended to 'breed true', with 4.7% risk for hebephrenia and zero risk for affective psychosis in the relatives. Use of DSM-III-R diagnoses tends to reduce considerably the estimates of schizophrenia (7.4%) and non-affective psychosis risk (3.7%) in the first-degree relatives of schizophrenics and to increase (24.7%) the estimates for mood disorders (Onstad *et al.*, 1991).

The data also suggest that aetiological (non-allelic) heterogeneity is entirely plausible in the genetics of schizophrenia. One might expect that a random sample of the schizophrenic population will contain a mix of predominantly genetic forms of schizophrenia, forms in which a gene–environment interaction is necessary to produce manifest disease, and cases of a primarily environmental causation. Due to the multiple pathways leading from genotype to phenotype, and from structural brain abnormalities to behavioural expression, these forms may be poorly distinguishable, if at all, at the level of clinical manifestations. To date, attempts to obtain 'pure' phenotypes for genetic analysis have mainly dichotomized the diagnostic category, for example: (i) process/reactive schizophrenia; (ii) paranoid/non-paranoid schizophrenia; (iii) mainly positive/mainly negative symptoms; (iv) type I/type II (Crow, 1985); (v) 'broad'/'narrow'; (vi) nuclear schizophrenia/ schizophrenia spectrum; (vii) remitting/non-remitting schizophrenia; (viii) definite/probable schizophrenia; and (ix) familial/sporadic schizophrenia. Few studies have used the classic Kraepelinian subtypes, presumably because of the small numbers that would result from distributing the sample over multiple categories, or because of doubts about the extent of genetic determination of the clinical subtypes of schizophrenia. The latter problem is illustrated by the case of four identical female twins (the Genain quadruplets), all concordant for schizophrenia but exhibiting different clinical subtypes and patterns of course (Rosenthal, 1963; DeLisi *et al.*, 1984).

Using the dichotomy of familial/sporadic schizophrenia, Reveley *et al.* (1984) and Murray *et al.* (1985) reported a relationship between negative family history and an increased VBR (interpreted as evidence of an early cerebral insult) in the affected cotwin from twin pairs discordant for schizophrenia. Ideally, comparisons between true familial and true sporadic cases should reveal differences that might pinpoint specific non-genetic aetiological factors. However, the feasibility of a familial/sporadic distinction on the basis of occurrence or non-occurrence of secondary cases in the families of schizophrenics has been questioned (Gottesman *et al.*, 1987). It has been pointed out that if a negative family history is restricted to first-degree relatives (as is usual in the majority of the family studies), 81% of the schizophrenics would fall into the sporadic category; if second-degree relatives are counted, the figure would still be around 60%. Assuming that a non-genetic form of the disorder is present in the majority of schizophrenics would clearly contradict the heritability estimates derived from twin data. However, the low frequency of manifest familial schizophrenia would be compatible with

the heritability estimates if an extended phenotype is assumed, including spectrum disorders and specified behavioural traits. In addition, any series of probands with a negative family history for schizophrenia is likely to contain both genetic cases which are 'chance isolates' and true non-genetic cases. Therefore, it would be reasonable to assume that the percentage of non-genetic cases is small (Gottesman *et al.*, 1987). Agreed sampling criteria will then be necessary for distinguishing not so much between 'genetic' familial and 'non-genetic' sporadic cases but rather between cases at high genetic risk and cases at low genetic risk.

A promising but laborious strategy is exemplified by the prospective high-risk (HR) case-control studies in the USA, Denmark and Israel (reviewed by Fish *et al.*, 1992). Between them, these nine studies comprise 230 offspring of schizophrenic parent(s), 248 offspring of parents with other psychiatric disorders and 392 control subjects. The main strength of this research emanates from the prospective design and the multiple repeated measurements at different points since birth. To date, only a minority of the offspring have passed through a significant proportion of the inception risk period; nevertheless, the available data permit certain conclusions. Fish (1977) has proposed an index of 'pandys-maturation' (PDM), defined as a transient retardation of motor and visual development, an abnormal pattern of functional test scores on cross-sectional developmental examinations, and a retardation of skeletal growth, as a marker of a 'neurointegrative defect' and a precursor of schizotypal traits measurable in the first 2 years of life. Seven out of 12 HR subjects, but only one of the 12 controls, all born in 1952, had exhibited PDM, and among the HR/PDM individuals one had developed schizophrenia and four schizo-typal disorder by the time of the last follow-up (compared with none in the control group). A reanalysis of the Israeli data (Fish *et al.*, 1992) produced very similar results. Obstetric complications do not lead to PDM in the absence of genetic risk. PDM can develop *in utero* and in such cases it is associated with low birth weight. The schizophrenic parent effect has been identified as the only 'robust and direct predictor of adult psychiatric outcomes' in another HR study in which 18% of the offspring of schizophrenic parent(s) had developed schizophrenic illnesses after 19 years of follow-up, compared with 7% psychosis in the offspring of parent(s) with affective disorders and 2% in the control group (Erlenmeyer-Kimling *et al.*, 1991).

In summary, the PDM syndrome seems to be a promising candidate for a developmental marker of the genetic liability to schizophrenia since it is: (i) diagnosable in the first year of life; (ii) a predictor of poor motor and cognitive functioning at age 10; (iii) associated with an increased risk for schizophrenia and schizotypal personality disorder; and (iv) relatively specific to the biological offspring of parent(s) with schizophrenia. However, it is not known whether PDM can be diagnosed reliably in larger samples and how frequently it occurs in non-HR subjects. Further research should clarify these issues and explore its potential usefulness as an intermediate phenotype which may be closer to the genotype than clinical schizophrenia.

Early antecedents and premorbid personality

A pattern of schizoid (Kretschmer, 1936) or schizotypal (Meehl, 1962) premorbid traits has been thought to be associated with a predisposition to schizophrenia. In a review of earlier German studies, Cutting (1985) noted that, on average, the schizoid trait complex was described in one-quarter of schizophrenic patients, and other abnormal personality traits (e.g. paranoid) in another one-sixth of the cases. Estimates of the frequency of schizotypal personality disorder among siblings of schizophrenic patients are in the order of 17% (Kendler *et al.*, 1984; Baron *et al.*, 1985), but epidemiological data on its occurrence in the general population are lacking. The discrimination between a schizoid and a schizotypal trait pattern remains a moot point, as is also the existence of subtypes of schizotypal personality disorder (Condray & Steinhauer, 1992).

Principal component analysis of key informant data collected retrospectively at the first-contact interview in the WHO 10-country study (Jablensky *et al.*, 1992) identified five premorbid trait patterns, of which one clearly corresponded to the description of the schizoid personality. Similarly collected data on 73 consecutive admissions diagnosed according to DSM-III as either schizophrenia or affective psychosis (Foerster *et al.*, 1991) indicated that a score on schizoid/schizotypal traits and a score on poor premorbid social adjustment in adolescence distinguished significantly between the two diagnostic groups (but only in men) and predicted an earlier age at first admission. Social underachievement, in the sense of failing to achieve the social status of the father [independently of intelligence quotient (IQ)], characterized the premorbid functioning of DSM-III schizophrenics but not of patients with affective psychoses.

Retrospective data tend to confirm the existence of characteristic personality traits prior to the manifest onset of schizophrenia but do not answer the questions: (i) whether abnormal personality traits occur more frequently in the premorbid history of schizophrenics than in their peers who do not develop the disease; and (ii) whether the schizoid/schizotypal trait complex is a risk factor proper which contributes independently to the onset of the disease, or is a preclinical expression of the dependent variable, i.e. the disease.

A follow-back search for any child guidance clinic records of 54 DSM-III schizophrenic men born in 1954–61 (Ambelas, 1992) revealed that 18 of them had a history of such contacts and that diagnoses of mixed emotional and conduct disorder, developmental (speech, language, reading) problems, peer relationship problems and a lower IQ (obtained at mean age 10 years and 3 months), distinguished significantly the schizophrenics from matched clinic controls. Future schizophrenics were twice as likely as their peers to have been perceived as in need of psychological help at an early age.

The evidence from prospective HR studies points to an increased incidence during childhood (Fish *et al.*, 1992) and adolescence (Dworkin *et al.*, 1991) of behavioural traits related to the schizoid/schizotypal complex in the offspring of schizophrenic parents. More specifically, Dworkin *et al.* (1991) found that poor social competence at age 7−12 years was specific to children at HR for schizophrenia compared with children at HR for affective disorder and normal controls.

A reanalysis of the Copenhagen HR study (Cannon *et al.*, 1990), in which 207 HR subjects and 104 controls were assessed at age 15 and reassessed 10 years later (at which time 15 of the HR subjects had developed schizophrenia), produced risk estimates for the manifestation of negative and positive symptoms. Behavioural traits of passivity and social isolation in adolescence, coupled with weak or absent electrodermal response to a conditioning task administered at age 15, were among the predictors of schizophrenia with predominantly negative symptoms at age 25, while overactive behaviour, aggressiveness, and high electrodermal reactivity predicted positive symptoms in those who eventually developed schizophrenia. While it is tempting to regard these predictors as continuous traits expressing at an early stage the genetic liability for schizophrenia in HR subjects, a possible role of non-genetic factors is suggested in this study by the increased incidence of birth trauma complications and enlarged third ventricle in the negative symptom subgroup and of a history of an unstable rearing environment during the first 5 years of life in the positive symptom subgroup. The Danish data therefore favour an interpretation of the premorbid trait complex in schizophrenia as a product of an interaction between genetic liability and possibly independent, developmental risk factors.

To sum up, there is a convergence of evidence for the occurrence during childhood and adolescence of an unspecified percentage of schizophrenics of a behavioural trait complex contiguous with the description of the schizoid/schizotypal personality and with the negative symptoms of schizophrenia. However, nothing conclusive can be said about the extent to which it is genetically or environmentally determined. In particular, the lack of population data on such traits and personality patterns is an obstacle to evaluating their contribution to the inception risk of schizophrenia (see also Chapter 7).

Psychosocial risk factors

There is a wealth of early research on the relationship between incidence and prevalence of schizophrenia on the one hand, and variables such as social class, occupation, education, urban/rural habitat, migration, unemployment, economic crises and similar adversities on the other hand (reviewed by Mischler & Scotch, 1983; Warner 1985; Jablensky, 1988).

Although the early studies have not been free from methodological flaws, such as reliance on admission statistics, poor control over diagnostic variation and weak operationalization of the key variables, the majority have consistently identified a significant relationship between macrosocial variables and the epidemiology of schizophrenia. However, many such significant relationships have turned out to be non-specific as regards schizophrenia, or to be the consequence of schizophrenic illness rather than its cause. As a result, the paradigm of schizophrenia research in the last decades has shifted away from macrosocial variables. However, it may be unwise to dismiss the potentially important conclusions of earlier research. The possibility that socioeconomic structures and processes are related to the occurrence of schizophrenia in a way we still fail to conceptualize should be retained, but more refined research tools will be needed before the issue is definitively settled.

More narrowly focused research has highlighted several groups of variables which either contribute to the risk of schizophrenia or may confer some protection.

Marital status is a powerful predictor of psychiatric hospitalization. In a statistical analysis based on 168 652 psychiatric admissions in England during 1986, Jarman *et al.* (1992) found that differences in marital status accounted for a major part of the variation in admission rates between health districts. In schizophrenia, marital status is associated with incidence, age at onset, and course and outcome. Single men, and to a lesser degree single women, tend to be overrepresented among first admissions or first contacts (68 and 39%, respectively, in the WHO

10-country study — Jablensky *et al.* 1992). Since both overt schizophrenia and the premorbid impairments associated with it reduce the probability of entering a marital relationship, married schizophrenics may be a positively selected group of milder forms of the disease (Ödegaard, 1946b); alternatively, marriage itself may prevent or delay the onset of schizophrenia.

In the absence of a prospectively conducted, controlled trial, it is difficult to reject either hypothesis solely on the basis of epidemiological age- and sex-incidence data. Riecher-Rossler *et al.* (1992) found a 12-fold higher first-admission rate for single men compared with married men, and a 3.3-times higher rate for single women compared with married women. On the other hand, the male—female difference in age at first admission in their sample decreased to a non-significant level when only single, divorced and widowed subjects were compared. Although the data seemed to suggest a protective effect of the married status, the correlation between age and marital state did not permit them to determine whether late-onset patients are more likely to be married just because they were older, or had the onset of their disorder at a later age because they were married and somehow protected. The issue certainly merits further research.

Migration and minority status have again surfaced as possible risk factors in schizophrenia in the light of the findings outlined above (see Ethnicity p. 234), which suggest an unusually high rate in Afro-Caribbeans in the UK, as well as data on increased morbidity in other immigrant ethnic groups (reviewed by Harrison, 1990). Current interpretations of such findings tend to focus primarily on hypothetical biological factors, such as viral infection and immune response, obstetric complications and foetal survival. Whether factors such as uprooting, refugee status and acculturation stress, which have dramatically increased in frequency, also increase the risk of developing schizophrenia remains to be determined by further research.

At the microsocial level, new data suggesting a possible role of the early rearing environment have emerged from the Copenhagen HR project (see Early antecendents and premorbid personality, p. 237). In contrast to the findings of Cannon *et al.* (1990), another Scandinavian study (Ohlund & Hultman, 1992) found that the electrodermal conditioning non-responders among 44 DSM-III schizophrenic in-patients had experienced significantly more parental loss (43.5% of non-responders compared with 9.5% of non-responders). The effect was particularly marked in females who had a history of early death of the father.

Support for an unspecified effect of the family environment is provided by the Finnish adoptive study (Tienari, 1991) in which extensive interviewing and other assessment procedures are being applied to 179 adopted-away offspring of schizophrenic mothers (pairwise matched with control adoptees), the biological parent(s), and the adoptive and control families. Psychosis or severe personality disorder had developed in 34 out of 121 HR subjects followed up for 5−7 years after the initial assessment, compared with 24 out of 150 controls. In both the HR and control groups the rates of disorder in the offspring were higher in dysfunctional or otherwise disturbed adoptive families than in normally functioning ones; this may be an indication of a modifying effect of the psychosocial environment on the expression of the schizophrenic genotype.

Recent additions to the literature on EE are not discussed here since the evidence does not suggest that its role extends beyond the prediction of psychotic relapse, i.e. a high-EE family environment does not increase the risk of inception of schizophrenia. Aetiological significance has been claimed for the elevated rate of life events during the 6 months preceding the onset of schizophrenia (Bebbington *et al.*, 1993), but similar increases have been found to precede the onset of mania and psychotic depression.

Non-psychosocial environmental factors

During the last decade the focus of the epidemiological search for environmental risk factors in schizophrenia has shifted towards non-psychosocial variables such as noxae and insults affecting brain development. The shift of focus reflects the increasing evidence of structural brain abnormalities in schizophrenic patients; this evidence is being supplied by neuroimaging histopathological studies.

Since the publication of data from one of the early HR studies (Mednick & Schulsinger, 1968) suggesting that obstetric complications (OCs) occur at an increased frequency in schizophrenic women, and that OCs predict developmental abnormalities and psychiatric illness in their offspring, the studies focusing on OCs fall into two groups: those reporting a higher than expected rate of OCs either in child-bearing schizophrenic women or in the perinatal history of schizophrenic patients; and those not finding an excess of OCs. In reviewing critically the evidence, McNiel (1991) stressed the importance of clearly separating: (i) the risk of OCs occurring in pregnant schizophrenic women; and (ii) the possible consequences of OCs, when such have occurred, for individuals at high genetic risk for schizophrenia. The review highlights the many sources of bias to which OC research is vulnerable, as well as the variation in the definitions and criteria of OCs employed by different investigators.

With regard to (i), when bias is taken into account, schizophrenic women do not appear to be at a higher risk of giving birth to low birth weight babies (on the contrary, the newborn may be unusually heavy); there is no excess of perinatal deaths; the rate of fetal distress is very low; and there is no excess of congenital malformations. However, schizophrenic women experience significantly more anxiety and other psychosocial complications during pregnancy; these have been found to be significantly related to the early development and psychosocial adjustment of their offspring at 6 years of age.

With regard to (ii), a recent Scottish study (McCreadie *et al.*, 1992) in which 51 mothers of 54 DSM-III-R schizophrenics and of 114 siblings were interviewed for a history of OCs, added to the negative results by finding no excess of OCs in the history of the patients, compared with their healthy siblings. Both the data from the Copenhagen HR study (Parnas *et al.*, 1982) and

the combined findings of nine other longitudinal HR studies reviewed by Fish *et al.* (1992) suggest that OCs produce an effect only through interaction with an existing genetic risk. If both OCs and HR for schizophrenia are present, the probability of an early developmental disorder with motor and cognitive deficits, as well as the risk of schizophrenia in later life are increased. However, the presence of genetic risk alone is sufficient to result in a schizophrenia spectrum disorder.

It should be pointed out that data on OCs in identical twins discordant for schizophrenia are at variance with the above trend emerging from HR studies. Reveley *et al.* (1984) found a significant excess of ventricle enlargement and history of birth injury in the affected members of twin pairs from families with no history of psychiatric illness (which they interpreted as evidence of a low genetic risk for schizophrenia). The implication of this finding is that OCs are sufficient to produce clinical schizophrenia in the absence of genetic risk, or in the presence of a low level of genetic risk. Such a radical conclusion would require a replication of the data taking into account the methodological difficulties in defining criteria for both negative family history of schizophrenia and OCs (see Familial and genetic risks, p. 234).

The phenomenon of seasonality of schizophrenic births, first described by Tramer (1929), has been the focus of a large number of studies (reviewed by Bradbury & Miller, 1985; Boyd *et al.*, 1986). An excess of schizophrenic births in winter, in both the northern and southern hemispheres, has been reported in the majority of these studies, so that on the strength of such reports birth seasonality might appear as one of the most robust findings in the epidemiology of schizophrenia. However, the evidence for a seasonal factor associated with the risk for schizophrenia has been seriously weakened by the argument that it could be an artefact of the so-called age-incidence and age-prevalence effect (Dalen, 1975; Lewis & Griffin, 1981): since the risk of onset of schizophrenia increases with age (in the younger age groups), individuals born in the early months of each calender year will have a higher rate of schizophrenia than individuals born late in the same year. The presence of an age-incidence effect in season of birth data is further suggested by reports that seasonality is not confined to schizophrenia but is found in depression, neurotic and personality disorders, as well as mental retardation (Häfner *et al.*, 1987). Lewis, M.S. (1989) has shown on at least one large dataset that the magnitude of the age-incidence effect is sufficient to simulate seasonality and has proposed statistical methods to correct for it.

The season of birth issue in schizophrenia has acquired an entirely new dimension following the publication of data indicating a statistically significant excess of schizophrenia (relative risk of 1.87) in Helsinki among individuals who prenatally had been in the second trimester of gestation during the A2 influenza pandemic in 1957 (Mednick *et al.*, 1988). A number of studies attempting to replicate these findings have been published or are in progress. Barr *et al.* (1990) have extended the evidence for a link between influenza epidemics and mean monthly schizophrenia births per 1000 live births to the total population of Denmark, 1911–50. Sham *et al.* (1992) have examined the data on all ICD schizophrenia patients born in England and Wales and admitted to hospital during 1970–79 (*n* = 14830). A generalized linear model took into account the number of births in the general population, the seasonality of births of schizophrenic patients and the number of deaths attributed to influenza in each month and each year of the 22-year period. The influenza factor was found to account, on average, for a 1.4% increase in the number of schizophrenic births per every 1000 influenza deaths in the population during the 2–3 preceding months. This effect was independent of season but the excess schizophrenic morbidity attributable to influenza tended to be highest in those born in April–May. Taking into account the time lag in influenza deaths relative to viral infection, the 'window of susceptibility' to this factor was estimated to be between the third and seventh month of gestation.

In a more general examination of the problem of temporal fluctuations in schizophrenia risk, Kendell and Adams (1991) calculated the year-to-year and month-to-month variation in schizophrenic births between 1914 and 1960 for patients admitted to hospitals in Scotland since 1963 (*n* = 13661). A Poisson distribution fitted to the data indicated significant deviations from the expected chance fluctuations. Time-lagged covariance analysis suggested that: (i) these deviations were linked to the curve of the mean monthly temperatures; and (ii) a time lag of 6 months pointed at the third month of gestation as a critical period for the effect of a temperature-related factor. The effect was almost entirely limited to the months February–May, in which the rates of schizophrenic births increased by 7% for every 1 °C temperature drop from the mean, or decreased by the same percentage for every 1 °C rise of temperature above the mean. While the first part of this relationship is compatible with an increased probability of a viral infection *in utero*, the second is difficult to interpret.

Although the statistical association between influenza epidemics and schizophrenic risk is highly suggestive, direct evidence of a cause-and-effect link has yet to be produced. To date, a study of the children of 945 mothers participating in the National Child Development Study in the UK, who had been in the second trimester of their pregnancies between September and November 1957 and were actually interviewed about viral infection at the time, did not show any excess of schizophrenia cases above the expected rate (Crow & Done, 1992). However, a follow-back study may not be the most appropriate design to test the influenza virus hypothesis and the issue is unlikely to be resolved unless the critical direct evidence is supplied.

Possible fetal vulnerability to maternal starvation during the first trimester and an increased subsequent risk of schizophrenia are suggested by a study of the offspring of Dutch women who had been exposed to wartime famine in 1944–45 (Susser & Lin, 1992). Severe food deprivation (<4200 kJ/day) during the first trimester was associated with an increased relative risk of 2.56 for narrowly defined schizophrenia in the female, but not the male, offspring (it should be noted that the suspected influenza effect referred to above is also slightly stronger in females).

Since the second gestational trimester is a critical period in fetal brain development (Lyon *et al.*, 1989), it is unlikely that the exogeneous factors which may in one way or another disrupt normal cerebral growth and differentiation would be restricted to the influenza virus. It is quite probable, therefore, that other noxae, in addition to starvation, will be added to the list (see also Chapters 12 & 16).

Conclusion: significance of epidemiological data for the evaluation of models of causation in schizophrenia

Models serve to organize large sets of observations into manageable, coherent structures of ideas and hypotheses which allow predictions to be made about the object of study, and usually specify the classes of evidence required for such predictions to be testable. The enormous heterogeneity and complexity of the observations relevant to understanding the nature of schizophrenia clearly calls for simplication and order, and there is no dearth of theoretical models proposed as representations of different facets of the disease: cognitive dysfunction models to deal with clinical symptomatology and with neuropsychological and psychophysiological data; neuroanatomical models to explain observed cerebral structural abnormalities; pharmacological models (e.g. the dopamine hypothesis) to link symptomatology and treatment response to brain structure and function; sociological and learning theory models to handle behavioural manifestations, etc.

Models of causation which depend, among other things, on epidemiological evidence for testing some of their predictions fall into three broad classes: (i) genetic transmission models; (ii) neurodevelopmental models; and (iii) environmental models.

With a few exceptions, the models grouped into these three classes are not mutually exclusive and almost none claim to predict all the conditions that are necessary and sufficient to explain the occurrence of schizophrenia. Some degree of complementarity with other partial models therefore characterizes each current model. For example, a significant genetic input into the aetiology of schizophrenia is assumed by all model types, but different net effects of such input on the observed phenotype are predicted, depending on the weights assigned to the other causal factors involved and the nature of their interaction. The main features of the three classes of models, and the predictions based on them, are outlined below.

Genetic transmission models

These have been summarized by Gottesman *et al.* (1987) as follows.

1 *Distinct heterogeneity model*: schizophrenia is a collection of several separate diseases, each associated with a single major locus (SML) that may be inherited either dominantly or recessively. In addition, there are sporadic, environmentally caused cases. *Predictions*: there should be individual pedigrees in which schizophrenia is transmitted as a dominant, recessive or X-linked trait; any collection of multiplex families is likely to contain different genetic forms of the disease and no common locus of susceptibility will be found; subtypes of schizophrenia, e.g. catatonia or hebephrenia, may be genetically different diseases.

2 *Monogenic model*: all cases of schizophrenia share the same SML but the penetrance of the trait is variable. The disease will always be expressed in homozygous individuals but only in variable proportions in heterozygous individuals. *Predictions*: Mendelian ratios will eventually be found if a sufficient number of pedigrees are analysed with appropriate corrections for mortality, sibship size, etc.

3 *Multifactorial-polygenic model (MFP), with or without a threshold effect*: schizophrenia is the result of a combined effect of multiple genes interacting with a variety of environmental factors, both biological and psychosial. The liability to schizophrenia is linked to one end of the distribution of a continuous trait, and there may be a threshold for the clinical expression of the disease. *Predictions*: there should be a detectable continuous trait capable of producing graded expressions of subclinical or compensated schizophrenia;

the expression of clinical schizophrenia will be a function of a HR combination of common genes; no specific environmental factor associated with the risk of schizophrenia is expected.

4 *A mixed or combined model* which includes the elements of some, or all, of the above three. For example, a two-component model (DeLisi, 1992) postulates.

(a) Multiple genes producing defective neuronal growth factors which result in an early developmental abnormality manifested in a cognitive and language-processing defect.

(b) An SML, possibly X-linked, becoming active in early adulthood and triggering the onset of clinical schizophrenia.

Predictions: heterogeneity and a very large number of genotypes; specific predictions (of expected risks, frequency of multiplex families, etc.) can be generated by computer simulation but the model seems to make no specific exclusions. However, involvement of an X-linked transmission should be testable.

Neurodevelopmental models

The principal assumption is that normal brain development is disrupted in specific ways at critical periods (*in utero* or postnatally) and the resulting lesion produces the symptoms of schizophrenia only through interaction with the normal maturational processes in the brain which occur in late adolescence or early adulthood (Weinberger, 1987). Normal brain ontogenesis may be disrupted by defective genes or environmental insult. A special variety of the neurodevelopmental model postulates that high degrees of homozygosity for a normally distributed brain developmental trait will produce phenotypes liable to increased 'developmental instability' (i.e. random vulnerability to environmental factors during development), manifested, among other things, in abberations from the normal lateralization of cerebral structure and function (Markow, 1992). Since sex dimorphism characterizes brain development and maturation, there will be gender differences in the manifestations of schizophrenia. *Predictions*: somatic, neurological and neurocognitive evi-

dence of developmental atypism ascertainable at an early age and preceding overt psychosis; deviations from the normal brain asymmetry and non-progressive structural lesions; liability to psychotic decompensation in response to everyday stress; period of highest risk in postpubertal age and early adulthood; male sex at greater risk because of longer CNS maturation; in addition to genetic forms of the disease, there will be non-genetic (sporadic) cases occurring at a frequency which varies in time and place, depending on exogeneous noxious factors.

Environmental models

The model of 'evocative influence of complex social demands' (Murphy, 1972) proposes four criteria for schizophrenia-evoking stress: (i) a situation demanding action or decision; (ii) complexity or ambiguity of the information supplied to deal with the task; (iii) unless resolved, the situation demanding action or decision persists; and (iv) the subject has no 'escape route' available. Most of the stresses of this nature will be non-pathogenic; a schizophrenia-evoking effect occurs only in conjunction with a specific genetic liability. *Predictions*: adverse social conditions will modify disease recurrence in families with the genetic predisposition by a factor of 2–2.5 (e.g. if the average risk for children of schizophrenics is 10%, social stress can push it up to about 25%; unusually favourable conditions may depress it to 5%).

Non-psychosocial environmental models (viral infection *in utero*, gluten sensitivity, brain malformations, obstetric complications, etc.) predict that an unspecified number and variety of physical factors will be sufficient to produce the specific cerebral lesions and dysfunctions thought to be characteristic of schizophrenia, regardless of the presence or absence of a genetic susceptibility. A substantial proportion of manifest schizophrenia will consist of phenocopies and 'genocopies' without evidence of familial transmission.

Table 13.8 Synopsis of key findings and conclusions about the epidemiology of schizophrenia

Incidence, prevalence and morbid risk

* No population has been found where schizophrenia is non-existent, or is extremely rare

* At the macro-level: incidence and morbid risk vary within narrow limits (incidence 0.16−0.42 per 1000; morbid risk 0.50−1.60%; ratio highest:lowest risk 4.9 or 2.9 in the WHO studies)

† At the micro-level: pockets of high incidence; small-area variation; non-random clustering of cases

* Non-random temporal fluctuations in the incidence can be detected over longer periods of time

‡ No single major environmental factor accounts for the variations in incidence and morbid risk

† The cumulated lifetime risk is about the same for men and women, or may be slightly higher for women

† The administrative incidence of schizophrenia may have been declining over the past four decades; the observed decline is more marked in women

‡ The mortality of schizophrenics is significantly above the population average; SMR > 2 is a conservative estimate; in some countries mortality has increased to SMR 5−8 in men and 2−5 in women; suicide accounts for most of the excess mortality

‡ The fertility of schizophrenic women and men is below the population average and below the replacement level

† No reproductive advantage has been shown to exist for siblings of schizophrenic patients

Manifestations and course of schizophrenia

‡ Manifest schizophrenia is often preceded by a characteristic premorbid handicap involving cognitive, language and social competence impairments; such dysfunction may be present early in life; the age-incidence of this handicap in preschizophrenics is unknown

* Onset of schizophrenia before puberty is extremely rare; there is no upper limit on the age of onset

‡ The age at onset is significantly lower in men than in women; this finding is specific to schizophrenia

† The age at onset is correlated within sibships

‡ The mode of onset is variable (acute/insidious) and significantly correlated with the pattern of course

† The symptomatology of schizophrenia 'breeds true' but the presenting symptoms show some variation related to the age at onset; there are no significant male−female differences at the level of symptoms

‡ The course of schizophrenia is highly variable; there is support for the 'rule of thumb': 1/3 recovery, 1/3 relapses and remissions, 1/3 chronic deterioration; complete recovery does occur in a minority of cases

† The frequency of relapses and remissions tends to increase over time; social impairment remains stable after the first 2−5 years; ageing brings about significant improvement

† Dichotomies such as paranoid−non-paranoid, systematic−unsystematic or positive−negative symptoms schizophrenia correlate significantly with course; the hebephrenic, paranoid and schizoaffective subtypes differ in overall prognosis

‡ Sex, marital status, mode of onset, premorbid social impairment and preindex chronicity are the best predictors of course and outcome; however, they account for a small proportion of the outcome variance; midcourse events and variables are at least equally important in predicting outcome

* The course and outcome of schizophrenia are significantly better in the developing countries than in Western societies; this effect is not specific to schizophrenia

Risk factors

‡ For any individual, the risk of schizophrenia is correlated with the proportion of genes shared with a person manifesting the disease; the schizophrenia parent effect is the only direct predictor of adult schizophrenia

‡ Familial schizophrenia is rare: 81% of schizophrenics have no affected parents or siblings; 60% of schizophrenics have no affected first- and second-degree relatives

† Familial risk may be higher for female probands with schizophrenia

* Schizoaffective disorder and catatonia show a significantly higher familial recurrence of any form of schizophrenia than do other subtypes

* Hebephrenia is associated with a lower familial risk than other schizophrenia subtypes but shows a high degree of homotypia

Continued

Table 13.8 (*Continued*)

---

‡ Schizophrenia shows a negative association with rheumatoid arthritis

* Schizophrenia is associated with an excess occurrence of minor physical anomalies and soft neurological signs

† Schizophreniform psychosis occurs with a number of rare genetic or idiopathic disorders; the association may be above chance expectancy

† Schizophrenia in the mother is not associated with an increased risk of low birth weight, congenital anomalies or perinatal mortality

† Obstetric complications do not increase the risk of schizophrenia in the absence of genetic risk

† An unstable early rearing environment may increase the risk of schizophrenia in the presence of genetic risk

* The incidence of schizophrenia shows fluctuations which are statistically associated with influenza epidemics and point to a possible maternal infection during the third to seventh gestational month

---

* Findings supported by adequate confirmatory evidence; ‡ 'robust', reliable and replicable findings; † findings in need of further confirmation.
SMR, standard mortality ratio.

The fit between epidemiological data and models

A summary of the main 'facts' that can be abstracted from epidemiological research described in the preceding sections is presented in Table 13.8.

Notwithstanding the complexity of the picture that emerges, and the likelihood that many of the 'facts' will eventually be revised or rejected and new ones added, it is possible to discern certain patterns which are compatible with some, but not with others, among the models outlined above. Viable models should leave room for environmental factors interacting with a genetic predisposition. Such interaction would accommodate practically most of the evidence underlying the neurodevelopmental theory, and 'neurodevelopmental schizophrenia' would be a subset within a more general, mixed model of the disease. However, whether environmental factors are at all necessary to explain the neurodevelopmental component of the disease remains an open question. A scrutiny of the results of studies published to date suggests that no hard, unequivocal evidence for a critical role of either perinatal complications or viral infection *in utero* has been produced, although an environmental contribution to the aetiology of schizophrenia is suggested by all heritability estimates produced up to this point. The role of gene–environment interaction in

schizophrenia is unlikely to be fully understood until the implications of new concepts such as genomic imprinting (Flint, 1992) for the study of the genetic epidemiology of psychiatric illness have been adequately explored.

Acknowledgements

This chapter was written while the author was a Fellow at the Center for Advanced Study in the Behavioral Sciences, Stanford, California. The financial support provided by the Andrew W. Mellon Foundation is gratefully acknowledged.

References

Achte, K.A. & Apo, M. (1967) Schizophrenic patients in 1950–52 and 1957–59: a comparative study. *Psychiatric Quarterly*, **41**, 422–441.

Adelstein, A.M., Downham, D.Y., Stein, Z. & Susser, M.W. (1968) The epidemiology of schizophrenia in an English city. *Social Psychiatry*, **3**, 47–59.

Adler, L.E. & Griffith, J.M. (1991) Concurrent medical illness in the schizophrenic patient. Epidemiology, diagnosis and management. *Schizophrenia Research*, **4**, 91–107.

de Alarcon, J., Seagroatt, V., Sellar, C. & Goldacre, M. (1992) Evidence for decline in schizophrenia (Abstract). *Schizophrenia Research*, **6**, 100–101.

Ambelas, A. (1992) Preschizophrenics: adding to the evidence, sharpening the focus. *British Journal of Psychiatry*, **160**, 401–404.

Anderson, C., Connelly, J., Johnstone, E.C. & Owens, D.G.C. (1991) V. Cause of death. In Johnstone, E.C. (ed.) Disabilities and circumstances of schizophrenic patients — a follow-up study. *British Journal of Psychiatry*, **159** (Suppl. 13), 30–33.

Angermeyer, M.C., Kuhn, L. & Goldstein, J.M. (1990) Gender and the course of schizophrenia: differences in treated outcomes. *Schizophrenia Bulletin*, **16**, 293–308.

Angst, J., Felder, W. & Lohmeyer, B. (1980) Course of schizoaffective psychoses: results of a followup study. *Schizophrenia Bulletin*, **6**, 579–585.

Baldwin, J.A. (1979) Schizophrenia and physical disease. *Psychological Medicine*, **9**, 611–618.

Bamrah, J.S., Freeman, H.L. & Goldberg, D.P. (1991) Epidemiology of schizophrenia in Salford, 1974–84. *British Journal of Psychiatry*, **159**, 802–810.

Baron, M., Gruen, R., Rainer, J.D., Kane, J., Asnis, L. & Lord, L. (1985) A family study of schizophrenic and normal control probands: implications for the spectrum concept of schizophrenia. *American Journal of Psychiatry*, **142**, 447–455.

Barr, C.E., Mednick, S.A. & Munk-Jorgensen, P. (1990) Exposure to influenza epidemics during gestation and adult schizophrenia. *Archives of General Psychiatry*, **47**, 869–874.

Bash, K.W. & Bash-Liechti, J. (1969) Psychiatrische epidemiologie in Iran. In Ehrhard, H.E. (ed.) *Perspektiven der heutigen Psychiatrie*. Gerhards, Frankfurt.

Bebbington, P., Wilkins, S., Jones, P. *et al.* (1993) Life events and psychosis. Initial results from the Camberwell collaborative psychosis study. *British Journal of Psychiatry*, **162**, 72–79.

Biehl, H., Maurer, K., Jung, E., Krumm, B. & Schubart, C. (1987) Zum 'natürlichen Verlauf' schizophrener Erkrankungen — Begriff und Beispiele zum beobachteten Verhalten in einer prospektiven Studie. *Nervenheilkunde*, **6**, 153–163.

Birchwood, M., Cochrane, R., Macmillan, F., Copestake, S., Kucharska, J. & Cariss, M. (1992) The influence of ethnicity and family structure on relapse in first-episode schizophrenia. A comparison of Asian, Afro-Caribbean, and white patients. *British Journal of Psychiatry*, **161**, 783–790.

Bland, H.C. & Orn, H. (1978) 14-year outcome in early schizophrenia. *Acta Psychiatrica Scandinavica*, **58**, 327–338.

Bleuler, E. (1911) *Dementia Praecox oder die Gruppe der Schizophrenien*. Deuticke, Leipzig.

Bleuler, M. (1972) *Die Schizophrenen Geistesstörungen im Lichte Langjährigen Kranken- und Familiengeschichten*. Thieme, Stuttgart.

Bleuler, M., Huber, G., Gross, G. & Schüttler, R. (1976) Der langfristige Verlauf schizophrener Psychosen. *Nervenarzt*, **47**, 477–481.

Bojholm, S. & Strömgren, E. (1989) Prevalence of schizophrenia on the island of Bornholm in 1935 and in 1983. *Acta Psychiatrica Scandinavica*, **79** (Suppl. 348), 157–166.

Böök J.A. (1953) A genetic and neuropsychiatric investigation of a North Swedish population (with special regard to schizophrenia and mental deficiency). *Acta Genetica*, **4**, 1–100.

Böök, J.A., Wetterberg, L. & Modrzewska, K. (1978) Schizophrenia in a North Swedish geographical isolate, 1900–1977: epidemiology, genetics and biochemistry. *Clinical Genetics*, **14**, 373–394.

Boyd, J.H., Pulver, A.E. & Stewart, W. (1986) Season of birth:

schizophrenia and bipolar disorder. *Schizophrenia Bulletin*, **12**, 173–185.

Bradbury, T.N. & Miller, G.A. (1985) Season of birth in schizophrenia: a review of the evidence, methodology and etiology. *Psychological Bulletin*, **98**, 569–594.

Breier, A., Schreiber, J.L., Dyer, J. & Pickar, D. (1991) National Institute of Mental Health longitudinal study of chronic schizophrenia. *Archives of General Psychiatry*, **48**, 239–246.

Bremer, J. (1951) A social–psychiatric investigation of a small community in Northern Norway. *Acta Psychiatrica et Neurologica Scandinavica*, Suppl. **62**.

Brockington, I.F., Kendell, R.E. & Leff, J.P. (1978) Definitions of schizophrenia. Concordance and prediction of outcome. *Psychological Medicine*, **8**, 387–398.

Brown, G.W. & Birley, J.L.T. (1968) Crises and life changes and the onset of schizophrenia. *Journal of Health and Social Behaviour*, **9**, 203–214.

Brugger, C. (1931) Versuch einer Geisteskrankenzählung in Thüringen. *Zeitschrift für dir gesamte Neurologie und Psychiatrie*, **133**, 252–390.

Brugger, C. (1933) Psychiatrische Ergebnisse einer medizinischen, anthropologischen und soziologischen Bevolkerungsuntersuchung. *Zeitschrift für die gesamte Neurologie und Psychiatrie*, **146**, 489–524.

Buck, C., Hobbs, G.E., Simpson, H. & Winokur, J.M. (1975) Fertility of the sibs of schizophrenic patients. *British Journal of Psychiatry*, **127**, 235–239.

Caldwell, C.B. & Gottesman, I.I. (1990) Schizophrenics kill themselves too: a review of risk factors for suicide. *Schizophrenia Bulletin*, **16**, 571–589.

Cannon, T.D., Mednick, S.A. & Parnas, J. (1990) Antecedents of predominantly negative- and predominantly positive-symptom schizophrenia in a high-risk population. *Archives of General Psychiatry*, **47**, 622–632.

Carone, B.J., Harrow, M. & Westermeyer, J.F. (1991) Posthospital course and outcome in schizophrenia. *Archives of General Psychiatry*, **48**, 247–253.

Castle, D. & Howard, R. (1992) What do we know about the aetiology of late-onset schizophrenia? *European Psychiatry*, **7**, 99–108.

Castle, D. & Murray, R.M. (1991) The neurodevelopmental basis of sex differences in schizophrenia. *Psychological Medicine*, **21**, 565–575.

Castle, D., Wessely, S., Der, G. & Murray, R.M. (1991) The incidence of operationally defined schizophrenia in Camberwell, 1965–84. *British Journal of Psychiatry*, **159**, 790–794.

Childers, S.E. & Harding, C.M. (1990) Gender, premorbid social functioning, and long-term outcome in DSM-III schizophrenia. *Schizophrenia Bulletin*, **16**, 309–318.

Ciompi, L. (1984) Is there really a schizophrenia? The long-term course of psychotic phenomena. *British Journal of Psychiatry*, **145**, 636–640.

Ciompi, L. & Muller, C. (1976) *Lebenslauf und Alter der Schizophrenen. Eine katamnestische Langzeitstudie bis ins Senium*. Springer-Verlag, Berlin.

Condray, R. & Steinhauer, S.R. (1992) Schizotypal personality disorder in individuals with and without schizophrenic relatives: similarities and contrasts in neurocognitive and clinical functioning. *Schizophrenia Research*, **7**, 33–41.

Cooper, J.E., Kendell, R.E., Gurland, B.J., Sharpe, L., Copeland, J.R.M. & Simon, R. (1972) *Psychiatric Diagnosis in New York and London*. Oxford University Press, Oxford.

Crocetti, G.J., Lemkau, P.V., Kulcar, Z. & Kesic, B. (1971) Selected aspect of the epidemiology of psychoses in Croatia, Yugoslavia. II. The cluster sample and the results of the pilot survey. *American Journal of Epidemiology*, **94**, 126–134.

Crow, T.J. (1985) The two-syndrome concept: Origins and current status. *Schizophrenia Bulletin*, **11**, 471–486.

Crow, T.J. & Done, D.J. (1992) Prenatal exposure to influenza does not cause schizophrenia. *British Journal of Psychiatry*, **161**, 390–393.

Cutting, J. (1985) *The Psychology of Schizophrenia*. Churchill Livingstone, Edinburgh.

Dalen, P. (1975) *Season of Birth. A Study of Schizophrenia and Other Mental Disorders*. North Holland, Amsterdam.

DeLisi, L.E. (1992) The significance of age of onset for schizophrenia. *Schizophrenia Bulletin*, **18**, 209–215.

DeLisi, L.E., Goldin, L.R., Maxwell, M.E., Kazuba, D.M. & Gershon, E.S. (1987) Clinical features of illness in siblings with schizophrenia or schizoaffective disorder. *Archives of General Psychiatry*, **44**, 891–896.

DeLisi, L.E., Mirsky, A.F., Buchsbaum, M.S. *et al.* (1984) The Genain quadruplets 25 years later: a diagnostic and biochemical follow-up. *Psychiatry Research*, **13**, 59–76.

Dencker, S.J., Malm, U. & Lepp, M. (1986) Schizophrenic relapse after drug withdrawal is predictable. *Acta Psychiatrica Scandinavica*, **73**, 181–185.

Der, G., Gupta, S. & Murray, R.M. (1990) Is schizophrenia disappearing? *Lancet*, **335**, 513–516.

Dohan, F.C. (1966) Cereals and schizophrenia: data and hypothesis. *Acta Psychiatrica Scandinavica*, **42**, 125–152.

Drake, R.E. & Wallach, M.A. (1989) Substance abuse among the chronically mentally ill. *Hospital and Community Psychiatry*, **40**, 1041–1046.

Dube, K.C. & Kumar, N. (1972) An epidemiological study of schizophrenia. *Journal of Biosocial Science*, **4**, 187–195.

Dupont, A., Jensen, O.M., Strömgren, E. & Jablensky, A. (1986) Incidence of cancer in patients diagnosed as schizophrenic in Denmark. In ten Horn, S.H., Giel, R. & Gubinat, W. (eds) *Psychiatric Case Registers in Public Health*. Elsevier, Amsterdam, 229–239.

Dworkin, R.H., Bernstein, G., Kaplansky, L.M. *et al.* (1991) Social competence and positive and negative symptoms: a longitudinal study of children and adolescents at risk for schizophrenia and affective disorder. *American Journal of Psychiatry*, **148**, 1182–1188.

Eagles, J.M. (1991) The relationship between schizophrenia and immigration. Are there alternatives to psychosocial hypotheses? *British Journal of Psychiatry*, **159**, 783–789.

Eagles, J.M. & Whalley, L.J. (1985) Decline in the diagnosis of schizophrenia among first admissions to Scottish mental hospitals from 1969–78. *British Journal of Psychiatry*, **146**, 151–154.

Eagles, J.M., Hunter, D. & McCance, C. (1988) Decline in the diagnosis of schizophrenia among first contacts with psychiatric services in North-East Scotland, 1969–1984. *British Journal of Psychiatry*, **152**, 793–798.

Eaton, J.W. & Weil, R.Y. (1955) *Culture and Mental Disorders*.

The Free Press, Illinois.

Eaton, W.W. (1985) Epidemiology of schizophrenia. *Epidemiologic Reviews*, **7**, 105–126.

Eaton, W.W., Romanoski, A., Anthony, J.C. & Nestadt, G. (1991) Screening for psychosis in the general population with a self-report interview. *Journal of Nervous and Mental Disease*, **179**, 689–693.

Erlenmeyer-Kimling, L. (1978) Fertility of psychotics: demography. In Cancro, R. (ed.) *Annual Review of the Schizophrenic Syndrome*, Vol. 5, pp. 298–333. Brunner/Mazel, New York.

Erlenmeyer-Kimling, L., Rock, D., Squires-Wheeler, E., Roberts, S. & Yang, J. (1991) Early life precursors of psychiatric outcomes in adulthood of subjects at risk for schizophrenia or affective disorders. *Psychiatry Research*, **39**, 239–256.

Essen-Möller, E. (1935) Untersuchungen über die Fruchtbarkeit gewisser Gruppen von Geisteskranken. *Acta Psychiatrica et Neurologica Scandinavica*, Suppl. **8**.

Essen-Möller, E., Larsson, H., Uddenberg, C.E. & White, G. (1956) Individual traits and morbidity in a Swedish rural population. *Acta Psychiatrica et Neurologica Scandinavica*, Suppl. **100**.

Fahy, T.A., Jones, P.B., Sham, P.C. & Murray, R.M. (1992) Schizophrenia in Afro-Caribbeans in the UK following prenatal exposure to the 1957 A2 influenza epidemic (Abstract). *Schizophrenia Research*, **6**, 98–99.

Feighner, J.P., Robins, E., Guze, S.B., Woodruff, R.A., Winokur, G. & Munoz, R. (1972) Diagnostic criteria for use in psychiatric research. *Archives of General Psychiatry*, **26**, 57–63.

Fenton, W.S. & McGlashan, T.H. (1991a) Natural history of schizophrenia subtypes. I. Longitudinal study of paranoid, hebephrenic, and undifferentiated schizophrenia. *Archives of General Psychiatry*, **48**, 969–977.

Fenton, W.S. & McGlashan, T.H. (1991b) Natural history of schizophrenia subtypes. II. Positive and negative symptoms and long-term course. *Archives of General Psychiatry*, **48**, 978–986.

Fish, B. (1977) Neurobiologic antecedents of schizophrenia in children: evidence for an inherited, congenital neurointegrative defect. *Archives of General Psychiatry*, **34**, 1297–1313.

Fish, B., Marcus, J., Hans, S.L., Auerbach, J.G. & Perdue, S. (1992) Infants at risk for schizophrenia: sequelae of a genetic neurointegrative defect. *Archives of General Psychiatry*, **49**, 221–235.

Flint, J. (1992) Implications of genomic imprinting for psychiatric genetics. *Psychological Medicine*, **22**, 5–10.

Foerster, A., Lewis, S.W., Owen, M. & Murray, R. (1991) Premorbid adjustment and personality in psychosis. Effects of sex and diagnosis. *British Journal of Psychiatry*, **158**, 171–176.

Francis, A. & Freeman, H. (1984) Psychiatric abnormality and brain calcification over four generations. *Journal of Nervous and Mental Disease*, **172**, 166–170.

Fremming, K.H. (1947) Sygdomsrisikoen for sindslidelser og andre sjaelelige abnormtilstande den Danske Genneshitbefolkning. Munksgaard, Copenhagen.

Gavrilova, S.I. (1979) Schizophrenic disorders not identified by the dispensary and revealed in a clinical and epidemiological study of advanced age groups in the general population (in Russian). *Zhurnal Nevropatologii i Psikhiatrii*, **79**, 1366–1372.

Goldstein, J.M., Faraone, S.V., Chen, W.J. & Tsuang, M.T. (1992) Gender and the familial risk for schizophrenia. Disentangling confounding factors. *Schizophrenia Research*, **7**, 135–140.

Gottesman, I.I. & Shields, J. (1982) *Schizophrenia. The Epigenetic Puzzle*. Cambridge University Press, Cambridge.

Gottesman, I.I., McGuffin, P. & Farmer, A.E. (1987) Clinical genetics as clues to the 'real' genetics of schizophrenia. *Schizophrenia Bulletin*, **13**, 23–47.

Green, M.F., Satz, P., Gaier, D.J., Ganzell, S. & Kharabi, F. (1989) Minor physical anomalies in schizophrenia. *Schizophrenia Bulletin*, **15**, 91–99.

Gruenberg, E.M. (1974) The epidemiology of schizophrenia. In Arieti, S. (ed.) *American Handbook of Psychiatry*, 2nd edn, Vol. 2, pp. 448–463. Basic Books, New York.

Gulbinat, W., Dupont, A., Jablensky, A. *et al.* (1992) Cancer incidence of schizophrenic patients. Results of linkage studies in three countries. *British Journal of Psychiatry*, **161**, (Suppl. 18), 75–85.

Häfner, H. & Reimann, H. (1970) Spatial distribution of mental disorders in Mannheim, 1965. In Hare, E.H. & Wing, J.K. (eds) *Psychiatric Epidemiology*, pp. 341–354. Oxford University Press, Oxford.

Häfner, H., Behrens, S., De Vry, & Gattaz, W.F. (1991a) Oestradiol enhances the vulnerability threshold for schizophrenia in women by an early effect on dopaminergic neurotransmission. *European Archives of Psychiatry and Clinical Neuroscience*, **241**, 65–68.

Häfner, H., Haas, S., Pfeifer-Kurda, M., Eichhorn, S. & Mitchisuji, S. (1987) Abnormal seasonality of schizophrenic births: a specific finding? *European Archives of Psychiatry and Neurological Sciences*, **236**, 333–342.

Häfner, H., Maurer, K., Löffler, W. & Riecher-Rössler, A. (1991b) Schizophrenie und Lebensalter. *Nervenarzt*, **62**, 536–548.

Häfner, H., Maurer, K., Löffler, W. & Riecher-Rössler, A. (1993) The influence of age and sex on the onset and early course of schizophrenia. *British Journal of Psychiatry*, **162**, 80–86.

Häfner, H., Riecher, A., Maurer, K. *et al.* (1991c) Geschlechtsunterschiede bei schizophrenen Erkrankungen. *Fortschritte der Neurologie und Psychiatrie*, **59**, 343–396.

Hagnell, O. (1966) *A Prospective Study of the Incidence of Mental Disorder*. Svenska Bokforlaget, Lund.

Hagnell, O. (1989) Repeated incidence and prevalence studies of mental disorders in a total population followed during 25 years. The Lundby study, Sweden. *Acta Psychiatrica Scandinavica*, **79** (Suppl. 348), 61–78.

Hambrecht, M., Maurer, K., Häfner, H. & Sartorius, N. (1992a) Transnational stability of gender differences in schizophrenia? *European Archives of Psychiatry and Clinical Neuroscience*, **242**, 6–12.

Hambrecht, M., Maurer, K. & Häfner, H. (1992b) Gender differences in schizophrenia in three cultures. Results of the WHO collaborative study on psychiatric disability. *Social Psychiatry and Psychiatric Epidemiology*, **27**, 117–121.

Hambrecht, M., Maurer, K. & Hafner, H. (1992c) Evidence for a gender bias in epidemiological studies of schizophrenia. *Schizophrenia Research*, **8**, 223–231.

Harding, C.M., Brooks, G.W., Ashikaga, T., Strauss, J.S. & Breier, A. (1987a) The Vermont longitudinal study of persons with severe mental illness. I. Methodology, study sample and overall status 32 years later. *American Journal of Psychiatry*, **144**, 718–726.

Harding, C.M., Brooks, G.W., Ashikaga, T., Strauss, J.S. & Breier, A. (1987b) The Vermont longitudinal study of persons with severe mental illness. II. Long-term outcome of subjects who retrospectively met DSM-III criteria for schizophrenia. *American Journal of Psychiatry*, **144**, 727–735.

Hare, E. (1983) Was insanity on the increase? *British Journal of Psychiatry*, **142**, 439–445.

Harris, A., Linker, I., Norris, V. & Shepherd, M. (1956) Schizophrenia. A prognostic and social study. *British Journal of Social and Preventive Medicine*, **10**, 107–114.

Harris, M.J. & Jeste, D.V. (1988) Late-onset schizophrenia: an overview. *Schizophrenia Bulletin*, **14**, 39–55.

Harrison, G. (1990) Searching for the causes of schizophrenia: the role of migrant studies. *Schizophrenia Bulletin*, **16**, 663–671.

Harrison, G., Cooper, J.E. & Gancarczyk, R. (1991) Changes in the administrative incidence of schizophrenia. *British Journal of Psychiatry*, **159**, 811–816.

Harrison, G., Owens, D., Holton, A., Neilson, D. & Boot, D. (1988) A prospective study of severe mental disorder in Afro-Caribbean patients. *Psychological Medicine*, **18**, 643–657.

Harvey, I., Williams, P., McGuffin, P. & Toone, B.K. (1990) The functional psychoses in Afro-Caribbeans. *British Journal of Psychiatry*, **157**, 515–522.

Haslam, J. (1809) *Observations on Madness and Melancholy*, 2nd edn. Callow, London.

Helgason, L. (1977) Psychiatric services and mental illness in Iceland. *Acta Psychiatrica Scandinavica*, Suppl. 268, 1–140.

Helgason, T. (1964) Epidemiology of mental disorders in Iceland. *Acta Psychiatrica Scandinavica*, Suppl. 173.

Helgason, T. & Magnusson, H. (1989) The first 80 years of life. A psychiatric epidemiological study. *Acta Psychiatrica Scandinavica*, **79** (Suppl. 348), 85–94.

Herrman, H.E., Baldwin, J.A. & Christie, D. (1983) A record-linkage study of mortality and general hospital discharge in patients diagnosed as schizophrenic. *Psychological Medicine*, **13**, 581–593.

Huber, G., Gross, G. & Schuttler, R. (1979) *Schizophrenie. Verlaufs- und Sozial-psychiatrische Langzeituntersuchungen an den 1945 bis 1959 in Bonn Hospitalisierten Schizophrenen Kranken*. Springer-Verlag, Berlin.

Huber, G., Gross, G., Schuttler, R. & Linz, M. (1980) Longitudinal studies of schizophrenic patients. *Schizophrenia Bulletin*, **6**, 592–605.

Huxley, J., Mayr, E., Osmond, H. & Hoffer, A. (1964) Schizophrenia as a genetic morphism. *Nature*, **204**, 220–221.

Israel, R.H. & Johnson, N.A. (1956) Discharge and readmission rates: 4,254 consecutive first admissions of schizophrenia. *American Journal of Psychiatry*, **112**, 903–909.

Jablensky, A. (1986) Epidemiology of schizophrenia: a

European perspective. *Schizophrenia Bulletin*, **12**, 52–73.

Jablensky, A. (1988) Schizophrenia and the environment. In Henderson, A.S. & Burrows, G. (eds) *Handbook of Social Psychiatry*. Elsevier, London, pp. 103–116.

Jablensky, A., Schwarz, R. & Tomov, T. (1980) WHO collaborative study of impairments and disabilities associated with schizophrenic disorders. A preliminary communication. Objectives and methods. *Acta Psychiatrica Scandinavica*, Suppl. 285, 152–163.

Jablensky, A., Hugler, H., von Cranach, M. & Kalinov, K. (1993) Kraepelin revisited: a reassessment and statistical analysis of dementia praecox and manic-depressive insanity in 1908. *Psychological Medicine*, **23**, 843–858.

Jablensky, A., Sartorius, N., Ernberg, G. *et al.* (1992) Schizophrenia: manifestations, incidence and course in different cultures. A World Health organization ten-country study. *Psychological Medicine*, Monograph Suppl. 20. Cambridge University Press, Cambridge.

Jarman, B., Hirsch, S., White, P. & Driscoll, R. (1992) Predicting psychiatric admission rates. *British Medical Journal*, **304**, 1146–1151.

Jaspers, K. (1963) *General Psychopathology*. Manchester University Press, Manchester.

Johnstone, E.C., Macmillan, J.F., Frith, C.D., Benn, D.K. & Crow, T.J. (1990) Further investigation of the predictors of outcome following first schizophrenic episodes. *British Journal of Psychiatry*, **157**, 182–189.

Jonsson, S.A.T. & Jonsson, H. (1992) Outcome in untreated schizophrenia: a search for symptoms and traits with prognostic meaning in patients admitted to a mental hospital in the preneuroleptic era. *Acta Psychiatrica Scandinavica*, **85**, 313–320.

Joyce, P.R. (1987) Changing trends in first admissions and readmissions for mania and schizophrenia in New Zealand, 1974 to 1984. *Australian and New Zealand Journal of Psychiatry*, **21**, 82–86.

Keith, S.J., Regier, D.A. & Rae, D.S. (1991) Schizophrenic disorders. In Robins, L.N. & Regier, D.A. (eds) *Psychiatric Disorders in America. The Epidemiologic Catchment Area Study*, pp. 33–52. The Free Press, New York.

Kendell, R.E. & Adams, W. (1991) Unexplained fluctuations in the risk for schizophrenia by month and year of birth. *British Journal of Psychiatry*, **158**, 758–763.

Kendler, K.S., Masterson, C.C., Ungaro, R. & Davis, K.L. (1984) A family history study of schizophrenia-related personality disorders. *American Journal of Psychiatry*, **141**, 424–427.

Klemperer, J. (1933) Zur Belastungsstatistik der Durchschnittsbevölkerung. Psychosehäufigkeit unter 1000 stichprobemassig ausgelesenen Probanden. *Zeitschrift für die gesamte Neurologie und Psychiatrie*, **146**, 277–316.

Kraepelin, E. (1904) *Psychiatrie*, 7th edn. Barth, Leipzig.

Kraepelin, E. (1919) *Dementia Praecox and Paraphrenia*. Livingstone, Edinburgh.

Kretschmer, E. (1936) *Physique and Character*, 2nd edn. Trubner, New York.

Lambo, T.A. (1965) Schizophrenia and borderline states. In De Reuck, A.V. & Porter, R. (eds) *Transcultural Psychiatry*. CIBA Foundation Symposium. Churchill, London, pp. 62–83.

Larson, C.A. & Nyman, G.E. (1973) Differential fertility in schizophrenia. *Acta Psychiatrica Scandinavica*, **49**, 272–280.

Leff, J., Sartorius, N., Jablensky, A., Korten, A. & Ernberg, G. (1992) The International Pilot Study of Schizophrenia: five-year follow-up findings. *Psychological Medicine*, **22**, 131–145.

Leff, J.P., Wig, N.N., Bedi, H. *et al.* (1990) Relatives' expressed emotion and the course of schizophrenia in Chandigarh: a two-year follow-up of a first-contact sample. *British Journal of Psychiatry*, **156**, 351–356.

Lemkau, P., Tietze, C. & Cooper, M. (1943) A survey of statistical studies on the prevalence and incidence of mental disorder in sample populations. *Public Health Reports*, **58**, 1909–1927.

Leonhard, K. (1957) *Die Aufteilung der Endogenen Psychosen*. Akademie Verlag, Berlin.

Lewis, M.S. (1989) Age incidence and schizophrenia. Part I. The season of birth controversy. Part II. Beyond age incidence. *Schizophrenia Bulletin*, **15**, 59–80.

Lewis, M.S. & Griffin, T. (1981) An explanation for the season of birth effect in schizophrenia and certain other diseases. *Psychological Bulletin*, **89**, 589–596.

Lewis, S.W. (1989) Congenital risk factors for schizophrenia. *Psychological Medicine*, **19**, 5–13.

Lewis, S.W. & Mezey, G.C. (1985) Clinical correlates of septum pellucidum cavities: an unusual association with psychosis. *Psychological Medicine*, **15**, 43–54.

Lewis, S.W., Reveley, A.M., David, A.S. & Ron, M.A. (1988) Agenesis of the corpus callosum and schizophrenia. *Psychological Medicine*, **18**, 341–347.

Lieberman, Y.I. (1974) The problem of incidence of schizophrenia: material from a clinical and epidemiological study (in Russian). *Zhurnal Nevropatologii i Psikhiatrii*, **74**, 1224–1232.

Lin, T.Y., Chu, H.M., Rin, H., Hsu, C., Yeh, E.K. & Chen, C. (1989) Effects of social change on mental disorders in Taiwan: observations based on a 15-year follow-up survey of general populations in three communities. *Acta Psychiatrica Scandinavica*, **79** (Suppl. 348), 11–34.

Lindelius, R. (1970) A study of schizophrenia. A clinical, prognostic and family investigation. *Acta Psychiatrica Scandinavica*, Suppl. **216**.

Link, B. & Dohrenwend, B.P. (1980) Formulation of hypotheses about the ratio of untreated to treated cases in the true prevalence studies of functional psychiatric disorders in adults in the United States. In Dohrenwend, B.P., Dohrenwend, B.S., Gould, M.S., Link, B., Neugebauer, R. & Wunsch-Hitzig, R. (eds) *Mental Illness in the United States: Epidemiologic Estimates*, pp. 133–148. Praeger, New York.

Lohr, J.B. & Flynn, K. (1992) Smoking and schizophrenia. *Schizophrenia Research*, **8**, 93–102.

Lyon, M., Barr, C.E., Cannon, T.D., Mednick, S.A. & Shore, D. (1989) Fetal neural development and schizophrenia. *Schizophrenia Bulletin*, **15**, 149–160.

McCreadie, R.G., Hall, D.J., Berry, I.J., Robertson L.J., Ewing, J.I. & Geals, M.F. (1992) The Nithsdale schizophrenia surveys. X. Obstetric complications, family history and abnormal movements. *British Journal of Psychiatry*, **161**, 799–805.

McGue, M., Gottesman, I.I. & Ras, D.C. (1983) The transmission of schizophrenia under a multi-factorial threshold model. *American Journal of Human Genetics*, 35, 1161–1178.

McNeil, T.F. (1991) Obstetric complications in schizophrenic patients. *Schizophrenia Research*, 5, 89–101.

Maj, M. (1985) Clinical course and outcome of schizoaffective disorders: a three-year follow-up study. *Acta Psychiatrica Scandinavica*, 72, 542–550.

Markow, T.A. (1992) Genetics and developmental stability: an integrative conjecture on aetiology and neurobiology of schizophrenia. *Psychological Medicine*, 22, 295–305.

Marneros, A., Deister, A. & Rohde, A. (1992) Comparison of long-term outcome of schizophrenic, affective and schizoaffective disorders. In Boker, W. & Brenner, H.D. (eds) Onset and course of schizophrenic disorders. *British Journal of Psychiatry*, 161 (Suppl. 18), 44–51.

Mathers, D.C. & Ghodse, A.H. (1992) Cannabis and psychotic illness. *British Journal of Psychiatry*, 161, 648–653.

Mednick, S.A. & Schulsinger, F. (1968) Some premorbid characteristics related to breakdown in children with schizophrenic mothers. In Rosenthal, D. & Kety, S.S. (eds) *The Transmission of Schizophrenia*, pp. 267–291. Pergamon Press, Oxford.

Mednick, S.A., Machon, R.A., Huttunen, M.O. & Bonett, D. (1988) Adult schizophrenia following prenatal exposure to an influenza epidemic. *Archives of General Psychiatry*, 45, 189–192.

Meehl, P.E. (1962) Schizotaxia, schizotypy, schizophrenia. *American Psychologist*, 17, 827–838.

Mischler, E.G. & Scotch, N.A. (1983) Sociocultural factors in the epidemiology of schizophrenia: a review. *Psychiatry*, 26, 315–351.

Mortensen, P.B. (1987) Neuroleptic treatment and other factors modifying cancer risk in schizophrenic patients. *Acta Psychiatrica Scandinavica*, 75, 585–590.

Munk-Jorgensen, P. (1986) Decreasing first-admission rates of schizophrenia among males in Denmark from 1970 to 1984. *Acta Psychiatrica Scandinavica*, 73, 645–650.

Munk-Jorgensen, P. & Mortensen, P.B. (1992) Incidence and other aspects of the epidemiology of schizophrenia in Denmark, 1971–87. *British Journal of Psychiatry*, 161, 489–495.

Murphy, H.B.M. (1972) The schizophrenia-evoking role of complex social demands. In Kaplan, A.R. (ed.) *Genetic Factors in Schizophrenia*. Charles C. Thomas, Springfield, pp. 407–422.

Murphy, H.B.M. (1980) European cultural offshoots in the new world: differences in their mental hospitalization patterns. Part II: German, Dutch and Scandinavian influences. *Archiv für Psychiatrie und Nervenheilkunde*, 228, 161–174.

Murphy, H.B.M. (1982) *Comparative Psychiatry*. Springer-Verlag, Berlin.

Murphy, H.B.M. & Raman, A.C. (1971) The chronicity of schizophrenia in indigenous tropical peoples. Results of a twelve-year follow-up survey in Mauritius. *British Journal of Psychiatry*, 118, 489–497.

Murray, R.M., Lewis, S. & Reveley, A.M. (1985) Towards an aetiological classification of schizophrenia. *Lancet*, I, 583.

Nicole, L., Lesage, A. & Lalonde, P. (1992) Lower incidence and increased male:female ratio in schizophrenia. *British Journal of Psychiatry*, 161, 556–557.

Nielsen, J. (1976) The Samsø project from 1967 to 1974. *Acta Psychiatrica Scandinavica*, 54, 198–222.

Ödegaard, Ö. (1946a) A statistical investigation of the incidence of mental disorder in Norway. *Psychiatric Quarterly*, 20, 381–401.

Ödegaard, Ö. (1946b) Marriage and mental disease: a study in social psychopathology. *Journal of Mental Science*, 92, 35–59.

Ödegaard, Ö. (1952) The incidence of mental diseases as measured by census investigations versus admission statistics. *Psychiatric Quarterly*, 26, 212–218.

Ödegaard, Ö. (1964) Patterns of discharge from Norwegian psychiatric hospitals before and after the introduction of psychotropic drugs. *American Journal of Psychiatry*, 120, 772–778.

Ödegaard, Ö. (1980) Fertility of psychiatric first admissions in Norway, 1936–75. *Acta Psychiatrica Scandinavica*, 62, 212–220.

Ohlund, L.S. & Hultman, C.M. (1992) Early parental death: relation to electrodermal orienting response and gender in schizophrenia. *Schizophrenia Research*, 7, 125–133.

Onstad, S., Skre, I., Edvardsen, J., Torgersen, S. & Kringlen, E. (1991) Mental disorders in first-degree relatives of schizophrenics. *Acta Psychiatrica Scandinavica*, 83, 463–467.

Österberg, E. (1978) Schizophrenia and rheumatic disease. *Acta Psychiatrica Scandinavica*, 58, 339–359.

Owen, M.J. (1992) Will schizophrenia become a graveyard for molecular geneticists? *Psychological Medicine*, 22, 289–293.

Parnas, J., Schulsinger, F., Teasdale, T.W., Schulsinger, H., Feldman, P.M. & Mednick, S.A. (1982) Perinatal complications and clinical outcome within the schizophrenia spectrum. *British Journal of Psychiatry*, 140, 416–420.

Perris, C. (1974) A study of cycloid psychoses. *Acta Psychiatrica Scandinavica*, Suppl. 253.

Pfeiffer, W.M. (1976) Psychiatrische Besonderheiten in Indonesien. In Petrilowitsch, N. (ed.) *Beiträge zur Vergleichenden Psychiatrie*. Karger, Basel, pp. 102–142.

Pinel, P. (1803) *Nosographie Philosophique, ou la Methode de l'Analyse Apliqueé à la Médecine*, 2nd edn, Vol. III. Brosson, Paris.

Propping, P. (1983) Genetic disorders presenting as 'schizophrenia'. Karl Bonhoeffer's early view of the psychosis in the light of medical genetics. *Human Genetics*, 65, 1–10.

Ram, R., Bromet, E.J., Eaton, W.W., Pato, C. & Schwartz, J. (1992) The natural course of schizophrenia: a review of first-admission studies. *Schizophrenia Bulletin*, 18, 185–207.

Raman, A.C. & Murphy, H.B.M. (1972) Failure of traditional prognostic indicators in Afro-Asian psychotics: results of a long-term follow-up survey. *Journal of Nervous and Mental Disorders*, 154, 238–247.

Reid, D.D. (1960) *Epidemiological Methods in the Study of Mental Disorders*. Public Health Papers, No. 2. World Health Organization, Geneva.

Reveley, A.M. & Reveley, M.A. (1983) Aqueduct stenosis

and schizophrenia. *Journal of Neurology, Neurosurgery and Psychiatry*, **46**, 18−22.

Reveley, A.M., Reveley, M.A. & Murray, R.M. (1984) Cerebral ventricular enlargement in nongenetic schizophrenia: a controlled twin study. *British Journal of Psychiatry*, **144**, 89−93.

Riecher-Rössler, A., Fatkenheuer, B., Löffler, W., Maurer, K. & Häfner, H. (1992) Is age of onset in schizophrenia influenced by marital status? *Social Psychiatry and Psychiatric Epidemiology*, **27**, 122−128.

Rimmer, J. & Jacobsen, B. (1976) Differential fertility of adopted schizophrenics and their half-siblings. *Acta Psychiatrica Scandinavica*, **54**, 161−166.

Rin, H. & Lin, T.Y. (1962) Mental illness among Formosan aborigines as compared with the Chinese in Taiwan. *Journal of Mental Science*, **198**, 134−146.

Roberts, J.K.A., Trimble, M.R. & Robertson, M. (1983) Schizophrenic psychosis associated with aqueduct stenosis in adults. *Journal of Neurology, Neurosurgery and Psychiatry*, **46**, 892−898.

Robins, L.N. (1989) Diagnostic grammar and assessment: translating criteria into questions. *Psychological Medicine*, **19**, 57−68.

Robins, L.N. & Regier, D.A. (eds) (1991) *Psychiatric Disorders in America. The Epidemiologic Catchment Area Study.* The Free Press, New York.

Robins, L.N., Helzer, J.E., Croughan, J., Williams, J.B.W. & Spitzer, R.L. (1981) National Institute of Mental Health Diagnostic Interview Schedule: its history, characteristics, and validity. *Archives of General Psychiatry*, **38**, 381−389.

Robins, L.N., Helzer, J.E., Weissman, M.M. *et al.* (1984) Lifetime prevalence of specific psychiatric disorders in three sites. *Archives of General Psychiatry*, **41**, 949−958.

Robins, L.N., Wing, J.K., Wittchen, H.U. *et al.* (1988) The Composite International Diagnostic Interview: an epidemiologic instrument suitable for use in conjunction with different diagnostic systems and in different cultures. *Archives of General Psychiatry*, **45**, 1069−1077.

Rosanoff, A.J. (1914) A statistical study of prognosis in insanity. *Journal of the American Medical Association*, **62**, 3−6.

Rosenthal, D. (ed.) (1963) *The Genain Quadruplets.* Basic Books, New York.

Rotstein, V.G. (1977) Material from a psychiatric survey of sample groups from the adult population in several areas of the USSR (in Russian). *Zhurnal Nevropatologii i Psikhiatrii*, **77**, 569−574.

Rüdin, E. (1916) *Zur Vererbung und Neuentstehung der Dementia praecox.* Springer-Verlag, Berlin.

Rupp, C. & Fletcher, E.K. (1940) A five- to ten-year follow-up study of 641 schizophrenic cases. *American Journal of Psychiatry*, **96**, 877−888.

Salokangas, R.K.R. (1983) Prognostic implications of the sex of schizophrenic patients. *British Journal of Psychiatry*, **142**, 145−151.

Sartorius, N., Jablensky, A., Korten, A., Ernberg, G., Anker, M., Cooper, J.E. & Day, R. (1986) Early manifestations and first-contact incidence of schizophrenia in different cultures. *Psychological Medicine*, **16**, 909−928.

Saugstad, L.F. (1989) Age at puberty and mental illness. Towards a neurodevelopmental aetiology of Kraepelin's endogenous psychoses. *British Journal of Psychiatry*, **155**, 536−544.

Saugstad, L.F. & Ödegaard, Ö. (1979) Mortality in psychiatric hospitals in Norway, 1950−74. *Acta Psychiatrica Scandinavica*, **59**, 431−447.

Scharfetter, C. & Nüsperli, M. (1980) The group of schizophrenias, schizoaffective psychoses, and affective disorders. *Schizophrenia Bulletin*, **6**, 586−591.

Schneier, F.R. & Siris, S.G. (1987) A review of psychoactive substance abuse in schizophrenia: patterns of drug choice. *Journal of Nervous and Mental Diseases*, **175**, 641−652.

Schubart, C., Schwarz, R., Krumm, B. & Biehl, H. (1986) *Schizophrenie und Soziale Anpassung. Eine Prospektive Langsschnittuntersuchung.* Springer-Verlag, Heidelberg.

Scottish Schizophrenia Research Group (1992) The Scottish first episode schizophrenia study. VIII. Five-year follow-up: clinical and psychosocial findings. *British Journal of Psychiatry*, **161**, 496−500.

Seeman, M.V. & Lang, M. (1990) The role of oestrogens in schizophrenia gender differences. *Schizophrenia Bulletin*, **16**, 185−194.

Sham, P.C., O'Callaghan, E., Takei, N., Murray, G.K., Hare, E.H. & Murray, R.M. (1992) Schizophrenia following prenatal exposure to influenza epidemics between 1939 and 1960. *British Journal of Psychiatry*, **160**, 461−466.

Sheldrick, C., Jablensky, A., Sartorius, N. & Shepherd, M. (1977) Schizophrenia succeeded by affective illness: catamnestic study and statistical enquiry. *Psychological Medicine*, **7**, 619−624.

Shepherd, M. (1957) *A Study of the Major Psychoses in an English County.* Oxford University Press, Oxford.

Shepherd, M., Watt, D., Falloon, I. & Smeeton, N. (1989) *The Natural History of Schizophrenia: A Five-Year Follow-up Study of Outcome and Prediction in a Representative Sample of Schizophrenics.* Cambridge University Press, Cambridge.

Shields, J. (1977) High risk for schizophrenia: genetic considerations. *Psychological Medicine*, **7**, 7−10.

Shmaonova, L.M., Lieberman, Y.I., Panicheva, E.V. & Rotstein, V.G. (1976) Family formation in schizophrenic and manic-depressive patients according to data from an epidemiological study − fertility (in Russian). *Zhurnal Nevropatologii i Psikhiatrii*, **76**, 754−759.

Sirota, P., Frydman, M. & Sirota, L. (1990) Schizophrenia and Marfan syndrome. *British Journal of Psychiatry*, **157**, 433−436.

Sjogren, T. (1948) Genetic-statistical and psychiatric investigations of a West Swedish population. *Acta Psychiatrica et Neurologica Scandinavica*, Suppl. **52**.

Stephens, J.H. & Astrup, C. (1963) Prognosis in 'process' and 'non-process' schizophrenia. *American Journal of Psychiatry*, **119**, 945−953.

Stephens, J.H., Astrup, C., Carpenter, W.T., Shaffer, J.W. & Goldberg, J. (1982) A comparison of nine systems to diagnose schizophrenia. *Psychiatry Research*, **6**, 127−143.

Strömgren, E. (1935) Zum Ersatz des Weinbergschen 'abgekurzten Verfahren'. Zugleich ein Beitrag zur Frage der Erblichkeit des Erkrankungsalters bei der Schizophrenie. *Zeitschrift für die gesamte Neurologie und Psychiatrie*, **153**, 784–797.

Strömgren, E. (1938) Beiträge zur psychiatrischen Erblehre, auf Grund von Untersuchungen an einer Inselbevölkerung. *Acta Psychiatrica et Neurologica Scandinavica*, Suppl. **19**.

Susser, E.S. & Lin, S.P. (1992) Schizophrenia after prenatal exposure to the Dutch hunger winter of 1944–1945. *Archives of General Psychiatry*, **49**, 983–988.

Temkov, I., Jablensky, A. & Boyadjieva, M. (1975) Use of reported prevalence data in cross-national comparisons of psychiatric morbidity. *Socialina Psihiatrija* (Zagreb), **3**, 111–117.

Tien, A.Y. & Eaton, W.W. (1992) Psychopathologic precursors and sociodemographic risk factors for the schizophrenia syndrome. *Archives of General Psychiatry*, **49**, 37–46.

Tienari, P. (1991) Interaction between genetic vulnerability and family environment: the Finnish adoptive family study of schizophrenia. *Acta Psychiatrica Scandinavica*, **84**, 460–465.

Torrey, E.F. (1980) *Schizophrenia and Civilization*. Jason Aronson, New York.

Torrey, E.F. (1987) Prevalence studies of schizophrenia. *British Journal of Psychiatry*, **150**, 598–608.

Tramer, M. (1929) Über die biologische Bedeutung des Geburtsmonats, insbesondere für die Psychosenerkrankung. *Schweizer Archiv für Neurologie, Neurochirurgie und Psychiatrie*, **24**, 17–24.

Treffert, D.A. (1978) Marijuana use in schizophrenia: a clear hazard. *American Journal of Psychiatry*, **135**, 1213–1215.

Tsuang, M.T. (1978) Suicide in schizophrenics, manics, depressives and surgical controls: a comparison with general population suicide mortality. *Archives of General Psychiatry*, **35**, 153–155.

Tsuang, M.T. & Dempsey, G.M. (1979) Long-term outcome of major psychoses. II. Schizoaffective disorder compared with schizophrenia, affective disorders, and a surgical control group. *Archives of General Psychiatry*, **36**, 1302–1304.

Vaillant, G.E. (1978) A 10-year followup of remitting schizophrenics. *Schizophrenia Bulletin*, **4**, 78–84.

Vaughn, C.E., Snyder, K.S., Jones, S., Freeman, W.B. & Falloon, I.R.H. (1984) Family factors in schizophrenic relapse: replication in California of British Research on expressed emotion. *Archives of General Psychiatry*, **41**, 1169–1177.

Vita, A., Dieci, M., Giobbio, G.M. *et al.* (1991) CT scan abnormalities and outcome of chronic schizophrenia. *American Journal of Psychiatry*, **148**, 1577–1579.

Walsh, D. (1969) Mental illness in Dublin — first admissions. *British Journal of Psychiatry*, **115**, 449–456.

Warner, R. (1985) *Recovery from Schizophrenia: Psychiatry and Political Economy*. Routledge & Kegan Paul, London.

Waxler, N.E. (1979) Is the outcome for schizophrenia better in non-industrial societies? The case of Sri Lanka. *Journal of Nervous and Mental Diseases*, **167**, 144–158.

Weeke, A. & Strömgren, E. (1978) Fifteen years later: A comparison of patients in Danish psychiatric institutions in 1957, 1962, 1967, and 1972. *Acta Psychiatrica Scandinavica*, **57**, 129–144.

Weeks, D.E., Brzustowicz, L., Squires-Wheeler, E. *et al.* (1990) Report of a workshop on genetic linkage studies in schizophrenia. *Schizophrenia Bulletin*, **16**, 673–686.

Weinberg, W. (1925) *Methoden und Technik der Statistik mit Besonderer Berücksichtigung der Sozialbiologie. Handbuch der Sozialen Hygiene und Gesundheitsfürsorge*, Vol. I. Springer-Verlag, Berlin.

Weinberger, D.R. (1987) Implications of normal brain development for the pathogenesis of schizophrenia. *Archives of General Psychiatry*, **44**, 660–669.

Wessely, S., Castle, D., Der, G. & Murray, R. (1991) Schizophrenia in Afro-Caribbeans. A case-control study. *British Journal of Psychiatry*, **159**, 795–801.

WHO (1973) *Report of the International Pilot Study of Schizophrenia*, Vol. I. World Health Organization, Geneva.

WHO (1979) *Schizophrenia. An International Follow-up Study*. Wiley, Chichester.

Wig, N.N., Menon, D.K. Bedi, H. *et al.* (1987) Expressed emotion and schizophrenia in North India. II. Distribution of expressed emotion components among relatives of schizophrenic patients in Aarhus and Chandigarh. *British Journal of Psychiatry*, **151**, 160–165.

Wing, J.K. (1975) Epidemiology of schizophrenia. In Silverstone, T. & Barraclough, B. (eds) *Contemporary Psychiatry. British Journal of Psychiatry Special Publication*, No. 9, 25–31.

Wing, J.K. & Brown, G.W. (1970) *Institutionalism and Schizophrenia*. Cambridge University Press. Cambridge.

Wing, J.K., Babor, T., Brugha, T. *et al.* (1990) SCAN: Schedules for Clinical Assessment in Neuropsychiatry. *Archives of General Psychiatry*, **47**, 589–593.

Wing, J.K., Cooper, J.E. & Sartorius, N. (1974) *The Measurement and Classification of Psychiatric Symptoms*. Cambridge University Press, Cambridge.

Wulff, E. (1976) Psychiatrischer Bericht aus Vietnam. In Petrilowitsch, N. (ed.) *Beiträge zur Vergleichenden Psychiatrie*. Karger, Basel, pp. 1–84.

Wyatt, R.J., Alexander, R.C., Egan, M.F. & Rirch, D.G. (1988) Schizophrenia, just the facts. What do we know, how well do we know it? *Schizophrenia Research*, **1**, 3–18.

Youssef, H.A., Kinsella, A. & Waddington, J.L. (1991) Evidence of geographical variations in the prevalence of schizophrenia in rural Ireland. *Archives of General Psychiatry*, **48**, 254–258.

P. ASHERSON, R. MANT AND P. McGUFFIN

Introduction

It has been recognized for a long time that schizophrenia runs in families, and there is compelling evidence from family twin and adoption studies that inherited genetic factors are important (McGue & Gottesman, 1991). Such evidence and the enormous rate of progress in molecular methods have together persuaded many that the time has arrived to pursue the molecular basis of schizophrenia. There is consequently a great deal of activity at present, with probably more researchers engaged in genetic studies than at any time in the history of the disorder. However, before discussing molecular genetics, a comparative recent arrival on the scene, it is necessary to review the 'classical' genetic methods of study.

Earlier family studies

The first systematic family study was published by Rudin in 1916, who found that dementia praecox was more common among the siblings of probands than in the general population. Following this, a large study of over 1000 schizophrenic probands was published by Kallman in 1938; this showed that both siblings and offspring had increased rates of the disorder.

These early workers recognized the need for systematically ascertaining index cases or probands for family studies in order to ensure as nearly as possible that the cases were representative of schizophrenia as a whole. In most studies this was achieved by taking consecutive admissions referred to a clinic. They also recognized that in order to make accurate estimates of the lifetime expectancy or morbid risk to various classes of relatives, they had to take account of the age of those being studied and make appropriate corrections. This is important when considering the status of unaffected relatives, some of whom will be too young to have entered the age of risk, while others who are within the age of risk may develop the disorder in the future. Only those who are beyond the age of risk can be unequivocally classified as unaffected. Lifetime expectancy for a particular class of relative can therefore be calculated by dividing the number of affecteds by an age-corrected total. The method most often used is Weinberg's shorter method, the denominator being known as the *Bezugsziffer* (BZ), but more complicated approaches include so-called life-table methods (Slater & Cowie, 1971).

The results of all western European studies from before the current era of operational diagnostic criteria, looking at the frequency of the disorder among various classes of relatives, have been summarized by Gottesman and Shields (Table 14.1). To interpret these data, comparisons must be made with the morbid risk in the general population. This is generally thought to be in the region of 1%. For example, Shields calculated a lifetime risk of 0.86% using the Camberwell register of all known hospital contacts within a borough of London, while Essen-Moller, who personally studied a small rural population in southern Sweden, found a lifetime risk of 1.39% (Gottesman & Shields, 1982).

These studies clearly show that the risk of developing schizophrenia is increased among the relatives of schizophrenic probands, but there are some apparent anomalies. The first is that while the risk to siblings and offspring of schizophrenia is in the order of 10%, the risk to the parent of a schizophrenic is only about 6%. This finding is likely to be explained by reduced fecundity which follows the development of schizophrenia, since illness among parents of index cases occurs mainly in those who developed the disease after they had children. It has been calculated that if this is taken into account the risk among parents would be about 11% (Essen-Moller, 1955). This decrease in reproduction may also account for the finding in some studies that mothers of schizophrenic probands are more likely to be affected than fathers, since women tend to have a later age of onset and tend to become parents at an earlier age than men. The alternative suggestions that affected women either are more 'schizophrenogenic' or pass on a greater genetic liability than affected men are both unlikely, since if we take as our starting point affected parents, the risk among the offspring is no greater for affected women than affected men (Gottesman & Shields, 1982).

Table 14.1 Lifetime expectancy (morbid risk) of schizophrenia in the relatives of schizophrenics. (From Gottesman & Shields, 1982)

Type of relative	Number at risk (BZ)	Lifetime expectancy (%)	r^*
First degree			
Parent	8020.0	5.6	0.30
Siblings	9920.7	10.1	0.48
Siblings with one parent schizophrenic	623.5	16.7	0.57
Children	1577.6	12.9	0.50
Children with both parents schizophrenic	134.0	46.3	0.85
Second degree			
Half siblings	499.5	4.2	0.24
Uncles/aunts	2421.0	2.4	0.14
Nephews/nieces	3965.5	3.0	0.18
Grandchildren	739.5	3.7	0.22
Third degree			
First cousins	1600.5	2.4	0.14

* Correlation in liability assuming general population morbid risk of 1%.
BZ, *Bezugsziffer*.

Recent family studies

Investigators studying the familiality of schizophrenia have more recently used standardized methods of assessment and explicit operationalized diagnostic criteria. They have also been rigorous in their methodology, using appropriate control samples and assessing relatives blind to proband diagnosis. The use of carefully collected control samples has proved to be important since there have been reports of lifetime risks for schizophrenia among first-degree relatives much lower than those found in earlier studies. For example, Kendler *et al.* (1985) reported a lifetime risk of only 3.7% among first-degree relatives using the *Diagnostic and Statistical Manual* DSM-III criteria of schizophrenia. However, this must be compared with a lifetime risk among controls of 0.2%. When other non-affective psychoses and schizoaffective disorder were considered, the lifetime risk in first-degree relatives of schizophrenics increased to 8.6%. Gershon *et al.* (1988) have reviewed the results of family studies using modern diagnostic criteria and found a wide range, from 3.1 to 16.9%, of lifetime risks reported in the first-degree relatives of schizophrenics probands. However, as in the study of Kendler *et al.*, where control samples had been collected there were substantially higher lifetime risks among the relatives of schizophrenics.

The reason for these highly variable results appears to be that different investigators have chosen to use different diagnostic criteria. This problem comes about because while there are numerous explicit diagnostic criteria which can all be reliably assessed, it is not at all clear which of these (if any) is the most valid. As can be seen in the study of Kendler *et al.*, when using DSM-III criteria the breadth of the criteria used to assign an individual as affected has a large impact upon the final result. It has been suggested that to overcome this problem researchers should collect data in such a way that they can apply many different operational criteria to the same dataset (McGuffin, 1991). This 'polydiagnostic' approach would enable researchers in different centres and countries to make direct comparisons between

their results. For this reason this approach has been adopted in Europe and the USA by many groups who are carrying out linkage and association studies of schizophrenia (Leboyer & McGuffin, 1991).

The studies just discussed clearly demonstrate that schizophrenia tends to cluster within families, but do not provide any evidence about the relative contributions of genetic vs. environmental components. To answer the question whether 'nature', 'nurture', or both bring about familial aggregation we have to turn to other 'classical' genetic approaches, twin and adoption studies.

Twin studies

The main strategy in twin studies is to compare the concordance for the disease between members of monozygotic (MZ) twin pairs and members of dizygotic (DZ) twin pairs. Since MZ twins are genetically identical, whereas DZ twins share on average 50% of their genes, greater MZ than DZ concordance will reflect genetic influence, providing both MZ and DZ twins share their environment to approximately the same extent.

Data from five twin studies which ascertained probands systematically from twin registrars are shown in Table 14.2. The results, while based on small samples, are consistent between studies showing MZ concordance rates about 3 times as high as DZ concordance rates. The twin registrars used consisted of national registrars (Fischer, 1971; Tienari, 1971; Kringlen, 1976), a consecutive hospital registrar of twins (Gottesman & Shields, 1972) and a registrar of US military veterans (Pollin *et al.*, 1969). Systematic ascertainment is essential in twin studies to avoid the substantial biases which can occur from selective ascertainment. These biases arise from the preferential selection of the most prominent twin pairs, which are likely to be MZ and corcordant for the disorder. The results are expressed as proband-wise concordance rates, which are calculated by dividing the number of affected cotwins by the total number of cotwins. On statistical grounds this method of calculating concordance rates is preferable to the pair-wise method which

Table 14.2 Studies of schizophrenia in monozygotic (MZ) and dizygotic (DZ) twins. (From Gottesman & Shields, 1982)

Study	Monozygotic			Dizygotic		
	No.	Proband-wise concordance (%)	r^*	No.	Proband-wise concordance (%)	r^*
Tienari (1971)	17	35	0.78	20	13	0.50
Kringlen (1976)	55	45	0.85	90	15	0.56
Fischer (1971)	21	56	0.90	141	27	0.70
Pollin *et al.* (1969)	95	43	0.83	125	9	0.41
Gottesman and Shields (1972)	22			33		
weighted		58	0.91		12	0.48
average		46	0.85		14	0.52

* Correlation in liability assuming morbid risk of 1% in general population.

Note Approximate broad heritability, $h^2 = (r\text{MZ} - r\text{DZ}) = 2 \times (0.85 - 0.52) = 0.66$.

calculates the proportion of affected pairs, since individuals within a twin pair may be ascertained independently as two separate probands. The proband-wise method has the effect of providing an unbiased assessment of morbid risk for each cotwin; this can then be compared with the morbid risk to other relatives and the general population.

As in early family studies, the diagnosis of individuals in these studies was not based upon modern operationalized diagnostic criteria, and they were therefore open to the criticism of diagnostic unreliability. This problem prompted a reassessment of the case material from the twin series studied by Gottesman and Shields (1972), applying operational criteria (McGuffin *et al.*, 1984; Farmer *et al.*, 1987). By using a poly-diagnostic approach these workers were able to compare the effect of different diagnostic criteria in producing the highest estimates of genetic parameters such as the MZ:DZ ratio and heritability (or proportion of variances accounted for by genes). Their results showed that Schneider's first-rank symptoms were excessively restrictive and gave no evidence of genetic determination, while the St Louis criteria (Feighner *et al.*, 1972) and research diagnostic criteria (Spitzer *et al.*, 1978) defined highly 'genetic' forms of the disease. Using DSM-III criteria, the best estimate of heritability was in the order of 80%.

More recently, a study was carried out in Norway using DSM-III-R criteria from the outset (Onstad *et al.*, 1991). The concordance rates found in this study are very close to those found when Farmer applied DSM criteria (Table 14.3). An attempt was also made to define the most genetically determined definition of schizophrenia by both research groups. They considered the effect of varying the definition of affected status on the MZ:DZ ratio by broadening the diagnosis to include other psychotic and affective disorders. Both groups found that including schizoaffective disorder, atypical psychosis and schizotypy gave the greatest difference between MZ and DZ concordance rates, whereas further broadening of the definition to include affective disorders and personality disorders greatly increased the DZ concordance rate, resulting in a lowering of the MZ:DZ ratio. These results are pertinent to the question of how to define the phenotype for genetic analysis, where the ability to define precisely what is being inherited greatly increases the chances of detecting genes. The MZ:DZ ratio is in fact a rather crude way of determining what is inherited, but in keeping with earlier observations of Gottesman and Shields (1972), the results suggest that the 'most genetic' definition is not restricted to tightly defined schizophrenia alone but, on the other hand, is not excessively broad.

Table 14.3 Proband-wise concordance for operationally defined schizophrenia

Reference	Criteria	Monozygotic		Dizygotic	
		No. of probands	Concordance (%)	No. of probands	Concordance (%)
Farmer *et al.* (1987)	DSM-III	21	48	21	10
Onstad *et al.* (1991)	DSM-III-R	31	48	28	4

DSM, *Diagnostic and Statistical Manual.*

Criticisms of twin studies

Twin studies have been criticized for making the assumption that the environments are equal between members of MZ and DZ twins. For example, MZ twins are more likely to dress alike, have similar interests and be treated in the same way than DZ twins. The argument is that the 'micro-environment' of MZ and DZ twins differs, and this could account for the increased concordance rates among MZ pairs. There is no direct evidence for this hypothesis, while on the other hand there is some evidence against if from data on MZ twins reared apart (MZA). Gottesman and Shields (1982) reviewed all systematic twin studies of schizophrenia and found 12 MZA pairs. Seven (58%) were concordant for the disorder, a rate similar to that for MZ twins reared together, suggesting that a shared environment contributed little to the development of the disorder.

An alternative hypothesis is that there are other non-genetic factors which occur more commonly between MZ twins. For example, it has been suggested that birth trauma, where the risk is higher in MZ than DZ twins, may predispose to schizophrenia. However, this is unlikely to account for greater MZ than DZ concordance since there is no evidence that twins in general have a higher risk for schizophrenia than other members of the population (Gottesman & Shields, 1982).

However, there has been continued interest in the relationship between the development of schizophrenia, subtle neurological signs and birth trauma. Twins discordant for schizophrenia have been examined for brain abnormalities using computerized tomography (CT) (Reveley *et al.*, 1982) and magnetic resonance imaging (MRI) (Suddath *et al.*, 1990). These studies show that individuals with schizophrenia have larger cerebral ventricles than do their unaffected cotwins. Other studies have examined series of unrelated schizophrenics and shown that ventricular enlargement is found in at least a proportion of acute-onset first-episode cases (Turner *et al.*, 1986). These observations have led some to propose that where there is evidence of such brain changes, schizophrenia is likely to be the result of intrauterine infection, birth complications or other trauma affecting neurodevelopment. Since it is no longer feasible to reject the view that inherited genetic factors are of major importance in the aetiology of schizophrenia, it has been proposed that there are in effect two separate mechanisms, one predominantly genetic and the other predominantly non-genetic (Murray *et al.*, 1985). If this was the case, we would expect that at least a proportion of those MZ twins discordant for schizophrenia would have the non-genetic form of schizophrenia. However, the evidence from the study of twins does not support this view. Early evidence was provided by Luxenberger (1928), who showed that the relatives of discordant MZ pairs had an equally high risk for schizophrenia as the relatives of concordant twin pairs. Further evidence was provided by Fisher (1971) and this work has been subsequently expanded and updated by

Gottesman and Bertelson (1989). The results are given in Table 14.4 and show that in discordant MZ pairs there is an equally high risk among the offspring of the affected cotwin as among the offspring of the unaffected cotwin. By contrast, discordant DZ twins show a marked difference in the risks of schizophrenia among the offspring.

Although a smaller but similar study by Kringlen and Cramer (1989) produced less clearcut results, the data of Gottesman and Bertelsen strongly argue for two important principles. First, that non-genetic forms of the disorder (phenocopies), if they exist, are relatively uncommon. Second, that genotypes which give susceptibility to schizophrenia may not be expressed. As we shall see later, this is important for linkage analysis where genetic parameters must be estimated.

Adoption studies

Adoption studies are also important in distinguishing inherited from non-inherited factors. Using various strategies, these studies give compelling evidence that schizophrenia has an important genetic component.

The first major adoption study was carried out by Heston (1966). He was able to study the adopted-away offspring of 47 schizophrenic mothers and compare them with an age- and sex-matched group of adopted-away offspring of psychiatrically well mothers. The schizophrenic mothers all gave birth within Oregon State mental hospitals at a time when it was the state law that their offspring must be fostered or adopted within 72 h of birth. At the time of the study the offspring

had all entered the age of risk for schizophrenia and Heston, along with two other psychiatrists, made diagnoses blind to the parental diagnosis. Among the offspring of the 47 schizophrenic mothers, five (10.6%; 16% after age correction) were themselves schizophrenic, compared with none of the offspring of the psychiatrically well mothers.

Rosenthal (1971), using a similar approach, was able to obtain subjects from Danish adoption registrars. This had the advantage over Heston's study that most of the affected parents gave up their children for adoption before their first admissions and about one-third of the affected parents were fathers. This provided safeguards against illness in adoptees being a result of either early contact with an overtly schizophrenic parent, or the intrauterine maternal environment. He thought that a variety of conditions, especially 'borderline schizophrenia' and schizoid or paranoid traits, might be biologically similar to more narrowly defined schizophrenia, and he used the term 'schizophrenia spectrum disorder' (SSD) to describe this group of disorders. The initial report found that three of the offspring of schizophrenic parents developed schizophrenia compared with none of 47 matched controls. When he later extended the study and considered SSD, they found that 13 (18.8%) of 69 adoptees of schizophrenic parents had SSD compared with eight (10.1%) of 79 matched controls.

The same research group was also able to employ a 'cross-fostering' study design (Wender *et al.*, 1974). Here, they considered the rate of SSD among the adopted offspring of affected parents. However, they were able to obtain a sample of 28 individuals whose biological parents were normal but who were adopted by parents one of whom later developed schizophrenia. In this comparison group 10.7% of the offspring were diagnosed as having SSD, a figure very close to that found among the 79 matched controls.

An alternative approach is the 'adoptees family study' design (Kety *et al.*, 1976), where the probands are individuals who were adopted in early life and subsequently developed schizophrenia. A comparison is then made between the rate of

Table 14.4 The offspring of twins discordant for schizophrenia. (From Gottesman & Bertelsen, 1989)

	Monozygotic		Dizogotic	
	Affected	Well	Affected	Well
Morbid risk of schizophrenia in offspring	16.8%	17.4%	17.2%	2.1%

schizophrenia among the biological and adoptive relatives. It was found that 20.3% of 118 biological parents of adopted-away schizophrenics had SSD compared with only 5.8% of 224 adoptive parents of schizophrenics and parents of control adoptees.

More recently, the results of the study by Kety *et al.* have been re-examined using more explicit and stricter criteria (Kendler & Gruenberg, 1984). This reanalysis served to emphasize the genetic relationship by increasing the separation between the different groups studied. Kendler took DSM-III schizophrenia and DSM-III schizotypal personality disorder as the definition of an affected case and found that 13.3% of 105 biological relatives of adopted-away schizophrenics were affected, compared with only 1.3% of the 224 adoptive parents.

The most recent adoption study is currently being carried out in Finland by Tienari (1990). Results so far are in line with previous adoptee studies in showing a lifetime prevalence of 9.4% in the adopted-away offspring of schizophrenic parents and a lifetime prevalence in control adoptees of 1.2%. In addition, this study attempts to measure environmental influences in detail. Interestingly, initial results show a significant association between the genetic predisposition to schizophrenia and psychological abnormalities in the adoptive parents; a result which it could be argued indicates the importance of psychological environmental factors in the aetiology of schizophrenia.

What is the mode of transmission?

It is clear from the preceding discussion that family, twin and adoption studies demonstrate the existence of inherited genetic factors in the aetiology of schizophrenia. However, analyses of families segregating schizophrenia and studies of the risks to various classes of relatives are unable to demonstrate a simple Mendelian mode of transmission. In other words, the pattern of inheritance is complex or irregular and it is not clear whether familial clustering in schizophrenia is due to one gene, a few genes or many genes. Attempts to

define the mode of transmission are important for two main reasons. First, the knowledge of how many genes are involved and the size of their effect determines the approach taken to their eventual isolation. Second, in order to perform linkage analysis the genetic parameters of penetrance and gene frequency must be defined.

Single gene models

In the simplest models single genes are considered to be the sole source of genetic influence resulting in resemblance among relatives. These are termed single major locus (SML) models. If this was the situation in schizophrenia, how can we account for the irregular pattern of transmission observed? One possible explanation is variable expressivity. An example of this is tuberous sclerosis, in which an affected individual may show occult skin lesions that are visible only with a Woods lamp, whereas in others a severe condition with multiple skin tumours and systemic involvement can occur. Likewise, it has been suggested that schizophrenia might be a single-gene dominant disorder with highly variable expression ranging from a 'core' syndrome through milder schizoid traits to a range of minor psychological characteristics among relatives (Heston, 1970). Another possible explanation for irregular transmission of a single-gene disorder is reduced penetrance. Indeed, as discussed above, evidence from the study of discordant MZ twin pairs strongly suggests that this is the case, since the risk in offspring of the unaffected cotwin is as high as that in the offspring of the affected twin (Table 14.4) (Gottesman & Bertelsen, 1989).

Slater (1958) proposed an intermediate gene for schizophrenia with 100% penetrance in homozygotes and 16% penetrance in heterozygotes. This 'intermediate' model, although a poor fit statistically (McGuffin, 1991), in fact turns out to be close to that suggested by the use of more sophisticated computer model fitting (Elston & Campbell, 1970).

However, it has been pointed out by James (1971) that attempts to fit a single gene model to data in pairs of relatives may give misleading results because of mathematical underidentification (i.e. there is not enough information to specify all the parameters which specify the model). This problem can be partly overcome by constraining parameter values to within biologically meaningful limits (i.e. between 0 and 1 for penetrances and gene frequencies). However, on doing this and testing a general SML model on published Western European data, O'Rourke et al. (1982) showed that single gene inheritance provided a mathematically unsatisfactory explanation, and McGue et al. (1985) showed that a SML model could be rejected statistically.

Multifactorial threshold model (MFT)

Under a polygenic or multifactorial liability/threshold model, genetic factors are assumed to be due to the additive effect of many genes at different loci. In other words, several or many genes, each of small effect, combine additively with the effects of non-inherited factors to influence the liability to schizophrenia. Liability to develop the disorder is considered to be a continuously distributed variable in the population, and individuals who develop the disorder are considered to have a liability which lies above a threshold value along that continuum (Falconer, 1965; Gottesman & Shields, 1967).

The MFT model of inheritance can account for the observed risks to different classes of relatives; these appear to decline exponentially as one passes from MZ twins to first-, second- and then third-degree relatives. This is explained by a reduction in the genetic risk due to a shift of the liability curve with successive generations, as the number of shared genes reduces from 1 to 1/2 to 1/4 to 1/8 and so on. There are several other observations which best fit an MFT model. For example, the risk for schizophrenia in an individual increases with the number of affected relatives, and schizophrenia persists in the population despite selective disadvantage conferred by the condition. Finally, if the severity of the condition is equated to the degree of liability for the disorder, this would explain the observation that concordance in twins or first-degree relatives increases with the severity of the disorder in the proband.

Mixed models

What is now referred to as a mixed model (Morton & Macclean, 1974) was first proposed as an explanation for the transmission of schizophrenia by Meehl (1973). He suggested that the expression of a single major gene is modified by interaction or coaction with a number of other genes, each having only a small effect on their own. There have been several studies of the mixed model in schizophrenia (Carter & Chung, 1980; Risch & Baron, 1984; Vogler et al., 1990), where iterative procedures have been used which define the model of 'best fit'. As mentioned above, these tests provide some evidence in favour of MFT over SML models, but they have been inconclusive and while they do not support SML models, they lack the power to differentiate mixed vs. MFT models.

Aetiological heterogeneity

So far it has proven impossible to demonstrate clearly which genetic model is most applicable to schizophrenia. Furthermore, most studies aimed at defining the mode of inheritance consider schizophrenia as a unitary disorder, whereas in reality there may well be genetic heterogeneity, as has now been demonstrated for a number of other common genetic disorders. One of the best examples is Alzheimer's disease, where genes on chromosome 21 (amyloid precursor protein) (Goate et al., 1991) and chromosome 14 (Van Broekhoven et al., 1992) have been detected and may be the main determinants of genetically different forms of the disease in individuals from multiply affected families. Interestingly, the illness differs in these familial Alzheimer's disease cases from that more commonly found by having an earlier age of onset and more rapidly progressive course. Other common disorders, such as non-insulin-dependent diabetes, coronary artery disease and breast cancer, also display this type of heterogeneity with a small proportion of multiply affected families characterized by an early age of onset resulting from a highly penetrant single gene defect.

In schizophrenia there are a number of pedigrees which are highly loaded with affected individuals and have a 'dominant-like' appearance (McGuffin & Owen, 1991). It is entirely possible that in these rare families single genes are the sole or main source of resemblance between relatives. There may of course be more than one mutation at a single genetic locus (allelic heterogeneity), and different pedigrees may segregate completely different disease genes (non-allelic heterogeneity). Furthermore, since single genes are unlikely to account for all cases of schizophrenia, aetiological heterogeneity might exist with different forms resulting from mixed genetic and environmental effects. The observation that affected individuals from multiply affected families show on average an earlier age of onset than among those with schizophrenia among the general population lends some support for the existence of major genes in such families, although this finding is equally compatible with polygenic inheritance (Walsh *et al.*, 1993).

Linkage and association studies

The two main strategies employed to locate disease genes with deoxyribonucleic acid (DNA) markers are positional cloning (linkage analysis) and association studies. To understand these methods it is essential to understand the concept of recombination (Fig. 14.1). Recombination events take place during meiosis (i.e. cell division in gametes resulting in the production of eggs or sperm) when there is crossing over between homologous chromosomes. If two genetic loci are on different chromosomes, the probability that they are inherited together will be 0.5. This phenomenon of independent assortment, as Mendel described it, is also true for two loci far apart on the same chromosome when there is an even chance that they will be separated by crossovers at meiosis. On the other hand, linkage is observed between two loci when they are in such close proximity on the same chromosome that their alleles are separated by crossing over less than half the time.

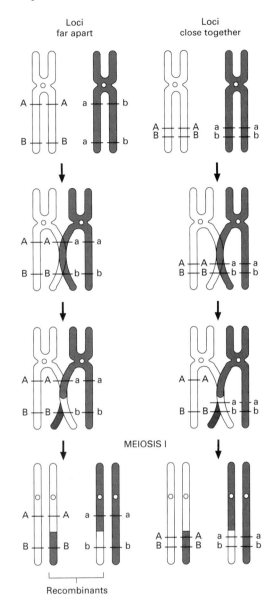

Fig. 14.1 Recombination between homologous chromosomes in meiosis. The left diagram illustrates two loci which are far apart on the same chromosome. These loci have an even chance that they will be separated by crossovers at meiosis. On the right, the two loci are close together so they are less likely to recombine.

In other words, there is a departure from the law of independent assortment (Fig. 14.2).

In linkage analysis the approximate distance

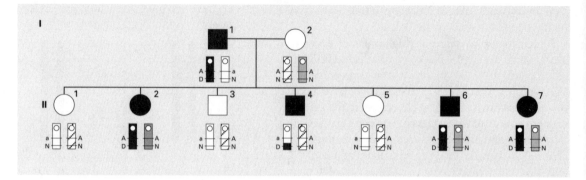

Fig. 14.2 Linkage between a disease gene and marker locus close together on the same chromosome. Allele D is a dominantly inherited disease gene, whereas N is the normal allele at the disease locus. A and a are alternative alleles at a marker locus. Individuals indicated by a solid symbol are affected by the disease. Among three of the four affected offspring the disease gene (D) is inherited with the marker allele A. The three unaffected offspring inherit the normal allele (N) along with the marker allele a. These individuals demonstrate linkage between the two loci. However, individual II-4 is a recombinant since D has been inherited along with a; crossover has occurred between the disease locus and marker locus in the paternal meiosis.

between two linked loci can be estimated by: (i) observing the number of individuals within a sibship where recombination has occurred; and (ii) calculating the recombination fraction (θ), i.e. the number of recombinants divided by the total number within the sibship. Thus, a value of θ equal to 1/2 indicates that there is independent assortment, but where θ is <1/2 the loci are linked. Genetic distance is usually expressed in centimorgans (cM), where 1 cM is equivalent to a 1% chance of recombination between two loci. The most common method of estimating the recombination fraction is to calculate the log of the odds (Lod) scores, as shown below.

$$\text{Lod score} = \log_{10} \frac{(\text{likelihood } (\theta < 0.5))}{(\text{likelihood } (\theta = 0.5))}$$

In practice, the Lod score is plotted for a range of possible values of θ between 0 and 0.5. Where the maximum Lod score is obtained provides the maximum likelihood (or best fit) estimate of θ. By convention, for simple Mendelian traits, a Lod score of 3 or more, corresponding to odds on linkage of 1000:1 or greater, is taken as acceptable evidence that linkage is present.

An alternative approach for detecting linkage is

the study of affected sibling pairs using non-parametric methods (Penrose, 1935; Green & Woodrow, 1977). This approach is much simpler and is based upon the assumption that two siblings both affected with the same disorder will share one or more susceptibility loci. This method compares the distribution of marker alleles inherited by the affected siblings with that expected under random segregation. Unlike the Lod score approach, it is not model dependent and therefore does not require the specification of genetic parameters. However, large samples are required, especially in the face of genetic heterogeneity, and the method cannot estimate the distance between the disease gene and the marker.

In contrast, association studies compare the frequencies of marker alleles in a group of affected individuals and a sample of controls without the disease or drawn from the general population. A statistically significant difference suggests either very tight linkage, resulting in linkage disequilibrium between a marker allele and the disease mutation, or that a marker allele itself confers susceptibility to disease. Linkage disequilibrium refers to the phenomenon when two loci are so close together on a chromosome (1 cM apart or less) that they are not separated by recombination over many generations. Alleles at the two loci will therefore appear to be associated, even in individuals from different families. A recent example of this is the population association between a marker near to the insulin gene and insulin-dependent diabetes mellitus. This finding has led to the identification within the insulin gene of mutations which have a definite role in the aetiology of diabetes.

Linkage studies are more difficult to carry out since they involve the study of multiply affected pedigrees, which are more difficult to collect than the unrelated individuals required for association studies. However, linkage is a powerful technique for locating genes of major effect and a single DNA marker may give information over a large genetic distance. In contrast, association studies are able to identify genes of small effect (Edwards, 1965; Nothen & Fimmers, 1992) if the mutation rates of both the DNA marker and the disease gene are sufficiently low.

DNA markers

Investigators working before DNA markers became readily accessible were restricted to the use of 'classical' genetic markers such as red blood cell antigens (ABO, MNS and rhesus) and the human leukocyte antigens (HLA) (McGuffin, 1991). However, these are limited in number and informativity and are unlikely to lead to the eventual location of disease genes. The revolution in molecular genetics, which has resulted in the localization of a host of disease genes, has followed the discovery of techniques for measuring variation within genomic DNA. Variation is in fact common in genomes and methods have been developed to exploit these differences. At loci where variation occurs there will be two or more different sequences or allelic variants which are inherited in a simple Mendelian fashion and behave as codominant markers. Loci at which two or more of the alleles have frequencies of at least 1% are described as polymorphisms. It is important that marker loci show a high degree of polymorphism, since this increases the chance of there being a different allelic variant on each of the parental

chromosomes (i.e. the parents are heterozygous at the marker locus). Where the parent is homozygous at a marker locus, the cosegregation of that locus and a putative disease locus cannot be examined, so that the meioses are not informative for linkage.

The detection of one class of DNA markers depends on the use of restriction endonucleases (REs), which are enzymes, isolated from bacteria, that cut DNA according to a specific base sequence; for example, one of these enzymes recognizes and cuts only at the sequence:
GAATTC
CTTAAG.

The specific sequences where REs cut are known as restriction sites. Where variation in the base sequence creates or deletes one of these restriction sites, DNA fragments of different lengths are produced; these are known as restriction fragment length polymorphisms (RFLPs). The standard method used to detect RFLPs is known as Southern blotting, named after its inventor E.M. Southern. In this technique, genomic DNA is incubated with the RE. The resulting fragments are then separated according to size on an agarose gel. The DNA is then transferred from the gel to a nylon membrane to produce a long-lasting copy of the DNA fragment pattern. A piece of DNA complimentary to the region of the polymorphism is then labelled with the isotope ^{32}P and used as a probe. The probe binds, or hybridizes, to the fragments on the nylon membrane to produce a pattern of bands on an autoradiogram.

More recently, it has been found that between restriction sites and within non-coding regions of genomic DNA there are multiple repeats of nucleotide sequences. The number of repeats of the core sequence can be highly variable and they are inherited in a Mendelian fashion. Some of these sequences are located only at one locus on a pair of homologous chromosomes — the so-called variable number of tandem repeats (VNTR). Most of these VNTR markers are located in the sub-telomeric region of the chromosome, so limiting their usefulness in mapping studies.

A subset of VNTR markers, consisting of 1−4

base pair (bp) repeat units, are now probably the most useful tool to genetic mappers, as they appear to be widely distributed throughout the human genome. These units are known as microsatellite DNA or simple sequence repeat (SSR) polymorphisms. These tandem repeats of di-, tri- or tetranucleotides often show length polymorphism. Generally, the longer the run of perfect repeat units the more polymorphic the marker, and sequences with 12 or fewer repeats are usually not polymorphic. On average, one microsatellite greater than 19 bp in length is found every 6000 bp (6 kb).

The most common of these repeat units is the AC repeat, one of which occurs approximately every 30 kb (Weber & May, 1989). All SSRs can be analysed relatively easily by amplifying a small segment of DNA which contains the repeat unit and a little sequence on either side. This is only possible using the polymerase chain reaction (PCR), a relatively recent innovation which has revolutionized molecular biology (Mullis & Faloona, 1987). In this technique, the starting material is total genomic DNA, which can be extracted easily from whole blood. Two primers are made; these are small stretches of about 20 DNA bases, complementary to sequences flanking the region to be amplified. The total DNA is heated and then cooled; this first separates the usually double-stranded DNA into single strands and then allows the primers to bind onto their complementary flanking sites. By adding a mixture of precursors for the four DNA bases (deoxynucleotides) and a heat-resistant polymerase (usually Taq polymerase), a new strand of DNA is synthesized between the two primers. The process is then repeated many times over, each step doubling the number of double-stranded target molecules, so that a rapid amplification of the target region is achieved. The amplified fragments can then be separated on a gel by electrophoresis so that different length fragments can be identified. The benefits of this method are that very small amounts of DNA are needed initially, and it results in the amplification of specified regions. In addition, the method is relatively easy, rapid and can be automated.

It has been calculated that the number of polymorphic AC repeat sequences in the human genome will number around 12 000. Assuming a total genetic length of 3300 cM, these markers would yield genetic maps with average resolution of approximately 0.3–0.5 cM (White & Lalouel, 1988).

Problems in linkage analysis

The current emphasis on linkage analysis in schizophrenia research assumes that genes of major effect exist in at least some families. However, as we have already described, we cannot be certain of this and even if major genes contribute to liability in schizophrenia in some multiply affected families, it seems likely that the commonest mode of transmission is either polygenic or oligogenic. In addition, to carry out linkage analysis, penetrance values and the frequency of the disease gene must be specified. Failure to specify these accurately reduces the power to detect linkage and leads to false-negative findings (Clerget-Darpoux, 1986; Ott, 1991). There are also the uncertainties, as discussed earlier, concerning aetiological heterogeneity. Interpretation of positive Lod scores under these circumstances is in fact very difficult (Ott, 1991), and as we shall see even seemingly very high Lod scores found in a schizophrenia linkage study have turned out to be false-positive results. On the other hand, it is equally difficult to interpret negative results, which can only exclude regions of the genome assuming specific genetic models.

These problems may at first sight seem to preclude the successful application of linkage analysis to schizophrenia. However, we have also seen that this disorder can occur in large pedigrees with multiple affected members, and these may be segregating single disease genes with more regular modes of transmission. These loaded families are atypical, and the resulting Mendelian appearance can be misleading (Sturt & McGuffin, 1985), but no bias with respect to the detection of linkage should be introduced (Ott, 1991).

Broadly, there are two approaches to searching for major genes conferring liability to schizophrenia. The first is to try to focus on a specific region or locus which appears promising. Several clues, such as cytogenetic abnormalities or other genetic disorders co-occurring with schizophrenia, as well as targeting genes which are a priori good candidates (i.e. search for proteins which might plausibly be involved in aetiology), have been followed up by investigators, and these will be described later. However, the issue of whether or not major genes for schizophrenia exist within these families may only be resolved following a second approach, which is to perform a systematic screening of the entire genome in a large sample of multiply affected families. To this end, many groups throughout Europe have come together under the auspices of the European Scientific Foundation (ESF) and a programme to complete this work by 1996 is under way (Leboyer & McGuffin, 1991). A similar collaboration is in progress in the USA, supported by the National Institute of Mental Health (NIMH).

Since the genome spans a genetic distance of approximately 3000 cM and each DNA marker should be informative for 10 cM either side of itself, it is planned to use a total of 300 markers evenly spaced throughout the genome. This is an enormous undertaking, which until very recently might have been viewed by many as unrealistic. However, the recent publication of a map of highly informative SSR markers throughout the genome and the use of automated PCR technology now makes this entirely possible (Weissenbach et al., 1992).

Linkage studies in schizophrenia

Early linkage studies before DNA markers became available used classical markers. Studies with HLA showed promise when a maximum Lod score of 2.57 was obtained at a recombination fraction of 0.15 between a broadly defined phenotype 'schizotaxia' (similar to Kety's SSD) and HLA (Turner, 1979). The analysis assumed an autosomal dominant mode of transmission. These findings were not, however, replicated by a further four linkage studies and a 'model-free' sibpair analysis which showed substantial evidence against

linkage. Studies with other classical markers have not provided evidence of linkage. Taken together, the exclusion of linkage to these markers has ruled out about 6% of the genome (see McGuffin & Sturt, 1986; Owen & McGuffin, 1991).

The segregation of a chromosomal abnormality, such as a translocation or deletion with the disorder, may provide clues to the localization of disease genes. This is because the altered segment of chromosome may contain the disease gene, which is itself disrupted, or because the disease gene is nearby and in linkage with the chromosomal lesion.

In 1988, Bassett et al. reported a Canadian family of oriental origin in which a young man who was schizophrenic and his schizophrenic uncle both had a partial trisomy of the long (q) arm of chromosome 5 due to an unbalanced translocation. This report stimulated a great deal of interest in this region of the genome, and genetic markers were used to map the area of the trisomy in other multiply affected pedigrees. The first study of this region published by Sherrington et al. (1988) resulted in much excitement after positive Lod scores were obtained with two genetic markers in their data set of five Icelandic and two British pedigrees. Lod scores of 2.45 were obtained when cases of schizophrenia alone were defined as affected, 4.33 when the phenotype was broadened to include mild schizophrenic-like syndromes and 6.49 when other psychiatric diagnoses (major and minor affective disorders, phobic disorder and alcoholism) were included. These results appeared to provide strong evidence for a dominant gene giving susceptibility to schizophrenia located on chromosome 5.

However, in the same edition of the journal another study was reported which gave evidence against such a locus being located within this region in a large Swedish pedigree (Kennedy et al., 1988). This study looked at eight markers along chromosome 5, and effectively excluded the trisomy region as a possible location for a major susceptibility locus in the pedigrees studied. Initial optimism was given a further dent when several subsequent studies were also unable to detect linkage between schizophrenia and DNA markers in this region (Detera-Wadleigh *et al.*, 1989; St Clair *et al.*, 1989; McGuffin *et al.*, 1990).

These conflicting results require some explanation and could have occurred by several means. Initially, it was suggested by many that linkage had been detected in the initial set of pedigrees studied and that subsequent failure to replicate this finding was due to non-allelic heterogeneity (Lander, 1988). In other words, it was proposed that a gene on 5q was acting in only a subset of all the families studied, so that many families showed no evidence of linkage to this locus. However, this conclusion was considered unlikely following a meta-analysis of world data which employed a test of heterogeneity but failed to find any evidence that a subset of 5q-linked families existed (McGuffin *et al.*, 1990). In this test, the evidence for linkage, assuming that the locus is linked in all families (linkage under homogeneity), is compared with the evidence for linkage assuming that only a proportion of the families are linked (linkage under heterogeneity). This study showed that the only families giving any evidence of linkage came from the initial 'positive' study and suggested that the very high Lod scores obtained must have arisen from some source of error. This is indeed likely since follow-up and reanalysis of the original 'linked' pedigrees, using more informative markers, has confirmed that the original results were falsely positive (Mankoo *et al.*, 1991).

Errors can be easily introduced by mistyping individuals, transferring incorrect genotype data onto computer files and a lack of strict blindness between investigators carrying out marker analysis and those making clinical diagnosis. As discussed above, there are many other problems which beset the study of complex disorders; these include unknown mode of inheritance, late age of onset and variable expressivity and uncertainties in diagnosis. To overcome these problems multiple tests using a range of parameters are often employed. In the study of Sherrington *et al.* this process may have acted to falsely inflate the Lod score, although it has been suggested that this alone could not have generated Lod scores of the size observed (McGuffin *et al.*, 1990; Ott, personal communication).

A further region where chromosomal abnormalities and other clues have initiated a number of linkage studies has been the long arm of chromosome 11 (11q). There are three independent reports of families in which psychotic illness is segregating with a balanced translocation of 11q (Smith *et al.*, 1989; Holland & Gosden, 1990; St Clair *et al.*, 1990). The D_2 dopamine receptor gene, a potentially strong candidate, maps close to this region (Grandy *et al.*, 1989). Baron (1976) reported a family in which schizophreniform psychosis is segregating with tyrosinase negative oculocutaneous albinism, which itself maps to 11q14−q21 (Barton *et al.*, 1988). In addition, the gene for porphobilinogen deaminase (PBGD), which gives rise to porphyria, is located on 11q23−qter (Wang *et al.*, 1981). This is of interest since patients with acute intermittent porphyria may present with psychotic symptoms, and allelic association between schizophrenia and one of the alleles of the *MspI* polymorphism at this locus was reported (Sanders *et al.*, 1991).

Unfortunately, despite the obvious interest in 11q there have been a number of negative linkage reports and no positive findings. Moises *et al.* (1991) studied a single large Swedish pedigree, which on its own is able to generate significant evidence of linkage, with markers close to the D_2 receptor gene; they obtained evidence to exclude linkage. A further large collaborative study examined a set of 24 pedigrees from Wales, London and Japan, using highly polymorphic markers covering the entire long arm of chromosome 11 at approximately 10 cM. These studies found no evidence of linkage and were able to exclude much of the region with a wide range of genetic parameters (Gill *et al.*, 1993). A further two studies with pedigrees from Ireland (Su *et al.*, 1993) and the USA (Wang *et al.*, 1993a) have come to similar conclusions.

Chromosome 21 has also been examined with highly polymorphic DNA markers spanning the long arm, with no evidence of linkage and exclusion of most of the long arm under a range of diagnostic and genetic parameters (Asherson *et al.*, 1993). In addition, this study employed a technique known as single-stranded conformational polymorphism (SSCP) to search directly for gene mutations in PCR products. In this case, SSCP was used to screen part of the coding sequence of the amyloid precurser protein, since it had been reported that a mutation in this gene had occurred in an individual with schizophrenia (Jones *et al.*, 1992). Sequence variations were not detected in a sample of 68 unrelated schizophrenics, indicating that the reported association had almost certainly occurred by chance. However, the approach of looking directly for mutations in candidate genes is important and we shall return to this in the section on association studies.

The pseudoautosomal region of the X chromosome has been proposed as a candidate region, based mainly on the observation that schizophrenic siblings are more often of the same sex than of opposite sex (Crow, 1988). Same-sex concordance would be expected if there was a major gene within this region and under dominant inheritance would occur following paternal transmission of the gene. However, evidence for this hypothesis has not been convincing following a number of linkage studies. Collinge *et al.* (1991), using a highly polymorphic marker from the telomeric end of the pseudoautosomal region, found that affected siblings shared alleles more often than expected under random segregation ($P < 0.05$). Although this finding was replicated ($P < 0.05$) in a sample of French families (d'Amato *et al.*, 1992), it is important to consider the fact that since the prior probability of linkage is only about 1:50, odds of 1000:1 ($P < 0.001$) are needed to reach the conventional level for acceptance of linkage (Morton, 1955; Ott, 1991). Furthermore, studies of pedigrees from Wales (Asherson *et al.*, 1992), the USA (Wang *et al.*, 1993b) and Canada (Sidenberg *et al.*, 1993), using both sibling pair and Lod score methods, have failed to find evidence of linkage.

Association studies

While linkage analysis enables the detection of genes of major effect, it will not detect genes of small effect that contribute in an additive or interactive way with other genes or with genes plus environment. However, genes of minor effect have

been successfully isolated, using association methods, in a number of other complex genetic disorders, such as the TGF α gene in cleft lip and palate (Holder *et al.*, 1992), the glucokinase and glycogen synthase genes in non-insulin-dependent diabetes (Chiu *et al.*, 1993) and insulin-dependent diabetes (Bell *et al.*, 1984), and the myelin basic protein gene in multiple sclerosis (Tienari *et al.*, 1992).

Association studies in schizophrenia using DNA markers have unfortunately thrown up a number of contradictory results. This has been in part because of the problems of diagnosis and the question of comparability of patient populations from different centres. However, the major confounding factor in these studies is the selection of controls which can result in so-called stratification effects. The problem is that there may be a section of the population in which a particular marker and a certain disorder are common, without there being any causal relationship. For example, HLA BW16 is more common in Ashkenazi Jews, so that an excess of Jewish patients in an affected sample could lead to the false conclusion that an association exists between the disorder and that antigen. A recent solution to this problem has been to compare the frequencies of the parental alleles not inherited by an affected individual with the alleles which are inherited, thus providing a perfectly matched internal control (Falk & Rubenstein, 1987). The samples for this approach are, however, less easy to collect than those for traditional association studies.

Another problem is the statistical handling of results. Since the prior probability of obtaining a true association is extremely remote, the conventional level of statistical significance ($P < 0.05$) is probably not sufficiently stringent. In addition, account must be made for the use of multiple markers in these studies. A conservative correction is to multiply the obtained P value by the number of markers tested.

The task of carrying out a systematic search for association throughout the entire genome would involve the use of a very series of markers, each showing linkage disequilibrium with its neighbour. While this at present would involve an impossibly large amount of work, it is likely to become increasingly feasible as automated technology is developed. For the moment, the best strategy is probably to focus upon markers that are close to, or within, candidate genes.

An alternative to the use of DNA markers, resulting from variations in non-coding sequences in the vicinity of candidate genes, is the study of sequence variations that affect protein structure or expression (VAPSEs) (Sobell *et al.*, 1992), and to look for these gene mutations directly among schizophrenic probands. This has the advantage that a VAPSE-disease association is not affected by recombination and directly identifies the pathogenic mutation. On the other hand, if the VAPSE is not the pathogenic mutation itself, it may well be very close to a mutation within the same gene that is pathogenic or in linkage disequilibrium with a mutation in a nearby gene. The problem here is that we understand little about the pathophysiology of schizophrenia and plausible candidate genes are few and far between.

Association studies in schizophrenia

Early association studies in schizophrenia used classical markers such as the ABO and other blood groups and the HLA system. The results of these studies are inconsistent but when considered overall no clear evidence for association has been found (McGuffin & Sturt, 1986). The main reasons for this, multiple testing and stratification, are discussed above.

An interesting finding was of an association between a subtype of schizophrenia (paranoid schizophrenia) and HLA9 in seven out of nine studies. Combining the data and applying a correction for multiple testing gave a *P* value of 0.0003 (McGuffin & Sturt, 1986). However, several conflicting findings have been found. Two groups found A9 to be decreased in paranoid schizophrenia compared with controls (Miyanga *et al.*, 1984; Rudduck, 1984), while others, using samples from the same countries, found A9 to be increased (Eberhard *et al.*, 1975; Asaka *et al.*, 1981). A9 consists of two subspecificities, AW23 and AW24. Two studies suggested an association

with AW23 (Crowe *et al.*, 1979; Asaka *et al.*, 1981), while others found a stronger relationship with AW24 (Ivanyi *et al.*, 1983). More recently, a study found no association between paranoid schizophrenia and either AW23 or AW24 (Alexander *et al.*, 1990). Another recent study of 33 pedigrees collected in France failed to find evidence of linkage between HLA and the schizophrenic phenotype (Campion *et al.*, 1992). In addition, these authors performed an association study using pooled data from six independent studies and were unable to show a significant excess of HLA9 in the affected group, but they did not subdivide their sample into paranoid vs. hebephrenic subforms.

A gene that has been of some interest is PBGD. As described above, this gene on the long arm of chromosome 11 is a candidate as a susceptibility locus in schizophrenia. Several RFLPs have been identified within this gene, and an initial report by Sanders *et al.* (1992) suggested strong association between schizophrenia and a restriction fragment produced by the restriction enzyme known as *Msp*I ($P = 0.00048$). In addition, it was noted that earlier age of onset, defined as first admission before the age of 30 years, was associated with homozygosity for this allele ($P = 0.019$). In seeking to replicate this finding, Owen *et al.* (1992) found no evidence for allelic association between the *Msp*I polymorphism in the PBGD gene and schizophrenia.

Disturbances in dopamine neurotransmission and dopamine receptors have long been postulated to underlie schizophrenia, and genes coding for dopamine receptors have been targeted as candidates. Until recently, two types of dopamine receptor had been identified, known as D_1 and D_2; these differ from each other functionally, with D_1 suppressing adenylate cyclase, whereas D_2 stimulates adenylate cyclase. However, recent work in this field has identified a further three dopamine receptor genes known as D_3, D_4 and D_5 (Sokoloff *et al.*, 1990; Sunahara *et al.*, 1991; Van Tol *et al.*, 1991). D_3 and D_4 have a similar structure to D_2 and bind D_2-selective ligands, while D_5 is similar in structure to D_1. It is thought that the therapeutic effects of antipsychotic drugs are related to their high affinity for D_2 receptors, and this view has been revised to include D_3 and D_4.

The D_3 receptor may be of particular interest since its expression is restricted to limbic regions implicated in schizophrenia. Furthermore, expression of D_3 in the brain is, unlike D_1 and D_2, increased by both typical and atypical neuroleptics (Buckland *et al.*, 1993) (see below). The gene for this receptor has been localized to the long arm of chromosome 3 (Le Conait *et al.*, 1991) and contains a polymorphic site in its coding region which gives rise to a glycine-to-serine substitution and results in a restriction site for the enzyme *Bal*I (Lannfelt *et al.*, 1992). Study of this polymorphism is an example of the VAPSE approach in a candidate gene (see above).

Initially, two independent groups from Wales and France carried out studies of this polymorphism in the dopamine D_3 receptor gene in samples of patients with DSM-III-R schizophrenia and normal controls (Crocq *et al.*, 1992). In both studies, more patients than controls were homozygotes of either type ($P = 0.005$, $P = 0.008$). Pooling of the data gave a highly significant result ($P = 0.0001$) with a relative risk of schizophrenia in homozygotes of 2.61 (95% confidence intervals $1.60-4.26$). The Welsh study has subsequently been extended and results suggest that this effect may be stronger in patients with a family history of mental illness, in males and in those who respond better to antipsychotic medication (Mant *et al.*, 1994). These later findings suggest that any attempt at replication must use a patient sample which is adequately matched for these clinical variables, if false-negative results are to be avoided.

These interesting findings may represent an example of heterozygote advantage (Cavalli-Sforza & Bodmer, 1971), perhaps because the presence of two different molecular forms of the receptor results in an increased ability to respond adaptively to variations in the environment occurring either during neural development or in adult life. If these results are confirmed, a locus contributing a small amount to the liability of developing schizophrenia has been identified. It is also possible that homozygosity at other loci influences genetic susceptibility to schizophrenia, and this mechanism may be of general relevance to the disorder.

Molecular neurobiology

Molecular techniques have also resulted in major advances to our understanding of neurobiology, much of which may be of relevance in schizophrenia. For example, the cloning of five separate dopamine receptor genes along with genes coding for enzymes and other proteins involved in dopaminergic transmission has opened up new approaches to examining hypotheses involving the dopamine system.

The expression of these genes can be studied in animals exposed to antipsychotic drugs in order to examine the mechanisms involved in the therapeutic action. Buckland *et al.* (1993) have studied the effect in rat brain of chronic treatment (32 days) with the 'atypical' antipsychotics sulpiride and clozapine. They demonstrated that dopamine D_3 receptor messenger ribonucleic acid (mRNA) levels increased by four-fold, whereas no effect was observed on the mRNA levels encoding D_1 or D_2 receptors, or tyrosine hydroxylase. They postulate that D_3 receptor mRNA may be associated with the therapeutic action of antipsychotic drugs. These results contrast with other studies which have shown increases in both D_2 and D_3 mRNA with 'typical' neuroleptics such as chlorpromazine and haloperidol.

A different approach is to look for variations within these genes that may be associated with drug responsiveness. Of recent interest has been the drug clozapine, which is widely reported to reduce symptoms of schizophrenia which are unresponsive to other antipsychotic medication (McKenna & Bailey, 1993). However, some patients remain unresponsive to clozapine and it has been suggested that response to this drug may be related to variation of the D_4 receptor. This view arises from observations that clozapine has a particularly high affinity for D_4 receptors, and that the D_4 receptor shows a high degree of variation (Van Tol *et al.*, 1992). The hypothesis is currently being tested by studying the relationship between particular allelic variants of the gene in patients who show a good response to clozapine and those who are clozapine unresponsive (Shaikh *et al.*, 1993).

Genetic counselling

At present, it is not possible to determine the specific risk that a particular individual will develop schizophrenia. Because of the complex mode of inheritance and variable expressivity of the disorder, the only reasonable information to provide to relatives regarding recurrence risks of the disorder in other family members is based upon the empirical data from family studies. Probably the most useful figures are those provided by Gottesman (1991) based upon a compilation of results from many Western European studies (see Table 14.1). Despite this, there is a definite role for counselling based upon an informed and responsible approach (see McGuffin *et al.*, 1994 for review).

There is now considerable experience in genetic counselling and the principal approaches are the same regardless of the disorder in question. Most counsellors take a non-directive educational approach (Harper, 1988). The aim is to impart accurate information and help the counsellee to understand fully the risks and potential burdens so that they can make an informed decision. It is important to emphasize that it is the counsellee who must make the ultimate decisions.

Most of those who seek counselling are concerned about the potential risks to their children, or if they are an unaffected relative, about their own chances of developing the disorder. At present, the only information which is useful to impart comes from empirical sources (i.e. family, twin and adoption studies). For example, a couple planning a family, one of whom has a parent with schizophrenia, would be informed that the average risk to each of their children is about 3% or 3 times that in the general population. In some rare cases the counsellee may come from a family which has multiple affected members and gives the appearance of Mendelian transmission.

However, with our current state of knowledge it would be wrong to assume that this is the case, since these loaded families would also be expected to exist as a result of multifactorial/polygenic inheritance. In these families the risk to relatives appears to increase in relation to the number of affected family members and to decrease in relation to the number of well family members (Gottesman, 1991).

Empirical data also tell us that schizophrenia is in most, if not all, cases a complex disease with both inherited and non-inherited causative factors. In schizophrenia the nature of these non-inherited factors remains controversial (McGuffin *et al.*, 1994) and some, such as exposure of the foetus to viral infections, are not easily avoided. On the other hand, it would be useful to advise relatives of patients with schizophrenia to avoid the 'experimental' use of drugs such as LSD, PCP, cocaine and amphetamine, since they may be especially vulnerable to drug-precipitated psychoses as a result of high genetic loading.

In the future, advances in our understanding of the molecular basis of schizophrenia may allow the use of prenatal and presymptomatic testing. The complexity of this disorder suggests that in most cases it will not be possible to attain high levels of predictive certainty, but, as mentioned previously, there may be rare families which show true single-gene inheritance and for whom accurate testing is a realistic possibility. The issues are best exemplified by work with relatives and patients from families with Huntington's disease. Until recently, risk calculations in this disorder relied upon DNA marker testing involving the genotyping of individuals in several generations, although the identification of the disease-causing mutation (Huntington's Disease Collaborative Research Group, 1993) makes possible a specific test in individuals. Predictive testing is usually carried out in specialist centres with expert counselling, and counsellees are given advice prior to testing to allow them to make an informed decision about the usefulness of such testing. In one series (Tyler *et al.*, 1992), out of 238 initial requests for testing, only 40 results were eventually given out as a result of such pretest counselling.

We would suggest that if presymptomatic or pre-natal testing were possible for schizophrenia, similar principles should be adopted. This would involve skilled counselling, with adequate consideration given to the severity of the disorder, the age of onset, variable expressivity and other aspects of the phenotype. This would allow counsellees to be fully informed before making any final decisions.

Conclusion

Family, twin and adoption studies provide compelling evidence that schizophrenia has an important genetic component, and quantitative analyses suggest that most of the variance in liability to the disorder (perhaps 80% or more) is accounted for by genetic factors. However, the pattern of transmission in families is complex and although some multi-generation pedigrees with a Mendelian-like appearance exist, they are very much the exception rather than the rule. It seems likely that schizophrenia at a molecular level will turn out to be heterogeneous, even though so far attempts to relate clinical heterogeneity to aetiological heterogeneity have failed. This may partly account for the disappointingly inconclusive results of attempts to resolve statistically the mode (or modes) of transmission. However, it now seems almost certain that if genes of major effect exist they will be localized by linkage strategies within the next few years. The search for such genes is premised not on any strong evidence that they occur, but rather on the fact that there is no convincing evidence against their existence. We therefore need to prepare for the eventuality that schizophrenia is transmitted by a few (oligo) genes, each of only moderate effect, or by many (poly) genes, each of only small effect. Such susceptibility loci will be more difficult to detect and localize using molecular genetic approaches but, nevertheless, their detection is now becoming feasible and it seems probable that schizophrenia, like many other common familial disorders, will have a molecular basis that will begin to be understood within the foreseeable future.

References

Alexander, R.C., Coggiano, M., Daniel, D.G. & Wyatt, R.S. (1990) HLA antigen in schizophrenia. *Psychiatry Research*, **31**, 221–223.

d'Amato, T., Campion, P., Gorwood, M. *et al.* (1992) Evidence for a pseudoautosomal locus for schizophrenia. II: a replication of non-random segregation of alleles at the DXYS14 locus. *British Journal of Psychiatry*, **161**, 59–62.

Asaka, A., Okazaki, Y., Namura, I. *et al.* (1981) Study of HLA antigens among Japanese schizophrenics. *British Journal of Psychiatry*, **138**, 498–500.

Asherson, P., Mant, R., Taylor, C. *et al.* (1993) Failure to find linkage between schizophrenia and genetic markers on chromosome 21. *American Journal of Medical Genetics (Neuropsychiatric Genetics)*, **48**, 161–165.

Asherson, P.J., Parfitt, E., Sargeant, M. *et al.* (1992) No evidence for a pseudo-autosomal locus for schizophrenia from linkage analysis of multiply affected families. *British Journal of Psychiatry*, **161**, 63–68.

Baron, M. (1976) Albinism and schizophreniform psychosis: a pedigree study. *American Journal of Psychiatry*, **133**, 1070–1073.

Barton, D., Kwon, B. & Francke, U. (1988) Human tyrosinase gene, mapped to chromosome 11(q14–q21) defines second region of homology with mouse chromosome 7. *Genomics*, **3**, 17–24.

Bassett, A.S., Jones, B.D., McGillivray, B.C. & Panztar, J.T. (1988) Partial trisomy chromosome 5 cosegregating with schizophrenia. *Lancet*, **1**, 799–801.

Bell, G.I., Horitas, S. & Karam, J.H. (1984) A polymorphic locus near the human insulin gene is associated with insulin-dependent diabetes mellitus. *Diabetes*, **33**, 176–183.

Buckland, P.R., O'Donovan, M.C. & McGuffin, P. (1993) Clozapine and sulpiride up-regulate dopamine D3 receptor mRNA levels. *Neuropharmacology*, **32**, 901–907.

Campion, D., Leboyer, M., Hillaire, D. *et al.* (1992) Relationship of HLA to schizophrenia not supported in multiplex families. *Psychiatry Research*, **41**, 99–105.

Carter, C.L. & Chung, C.S. (1980) Segregation analysis of schizophrenia under a mixed model. *Human Heredity*, **30**, 350–356.

Cavalli-Sforza, L.L. & Bodmer, W.F. (1971) *The Genetics of Human Populations*. Freeman, San Francisco.

Chiu, K.C., Tanizawa, Y., & Permott, M.A. (1993) Glucokinase gene variants in the common form of NIDDM. *Diabetes*, **42**, 579–582.

Clerget-Darpoux, F. (1986) Effects of misspecifying genetic parameters in lod score analysis. *Biometrics*, **42**, 393–399.

Collinge, J., DeLisi, L.E., Boccio, A. *et al.* (1991) Evidence for a pseudo-autosomal locus for schizophrenia using the method of affected sibling pairs. *British Journal of Psychiatry*, **158**, 624–629.

Crocq, M.A., Mant, R., Asherson, P. *et al.* (1992) Association between schizophrenia and homozygosity at the dopamine D3 receptor gene. *Journal of Medical Genetics*, **29**, 858–860.

Crow, T.J. (1988) Sex chromosomes and psychosis. The case for a pseudoautosomal locus. *British Journal of Psychiatry*, **153**, 675–683.

Crowe, R.R., Thompson, I.S., Flink, R.F. *et al.* (1979) HLA antigens and schizophrenia. *Archives of General Psychiatry*, **36**, 231–233.

Detera-Wadleigh, S.D., Goldin, L.R., Sherrington, R. *et al.* (1989) Exclusion of linkage to 5q11–q13 in families with schizophrenia and other psychiatric disorders. *Nature*, **340**, 391–393.

Eberhard, G., Franzen, G. & Low, B. (1975) Schizophrenia susceptibility and HLA antigens. *Neuropsychobiology*, **1**, 211–217.

Edwards, T.H. (1965) The meaning of the associations between blood groups and disease. *Annals of Human Genetics*, **29**, 77–83.

Elston, R.C. & Campbell, A.A. (1970) Schizophrenia. Evidence for a major gene hypothesis. *Behavioural Genetics*, **1**, 101–106.

Essen-Moller, E. (1955) The calculation of morbid risk in parents of index cases, as applied to a family sample of schizophrenics. *Acta Genetica et Statistica Medica*, **5**, 334–342.

Falconer, D.S. (1965) The inheritance of liability to certain diseases, estimated from the incidence among relatives. *Annals of Human Genetics*, **29**, 51–76.

Falk, C.T. & Rubinstein, P. (1987) An easy, reliable way to construct control sample for risk calculation. *Annals of Human Genetics*, **51**, 227–233.

Farmer, A.E., McGuffin, P. & Gottesman, I.I. (1987) Twin concordance for DSM-III schizophrenia: scrutinising the validity of the definition. *Archives of General Psychiatry*, **44**, 634–641.

Feighner, J.P., Robins, E., Guze, S.B., Woodruff, R.A., Winokur, G. & Munoz, R. (1972) Diagnostic criteria for use in psychiatric research. *Archives of General Psychiatry*, **26**, 57–63.

Fischer, M. (1971) Psychoses in the offspring of schizophrenic monozygotic twins and their normal co-twins. *British Journal of Psychiatry*, **118**, 43–52.

Gershon, E.S., Delisi, L.E., Hamovit, J., Nurnberger, J.L., Maxwell, M.E. & Schreiber, J. (1988) A controlled study of chronic psychoses. Schizophrenia and schizoaffective disorder. *Archives of General Psychiatry*, **45**, 328–336.

Gill, M., McGuffin, P., Parfitt, E., Mant, R., Asherson, P. & Collier, D. (1993) A linkage study of schizophrenia with DNA markers from the long arm of chromosome 11. *Psychological Medicine*, **23**, 27–44.

Goate, A.M., Chartier-Harlin, M-C., Mullan, M. *et al.* (1991) Segregation of a misense mutation in the amyloid precursor protein gene with familial Alzheimer's Disease. *Nature*, **349**, 704–706.

Gottesman, I.I. (1991) *Schizophrenia Genesis. Origins of Madness.* W.H. Freeman, San Francisco.

Gottesman, I.I. & Bertelsen, A. (1989) Confirming unexpressed genotypes for schizophrenia-risks in the offspring of Fischer's Danish identical and fraternal discordant twins. *Archives of General Psychiatry*, **46**, 867–872.

Gottesman, I.I. & Shields, J. (1967) A polygenic theory of schizophrenia. *Proceedings of the National Academy of Sciences (USA)*, **58**, 199–205.

Gottesman, I.I. & Shields, J. (1972) *Schizophrenia and Genetics.*

A *Twin Vantage Point.* Academic Press, New York.

Gottesman, I.I. & Shields, J. (1982) *Schizophrenia: The Epigenetic Puzzle.* Cambridge University Press, Cambridge.

Grandy, D.K., Litt, M., Allen, N. *et al.* (1989) The human dopamine D2 receptor gene is located on chromosome 11 at q22–q23 and identifies a Taq I RFLP. *American Journal of Human Genetics*, **45**, 778–785.

Green, J.R. & Woodrow, J.C. (1977) Sibling method for detecting HLA-linked genes in the disease. *Tissue Antigens*, **9**, 31–35.

Harper, P.S. (1988) *Practical Genetic Counselling*, 3rd edn. Wright & Sons, Bristol.

Heston, L.L. (1966) Psychiatric disorders in foster home reared children of schizophrenic mothers. *British Journal of Psychiatry*, **122**, 819–825.

Heston, L.L. (1970) The genetics of schizophrenia and schizoid disease. *Science*, **167**, 249–256.

Holder, S.E., Vintiner, G.M. & Farren, B. (1992) Confirmation of an association between RFLPs at the transforming growth factor-alpha locus and non-syndromic cleft lip and palate. *Journal of Medical Genetics*, **29**, 390–392.

Holland, A. & Gosden, C. (1990) A balanced translocation partially co-segregating with psychotic illness in a family. *Psychiatric Research*, **32**, 1–8.

Huntington's Disease Collaborative Research Group (1993) A novel gene containing a trinucleotide repeat that is expanded and unstable on Huntington's disease chromosomes. *Cell*, **72**, 971–983.

Ivanyi, D., Droes, J., Schreuder, G.M.T. *et al.* (1983) A search for association of HLA antigens with paranoid schizophrenia. *Tissue Antigens*, **22**, 186–193.

James, J.W. (1971) Frequency in relatives for an all-or-none trait. *Annals of Human Genetics*, **35**, 47–49.

Jones, C.T., Morris, S., Yates, C.M. *et al.* (1992) Mutation in codon 713 of the beta amyloid precursor gene presenting with schizophrenia. *Nature Genetics*, **1**, 306–309.

Kallman, F.J. (1938) *The Genetics of Schizophrenia.* Augustin, New York.

Kendler, K.S. & Gruenberg, A.M. (1984) An independent antigen of the Danish adoption study of schizophrena, VI. *Archives of General Psychiatry*, **41**, 555–564.

Kendler, K.S., Gruenberg, A.M. & Tsuang, M.T. (1985) Psychiatric illness in first degree relatives of schizophrenics and surgical controls patients. *Archives of General Psychiatry*, **42**, 770–779.

Kennedy, J.L., Guiffra, L.A., Moises, H.W. *et al.* (1988) Evidence against linkage of schizophrenia to markers on chromosome 5 in a Northern Swedish pedigree. *Nature*, **336**, 167–169.

Kety, S.S., Rosenthal, D., Wender, P.H. *et al.* (1976) Mental illness in the biological and adoptive families of individuals who have become schizophrenic. *Behaviour Genetics*, **6**, 219–225.

Kringlen, E. (1976) Twins — still our best method. *Schizophrenic Bulletin*, **2**, 429–433.

Kringlen, E. & Cramer, G. (1989) Offspring of monozygotic twins discordant for schizophrenia. *Archives of General Psychiatry*, **46**, 873–877.

Lander, E.S. (1988) Splitting schizophrenia. *Nature*, **336**,

105–106.

Lannfelt, L., Sokoloff, P. & Martres, M.P. (1992) Amino-acid substitution in the dopamine D3 receptor as a useful polymorphism for investigating psychiatric disorders. *Psychiatric Genetics*, **2**, 249–256.

Le Conait, M., Sokoloff, P., Hillion, J., Matres, M.P., Gires, B. & Pilon, C. (1991) Chromosomal localization of the human D3 dopamine receptor gene. *Human Genetics*, **87**, 618–620.

Leboyer, M. & McGuffin, P. (1991) Collaborative strategies in the molecular genetics of major psychoses. *British Journal of Psychiatry*, **158**, 605–610.

Luxenberger, H. (1928) Vorlaufizer Bericht über psychiatrische Serien Untersuchungen an Zwillinger. *Zeitschift für gesamte Neurologie und Psychiatrie*, **116**, 297–326.

McGue, M. & Gottesman, I.I. (1991) The genetic epidemiology of schizophrenia and the design of linkage studies. *European Archives of Clinical Psychiatry*, **240**, 174–181.

McGue, M., Gottesman, I.I. Rao, D.C. *et al.* (1985) Resolving genetic models for the transmission of schizophrenia. *Genetic Epidemiology*, **2**, 99–110.

McGuffin, P. (1991) Genetic models of madness. In McGuffin, P. & Murray, R. (eds) *The New Genetics of Mental Illness*, pp. 27–43. Butterworth-Heinemann, Oxford.

McGuffin, P. & Owen, M. (1991) The molecular genetics of schizophrenia: an overview and forward view. *European Archives of Clinical Neuroscience*, **240**, 169–173.

McGuffin, P. & Sturt, E. (1986) Genetic markers in schizophrenia. *Human Heredity*, **36**, 65–88.

McGuffin, P., Asherson, P., Owen, M. & Farmer, A.E. (1994a) The strength of the genetic effect — is there room for an environmental influence in the aetiology of schizophrenia? *British Journal of Psychiatry*, **164**, 593–599.

McGuffin, P., Owen, M., O'Donovan, M., Thapar, A. & Gottesman, I.I. (1994b) Genetic counselling and ethical issues. *Seminars in Psychiatric Genetics* (in press). Gaskell Press, London.

McGuffin, P., Farmer, A.E., Gottesman, I.I. *et al.* (1984) Twin concordance for operationally defined schizophrenia. Confirmation of familiality and heritability. *Archives of General Psychiatry*, **41**, 541–545.

McGuffin, P., Sargeant, M.P., Hett, G. *et al.* (1990) Exclusion of a schizophrenia susceptibility gene from the chromosome 5q11–q13 region: new data and a reanalysis of previous reports. *American Journal of Human Genetics*, **47**, 524–535.

McKenna, P.J. & Bailey, P.E. (1993) The strange story of clozapine. *British Journal of Psychiatry*, **162**, 32–37.

Mankoo, B., Sherrington, R., Brynjolfsson, J. *et al.* (1991) New microsatellite polymorphisms provide a highly polymorphic map of chromosome 5 bands q11.2–q13.3 for linkage analysis of Icelandic and English families affected by schizophrenia. *Psychiatric Genetics*, **2**, 17.

Mant, R., Williams, J., Asherson, P. *et al.* (1994) The relationship between homozygosity at the dopamine D3 receptor gene and schizophrenia. *American Journal of Medical Genetics (Neuropsychiatric Genetics)*, **54**, 21–26.

Meehl, P.E. (1973) *Psychodiagnosis: Selected Papers*. University of Minnesota Press, Minneapolis.

Miyanga, K., Machiymaya, Y. & Juji, T. (1984) Schizophrenic disorders and HLA-DR antigens. *Biological Psychiatry*, **19**, 121–129.

Moises, H.W., Gelernter, J., Giuffra, L. *et al.* (1991) No linkage between D2 dopamine receptor gene region and schizophrenia. *Archives of General Psychiatry*, **48**, 643–647.

Morton, N.E. (1955) Sequential tests for the detection of linkage. *American Journal of Human Genetics*, **7**, 277–318.

Morton, N.E. & Macclean, C.J. (1974) Analysis of family resemblance. III. Complex segregation analysis of quantitative traits. *American Journal of Human Genetics*, **26**, 489–503.

Mullis, K.B. & Faloona, F.A. (1987) Specific synthesis of DNA *in vitro* via a polymerase catalysed chain reaction. *Methods in Enzymology*, **155**, 335–350.

Murray, R.M., Lewis, S.W. & Reveley, A.M. (1985) Towards an aetiological classification of schizophrenia. *Lancet*, **i**, 1023–1026.

Nothen, M.M. & Fimmers, R. (1992) Association versus linkage studies in psychosis genetics. *Journal of Medical Genetics*, **30**, 634–637.

Onstad, S., Skre, I., Torgrersen, S. & Kringlen, E. (1991) Twin concordance for DSM-IIIR schizophrenia. *Acta Psychiatrica Scandinavica*, **83**, 395–402.

O'Rourke, D.H., Gottesman, I.I., Suarez, B.K. *et al.* (1982) Refutation of the single locus model in the aetiology of schizophrenia. *American Journal of Human Genetics*, **33**, 630–649.

Ott, J. (1991) *Analysis of Human Genetic Linkage*. John Hopkins University Press, Baltimore.

Owen, M. & McGuffin, P. (1991) DNA and classical genetic markers in schizophrenia. *European Archives of Psychiatry and Clinical Neuroscience*, **240**, 197–203.

Owen, M.J., Mant, R., Parfitt, E. *et al.* (1992) No association between RFLPs at the porphobilinogen deaminase gene and schizophrenia. *Human Genetics*, **90**, 131–132.

Penrose, L.S. (1935) The detection of autosomal linkage in data which consists of pairs of brothers and sisters of unspecified parentage. *Annals of Eugenics*, **6**, 133–138.

Pollin, W., Allen, M.G., Hoffer, A., Stabenau, J.R. & Hrubec, Z. (1969) Psychopathology in 15 909 pairs of veteran twins: evidence for a genetic factor in the pathogenesis of schizophrenia and its relative absence in psychoneurosis. *American Journal of Psychiatry*, **126**, 597–610.

Reveley, A.M., Reveley, M.A., Clifford, C.A. & Murray, R.M. (1982) Cerebral ventricular size is twins discordant for schizophrenia. *Lancet*, **March**, 540–541.

Risch, N. & Baron, M. (1984) Segregation analysis of schizophrenia and related disorders. *American Journal of Human Genetics*, **36**, 1039–1059.

Rosenthal, D. (1971) Two adoption studies of heredity in the schizophrenic disorders. In Bleuler, M. & Angst, J. (eds) *The Origins of Schizophrenia*, pp. 21–34. Huber, Bern.

Rudduck, C. (1984) *Genetic markers and schizophrenia*. PhD Thesis, University of Lund.

Rudin, E. (1916) *Zur Vererbung und Nuenentstehung der Dementia Praecox*. Springer-Verlag, Berlin.

Sanders, A., Hamilton, J., Chakraborty, R. *et al.* (1993) Association of genetic variation at the porphobilinogen deaminase gene with schizophrenia. *Schizophrenia Research*,

8, 211–221.

Shaikh, S., Collier, D. & Kerwin, R.W. (1993) Dopamine D4 receptor subtypes and response to clozapine. *Lancet*, **341**, 116.

Sherrington, R., Brynjolffson, J., Petersson, H. *et al.* (1988) Localization of a susceptibility locus for schizophrenia on chromosome 5. *Nature*, **336**, 164–167.

Sidenberg, D.G., Bassett, A., Cavallini, M.C. *et al.* (1993) Lack of linkage of the pseudoautosomal region in five Canadian pedigrees. (in press).

Slater, E. (1958) The monogenic theory of schizophrenia. *Acta Genetica*, **8**, 50–56.

Slater, E. & Cowie, V. (1971) *The Genetics of Mental Disorder*. Oxford University Press, Oxford.

Smith, M., Wasmuth, J., McPherson, J.D. *et al.* (1989) Cosegregation of an 11q22-9p22 translocation with affective disorder: proximity of the dopamine D2 receptor gene relative to the translocation breakpoint. *American Journal of Human Genetics*, **45**, A220.

Sobell, J.C., Heston, L.L. & Sommer, S.S. (1992) Delineation of genetic predisposition to multifactorial disease; a general approach on the threshhold of feasibility. *Genomics*, **12**, 1–6.

Sokoloff, P., Giros, B., Martres, M.P., Bouthenet, M.L. & Schwartz, J.C. (1990) Molecular cloning and characterisation of a novel dopamine receptor (D3) as a target for neuroleptics. *Nature*, **347**, 146–151.

Spitzer, R.L., Endicott, J. & Robins, E. (1978) Research Diagnostic Criteria: rationale and reliability. *Archives of General Psychiatry*, **35**, 773–782.

St Clair, D., Blackwood, D., Muir, W. *et al.* (1989) No linkage of 5q11–q13 markers to schizophrenia in Scottish families. *Nature*, **339**, 305–309.

St Clair, D., Blackwood, D., Muir, W. *et al.* (1990) Association within a family of a balanced autosomal translocation with major mental illness. *Lancet*, **336**, 13–16.

Sturt, E. & McGuffin, P. (1985) Can linkage and marker association resolve the genetic aetiology of psychiatric disorders: review and argument. *Psychological Medicine*, **15**, 455–462.

Su, Y., Burke, J. & O'Neill, A. (1993) Exclusion of linkage between schizophrenia and the D2 dopamine receptor gene region of chromosome 11q in 112 Irish multiplex families. *Archives of General Psychiatry*, **50**, 205–211.

Suddath, R.L., Christison, G.W., Torrey, F., Cassonova, M.F. & Weinleigh, D.R. (1990) Anatomic abnormalities in the brains of monozygotic twins discordant for schizophrenia. *New England Journal of Medicine*, **322**, 789–794.

Sunahara, R.K., Guan, H.C., O'Dowd, B.F. *et al.* (1991) Cloning of the gene for a human D5 receptor with higher affinity for dopamine than D1. *Nature*, **350**, 614–619.

Tienari, P. (1971) Schizophrenia and monozygotic twins. *Psychiatrica Fennica*, 97–104.

Tienari, P. (1990) Gene–environment interaction in adoptive families. In Hafner, H. & Gattaz, W. (eds) *Search for the Causes of Schizophrenia*, pp. 126–143. Springer-Verlag, Berlin.

Tienari, P., Wikstrom, J., Sajantila, A., Palo, J. & Peltonen, L. (1992) Genetic susceptibility to multiple sclerosis linked myelin basic protein gene. *Lancet*, **340**, 987–991.

Turner, S.W., Toone, B.K. & Brett-Jones, J.R. (1986) Preliminary communication. Computerised tomographic scan changes in early schizophrenia – preliminary findings. *Psychological Medicine*, **16**, 219–225.

Turner, W.J. (1979) Genetic markers for schizophrenia. *Biological Psychiatry*, **14**, 177–205.

Tyler, A., Morris, M., Lazarou, L., Meredith, L., Myring, J. & Harper, P. (1992) Presymptomatic testing for Huntington's Disease in Wales, 1987–90. *British Journal of Psychiatry*, **161**, 481–488.

Van Broekhoven, C., Backhovens, H., Cruts, M. *et al.* (1992) Mapping of a gene predisposing to early-onset Alzheimer's Disease to chromosome 14q24.3. *Nature Genetics*, **2**, 335–339.

Van Tol, H.H., Bunzow J.R., Guan, H.C. *et al.* (1991) Cloning of the gene for a human dopamine D4 receptor with high affinity for the antipsychotic clozapine. *Nature*, **350**, 610–614.

Van Tol, H.H., Wu, C.M., Guan, H.C. *et al.* (1992) Multiple D4 receptor variants in the human population. *Nature*, **358**, 149–152.

Vogler, G.P., Gottesman, I.I. McGue, M.K. & Rao, D.C. (1990) Mixed model segregation analysis of schizophrenia in the Lindelius Swedish pedigrees. *Behavior Genetics*, **20**, 461–472.

Walsh, C., Asherson, P., Sham, P. *et al.* (1993) Familial schizophrenia shows no gender difference in age of onset. *Schizophrenia Research*, **9**, 127.

Wang, A.L., Arredondo-Vega F.X., Giampetro, P.F. *et al.* (1981) Regional gene assignment of human porpholilinogen deaminase and esterase A4 to chromosome 11q 23-11qter. *Proceedings of the National Academy of Science (USA)*, **78**, 5734–5738.

Wang, Z.W., Black, D., Andreasen N. & Crowe, R.R. (1993a) A linkage study of chromosome 11q in schizophrenia. *Archives of General Psychiatry*, **50**, 212–216.

Wang, Z.W., Black, D., Andreasen, N. & Crowe, R.R. (1993b) Pseudoautosomal locus for schizophrenia is excluded in 12 pedigrees. *Archives of General Psychiatry*, **50**, 199–204.

Weber J. & May, P.E. (1989) Abundant class of human DNA polymorphisms which can be typed using the polymerase chain reaction. *American Journal of Human Genetics*, **14**, 388–396.

Weissenbach, J., Gyapay, G., Dib, C. *et al.* (1992) A second-generation linkage map of the human genome. *Nature*, **359**, 794–801.

Wender, P.H., Rosenthal, D., Kety, S.S., Schulsinger, F. & Welner, J. (1974) Crossfostering. A research strategy for clarifying the role of genetic and experimental factors in the aetiology of schizophrenia. *Archives of General Psychiatry*, **31**, 121–128.

White, R. & Lalouel J.M. (1988) Sets of linked genetic markers for human chromosomes. *Annual Review of Genetics*, **22**, 259–279.

Chapter 15
The Neuropathology of Schizophrenia

P. FALKAI AND B. BOGERTS

Historical considerations

At the turn of the century, the development of new methods in the histopathology of the central nervous system essentially resulted from the search for anatomical substrates of mental disorders. This early stage of neuropathological research mainly was initiated by the two psychiatrists Franz Nissl and Alois Alzheimer, who, under the influence of their powerful mentor Emil Kraepelin, performed the first neurohistopathological studies in a variety of psychiatric disorders. After Nissl had developed for the first time a specific and reliable staining procedure for nerve cells, this method was applied by Alzheimer to investigate at first the cortex of psychotic patients, including those we would today diagnose as schizophrenics. In 1887 (9 years before his famous discovery of the typical neurohistological alterations in senile dementia), Alzheimer published a paper in which he described abnormal cortical nerve cells in younger psychotic patients who did not have a known organic brain disease. Alzheimer emphasized that the cortical alterations in some of these psychotic patients were not associated with

gliosis and, therefore, this type of brain disease principally could have a benign outcome. This paper can be regarded as the first neurohistological study in schizophrenics. Alzheimer later wrote: 'everybody who doubts that dementia precox and epilepsy are diseases associated with severe organic alterations, now easily can set aside his doubts'. He believed that senile dementia, dementia praecox and epilepsies, but not manic-depressive disorder and hysteria, were organic brain diseases. This was one of the reasons why in the first half of the 20th century there were numerous neuropathological reports on schizophrenia and epilepsy, but none on affective disorders.

Cortical atrophy also was reported by Southard (1915), who mentioned the association areas of the cerebral cortex as being most affected. Buscaino (1920) described various histopathological changes, mainly in the basal ganglia, which he assumed to be responsible for catatonia-like and stereotyped behaviour. Another approach to the neuropathology of psychiatric diseases had been made by Vogt and Vogt and their coworkers, who reported cellular alterations in the cortex, thalamus and basal ganglia of schizophrenics (Fünfgeld, 1925, 1952; Vogt & Vogt, 1948, 1952; Bäumer, 1954; Hopf, 1954; Buttlar-Brentano, 1956; Treff & Hempel, 1958).

The early neuropathological findings in the cortex, basal ganglia and thalamus of schizophrenics later were heavily criticized by the influential neuropathologist Peters (1967), who regarded the reported neuroanatomical changes, especially the so-called dwarf cells (*Schwundzellen*), as postmortem artefacts or normal variants.

The early neurohistological findings in schizophrenia, although never conclusively disproven, remained controversial and finally were widely forgotten. This might become more understandable in view of the fact that, traditionally, the relation between psychiatry and neuropathology has always been much more problematic than the relation between neurology and neuropathology. With the exception of dementias and the so-called organic psychoses, no such obvious and homogeneous types of brain pathology as seen in neurological disorders have been detected for the major psychiatric illnesses such as schizophrenia, manic-depressive illness, personality disorders and neuroses. This is not surprising for neuroses and personality disorders, which traditionally are thought to be caused by psychosocial factors or to represent variations of normal personality traits and were therefore never the subject of systematic neuropathological studies. Similarly, affective disorders, which are believed by many psychiatrists to be caused by deficits or functional imbalances of neurotransmitter systems, never gained much interest from neuropathologists.

Methodological problems in neuropathological studies in schizophrenia

In addition to the traditional approaches of qualitative neuropathological description, which have proved largely inadequate to characterize psychiatric disorders, the most frequently applied research strategies in modern neuropathological investigations have been volume determinations, cell counts, laterality measures and investigations of glial cells (Bogerts & Lieberman, 1993). There are several critical reviews of the methods applied in anatomical postmortem research in psychiatric diseases (Jellinger, 1985; Benes, 1988; Pakkenberg & Gundersen, 1988; Casanova & Kleinman, 1990; Bogerts & Lieberman, 1993). Some of these methodological problems are now discussed.

Postmortem artefacts

Among the possible sources of error are brain changes secondary to complicating neurological or vascular diseases, preagonal conditions such as protracted coma, chronic diseases of peripheral organs, paraneoplastic limbic encephalopathy (Newman *et al.*, 1990), drugs known to affect brain structures [e.g. corticosteroids (McEwen *et al.*, 1992)], time to fixation, postmortem shrinkage and swelling of brain tissue. In order to exclude brains showing signs of dementia or vascular damage or other neurological diseases, a neuropathological examination on any case under study is necessary.

Validity of diagnosis

If diagnostic constructs such as schizophrenia and affective disorders are composed of various clinical and biological subtypes, large samples of patients are necessary to obtain representative data by which subgroups can be characterized in terms of their brain morphology. This is not an easy task, because it is difficult to collect brains of clinically well-characterized patients that have met all the requirements for provision of optimal material (e.g. the postmortem delay should not exceed a critical time frame, there should be an absence of potentially confounding comorbid conditions, etc.). However, to establish the diagnosis of schizophrenia based on the *Diagnostic and Statistical Manual* DSM-III-R or *International Classification of Disease* ICD-10 criteria is vital and this should be done by two independent psychiatrists by retrospective chart review, or prospectively if possible (e.g. Crow *et al.*, 1989; Bruton *et al.*, 1990).

Control groups

It is important to match patients and control subjects, not only for age and sex, but also as closely as possible for all relevant ante- or post-mortem factors. If all confounding variables cannot be controlled for, multivariate statistical methods (i.e. analysis of covariance, partial correlations, stepwise regression analysis) should be applied to determine whether factors unrelated to the disease have contributed to the group differences.

Is it worthwhile to perform postmortem studies in schizophrenia at all?

One of the main criticisms facing postmortem studies in schizophrenia is that owing to all the shortcomings and artefacts mentioned above, it is impossible to tell from any finding if it is really specific for the disease or only an epiphenomenon. We believe that this is a problem of most research carried out in schizophrenia, but today there is no real alternative to this approach as brain imaging is far beyond visualization, e.g. neurones or glial cells. At the moment, neuropathology with all its problems is one powerful tool in the search for mechanisms causing morphological abnormalities in the brains of schizophrenic patients.

Recent neuropathological findings in schizophrenia

A new era of neuromorphological schizophrenia research was started in the 1980s and received strong impetus from the new brain-imaging techniques. Since then, more than 50 morphometric postmortem studies have been performed. The most prominent pathomorphological findings in schizophrenia are:

ventricular enlargement and regional cortical sulcal enlargement;

limbic system pathology (reduced tissue components, disturbed cytoarchitecture);

thalamic pathology (volume reductions, cell loss);

cytoarchitectural changes in frontal and temporal areas; and

absence of normal structural asymmetry in some cortical regions.

The purpose of this chapter is to list briefly the most important findings in different brain regions of interest and then turn to the question of whether there is a more focal brain pathology in certain brain regions or a diffuse process affecting the whole brain.

Limbic system structures

Since the first report 10 years ago of reduced tissue volume in temporolimbic structures of schizophrenics (Bogerts *et al.*, 1983c), some 30 quantitative or qualitative anatomical postmortem studies in limbic structures of schizophrenics have been published. About 25 of these studies found subtle structural changes in at least one of the investigated areas (Bogerts, 1984, 1985; Kovelman & Scheibel, 1984; Brown *et al.*, 1986; Falkai & Bogerts, 1986, 1989, 1992; Jakob & Beckmann, 1986; Benes & Bird, 1987; Benes *et al.*, 1987, 1991a,b; Colter *et al.*, 1987; Falkai *et al.*, 1988; Crow *et al.*, 1989; Jeste & Lohr, 1989; Altshuler *et al.*, 1990; Bogerts *et al.*, 1990a–c; Arnold *et al.*, 1991; Casanova *et al.*, 1991b; Conrad *et al.*, 1991; Heckers *et al.*, 1991b; Senitz & Winkelmann, 1991; Akbarian *et al.*, 1993b), while four studies yielded entirely negative results (Rosenthal & Bigelow, 1972; Christison *et al.*, 1989; Heckers *et al.*, 1990a,b). The findings comprise reduced volumes or cross-sectional areas of the hippocampus, amygdala and parahippocampal gyrus (Bogerts, 1984, 1985; Brown *et al.*, 1986, Falkai & Bogerts, 1986; Colter *et al.*, 1987; Falkai *et al.*, 1988; Jeste & Lohr, 1989; Bogerts *et al.*, 1990b; Altshuler *et al.*, 1990), which were later corroborated by morphometric magnetic resonance imaging (MRI) studies of mesio-temporal structures (DeLisi *et al.*, 1988; Suddath *et al.*, 1989, 1990; Barta *et al.*, 1990; Becker *et al.*, 1990; Bogerts *et al.*, 1990c; Dauphinais *et al.*, 1990; Rossi *et al.*, 1990; Jernigan *et al.*, 1991). Other findings in limbic brain regions are left temporal horn enlargement (Bogerts, 1985; Brown *et al.*, 1986; Crow *et al.*, 1989), reduced cell numbers or cell size in the hippocampus or parahippocampal gyrus/entorhinal cortex (Falkai & Bogerts, 1986; Jakob & Beckmann, 1986; Falkai *et al.*, 1988; Jeste & Lohr, 1989; Benes *et al.*, 1991b; Casanova *et al.*, 1991b), white matter reductions in the parahippocampal gyrus or hippocampus (Colter *et al.*, 1987; Heckers *et al.*, 1991b), disturbed cytoarchitecture, increased vertical axon numbers and deficits in small interneurones in the cingulate gyrus (Benes *et al.*, 1987, 1991b; Benes & Bird, 1987), abnormal cell arrangements in the hippocampus or entorhinal cortex (Kovelman & Scheibel, 1984; Jakob & Beckmann, 1986; Falkai & Bogerts, 1989, 1992; Arnold *et al.*, 1991; Conrad *et al.*, 1991) and an increased incidence of a cavum septi pellucidi (Degreef *et al.*, 1992). Two groups could not confirm cellular disarray in the hippocampus (Christison *et al.*, 1989; Benes *et al.*, 1991b) and one group could not find significant volume and cell number reductions in the hippocampus and entorhinal cortex (Heckers *et al.*, 1990a,b, 1991b).

Cortex

Alzheimer (1897) was the first to describe pallor and loss of pyramidal cells in the cortex of patients with dementia praecox. In the new era of neuropathological schizophrenia research, there are reports of a reduction of cortical thickness and cell loss in deep cortical layers (Colon, 1972), lower neuronal densities and deficits in small interneurones in the prefrontal cortex and anterior cingulate gyrus (Benes *et al.*, 1986, 1991a), and higher neuronal and glial densities in prefrontal areas 9 and 46 (Selemon *et al.*, 1993).

Three planimetric postmortem studies of the whole cortex have been performed: one reported significant reductions of cortical volume (12%) and central grey matter (6%) (Pakkenberg, 1987); the other two reported virtually identical volumes of cortex, white matter and whole hemispheres in schizophrenics and controls (Rosenthal & Bigelow, 1972; Heckers *et al.*, 1991a). Taking the large biological and clinical heterogeneity of schizophrenia into account, the contradicting results of these planimetric studies are possibly a sampling artefact, which means that much larger samples are required to clarify all, or at least a subgroup of schizophrenics show reduced whole brain measures. A postmortem study of a large number of patients and control subjects will quickly reach limits as the collection and preparation of postmortem brain tissue is costly and time consuming. It is therefore easier to approach this question by using brain-imaging techniques like MRI and computerized tomography (CT) scanning. For further discussion of this question see the section Brain size and weight on p. 280–283.

Basal ganglia

Unchanged volumes of the striatum and external pallidum, a subtle volume decrease in the internal pallidal segment and decreased diameter of the microneurones in the striatum (but only in those with catatonic schizophrenia) (Dom *et al.*, 1981; Stevens, 1986) were found in brains from the preneuroleptic era (Bogerts *et al.*, 1985). A study of patients chronically treated with neuroleptics found bilaterally increased striatal volumes reaching a significant level on the left side (Heckers *et al.*, 1991a); this finding was corroborated in two MRI studies (Jernigan *et al.*, 1991; Swayze *et al.*, 1992). Recently, a follow-up MRI study of first-episode schizophrenics showed that caudate volume might increase under the influence of continuous neuroleptic treatment (Chakos *et al.*, 1993). Thus, the discrepancy in the results of basal ganglia volume measurements might be due to the fact that some patient samples were from the preneuroleptic era and demonstrated no difference, while others had chronic neuroleptic drug treatment, possibly inducing synaptic overgrowth and resulting in a volume increase.

Corpus callosum

Structural anomalies of the midline area of the corpus callosum have been demonstrated by several MRI scanning and postmortem studies (Rosenthal & Bigelow, 1972; Bogerts *et al.*, 1983b; Nasrallah *et al.*, 1983, 1986a; Mathew & Partain, 1985; Uematso & Kaiya, 1988; Günther *et al.*, 1989; Rossi *et al.*, 1989; Raine *et al.*, 1990). The findings, however, are inconsistent; there are reports of increased (Rosenthal & Bigelow, 1972) as well as of decreased (Bogerts *et al.*, 1983b; Rossi *et al.*, 1989) midline areas. More consistent are reports of shape abnormalities, in that the sex difference in anterior and posterior callosal thicknesses in normal controls seems to be reversed in schizophrenics (Nasrallah *et al.*, 1986a; Raine *et al.*, 1990), and the mean curvature in the corpus callosum is more marked in schizophrenics (Casanova *et al.*, 1991a), with the corpus callosum being thicker in female schizophrenics and thinner in male schizophrenics.

Thalamus

Cell loss and reduced tissue volume of medial thalamic structures have already been described several decades ago in schizophrenics of the Vogt collection (Fünfgeld, 1925; Bäumer, 1954; Treff & Hempel, 1958), although these could not later be replicated on the same brain material (Dom *et al.*, 1981; Lesch & Bogerts, 1984). However, two controlled morphometric investigations using different brain collections have again found volume and cell number reductions in the mediodorsal nucleus of the thalamus (Pakkenberg, 1990), or smaller whole thalamic volumes (Bogerts *et al.*, 1993).

Brain-stem transmitter systems

A qualitative report on degenerative changes in the cholinergic basal nucleus of schizophrenics has been published (Averback, 1981). More recent quantitative studies found normal cell numbers in the basal nucleus (Arendt *et al.*, 1983), substantia nigra (Bogerts *et al.*, 1983a) and locus coeruleus of schizophrenics (Lohr & Jeste, 1988). There was, however, a reduced nigral volume and a trend for reduced locus coeruleus volume, taken as indicative of a dopaminergic/noradrenergic underactivity rather than overactivity of these cells in schizophrenics.

Investigating the brain-stem reticular formation in four patients and five controls, Karson *et al.* (1991) found a twofold increase in the number of cholinergic neurones of the pedunculopontine nucleus and the dorsal tegmental nucleus as well as a reduced cell size in the locus coeruleus.

Brain size and weight

A very important issue is whether the neuropathological findings reported above are localized in a few brain regions or reflect only different aspects of a generalized process affecting the whole brain. A considerable number of postmortem, CT and MRI studies have addressed this question, determining whole brain parameters such as brain weight and whole brain or cortical volumes.

Four recent controlled quantitative postmortem studies found significant decreases in brain weight by 5–8% (Brown *et al.*, 1986; Pakkenberg, 1987; Bruton *et al.*, 1990) and a significant reduction (4%) of brain anterior–posterior length (Crow *et al.*, 1989; Bruton *et al.*, 1990), while seven studies found nearly identical brain weight and/or hemispheric volumes in schizophrenics and controls (Rosenthal & Bigelow, 1972; Weinberger *et al.*, 1980; Bogerts *et al.*, 1990c; Heckers *et al.*, 1990a, 1991a,b; Pakkenberg, 1990; Table 15.1). These 11 studies were performed on six different brain collections, three of which gave positive results and three negative results; thus, sampling artefacts may play a role.

In addition to the postmortem studies, we found 21 CT and MRI studies in the literature specifically addressing the question of whole brain, hemispheric or cortical volumes; 14 of them revealed entirely negative results (Table 15.2). Five of these studies found a decrease in cerebral and cranial area, whole brain area, brain slice area, cerebral hemisphere volume and brain volume in schizophrenics (Andreasen *et al.*, 1986; Johnstone *et al.*, 1989a,b; Pearlson *et al.*, 1989; Dauphinais *et al.*, 1990; Zipursky *et al.*, 1991). One paper described reduced cranial and cerebral areas without ventricular enlargement in familial schizophrenia, but the reverse in sporadic schizophrenia (Schwarzkopf *et al.*, 1991).

The postmortem studies presented give equivocal results, whereas the majority of CT and MRI studies dismiss the idea of reduced brain size in a

Table 15.1 Postmortem studies employing whole brain measurements

Reference	Number of patients (and controls)	Findings
Rosenthal and Bigelow (1972)	10(10)	No difference in fresh brain weight; increase in corpus callosum width
Weinberger et al. (1980)	12(35)	Increase in formalin-fixed brain weight in schizophrenics
Brown et al. (1986)	41(29)	Reduction of brain weight; bilateral reduction of parahippocampal thickness; ventricular, especially temporal horn enlargement bilaterally
Pakkenberg (1987)	12(12)	Reduction of total brain weight, hemispheric volumes, cortical volume and central grey matter; increase of ventricular volume
Crow et al. (1989)	56(56)	Reduction of brain length; selective left temporal horn enlargement
Bogerts et al. (1990c)	18(21)	No difference in fresh brain weight; left and right reduced hippocampal volume (new Düsseldorf brain collection)
Bruton et al. (1990)	56(56)	Reduction of fixed brain weight and length; increase of ventricular size; periventricular fibrous gliosis in 50% of schizophrenic patients
Heckers et al. (1990a)	20(20)	No difference in hemispheric volumes; unchanged volume of hippocampus amygdala and ventricular system; significant increase of left ventricular volume in paranoid schizophrenics
Pakkenberg (1990)	12(12)	No difference in brain weight; reduction of total neurone and glial cell numbers in the mediodorsal thalamic nucleus and nucleus accumbens
Heckers et al. (1991b)	13(13)	No difference in hemispheric volumes; reduction of hippocampal white matter; no difference in total cell numbers, cell density and volume of hippocampus; non-significant decrease of absolute cell numbers in the left CA1 region
Heckers et al. (1991a)	23(23)	No difference in fresh and fixed brain weight, volumes of the hemispheres, cortex and white matter; bilateral increase of striatal volume; right-sided increase of pallidal volume

Table 15.2 Computerized tomography (CT) and magnetic resonance imaging (MRI) studies to determine brain volume, length and whole brain area

Reference	Number of patients (and controls)	Imaging technique	Findings
Andreasen *et al.* (1986)	38(49)	MRI	Decreased cerebral and cranial area
Johnstone *et al.* (1989a)	21(20/21)*	MRI	No difference in total brain area
Johnstone *et al.* (1989b)	127(17/38)[†]	CT	Reduction of whole brain area comparing all schizophrenics vs. non-schizophrenics, and chronic schizophrenics vs. neurotics
Pearlson *et al.* (1989)	50(87)	CT	Smaller brain slice area
Barta *et al.* (1990)	15(15)	MRI	No difference in overall brain volume
Rossi *et al.* (1990)	17(13)	MRI	No difference in cerebral area
Andreasen *et al.* (1990)	55(47)	MRI	No difference in cranial and cerebral areas
Dauphinais *et al.* (1990)	28(28)	MRI	Reduction to cerebral hemisphere volume due to volume decrease of the temporal lobes
Shenton *et al.* (1991)	10(12)	MRI	No difference in brain volume
Jernigan *et al.* (1991)	42(24)	MRI	Supratentorial cranial volume non-significantly smaller
Schwarzkopf *et al.* (1991)	31(14)	MRI	Reduced cranial and cerebral areas without ventricular enlargement in familial schizophrenia
Gur *et al.* (1991)	42(43)	MRI	No difference in brain volume
DeLisi *et al.* (1991)	45(20)	MRI	No difference in total brain volume
Zipursky *et al.* (1991)	45(37/37)[‡]	CT	Smaller brain volume
Shenton *et al.* (1991)	15(15)	MRI	No difference in different measurements of whole brain volumes
Breier *et al.* (1992)	44(29)	MRI	No difference in total cranial volume
Zipursky *et al.* (1992)	22(20)	MRI	Less grey matter; no change in white matter; ventricular volume increased by 34%
McCarley *et al.* (1993)	15(14)	MRI	No difference in total intracranial content
Buchanan *et al.* (1993)	41(30)	MRI	No difference in cranial volume
Colombo *et al.* (1993)	18(18)	MRI	No difference for whole brain area
Bilder *et al.* (1993)	70(51)	MRI	No difference in hemispheric volumes

* 20 patients with manic-depressive psychosis and 21 non-psychiatric control subjects.

[†] 17 neurotics and 38 patients with manic-depressive psychosis.

[‡] 37 non-psychiatric control subjects and 37 alcoholics.

substantial number of schizophrenic patients, and therefore rather support the idea of focal pathology in schizophrenia. Subtyping schizophrenia, e.g. in a familial and sporadic subgroup, might help to overcome this problem (Schwarzkopf *et al.*, 1991). However, a lot of the studies presented have their methodological problems and therefore further MRI studies are required to answer this question more definitively.

It is widely believed that during prenatal and postnatal development, brain growth drives skull growth (Davis & Wright, 1977). If the whole brain is smaller in schizophrenics, one might expect reduced head size in some patients with schizophrenia. In a recent investigation (McNeil *et al.*, 1993) it was shown that schizophrenics have disproportionately small head circumferences at birth, providing evidence of disturbed prenatal cerebral development. The finding was significantly related to an absence of a family history of psychosis.

In summary, recent postmortem studies in schizophrenics point to the limbic system as one major locus of pathology. While microscopic changes in the cortex and shape distortion in the corpus callosum were replicable, basal ganglia, thalamus and brain-stem transmitter structures have so far yielded equivocal results. Whole brain parameters support the notion of a focal pathology rather than a generalized process. More studies are required to examine different parts of the brain on the same sample to reach a conclusion on where and to what extent there are neuropathological changes in schizophrenia.

Clues to mechanisms underlying the neuropathological changes

Atrophy or hypoplasia?

According to Kraepelin's concept, dementia praecox is a chronic progressive disease with a poor outcome. Kraepelin therefore assumed a progressive neuropathological process in this disease. Several lines of evidence, however, argue against this assumption and demonstrate that the majority of patients, if not all, have static, non-progressive subtle brain abnormalities resulting from disturbed prenatal brain development. Anatomical findings in favour of subtle abnormalities of prenatal brain development are: (i) a lack of gliosis in affected brain regions, such as limbic structures and thalamus; (ii) cytoarchitectural abnormalities in limbic, frontal and temporal cortical areas; (iii) the absence of normal cortical lateralization; and (iv) a lack of progressive ventricular enlargement in CT and MRI follow-up studies.

Lack of gliosis in limbic structures

The neuroglia, sometimes known as macroglia, consist of the astrocytes, oligodendroglia and ependymal cells. The astrocytes form the majority and are classified as protoplasmic or fibrous forms. Although astrocytes clearly play a structurally supportive role in the nervous system, there are specialized subclasses of astrocytes performing different functions, such as reaction to injury (reactive gliosis). Astrocytes show changes in response to almost every type of injury or disease in the central nervous system. This may take the form of degeneration, hypertrophy or hyperplasia. The capacity of astrocytes to react with proliferation and hypertrophy develops during the last trimester of gestation, and is already evident in the mature newborn. Astrocytosis is not a static process but rather one that evolves with time. Immediately after injury, astrocytes undergo both hyperplasia and hypertrophy in an attempt to repair the damage. These plump cellular elements stain with the glial fibrillary acid protein (GFAP) antibody. As the tissue repair response matures, astrocytic bodies diminish in number, while their fibrils become more prominent. The resultant chronic fibrillary gliosis is best detected by special stains such as the Holzer technique.

From about 50 postmortem studies on schizophrenics published in the last 20 years, 18 specifically addressed the question of gliosis.

Fibrous gliosis. Taking the chronic, sometimes disabling, course in most schizophrenics into account, some researchers have looked for diffuse gliosis. Applying stains, like Holzer staining, for glial fibres, glial knots in the brain stem (Fisman, 1975), diffuse gliosis in the diencephalon, mesencephalon and hippocampus, and fibrous gliosis in the hypothalamus, midbrain tegmentum, bed nucleus of the stria terminalis, basal nucleus, medial thalamus, amygdala and hippocampus were described (Stevens, 1982). Examination of all brain regions using Holzer stain revealed no evidence for gliosis in a brain sample, where cases with focal pathology were excluded (Bruton *et al.*, 1990).

Glial cell counts (astrocytes and oligodendroglia). As outlined before, GFAP staining makes the body of the astroglial cell apparent. Therefore, increased or decreased astroglial cell density can easily be picked up by this staining method. Using GFAP staining, three studies failed to find a significant increase in astrocytes in temporal lobe structures using densitometry — an automated measuring method — (Roberts *et al.*, 1986, 1987) and manual cell counts (Stevens *et al.*, 1988). Astroglial cell densities were unchanged in the anterior cingulate and prefrontal cortex (Benes *et al.*, 1986; Benes & Bird, 1987). An assay of diazepam-binding inhibitor-like immunoreactivity, which is regarded as another marker for gliosis, was applied in one study, parallel to using the Holzer technique in the contralateral hemisphere; however, neither technique showed a difference between groups in any brain region (Crow *et al.*, 1989). Glial cells in general were determined on Nissl-stained sections in five studies. No significant difference between schizophrenics and controls for glial cell densities or absolute glial counts could be detected in the mesencephalon (Bogerts *et al.*, 1983a), prefrontal, anterior cingulate and primary motor cortex (Benes *et al.*, 1986), corpus callosum (Nasrallah *et al.*, 1986a), hippocampus (Falkai & Bogerts, 1986) or entorhinal cortex (Falkai *et al.*, 1988).

The density of astrocytes and oligodendroglia was reduced in the mediodorsal thalamic nucleus and the nucleus accumbens, but was unchanged in the ventral pallidum and basolateral nucleus of the amygdala (Pakkenberg, 1990).

Using Holzer staining, Casanova *et al.* quantified the number of astrocytic markers within the terminal fields of the perforant pathway originating from the entorhinal cortex in schizophrenics, patients with Alzheimer's disease and healthy control subjects. While patients with Alzheimer's disease had astrocytosis, there was an absence of similar changes in the schizophrenic group. The authors concluded that anomalies in the entorhinal cortex are therefore static in nature and occurred many years before the patients were autopsied (Casanova *et al.*, 1991c).

Neurone:glia ratio. The neurone:glia ratios for each layer of the prefrontal, anterior cingulate and primary motor cortex were calculated but showed no difference between schizophrenics and controls (Benes *et al.*, 1986).

Thus, the majority of studies involving glial cell counts, neurone:glial ratios and glial cell nuclei volumes found no difference in temporolimbic structures, thalamus and cingulate gyrus. Although the question of fibrous gliosis (i.e. an increase in glial cell fibres) remains more controversial, in general most studies examining glial cells in schizophrenia dismiss a chronic progressive disease, but support the idea of a static lesion occurring prior to the 20th week of gestation.

Neurohistological indicators of subtle anomalies of prenatal brain development

General considerations. There are three stages in the embryonic development of the cellular elements of the cerebral cortex (Bayer & Altman, 1991).

1 Growth of a large pool of proliferative precursor cells of neurones and glia. This takes place in the germinal matrix (primarily the neuroepithelium and to a lesser extent the subventricular zone) of the cortical primordium.

2 Translocation of differentiating cells into the intermediate zone. The migrating young neurones begin to sprout their axons before they proceed towards the surface of the cortex.

3 Settling of neurones in the future cerebral

cortex, composed of the primordial plexiform layer and the cortical plate.

It is at the latter sites that the final differentiation of neurones, including their dendritic development and synaptic organization, takes place.

Substantial disability may result from disorders of development which do not lead to deformities that are grossly evident at birth. Large numbers of these lesser disturbances may be ascertained only by their functional consequences, such as disturbances of learning, language disorders, autism and recurrent seizures. It is probable that in most instances these milder disorders reflect disturbances of the processes of growth and differentiation (Caviness, 1989).

The findings of abnormal cortical architecture in schizophrenics (reviewed below) are strong indicators that many patients have a disorder of the third stage of brain development, that is the settling of neurones in the cerebral cortex.

Cytoarchitectural abnormalities in schizophrenia. Subtle cytoarchitectural anomalies were described in the hippocampal formation (McLardy, 1974; Scheibel & Kovelman, 1981; Kovelman & Scheibel, 1984; Conrad *et al.*, 1991), frontal cortex, cingulate gyrus (Benes *et al.*, 1986; Benes & Bird, 1987) and entorhinal cortex (Jakob & Beckmann, 1986; Falkai & Bogerts, 1989, 1992; Arnold *et al.*, 1991) of patients suffering from schizophrenia compared with control subjects.

McLardy (1974) found a significant thinning of the granular layer of the dentate gyrus in 30% of schizophrenic patients, 100% of chronic alcoholics and in none of the controls. The cell picture in schizophrenia did not have a degenerative appearance, but was fully consistent with developmental arrest.

Qualitatively, and later quantitatively, a significant cellular disarray in the CA3/CA4 interface was described in the left hippocampus (Scheibel & Kovelman, 1981; Kovelman & Scheibel, 1984) and replicated in the right hippocampus (Conrad *et al.*, 1991). This was interpreted as a bilateral migrational abnormality and broadly correlated with the degree of disease severity. Altshuler *et al.* (1987) were not able to fully replicate the study,

but did confirm a within-case correlation with severity, whereas Christison *et al.* (1989) did not find a significant disarray in schizophrenics.

On Nissl-stained sections the neuronal density was significantly lower in layer VI of the prefrontal, layer V of the cingulate and layer III of the motor cortex (Benes *et al.*, 1986). In a subsequent study, clusters of cells were found in the anterior cingulate cortex of schizophrenic patients; these cells were smaller in size and separated by wider distances than those observed in the control group (Benes & Bird, 1987). This finding was supported by a 25% increase of vertical axons in the cingulate cortex in schizophrenics (Benes *et al.*, 1987).

An abnormal sulcogyral pattern or abnormal gross configuration of the temporal lobe and cytoarchitectonic abnormalities of the rostral entorhinal region as well as of the ventral insular cortex of schizophrenics have been recently described (Jakob & Beckmann, 1986, 1989). The cytoarchitectonic abnormalities of the rostral entorhinal region consisted of heterotopic pre-alpha cells in the pre-beta layer (third layer), which would normally belong to the pre-alpha layer (second layer).

Rating abnormally positioned (heterotopic) pre-alpha cell clusters in the entorhinal cortex, we found a significant increase in the mean rating values in schizophrenics on the left side by 43% ($P < 0.03$). Patients with a family history of psychiatric illness, compared with schizophrenics without such a history, had significantly more heterotopic clusters on the left side ($+49\%$, $P < 0.01$), but did not differ on the right side. There was a trend for an inversive correlation between onset of the disease and the heterotopic ratings in the left entorhinal cortex ($r = -0.298$; $P < 0.10$), suggesting that earlier onset of the disease is associated with more heterotopias in the left entorhinal cortex (Falkai & Bogerts, 1992; Falkai *et al.*, 1993a).

In a recent study on the dorsolateral prefrontal area of five schizophrenics, a significant decline in nicotinamide adenine dinucleotide phosphate diaphorase (NADPH-d) neurones in the superficial white matter and in the overlying cortex, but a significant increase in these neurones in the deeper white matter, was demonstrated compared with the same number of matched controls (Akbarian *et al.* 1993a). Subsequently, the same group analysed the distribution of NADPH-d-expressing neurones in the lateral and medial temporal lobes of seven schizophrenics and seven matched controls. The schizophrenics had significantly lower numbers of NADPH-d neurones in the hippocampal formation and in the neocortex of the lateral temporal lobe but significantly greater numbers of these neurones in the adjacent white matter (Akbarian *et al.*, 1993b).

The cytoarchitectonic abnormalities recently described in different limbic structures, prefrontal and temporal cortex of schizophrenics are very subtle and will easily be missed using classical neuropathological methods. It is unlikely that the subtle differences seen in a substantial subgroup of the patients are due to disturbances in the proliferative or early migrational phase, but rather are caused by disturbances in the late migration or final differentiation of neurones that takes place in the second and third trimesters of pregnancy.

Absence of normal cortical lateralization

Development of normal cerebral lateralization. The two hemispheres of the human brain are neither functional nor structural mirror images of each other. The extent of data now available indicating reliable right–left neuroanatomical asymmetry is growing. The asymmetry is most marked in the temporoparietal region, the same region noted by the classical neuroanatomists to show the greatest variation among individuals. Morphological asymmetries are visible very early on in brain development, e.g. Sylvian fissure (SF) asymmetry can be traced in the 29th week of gestation (Wada *et al.*, 1975).

From the 50 postmortem studies reviewed above, 22 examined both brain hemispheres; eight found changes in the left side, two changes in the right side, five bilateral changes and in seven studies there either were negative findings or it was not clear which hemisphere had been investigated. Four studies (Brown *et al.*, 1986; Crow *et al.*, 1989; Falkai & Bogerts, 1992; Falkai *et al.*,

1992b) examined diagnosis-by-side interactions and three (Brown *et al.*, 1986; Crow *et al.*, 1989; Falkai *et al.*, 1992b) found a significant interaction for the left hemisphere.

Crow *et al.* (1989) reported that in schizophrenia the size of the posterior, and particularly the temporal, horn was increased (by 28 and 82%, respectively), while in Alzheimer-type dementia a relatively uniform increase in area of the ventricular components was observed. Diagnosis-by-side interaction revealed a selective enlargement of the left temporal horn in schizophrenics compared with normal controls and the Alzheimer patients. Excluding all brains with neuropathological signs of significant disease, the brains of 22 schizophrenics and 26 controls were reanalysed and yielded the same result. The authors concluded that these findings are consistent with the view that schizophrenia is a disorder of the genetic mechanism that controls the development of cerebral asymmetry.

We examined the SF and planum temporale in two subsequent postmortem studies (Falkai *et al.*, 1992a). Both structures belong to the most asymmetrical anatomical areas in the human brain, are usually longer or bigger in the left compared with the right hemisphere and seem to represent the morphological correlate for lateralized functions in humans, e.g. language and handedness.

In the first study the SF length was measured postmortem in the brains of 35 schizophrenic patients and 33 matched non-psychiatric control subjects of the new Düsseldorf brain collection. The schizophrenics showed a significantly reduced length of the left SF (-16%, $P < 0.0001$) compared with the control subjects, while the right SF length was unchanged. SF asymmetry, expressed as left:right SF length ratio, was more reduced in male schizophrenics (-24%, $P < 0.001$) than in female patients (-16%, $P < 0.03$; Falkai *et al.*, 1992b).

Recently, a significant ($P < 0.002$) reduction in brain length, a relative reduction in SF length on the left side and a reduction in the vertical distance between the Sylvian point and the dorsal surface of the brain on the left side were found, thereby replicating the finding mentioned above

(Crow *et al.*, 1992).

As there is a correlation between the area of the planum temporale and the length of the SF (Steinmetz, personal communication), we determined in a second study the volume of the cortical structures underlying the planum temporale by use of planimetry on serial sections of Nissl- and myelin-stained whole brain coronal sections of postmortem brains from 29 schizophrenic patients and 30 matched non-psychiatric control subjects. The underlying cortical volume of the planum temporale was significantly reduced on the left side (-17%, $P < 0.03$) but unchanged on the right side in female patients and even increased in male patients. The mean anterior−posterior diameter of the planum temporale was significantly reduced in the left hemisphere (-16%, $P < 0.017$) but unchanged on the right side. Planum temporale asymmetry expressed as a laterality index, introduced by Galaburda *et al.* (1987), was significantly reduced in schizophrenics ($P < 0.04$); this was more obvious in male patients (Falkai *et al.*, 1992a).

Further evidence for asymmetrical findings in schizophrenia comes from MRI and CT scan studies. Bogerts *et al.* (1990a) found a significant volume reduction of the left hippocampus accompanied by a significant increase of the left temporal horn in first-episode schizophrenia. Determining the volumes of all major cortical regions from the MRI scans of 70 schizophrenic patients and 51 control subjects, Bilder *et al.* (1993) found a lack of normal hemispheral asymmetries in the posterior, premotor and prefrontal regions. Likewise, on the CT scans of 135 schizophrenic patients, 131 non-psychiatric control subjects and 102 psychiatric controls — including patients with affective psychosis, addiction and personality disorders — a significant reduction of frontal (5%, $P < 0.0001$) and occipital (3%, $P < 0.022$) asymmetry was found in schizophrenics compared with both control groups. There was no difference between the two control groups, suggesting a specific reduction of hemispheral asymmetries in schizophrenia (Falkai *et al.*, 1993).

The growing evidence from postmortem, MRI

scanning and CT scanning studies indicating an absence of normal cerebral asymmetry in cortical and limbic areas suggests disturbed brain lateralization at early stages of brain development. This does not seem unique for schizophrenia. Functional studies suggest that abnormal functioning of the left hemisphere is also present in autism, a disease which has several symptoms in common with schizophrenia. This evidence is based on studies of cognitive abilities (Dawson & Adams, 1984), handedness (Colby & Parkinson, 1977), clinical electroencephalograms (Small, 1975), neuropsychological testing and measures of hemispheric activity during speech and other stimuli (Blackstock, 1978).

Lack of progressive ventricular enlargement in CT and MRI follow-up studies

The evidence for a neurodevelopmental basis to schizophrenia is substantial; whether structural abnormalities progress over the course of chronic illness is an independent issue. To date, six studies have examined the progressive nature of lateral ventricular enlargement in schizophrenic patients by performing follow-up CT or MRI scans on two occasions. Four prospective CT-scan studies found no evidence of progressive lateral ventricular enlargement (Nasrallah *et al.*, 1986b; Illowsky *et al.*, 1988; Vita *et al.*, 1988; Sponheim *et al.*, 1991). Using MRI, Degreef *et al.* (1991) have reported no overall change in ventricular or cortical volume on re-examination of first-episode patients and controls 1−2 years later. On the other hand, one prospective study found a significant increase in ventricular size among 18 schizophrenic patients over a 3-year period, with the increase being especially prominent in four of the patients (Kemali *et al.*, 1989).

In addition to the prospective studies, Woods *et al.* (1990) carried out a retrospective analysis using hospital files and reported a significant increase in ventricular size for nine schizophrenic patients and no increase for nine bipolar patients. In sum, four out of five prospective CT and MRI studies show no progressive ventricular enlargement in schizophrenia, suggesting a neurodevelopmental aetiology and not a chronic progressive disease underlying schizophrenia.

In summary, when looking for possible mechanisms underlying the pathomorphological changes in the brains of schizophrenics, a neurodevelopmental model is presently favoured. Lack of a significant degree of gliosis, the presence of neurohistological indicators of disturbed prenatal brain development, reduced normal cortical lateralization and the lack of progressive ventricular enlargement rather dismiss the idea of a chronic progressive brain lesion, but point to a disturbance of brain development at an early stage in schizophrenia.

Conclusion

After the early stages of neuropathological research in schizophrenia proved largely unsuccessful, substantial progress in unravelling the anatomical correlates of the disease have been made in the last 10 years. Recent postmortem studies on schizophrenics described a multitude of morphological changes in different brain structures. The most often reported structural alterations are in the limbic system, mainly in the hippocampal formation and parahippocampal and cingulate gyri. However, other structures such as the thalamus, frontal and temporal cortex and basal ganglia seem to be affected too. These changes represent focal rather than general brain pathology and, at least in the majority of patients, are non-progressive and notably neurodevelopmental in origin. Disturbed cerebral lateralization is present in a substantial proportion of schizophrenic patients and can be taken as an additional indicator of abnormal early brain development. Despite the increasing number of postmortem and brain-imaging studies demonstrating various types of subtle brain anomalies in schizophrenics, there is as yet no evidence for a specific and homogeneous pathoanatomical substratum characteristic for all patients diagnosed as schizophrenic. Brain-imaging and postmortem studies show considerable overlap of the neuroanatomical data with control subjects; most patients have values in the normal range, even if the means are statistically different. There is now evidence that the anatomical anomalies in at least a substantial subgroup of schizophrenics are localized in brain systems; the functional significance became known relatively late and therefore was overlooked in the first half of this century. The best example is the limbic system, the function of which was first proposed by McLean in 1952.

The pathomorphological changes in schizophrenia are subtle and not comparable in magnitude with the brain tissue loss seen in the well-known degenerative brain disorders. An additional difference from the neurodegenerative disorders is that, at least in most patients, the structural changes are not progressive and were acquired very early in life (Weinberger, 1987; Bogerts, 1989; Bogerts *et al.*, 1990a; Crow, 1990; Jones & Murray, 1991; Roberts, 1991; Waddington, 1993).

A problem in relating the pathomorphological findings with the clinical subtypes of schizophrenia is that different types of symptoms (e.g. positive and negative symptoms, catatonic behaviour and hallucinations) can occur simultaneously or in alternating periods in the same patient. The reported neuroanatomical changes, however, are believed by most authors to be stable over time and not as mutable as the psychopathology is. One answer to this problem is that the neuroanatomical findings can be considered as only one component of many pathophysiological and psychosocial factors which contribute to the clinical picture of schizophrenia. There are convincing arguments linking positive and negative psychotic symptoms to biochemical factors such as an imbalance of cerebral dopaminergic (Meltzer & Stahl, 1976; McKenna, 1987) and cholinergic (Tandon & Greden, 1990) mechanisms. Moreover, the role of psychosocial factors, e.g. stress, in precipitating acute psychotic symptoms (Zubin & Spring, 1977; Curran & Cirelli, 1988), and the consequences of long-term hospitalization and social depravation for the development of syndromes similar to negative schizophrenia are well known.

We believe that the various types of structural abnormalities in the brains of schizophrenics are vulnerability or trait markers. These predispose the brain to decompensate under the influence of additional factors related to the vulnerable age period between puberty and old age; these factors include late myelination in the frontal or limbic cortex (Weinberger, 1987; Benes, 1989), steroid hormones (Bogerts, 1989), abnormal synaptic sprouting (Stevens, 1992) or psychosocial stressors (Zubin & Spring, 1977) and lead to the development of the typical clinical picture of schizophrenia.

Acknowledgements

We acknowledge support by the Deutsche Forschungsgemeinschaft (Bo 799/1–4) and the Stanley Foundation.

References

Akbarian, S., Bunney, W.E., Potkin, S.G. *et al.* (1993a) Altered distribution of nicotinamide-adenine dinucleotide phosphate-diaphorase cells in frontal lobe of schizophrenics implies disturbances of cortical development. *Archives of General Psychiatry*, **50**, 169–177.

Akbarian, S., Vinuela, A., Kim, J.J., Potkin, S.G., Bunney, W.E. & Jones, E.G. (1993b) Distorted distribution of nicotinamide-adenine dinucleotide phosphate-diaphorase neurons in temporal lobe in schizophrenics implies anomalous cortical development. *Archives of General Psychiatry*, **50**, 178–187.

Altshuler, L.L., Casanova, M.F., Goldberg, T.E. & Kleinman, J.E. (1990) The hippocampus and parahippocampus in schizophrenic, suicide, and control brains. *Archives of General Psychiatry*, **47**, 1029–1034.

Altshuler, L.L., Conrad, A., Kovelman, J.A. & Scheibel, A. (1987) Hippocampal pyramidal cell orientation in schizophrenia. *Archives of General Psychiatry*, **44**, 1094–1098.

Alzheimer, A. (1897) Beiträge zur pathologischen Anatomie der Hirnrinde und zur anatomischen Grundlage der Psychosen. *Monatsschrift Psychiatrie und Neurologie*, **2**, 82–120.

Andreasen, N., Ehrhardt, J.C., Swayze, V.W. *et al.* (1990) Magnetic resonance imaging of the brain in schizophrenia. *Archives of General Psychiatry*, **47**, 35–44.

Andreasen, N., Nasrallah, H.A., Dunn, V. *et al.* (1986) Structural abnormalities in the frontal system in schizophrenia. *Archives of General Psychiatry*, **43**, 136–144.

Arendt, T., Bigl, Y., Arendt, A. & Tennstedt, A. (1983) Loss of neurons in the nucleus basalis of Meynert in Alzheimer's disease, paralysis agitans and Korsakoff's disease. *Acta Neuropathologica*, **61**, 101–108.

Arnold, S.E., Hyman, B.T., Van Hösen, G.W. & Damasio, A.R. (1991) Some cytoarchitectural abnormalities of the entorhinal cortex in schizophrenia. *Archives of General Psychiatry*, **48**, 625–632.

Averback, P. (1981) Lesions of the nucleus ansae peduncularis in neuropsychiatric disease. *Archives of Neurology*, **38**, 230–235.

Barta, P.E., Pearlson, G.D., Powers, R.E., Richards, S.S. & Tune, L.E. (1990) Auditory hallucinations and smaller superior temporal gyral volume in schizophrenia. *American Journal of Psychiatry*, **147**, 1457–1462.

Bäumer, H. (1954) Veränderungen des Thalamus bei Schizophrenie. *Journal für Hirnforschung*, **1**, 157–172.

Bayer, S.A. & Altman, J. (1991) *Neocortical Development*, pp. 3–10. Raven Press, New York.

Becker, T., Elmer, K., Mechela, B. *et al.* (1990) MRI findings in medial temporal lobe structures in schizophrenia. *European Neuropsychopharmacology*, **1**, 83–86.

Benes, F.M. (1988) Post-mortem structural analyses of schizophrenic brain: study designs and the interpretation of data. *Psychiatric Developments*, **3**, 213–226.

Benes, F.M. (1989) Myelination of cortical–hippocampal relays during late adolescence. *Schizophrenic Bulletin*, **15**, 585–593.

Benes, F.M. & Bird, E.D. (1987) An analysis of the arrangement of neurons in the cingulate cortex of schizophrenic patients. *Archives of General Psychiatry*, **44**, 608–616.

Benes, F.M., Davidson, B. & Bird, E.D. (1986) Quantitative cytoarchitectural studies of the cerebral cortex of schizophrenics. *Archives of General Psychiatry*, **43**, 31–35.

Benes, F.M., Sorensen, I. & Bird, E.D. (1991b) Reduced neuronal size in posterior hippocampus of schizophrenic patients. *Schizophrenia Bulletin*, **17(4)**, 597–608.

Benes, F.M., Majocha, R., Bird, E.D. & Marotta, C.A. (1987) Increased vertical axon numbers in cingulate cortex of schizophrenics. *Archives of General Psychiatry*, **44**, 1017–1021.

Benes, F.M., McSparren, J., Bird, E.D., SanGiovanni, J.P. & Vincent, S.L. (1991a) Deficits in small interneurons in prefrontal and cingulate cortices of schizophrenic and schizoaffective patients. *Archives of General Psychiatry*, **48**, 996–1001.

Bilder, R.M., Wu, H., Degreef, G. *et al.* (1993) Yakovlevian Torque is absent in first-episode schizophrenia. *Schizophrenia Research*, **9(2,3)**, 193.

Blackstock, E.G. (1978) Cerebral asymmetry and the development of early infantile autism. *Journal of Autism and Childhood Schizophrenia*, **8**, 339–353.

Bogerts, B. (1984) Zur Neuropathologie der Schizophrenien. *Fortschritte der Neurologie-Psychiatrie*, **52**, 428–437.

Bogerts, B. (1985) Schizophrenien als Erkrankungen des limbischen Systems. In Huber, G. (ed.) *Basisstadien Endogener Psychosen und das Borderline-Problem*, pp. 163–179. Schattauer, Stuttgart.

Bogerts, B. (1989) Limbic and paralimbic pathology in schizophrenia: interaction with age and stress-related factors. In Schulz, S.C. & Tamminga, C.A. (eds) *Schizophrenia: Scientific Progress*, pp. 216–227. Oxford University Press, Oxford.

Bogerts, B. & Lieberman, J. (1993) Neuropathology in the study of psychiatric disease. In Andreasen, N.A. & Sato, M.

(eds) *International Review of Psychiatry*, Vol. 1, pp. 515–555. American Psychiatric Press, Washington DC.

Bogerts, B., Häntsch, H. & Herzer, M. (1983a) A morphometric study of the dopamine-containing cell groups in the mesencephalon of normals, Parkinson patients and schizophrenics. *Biological Psychiatry*, **18**, 951–971.

Bogerts, B., Meertz, E. & Schönfeldt-Bausch, R. (1983c) Limbic system pathology in schizophrenia: a controlled post mortem study VII: World Congress of Psychiatry, [Abstract F6], Vienna, Austria, p. 267.

Bogerts, B., Meertz, E. & Schönfeld-Bausch, R. (1985) Basal ganglia and limbic system pathology in schizophrenia. *Archives of General Psychiatry*, **42**, 784–791.

Bogerts, B., David, S., Falkai, P. & Tapernon-Franz, U. (1990b) Quantitative evaluation of astrocyte densities in schizophrenia (Abstract P-13-1-22). Presented at the *17th Congress of the Collegium Internationale Neuro-Psychopharmacologicum, Kyoto*, Japan, Vol. II, p. 272.

Bogerts, B., Falkai, P., Greve, B., Pfeiffer, U. & Schneider, T. (1993) Volumes of thalamic, limbic structures and basal ganglia in chronic schizophrenia. A controlled post-mortem study from the New Düsseldorf Brain Collection. *Schizophrenia Research*, **9**(2–3), 146–147.

Bogerts, B., Lesch, A., Lange, H., Zech, M. & Tutsch, J. (1983b) Hypotrophy of the corpus callosum in schizophrenia. *Neuroscience Letters*, (Suppl. 14), **34**, 534.

Bogerts, B., Ashtari, M., Degreef, G., Alvir, J.Ma.J., Bilder, R.M. & Lieberman, J.A. (1990a) Reduced temporal limbic structure volumes on magnetic resonance images in first-episode schizophrenia. *Psychiatry Research: Neuroimaging*, **35**, 1–13.

Bogerts, B., Falkai, P., Haupts, M. *et al.* (1990c) Post-mortem volume measurements of limbic system and basal ganglia structures in chronic schizophrenics. *Schizophrenia Research*, **3**, 295–301.

Breier, A., Buchanan, R.W., Elkashef, A., Munson, R.C., Kirkpatrick, B. & Gellad, F. (1992) Brain morphology and schizophrenia. A magnetic resonance imaging study of limbic, prefrontal cortex and caudate structures. *Archives of General Psychiatry*, **49**, 921–926.

Brown, R., Colter, N., Corsellis, J.A.N. *et al.* (1986) Post-mortem evidence of structural brain changes in schizophrenia. Differences in brain weight, temporal horn area and parahippocampal gyrus compared with affective disorder. *Archives of General Psychiatry*, **43**, 36–42.

Bruton, C.J., Crow, T.J. Frith, C.D., Johnstone, E.C., Owens, D.G.C. & Roberts, G.W. (1990) Schizophrenia and the brain: a prospective cliniconeuropathological study. *Psychological Medicine*, **20**, 285–304.

Buchanan, R.W., Breier, A., Kirkpatrick, B. *et al.* (1993) Structural abnormalities in deficit and nondeficit schizophrenia. *American Journal of Psychiatry*, **150**, 59–65.

Buscaino, V.M. (1920) Le cause anatoma-patologiche della manifestatione schizophrenic delle demenza precoce. *Rivista Patol Nerv Ment*, **25**, 197–226.

Buttlar-Brentano, K. (1956) Zur weiteren Kenntnis der Veränderungen des Basalkerns bei Schizophrenen. *Journal für Hirnforschung*, **2**, 271–291.

Casanova, M.F. & Kleinman, J.E. (1990) The neuropathology of schizophrenia: a critical assessment of research methodologies. *Biological Psychiatry*, **27**, 353–362.

Casanova, M.F., Stevens, J.R. & Kleinman, J.E. (1991c) Quantitation of astrocytes in the molecular layer of the dentate gyrus: a study in schizophrenia and Alzheimer's disease patients. *Psychiatry Research* (in press).

Casanova, M., Atkinson, D., Goldberg, T. *et al.* (1991a) A quantitative morphometric study of the corpus callosum and cingulate cortex in schizophrenia. In Racagni, G. *et al.* (eds) *Biological Psychiatry*, pp. 373–375. Elsevier, Amsterdam.

Casanova, M.F., Saunder, R., Altshuler, L. *et al.* (1991b) Entorhinal cortex pathology in schizophrenia and affective disorders. In Racagni, G. *et al.* (eds) *Biological Psychiatry*, pp. 504–506. Elsevier, Amsterdam.

Caviness, V.S. (1989) Normal development of cerebral neocortex. In Evrard, P. & Minkowski, A. (eds) *Developmental Neurobiology*. Nestle Nutrition Workshop Series, Vol. 12, pp. 1–10. Raven Press, New York.

Chakos, M.H., Lieberman, J.A., Bilder, R.M., Lerner, G., Bogerts, B. & Ashtari, M. (1993) Prospective MRI study of caudate pathomorphology in first episode schizophrenia. *Schizophrenia Research*, **9**, 196.

Christison, G.W., Casanova, M.F., Weinberger, D.R., Rawlings, R. & Kleinman, J.E. (1989) A quantitative investigation of hippocampal pyramidal cell size, shape and variability of orientation in schizophrenia. *Archives of General Psychiatry*, **46**, 1027–1032.

Colby, K.M. & Parkinson, C. (1977) Handedness in autistic children. *Journal of Autism and Childhood Schizophrenia*, **7**, 3–9.

Colombo, C., Abbruzzese, M., Livian, S. *et al.* (1993) Memory functions and temporal-limbic morphology in schizophrenia. *Psychiatry Research*, **243**, 244–248.

Colon, E.J. (1972) Quantitative cytoarchitectonics of the human cerebral cortex in schizophrenic dementia. *Acta Neuropathologica*, **20**, 1–10.

Colter, N., Battal, S., Crow, T.J., Johnstone, E.C., Brown, R. & Bruton, C.L. (1987) White matter reduction in the parahippocampal gyrus of patients with schizophrenia. *Archives of General Psychiatry*, **44**, 1023.

Conrad, A.J., Abebe, T., Austin, R., Forsythe, S. & Scheibel, A.B. (1991) Hippocampal cell disarray in schizophrenia. *Archives of General Psychiatry*, **48**, 413–417.

Crow, T.J. (1990) Temporal lobe asymmetries as the key to the etiology of schizophrenia. *Schizophrenia Bulletin*, **16**(3), 434–443.

Crow, T.J., Brown, R., Bruton, C.J., Frith, C.D., & Gray, V. (1992) Loss of Sylvian fissure asymmetry in schizophrenia: findings in the Runwell 2 series of brains. *Schizophrenia Research*, **6**(2), 152–153.

Crow, T.J., Ball, J., Bloom, St R. *et al.* (1989) Schizophrenia as an anomaly of development of cerebral asymmetry. *Archives of General Psychiatry*, **46**, 1145–1150.

Curran, J.P. & Cirelli, V.A. (1988) The role of psychosocial factors in the etiology, course and outcome of schizophrenia. In Tsuang, M.T. & Simpson, J.C. (eds) *Handbook of Schizophrenia*, Vol. 3, pp. 275–297. Elsevier, Amsterdam.

Dauphinais, D.I., DeLisi, L.E., Crow, T.J. *et al.* (1990)

Reduction in temporal lobe size in siblings with schizo-phrenia: a magnetic resonance imaging study. *Psychiatry Research: Neuroimaging*, **35**, 137–147.

Davis, P.J.M. & Wright, E.A. (1977) A new method for measuring cranial cavity volume and its application to the assessment of cerebral atrophy at autopsy. *Neuropathology and Applied Neurobiology*, **3**, 341–358.

Dawson, G. & Adams, A. (1984) Imitation and social respon-siveness in autistic children. *Journal of Abnormal Child Psychiatry*, **12**, 209–225.

Degreef, G., Ashtari, M., Wu, H., Borenstein, M., Geisler, S. & Lieberman, J. (1991) Follow up MRI study in first-episode schizophrenia. *Schizophrenia Research*, **5**, 204–206.

Degreef, G., Bogerts, B., Falkai, P. *et al.* (1992) Increased prevalence of the cavum septum pellucidum in MRI scans and postmortem brains of schizophrenic patients. *Psychiatry Research: Neuroimaging*, **45**, 1–13.

DeLisi, L.E., Dauphinais, I.D. & Gershon, E. (1988) Perinatal complications and reduced size of brain limbic structures in familial schizophrenia. *Schizophrenia Bulletin*, **14**, 185–191.

DeLisi, L.E., Hoff, A.L., Schwartz, J.E. *et al.* (1991) Brain morphology in first-episode schizophrenic-like psychotic patients: a quantitative magnetic resonance imaging study. *Biological Psychiatry*, **29**, 159–175.

Dom, R., de Saedeler, J., Bogerts, B. & Hopf, A. (1981) Quantitative cytometric analysis of basal ganglia in catatonic schizophrenics. In Perris, C., Strauwe, G., Jonsson, B. *et al.* (eds) *Biological Psychiatry*, pp. 723–726. Elsevier, Amsterdam.

Falkai, P. & Bogerts, B. (1986) Cell loss in the hippocampus of schizophrenics. *European Archives of Psychiatry and Neuro-logical Sciences*, **236**, 154–161.

Falkai, P. & Bogerts, B. (1989) Morphometric evidence for developmental disturbances in brains of some schizo-phrenics. *Schizophrenia Research*, **2(1–2)**, 99.

Falkai, P. & Bogerts, B. (1992) The neuropathology of schizo-phrenia. Limbic system, brain development and cerebral dominance. *European Neuropsychopharmacology*, **2(3)**, 235–236.

Falkai, P., Bogerts, B. & Rozumek, M. (1988) Cell loss and volume reduction in the entorhinal cortex of schizophrenics. *Biological Psychiatry*, **24**, 515–521.

Falkai, P., Bogerts, B., Schneider, Th. & Greve, B. (1993b) Reduced frontal and occipital lobe asymmetry on the CT-scans of schizophrenic patients. Its specifity and clinical significance. *Schizophrenia Research*, **9(2,3)**, 198.

Falkai, P., Bogerts, B., Greve, B. *et al.* (1992a) Reduced Sylvian fissure and planum temporale asymmetry in schizo-phrenia. Evidence for disturbed left hemispheric neuro-development? *Schizophrenia Research*, **6(2)**, 152.

Falkai, P., Bogerts, B., Greve, B. *et al.* (1992b) Loss of Sylvian fissure asymmetry in schizophrenia. A quantitative post mortem study. *Schizophrenia Research*, **7**, 23–32.

Fisman, M. (1975) The brain stem in psychosis. *British Journal of Psychiatry*, **126**, 414–422.

Fünfgeld, E.W. (1925) Pathologische-anatomische Unter-suchungen bei Dementia praecox mit besonderer Berück-sichtigung des Thalamus opticus. *Zeitschrift für Gesellschaft Neurologie und Psychiatrie*, **95**, 411–463.

Fünfgeld, E.W. (1952) Der Nucleus anterior thalami bei Schizophrenie. *Journal für Hirnforschung*, **1**, 147–155.

Galaburda, A.M. Corsiglia, J., Rosen, G.D. & Sherman, G.F. (1987) Planum temporale asymmetry, reappraisal since Geschwind and Levitsky. *Neuropsychologia*, **25**, 853–868.

Günther, W., Moser, E., Petsch, R., Brodie, J.D., Steinberg, R. & Streck, P. (1989) Pathological cerebral blood flow and corpus callosum abnormalities in schizophrenia: relations to EEG mapping and Pet data. *Psychiatry Research*, **29**, 453–455.

Gur, R.E., Mozley, D.P., Resnick, S.M. *et al.* (1991) Magnetic resonance imaging in schizophrenia. *Archives of General Psychiatry*, **48**, 407–412.

Heckers, S., Heinsen, H., Geiger, B. & Beckmann, H. (1991a) Hippocampal neuron number in schizophrenia. *Archives of General Psychiatry*, **48**, 1002–1008.

Heckers, S., Heinsen, H., Heinsen, Y. & Beckmann, H. (1990a) Morphometry of the parahippocampal gyrus in schizophrenics and controls. Some anatomical consider-ations. *Journal of Neural Transmission*, **80**, 151–155.

Heckers, S., Heinsen, H., Heinsen, Y.C. & Beckmann, H. (1990b) Limbic structures and lateral ventricle in schizo-phrenia. *Archives of General Psychiatry*, **47**, 1016–1022.

Heckers, S., Heinsen, H., Heinsen, Y. & Beckmann, H. (1991b) Cortex, white matter, and basal ganglia in schizo-phrenia: a volumetric post mortem study. *Biological Psy-chiatry*, **29**, 556–566.

Hopf, A. (1954) Orientierende Untersuchung zur Frage patho-anatomischer Veränderungen im Pallidum und Striatum bei Schizophrenie. *Journal für Hirnforschung*, **1**, 97–145.

Illowsky, B.P., Juliano, D.M., Bigelow, L.B. & Weinberger, D.R. (1988) Stability of CT scan findings in schizophrenia: results of an 8-year follow-up study. *Journal of Neurology, Neurosurgery and Psychiatry*, **56**, 209–213.

Jackob, H. & Beckmann, H. (1986) Prenatal developmental disturbances in the limbic allocortex in schizophrenics. *Journal of Neural Transmission*, **65**, 303–326.

Jakob, H. & Beckmann, H. (1989) Gross and histological criteria for developmental disorders in brains of schizo-phrenics. *Journal of the Royal Society of Medicine*, **82(8)**, 466–469.

Jellinger, K.A. (1985) Neuromorphological background of pathochemical studies in major psychoses. In Beckmann, H. & Riederer, P. (eds) *Pathochemical Markers in Major Psychoses*, 1–23. Springer-Verlag, Heidelberg.

Jernigan, T.L., Zisook, S., Heaton, R.K., Moranville, J.T., Hellelink, J.R. & Braff, D.L. (1991) Magnetic resonance imaging abnormalities in lenticular nuclei and cerebral cortex in schizophrenia. *Archives of General Psychiatry*, **48**, 881–890.

Jeste, D.V. & Lohr, J.B. (1989) Hippocampal pathologic findings in schizophrenia. A morphometric study. *Archives of General Psychiatry*, **46**, 1019–1024.

Johnstone, E.C., Owens, D.G., Crow, T.J. *et al.* (1989a) Temporal lobe structure as determined by nuclear magnetic resonance in schizophrenia and bipolar affective dis-order. *Journal of Neurology, Neurosurgery and Psychiatry*, **52**, 736–741.

Johnstone, E.C., Owens, D.G.C., Bydder, G.M., Colter, N.,

Crow, T.J. & Frith, C.D. (1989b) The spectrum of structural brain changes in schizophrenia: age of onset as a predictor of cognitive and clinical impairments and their cerebral correlates. *Psychological Medicine*, **19**, 91–103.

Jones, P. & Murray, R.M. (1991) The genetics of schizophrenia is the genetics of neurodevelopment. *British Journal of Psychiatry*, **158**, 615–623.

Karson, C.N., Garcia-Rill, E., Biedermann, J.A., Mrak, R.E., Husain, M.M. & Skinner, R.D. (1991) The brain stem reticular formation in schizophrenia. *Psychiatry Research: Neuroimaging*, **40**, 31–48.

Kemali, D., Maj, M., Galderisi, S., Milici, N. & Salvati, A. (1989) Ventricle-to-brain ratio in schizophrenia: a controlled follow-up study. *Biological Psychiatry*, **26**, 753–756.

Kovelman, J.A. & Scheibel, A.B. (1984) A neurohistological correlate of schizophrenia. *Biological Psychiatry*, **19**, 1601–1621.

Lesch, A. & Bogerts, B. (1984) The diencephalon in schizophrenia: evidence for reduced thickness of the periventricular grey matter. *European Archives of Psychiatry and Neurological Sciences*, **234**, 212–219.

Lohr, J.B. & Jeste, D.V. (1988) Locus ceruleus morphometry in aging and schizophrenia. *Acta Psychiatrica Scandinavica*, **77**, 689–697.

McCarley, R.W., Shenton, M.E., O'Donnell, F.B. *et al.* (1993) Auditory P300 abnormalities and left posterior superior temporal gyrus volume reduction in schizophrenia. *Archives of General Psychiatry*, **50**, 190–197.

McEwen, B.S., Gould, E.A. & Sakai, R.R. (1992) The vulnerability of the hippocampus to protective and destructive effects of glucocorticoids in relation to stress. *British Journal of Psychiatry*, **160** (Suppl. 15), 18–24.

McKenna, P.J. (1987) Pathology, phenomenology and the dopamine hypothesis of schizophrenia. *British Journal of Psychiatry*, **151**, 288–301.

McLardy, T. (1974) Hippocampal zinc and structural deficit in brains from chronic alcoholics and some schizophrenics. *Journal of Orthomolecular Psychiatry*, **4**(1), 32–36.

McLean, P.D. (1952) Some psychiatric implications of physiological studies on frontotemporal portion of limbic system (visceral brain). *Electroencephalography and Clinical Neurophysiology*, **4**, 407–418.

McNeil, T.F., Cantor-Graae, E., Nordström, L.G. & Rosenlund, T. (1993) Head circumference in 'preschizophrenics' and control neonates. *British Journal of Psychiatry*, **162**, 517–523.

Mathew, P.J. & Partain, C.L. (1985) Midsagittal sections of the cerebellar vermis and fourth ventricle obtained with magnetic resonance imaging in schizophrenic patients. *American Journal of Psychiatry*, **142**(8), 970–971.

Meltzer, H.Y. & Stahl, S.M. (1976) The dopamine hypothesis of schizophrenia: a review. *Schizophrenia Bulletin*, **2**, 19–76.

Nasrallah, H.A., Olson, S.C., McCalley-Whitters, M., Chapman, S. & Jacoby, C.G. (1986b) Cerebral ventricular enlargement in schizophrenia: a preliminary follow-up study. *Archives of General Psychiatry*, **43**, 157–159.

Nasrallah, H.A., Andreasen, N.C., Coffmann, J.A. *et al.* (1986a) A controlled magnetic resonance imaging study of corpus callosum thickness in schizophrenia. *Biological Psychiatry*, **21**, 274–282.

Nasrallah, H.A., McCalley-Whitters, M., Rauscher, F.P. *et al.* (1983) A histological study of the corpus callosum in chronic schizophrenia. *Psychiatry Research*, **8**, 151–160.

Newman, N.J., Bell, I.R. & McKee, A.C. (1990) Paraneoplastic limbic encephalitis: neuropsychiatric presentation. *Biological Psychiatry*, **27**, 529–542.

Pakkenberg, B. (1987) Post-mortem study of chronic schizophrenic brains. *British Journal of Psychiatry*, **151**, 744–752.

Pakkenberg, B. (1990) Pronounced reduction of total neuron number in mediodorsal thalamic nucleus and nucleus accumbens in schizophrenics. *Archives of General Psychiatry*, **47**, 1023–1028.

Pakkenberg, B. & Gundersen, H.J.G. (1988) Total number of neurons and glial cells in human brain nuclei estimated by the dissector and the fractionator. *Journal of Microscopy*, **150**, 1–20.

Pearlson, G.D., Kim, W.S., Kubos, K.L. *et al.* (1989) Ventricle-brain ratio, computed tomographic density, and brain area in 50 schizophrenics. *Archives of General Psychiatry*, **46**, 690–697.

Peters, G. (1967) Die symptomatischen Schizophrenien. In Gruhle, H.W., Jung, R., Mayer-Gross, W. & Müller, M. (eds) *Psychiatrie der Gegenwart*, Vol. I/1A, pp. 298–305. Springer-Verlag, Berlin.

Raine, A., Harrison, G.N., Reynolds, G.P., Sheard, Ch., Cooper, J.E. & Medley, I. (1990) Structural and functional characteristics of the corpus callosum in schizophrenics, psychiatric controls and normal controls. *Archives of General Psychiatry*, **47**, 1060–1064.

Roberts, G.W. (1991) Schizophrenia: a neuropathological perspective. *British Journal of Psychiatry*, **158**, 8–17.

Roberts, G.W., Colter, N., Lofthouse, R., Johnstone, E.C. & Crow, T.J. (1987) Is there gliosis in schizophrenia? Investigations of the temporal lobe. *Biological Psychiatry*, **22**, 1459–1468.

Roberts, G.W., Colter, N., Lofthouse, R., Bogerts, B., Zech, M. & Crow, T.J. (1986) Gliosis in schizophrenia: a survey. *Biological Psychiatry*, **21**, 1043–1050.

Rosenthal, R. & Bigelow, L.B. (1972) Quantitative brain measurements in chronic schizophrenia. *British Journal of Psychiatry*, **121**, 259–264.

Rossi, A., Stratta, P., Gallucci, M., Passarellio, R. & Cassachia, M. (1989) Quantification of corpus callosum and ventricles in schizophrenia with nuclear magnetic resonance imaging: a pilot study. *American Journal of Psychiatry*, **146**, 99–101.

Rossi, A., Stratta, P., D'Albenzio, L. *et al.* (1990) Reduced temporal lobe areas in schizophrenia: preliminary evidences from a controlled multiplanar magnetic resonance imaging study. *Biological Psychiatry*, **27**, 61–68.

Scheibel, A.B. & Kovelman, J.A. (1981) Disorientation of the hippocampal pyramidal cells and its processes in the schizophrenic patient. *Biological Psychiatry*, **16**, 101–102.

Schwarzkopf, S.B., Nasrallah, H.A., Olson, S.C., Bogerts, B., McLaughlin, J.A. & Mitra, T. (1991) Family history and brain morphology in schizophrenia: an MRI study. *Psychiatry Research: Neuroimaging*, **40**, 49–60.

Selemon, L.D., Rajkowska, G. & Goldman-Rakic, P.S. (1993) A morphometric analysis of prefrontal areas 9 and 46 in the schizophrenic and normal human brain. *Schizophrenia Research*, 9, 151.

Senitz, D. & Winkelmann, E. (1991) Neuronale Struktura-normalität im orbito-frontalen Cortex bei Schizophrenien. *Journal für Hirnforschung*, 32(2), 149–158.

Shenton, M.E., Kikinis, R., McCarley, R.W., Metcalf, D., Tieman, J. & Jolesz, F. (1991) Application of automated MRI volumetric measurement techniques to the ventricular system in schizophrenics and normal controls. *Schizophrenia Research*, 5, 103–113.

Small, J.G. (1975) EEG and neurophysiological studies of early infantile autism. *Biological Psychiatry*, 10, 385–389.

Southard, E.E. (1915) On the topographic distribution of cortex lesions and anomalies in dementia praecox with some account of their functional significance. *American Journal of Insanity*, 71, 603–671.

Sponheim, S.R., Iacono, W.G. & Beiser, M. (1991) Stability of ventricular size after the onset of psychosis in schizophrenia. *Psychiatry Research: Neuroimaging*, 40, 21–29.

Stevens, C.D., Altshuler, L.L., Bogerts, B. & Falkai, P. (1988) Quantitative study of gliosis in schizophrenia and Huntingston's chorea. *Biological Psychiatry*, 24, 697–700.

Stevens, J.R. (1982) Neuropathology of schizophrenia. *Archives of General Psychiatry*, 39, 1131–1139.

Stevens, J.R. (1986) Clinicopathological correlations in schizophrenia. *Archives of General Psychiatry*, 43, 715–716.

Stevens, J.R. (1992) Abnormal reinnervation as a basis for schizophrenia: a hypothesis. *Archives of General Psychiatry*, 49, 238–243.

Suddath, R.L., Casanova, M.F., Goldberg, T.E., Daniel, D.G., Kelsoe, J. & Weinberger, D.R. (1989) Temporal lobe pathology in schizophrenia: a quantitative magnetic resonance imaging study. *American Journal of Psychiatry*, 146, 464–472.

Suddath, R.L., Christison, G.W., Torrey, E.F., Casanova, M.F. & Weinberger, D.R. (1990) Anatomical abnormalities in the brains of monozygotic twins discordant for schizophrenia. *New England Journal of Medicine*, 322(12), 62–67.

Swayze, V.W., Andreasen, N.C., Alliger, R.J., Yuh, W.T.C. & Ehrhard, J.C. (1992) Subcortical and temporal structures in affective disorder and schizophrenia: a magnetic resonance imaging study. *Biological Psychiatry*, 31, 221–240.

Tandon, R. & Greden, J.F. (1990) Cholinergic hyperactivity and negative schizophrenic symptoms. *Archives of General*

Psychiatry, 46, 745–753.

Treff, W.M. & Hempel, K.J. (1958) Die Zelldichte bei Schizophrenen und klinische Gesunden. *Journal für Hirnforschung*, 4, 314–369.

Uematso, M. & Kaiya, H. (1988) The morphology of the corpus callosum in schizophrenia: an MRI study. *Schizophrenie Research*, 1, 391–398.

Vita, A., Sacchetti, G. & Cazullo, C.L. (1988) Brain morphology in schizophrenia: a 2- to 5-year follow-up study. *Acta Psychiatrica Scandinavica*, 78, 618–621.

Vogt, C. & Vogt, O. (1948) Über anatomische Substrate. Bemerkungen zu pathoanatomischen Befunden bei Schizophrenie. *Ärztliche Forschung*, 3, 1–7.

Vogt, C. & Vogt, O. (1952) Resultats de l'etude anatomique de la schizophrenie et d'autres psychoses dites fontionelles faite a l'institut du cerveau de Neustadt (Schwarzwald). In Rosenberg, & Sellier, (eds) *Proceedings of the First International Congress of Neuropathology, Turin*, Vol. 1, S. 515–532.

Wada, J.A., Clarke, R. & Hamm, A. (1975) Cerebral hemispheric asymmetries in humans. *Archives of Neurology*, 32, 239–246.

Waddington, J.L. (1993) Neurodynamics of abnormalities in cerebral metabolism and structure in schizophrenia. *Schizophrenia Bulletin*, 19, 55–69.

Weinberger, D.R. (1987) Implications of normal brain development for the pathogenesis of schizophrenia. *Archives of General Psychiatry*, 44, 660–669.

Weinberger, D.R., Kleinman, J.E., Luchins, D.J., Bigelow, L.B. & Wyatt, R.J. (1980) Cerebellar pathology in schizophrenia: a controlled post mortem study. *American Journal of Psychiatry*, 137, 359–361.

Woods, B.T., Douglass, A. & Gescuk, B. (1990) Is the VBR still a useful measure of changes in the cerebral ventricles? *Psychiatry Research: Neuroimaging*, 40, 1–10.

Zipursky, R.B., Lim, K.O. & Pfefferbaum, A. (1991) Brain size in schizophrenia. *Archives of General Psychiatry*, 48, 179–180.

Zipursky, R.B., Lim, K.O., Sullivan, E.V., Brown, B.W. & Pfefferbaum, A. (1992) Widespread cerebral gray matter volume deficits in schizophrenia. *Archives of General Psychiatry*, 49, 195–205.

Zubin, J. & Spring, B. (1977) Vulnerability — a new view of schizophrenia. *Journal of Abnormal Psychology*, 86, 103–126.

Chapter 16
Schizophrenia as a Neurodevelopmental Disorder

D. R. WEINBERGER

Introduction

After many decades of speculation that schizophrenia occurs because of cerebral pathological events that happen or are expressed around early adult life, there has been a dramatic conceptual shift in thinking about the neurobiology of schizophrenia. Schizophrenia is now regarded as a neurodevelopmental disorder in which the primary cerebral insult or pathological process occurs during brain development long before the illness is clinically manifest (Weinberger, 1986, 1987; Murray & Lewis, 1987; Bogerts, 1989; Crow et al., 1989; Lewis, 1989; Waddington, 1990; Mednick et al., 1991; Murray et al., 1992; Bloom, 1993).

The hypothesis that schizophrenia is neurodevelopmental in origin is not new. Indeed, Kraepelin and others throughout the 20th century argued that some cases of schizophrenia probably resulted from insults that cause cerebral maldevelopment (Southard, 1915; Kraepelin, 1919). However, the predominant view that has guided most research and clinical practice until very recently emerged from Kraepelin's concept of a premature dementia and a clinical deterio-

ration over the course of the illness. From this conceptual framework, it was logical to assume that in most cases the brain was relatively normal until the illness struck in early adulthood. Moreover, it followed that any pathological changes inflicted on the brain by the illness would become more apparent as the illness progressed. This conceptual model was consistent with most known adult-onset brain disorders, including metabolic and infectious encephalopathies (both genetic and sporadic) and degenerative conditions, which have often been used as analogies for explaining the pathophysiology of schizophrenia. The effort to attribute schizophrenia to such processes is far from exhausted, and with respect to the viro-immunological hypothesis, research is still in progress (Yolken & Torrey, 1995; see also Chapter 13, this volume).

In this historical context, the seemingly widespread conceptual shift away from models of adult-onset pathology to the presumption of pathological neurodevelopment is especially remarkable. The reasons for this shift are primarily threefold: scientific data confirming adult-onset pathological cerebral changes have remained elusive; replicable evidence of cortical maldevelopment has emerged;

and neurobiological models that may explain the relationships between such maldevelopment and the clinical features of the illness exist. This chapter will review several issues underlying this conceptual reorientation about schizophrenia (see also Chapters 12 & 15, this volume). First, a brief overview of normal brain development will be presented, with particular reference to how and when the putative abnormalities associated with schizophrenia might occur. Second, the research data interpreted to represent cerebral maldevelopment will be discussed. The third section will review recent studies that have attributed maldevelopment to specific aetiological factors. Finally, the last sections will discuss several mechanisms that have been proposed to explain how the onset of the illness might be delayed until long after the pathology occurs. Clarification of these mechanisms will draw on relevant neurological and animal models. Portions of this chapter have appeared elsewhere (Weinberger, 1995).

Normal brain development

The human brain develops from the embryological ectoderm as a result of a highly complex and mostly orderly sequence of changes. Initially, these changes are progressive in nature, involving proliferation and migration of cells and expansion of cellular processes, but later progressive events become confined to modifications in cellular elements while major regressive changes in neuronal populations and neuronal processes appear. Though the most dramatic changes occur during gestation, important changes continue to occur after birth and probably continue to some degree throughout life. In general, normal brain development depends on both genetic and environmental influences, with the former dominating during the earlier stages and the later becoming more of a factor during the later stages. Information about human brain development has come from a number of archival histological studies of human embryos and fetuses and more recently from studies of non-human primates utilizing radiolabelled amino acid incorporation, electron microscopy and immunohistochemical

and recombinant deoxyribonucleic acid (DNA) techniques.

The traditional scheme of mammalian central nervous system development highlights several discrete stages or milestones (Sidman & Rakic, 1982; Nowakowski, 1991a). These include neurulation or formation of the primitive neural tube, cellular proliferation or neurogenesis, cellular migration and cellular and regional differentiation. Each of these involves complicated molecular events that occur intracellularly as well as at the level of cell-to-cell interactions.

Neurulation

The formation of the primitive neural tube is the first obvious step in the formation of the nervous system. It begins near the end of the third week following conception with the invagination of the embryological ectoderm into a groove, and the subsequent closing of the groove into a tube. The tube differentiates along its longitudinal axis so that by the fourth week three bulges are visible at its rostral end. These represent the primary brain vesicles, which ultimately give rise to the cerebrum, cerebellum and brain stem. In cross-section, the vesicles consist of undifferentiated pseudostratified epithelial cells clumped around the lumen and a thin, acellular matrix zone near the pial surface. Defects in neural tube formation if major are usually incompatible with life (e.g. anencephaly) or if minor produce gross midline defects (e.g. cysts, spina bifida) that are not associated with schizophrenia *per se*.

Proliferation

The neuronal and glial cell precursors that are the ancestors of all brain cells cluster near the lumen of the brain vesicles, which soon become the ventricular walls. This cellular region is called the ventricular proliferative zone. In some parts of the developing brain, an additional layer of precursor cells separates from the ventricular zone and becomes a separate proliferative region, the subventricular zone. All mature brain cells originate from precursors in one of these two periventricular zones. Cell division continues in the subventricular zone after it ceases in the ventricular zone, so the last cellular elements to be formed in the brain come from this subventricular zone. This latter proliferative centre has been considered the more highly evolved element (Nowakowski & Rakic, 1981; Nowakowski, 1987). In keeping with this possibility, most neocortical regions are formed from cells originating in both ventricular and subventricular zones, while the rostral hippocampus, subiculum and diencephalon are formed only from ventricular zone precursors (Nowakowski & Rakic, 1981; Nowakowski, 1987).

The process of cortical neurogenesis takes place in humans over a period of 85 days (i.e. days 40–125), ending by the middle of the second trimester (Rakic, 1988a). Interestingly, in mammals other than primates, cortical neurogenesis is a more protracted process. In rats, for example, hippocampal granule cells continue to divide after birth and may even increase in number throughout life (Stanfield & Cowan, 1988). It is uncertain whether postnatal neural proliferation occurs anywhere in primates.

The degree to which eventual cerebral specialization is related to events during neurogenesis has been the subject of a long-standing controversy. Early speculation emphasized that proliferating neurones were pluripotential and that their eventual phenotypic attributes were determined after they reached their targets and interacted with other neurones (O'Leary, 1989). Recently, greater emphasis has been placed on the importance of genetic mechanisms in the early stages of cortical development. For example, Rakic (1988b) has hypothesized that a genetically programmed 'protomap' of eventual cortical regional topography exists in the periventricular proliferative zones in the guise of spatially designated 'proliferative units'. His 'radial unit hypothesis' proposes further that these proliferative units, consisting of groups of stem cells separated by glial septa that are formed by day 45, give rise over the next 85 days to successive generations of young neurones that migrate radially to form spatially defined ontogenic columns. Within these columns, young neurones differentiate into cortical neuronal phenotypes, while arrays of columns differentiate into cortical cytoarchitectonic regions. According to this hypothesis, cortical surface area is related to the number of proliferative units; the size of a cortical cytoarchitectonic region is a function of the number of units genetically programmed to generate the columns of neurones that will make up the region; and cortical thickness is related to the size of an ontogenic column (i.e. the number of neurones formed from stem cells in a proliferative unit). As an illustration, area 17 of rhesus monkey visual cortex is comprised of approximately 3 million ontogenic columns of neurones, presumably generated by 3 million proliferative units from the area of the periventricular protomap genetically designated as the area 17 precursor zone. Though a compelling and heuristically profound hypothesis, the notion of a genetic protomap and spatially predestined proliferative units in the periventricular zone may be overly reductionistic. Recent data using molecular cloning techniques to map the migratory targets of periventricular stem cells suggest that their eventual spatial domains are not as specifically programmed as the hypothesis would predict (Walsh & Cepko, 1992).

In spite of its few limitations, the radial unit hypothesis has far-reaching implications for understanding evolutionary aspects of cortical development, for identifying early factors in the regulation of cortical regional specialization and for understanding the abnormalities of cortical development that have been implicated in schizophrenia. This hypothesis proposes that the cortex has expanded in evolution by virtue of a phylogenetic increase in the number of proliferative units. It predicts correctly that since the number of neuronal generations formed by a proliferative unit appears to be relatively constant, cortical thickness varies little from one region of cortex to another, and in fact, it varies little from one mammalian species to another (Rakic, 1988b). Moreover, the radial unit hypothesis predicts the impact of the timing of abnormalities in cell proliferation. Aberrations that occur prior to day 45 will affect the formation of proliferative units and thus their number. The result will be reduced cortical surface area, or a lissencephalic brain. This anomaly has not been linked to schizophrenia. Aberrations that occur after day 45 will affect the number of stem-cell divisions associated with a particular ontogenic column (i.e. the number of neurones per column). This should lead to a thinner cortex and possibly to the existence of heterotopic neurones, both of which have been associated with schizophrenia (see below). Because the ultimate neuronal phenotype and laminar location of cortical neurones depends to some degree on their time of origin in the generation of an ontogenic column, abnormal gestational events, depending on their timing, might selectively affect specific populations of cortical neurones. For example, neocortical neurones that end up in deeper layers are older than neurones destined for superficial layers (Rakic, 1988b, 1990); entorhinal neurones are spawned before subicular neurones (Stanfield & Cowan, 1988). Such timing differences could conceivably account for some of the specific neuropathological findings described below.

Migration

Soon after a neurone has stopped dividing in the periventricular zone, it attaches itself to a transient radial glial fibre, which guides it on a migratory path towards its eventual target (Rakic, 1990). The apposition of young neurones to glial fibres is the best characterized form of cell-to-cell interaction in the developing brain (Rakic, 1971). A variety of genetic and molecular processes have been identified as being important in this process, including the regulation of cell-surface adhesion molecules and activation of glutamate receptors and calcium channels (Komuro & Rakic, 1993). Once they start their journey, neurones move at the rate of $0.5-10\,\mu m/h$ (Nowakowski & Rakic, 1981; Rakic, 1990). Those that travel to the neocortex have a much longer journey and arrive later than do those that are destined for periventricular structures such as the hippocampus or basal ganglia (Brand & Rakic, 1979; Rakic, 1988b, 1990). Since postmitotic neurones leave the proliferative zones while new neurones are still being

generated, the first neurones to reach their targets are the oldest neurones. In fact, the process of migration to cortex involves an 'inside-to-outside' spatial–temporal gradient where older neurones settle in relatively deeper layers and younger neurones pass over them on their way to more superficial layers (Rakic, 1988b). This probably allows for cell–cell interactions and communication among neurones of different generations and trajectories before they form synapses (Rakic, 1990).

The arrival of neurones to the pial side of the vesicular wall marks the appearance of the cortical plate, the primitive structure that eventually differentiates into the cortex. Two cellular zones, which are formed by the earliest arriving neurones, are split off as the cortical plate expands: a superficial marginal zone which eventually becomes cortical layer I; and a deep layer called the subplate zone, which eventually becomes the sparse cortical layer VII (Marin-Padilla, 1988). This primitive laminarity is apparent by day 54. As the cortical plate expands, these layers get farther apart. Neocortical layers II–VI are formed from the rest of the cortical plate. Neurones that contribute to the growing cortical plate during the remainder of the period of neuronal migration must pass through the subplate zone. This passage and the development of the subplate zone has become a subject of increasing interest. The subplate zone is thought to afford an opportunity for migrating neurones to intermingle with afferents from subcortical, thalamic and intracortical regions. Such intermingling may be important for further neuronal and regional differentiation. Moreover, the subplate zone is phylogenetically most developed in the human brain and especially in highly evolved regions such as prefrontal cortex (Kostovic *et al.*, 1989). While it has been proposed that many of the phenotypic features of neurones are probably determined before they enter the cortical plate (Rakic, 1988b), their laminar location within the cortex is determined by their time of arrival (i.e. layer VI neurones arrive before layer V, etc.).

Neuronal migration appears to be sensitive to a number of genetic and environmental insults and can easily be disrupted. Evidence of faulty migration includes ectopic neurones, other cytoarchitectural anomalies and hypocellular areas. Since such anomalies have been reported in several developmental disorders, such as mental retardation, dyslexia, autism, fetal alcohol syndrome, as well as schizophrenia, a fault in migration has been implicated in each instance as an explanation for the neuropathological findings (Nowakowski, 1987, 1991a). The causes of neuronal migratory abnormalities are legion, and include genetic mutations, heat, various toxins, alcohol, viruses and radiation (Rakic, 1988a, 1990; Nowakowski, 1991b). For example, in animals, prenatal administration of 6-OH-dopamine results in superficial cortical ectopias (Rakic, 1988b). Faulty migration in mutant rat strains has been attributed to genetic abnormalities that affect the regulation of neuronal–glial interactions (Nowakowski, 1991b). In humans, mental retardation following the Hiroshima nuclear blast was most frequent and most clearly dose related if exposure occurred during neuronal migration (i.e. the eighth to 15th week of gestation) (Otake & Schull, 1984). As will be discussed below, the characteristics of certain neuropathological deviations associated with schizophrenia and the timing of certain prenatal adverse events that may be associated with schizophrenia have encouraged speculation that neuronal migration is disrupted in this illness.

Differentiation

The final and most protracted stage of brain development involves cellular and regional anatomical and functional differentiation. This stage, which continues at least into the second decade of life, is characterized by intracellular molecular changes and refinements of interneuronal connectivity. In addition to the localization of neurones as a factor in their phenotypic specialization, the impact of their connections and of the neurotransmitters that interact with them are very important in regulating dendritic and axonal development, the cell surface molecules and receptors that they express and the neurotransmitters they use (Lipton & Kater, 1989). How does a neurone know what neurotransmitter

or which receptors to synthesize? It possesses the genetic information to make them all. The answer to such questions likely involves interactions between genetic and epigenetic factors, and such interactions appear to permit considerable flexibility. As an example, when catecholeaminergic neurones are placed in cell culture with only cholinoceptive neurones, they change their phenotype and synthesize acetylcholine (Landis, 1990).

Afferent contacts are clearly important for the further specialization of cortical regions beyond that programmed into the putative periventricular 'protomaps'. This has been demonstrated in studies of the long-term effects of deafferentation lesions produced during development. For instance, lateral geniculate lesions that abolish developing thalamostriate cortical afferents in monkeys not only diminish the size of visual cortex area 17 but alter qualitatively the cytoarchitecture of area 18 as well (Rakic, 1991; Rakic et al., 1991).

Afferent fibres from distant neurones first appear before cortical neurogenesis. In the monkey, catecholeaminergic afferents can be seen in the ventromesial vesicular wall 3 weeks after conception (Stanfield & Cowan, 1988). Early in the first trimester, primitive axonal processes, called growth cones, begin to branch out, probably under genetic direction at the start. Soon, however, they expand, retract and reroute in response to contacts with other elements in their environment. The first cortical synapses become apparent by approximately day 53, when they can be found in both the marginal and subplate zones (Marin-Padilla, 1988; Zecevic et al., 1989). Thereafter, afferents from subcortical nucleii (e.g. cholinergic, catecholeaminergic), thalamic and other cortical regions arrive at the subplate region, make synapses with neurones staying there and passing through, and continue to grow into the cortical plate to make additional synaptic contacts. The timing of arrival of these afferents corresponds roughly with the timing of cortical laminar differentiation. Cortical layers V and VI differentiate first with the arrival of thalamocortical projections, followed by differentiation of layer III with the arrival of interhemispheric connections, and then by layer II with the arrival of intracortical fibres (Marin-Padilla, 1988). The ipsilateral and contralateral intracortical afferents are the last fibres to reach the subplate zone; they remain there the longest, and they are the last to leave. The size of the subplate itself is proportional to the number of corticocortical afferents that reach it, perhaps explaining why it is most prominent and persists longest in prefrontal cortex (Kostovic & Rakic, 1990).

The development of cortical connectivity also parallels the beginning of the buckling of the cortical surface and the appearance of cortical gyri and sulci. The Sylvian and longitudinal fissures begin to develop around 20 weeks. The fact that these fissures appear in the right hemisphere about 2 weeks before they are clearly seen in the left (Chi *et al.*, 1977) has prompted some to speculate that there is a lateralized gradient in brain development which may render the left hemisphere more susceptible to injury *in utero* (Roberts, 1991). Whether this can explain the tendency for neuropathological changes in schizophrenia to involve the left hemisphere more than the right when such changes are reported to be lateralized is unclear.

In the last trimester of gestation, there is a dramatic increase in the number of synaptic contacts formed throughout the brain. In monkeys, this programmed overproduction of mostly collateral connections, which involves all cortical regions and lamina equally, continues postnatally and accelerates almost 10-fold during the first 2 postnatal months until reaching a plateau in which the number of synapses is virtually twice that found in the adult brain (Brand & Rakic, 1984; Rakic *et al.*, 1986; Zecevic *et al.*, 1989; Zecevic & Rakic, 1991). An analogous process has been observed in human brain, where synaptic numbers increase 10-fold in visual and prefrontal cortices until reaching a peak by 8–12 postnatal months (Huttenlocher *et al.*, 1982) and 1–2 postnatal years (Huttenlocher, 1979), respectively. Synaptic proliferation seems to involve numerous neurotransmitter receptor types, including various subtypes of dopaminergic, adrenergic, gamma-aminobutyric acidergic (GABAergic) and serotonergic receptors

(Lidow *et al.*, 1991; Lidow & Rakic, 1992).

Following this explosion of synaptic synthetic activity, a gradual and protracted period of regression of axonal processes and pruning of synaptic contacts begins and continues at least through puberty and into early adult life. The reduction in axonal and synaptic numbers probably occurs by a combination of cell death, axonal retraction and synaptic elimination. Programmed cell death is seen throughout the nervous system prenatally (Oppenheim, 1985). The mechanisms responsible are unknown, but probably are random to some extent, genetic to some extent, and also involve target-associated factors such as neuronal growth factors which are taken up at terminals and transported back to the cell nucleus (Changeux & Danchin, 1976; Oppenheim, 1985). In monkeys, cell death continues to a small degree after birth (e.g. 15% of visual cortex neurones are lost from birth to maturity) (O'Kusky & Colonnier, 1982). In humans, the extent of postnatal cell death is uncertain (Huttenlocher, 1992). One region of human brain that clearly undergoes regression and probably neuronal degeneration is the subplate zone. This changes from being markedly cellular in the last trimester, particularly in association with cortical areas such as prefrontal cortex, to being represented in adulthood by rare neurones scattered through subcortical white matter (Kostovic & Rakic, 1990).

In contrast to cell death, synaptic elimination and axonal retraction are primarily postnatal phenomena. Studies in monkeys indicate that synaptic elimination proceeds throughout the cortex at a gradual but consistent pace until around puberty, when it may briefly accelerate before levelling off (Zecevic & Rakic, 1991). Electron microscopy studies have revealed that synaptic elimination involves specifically asymmetrical, axospinous synapses. The numbers of axosomatic synapses and synapses not on spines remain stable after they are formed (Zecevic & Rakic, 1991). These observations suggest that the process of synaptic elimination is selective for excitatory inputs. However, studies of receptor binding have raised questions about this conclusion. While a postnatal decline in the density of neurotransmitter receptors has been observed analogous to that of synaptic elimination, multiple receptor types, both excitatory and inhibitory, are affected (Lidow *et al.*, 1991; Lidow & Rakic, 1992). This has prompted speculation that some of the receptors that are lost may be extrasynaptic (Lidow *et al.*, 1991). Studies in human cortex also demonstrate that synapses are gradually eliminated after the second year of life until the process levels off in the second decade (Huttenlocher, 1979, 1992). At age 7 years, when the human brain is almost fully grown, synaptic numbers in prefrontal cortex are still 36% above adult levels (Huttenlocher, 1979). In contrast to monkeys, however, the data in humans suggest that synaptic elimination may have run its course by the time puberty occurs.

The mechanisms responsible for which axons and synapses survive are undoubtedly complex and probably include target feedback in the form of humoral growth factors (Changeux & Danchin, 1976), neuronal electrical activity (Nowakowski, 1987), glutamate receptor stimulation (Rabacchi *et al.*, 1992) and a spectrum of putative trophic effects of many classical neurotransmitters (Mattson, 1988; Lipton & Kater, 1989). Overall, the process seems to represent the maturational refinement and functional validation of cortical connectivity and organization. Numerous explanations have been advanced to explain why exuberant neuronal contacts would predominate early in cortical development only to have most of them disappear later. The emphases have been on the idea of selective stabilization of functionally meaningful connections, on the notion of synaptic competition for survival, and on connectivity that endures because it is reinforced by experience (Purves, 1988).

Studies of synaptic proliferation and pruning strongly suggest that the cortex matures as an integrated system, not as the result of a sequential or hierarchical march of functionally independent regions (Zecevic & Rakic, 1991; Lidow & Rakic, 1992). While the basic circuitry appears to be laid down at the direction of genetic and humoral factors, which control the fundamental behaviour of individuals cells and interactions between cat-

egories of cells, fine tuning depends on functional reinforcement (Changeux & Danchin, 1976). One might imagine that genetic programmes tell neurones how to divide, how many divisions to make, how to migrate, what it takes to survive, how to make connections and what it takes to have a connection survive (Williams & Herrup, 1988). Beyond these fundamental principles, the final shaping of cortical organization is affected by, if not dependent upon, experience.

Lesion studies in animals and in humans demonstrate unequivocally that synaptic remodelling is affected by function and by afferent input (Schwartz & Goldman-Rakic, 1990; Huttenlocher, 1992). This has led to the concept that functional plasticity or 'sparing' after early developmental injury occurs because exuberant synapses are available to compensate. Huttenlocher has remarked that 'plasticity appears to be mediated by structures that are normally transient' (Huttenlocher, 1992). The adaptive advantage of this capability for developmental compensation and variation is obvious. It also should be considered that if it is possible to compensate for defective circuits by recruiting connections that might otherwise regress, it might also be possible to enhance neuronal and synaptic survivability by enriching experience. This possibility has been demonstrated in laboratory animals (Greer *et al.*, 1982; Meaney *et al.*, 1988).

During the years of synaptic pruning and probably beyond, progressive maturational changes also take place, and many of these continue after the regressive processes appear to have ceased. Those synapses that survive become much more complex by adulthood (Zecevic & Rakic, 1991). Cortical laminations become more clearly defined. Long projecting afferents expand and arborize in more complex patterns. Neuronal dendritic trees also become more complex and larger. Myelination of selected axons proceeds well into the third decade, especially in association cortex. Despite the massive regression of synapses, neuropil actually expands, and the overall growth of the brain continues through adolescence. In fact, the last growth spurt in brain size occurs around the age of 13–15 years (Epstein, 1986).

Various aspects of neuronal and regional differentiation have been implicated in neurodevelopmental models of schizophrenia. Feinberg (1982), in citing phenomenological characteristics of patients with schizophrenia that might be interpreted as developmentally immature, proposed that schizophrenia is caused by a primary fault in synaptic pruning. This hypothesis, in addition to not accounting for the neuropathological changes that have been associated with schizophrenia (discussed below), raises the question of whether pruning *per se* can go awry, or whether it almost by definition results from other primary developmental phenomena. It has also been proposed that schizophrenia might be the result of abnormalities of myelination or might be expressed because of variations in myelogenesis (Benes, 1989). Progressive changes in synaptic contacts and abnormalities of neuronal sprouting have been offered as an explanation for the onset of the disorder in late adolescence (Stevens, 1992). An alternative perspective is that rather than an abnormality of postnatal maturational processes being responsible for the illness or its onset, the latter might correspond to the relative cessation of these normal processes and the resulting functional stabilization of neuronal circuitry (Weinberger, 1987). These largely speculative possibilities will be discussed in more detail below.

Developmental neuropathology

An association between putative abnormalities in intrauterine development and schizophrenia has been reported throughout the 20th century. The evidence ranges from circumstantial and weak (e.g. slight overrepresentation of minor physical anomalies), to at least compelling (e.g. replicated cytoarchitectural anomalies). When viewed *in toto*, the evidence might be interpreted to weave a coherent story of developmental abnormalities; however, at the level of individual findings, there are many inconsistencies and methodological problems. The most important research questions at the present time are whether evidence of cytoarchitectural deviations can be more widely replicated and whether lingering methodological

uncertainties can be resolved. If these questions are answered positively, most of the research controversies and theoretical speculation considered below (e.g. obstetric complications, pruning defects) will be irrelevant, because a 'smoking gun' will have been found.

Minor physical abnormalities

Since abnormal intrauterine events might also be expected to affect the development of extracerebral tissues, reports of somatic morphological variations are of potential relevance. The spectrum of potential minor physical abnormalities (MPA) and their relationship to abnormal brain development is not clearly defined. In the schizophrenia literature, there is no consistent pattern of associations and often the samples have to be broken down *post hoc* into putative subgroups for any associations to be found (Torrey *et al.*, 1994). Kraepelin (1919) cited a high palate and low-set ears as being overrepresented in patients with schizophrenia. Since that observation, other anomalies have been noted, including variations in limb length and angle, finger-print patterns and ridge counts, webbed digits, etc. (Green *et al.*, 1989). Proponents of the relevance of MPAs have stressed that many of these abnormalities are seen as a result of second trimester insults, timing that is consistent with a putative defect in neuronal migration. They also stress that MPAs are seen in other neurodevelopmental disorders, such as intrauterine viral encephalopathies, and in other psychiatric disorders of presumed developmental origin (e.g. autism) (Torrey *et al.*, 1994).

However, the circumstantial nature of these arguments notwithstanding, they are undermined further by problems with the fundamental database. The true frequency of MPAs in patients with schizophrenia is not known, as large unselected samples of patients and well-matched controls have not been studied. Whether all the morphological characteristics reported are actually pathological is also uncertain. Moreover, few of the studies have used the same methods of assessment, and it is uncertain whether any of the studies were truly blind comparisons. The studies that report increases in MPAs tend to lump them all together as if each signified the same thing, when, in fact, their relative frequencies seem not to correlate with each other (Torrey *et al.*, 1994). Because the search for MPAs has not been a centrepiece of schizophrenia research, it is doubtful that investigators who failed to find MPAs in their samples reported the negative results. Another uncertainty is that the timing of events that cause MPAs is not well established and considerable variability exists. In light of these questions and other contradictory data [e.g. no difference in MPAs within pairs of discordant monozygotic twins (Torrey *et al.*, 1994), no consistent abnormalities in birth weights of schizophrenic births compared with healthy sibling births (McNeil, 1988) and no relationship of MPAs to birth weight or other clinical signs of intrauterine adversity (McNeil, 1988; Torrey *et al.*, 1994)], the relevance of MPAs to understanding potential cerebral maldevelopment in schizophrenia is weak.

Premorbid neurological abnormalities

If the brains of patients with schizophrenia have not developed normally, it might be expected that some evidence of subtle abnormalities of neural function would be apparent during childhood before individuals became clinically ill. Several lines of circumstantial data support this possibility. Studies of premorbid neuropsychological test performance and school achievement have tended to report that individuals who later manifest schizophrenia did worse than their healthy siblings (Aylward *et al.*, 1984). Reports of no difference have also appeared (Torrey *et al.*, 1994). Four series of reports of high-risk subjects, that is children with at least one schizophrenic parent, have found various abnormalities of motor function (Mednick & Silverton, 1988; Fish *et al.*, 1992), autonomic responsivity (Mednick & Silverton, 1988) and attention (Erlenmeyer-Kimling, 1987; Asarnow, 1988; Fish *et al.*, 1992). The abnormalities vary somewhat from one study to another and are not linked with schizophrenia *per se*. Fish (1977) has provided a detailed description of what she refers to as a 'pandysmaturational defect' in

high-risk children, consisting of gross abnormalities of gait, posture, muscle tone and reflexes in early childhood. It is uncertain how representative these relatively dramatic findings are of most children who subsequently manifest the illness. Moreover, the findings disappear to some degree over time, further complicating their interpretation. Finally, Walker and Lewine (1990) recently reported a novel study of home movies of families having a child who later developed schizophrenia. In a blind comparison of affected and unaffected siblings in four sibships, they reported clear differences in bimanual dexterity, gait and other gross motor functions that allowed them to invariably identify the affected family member even in the first few years of life. To clinicians, the severity of the observations of Fish, and the severity and consistency of the observations of Walker and Lewine may seem surprising. Clearly, further replication is needed. Nevertheless, the results of these studies, while open to other lines of interpretation, are consistent with the possibility of brain maldevelopment.

Cerebral morphometric abnormalities

In vivo *studies*

Beginning in 1976 with an *in vivo* study of cerebral ventricular size using the novel method of computerized axial tomography (CAT) scanning (Johnstone *et al.*, 1976), literally hundreds of reports have appeared of subtle variations in cerebral anatomy associated with schizophrenia. The CAT database established that, as a group, patients with schizophrenia have slightly enlarged ventricles and wider cortical fissures and sulci (Shelton & Weinberger, 1987). These findings suggested a non-focal reduction in cerebral and probably cortical volume. Moreover, the data did not support the widely expressed assumption that morphological abnormalities characterized only a subgroup of patients (Meltzer, 1979). Instead, they seemed to describe a continuum of pathological change (Weinberger *et al.*, 1981; Reveley *et al.*, 1982; Daniel *et al.*, 1991; Roberts, 1991) that characterized the majority patient population.

Recently, using magnetic resonance imaging (MRI), which produces images of much greater tissue contrast and resolution, the CAT data have been confirmed and refined. Evidence of cortical volume loss, most frequently replicated in, but not confined to, mesial temporal cortex in the area of the rostral hippocampus, has been a relatively consistent finding (Zigun & Weinberger, 1992). Again, the data do not implicate only a subgroup of patients (Suddath *et al.*, 1990; Zigun & Weinberger, 1992).

In some studies, evidence of pathological changes appears to favour the left side of the brain. This has been especially true for the size of the ventricles (Crow *et al.*, 1989) and for the volume of the superior temporal gyrus (Shenton *et al.*, 1992). Reports of relatively greater reductions in other regions of left temporal cortex have also appeared (Suddath *et al.*, 1990). Indeed, when asymmetrical findings have been reported, they usually involve the left hemisphere. This has prompted some to suggest that this lateralization tendency is consistent with a putative delay in the development of the left hemisphere during the second trimester, leaving it more vulnerable to adverse events that might otherwise affect the brain diffusely (Crow *et al.*, 1989; Roberts, 1991). This is an interesting hypothesis, but it depends on a number of assumptions and probably over-interprets the morphometric literature. Whether the slight delay in the appearance of surface gyri means that the left hemisphere is developing slower or that it is more vulnerable to injury or vulnerable for a longer period is unknown. More-over, most of the morphometric studies, even those that report unilateral findings (Crow *et al.*, 1989; Shenton *et al.*, 1992), have observed bilateral changes as well.

While *in vivo* evidence of subtle morphometric deviations might implicate a neuropathological process as being related to schizophrenia, it does not by itself implicate a neurodevelopmental one. However, beginning with the results of the second CAT study of schizophrenia, the correlative data have not been consistent with what would be expected of a degenerative condition of adult onset, and have been consistent with what would be expected of a neurodevelopmental one. Weinberger *et al.* (1979) reported, to their surprise, that ventricular size did not correlate with duration of illness, as would have been expected if the neuropathological process responsible for ventricular enlargement advanced as the illness progressed. They raised the possibility that the underlying process was no longer active. This finding has been replicated by the majority of cross-sectional correlation studies (Marsh *et al.*, 1994), highlighted in meta-analytical reviews (Raz & Raz, 1990), and more recently confirmed by several prospective studies that have followed the same individuals for up to 10 years from the time of the first psychotic episode (Abi-Dargham *et al.*, 1991). It thus appears that for most patients the pathological process responsible for the *in vivo* morphometric changes associated with schizophrenia has been arrested at least by the time their clinical illness is diagnosed.

Circumstantial and correlational evidence that the pathological process might have been arrested early in life, if not during early development, also emerged from *in vivo* imaging studies. Ventricular enlargement has been found in most studies of patients at the onset of the clinical illness in early adulthood (Weinberger *et al.*, 1982a; DeLisi *et al.*, 1991; Lieberman *et al.*, 1993) and reduced hippo-campal volume has been observed in at least one first-break study (Bogerts *et al.*, 1990). This suggests that these findings do not develop during the early phases of illness and probably predate the onset of the illness. There have been isolated case reports of ventriculomegaly and cortical sulcal dilatation in asymptomatic patients scanned for unrelated reasons and who many months later have a schizophreniform episode (Weinberger, 1988). Several, though not all, studies have found an unexpected correlation between ventricular enlargement in patients with schizophrenia and poor premorbid social and educational adjust-ment during early childhood (Weinberger *et al.*, 1980; Kolakowska *et al.*, 1985; Keefe *et al.*, 1989; Erel *et al.*, 1991). This finding further suggests the possibility that the morbid pathology had occurred early in life and manifested itself in different ways at different times of life (Weinberger *et al.*, 1980).

Postmortem studies

Data from postmortem morphometric studies of brains of patients who died with schizophrenia are generally consistent with the conclusions from the *in vivo* studies (Hyde *et al.*, 1991). In general, volumetric assessments of cerebral ventricular size (Brown *et al.*, 1986; Pakkenberg, 1987; Crow *et al.*, 1989; Bruton *et al.*, 1990), of various cortical regions, the hippocampal formation (including the parahippocampal cortex), and of various peri-ventricular subcortical nucleii have found differences between patients and normals (Bogerts *et al.*, 1985; Pakkenberg, 1987; Crow *et al.*, 1989; Altshuler *et al.*, 1990). Likewise, neuronal counts have been reported to be reduced in patients in selected cortical and periventricular regions (Bogerts *et al.*, 1985; Benes *et al.*, 1986; Jeste & Lohr, 1989). These studies, like the *in vivo* studies, implicate a fairly widespread neuropatho-logical process. It should be noted, however, that there have also been negative reports (Heckers *et al.*, 1990; Benes *et al.*, 1991b), and the reasons for the inconsistencies are unclear.

One observation that has been relatively con-sistent is a lack of gliosis. In fact, it was the absence of gliosis that prompted many classical neuropathologists during the first half of the 20th century to dismiss reports of neuropathological changes in schizophrenic brain specimens. With the exception of one study that was non-blind and probably included cases of secondary encephalo-pathies (Stevens, 1982), recent studies, whether in neocortex (Benes *et al.*, 1986; Bruton *et al.*, 1990), hippocampus (Roberts *et al.*, 1986) or parahippocampal cortex (Falkai *et al.*, 1988), have not found evidence of either acute or chronic gliosis. Since proliferation of glial cells is seen in most degenerative brain conditions and encepha-lopathies that arise after birth, this negative result would seem more consistent with neuropath-ological events that predate the responsivity of

glial cells to injury, which is before the third trimester of gestation (Larroche, 1984).

It is also interesting to note that as in the *in vivo* morphometry data, correlational results are not consistent with a neuropathological process that progresses once the illness is manifest. Ventricular size and cortical volume have not been correlated with duration of illness (Pakkenberg, 1987; Crow *et al.*, 1989). Pakkenberg (1987) reported, more-over, that ventricular size did not correlate with cognitive deficits noted in the hospital records at the time of death, but instead, correlated with those noted at the time of onset of the illness. This curious finding is more consistent with an underlying pathological defect that set the neuro-biological stage for an illness rather than one that evolved over the course of the illness.

Anomalous lateralization

The possibility that normally lateralized aspects of the brain might be anomalous in patients with schizophrenia has come from several experimental directions. Studies of lateralized cerebral function, such as handedness, dichotic listening asym-metries and lateralized cognitive tasks, have suggested that patients with schizophrenia may be less completely lateralized than normal individuals (Gruzelier *et al.*, 1988). If these functional asymmetries are related to mechanisms of the development of normal anatomical asymmetries, the findings may have implications for abnormal cerebral development in schizophrenia. In a sense, normal anatomical asymmetries are closer to the issue of intrauterine development than are other morphometric assessments. They inherently control for individual differences in state variables and other artefacts that can confound measure-ments of *in vivo* and postmortem specimens, presumably because such variables should not be lateralized. In contrast to asymmetrical findings (referred to above), findings of anomalous asym-metries are potentially more understandable. The research question involved is not whether a pathological process is distributed or affects the brain asymmetrically, but whether the normal programmes that determine healthy asymmetry have been disrupted. Since the times of origin of many of the well-characterized normal anatomical asymmetries are known, the time of disruption might be inferred. For instance, normal asymmetries of the Sylvian fissures (Chi *et al.*, 1977), of the planum temporale (Wada *et al.*, 1975), of the frontal operculum (Chi *et al.*, 1977) and of the frontal and occipital lobes (Weinberger *et al.*, 1982b) appear during the second trimester of gestation. Therefore, if consistent variations in the appearance of such asymmetries are seen in patients with schizophrenia, this might provide further evidence of adverse development during that period. This is a big 'if', however, and the data in schizophrenia are not consistent.

In the first CAT study of anatomical asymmetries in schizophrenia, Luchins *et al.* (1979) reported reduced asymmetries of the widths of the occipital lobes. While there have been replications of this observation by several groups, at least as many have failed to do so (Shelton & Weinberger, 1987). The same inconsistency appears to characterize the majority of the other literature on cerebral anatomical asymmetries in schizophrenia. For example, while some groups have reported less asymmetry of normally asymmetrical perisylvian structures, such as the Sylvian fissure (Falkai *et al.*, 1992) and the planum temporale (Rossi *et al.*, 1992), other groups have failed to replicate these findings (Bartley *et al.*, 1993; Kulynych *et al.*, 1995). Based on a finding of asymmetry of the ventricles seen in two-dimensional X-ray films of postmortem brain specimens, Crow *et al.* (1989) went so far as to hypothesize that schizophrenia is caused by a gene that controls the normal development of temporal lobe asymmetries. Tests of this hypothesis in discordant monozygotic twins, where the abnormalities of asymmetry would be expected in the unaffected twin as well as in the affected twin, have been negative (Weinberger *et al.*, 1991; Bartley *et al.*, 1993).

One possible explanation for these various discrepancies may relate to the fact that many of these asymmetries are less obvious in normal individuals who are incompletely right handed. If mixed dominance is overrepresented in populations of patients with schizophrenia, as has been reported (Myslobodsky & Weinberger, 1987), it is conceivable that positive studies did not adequately control for this variable. In other words, incomplete anatomical asymmetries may be a non-specific sign of developmental variance that is not associated with schizophrenia *per se*, and that may or may not reflect pathological intrauterine development. The fact that incomplete asymmetries are associated with left handedness, presumably even if genetic and not pathological (Bartley *et al.*, 1993), and have been reported in other patients with putative developmental disorders (e.g. autism, dyslexia) supports this possibility.

In summary, notwithstanding the uncertainties about lateralization, the data from morphometric studies have in general a considerable degree of internal consistency and tend towards the interpretation of neurodevelopmental deviance, most likely occurring before the end of the second trimester. The strongest feature of the morphometric data is the replicability. Moreover, the weight of the evidence does not fit into the model of adult-onset brain disorders. Unfortunately, measurements of the size of various cerebral structures and counts of cell numbers are not conclusive evidence of any neuropathological condition, developmental or otherwise, and could conceivably be accounted for by other explanations (e.g. non-pathological volume changes on *in vivo* scanning, e.g. because of dehydration, or coincidental neuronal loss or other artefacts unrelated to illness in postmortem studies, which usually involve elderly subjects). The possibility that the development of normal anatomical asymmetries is disrupted in patients with schizophrenia also is inconclusive and does not necessarily implicate a specific neuropathological condition. The most conceptually unimpeachable evidence comes from qualitative studies of cytoarchitecture.

Cytoarchitectural abnormalities

Consistent with the discussion above about normal brain development, the laminar patterns of neurones in cortex, the orientation of neurones and their internal relationships are fixed during the second trimester of gestation. It is generally assumed that such relationships and patterns do not change during life, even if cells are lost or secondary pathological conditions arise. If this assumption is correct, and this is not certain, then abnormalities of cytoarchitecture would strongly implicate pathological development.

Kovelman and Sheibel reported in 1984 that the orientation of hippocampal pyramidal cells in Nissl-stained sections of left hemispheres from 10 patients with chronic schizophrenia was abnormal in most of the specimens as compared with eight normal controls. Conrad *et al.* (1991) subsequently reported identical findings in the right hemispheres of mostly the same subjects. They interpreted their findings as consistent with a defect in neural migration, arguing that disorientation reflected a fault of neuronal settling into the target sites. Unfortunately, this finding has not been independently replicated. Three groups have reported negative results. Altshuler *et al.* (1987) could not replicate the observation in a sample of brains from the Yakovlev collection, although the authors claimed that within the normal range of orientation, those specimens that showed the most disorientation had clinical histories suggestive of more florid paranoid symptoms. In a larger study on the same brain collection, Christison *et al.* (1989) found no evidence of hippocampal cell disorientation. Benes *et al.* (1991b) evaluated subjectively pyramidal cell orientation and found no differences between patients and controls.

In contrast to the data on pyramidal cell orientation, the data on laminar organization in neocortex and limbic cortex are more consistent, though still far from ideal. Jakob and Beckmann (1986) made a potentially landmark observation in the entorhinal cortex. In Nissl-stained sections of 64 brains of patients with the diagnosis of schizophrenia and 10 controls, they reported that in the majority of ill cases there were cytoarchitectural anomalies of laminar organization. Specifically, they described attenuation of cellularity in superficial layers I and II, incomplete clustering of neurones into normal glomerular structures in layer II and the inclusion of such clusters in deeper layers where they are not normally found. They studied the rostral entorhinal cortex in the region of the amygdala and pes hippocampus. Interestingly, this is similar to the area of mesial temporal cortex where the most consistent morphometric abnormalities have been found in both *in vivo* and postmortem studies (Jeste & Lohr, 1989; Altshuler *et al.*, 1990; Brown *et al.*, 1986; Suddath *et al.*, 1990). They interpreted the findings as the result of a failure of cortical development, probably an arrest of migration, whereby relatively recent generation neurones destined for the superficial cortical lamina were held up in deeper layers. Perhaps the most compelling aspect of their observations is that they are difficult, if not impossible, to attribute to an insult that occurred to an already developed brain. The major uncertainties about the findings are: (i) are they artefacts of localization within entorhinal cortex?; (ii) are they related to schizophrenia *per se*?; and (iii) are they replicable? Other problems with the study included that it was not blind, that the controls were neurologically impaired in nine of the cases and that the patient population was probably atypical (e.g. mean age of illness onset was 36 years).

Normal entorhinal cortex anatomy is characterized by remarkable regional variability. In fact, as one moves caudal in entorhinal cortex, the normal appearance looks increasingly like what Jakob and Beckmann reported in schizophrenia (Hyde & Saunders, 1991). Therefore, it is critical that patients and controls are very carefully examined in the same cytoarchitectonic areas. The possibility that what Jakob and Beckmann observed may not be related to schizophrenia *per se* also must be considered. They subsequently reported the identical abnormalities in four patients with bipolar disorder, although two of these patients had originally been diagnosed with schizophrenia (Beckmann & Jakob, 1991). Moreover, additional questions exist about the schizophrenia sample, because they have also described gross cortical abnormalities [e.g. vertical temporal gyri, hypoplastic frontal gyri (Jakob & Beckmann, 1989)] that have not been associated with schizophrenia by other recent investigations.

In spite of these questions, the basic findings of Jakob and Beckmann have been independently replicated using the same methods and further supported by other recent data from different approaches to cortical cytoarchitecture. Arnold *et al.* (1991) studied Nissl-stained sections of six brains of patients with schizophrenia from the Yakovlev collection and 16 controls. They observed essentially the same abnormalities as described by Jakob and Beckmann and in addition reported anomalous mesial temporal sulci in their specimens. They felt that all six cases were abnormal, but in five the abnormalities were dramatic and unequivocal. None of the controls had similar findings. The authors acknowledged the importance of location within entorhinal cortex and attempted to control for this. Moreover, they reported that as they moved caudally, the differences between patients and controls disappeared, an observation that again corresponds to reports from the morphometric literature. The authors believed that their findings indicated an abnormality of entorhinal cortex development, probably a migration failure, that would render normal neocortical–hippocampal communication impossible. In addition to its small sample size, this study suffered from one other obvious problem. The entire patient sample had undergone prefrontal leucotomies. To control for the possible effect of this, they had included three controls who underwent leucotomy for non-psychiatric indications (e.g. chronic pain). Though the potential confound of leucotomy cannot be conclusively ruled out by this control group, it is difficult to imagine how the pattern of changes could be explained by this procedure.

Akbarian *et al.* (1993a) took a different approach to studying cytoarchitecture, but their results suggest the same defect as do those of Jakob and Beckmann (1986) and Arnold *et al.* (1991). Using a histochemical stain for cortical neurones that express the enzyme nicotinamide adenine dinucleotide phosphate diaphorase (NADPH-d), a neuronal population said to be remnants of the embryological subplate zone and particularly resistant to degeneration from ischaemia, infection,

etc., they studied the superior frontal gyrus region of dorsolateral prefrontal cortex in five brains of patients with schizophrenia and five controls matched for age, gender and postmortem interval before fixation. They found reduced numbers of these neurones in superficial cortical layers I–III and increased numbers in deep layers, especially in subcortical white matter, the putative vestigial subplate neurones. In essence, they observed a qualitative shift in the representation of NADPH-d positive neurones, as though the younger neurones destined to migrate last from the subplate zone got held up and never made it to their superficial cortical targets. The interpretations of the findings are remarkably similar to those of Jakob and Beckmann (1986) and Arnold *et al.* (1991).

It is also possible that the underlying defect reflected in the findings of Akbarian *et al.* is the same as that of yet another recent report, a study of Nissl-stained sections of cingulate cortex by Benes *et al.* (1991a). They found decreased numbers of small, presumably gabaergic neurones in superficial layers of prefrontal cortex of patients with schizophrenia and larger numbers of pyramidal cells in deeper layers. This finding also might suggest a failure of completion of the normal inside-out migratory gradient. The potential coherence of these two studies may be underscored by the fact that NADPH-d positive neurones appear to be gabaergic. Unfortunately, there are some inconsistencies. Subsequent cell counts of small, presumably gabaergic neurones in Nissl-stained sections of the samples used by Akbarian *et al.* could not directly confirm the finding of Benes *et al.* of a reduction in the small neurone population (Bunney *et al.*, 1993).

In a subsequent study of NADPH-d neurones of temporal lobe, including lateral temporal neocortex and mesial limbic cortex, Akbarian *et al.* (1993b) extended their abnormal findings to this region, suggesting a more widespread cortical developmental defect. This also would be consistent with the morphometric data. However, this second study presented some new inconsistencies. While they did find gradient abnormalities in hippocampus and lateral temporal neocortex, entorhinal cortex was normal. It is conceivable that the abnormalities of entorhinal cortex observed by Jakob and Beckmann and by Arnold *et al.* did not involve the subset of neurones that express NADPH-d. This might be consistent with the latter neurones being primarily GABAergic and the layer-II entorhinal cortex neurones being primarily glutamatergic. On the other hand, the involvement of NADPH-d neurones in each of the other cortical areas examined by Akbarian *et al.* make this explanation seem a bit strained. It also should be noted that the small sample size of the studies by Akbarian *et al.* necessitated a matched pair statistical analysis. It is unclear whether the findings would have held up if the matching had been done differently. Clearly, further studies of this type are needed before these uncertainties can be resolved.

In summary, if one looks at the research data about brain abnormalities in schizophrenia as a whole, one gets the impression of a convergence towards a story of subtle multifocal or diffuse anatomical deviations that appear to predate the onset of the illness and to be static, that are most consistent with the notion of a developmental defect, and that may implicate a failure of second trimester neuronal migration, leading to cortical maldevelopment. The most potentially incriminating evidence comes from studies of cortical cytoarchitecture. The possibility of cortical maldevelopment in the second trimester is also critical to a discussion of the additional speculation about neurodevelopmental factors and models that follow.

Aetiological considerations

Obstetric abnormalities

The possibility that obstetric complications (OCs) could contribute to, or even cause, schizophrenia has been the subject of a surprisingly large number of investigations over the past three decades. The literature on this issue is difficult to interpret, as the same methods are rarely used, the same findings are rarely reported and the implications of the data are rarely critically addressed. An illus-

tration of the tendency for uncritical acceptance of this literature is seen in frequent references to the work of Rosanoff *et al.* (1934). With rare exception, recent studies and reviews of OCs prominently cite Rosanoff *et al.* as being the first to draw attention to this subject. They are often credited with the supposedly prescient conclusion that 'a large proportion of such psychoses originate in cerebral trauma at birth', as if the existence of such a statement for six decades gives validity to the conclusion. In fact, Rosanoff *et al.* made this comment without presenting any objective data whatsoever. They offered it as an explanation for anecdotal postmortem observations that have subsequently turned out to be spurious. They claimed that the brains of patients with schizophrenia had pial haemorrhages and partial pial avulsions, and they argued that these injuries caused 'interference with blood supply, slow atrophy, and progressive impairment of mental function'. In other words, the 'prescient' belief of Rosanoff *et al.* was that pial trauma at birth caused progressive ischaemia of the cerebral cortex that continued throughout life!

The flip side of the OC literature is that the weight of the evidence suggests that there is a statistical association between OCs and schizophrenia. In the first controlled study of OCs, Pollack *et al.* (1966) compared maternal recollections of pregnancy and delivery complications of 33 patients with schizophrenia and their unaffected siblings. They found a trend for more frequent and severe complications in the affected siblings, which was subsequently found to be significant in a latter report of a larger sample (Woerner *et al.*, 1973). While there have been negative reports (e.g. Parnas *et al.*, 1982; Done *et al.*, 1991; McCreadie *et al.*, 1992), the majority of studies have found more frequent complications during both pregnancy and delivery in births of individuals who later manifest schizophrenia (McNeil, 1988). An overview of the literature in which birth histories of patients were compared with those of their unaffected siblings is shown in Tables 16.1 and 16.2. Sibship studies are particularly important because uncertainty about the validity of maternal recall is less problematic.

Table 16.1 Obstetric complications in adult schizophrenics and sibling controls

Study	Sample	Recall/records	Findings
Pollack *et al.* (1966)	33 patients 33 sibs	Recall	NS differences
Woerner *et al.* (1973)	52 patients 54 sibs	Both	Increase in OCs in schizophrenic and other abnormal sibs
McCreadie *et al.* (1992)	54 patients 114 sibs	Recall	No differences
DeLisi *et al.* (1988)	123 patients 148 sibs	Recall	Increase in OCs
Eagles *et al.* (1990)	27 patients 27 sibs	Records	Increase in OCs

OC, obstetric complication; NS, not significant.

Table 16.2 Obstetric complications in monozygotic twins with schizophrenia

Study	Sample	Recall/records	Findings
Torrey *et al.* (1994)	26 discordant pairs	Recall	No differences between affected and unaffected twins
Pollin and Stabenau (1968)	100 discordant pairs	Both	Increase in OCs in affected twin
Reveley *et al.* (1984)	21 schizophrenic MZ pairs 18 normal MZ pairs	Recall	Complex interactions with family history
Onstad *et al.* (1992)	16 discordant pairs 8 concordant pairs	Recall	No differences

OC, obstetric complications; MZ, monozygotic.

While the twin studies tend to be less conclusive, perhaps because twin pregnancies are often complicated, the sibling data suggest an association.

The controversial aspects of the OC literature concern the specific nature of the complications themselves, their neuropathological correlations and their overall significance. For example, McNeil (1988) has argued that schizophrenia is associated primarily with an increased frequency of delivery, and not pregnancy, complications, though clearly the latter have also been found (e.g. Woerner *et al.*, 1973). The possibility cannot be excluded that the amount of routine historical information about delivery is greater than about pregnancy, spuriously biasing the historical database. Another problem is that the nature of the delivery complications tends to vary from one study to another (e.g. some find prolonged labour, others premature membrane rupture, abnormal position or use of forceps, etc.), raising questions about the role of chance in some of the reports. Furthermore, the neuropathological implications that have been attributed to OCs are difficult to reconcile with the neuropathological findings associated with schizophrenia. Murray and Lewis (1987) and Cannon and Mednick (1991) have suggested that OCs result in periventricular haemorrhages, hypoxic–ischaemic injury and, ultimately, abnormalities of pruning, cell death and developmental connectivity. McNeil (1988) also suggests that delivery complications result in brain damage by virtue of hypoxic–ischaemic injury. Such injuries are typically characterized by gliosis (Roberts, 1991) and could not account for the cytoarchitectural changes described above, which presumably occur at least 3 months before delivery. If cytoarchitectural abnormalities and a lack of gliosis are a neuropathological signature of schizophrenia, it is virtually certain that these occur independent of delivery events.

Other inconsistencies in the OC literature have to do with the overall pathogenic significance of the findings. Mednick *et al.* have proposed that OCs are related to the genetic risk for schizophrenia and that somehow the gene for schizophrenic liability increases the neuropathological effects of OCs, including the effects of anaesthesia used during delivery (Cannon & Mednick, 1991; Cannon *et al.*, 1993). This complex hypothesis emerged as a result of correlational data from arbitrarily defined patient subgroups, when in fact, these investigators did not find an absolute increase of OCs in their entire sample of patients with schizoprenia (Parnas *et al.*, 1982) or in their entire high-risk population (Cannon *et al.*, 1993). Moreover, the interpretation of OCs being related to increased genetic risk is exactly the opposite interpretation of Murray *et al.* (1992), who argued from their data that OCs are especially relevant to non-genetic forms of schizophrenia (Reveley *et al.*, 1984).

A sober perspective on the OC literature and the pathogenic implications of OCs was offered by Goodman (1988) in an enlightening critique of the subject. He pointed out that even if one accepts the frequency data, OCs increase the risk of schizophrenia by, at most, 1%. Moreover, OCs are much more common in certain environments, but the frequency of schizophrenia does not parallel this geographical and cultural distribution. Thus, OCs appear to be 'very poor predictors' of

schizophrenia. Finally, he suggested that a more likely scenario for a relationship between OCs and schizophrenia was that the latter caused the former, and not the other way around. It has become increasingly apparent, as first proposed by Freud in reference to cerebral palsy (Freud, 1968), that pre-existing fetal abnormalities predispose to OCs. This synthesis of the OC literature also would be more compatible with the neuropathological data.

Prenatal viral exposure

Another potential cause of developmental injury that has occasionally been considered as a pathogenic factor in schizophrenia is prenatal viral exposure. Recently, interest in this potential aetiology has mushroomed as a result of a remarkable result reported by Mednick *et al.* (1988). They examined the hospital admission records of 1781 adult individuals in Finland, some of whom were born around the time of the Helsinki influenza A2 epidemic of 1957 (the index cases) and others who were born before the epidemic (control cases). They found that both males and females who had been in their second trimester of gestation during the height of the epidemic had a significantly higher percentage of subsequent admission diagnosis of schizophrenia than either the control cases or the index cases exposed during other trimesters. The implications were that influenza itself or related phenomena (e.g. fever) interfered with second trimester brain development, and that such interference was an aetiological risk factor for schizophrenia. This study has spawned at least six other studies (summarized in Table 16.3), opening a new area of research controversy. While there have been positive reports supporting the findings of Mednick *et al.* negative reports are virtually as frequent, and methodological uncertainties cloud the interpretation of the results.

Kendell and Kemp (1989) compared hospital admission records throughout Scotland of individuals who had been *in utero* during the influenza A epidemics of 1918–19 and 1957. Although they did find an increased risk of schizophrenia

Table 16.3 Prenatal influenza and adult schizophrenia

Study	Sample	Findings
Mednick *et al.* (1988)	Pregnancies coincident with Helsinki 1957 A2 epidemic	Increase in schizophrenia in second trimester cohort, especially at 6 months gestation
Kendell and Kemp (1989)	Pregnancies coincident with Scottish 1918, 1919 and 1957 A2 epidemics	Increase in Edinburgh samples for 1957, second trimester; no increase in association in entire sample
Torrey *et al.* (1994)	43 814 schizophrenic births between 1950 and 1959 in USA	No increase in association with 1957 A2
Barr *et al.* (1990)	Danish schizophrenic samples born between 1911 and 1950 ($n = 7239$)	Increase in schizophrenia in $6-7$ months gestational group coincident with high incidence of influenza compared with group coincident with low incidence
O'Callaghan *et al.* (1991)	339 schizophrenic patients born around English 1957 A2 epidemic	Abnormal distribution of schizophrenia births in index year in women only, *appearance* of increased risk in fifth gestational month
Sham *et al.* (1992)	British hospital first admission $1970-79$ with schizophrenia; n not specified	Weak statistical association between frequency pattern of influenza deaths $1939-60$ and second trimester of schizophrenic births
Crow and Done (1992)	1620 pregnancies with history of 1957 A2 influenza *infection* in Great Britain	No increased risk of schizophrenia
Adams *et al.* (1993)	Reanalysis of data from studies of Kendell and Kemp; Sham *et al.* and Barr *et al.*	Increased risk in all populations for 1957 A2; no increase in association with other epidemics

for those in the second trimester in 1957 in a sample from Edinburgh, the overall Scottish admission data revealed no such effect. These authors tended to dismiss the Edinburgh data and emphasized their negative findings. Moreover, they have argued that a reanalysis of the data of Mednick *et al.* using absolute numbers of patients with schizophrenia rather than proportions of such patients relative to other diagnoses is also negative (Kendell & Kemp, 1990).

Subsequent studies have only added to the controversy. Torrey *et al.* (1988) looked at a large birth cohort in the USA and found no association of increased risk with the US influenza A2 epidemic of 1957. Barr *et al.* (1990) attempted to replicate the study of Mednick *et al.* (1988) in a Danish sample. Regrettably, they chose a different approach to data collection and analysis. They collected hospital admission data about all patients

in Denmark with a diagnosis of schizophrenia born between 1911 and 1951, divided them into three groups based on the relative frequency of influenza infections in the general population during their birth month, as recorded in public health infectious disease records, and analysed the birth-rate data as a deviation score from the expected schizophrenia birth rate for a particular month. This complex analysis was justified as an attempt to control for spurious associations that might result from seasonal variations in influenza exposure and in schizophrenia birth rates. The authors reported that in the high seasonal influenza exposure subgroup, those exposed during the sixth month of gestation had the highest rates of schizophrenia. Unfortunately, the data also appear to show that the other two groups have lower than expected schizophrenia birth rates during the same month (i.e. the sixth) of gestation.

Moreover, it appears, though this analysis is not reported, that unless the tripartite approach to subgrouping is used, there is no overall association between schizophrenia birth rate and exposure to influenza A2. Indeed, the authors acknowledge that even in their positive subgroup, the association between schizophrenia and influenza is weak, accounting for at most 4% of the variance.

Another example of the confusing nature of this literature is the study of O'Callaghan *et al.* (1991). These investigators compared admission diagnoses in eight health regions of England and Wales with birth records around the time of the 1957 influenza epidemic. They reported that for patients *in utero* during the second trimester (especially the fifth month) 'the number of births of individuals who later developed schizophrenia was 88% higher' than expected. In fact, what they actually found was that the overall monthly distribution of affected births (i.e. subsequent schizophrenics) was different in the exposure and the control years. Since they did not perform *post hoc* tests on individual months, they did not statistically determine what month(s) accounted for the overall distribution differences. Indeed, their data also show a peak at around 3 months and a trough at around 8 months, both of which may have been important factors in the overall distribution analysis. In a related study, Sham *et al.* (1992) examined the numbers of first-time admissions with a diagnosis of schizophrenia throughout England and Wales from 1970−79 and compared them with the number of deaths from influenza during the period 1930−69. Arguing that the latter was a relative index of likelihood of influenza exposure *in utero* for the former, they found a statistical relationship using a complex model-fitting paradigm of the two frequency distributions, with greatest correspondence during the third and seventh months of gestation. The data suggested, however, that at most 1−2% of schizophrenic births could be explained by this relationship.

A recent report by Adams *et al.* (1993) both clarifies and confuses the picture even further. They performed an extensive epidemiological analysis of cohorts of English, Scottish, and Danish samples that included but enlarged upon those of Sham *et al.* (1992); Kendell and Kemp (1989; Barr *et al.* (1990), respectively. They tested two questions: (i) the association of incidence rates of schizophrenia with incidence rates of influenza throughout this century, analogous to the studies of Sham *et al.* and Barr *et al.* and (ii) the risk of developing schizophrenia associated with gestation during the Influenza A2 epidemic of 1957. With respect to (i), they confirmed an association in the English sample, but failed to do so in the Danish or Scottish samples. Of note, they failed to replicate the study of Barr *et al.* (1990), using the same sample but more appropriate statistics. With respect to (ii), they confirmed an association of increased risk of schizophrenia with second trimester of gestation during the 1957 epidemic. An association was found in each sample, though only for women. Also of note, using a larger control sample and a different statistical procedure than previously (Kendell & Kemp 1989), they found a positive association in the Scottish sample that had not been observed in the earlier report. While the study of Adams *et al.* (1993) appropriately stresses this newly positive result, it tended to overlook some of the inconsistencies in the same Scottish dataset. For example, while significantly increased risk for schizophrenia was now found in association with the Scottish influenza epidemic during the fifth month of gestation, a significantly *decreased* risk was found during the sixth month!

An important limitation of each of the perinatal exposure studies is that none of them documented actual maternal, let alone intrauterine, infection. In the only study to attempt this, Crow and Done (1992) investigated psychiatric admissions of individuals born around the 1957 epidemic who had been enrolled in a perinatal injury and child development research project in England. They identified 945 individuals whose mothers had been diagnosed during their second trimester of pregnancy as having influenza. They did not find an increased risk of subsequent schizophrenia in the offspring of these mothers. This study has been criticized, however, for possibly having a low ascertainment rate of cases of schizophrenia (Cooper, 1992).

In summary, the perinatal viral exposure litera-ture is provocative but inconclusive. The 1957 influenza data from Europe are the most compel-ling, but important inconsistencies remain. The reasons for the inconsistencies are uncertain, and it is doubtful that they will be resolved in the near future. Even if the inconsistencies can be resolved and the positive results prevail, exposure to influ-enza will account for at most a very small minority of cases. Moreover, while the positive results may add circumstantially to the notion that second trimester maldevelopment increases the risk of schizophrenia, the mechanisms by which this happens will be difficult to establish from epi-demiological studies of potential viral exposure.

Other aetiological factors

Because of the possibility that neural development may be disrupted by a number of adverse events in addition to viral exposure, other causes have been considered. For example, alcohol can adversely affect fetal development, causing some changes that have been described in schizophrenia (e.g. migrational defects, reduced cortical volume) (Lohr & Bracha, 1989). Epidemiological data, however, do not suggest that maternal alcoholism is an important risk factor for schizophrenia. In a recent study of the potential impact of maternal malnutrition, Susser and Lin (1992) studied the effects of starvation in occupied Holland during World War II and found that first- but not second-trimester starvation was associated with an increased risk of schizophrenic births. Since the implications of this finding for the neuro-pathological changes associated with schizo-phrenia are unclear, if not contradictory, this study is difficult to integrate with the rest of the neurodevelopmental database. This study also did not control for the implication of social class both in access to food and on risk for schizophrenia.

In light of the widely accepted data that genetic factors convey susceptibility to schizophrenia, it is not surprising that there has been speculation about genetic factors that may affect brain devel-opment in schizophrenia. Since approximately 30% of the genome is expressed in brain (Sutcliffe

et al., 1984), and many genes are turned on and off during discrete phases of brain development, there are many potential candidates. No existing data link schizophrenia with a defect in any known gene related to brain development. Nevertheless, Murray *et al.* (1992) have hypothesized that the fundamental neuropathological deviations in the schizophrenic brain arise because of a primary genetic defect in at least a substantial subgroup of patients. Mednick *et al.* (1991) have hypothesized that a genetic defect predisposes the schizophrenic brain to being adversely affected by intrauterine or perinatal environmental events. Another poss-ibility is that the genetic control of brain develop-ment, such as genes that regulate trophic factors, may be disrupted by adverse environmental events (e.g. fever, toxins, etc.) (Bloom, 1993). These hypotheses, and undoubtedly many others that will be advanced, must await the discovery and practicability of scientific methods to test them.

Mechanisms of delayed onset

The possibility that schizophrenia is related to an abnormality of early brain development poses yet another interesting challenge, for the clinical expression of the illness is delayed typically for about two decades after birth. If the neurological abnormality is present at birth, why is the illness itself not manifested earlier in life and what accounts for its predictable clinical expression in early adulthood? Speculation about the answers to these questions has come primarily from two perspectives: (i) the possibility of an additional pathological process occurring around the time of onset of the clinical illness; and (ii) an interaction between a static developmental defect and normal developmental programmes or events that occur in early adult life.

As the foremost proponent of the first perspec-tive, Feinberg (1982) focused on the age of onset of schizophrenia as a clue to neurodevelopmental abnormalities that might explain the illness. He posited that schizophrenia is caused by a defect in adolescent synaptic reorganization, because either 'too many, too few, or the wrong synapses are eliminated'. In effect, he argues for a second pathological process, a specific pathology of synaptic elimination not necessarily related to possible maldevelopment *in utero*. His hypothesis does not take into account the neuropathological database (most of which did not exist at the time of his original proposal), and he does not address the biological mechanisms that might be responsible for this putative disorder of synaptic elimination. In light of the neuropathological database that implicates maldevelopment *in utero*, this hypothesis would require the unlikely scenario of a second primary pathology. Another problem with this hypothesis is that it is unclear how one could directly test it, especially because it accommodates all potential variations (i.e. too much, too little or the 'wrong' pruning).

An alternative scenario that might be considered is that maldevelopment *in utero* sets the stage for secondary synaptic disorganization that has its greatest neurobiological and clinical impact in adolescence. This integration of the neuropathological data with the 'Feinberg hypothesis' would tend to regard irregularities of synaptic pruning as epiphenomena. It would be consistent with the notion that neuronal circuitry that is anomalous from early in development may have particularly profound implications for eventual connectivity (Schwartz & Goldman-Rakic, 1990). In other words, perhaps primary migratory or other developmental defects lead to the creation of abnormal circuits which compete successfully for survival, while certain normal circuits either do not form or are structurally disadvantaged so that they cannot avoid elimination.

Despite the theoretical improbability of a primary pathology of synaptic elimination in late adolescence, this hypothesis is frequently recruited as an explanation for counterintuitive findings in the research literature [e.g. an unexpected pattern of degenerative abnormalities of phospholipid concentrations measured with magnetic resonance spectroscopy (Pettegrew *et al.*, 1993), and increased basal ganglia size on MRI imaging (Jernigan *et al.*, 1991)]. These latter two examples from MRI also illustrate that the abnormal pruning hypothesis is sometimes cited as positing too much pruning (Pettegrew *et al.*,

1993) and sometimes cited as implicating too little pruning (Jernigan *et al.*, 1991).

Other mechanisms for delayed onset that emphasize a new process going wrong around the time of clinical onset have been proposed. These include abnormalities of myelination (Benes, 1989) or neuronal sprouting (Stevens, 1992), and of adverse effects of stress-related neural transmission (Bogerts, 1989). Each of these involves a variation on the theme of another abnormality taking place in early adult life. In essence, they are dual pathology hypotheses, positing either that maldevelopment *in utero* is not sufficient pathology, or is coincidental, or that it is only one of two relatively independent pathologies that characterize the illness.

The second perspective maintains that it might be possible to accommodate both maldevelopment *in utero* and delayed clinical onset without positing an additional abnormal process in adolescence. This perspective involves an interaction between cortical maldevelopment *in utero* and normal developmental events that occur much later (Weinberger, 1987). This view rests on several assumptions: that the clinical implications of a developmental defect vary with the maturational state of the brain; that the neural systems disrupted by the defect in early brain development in schizophrenia are normally late-maturing neural systems; and that a defect in the function of these neural systems will not be reliably apparent until their normal time of functional maturation. In other words, it is posited that certain neural systems are destined from early development to malfunction in a manner that accounts for the illness, but until a certain state of postnatal brain development either they do not malfunction to a clinically significant degree, or their malfunctioning can be compensated for by other systems. The first of these assumptions has been repeatedly validated in developmental neurobiology. Indeed, a fundamental principle of the clinical impact of developmental neuropathology, as exemplified by the work of Kennard (1936), is that in general, early brain damage is apparent early and tends to become less so over time. The young brain has a greater capacity for functional compensation than does the old brain (Kolb & Whishaw, 1989). It is also a fundamental principle of paediatric neurology that in some cases congenital brain damage can have delayed or varying clinical effects if the neural systems involved are neurologically immature at birth (Adams & Lyons, 1982).

In the case of schizophrenia, the 'Kennard principle' appears to be inverted, in that the impact of putative early damage is less apparent early and more apparent later. In this respect, the other two assumptions of this perspective are much more speculative. It is not known whether the principle of clinical effects being delayed until the affected neural systems reach functional maturity applies to those neural systems implicated in schizophrenia. More data are needed about the neural systems that develop abnormally in schizophrenia and about their normal course of functional maturation. Nevertheless, in the absence of such data, the following speculation seems appropriate. The neuropathological database about schizophrenia has highlighted subtle maldevelopment of cerebral cortex. The clinical implications of such changes are likely to be in the realm of cortical malfunction. Correlative data from studies of cortical function in patients with schizophrenia, including neuropsychological testing results (Goldberg *et al.*, 1991) and studies of cortical physiology using functional brain-imaging techniques (Berman & Weinberger, 1991), indicate that cortical dysfunction is a prominent characteristic of the illness and that prefrontal–temporal functional connectivity is especially impaired. Even if cortical maldevelopment is widespread, the functional neural systems that appear to be particularly relevant to the clinical characteristics of schizophrenia are those involved in prefrontal–temporal connectivity (Berman & Weinberger, 1991; Weinberger, 1991; Weinberger *et al.*, 1992). This pattern is consistent with the developmental neuropathology reviewed above. If the function of systems that subserve such connectivity is late maturing, as a number of lines of evidence suggest (Bachevalier & Mishkin, 1984; Chelune & Baer, 1986; Thatcher *et al.*, 1987; Weinberger, 1987; Buchsbaum *et al.*, 1992), then this would fit the model of this perspective about delayed onset.

The molecular events that account for the functional maturation of these systems are probably complex, and may involve stabilization of synapses, levelling off of the growth of dendritic arbours, and other processes related to the refinement of cortical connectivity, all of which seem to plateau in early adult life. This is consistent with the notion that it is the stabilization of dynamic processes involved in postnatal cortical differentiation that signals the functional maturation of cortex (Rakic *et al.*, 1986; Lidow & Rakic, 1992).

In a more psychological vein, prefrontal–temporal connectivity has been viewed as facilitating the use of past experience to guide purposeful behaviour when environmental cues are inadequate or maladaptive (Goldman-Rakic, 1987; Weinberger, 1993). The stresses of independent adult living might be especially likely to place a premium on this manner of neural function. If the neural systems that permit such highly evolved behaviours are developmentally defective, their malfunction might be occult until either they alone are meant to subserve such functions, so other systems can no longer compensate, or the environmental demands for such behaviour overwhelm their diminished capacity.

These alternative perspectives on mechanisms of delayed onset, though differing on the question of whether neurodevelopmental processes of adolescence are abnormal, share an emphasis on cortical connectivity being abnormal, as do the *in vivo* imaging, neuropsychological and postmortem data (Weinberger, 1991). This raises an additional problem for the explanatory power of neurodevelopmental models of schizophrenia, in that the diagnostic symptoms of the illness, i.e. hallucinations and delusions, have not been classically imputed to cortical dysfunction (Jaskiw & Weinberger, 1992). Moreover, it is unclear how this apparent inconsistency could be resolved by the added complexity of the neurodevelopmental frame of reference. Potential insights into these issues have come from studies of neurological illnesses associated with developmental neuropathology and psychosis, and from animal models of delayed effects of perinatal injury.

Neurobiological models

Neurological analogies

Hallucinations and delusions are not unique to schizophrenia. They are encountered in a number of neurological conditions, involving many areas of the brain (Davison & Bagley, 1969). It has been pointed out that one of the better predictors of whether a neurological condition presents with psychosis is the age at which it presents (Weinberger, 1987). Of those disorders that may have psychopathology as a prominent clinical feature, psychosis is much more likely to be manifest in late adolescence and early adulthood than at other times of life. This is true even if the neuropathological changes do not vary with age. In other words, simply disrupting the neural systems related to psychosis is not necessarily sufficient to cause the syndrome. The brain needs to be at a certain state of development for the maximum likelihood of psychosis.

Metachromatic leucodystrophy (MLD) is an informative example of this age association and also of the potential importance of functional 'dysconnection' of cortical regions. Hyde *et al.* (1992) have demonstrated that when MLD presents between the ages of 13 and 30 years, it presents in the majority of cases as a schizophrenia-like illness. Moreover, the clinical presentation is probably more similar to schizophrenia than is seen in any other neurological disease. Patients have disorganized thinking, act bizarrely, have complex delusions and, when hallucinating, invariably have complex, Schneiderian-type auditory hallucinations. The condition is often misdiagnosed as schizophrenia, sometimes for years, before neurological symptoms appear. Interestingly, MLD is not a disease of mesial temporal cortex or of frontal cortex. It is a pure connectivity disorder in that the neuropathological changes involve white matter. In its early neuropathological stages, when it is most likely to present with psychosis, the changes are especially prominent in subprefrontal white matter. This suggests that a neural dysfunction with a high valence for producing psychotic symptoms is a failure of some aspects of prefrontal connectivity, analogous functionally to what has been implicated in schizophrenia.

In the case of MLD, however, this functional 'dysconnection' does not appear to be enough. When MLD presents outside of this critical age range, it almost never presents with psychosis, even though the location of the neuropathology is not age dependent. In other words, the involvement of critical neural systems is not by itself sufficient for the expression of psychosis. An age-related factor that appears to be independent of the illness is also required. Since this age association is seen in other diseases, and thus transcends specific illness boundaries, it is probably a function of normal postnatal brain maturation. Thus, the example of MLD supports the theoretical perspective that psychosis may reflect a cortical defect that interacts with developmental programmes normally linked to a late adolescent brain.

The MLD example also provides another potential insight into how cortical maldevelopment might be a crucial factor in schizophrenia. The distribution of white matter pathology in MLD is not unique to this illness. For example, a similar distribution of changes was produced by prefrontal leucotomies which did not worsen psychosis. Subfrontal white matter lesions also are seen in multiple sclerosis (MS), but psychosis is rare. However, MS plaques and leucotomy lesions spare intracortical fibres which are affected in MLD, suggesting that intracortical 'dysconnection' is closer to the source of psychosis. It also suggests, particularly with reference to leucotomy, that 'dysconnection' is more problematic than no connection. The developmental neuropathology described above in association with schizophrenia is much more consistent with the possibility of dysconnection than of no connection. Further support for this possibility comes from studies of epilepsy and psychosis in which congenital malformations of the mesial temporal lobe are more likely to be associated with psychosis than are sclerotic lesions (Roberts *et al.*, 1990). The former are also more consistent with the possibility of dysconnection than are the latter. Moreover, temporal lobectomy does not cure psychosis associated with epilepsy, further suggesting that the source of the psychosis is represented as a distributed abnormality.

Animal models

The neurological analogies cited suggest that a putative defect in intracortical connectivity occurring at a critical period in postnatal brain maturation may be clinically manifest as psychosis. They do not, however, suggest that a defect in such connectivity existing at birth could remain clinically silent until late adolescence. Studies in animals have supported this possibility.

Goldman (1971) showed that a perinatal ablation of the dorsolateral prefrontal cortex did not impair performance on delayed response tasks in animals before adolescence as a similar lesion placed in adult animals did. However, when animals with perinatal lesions of this cortical region reached adolescence, their performance on these tests actually became impaired. Goldman suggested that prior to puberty other brain regions (e.g. caudate) took responsibility for this behaviour, but by adolescence the brain was developmentally committed to use the cortex for this activity. In other words, the other neural strategies or systems were no longer available or were incapable of performing normally in the context of a more developed brain. She also showed that this delay in presentation of the cognitive deficit was a characteristic of some neural systems and not others. In animals with ablations of orbital frontal cortex, a phylogenetically older cortical region, the Kennard principle seemed to hold. The animals manifested their deficits early in life, and if anything, they improved as they got older.

Recently, Beauregard *et al.* (1992) reported preliminary data suggesting that an analogous delay in the appearance of certain cognitive deficits can be seen after perinatal hippocampal ablations. In rhesus monkeys with selective ablations of the rostral hippocampus, performance on delayed non-matching to sample tests, tests that are sensitive to hippocampal dysfunction in adult monkeys, are only mildly impaired until after puberty, when they become more profoundly so.

These studies indicate that perinatal injury to prefrontal and limbic cortices, two regions that are strongly implicated in schizophrenia, can have minimal impact on cognitive function before puberty and clinically significant impact afterwards. This suggests that the apparent deterioration in cognitive function seen in patients with schizophrenia around the time of onset of their illness (Goldberg *et al.*, 1993) could conceivably be the result of early developmental brain injury as the sole pathological event. However, these studies do not suggest that psychotic symptoms, symptoms that tend to respond to antipsychotic drugs, presumably through the blockade of dopamine receptors, also could suddenly emerge during early adulthood as a result of early developmental brain injury. Recent studies in the rat, however, have made it possible to conceive of this as well.

In a series of studies, Lipska *et al.* (Lipska *et al.*, 1993; Lipska & Weinberger, 1993a,b) have shown that perinatal excitotoxic damage of the ventral hippocampus of the rat represents an interesting model of delayed emergence of hyperdopaminergic behaviours. These animals show no evidence of abnormalities of mesolimbic or nigrostriatally mediated behaviours until after puberty, whereupon they become hyperresponsive to dopaminergic drugs, and to a variety of experiential stresses. They also manifest the delayed emergence of other abnormalities associated with schizophrenia, such as abnormal prepulse inhibition of startle. Moreover, in some respects they grow up to look like animals with adult prefrontal lesions, suggesting that the neonatal hippocampal lesion has affected prefrontal development as well. Their abnormal dopaminergic behaviours are ameliorated by antipsychotic drugs.

This provocative animal model illustrates that early developmental damage to cortical systems that have been implicated in schizophrenia may also have delayed effects on the regulation of brain dopamine systems. These delayed effects may have something to do with the maturation of these dopamine systems. They might also reflect the maturation of experience-based cortical systems which are programmed to take responsibility in early adulthood for regulating subcortical dopamine systems when they are needed. It seems theoretically possible that if these cortical systems developed abnormally, they may be unable to appropriately regulate subcortical dopamine systems when it is time to do so.

Overview

The research summarized in this chapter tends, on the whole, towards the interpretation that individuals who manifest schizophrenia in early adult life have suffered some form of subtle cerebral maldevelopment *in utero*. This assumption is based on imperfect studies and inconclusive data. Nevertheless, there are a number of converging lines of evidence. The morphometric anatomical data from *in vivo* and postmortem investigations are difficult to attribute to a neuropathological process of adult life. The static nature of the structural findings, the correlations with early life adaptation and the absence of gliosis are much more consistent with the possibility of a developmental anomaly. By far the most important anatomical data concern the evidence of cytoarchitectural disorganization of cortex. These findings are virtually pathognomonic of a defect in cortical development occurring during the second trimester of gestation. If these data can be replicated in methodologically unimpeachable studies, a 'smoking gun' will have been identified. Further efforts in this regard should be at the top of the list of priorities in schizophrenia research.

The other issues in thinking about schizophrenia as a neurodevelopmental disorder pivot on the validity of the cytoarchitectural findings. If these postmortem results are valid, then the aetiology is one that affects brain development during this critical period. The question of why the clinical manifestations of such congenital damage are not present in recognizable form until early adulthood is reached is important because answering it may hold clues to the mechanisms of clinical compensation and decompensation. The scenario stressed in this chapter involves an interaction of cortical maldevelopment with normal programmes of postnatal functional development of critical intracortical neural systems. The systems that appear to be especially relevant to the cortical functional impairments of schizophrenia involve prefrontal and limbic cortices and their connectivity. Such highly evolved, late-maturing systems may be especially important in coping with the vicissitudes of independent psychosocial functioning and may be critical as well for stress-related management of subcortical dopamine activity. As recently demonstrated in a new wave of heuristically meaningful animal models, it is conceivable that a congenital defect in such systems would remain submerged until early adult life and then fail to properly regulate subcortical dopamine activity in the context of environmental stress. It is further conceivable that genetically determined variations in intracortical connectivity or in limbic dopamine-system responsivity, which would not be clinically significant by themselves, could become clinically devastating when combined with the cortical maldevelopment implicated above.

References

Abi-Dargham, A., Jaskiw, G., Suddath, R.L. & Weinberger, D.R. (1991) Evidence against progression of *in vivo* anatomical abnormalities in schizophrenia. *Schizophrenia Research*, 5, 210.

Adams, R.D. & Lyons, G. (1982) *Neurology of Hereditary Metabolic Diseases of Children*. McGraw-Hill, New York.

Adams, W., Kendell, R.E., Hare, E.H. & Munk-Jørgensen, P. (1993) Epidemiological evidence that maternal influenza contributes to the aetiology of Schizophrenia: an analysis of Scottish, English and Danish data. *British Journal of Psychiatry*, 163, 169–177.

Akbarian, S., Bunney, W.E. Jr, Potkin, S.G. *et al.* (1993a) Altered distribution of nicotinamide-adenine dinucleotide phosphate-diaphorase cells in frontal lobe of schizophrenics implies disturbances of cortical development. *Archives of General Psychiatry*, 50, 169–177.

Akbarian, S., Viñuela, A., Kim, J.J., Potkin, S.G., Bunney, W.E. Jr & Jones, E.G. (1993b) Distorted distribution of nicotinamide-adenine dinucleotide phosphate-diaphorase neurons in temporal lobe of schizophrenics implies anomalous cortical development. *Archives of General Psychiatry*, 50, 178–187.

Altshuler, L.L., Casanova, M.F., Goldberg, T.E. & Kleinman, J.E. (1990) The hippocampus and parahippocampus in schizophrenic, suicide, and control brains. *Archives of General Psychiatry*, 47, 1029–1034.

Altshuler, L.L., Conrad, A., Kovelman, J.A. & Scheibel, A. (1987) Hippocampal pyramidal cell orientation in schizophrenia. A controlled neurohistologic study of the Yakovlev collection. *Archives of General Psychiatry*, **44**, 1094–1098.

Arnold, S.E., Hyman, B.T., van Hoesen, G.W. & Damasio, A.R. (1991) Some cytoarchitectural abnormalities of the entorhinal cortex in schizophrenia. *Archives of General Psychiatry*, **48**, 625–632.

Asarnow, J.R. (1988) Children at risk for schizophrenia: converging lines of evidence. *Schizophrenia Bulletin*, **14**, 613–631.

Aylward, E., Walker, E. & Bittes, B. (1984) Intelligence in schizophrenia. *Schizophrenia Bulletin*, **10**, 430–459.

Bachevalier, J. & Mishkin, M. (1984) An early and a late developing system for learning and retention in infant monkeys. *Behavioral Neuroscience*, **98**, 770–778.

Barr, C.E., Mednick, S.A. & Munk-Jorgensen, P. (1990) Exposure to influenza epidemics during gestation and adult schizophrenia. A 40-year study. *Archives of General Psychiatry*, **47**, 869–874.

Bartley, A.J., Jones, D.W., Torrey, E.F., Zigun, J.R. & Weinberger, D.R. (1993) Sylvian fissure asymmetries in monozygotic twins: a test of laterality in schizophrenia. *Biological Psychiatry*, **34**, 853–863.

Beauregard, M., Malkova, L. & Bachevalier, J. (1992) Is schizophrenia a result of early damage to the hippocampal formation? A behavioral study in primates. *Society of Neuroscience Abstracts*, **18**, 872.

Beckmann, H. & Jakob, H. (1991) Prenatal disturbances of nerve cell migration in the entorhinal region: a common vulnerability factor in functional psychoses? *Journal of Neural Transmission*, **84**, 155–164.

Benes, F.M. (1989) Myelination of cortical–hippocampal relays during late adolescence. *Schizophrenia Bulletin*, **15**, 585–593.

Benes, F.M., Davidson, J. & Bird, E.D. (1986) Quantitative cytoarchitectural studies of the cerebral cortex of schizophrenics. *Archives of General Psychiatry*, **43**, 31–35.

Benes, F.M., McSparren, J., Bird, E.D., SanGiovanni, J.P. & Vincent, S.L. (1991a) Deficits in small interneurons in prefrontal and cingulate cortices of schizophrenic and schizoaffective patients. *Archives of General Psychiatry*, **48**, 996–1001.

Benes, F.M., Sorensen, I. & Bird, E.D. (1991b) Reduced neuronal size in posterior hippocampus of schizophrenic patients. *Schizophrenia Bulletin*, **17**, 597–608.

Berman, K.F. & Weinberger, D.R. (1991) Functional localization in the brain in schizophrenia. In Tasman, A. & Goldfinger, S.M. (eds) *American Psychiatric Press Review of Psychiatry*, Vol. 10 pp. 24–59. American Psychiatric Association, Washington DC.

Bloom, F.E. (1993) Advancing a neurodevelopmental origin for schizophrenia. *Archives of General Psychiatry*, **50**, 224–227.

Beckmann, H. & Jakob, H. (1991) Prenatal disturbances of nerve cell migration in the entorhinal region: a common vulnerability factor in functional psychoses? *Journal of Neural Transmission*, **84**, 155–164.

Benes, F.M. (1989) Myelination of cortical–hippocampal relays during late adolescence. *Schizophrenia Bulletin*, **15**, 585–593.

Benes, F.M., Davidson, J. & Bird, E.D. (1986) Quantitative cytoarchitectural studies of the cerebral cortex of schizophrenics. *Archives of General Psychiatry*, **43**, 31–35.

Benes, F.M., McSparren, J., Bird, E.D., SanGiovanni, J.P. & Vincent, S.L. (1991a) Deficits in small interneurons in prefrontal and cingulate cortices of schizophrenic and schizoaffective patients. *Archives of General Psychiatry*, **48**, 996–1001.

Benes, F.M., Sorensen, I. & Bird, E.D. (1991b) Reduced neuronal size in posterior hippocampus of schizophrenic patients. *Schizophrenia Bulletin*, **17**, 597–608.

Berman, K.F. & Weinberger, D.R. (1991) Functional localization in the brain in schizophrenia. In Tasman, A. & Goldfinger, S.M. (eds) *American Psychiatric Press Review of Psychiatry*, Vol. 10 pp. 24–59. American Psychiatric Association, Washington DC.

Bloom, F.E. (1993) Advancing a neurodevelopmental origin for schizophrenia. *Archives of General Psychiatry*, **50**, 224–227.

Bogerts, B. (1989) Limbic and paralimbic pathology in schizophrenia: interaction with age- and stress-related factors. In Schulz, S.C. & Tamminga, C.A. (eds) *Schizophrenia: Scientific Progress*, pp. 216–226. Oxford University Press, Oxford.

Bogerts, B., Ashtari, M., Degreef, G., Alvir, J.M.J., Bilder, R.M. & Lieberman, J.A. (1990) Reduced temporal limbic structure volumes on magnetic resonance images in first-episode schizophrenia. *Psychiatry Research: Neuroimaging*, **35**, 1–13.

Bogerts, B., Meertz, E. & Schönfeldt-Bausch, R. (1985) Basal ganglia and limbic system pathology in schizophrenia. A morphometric study of brain volume and shrinkage. *Archives of General Psychiatry*, **42**, 784–791.

Brand, S. & Rakic, P. (1979) Genesis of the primate neostriatum: [^{3}H]thymidine autoradiographic analysis of the time of neuron origin in the rhesus monkey. *Neuroscience*, **4**, 767–778.

Brand, S. & Rakic, P. (1984) Cytodiffentiation and synaptogenesis in the neostriatum of fetal and neonatal rhesus monkeys. *Anatomy and Embryology* **169**, 21–34.

Brown, R., Colter, N., Corsellis, J.A.N. *et al.* (1986) Postmortem evidence of structural brain changes in schizophrenia. *Archives of General Psychiatry* **43**: 36–42.

Bruton, C.J., Crow, T.J., Frith, C.D., Johnstone, E.C., Owens, D.G.C. & Roberts, G.W. (1990) Schizophrenia and the brain: a prospective clinico-neuropathological study. *Psychological Medicine*, **20**, 285–304.

Buchsbaum, M.S., Mansour, C.S., Teng, D.G., Zia, A.D., Siegel, B.V. Jr & Rich, D.M. (1992) Adolescent developmental changed in topography of EEG amplitude. *Schizophrenia Research*, **7**, 101–107.

Bunney, W.E. Jr, Akbarian, S., Kim, J.J., Hagman, J.O., Potkin, S.G. & Jones, E.G. (1993) Gene expression for glutamic acid decarboxylase is reduced in prefrontal cortex of schizophrenics. *Neuroscience Abstracts* **19**, 199.

Cannon, T.D. & Mednick, S.A. (1991) Fetal neural development and adult schizophrenia: an elaboration of the paradigm. In Mednick, S.A., Cannon, T.D., Barr, C.E. & Lyon, M. (eds) *Fetal Neural Development and Adult Schizophrenia*, pp. 227–237. Cambridge University Press, Cambridge.

Cannon, T.D., Mednick, S.A., Parnas, J., Schulsinger, F., Praestholm, J. & Vestergaard, A. (1993) Developmental brain abnormalities in the offspring of schizophrenic mothers. I. Contributions of genetic and perinatal factors. *Archives of General Psychiatry*, **50**, 551–564.

Changeux, J.-P. & Danchin, A. (1976) Selective stabilisation of developing synapses as a mechanism for the specification of neuronal networks. *Nature*, **264**, 705–712.

Chelune, G.J. & Baer, R.A. (1986) Developmental norms for the Wisconsin Card Sorting Test. *Journal of Clinical Experimental Neuropsychology*, **8**, 219–228.

Chi, J.G., Dooling, E.C. & Gilles, F.H. (1977) Gyral development of the human brain. *Annals of Neurology*, **1**, 86–93.

Christison, G.W., Casanova, M.F., Weinberger, D.R., Rawlings, R. & Kleinman, J.E. (1989) A quantitative investigation of hippocampal pyramidal cell size, shape, and variability of orientation in schizophrenia. *Archives of General Psychiatry*, **46**, 1027–1032.

Conrad, A.J., Abebe, T., Austin, R., Forsythe, S. & Scheibel, A.B. (1991) Hippocampal pyramidal cell disarray in schizophrenia as a bilateral phenomenon. *Archives of General Psychiatry*, **48**, 413–417.

Cooper, S.J. (1992) Schizophrenia after prenatal exposure to 1957 A2 influenza epidemic. *British Journal of Psychiatry*, **161**, 394–396.

Crow, T.J. & Done, D.J. (1992) Prenatal exposure to influenza does not cause schizophrenia. *British Journal of Psychiatry*, **161**, 390–393.

Crow, T.J., Ball, J., Bloom, S.R. *et al.* (1989) Schizophrenia as an anomaly of development of cerebral asymmetry. A postmortem study and a proposal concerning the genetic basis of the disease. *Archives of General Psychiatry*, **46**, 1145–1150.

Daniel, D.G., Goldberg, T.E. & Weinberger, D.R. (1991) Lack of a bimodal distribution of ventricular size in patients with schizophrenia. *Biological Psychiatry*, **30**, 887–903.

Davison, K. & Bagley, C.R. (1969) Schizophrenia-like psychoses associated with organic disorders of the central nervous system. *British Journal of Psychiatry*, **113**, 18–69.

DeLisi, L.E., Dauphinais, I.D. & Gershon, E.S. (1988) Perinatal complications and reduced size of brain limbic structures in familial schizophrenia. *Schizophrenia Bulletin*, **14**, 185–191.

DeLisi, L.E., Hoff, A.L., Schwartz, J.E., *et al.* (1991) Brain morphology in first-episode schizophrenic-like psychotic patients: a quantitative magnetic resonance imaging study. *Biological Psychiatry*, **129**, 159–175.

Done, D.J., Johnstone, E.C., Frith, C.D., Golding, J., Shepherd, P.M. & Crow, T.J. (1991) Complications of pregnancy and delivery in relation to psychosis in adult life: data from the British perinatal mortality survey sample. *British Medical Journal*, **302**, 1576–1580.

Eagles, J.M., Gibson, I., Bremner, M.H., Clunie, F., Ebmeier, K.P. & Smith, N.C. (1990) Obstetric complications in DSM-III schizophrenics and their siblings. *Lancet*, **335**, 1139–1141.

Erel, O., Cannon, T.D., Hollister, J.M., Mednick, S.A. & Parnas, J. (1991) Ventricular enlargement and premorbid deficits in school-occupational attainment in a high risk sample. *Schizophrenia Research*, **4**, 49–52.

Erlenmeyer-Kimling, L. (1987) High-risk research in schizophrenia: a summary of what has been learned. *Journal of Psychiatric Research*, **21**, 401–411.

Epstein, H.T. (1986) Stages in human brain development. *Developments in Brain Research*, **30**, 114–119.

Falkai, P., Bogerts, B., Greve, B. *et al.* (1992) Loss of Sylvian fissure asymmetry in schizophrenia. A quantitative postmortem study. *Schizophrenia Research*, **7**, 23–32.

Falkai, P., Bogerts, B. & Rozumek, M. (1988) Limbic pathology in schizophrenia: the entorhinal region — a morphometric study. *Biological Psychiatry*, **24**, 515–521.

Feinberg, I. (1982) Schizophrenia: caused by a fault in programmed synaptic elimination during adolescence? *Journal of Psychiatric Research*, **17**, 319–334.

Fish, B. (1977) Neurobiological antecedents of schizophrenia in childhood. *Archives of General Psychiatry*, **34**, 1297–1313.

Fish, B., Marcus, J., Hans, S.L., Auerbach, J.G. & Perdue, S. (1992) Infants at risk for schizophrenia: sequelae of a genetic neurointegrative defect. A review and replication analysis of pandysmaturation in the Jerusalem infant development study. *Archives of General Psychiatry*, **49**, 221–235.

Freud, S. (1968) *Infantile Cerebral Paralysis.* University of Miami Press, Florida. Translated by Russin, L.A.

Goldberg, T.E., Gold, J.M. & Braff, D.L. (1991) Neuropsychological functioning and time-linked information processing in schizophrenia. In Tasman, A. & Goldfinger, S.M. (eds) *American Psychiatric Press Review of Psychiatry*, Vol. 10, pp. 60–78. American Psychiatric Association, Washington DC.

Goldberg, T.E., Gold, J.M., Greenberg, R. *et al.* (1993) Contrasts between patients with affective disorder and patients with schizophrenia on a neuropsychological screening battery. *American Journal of Psychiatry*, **150**, 1355–1362.

Goldman, P.S. (1971) Functional development of the prefrontal cortex in early life and the problem of neuronal plasticity. *Experimental Neurology*, **132**, 366–387.

Goldman-Rakic, P. (1987) Circuitry of primate prefrontal cortex and regulation of behavior by representation knowledge. In Plum, F. & Mountcastle, V. (eds) *Higher Cortical Function: Handbook of Physiology*, Vol. 5., pp. 373–417. American Physiological Society, Washington DC.

Goodman, R. (1988) Are complications of pregnancy and birth causes of schizoprenia? *Developmental Medicine Child Neurology*, **30**, 391–395.

Green, M.F., Satz, P., Gaier, D.J., Ganzell, S. & Kharabi, F. (1989) Minor physical anomalies in schizophrenia. *Schizophrenia Bulletin*, **15**, 91–99.

Greer, E.R., Diamond, M.C. & Tang, J.M. (1982) Environmental enrichment in Brattleboro rats: brain morphology. *Annals of the New York Academy of Sciences*, **394**, 749–752.

Gruzelier, J.H., Seymour, K., Wilson, L., Jolley, T. & Hirsch, S. (1988) Impairments on neuropsychological tests of temporo-hippocampal and fronto-hippocampal functions and word fluency in remitting schizophrenia and affective disorders. *Archives of General Psychiatry*, **45**, 623–629.

Heckers, S., Heinsen, H., Heinsen, Y.C. & Beckmann, H. (1990) Limbic structures and lateral ventricle in schizophrenia. *Archives of General Psychiatry*, **47**, 1016–1022.

Huttenlocher, P.R. (1979) Synaptic density in human frontal cortex — developmental changes and effects of aging. *Brain Research*, **163**, 195–205.

Huttenlocher, P.R. (1992) Neural plasticity. In Asbury, A.K., McKhann, G.M. & McDonald, W.I. (eds) *Diseases of the Nervous System: Clinical Neurobiology*, Vol. 1, pp. 63–71. WB Saunders, Philadelphia.

Huttenlocher, P.R., de Courten, C., Garey, L.J. & van der Loos, H. (1982) Synaptogenesis in human visual cortex — evidence for synapse elimination during normal development. *Neuroscience Letters*, **33**, 247–252.

Hyde, T.M. & Saunders, R.C. (1991) The entorhinal cortex in humans: a cytoarchitectonic and comparative study with non-human primates. *Neuroscience Abstracts*, **17**, 134.

Hyde, T.M., Casanova, M.F., Kleinman, J.E. & Weinberger, D.R. (1991) Neuroanatomical and neurochemical pathology in schizophrenia. In Tasman, A. & Goldfinger, S.M. (eds) *American Psychiatric Press Review of Psychiatry*, Vol. 10, pp. 7–23. American Psychiatric Association, Washington DC.

Hyde, T.M., Ziegler, J.C. & Weinberger, D.R. (1992) Psychiatric disturbances in metachromatic leukodystrophy: insight into the neurobiology of psychosis. *Archives of Neurology*, **49**, 401–406.

Jakob, H. & Beckmann, H. (1986) Prenatal developmental disturbances in the limbic allocortex in schizophrenics. *Journal of Neural Transmission*, **65**, 303–326.

Jakob, H. & Beckmann, H. (1989) Gross and histological criteria for developmental disorders in brains of schizophrenics. *Journal of the Royal Society of Medicine*, **82**, 466–469.

Jaskiw, G.E. & Weinberger, D.R. (1992) Dopamine and schizophrenia: a cortically corrective perspective. *Seminars in Neuroscience*, **4**, 179–188.

Jernigan, T.L., Zisook, S., Heaton, R.K., Moranville, J.T., Hesselink, J.R. & Braff, D.L. (1991) Magnetic resonance imaging abnormalities in lenticular nuclei and cerebral cortex in schizophrenia. *Archives of General Psychiatry*, **48**, 881–890.

Jeste, D.V. & Lohr, J.B. (1989) Hippocampal pathologic findings in schizophrenia. *Archives of General Psychiatry*, **46**, 1019–1024.

Johnstone, E.C., Crow, T.J., Frith, C.D., Husband, J. & Kreel, L. (1976) Cerebral ventricular size and cognitive chronic schizophrenia. *Lancet*, **2**, 924–926.

Keefe, R.S.E., Mohs, R.C., Losonczy, M.F. *et al.* (1989) Premorbid sociosexual functioning and long-term outcome in schizophrenia. *American Journal of Psychiatry*, **146**, 206–211.

Kendell, R.E. & Kemp, I.W. (1989) Maternal influenza in the etiology of schizophrenia. *Archives of General Psychiatry*, **46**, 878–882.

Kendell, R.E. & Kemp, I.W. (1990) Influenza and schizophrenia: Helsinki vs Edinburgh. *Archives of General Psychiatry*, **47**, 877–878.

Kennard, M.A. (1936) Age and other factors in motor recovery from precentral lesions in monkeys. *American Journal of Physiology*, **115**, 138–146.

Kolakowska, T., Williams, A.O., Ardern, M. *et al.* (1985)

Schizophrenia with good and poor outcome. I. Early clinical features, response to neuroleptics and signs of organic dysfunction. *British Journal of Psychiatry*, **146**, 229–246.

Kolb, B. & Whishaw, I.Q. (1989) Plasticity in the neocortex: mechanisms underlying recovery from early brain damage. *Progress in Neurobiology*, **32**, 235–276.

Komuro, H. & Rakic, P. (1993) Modulation of neuronal migration by NMDA receptors. *Science*, **260**, 95–97.

Kostovic, I. & Rakic, P. (1990) Developmental history of the transient subplate zone in the visual and somatosensory cortex of the Macaque monkey and human brain. *Journal of Comparative Neurology*, **287**, 441–470.

Kostovic, I., Lukinovic, N., Judas, M. *et al.* (1989) Structural basis of the developmental plasticity in the human cerebral cortex: the role of transient subplate zone. *Metabolic Brain Disease*, **4**, 17–23.

Kovelman, J.A. & Scheibel, A.B. (1984) A neurohistological correlate of schizophrenia. *Biological Psychiatry*, **19**, 1601–1621.

Kraepelin, E. (ed.) (1919) *Dementia Praecox and Paraphrenia*. Livingstone, Edinburgh.

Kulynych, J.J., Vladar, K., Fantie, B.D., Jones, D.W. & Weinberger, D.R. (1994) Normal asymmetry of the planum temporale in patients with schizophrenia: three-dimensional cortical morphometry with MRI. *British Journal of Psychiatry* (in press).

Landis, S.C. (1990) Target regulation of neurotransmitter phenotype. *Trends in Neuroscience*, **13**, 344–350.

Larroche, J.C. (1984) Malformations of the nervous system. In Adams, J.M., Corsellis, J.A.N. & Duchen, L.W. (eds) *Greenfields Neuropathology*, 4th edn, p. 85. Edward Arnold, London.

Lewis, S.W. (1989) Congenital risk factors for schizophrenia. *Psychological Medicine*, **19**, 5–13.

Lidow, M.S. & Rakic, P. (1992) Scheduling of monoaminergic neurotransmitter receptor expression in the primate neocortex during postnatal development. *Cerebral Cortex*, **2**, 401–416.

Lidow, M.S., Goldman-Rakic, P.S. & Rakic, P. (1991) Synchronized overproduction of neurotransmitter receptors in diverse regions of the primate cerebral cortex. *Proceedings of the National Academy of Science*, **88**, 10218–10220.

Lieberman, J., Jody, D., Geisler, S. *et al.* (1993) Time course and biologic correlates of treatment response in first-episode schizophrenia. *Archives of General Psychiatry*, **50**, 369–376.

Lipska, B.K. & Weinberger, D.R. (1993a) Cortical regulation of the mesolimbic dopamine system: implications for schizophrenia. In Kalivas, P.W. (ed.) *The Mesolimbic Motor Circuit and its Role in Neuropsychiatric Disorders*, pp. 329–349. CRC Press, Boca Raton.

Lipska, B.K. & Weinberger, D.R. (1993b) Delayed effects of neonatal hippocampal damage on the haloperidol-induced catalepsy and apomorphine-induced stereotypic behaviors in the rat. *Developments in Brain Research*, **75**, 213–222.

Lipska, B.K., Jaskiw, G.E. & Weinberger, D.R. (1993) Post-pubertal emergence of augmented exploration and amphetamine supersensitivity after neonatal deafferentation of the rat ventral hippocampus: a potential animal model of schizophrenia. *Neuropsychopharmacology*, **9**, 67–75.

Lipton, S.A. & Kater, S.B. (1989) Neurotransmitter regulation of neuronal outgrowth, plasticity and survival. *Trends in Neuroscience*, **12**, 265–270.

Lohr, J.B. & Bracha, S. (1989) Can schizoprenia be related to prenatal exposure to alcohol? Some speculations. *Schizophrenia Bulletin*, **15**, 595–603.

Luchins, D.J., Weinberger, D.R. & Wyatt, R.J. (1979) Schizophrenia evidence for a subgroup with reversed cerebral asymmetry. *Archives of General Psychiatry*, **36**, 1309–1311.

McCreadie, R.G., Hall, D.J., Berry, I.J., Robertson, L.J., Ewing, J.I. & Geals, M.F. (1992) The Nithsdala schizophrenia surveys. X. Obstetric complications, family history and abnormal movements. *British Journal of Psychiatry*, **161**, 799–805.

McNeil, T.F. (1988) Obstetric factors and perinatal injuries. In Tsuang, M.T. & Simpson, J.C. (eds) *Handbook of Schizophrenia, Vol. 3, Nosology, Epidemiology and Genetics*, pp. 319–344. Elsevier, Amsterdam.

Marin-Padilla, M. (1988) Early ontogenesis of the human cerebral cortex. In Peters, A. & Jones, E.G. (eds) *Cerebral Cortex*, Vol. 7, pp. 1–34. Plenum Press, New York.

Marsh, L., Suddath, R.L., Higgins, N. & Weinberger, D.R. (1994) Medial temporal structures in schizophrenia: lack of correlation between size reduction and normal age-related changes. *Schizophrenia Research*, **11**, 225–238.

Mattson, M.P. (1988) Neurotransmitters in the regulation of neuronal cytoarchitecture. *Brain Research Reviews*, **13**, 179–212.

Meaney, M.J., Aitken, D.H., van Berkel, C., Bhatnagar, S. & Sapolsky, R.M. (1988) Effect of neonatal handling on age-related impairments associated with the hippocampus. *Science*, **239**, 766–768.

Mednick, S.A. & Silverton, L. (1988) High-risk studies of the etiology of schizophrenia. In Tsuang, M.T. & Simpson, J.C. (eds) *Handbook of Schizophrenia, Vol. 3, Nosology, Epidemiology and Genetics of Schizophrenia*, pp. 543–562. Elsevier, Amsterdam.

Mednick, S.A., Cannon, T.D., Barr, C.E. & Lyon, M. (eds) (1991) *Fetal Neural Development and Adult Schizophrenia*. Cambridge University Press, Cambridge.

Mednick, S.A., Machon, R.A., Huttunen, M.O. & Bonett, D. (1988) Adult schizophrenia following prenatal exposure to an influenza epidemic. *Archives of General Psychiatry*, **45**, 189–192.

Meltzer, H.Y. (1979) The biology of schizophrenic subtypes: a review and proposal for methods of study. *Schizophrenia Bulletin*, **5**, 460–472.

Murray, R.M. & Lewis, S.W. (1987) Is schizophrenia a neurodevelopmental disorder? *British Medical Journal*, **295**, 681–682.

Murray, R.M., O'Callaghan, E., Castle, D.J. & Lewis, S.W. (1992) A neurodevelopmental approach to the classification of schizophrenia. *Schizophrenia Bulletin*, **18**, 319–332.

Myslobodsky, M.S. & Weinberger, D.R. (1987) Brain CT asymmetry in schizophrenia and sighting dominance. In Takahashi, R., Flor-Henry, P., Gruzelier, J. & Niwa, S. (eds) *Cerebral Dynamics, Laterality and Psychopathology*, pp. 439–448. Elsevier, Amsterdam.

Nowakowski, R.S. (1987) Basic concepts of CNS development. *Child Development*, **58**, 568–595.

Nowakowski, R.S. (1991a) Some basic concepts of the development of the central nervous system. In Mednick, S.A., Cannon, T.D., Barr, C.E. & Lyon, M. (eds) *Fetal Neural Development and Adult Schizophrenia*, pp. 17–39. Cambridge University Press, Cambridge.

Nowakowski, R.S. (1991b) Genetic disturbances of neuronal migration: some examples from the limbic system of mutant mice. In Mednick, S.A., Cannon, T.D., Barr, C.E. & Lyon, M. (eds) *Fetal Neural Development and Adult Schizoprenia*, pp. 69–96. Cambridge University Press, Cambridge.

Nowakowski, R.S. & Rakic, P. (1981) The site of origin and route and rate of migration of neurons to the hippocampal region of the rhesus monkey. *Journal of Comparative Neurology*, **196**, 129–154.

O'Callaghan, E., Sham, P., Takei, N., Glover, G. & Murray, R.M. (1991) Schizophrenia after prenatal exposure to 1957 A2 influenza epidemic. *Lancet*, **337**, 1248–1250.

O'Kusky, J. & Colonnier, M. (1982) Postnatal changes in the number of neurons and synapses in the visual cortex (A17) of the Macaque monkey. *Journal of Comparative Neurology*, **210**, 291–306.

O'Leary, D.D.M. (1989) Do cortical areas emerge from a protocortex? *Trends in Neuroscience*, **12**, 400–406.

Onstad, S., Skre, I., Torgersen, S. & Kringlen, E. (1992) Birthweight and obstetric complications in schizophrenic twins. *Acta Psychiatrica Scandinavica*, **185**, 70–73.

Oppenheim, R.W. (1985) Naturally occurring cell death during neural development. *Trends in Neuroscience*, **17**, 487–493.

Otake, M. & Schull, W.J. (1984) *In utero* exposure of A-bomb radiation and mental retardation: a reassessment. *British Journal of Radiology*, **57**, 409–414.

Pakkenberg, B. (1987) Post-mortem study of chronic schizophrenic brains. *British Journal of Psychiatry*, **151**, 744–752.

Parnas, J., Schulsinger, F., Teasdale, T.W., Schulsinger, H., Feldman, P.M. & Mednick, S.A. (1982) Perinatal complications and clinical outcome within the schizophrenia spectrum. *British Journal of Psychiatry*, **140**, 416–420.

Pettegrew, J.W., Keshavan, M.S. & Minshew, N.J. (1993) ^{31}P nuclear magnetic resonance spectroscopy: neurodevelopment and schizophrenia. *Schizophrenia Bulletin*, **19**, 35–53.

Pollack, M., Woerner, M.G., Goodman, W. & Greenberg, I.M. (1966) Childhood development patterns of hospitalized adult schizophrenic and nonschizophrenic patients and their siblings. *American Journal of Orthopsychiatry*, **36**, 510–517.

Pollin, W. & Stabenau, J.R. (1968) Biological, psychological and historical differences in a series of monozygotic twins discordant for schizophrenia. In Rosenthal, D. & Kety, S. (eds) *The Transmission of Schizophrenia*, pp. 317–322. Pergamon Press, Oxford.

Purves, D. (1988) *Body and brain: A trophic theory of neuronal connections*, Harvard University Press, Cambridge.

Rabacchi, S., Bailly, Y., Delhay-Bouchaud, N. & Mariani, J. (1992) Involvement of the *N*-methyl D-aspartate (NMDA) receptor in synapse elimination during cerebellar development. *Science*, **256**, 1823–1825.

Rakic, P. (1971) Guidance of neurons migrating to the fetal monkey neocortex. *Brain Research*, **33**, 471–476.

Rakic, P. (1988a) Defects of neuronal migration and the

pathogenesis of cortical malformations. In Boer, G.J., Feenstra, M.G.P., Mirmiran, M., Swaab, D.F. & Van Haaren, F.V. (eds) *Progress in Brain Research*, Vol. 73, pp. 15–37. Elsevier, Amsterdam.

Rakic, P. (1988b) Specification of cerebral cortical areas. *Science*, **241**, 170–176.

Rakic, P. (1990) Principles of neural cell migration. *Experientia*, **46**, 882–891.

Rakic, P. (1991) Experimental manipulation of cerebral cortical areas in primates. *Philosophical Transactions of the Royal Society of London, Series B*, **331**, 291–294.

Rakic, P., Suñer, I. & Williams, R.W. (1991) A novel cytoarchitectonic area induced experimentally within the primate visual cortex. *Proceedings of the National Academy of Science*, **88**, 2083–2087.

Rakic, P., Bourgeois, J.-P., Eckenhoff, M.F., Zecevic, N. & Goldman-Rakic, P.S. (1986) Concurrent overproduction of synapses in diverse regions of the primate cerebral cortex. *Science*, **232**, 232–235.

Raz, S. & Raz, N. (1990) Structural brain abnormalities in the major psychoses: a quantitative review of the evidence from computerized imaging. *Psychological Bulletin*, **108**, 93–108.

Reveley, A.M., Reveley, M.A. & Murray, R.M. (1984) Cerebral ventricular enlargement in non-genetic schizophrenia: a controlled twin study. *British Journal of Psychiatry*, **144**, 89–93.

Reveley, A.M., Reveley, M.A., Clifford, C.A. & Murray, R.M. (1982) Cerebral ventricular size in twins discordant for schizophrenia. *Lancet*, **2**, 540–541.

Roberts, G.W. (1991) Schizophrenia: a neuropathological perspective. *British Journal of Psychiatry*, **158**, 8–17.

Roberts, G.W., Done, D.J., Bruton, C. & Crow, T.J. (1990) A 'mock up' of schizophrenia: temporal lobe epilepsy and schizophrenia-like psychosis. *Biological Psychiatry*, **28**, 127–143.

Roberts, G.W., Colter, N., Lofthouse, R., Bogerts, B., Zech, M. & Crow, T.J. (1986) Gliosis in schizophrenia: a survey. *Biological Psychiatry*, **21**, 1043–1050.

Rosanoff, A.J., Handy, L.M., Rosanoff-Plesset, I.R. & Brush, S. (1934) The etiology of so-called schizophrenic psychoses. *American Journal of Psychiatry*, **91**, 247–286.

Rossi, A., Stratta, P., Mattei, P. *et al.* (1992) Planum temporale in schizophrenia: a magnetic resonance study. *Schizophrenia Research*, **7**, 19–22.

Schwartz, M.L. & Goldman-Rakic, P. (1990) Development and plasticity of the primate cerebral cortex. *Clinical Perinatology*, **17**, 83–102.

Sham, P.C., O'Callaghan, E., Takei, N., Murray, G.K., Hare, E.H. & Murray, R.M. (1992) Schizophrenia following prenatal exposure to influenza epidemics between 1939 and 1960. *British Journal of Psychiatry*, **160**, 461–466.

Shelton, R. & Weinberger, D.R. (1987) Brain morphology in schizophrenia. In Meltzer, H., Bunney, W., Coyle, J. *et al.* (eds) *Psychopharmacology, The Third Generation of Progress*, pp. 773–781. Raven Press, New York.

Shenton, M.E., Kirkinis, R., Jolesz, F.A. *et al.* (1992) Abnormalities of the left temporal lobe and thought disorder in schizophrenia. A quantitative magnetic resonance imaging study. *New England Journal of Medicine*, **327**, 604–612.

Sidman, R.L. & Rakic, P. (1982) Development of the human central nervous system. In Haymaker, W. & Adams, R.D. (eds) *Histology and Histopathology of the Nervous System*, pp. 3–145. Charles C. Thomas, Springfield.

Southard, E.E. (1915) On the topographical distribution of cortex lesions and anamolies in dementia praecox, with some account of their functional significance. *American Journal of Insanity*, **71**, 603–671.

Stanfield, B.B. & Cowan, W.M. (1988) The development of the hippocampal region. In Peters, A. & Jones, E.G. (eds) *Cerebral Cortex*, Vol. 7, pp. 91–131. Plenum Press, New York.

Stevens, J.R. (1982) Neuropathology of schizophrenia. *Archives of General Psychiatry*, **39**, 1131–1139.

Stevens, J.R. (1992) Abnormal reinnvervation as a basis for schizophrenia: a hypothesis. *Archives of General Psychiatry*, **49**, 238–243.

Suddath, R.L., Christison, G.W., Torrey, E.F. & Weinberger, D.R. (1990) Cerebral anatomical abnormalities in monozygotic twins discordant for schizophrenia. *New England Journal of Medicine*, **322**, 789–794.

Susser, E.S. & Lin, S.P. (1992) Schizophrenia after prenatal exposure to the Dutch Hunger Winter of 1944–1945. *Archives of General Psychiatry*, **49**, 983–988.

Sutcliffe, J.G., Milner, R.J., Gottesfeld, J.M. & Reynolds, W. (1984) Control of neuronal gene expression. *Science*, **225**, 1308–1315.

Thatcher, R.W., Walker, R.A. & Giudice, S. (1987) Human cerebral hemispheres develop at different rates and ages. *Science*, **236**, 1110–1113.

Torrey, E.F., Rawlings, R. & Waldman, I.N. (1988) Schizophrenic births and viral diseases in two states. *Schizophrenia Research*, **1**, 73–77.

Torrey, E.F., Bowler, A.E., Taylor, E.H. & Gottesman, I.I. (1994) *Schizophrenia and Manic Depression Disorders: The Biological Roots of Mental Illness as Revealed by a Landmark Study of Identical Twins*. Basic Books, New York.

Wada, J.A., Clarke, R. & Hamm, A. (1975) Cerebral hemisphere asymmetry in humans: cortical speech zones in 100 adult and 100 infant brains. *Archives of Neurology*, **32**, 239–246.

Waddington, J.L. (1990) Sight and insight: regional cerebral metabolic activity in schizophrenia visualized by positron emission tomography, and competing neurodevelopmental perspectives. *British Journal of Psychiatry*, **156**, 615–619.

Walker, E. & Lewine, R.J. (1990) Prediction of adult-onset schizophrenia from childhood home movies of the patients. *American Journal of Psychiatry*, **147**, 1052–1056.

Walsh, C. & Cepko, C.L. (1992) Widespread dispersion of neuronal clones across functional regions of the cerebral cortex. *Science*, **255**, 434–440.

Weinberger, D.R. (1986) The pathogenesis of schizophrenia: a neurodevelopmental theory. In Nasrallah, H.A. & Weinberger, D.R. (eds) *The Neurology of Schizophrenia*, pp. 397–406. Elsevier, Amsterdam.

Weinberger, D.R. (1987) Implications of normal brain development for the pathogenesis of schizophrenia. *Archives of General Psychiatry*, **44**, 660–669.

Weinberger, D.R. (1988) Premorbid neuropathology in

schizophrenia. *Lancet*, **ii**, 445.

Weinberger, D.R. (1991) Anteriormedial temporal-prefrontal connectivity: a functional anatomical system implicated in schizophrenia. In Carrol, B.J. & Barnett, J.E. (eds) *Psychopathology and the Brain*, pp. 25–42. Raven Press, New York.

Weinberger, D.R. (1993) A connectionist approach to the prefrontal cortex. *Journal of Neuropsychiatry and Clinical Neuroscience*, **5**, 241–253.

Weinberger, D.R. (1995) Neurodevelopmental perspectives on schizophrenia. In Kupfer, D. & Bloom, F. (eds) *Psychopharmacology: A Fourth Generation of Progress*. Raven Press, New York (in press).

Weinberger, D.R., Berman, K.F., Suddath, R. & Torrey, E.F. (1992) Evidence for dysfunction of a prefrontal-limbic network in schizophrenia: An MRI and rCBF study of discordant monozygotic twins. *American Journal of Psychiatry*, **149**, 890–897.

Weinberger, D.R., Cannon-Spoor, E., Potkin, S.G. & Wyatt, R.J. (1980) Poor premorbid adjustment and CT scan abnormalities in chronic schizophrenia. *American Journal of Psychiatry*, **137**, 1410–1413.

Weinberger, D.R., DeLisi, L.E., Neophytides, A.N. & Wyatt, R.J. (1981) Familial aspects of CT abnormalities in chronic schizophrenic patients. *Psychiatry Research*, **4**, 65–71.

Weinberger, D.R., Luchins, D.J., Morihisa, J. & Wyatt, R.J. (1982b) Asymmetric volumes of the right and left frontal and occipital regions of the human brain. *Annals of Neurology*, **11**, 97–100.

Weinberger, D.R., Torrey, E.F., Neophytides, A. & Wyatt, R.J. (1979) Lateral cerebral ventricular enlargement in chronic schizophrenia. *Archives of General Psychiatry*, **36**, 735–738.

Weinberger, D.R., DeLisi, L.E., Perman, G., Targum, S. & Wyatt, R.J. (1982a) Computed tomography scans in schizophreniform disorder and other acute psychiatric patients. *Archives of General Psychiatry*, **39**, 778–783.

Weinberger, D.R., Suddath, R.L., Casanova, M.F., Torrey, E.F. & Kleinman, J.E. (1991) Crow's 'lateralization hypothesis' for schizophrenia. *Archives of General Psychiatry*, **48**, 85.

Williams, R.W. & Herrup, K. (1988) The control of neuron number. *Annual Review of Neuroscience*, **11**, 423–453.

Woerner, M.G., Pollack, M. & Klein, D.F. (1973) Pregnancy and birth complications in psychiatric patients: a comparison of schizophrenic and personality disorder patients with their siblings. *Acta Psychiatrica Scandinavica*, **49**, 712–721.

Yolken, R.H. & Torrey, E.F. (1995) Viruses and serious mental diseases. *Clinical Microbiology Reviews* (in press).

Zecevic, N., & Rakic, P. (1991) Synaptogenesis in monkey somatosensory cortex. *Cerebral Cortex*, **1**, 510–523.

Zecevic, N., Bourgeois, J.-P. & Rakic, P. (1989) Changes in synaptic density in motor cortex of rhesus monkey during fetal and postnatal life. *Developments in Brain Research*, **50**, 11–32.

Zigun, J. & Weinberger, D.R. (1992) *In vivo* studies of brain morphology in patients with schizophrenia. In Lindenmayer, J.-P. & Kay, S.R. (eds) *New Biological Vistas on Schizophrenia*, pp. 57–81. Brunner Mazel, New York.

Chapter 17
The Secondary Schizophrenias

S. W. LEWIS

Introduction

For as long as the syndrome of schizophrenia has been recognized, the possibility that coarse brain disease can produce similar or identical symptoms has also been acknowledged. This was explicitly recognized by Kraepelin, Bleuler and particularly Schneider, as a caveat in the delineation of his first-rank symptoms. The existence of a disparate range of brain disorders which can, uncommonly, give rise to schizophrenia-like symptomatology presents psychiatry with a problem and an opportunity. On the one hand, it poses nosological dilemmas about the limits of the definition of schizophrenia. On the other hand, it provides a model for possible insights into mechanisms underlying the generation of schizophrenic symptoms.

This chapter will outline first the nosological challenges and how recent classificatory systems have dealt with these, distinguishing secondary schizophrenias arising out of unsuspected brain lesions and those secondary to cerebral complications of systemic illness. Second, it will attempt to estimate the prevalence of such secondary

schizophrenias in relation to schizophrenia in general. Third, it will examine the evidence for symptomatic differences between secondary and primary schizophrenia and discuss their clinical diagnosis. Finally, the chapter will review broadly which specific brain diseases seem to present a particularly increased risk of schizophrenic symptoms.

Terminology and classification

In the past, schizophrenia has belonged to a class of disorders conventionally known as 'functional psychoses' and this was the terminology which held sway in the *International Classification of Disease* ICD-9 (WHO, 1978). Although ICD-9 had several disadvantages, most particularly the absence of clearly defined, reliable operational diagnostic criteria, one potential advantage was the adherence to a *descriptive* pattern of phenomenological definition. Thus, the term 'organic', as opposed to 'functional', was not intended to imply an organic aetiology, but specifically to describe a set of symptoms of cognitive impairment such as disorientation, reduced level of consciousness and impairments of memory. This allowed schizophrenia secondary to coarse brain disease to be classed under the rubric of schizophrenia, with appropriate subdiagnosis according to the pathology of the causative agent or disease.

In the *Diagnostic and Statistical Manual* DSM-III and DSM-III-R, the term organic was redefined in an important way, so as to imply an organic *aetiology*, rather than to describe particular symptoms in the mental state. Thus, separate categories of 'organic mental disorders' were introduced. Cases of psychosis without cognitive impairment, but in the presence of 'evidence from the history, physical examination, or laboratory tests of a specific organic factor judged to be aetiologically related', were now called 'organic delusional syndrome' or 'organic hallucinosis', depending on the predominant symptoms. Nevertheless, in DSM-III it was acknowledged that symptoms in these organic mental disorders can be 'essentially identical with schizophrenia'. This convention put the diagnostician in the problematic position of having to rename a syndrome whenever a likely organic case became apparent (Lewis *et al.*, 1987).

Potential problems with the term organic are highlighted by treatment of the term in the ICD-10 (WHO, 1992), particularly in the section on 'Other Organic Mental Disorders' (F06). It is worthwhile examining this in a little detail so as to advance the argument that the term organic should be abandoned as a descriptor for schizophrenias caused by coarse brain disease. The ICD-10 use of the term organic introduces a paradox which is referred to in the text thus: 'use of the term organic does not imply that conditions elsewhere in this classification are non-organic'. Moreover, the criteria put forward in ICD-10 by which to identify disorders such as organic schizophrenialike disorder are not strictly logical. One of the two requirements to justify a diagnosis is 'a temporal relationship (weeks or a few months) between the development of the underlying disease and the onset of the syndrome'. In reality, this time scale limits inclusion to what are essentially precipitating factors rather than true causes which, as will be discussed later in the chapter, seem often to take several years before generating schizophrenia-like symptoms. A further limitation of the notion of splitting off organic schizophrenias from schizophrenia in general is that our knowledge base as to the epidemiology of the first group, and of the relationship in general between the two groups, is very limited. The greatest difficulty in confidently diagnosing a case of organic schizophrenia-like disorder is in the attribution of the symptoms to a particular organic cause. This is seldom simple, particularly since there may be little time congruence between onset of the physical disorder and onset of the schizophrenic symptoms.

Spitzer *et al.* (1992) have argued cogently for retiring the term organic mental disorders and in this review their lead will be followed. They assert that the term organic has insoluble problems attached to it and for this reason another term should be chosen. They consider the term 'symptomatic', but note that this can be ambiguous. They propose that the term 'secondary' should be used instead. Secondary disorders should be distinguished from substance-induced disorders, and are recognized if they are due to medical disorders that are classified outside the mental disorder section of the ICD. Schizophrenic symptoms can thus be categorized in any individual case to being primary, or secondary 'to a non-psychiatric medical disorder' or substance induced.

The DSM-IV criteria (APA, 1993) have indeed adopted this approach, which harks back to the phenomenological basis of classification in ICD-9. Sensibly, the introduction to the organizational plan in DSM-IV states that 'the term organic mental disorder is no longer used in DSM-IV because it incorrectly implies that the other mental disorders in the manual do not have a biologic basis'. Thus, schizophrenic symptoms secondary to a non-psychiatric medical disorder are now headed 'Psychotic Disorder due to a General Medical Condition'.

Secondary schizophrenias can be thought of as falling into two categories. The first is where the psychotic symptoms arise from the cerebral involvement of a named physical disease known to affect the central nervous system (CNS). This is the category headed 293.8 in DSM-IV draft. The second category is where schizophrenic symptoms arise in the context of a demonstrable, often clinically unsuspected brain lesion which is not part of an ongoing, systemic disease process. This latter area has become considerably more important since the advent of computerized neuro-imaging techniques in the past 20 years. In DSM-IV draft, this category is subsumed back into the general class of schizophrenia.

How common are secondary schizophrenias?

Given the disputes over definition and diagnosis, it is not surprising that the epidemiology of secondary schizophrenia has been little researched. As noted, one difficulty in estimating prevalence is the problem of definition: how confident can one be that an uncovered brain lesion is truly responsible for the presenting schizophrenic symptoms? A second difficulty is that the closer one looks, the more likely it is that organic pathology will be revealed. The increasingly widespread availability of non-invasive brain-imaging techniques has shown that unsuspected cerebral lesions occur in a small but significant number of patients with schizophrenic symptoms. Most structural brain-imaging research in psychosis has concentrated rather on minor, quantitative changes involving widened fluid spaces and reduced volume of particular structures in the medial temporal lobe (Chapter 15).

These minor, quantitative changes would not usually be reported as abnormal by most clinical radiologists. However, there are a handful of reports in the literature of gross focal brain lesions in schizophrenia. Three larger imaging studies using X-ray computerized tomography (CT) enable an estimate to be made of the prevalence of such unequivocal, focal lesions in schizophrenia. Owens *et al.* (1980), in their series of 136 schizophrenic patients, found 'unsuspected intra-cranial pathology' as a focal finding on CT in 12 cases (9%), after excluding lesions due to leucotomy. This was a relatively elderly sample: five of these 12 cases were aged over 65. Lewis

(1990) examined a series of 228 Maudsley Hospital patients who met research diagnostic criteria (RDC) for schizophrenia and who had been consecutively scanned for clinical reasons. Patients with a history of epilepsy or intracranial surgery, or who were aged over 65 at the time of scan, were excluded. The original scan reports were examined and the films of those not unequivocally normal were reappraised by a neuro-radiologist blind to the original report. In 41 patients the scan showed a definite intracranial abnormality. This was in the nature of enlarged fluid spaces in 28 cases, but in 13 patients (6%) there was a discrete focal lesion. These lesions varied widely in location and probable pathology (Table 17.1), although left temporal and right parietal regions were most commonly implicated.

The third study (Lewis and Reveley, in preparation) was an attempt to examine a geographically defined sample of schizophrenic patients, ascertained as part of a large, multidisciplinary survey (Brugha *et al.*, 1988). All Camberwell residents who, on a particular census day, were aged between 18 and 65 and were in regular contact with any psychiatric day service were approached. Of 120 eligible people, 83 consented to CT and psychiatric interview. Fifty of these met RDC for schizophrenia or schizoaffective disorder. In four of these 50 patients (8%) clinically unsuspected focal lesions were found: low density in the right caudate head; a left occipito-temporal porencephalic cyst; low-density regions in the right parietal lobe; agenesis of the corpus callosum (see below). None of 50 matched healthy volunteers showed focal pathology on CT.

Given the differences in the nature of the patient samples, these three studies are in rough agreement about the prevalence of unexpected focal abnormalities on CT: between 6 and 9%. One magnetic resonance imaging (MRI) study has also examined the issue of the prevalence of focal abnormalities in schizophrenia. O'Callaghan *et al.* (1992) scanned 47 patients under the age of 65 meeting DSM-III criteria for schizophrenia, with 25 matched controls. Four patients (9%) were revealed to have unsuspected lesions of a neurodevelopmental type: one partial agenesis

Table 17.1 Laterality, locus and nature of focal lesions found on computerized tomography in 13 of 228 schizophrenic patients. (From Lewis, 1990)

Site	Number	Nature of lesion
Right-sided		
Frontal	1	Low attenuation
Parietal	3	Calcified mass (1), porencephalic cyst (1), low attenuation (1)
Temporal	1	Old abscess cavity
Left-sided		
Frontoparietal	1	Low attenuation
Temporal	3	Arachnoid cyst (2), calcification (1)
Occipitotemporal	1	Arachnoid cyst
Midline	1	Septal cyst
Bilateral	2	Occipital low attenuation (1), parasagittal calcification (1)

of the corpus callosum; two cases of marked asymmetrical dilatation of the left lateral ventricle (one with an associated porencephalic cyst); and one cerebellar hypoplasia.

The only epidemiologically sound and well-executed study to report prevalence figures for secondary schizophrenias of the type secondary to systemic physical illness is the important study of Johnstone *et al.* (1987). The study examined a sample of 328 consecutive patients presenting with a first episode of schizophrenia between the age of 15 and 70 years. Patients were screened clinically, without routine diagnostic neuro-imaging, for the presence of organic illnesses which the authors judged to be 'of definite or possible aetiological significance'. Thirteen patients fell into the category of substance-induced schizophrenia, including one patient who was judged to have developed schizophrenia-like symptoms secondary to treatment with steroids. Nine patients (3%) were regarded as falling into the category of schizophrenia secondary to non-psychiatric medical disorder. These comprised three cases of tertiary syphilis, two cases of sarcoidosis, one case of multisystem autoimmune disease including systemic lupus erythematosus (SLE), one case of carcinoma of the bronchus

with a secondary right parietal and frontal brain infarction, one cerebral cysticercosis and one chronic thyrotoxicosis. In these cases, neurological signs were the exception rather than the rule and a history of epilepsy was noted in only one case. Over 50% of the cases had migrated from developing countries and had presumably been at increased risk of untreated infections and other disorders. No case had a family history of schizophrenia. Two additional aspects of the data which were not specifically commented on by the authors were the relatively late age at onset of these nine cases (range 29–59 years) and, curiously, that all nine cases were female.

Inferring cause and effect

The attribution of a cause–effect relationship to a particular organic disease or lesion with regard to schizophrenic symptoms in clinical practice can be very difficult. Table 17.2 gives general criteria by which observations are used in disease models to support the existence of a causal relationship. As can be seen, in the case of secondary schizophrenias several of these criteria are difficult to fulfil. Neurodevelopmental formulations of aetiology in schizophrenia generally are relatively

Table 17.2 General criteria to support causal relationships used in disease models

Criterion	Observation	Comments regarding schizophrenia
Temporality	Cause precedes effect	Cause may be several years earlier. Problem with cross-sectional surveys of schizophrenic patients: temporality must be inferred
Consistency	Repeatedly observed	Many observations are anecdotal, single-case reports
Strength	Large relative risk	Relative risk difficult to evaluate because associations are often rare; best established for epilepsy
Dose–response	Larger exposure to cause associated with larger effect	May not hold for schizophrenia where specific, subtle lesion may be important
Reversibility	Reduced exposure to cause associated with reduced effect	Not shown
Specificity	One cause leads to one effect	Several different causes with no clear common pathology; each cause can have different neuropsychiatric effects
Analogy	Similar exposure gives known effects	Closest analogy probably epilepsy: variety of causes, latent period, pleiomorphic behavioural syndrome
Biological plausibility	Makes sense	Neurodevelopmental model facilitates understanding of mechanisms; but what about non-neurodevelopmental causes?

recent, but mean that the temporality criterion can be difficult to demonstrate if the cause arises many years before the schizophrenic symptoms. Nonetheless, there are clear instances in the literature of cause being attributed where it is by no means clear that the lesion predated the schizophrenia: one example of this is several old post-mortem studies disclosing brain tumours in schizophrenic patients without evidence that the tumour predated the psychiatric symptoms (Davison & Bagley, 1969). In addition to the problems noted in Table 17.2, there are other difficulties in many cases. In some instances both the physical disease and the schizophrenic symptoms may result from another, underlying cause.

Epilepsy might be the best example of this, where the symptoms of both epilepsy, itself a syndrome, and schizophrenia may arise from some underlying brain disease, rather than epilepsy causing schizophrenia directly. Drug treatments of the physical disorder can also predispose to psychotic symptomatology; steroids (for SLE) and amphetamines (in the case of narcolepsy), for instance. A further possible confounder is that some aspect of pre-schizophrenic personality might predispose to healthendangering behaviours, for example head injury.

Despite all these caveats a number of different physical disorders have, down the years, been linked to the emergence of secondary schizophrenia.

The co-occurrence of schizophrenia-like symptoms and organic brain disease

In 1969, Davison and Bagley published a review of the world literature, backed with some 800 references, of the co-occurrence of schizophrenia-like symptoms and organic disease. This review remains a landmark in the field. It took as its starting point the operational criteria for schizophrenia of the 1957 WHO Committee; these were adapted slightly by Davison and Bagley so that their case material included cases which today would broadly be headed under the rubric of schizophrenia and paranoid psychosis. Criteria also included the absence of impaired consciousness and the absence of prominent affective symptoms. The authors concluded that the occurrence of schizophrenia-like symptoms exceeded chance expectation in many organic CNS disorders and that, where a discrete lesion was present, those in the temporal lobe and diencephalon seemed to be particularly significant.

Davison and Bagley reviewed the evidence for schizophrenia being linked to a large range of individual CNS disorders. Epilepsy was statistically associated with schizophrenia-like psychosis, particularly where a temporal lobe lesion existed. Head injury was also a risk factor for psychosis, again with a possible association with temporal lobe lesions. Severe closed head injury with diffuse cerebral damage was related to early development of psychotic symptoms. Encephalitic disorders, cerebral syphilis, Wilson's disease, Huntington's disease, Friedreich's ataxia, vitamin B_{12} deficiency, subarachnoid haemorrhage and cerebral tumour also seemed to be associated with an increased risk of schizophrenia-like symptoms. They found much less evidence to implicate other CNS disorders such as multiple sclerosis (MS), motor neurone disease and Parkinson's disease.

It should not be surprising that, 20 years later, a few of Davison and Bagley's conclusions might be amended. For example, their finding of an association between narcolepsy and psychosis would now be explained by most authorities on the basis of the use of amphetamines in treatment, rather than the disease itself. As noted above, the correlation between cerebral tumour and schizophrenia-like symptoms is probably overestimated. Many such instances could be better explained as chance association, unless the tumours were of the type whose natural history was very long standing. Conversely, new evidence for these and other disorders being associated is now available, and is reviewed below.

Epilepsy

Estimates of the incidence of schizophrenic symptoms in temporal lobe epilepsy vary widely (reviewed in Hyde *et al.*, 1992), and are obviously sensitive to artefacts of ascertainment. Roberts *et al.* (1990) reported that 25 out of his consecutive autopsy series of 249 cases (10%) had a lifetime history of psychotic symptoms. Trimble (1988) estimated that patients with epilepsy were at three- to ninefold increased risk of schizophrenia-like psychoses.

The definitive case series of 69 patients by Slater and Beard (1963) noted classical Schneiderian 'positive' symptoms in these schizophrenias, but often without negative symptoms and in the context of a normal premorbid personality, without a family history of schizophrenia. An association between medial temporal lobe, perhaps particularly dominant temporal lobe, epilepsy and Schneiderian symptoms does seem to exist. Flor-Henry's initial report (1969) about laterality actually contained 19 cases of left and 12 cases of right temporal lobe involvement (most cases had bilateral involvement), a similar proportion to Slater and Beard's original series (36 left, 32 right). The 10 independent series to examine the laterality issue do show a trend towards left-sided predominance, as reviewed by Trimble (1990). Nonetheless, the observation that about one-sixth of patients with schizophrenic psychoses of epilepsy had only right temporal lobe involvement detracts from the hypothesis that left temporal involvement is necessary: involvement of either side may be sufficient.

In temporal lobe epilepsy with schizophrenia, neurodevelopmental lesions in the temporal lobe such as hamartomata, rather than the early acquired lesion of mesial temporal sclerosis, are overrepresented (Taylor, 1975). Roberts *et al.* (1990) noted that in 16 of 249 cases of TLE coming to temporal lobectomy; schizophrenic symptoms were present preoperatively; in a further nine they emerged postoperatively. Schizophrenic symptoms were more commonly found in those epilepsies associated with lesions originating in the fetus or perinatally and which were physiologically active at a relatively early age, as inferred from a comparatively early age at first seizure. The medial temporal lobe was most often involved. A neurodevelopmental tumour, the ganglioglioma, was specially associated with risk of psychosis.

The two competing hypotheses to explain the association between epilepsy and schizophrenic symptoms are either that both sets of symptoms arise from a common underlying cerebral pathology, usually in the temporal lobe, or, more intriguingly, that the schizophrenic symptoms arise out of a process of progressive facilitation of subthreshold electrical activity ('kindling'). The relationship between the timing of seizures and the emergence of schizophrenic symptoms can vary. Classically, the schizophrenic symptoms emerge as interictal phenomena, although occasionally schizophreniform symptoms are part of a postictal psychosis or even an ictal phenomenon during partial complex seizures (Mace, 1993). The scalp electroencephalogram (EEG) usually shows no change during interictal schizophrenic psychosis, which somewhat argues against the notion of kindling being an important mechanism. Stevens (1992) has advanced a third, neurodevelopmental explanation of the link between epilepsy and schizophrenia, proposing that it is abnormal neuronal regeneration in adolescence in some individuals with epilepsy that predisposes to schizophrenic symptoms. Further depth electrophysiological studies, perhaps using magnetoencephalography, may be the most promising avenue to explore the links between schizophrenic symptoms and epilepsy (Mace, 1993).

Cerebral trauma

The largest cohort of brain-injured patients followed up psychiatrically is the national Finnish cohort of approximately 10 000 cases described by Achte *et al.* (1991). Of these, 762 (7.6%) were described as having psychotic disorders, although systematic evaluation was lacking. Delusional disorder appeared to be the most common psychosis. Gualtieri and Cox (1991) estimated that traumatic brain injury increases the risk of psychosis by two- to fivefold. Many years often elapse between the head injury and the emergence of psychotic symptoms.

Buckley *et al.* (1993) ascertained three cases of schizophrenia and two cases of schizoaffective disorder in whom the psychosis followed a severe (loss of consciousness greater than 4 hours) head injury. MRI showed no abnormality in the two schizoaffective patients. Left temporal gliosis and/or atrophy were consistently found in the three schizophrenic patients. Psychosis followed injury at intervals of 1, 7 and 19 years in these patients.

Cerebrovascular disease

Schizophrenias arising in late life are fertile but underresearched areas in which to explore pathogenetic mechanisms of secondary schizophrenias. Miller *et al.* (1991) assessed 24 consecutively ascertained patients with 'late-life psychosis', defined as DSM-III-R schizophrenia, schizophreniform or delusional disorder or unspecified psychosis of at least 4 weeks duration, beginning over the age of 45. Brain disease was sought with MRI and compared with a series of 72 healthy controls. A known history of neurological disease was an exclusion criterion in all subjects. Unsuspected cortical or subcortical white matter infarcts were seen in 25% of the patients compared with 6% of controls. The largest regional difference between patients and controls was in the temporal region. Another two patients showed radiological changes of dementia, one a cerebellar tumour and one post-traumatic brain injury. Delusions and hallucinations occur in early Alzheimer's disease in about 50% of cases (Chen *et al.*, 1991). Again, this is a fertile area for research into the pathogenesis of psychotic symptoms (Zubencko *et al.*, 1991).

In a previous report, Miller *et al.* (1989)

described five cases of subfrontal white matter infarction leading to psychosis. Vascular subfrontal damage can seemingly lead to psychosis in young adults also. Hall and Young (1992) described an acute schizophreniform psychosis with blunted affect, thought disorder and auditory hallucinations in a 23-year-old man, secondary to a ruptured cerebral aneurysm in the left frontal lobe.

Demyelinating diseases

Multiple sclerosis (MS) has been associated with a variety of psychiatric sequelae, most commonly affective disorders. Stevens (1988) noted epidemiological similarities between MS and schizophrenia, taking this as circumstantial evidence that both disorders might have a similar immunological cause. Davison and Bagley (1969) considered that there was little evidence for increased risk of schizophrenic symptoms in MS. However, recent reports suggest that schizophrenia can arise secondary to MS in some rare cases. Temporal lobe demyelination could be the mediating link (Ron & Logsdail, 1989). Feinstein *et al.* (1992) compared MRI findings in 10 psychotic and 10 non-psychotic MS patients: the psychotic patients tended to show more lesions around the temporal horns bilaterally, a similar finding to that of Honer *et al.* (1987) and Reischies *et al.* (1988). Feinstein *et al.* noted that the symptoms of schizophrenia began relatively late (mean age 36) in their sample, although were typical of schizophrenia thereafter, and postulated that longstanding strategically placed lesions were crucial in the development of psychosis.

Schizophrenic symptoms have also been noted in rarer demyelinating syndromes (e.g. Neumann *et al.*, 1988). Schilder's disease is a progressive, usually fatal demyelinating disease of children and adolescents which is sporadic and probably related to MS. Occasional reports with schizophrenic symptoms exist (Davison & Bagley, 1969; Ramani, 1981). A review of reported cases (Ramani, 1981) confirmed primary frontal lobe involvement in those cases presenting with psychoses.

Metachromatic leucodystrophy (MLD) is a rare, autosomal recessive demyelinating disorder with a particularly strong association with psychosis. Deficiency of arylsulphatase-A is the basic biochemical lesion, which leads to progressive demyelination. The inheritance shows incomplete penetrance and the extent of arylsulphatase-A deficiency seems to dictate age at onset. Hyde *et al.* (1992) reviewed the world literature of MLD, 129 definite cases, and noted that when the onset was timed in adolescence or early adulthood (10–30 years), hallucinations or delusions occurred in over 50% of cases and a clinical diagnosis of schizophrenia was made in 35%. Complex auditory hallucinations typical of schizophrenia were commonly reported, and other motor as well as negative symptoms also occurred. Hyde *et al.* argued that the high frequency of schizophrenic symptoms seen in MLD reflected its neuropathological origins in the periventricular frontal white matter. Progressive extension posteriorly heralds the appearance of more formal neurological signs. These observations led to the authors' hypothesis that dysfunctional subcortical pathways linking frontal cortex with normally functioning temporolimbic cortex are crucial to the production of schizophrenic symptoms.

Arylsulphatase-A deficits in the absence of clinical MLD have occasionally been reported in schizophrenic patients (Manowitz *et al.* 1981). Adrenoleucodystrophy (ALD) is a separate group of disorders, the main subtype of which involves an X-linked deficit in the breakdown of very long-chain fatty acids. Three cases have been described with schizophrenic symptoms (Kitchin *et al.*, 1987).

Metabolic and autoimmune disorders

Thyroid-related psychoses are most usually affectively based (Davis, 1989). Hyperparathyroidism, usually an adenoma leading to hypercalcaemia, often causes psychiatric symptoms, although again convincing schizophrenic symptoms seem to be rare (Johnson, 1975; Alarcon & Franceschini, 1984; Ebel *et al.*, 1991). Organic mental states with delirium, or depressive symptoms are the rule (Gatewood *et al.*, 1975).

Vitamin B_{12} deficiency can present with mental changes, although psychosis is unusual. Zucker *et al.* (1981) reviewed the literature and found only 15 cases of 'B$_{12}$ psychosis' responding to B$_{12}$ replacement: most of these were depressive disorders. B$_{12}$ deficiency may more often be an effect, rather than a cause, of schizophrenic symptoms.

It has been recognized only relatively recently (MacNeil *et al.*, 1976) that cerebral SLE can give schizophrenia-like symptoms. Attributing causation in individual cases can be difficult: SLE is common, with variable course and symptoms, and its first-line treatment, steroids, can cause psychotic symptoms.

Encephalitis and other infections

Limbic encephalitis is most often associated with psychotic symptoms. Many viruses are known to cause limbic encephalitis (Glaser & Pincus, 1969; Damasio & Hoesen, 1985). In a review of 22 cases, Torrey (1986) noted reports of a variety of neuropathic viruses causing encephalitis leading to psychotic symptoms: Epstein–Barr, cytomegalovirus, rubella, herpes simplex and measles. Nunn *et al.* (1986) reported four cases of adult-type arising in children after viral encephalitic illnesses of varying pathology: rubella, measles, varicella and herpes. Psychosis in Epstein–Barr viral infection is unusual (Leavell *et al.*, 1986) and most commonly depressive in form (Rubin, 1978; White & Lewis, 1987).

Subacute sclerosing panencephalitis (SSPE) is a rare, slow-virus-like presentation of measles infection. It presents as a progressive neurological disorder (Koehler & Jakumeit, 1976) with a clinical onset usually in early adult life or before, although often years after the initial measles infection. Two recently reported case histories are typical: symptoms of schizophrenia (Duncalf *et al.*, 1989) or delusional disorder (dysmorphophobia: Salib, 1988) presenting in young adults, with the emergence of rapidly progressive neurological signs several months later and death within a year. A report of schizophreniform psychosis more directly following measles infection (Stoler *et al.*, 1987) was criticized for failing conclusively to demonstrate brain involvement with the virus (McCune, 1987).

Sporadic reports of schizophrenia in other infective and inflammatory conditions exist. Borellia encephalitis is a recently described cause of schizophrenic symptoms which apparently responds to chemotherapy (Barnett *et al.*, 1991). Childhood Sydenham's chorea, a complication of rheumatic fever with basal ganglia pathology, may predispose to later schizophrenia (Wilcox & Nasrallah, 1986).

Paraneoplastic encephalopathies are uncommon, poorly understood complications of non-CNS tumours. They can, rarely, cause schizophrenic symptoms, seemingly mediated by limbic inflammation (Van Sweden & Van Peteghem, 1986). Neurocysticercosis results from invasion of the CNS with *Taenia solium* larvae, producing cysts, nodules and fibrosis. Schizophrenia-like complications are apparently not uncommon, although the disease deserves more research (Tavares *et al.*, 1993).

Psychotic symptoms can arise in the context of human immunodeficiency virus (HIV) disease, usually acquired immune deficiency syndrome (AIDS). Harris *et al.* (1991) reviewed the literature, as well as the histories of a cohort of 124 HIV-infected patients followed up for 6 years, for new-onset psychosis, after excluding cases where psychotic symptoms arose out of substance misuse or delirium. Psychotic symptoms usually took the form of acute-onset delusions, hallucinations and bizarre behaviour, most often in the context of a mood disturbance, particularly hypomania. Typical schizophrenic symptoms in clear consciousness were rarely described. The pathogenesis of such psychoses has yet to be established.

Sex chromosome abnormalities

Turner's syndrome (45 XO) in association with schizophrenia has been reported in about 10 cases. Studies of large samples (Nielsen & Stradiot, 1987) have not disclosed a raised incidence of schizophrenia in Turner's syndrome: two cases in 968 female schizophrenic patients (Kaplan & Cotton, 1968); or one case in 3558 (Akesson & O'Landers, 1969), with the likely incidence rate for Turner's syndrome being 0.01% of live female births. Bamrah and MacKay (1989) speculated whether Turner's syndrome was actually protective against schizophrenia. The issue is complicated by the heterogeneity of the syndrome: only half of cases are 45 XO, the rest being mosaics or having a structurally abnormal X chromosome (Fishbain, 1990).

Other sex chromosome abnormalities reported with schizophrenia include an XX male (Muller & Endres, 1987) and an XO/XY mosaic with basal ganglia calcification (Deckert *et al.*, 1992).

Schizophrenia has been described in Noonan's syndrome (Turner's syndrome phenotype with normal karyotype: Krishna *et al.*, 1977) and in 47 XYY males (Faber & Abrams, 1975; Dorus *et al.*, 1977). Of 20 psychotic males with Klinefelter's syndrome (47 XXY), described by Sørensen and Nielsen (1977), five fulfil criteria for schizophrenia. The authors nonetheless conclude that this was insufficient evidence for a genuine association.

In his review of the area, Propping (1983) considered that the Klinefelter karyotype and the XXX karyotype were the two sex chromosomal abnormalities which had the strongest association with schizophrenia. From the data available, Propping estimated that for both XXY and XXX the risk of schizophrenia was increased threefold. DeLisi and Crow (1991) concurred with this conclusion, citing it as evidence for possible linkage of schizophrenia to the X chromosome.

Associations with Mendelian disorders

Propping's review (1983) discussed possible associations between a variety of Mendelian disorders and schizophrenia. Table 17.3 summarizes Propping's conclusions, dividing such disorders into probable and possible associations with an increased risk of schizophrenia. Interest in reports in this area has increased over the past 5 years as it has become apparent that cosegregation in pedigrees with a disorder whose inheritance is understood offers the identification of candidate chromosomes or chromosomal regions to explore in linkage studies.

The association of Huntington's disease with an increased risk of schizophrenia is well established. Schizophrenic symptoms were reported in

Table 17.3 Mendelian disorders with an increased risk of schizophrenia. (Adapted from Propping, 1983)

Very probable
Huntington's disease
Acute intermittent porphyria
Porphyria variegata
Metachromatic leucodystrophy
Familial basal ganglia calcification

Possible
Erythropoetic porphyria
Niemann–Pick's disease
Gaucher's disease, adult type
Fabry disease
Kuf's disease
Congenital adrenal hyperplasia
Homocystinuria
Wilson's disease
Haemochromatosis
Ichthyosis vulgaris
Laurence–Moon–Biedl syndrome
G-6-PD deficiency
Phenylketonuria
Oculocutaneous albinism
Kartaneger's syndrome
Familial ataxia
Hyperasparaginaemia

5–11% of patients with Huntington's disease in six series, each comprising at least 50 cases and reviewed in Hyde *et al.* (1992). The review by Davison (1983) quotes similar prevalence figures. Weinberger (1987) noted the age-related risk of psychosis in Huntington's disease.

Further case reports have elucidated the link between some of the disorders noted previously by Propping. The link between the autosomal dominant acute intermittent porphyria and psychosis has fuelled recent searches for linkage of schizophrenia to chromosome 11, home of the porphyrin deaminase gene. Cosegregation of schizophrenia and oculocutaneous albinism has repeatedly been described (Baron, 1976; Clarke & Buckley, 1989); interestingly, neurodevelopmental abnormalities, particularly of projections to the visual association cortex, are known to occur in albinism (Clarke & Buckley, 1989).

It is likely that the alleged association between Wilson's disease and schizophrenic symptoms has been overemphasized. Although Wilson's original series included two patients with schizophrenic symptoms, the 520 case reports up to 1959 included only eight convincing cases (Davison & Bagley, 1969). Dening and Berrios (1989) reviewed psychiatric symptomatology in a series of 195 cases. Hallucinations occurred in only two cases and delusions in three.

Further case reports of Mendelian disorders convincingly associated with schizophrenia have emerged since Propping's review. Two families in which the autosomal dominant connective tissue disorder Marfan's syndrome cosegregated with schizophrenia have been described (Sirota *et al.*, 1990), plus a further case (Romano & Linares, 1987). Usher's syndrome, an autosomal recessive syndrome causing progressive sensorial deafness and blindness has been described in large pedigrees cosegregating with schizophrenia (Sharp *et al.*, 1993). A family with multiple instances of the X-linked Alport's syndrome and psychosis has been described (Shields *et al.*, 1990). Recent interest has also focused on the risk of psychoses in families affected by Wolfram syndrome (Swift *et al.*, 1990). Tuberous sclerosis is an autosomal dominant condition giving rise to slow-growing intercerebral lesions in some cases. Schizophrenia-like symptoms have been reported and seem to be linked with tumours affecting the medial temporal lobe (Heckert *et al.*, 1972). Bilateral calcification in the temporal lobe was probably the mediating link in a patient with psychotic symptoms in the context of a longstanding autosomal illness, lipoid proteinosis (Emsley & Paster, 1985).

The status of schizophrenic disorders when found to cosegregate with named Mendelian disorders is difficult to evaluate. In some instances it is possible that, rather than the schizophrenia being directly secondary to the genetic disorder, this is a familial subtype of schizophrenia inherited in an autosomal dominant manner and showing genetic linkage to the medical disorder, but having no true aetiological association.

Unsuspected intracranial lesions

Routine non-invasive imaging in the clinical assessment of schizophrenia, as well as prospective research, has led to increasing numbers of case reports of more or less unusual cerebral lesions in schizophrenia (Lewis, 1989). In most cases these are clinically unsuspected, in that there was no history of neurological symptoms or neurological signs on examination. Such lesions have been described in many parts of the brain and are of different pathologies. Some lesions reported are likely to be coincidental. Lesions falling into this category include the small cerebral infarcts and white-matter abnormalities on MRI that are seen predominantly in older patients; these are also seen in normal controls. These are often linked to a history of cerebrovascular disease.

Very rarely, unsuspected, slow-growing cerebral tumours can present with schizophrenic symptoms. In the series reported by Malamud (1967), these symptoms were most common in tumours affecting the temporal lobe and cingulate gyrus. However, unsuspected brain lesions found in association with schizophrenia are often those which can be classified as neurodevelopmental anomalies of one type or another. These include aqueduct stenosis (Reveley & Reveley, 1983), arachnoid cysts (Lanczik *et al.*, 1989), porencephalic cysts (O'Callaghan *et al.*, 1992), and cerebrovascular malformations including congenital arteriovenous malformations in the temporal lobe (Vaillant, 1965) and the midline great vein of Galen (Remington & Jeffries, 1984). Despite cases of familial basal ganglia calcification being reported in association with schizophrenia (Propping, 1983), two large studies have found no association in general between basal ganglia calcification and schizophrenia in large samples of psychiatric patients (Casanova *et al.*, 1990; Philpot & Lewis, 1990).

Probably the most intriguing subclass of neurodevelopmental lesions reported in association with schizophrenia are midline anomalies associated with the septum pellucidum and adjacent corpus callosum. The first case description of complete agenesis of the corpus callosum (Lewis *et al.*, 1987) has been followed by further cases of callosal agenesis, usually involving partial agenesis of the anterior part of the corpus callosum (Vellek *et al.*, 1988; O'Callaghan *et al.*, 1992; Swayze *et al.*, 1992). An initial CT report of six cases of developmental cavum septum pellucidum (Lewis & Mezey, 1985) has been complemented by a combined MRI and postmortem study reporting a surprisingly high prevalence of varying degrees of this anomaly in schizophrenic patients compared with controls (Degreef *et al.*, 1992). Congenital absence of the septum pellucidum has also been described in schizophrenia (George *et al.*, 1989). More work is needed in this area. It is unclear whether such neurodevelopmental lesions are in some way directly conferring an increased risk of schizophrenia or whether they are merely signals of a more general neurodevelopmental brain abnormality, whose critical site of action is actually elsewhere, or more generalized.

Phenomenology of primary vs. secondary schizophrenia

As reviewed above, both brain imaging and clinical studies point to a prevalence rate of 5−8% for psychoses of likely identifiable organic aetiology among series of relatively unselected patients. If this is the case, is it possible to distinguish the minority of organic cases on clinical grounds alone? The short answer is no, in that there is a large overlap in presenting symptoms between functional and organic psychoses. Nonetheless, several studies have compared symptom profiles in the two groups and some general differences do emerge.

In their review of the literature, Davison and Bagley (1969) compared rates of individual psychotic symptoms in 150 reported cases of various organic schizophrenia-like psychoses with a series of 475 patients with functional schizophrenia reported by other authors. Of 14 clinical features compared, seven occurred significantly less frequently in the organic group: flat or incongruous affect, passivity feelings, thought disorder, auditory hallucinations, tactile hallucinations, schizoid premorbid personality and family history of schizophrenia. Catatonic symptoms were reported more frequently in organic cases; 64% of the organic group showed

Schneiderian first-rank symptoms, although this feature was not recorded in the control group. These results are intriguing, although they represent a retrospective survey of a varied collection of different case reports.

Cutting (1987) compared the Present State Examination (PSE)-rated symptomatology of 74 cases of organic psychosis with 74 cases of RDC acute schizophrenia, all prospectively interviewed. Like Davison and Bagley, he found auditory hallucinations to be less common in the organic group. Delusions were also less frequently found, although simple persecutory delusions were actually more common in the organic group. Contrary to the findings of Davison and Bagley, Schneiderian symptoms were rare in the organic group (3%). Thought disorder and visual hallucinations were more common. Cutting also noted a difference in the content of the phenomenology. Whereas delusions of the first rank were unusual in organic cases, in nearly 50% of the deluded organic patients, two delusional themes were apparent: belief of imminent misadventure to others, or bizarre occurrences in the immediate vicinity. Few non-organic schizophrenic patients showed these features. Cutting offers possible explanations for these organic themes as being delusional elaborations of deficits of perception or memory. In the area of perceptual disturbance, the mistaken identity of other people was another theme found more commonly in the organic group.

In the study of Johnstone *et al.* (1988), PSE-rated symptomatology was compared between 23 cases of so-called organic psychosis and 92 non-organic psychoses matched for age, sex and ethnicity and conforming to DSM-III criteria for schizophrenia, mania and psychotic depression. The authors found considerable overlap in symptoms. Comparing the organic and schizophrenic ($n = 43$) groups, nuclear (first-rank) schizophrenic symptoms tended to be less frequent in the organic group (50 vs. 74%; $P < 0.06$). Visual hallucinations were more common in the organic group only if consciousness was clouded.

In the series of RDC schizophrenia patients

under 65 years, referred to above, Lewis (1987) compared clinical features of those 41 patients with unequivocally abnormal CT scans with features in the 166 with a normal CT scan. Those with abnormal CT scans had significantly less evidence of a family history of schizophrenia among first-degree relatives, were more likely to have demonstrated formal thought disorder and more often had EEG abnormalities. Clinical presentation also seemed more atypical in the abnormal scan group, in that these patients were significantly more likely to have received alternative prior hospital diagnoses, and a longer interval had intervened before a diagnosis of schizophrenia was made.

Most recently, Feinstein and Ron (1990) examined the symptomatology in a series of 53 schizophrenic patients, ascertained retrospectively, in whom psychotic symptoms arose secondary to overt brain disease. Symptom patterns were compared with normative data derived from the International Pilot Study of Schizophrenia. The only individual symptom difference was an excess of visual hallucinations in the secondary schizophrenia group. Feinstein and Ron noted a relatively old age at onset (mean of 34 years), and a family history of schizophrenia in first-degree relatives was present in only three of 53 cases. A wide variety of organic disease was

represented. Overall, 50% of cases had epilepsy, reflecting a referral bias compared with the more representative series of Johnstone *et al.* (1987). Individual cases included frontal meningioma, cerebral lymphoma, tuberous sclerosis, MS, Huntington's disease, encephalitis, cerebral abscess and hyperparathyroidism. Three cases of schizophrenic symptoms arising after neurosurgical operation were also included. The authors noted the wide variability in brain regions involved with, in particular, no consistent lateralized temporal pathology.

Excluding secondary schizophrenia in practice: physical investigations

Table 17.4 outlines first- and second-line physical investigations which should be considered in new cases of psychosis, including schizophrenia. Of the first-line investigations, some may dispute the need always for syphilis serology and EEG. However, tertiary syphilis still occasionally presents as a psychosis in clinical practice. The EEG is carried out to exclude the generalized slowing indicative of diffuse brain disease, or the focal paroxysmal spike-and-wave discharges of an epileptic focus.

The second-line investigations are dependent on other abnormal findings (autoantibodies if

Table 17.4 Secondary schizophrenias: suggested screening procedures

Physical investigations	
First line	Second line
Neurological examination	Autoantibodies
Full blood count	Computerized tomography/magnetic resonance imaging
Erythrocyte sedimentation rate	Serum calcium
Electrolytes	Human immunodeficiency virus serology
Syphilis serology	Arylsulphatase-A
Thyroid function	
Liver function	Chromosome studies
Electroencephalogram	Serum copper studies
Urinary drug screen	Cerebrospinal fluid examination

raised erythrocyte sedimentation rate, chromosome studies if developmental delays or unusual body morphology). In particular, a CT or MRI scan is probably only warranted in clinical practice if there are neurological symptoms in the history (e.g. epilepsy), neurological signs on examination or with an abnormal EEG.

Conclusion

Clinically unsuspected, usually neurodevelopmental, brain lesions of aetiological relevance occur in 5−10% of schizophrenic illness. Cases among males seem to predominate. There is no indication that the discovery of such a lesion influences treatment in any specific way. The more classical variants of secondary schizophrenia are those psychotic disorders arising in the context of systemic physical disease. The best evidence available is that these account for about 3% of newly presenting schizophrenias. Clinically, it is important to detect this subtype, since recognition and treatment of primary disorder is needed. The existence of secondary schizophrenias offers several potential avenues to illuminate the cause of primary schizophrenia. The observation of neurodevelopmental lesions was one of the building blocks of the neurodevelopmental model of schizophrenia. Those disorders which remain unexplained by this model are adult-onset physical disorders which produce secondary schizophrenic symptoms, although the notion of a developmental window may prove important in understanding the onset of these disorders.

References

Achte, K., Jarho, L., Kyykka, T. & Vesterinen, E. (1991) Paranoid disorders following war brain damage. *Psychopathology*, **24**, 309−315.

Akesson, H.O. & O'Landers, S. (1969) Frequency of negative sex chromatin among women in mental hospitals. *Human Heredity*, **19**, 43−47.

Alarcon, R.D. & Franceschini, J.A. (1984) Hyperparathyroidism and paranoid psychosis case report and review of the literature. *British Journal of Psychiatry*, **145**, 477−486.

APA (1993) *Diagnostic and Statistical Manual of Mental Disorders*, 4th edn. American Psychiatric Association, Washington.

Bamrah, J.S. & MacKay, M.E. (1989) Chronic psychosis in Turner's syndrome. *British Journal of Psychiatry*, **155**, 857−859.

Barnett, W., Sigmund, D., Roelcke, U. & Mundt, C. (1991) Endogenous-like paranoid-hallucinatory syndrome due to borrelia encephalitis. *Nervenarzt*, 445−447.

Baron, M. (1976) Albinism and schizophreniform psychosis: a pedigree study. *American Journal of Psychiatry*, **133**, 1070−1073.

Brugha, T.S., Wing, J.K., Brewin, L.R. *et al.* (1988) The problems of people in long-term psychiatric care. An introduction to the Camberwell High Contact Survey. *Psychological Medicine*, **18**, 457−468.

Buckley, P., Stack, J.P., Madigan, C. *et al.* (1993) Magnetic resonance imaging of schizophrenia-like psychoses associated with cerebral trauma: clinicopathological correlates. *American Journal of Psychiatry*, **150**, 146−148.

Casanova, M.F., Prasad, C.N., Waldman, I. *et al.* (1990) No difference in basal ganglia mineralization between schizophrenic and non-schizophrenic patients: a quantitative CT study. *Biological Psychiatry*, **27**, 138−142.

Chen, J., Stern, Y., Sano, M. & Mayeux, R. (1991) Cumulative risks of developing extrapyramidal signs, psychosis, or myoclonus in the course of Alzheimer's disease. *Archives of Neurology*, **48**, 1141−1143.

Clarke, D.J. & Buckley, M. (1989) Familial association of albinism and schizophrenia. *British Journal of Psychiatry*, **155**, 551−553.

Cutting, J. (1987) The phenomenology of acute organic psychosis: comparison with acute schizophrenia. *British Journal of Psychiatry*, **151**, 324−332.

Damasio, A.R. & Van Hoesen, G.W. (1985) The limbic system and the localization of herpes simplex encephalitis. *Journal of Neurology, Neurosurgery and Psychiatry*, **48**, 279−301.

Davis, A.T. (1989) Psychotic states associated with disorders of thyroid function. *International Journal of Psychiatry in Medicine*, **19**, 47−56.

Davison, K. (1983) Schizophrenia-like psychoses associated with organic cerebral disorders: a review. *Psychiatric Developments*, **1**, 1−34.

Davison, K. & Bagley, C.R. (1969) Schizophrenia-like psychoses associated with organic disorders of the central nervous system. In Herrington, R. (ed.) *Current Problems in Neuropsychiatry: Schizophrenia, Epilepsy, the Temporal Lobe*, special publication No. 4. British Journal of Psychiatry, London.

Deckert, J., Strik, W.K. & Fritze, J. (1992) Organic schizophrenic syndrome associated with symmetrical basal ganglia sclerosis and XO/XY-mosaic. *Biological Psychiatry*, **31**, 401−403.

Degreef, G., Bogerts, B., Falkai, P. *et al.* (1992) Increased prevalence of cavum septum pellucidum in schizophrenic patients. *Psychiatry Research*, **45**, 1−13.

DeLisi, L.E. & Crow, T.J. (1991) Sex chromosome anomalies and schizophrenia. *Schizophrenia Research*, **3**, 72−83.

Dening, T.R. & Berrios, G.E. (1989) Wilson's disease: psychiatric symptoms in 195 cases. *Archives of General Psychiatry*, **46**, 1126−1134.

Dorus, E., Dorus, W. & Telfer, M.A. (1977) Paranoid schizophrenia in a 47,XYY male. *American Journal of Psychiatry*, **134**, 687–689.

Duncalf, C.M., Kent, J.N., Harbord, M. & Hicks, E.P. (1989) Subacute sclursing ponecenphalitis presenting as schizophreniform psychosis. *British Journal of Psychiatry*, **155**, 557–559.

Ebel, H., Schlegel, U. & Klosterkotter, J. (1991) Chronic schizophreniform psychoses in primary hyperparathyroidism. *Nervenarzt*, **63**, 180–183.

Emsley, R.A. & Paster, L. (1985) Lipoid proteinosis presenting with neuropsychiatric manifestations. *Journal of Neurology, Neurosurgery and Psychiatry*, **48**, 1290–1292.

Faber, R. & Abrams, R. (1975) Schizophrenia in a 47,XYY male. *British Journal of Psychiatry*, **127**, 401–403.

Feinstein, A. & Ron, M.A. (1990) Psychosis associated with demonstrable brain disease. *Psychological Medicine*, **20**, 793–803.

Feinstein, A., du Boulay, G. & Ron, M.A. (1992) Psychotic illness in multiple sclerosis. A clinical and magnetic resonance imaging study. *British Journal of Psychiatry*, **161**, 680–685.

Fishbain, D.A. (1990) Chronic psychoses in Turner's syndrome. *British Journal of Psychiatry*, **156**, 745–746.

Flor-Henry, P. (1969) Psychosis and temporal lobe epilepsy. *Epilepsia*, **10**, 363–395.

Gatewood, J.W., Organ, C.H. & Mead, B.T. (1975) Mental changes associated with hyperparathyroidism. *American Journal of Psychiatry*, **132**, 129–132.

George, M.S., Scott, T., Kellner, C.H. & Malcolm, R. (1989) Abnormalities of the septum pellucidum in schizophrenia. *Journal of Neuropsychiatry and Clinical Neurosciences*, **1**, 385–390.

Glaser, G.H. & Pincus, J.H. (1969) Limbic encephalitis. *Journal of Nervous and Mental Disease*, **149**, 59–67.

Gualtieri, T. & Cox, D.R. (1991) The delayed neurobehavioural sequelae of traumatic brain injury. *Brain Injury*, **5**, 219–232.

Hall, D.P. & Young, S.A. (1992) Frontal lobe cerebral aneurysm rupture presenting as psychosis. *Journal of Neurology, Neurosurgery and Psychiatry*, **55**, 1207–1208.

Harris, M.J., Jeste, D.V., Gleghorn, A. & Sewell, D.D. (1991) New-onset psychosis in HIV-infected patients. *Journal of Clinical Psychiatry*, **52**, 369–376.

Heckert, E.E., Wald, A. & Romero, O. (1972) Tuberous sclerosis and schizophrenia. *Diseases of the Nervous System*, **33**, 439–445.

Honer, W.G., Hurwitz, T., Li, D.K.B., Palmer, M. & Paty, D.W. (1987) Temporal lobe involvement in multiple sclerosis patients with psychiatric disorders. *Archives of Neurology*, **44**, 187–190.

Hyde, T.M., Ziegler, J.C. & Weinberger, D.R. (1992) Psychiatric disturbances in metachromatic leukodystrophy: insights into the neurobiology of psychosis. *Archives of Neurology*, **49**, 401–406.

Johnson, J. (1975) Schizophrenia and Cushing's syndrome cured by adrenalectomy. *Psychological Medicine*, **5**, 165–168.

Johnstone, E., MacMillan, F. & Crow, T.J. (1987) The occurrence of organic disease of aetiological significance in a population of 268 cases of first episode schizophrenia.

Psychological Medicine, **17**, 371–379.

Johnstone, E. *et al.* (1988) Phenomenology of organic and functional psychoses and the overlap between them. *British Journal of Psychiatry*, **153**, 770–776.

Kaplan, A.R. & Cotton, J.E. (1968) Chromosomal abnormalities in female schizophrenics. *Journal of Nervous and Mental Diseases*, **147**, 402–417.

Kitchin, W., Cohen-Cole, S.A. & Mickel, S.F. (1987) Adrenoleukodystrophy: frequency of presentation as a psychiatric disorder. *Society of Biological Psychiatry*, **22**, 1375–1387.

Koehler, K. & Jakumeit, U. (1976) Subacute sclerosing panencephalitis presenting as Leonhard's speech-prompt catatonia. *British Journal of Psychiatry*, **129**, 29–31.

Krishna, N.R., Abrams, R., Taylor, M.A. & Behar, D. (1977) Schizophrenia in a 46,XY male with the Noonan syndrome. *British Journal of Psychiatry*, **130**, 570–572.

Lanczik, M., Fritze, J., Classen, W., Ihl, R. & Maurer, K. (1989) Schizophrenia-like psychosis associated with an arachnoid cyst visualized by mapping of EEG and P300. *Psychiatry Research*, **29**, 421–423.

Leavell, R., Ray, C.G., Ferry, P.C. & Minnich, L.L. (1986) Unusual acute neurologic presentations with Epstein–Barr virus infection. *Archives of Neurology*, **43**, 186–188.

Lewis, S.W. (1987) *Schizophrenia with and without intracranial abnormalities on CT scan.* MPhil Thesis, University of London.

Lewis, S.W. (1989) Congenital risk factors for schizophrenia. *Psychological Medicine*, **19**, 5–13.

Lewis, S.W. (1990) Computed tomography in schizophrenia fifteen years on. *British Journal of Psychiatry*, **157** (Suppl. 9), 16–24.

Lewis, S.W. & Mezey, G. (1985) Clinical correlates of septum pellucidum cavities: an unusual association with psychosis. *Psychological Medicine*, **15**, 43–54.

Lewis, S.W., Reveley, A.M., Reveley, M.A., Chitkara, B. & Murray, R.M. (1987) The familial-sporadic distinction in schizophrenia research. *British Journal of Psychiatry*, **151**, 306–313.

McCune, N. (1987) Schizophreniform episode following measles infection. *British Journal of Psychiatry*, **151**, 558–559.

Mace, C.J. (1993) Epilepsy and schizophrenia. *British Journal of Psychiatry*, **163**, 439–445.

MacNeil, A., Grennan, D.M., Ward, D. & Dick, W.C. (1976) Psychiatric problems in systemic lupus erythematosus. *British Journal of Psychiatry*, **128**, 442–445.

Malamud, N. (1967) Psychiatric disorder with intracranial tumours of limbic system. *Archives of Neurology*, **18**, 113–123.

Manowitz, P., Goldstein, L. & Nora, R. (1981) An arylsulfatase A variant in schizophrenic patients: preliminary report. *Biological Psychiatry*, **16**, 1107–1113.

Miller, B.L., Lesser, I.M., Boone, K. *et al.* (1989) Brain white-matter lesions and psychosis. *British Journal of Psychiatry*, **155**, 73–78.

Miller, B.L., Lesser, I.M., Boone, B.K., Hill, E., Mehringer, C.M. & Wong, K. (1991) Brain lesions and cognitive function in late-life psychosis. *British Journal of Psychiatry*,

158, 76–82.

Muller, N. & Endres, M. (1987) An XX male with schizophrenia: a case of personality development and illness similar to that in XXY males. *Journal of Clinical Psychiatry*, **48**, 379–380.

Neumann, P.E., Mehler, M.F., Horoupian, D.S. & Merriam, A.E. (1988) Atypical psychosis with disseminated subpial demyelination. *Archives of Neurology*, **45**, 634–636.

Nielsen, J. & Stradiot, M. (1987) Transcultural study of Turner's syndrome. *Clinical Genetics*, **32**, 260–270.

Nunn, K.P. *et al.* (1986) *Journal of Child Psychology and Psychiatry*, **27**, 55–64.

O'Callaghan, E., Buckley, P., Redmond, O. *et al.* (1992) Abnormalities of cerebral structure on MRI: interpretation in relation to the neurodevelopmental hypothesis. *Journal of the Royal Society of Medicine*, **85**, 227–231.

Owens, D.G.C., Johnstone, E.C., Bydder, G.M. *et al.* (1980) Unsuspected organic disease in chronic schizophrenia demonstrated by computed tomography. *Journal of Neurology, Neurosurgery and Psychiatry*, **43**, 1065–1069.

Philpot, M. & Lewis, S.W. (1990) Psychopathology of basal ganglia calcification. *Behavioural Neurology*, **2**, 227–234.

Propping, P. (1983) Genetic disorders presenting as schizophrenia. Karl Bonhoffers early view of the psychoses in the light of medical genetics. *Human Genetics*, **65**, 1–10.

Ramani, S.V. (1981) Psychosis associated with frontal lobe lesions in Schilder's cerebral sclerosis: a case report with CT scan evidence. *Journal of Clinical Psychiatry*, **42**, 250–252.

Reischies, F.M., Baum, K., Brau, H. *et al.* (1988) Cerebral magnetic resonance imaging findings in multiple sclerosis. Relation to disturbance of affect, drive and cognition. *Archives of Neurology*, **45**, 1114–1116.

Remington, G. & Jeffries, J.J. (1984) The role of cerebral arteriovenous malformations in psychiatric disturbances: case report. *Journal of Clinical Psychiatry*, **45**, 226–229.

Reveley, A.M. & Reveley, M.A. (1983) Aqueduct stenosis and schizophrenia. *Journal of Neurology, Neurosurgery and Psychiatry*, **46**, 18–22.

Roberts, C.W., Dane, D.J., Bauton, C. & Crow, T.J. (1990) A 'mock-up' of schizophrenia: temporal lobe epilepsy and schizophrenia-like psychosis. *Biological Psychiatry*, **1990**, 127–143.

Romano, J. & Linares, R.L. (1987) Marfan syndrome and schizophrenia: a case report. *Archives of General Psychiatry*, **44**, 190–192.

Ron, M.A. & Logsdail, S.J. (1989) Psychiatric morbidity in multiple sclerosis: a clinical and MRI study. *Psychological Medicine*, **19**, 887–895.

Rubin, R.L. (1978) Adolescent infectious mononucleosis with psychosis. *Journal of Clinical Psychiatry*, **39**, 773–775.

Salib, E.A. (1988) SSPE presenting as a schizophrenia-like state with bizarre dysmorphophic features. *British Journal of Psychiatry*, **152**, 709–710.

Sharp, C.W., Muir, W.J., Blackwood, D.H. *et al.* (1993) Schizophrenia: a neuropsychiatric phenotype of the Usher syndrome type 3 allele. *Schizophrenia Research*, **9**, 125.

Shields, G.W., Pataki, C. & DeLisi, E. (1990) A family with Alport syndrome and psychosis. *Schizophrenia Research*, **3**,

235–239.

Sirota, P., Frydman, M. & Sirota, L. (1990) Schizophrenia and Marfan syndrome. *British Journal of Psychiatry*, **157**, 433–436.

Slater, E. & Beard, A.W. (1963) The schizophrenia-like psychoses of epilepsy. *British Journal of Psychiatry*, **109**, 95–112.

Sørensen, K. & Nielsen, J. (1977) Twenty psychotic males with Klinefelter's syndrome. *Acta Psychiatrica Scandinavica*, **56**, 249–255.

Spitzer, R.H., First, M.B., Williams, J.B.W., Kendler, K., Pincus, H.A. & Tucker, G. (1992) Now is the time to retire the term 'organic mental disorders'. *American Journal of Psychiatry*, **149**, 240–244.

Stevens, J.R. (1988) Schizophrenia and multiple sclerosis. *Schizophrenia Bulletin*, **14**, 231–241.

Stevens, J.R. (1992) Abnormal reinnervation as a basis for schizophrenia: a hypothesis. *Archives of General Psychiatry*, **49**, 235–243.

Stoler, M., Meshulam, B., Zoldan, J. & Zirota, P. (1987) Schizophreniform episode following measles infection. *British Journal of Psychiatry*, **150**, 861–863.

Swayze, V.W., Andreasan, N.C., Ehrhardt, J. *et al.* (1990) Developmental abnormalities of the corpus callosum in schizophrenia. *Archives of Neurology*, **47**, 805–808.

Swift, R.G., Sadler, D.B. & Swift, M. (1990) Psychiatric findings in Wolfram syndrome homozygotes. *Lancet*, **336**, 667–669.

Tavares, A.R., Pinto, D.C., Lemow, A. & Nascimento, E. (1993) Lesion localization in schizophrenia-like disorder associated with neurocysticerosis. *Schizophrenia Research*, **9**, 111.

Taylor, D. (1975) Factors influencing the occurrence of schizophrenia-like psychoses in temporal lobe epilepsy. *Psychological Medicine*, **1**, 247–253.

Torrey, E.F. (1986) Functional psychosis and viral encephalitis. *Integrated Psychiatry*, **4**, 224–236.

Trimble, M.R. (1988) *Biological Psychiatry*. Wiley, Chichester.

Trimble, M.R. (1990) First-rank symptoms of Schneider. A new perspective? *British Journal of Psychiatry*, **156**, 195–200.

Vaillant, G. (1965) Schizophrenia in a woman with temporal lobe arterio-venous malformations. *British Journal of Psychiatry*, **111**, 307–308.

Van Sweden, B. & Van Peteghem, P. (1986) Psychopathology in paraneoplastic encephalopathy: an electroclinical observation. *Journal of Clinical Psychiatry*, **47**, 267–268.

Velek, M., White, L.E. Jr, Williams, J.P., Stafford, R.L. & Marco, L.A. (1988) Psychosis in a case of corpus callosum agenesis. *Alabama Medicine*, **58**, 27–29.

Weinberger, D.R. (1987) Implications of normal brain development for pathogenesis of schizophrenia. *Archives of General Psychiatry*, **44**, 660–669.

White, P.D. & Lewis, S.W. (1987) Delusional depression following infectious mononucleosis. *British Medical Journal*, **295**, 297–298.

WHO (1978) *The ICD-9 Classification of Mental and Behavioural Disorders*. World Health Organization, Geneva.

WHO (1992) *The ICD-10 Classification of Mental and Behav-*

ioural Disorders. World Health Organization, Geneva.

Wilcox, J.A. & Nasrallah, H.A. (1986) Sydenham's chorea and psychosis. *Neuropsychobiology*, **15**, 13–14.

Zubencko, G.S., Moossy, J., Martinez, A.J. *et al.* (1991) Neuropathologic and neurochemical correlates of psychosis in primary dementia. *Archives of Neurology*, **48**, 619–624.

Zucker, D.K., Livingston, R.L., Nakra, R. & Clayton, P.J. (1981) B12 deficiency and psychiatric disorders: case report and literature review. *Biological Psychiatry*, **16**, 197–205.

Chapter 18
The Clinical Psychopharmacology of Antipsychotic Drugs in Schizophrenia

J. L. WADDINGTON

Historical origins of contemporary formulations

The discovery of neuroleptic drugs and their introduction for the treatment of psychotic illness (see Deniker, 1983) has been of such profound significance that we have entered recently the fifth decade of an incremental search for the fundamental basis of their antipsychotic activity (Waddington, 1993a), while their evident imperfections have resulted in a similarly prolonged quest for improved agents (Johnstone, 1993). More than 35 years after its identification as the progenitor neuroleptic, the phenothiazine chlorpromazine has remained among the most widely prescribed of such drugs, at least in the USA (Wysowski & Baum, 1989), yet several fundamental clinical issues regarding the nature of their antipsychotic action have remained controversial; diagnostic specificity (Johnstone *et al.*, 1988), time

course of therapeutic effect (Keck *et al.*, 1989) and optimal dosage (McEvoy *et al.*, 1991) have all required renewed investigation, consequent to imprecise specification over several previous decades, despite such extensive usage. Recent studies have thrown light not only on further aspects of the mechanism(s) of action of neuroleptics but also on a number of these enduring clinical controversies, and the present article seeks to document the advances that have derived therefrom.

Over the early years following the initial identification of chlorpromazine, application of the classical laboratory neuropharmacological techniques available in that era generated hypotheses of neuroleptic drug action centred around their presumed modulation of the reticular activating system. Though such hypotheses are no longer to the forefront of current theorizing, they are not without contemporary interest. However, the proposal that neuroleptic drugs might act via blockade of dopamine (DA) receptors in the brain (Carlsson & Lindqvist, 1963) has had greater impact because of perceived aetiological implications. Furthermore, the concept of 'atypical' antipsychotics (i.e. those having a low propensity to induce extrapyramidal side effects with or without greater efficacy to alleviate the symptoms of schizophrenia relative to their more typical counterparts) has prompted a search for the pharmacological basis(es) of such properties. A critical issue that remains to be resolved is the extent to which the putative basis(es) of such atypicality can be accommodated within, or else prove supplementary to (or even contradictory of), the DA receptor blockade hypothesis (Meltzer, 1992).

The classical D_2 receptor blockade hypothesis

It is well established that typical neuroleptic drugs have in common an ability to block brain DA receptors; this effect in the mesostriatal system has been held to account for their induction of extrapyramidal side effects, and blockade in the mesocorticolimbic system to account for their antipsychotic efficacy (Niemegeers & Janssen, 1978; see Chapter 21, this volume). One particularly important study in this regard was the demonstration that the antipsychotic activity of flupenthixol resided in its α [i.e. *cis*(Z) and DA receptor-blocking] rather than its β [i.e. *trans*(E) and non-DA receptor-blocking] geometric isomer (Johnstone *et al.*, 1978).

The relationship of this property to therapeutic efficacy in schizophrenia received powerful support from data indicating that the *in vitro* affinities of a broad range of neuroleptic drugs for DA antagonist-binding sites in the brain were highly correlated with their clinical potencies to control psychotic symptoms. Subsequently, it was recognized that DA receptors existed as at least two major subtypes, D_1 and D_2, defined by whether they do or do not stimulate adenylyl cyclase as a second messenger (Kebabian & Calne, 1979). Subsequent re-evaluation of the above relationship in terms of this D_1/D_2 schema indi-

cated a very high correlation between the affinity of neuroleptics for the D_2 receptor and clinical antipsychotic potency that was not evident in relation to their D_1 receptor affinities; this relationship held using both rat striatal *and* human postmortem putamen tissue (Seeman, 1980; Richelson & Nelson, 1984), and no differences were apparent between the affinities of such drugs for D_2 receptors in putamen (presumably related to parkinsonian side effects) vs. nucleus accumbens (presumably related to antipsychotic efficacy) of human postmortem brain (Reynolds *et al.*, 1982; Seeman & Ulpian, 1983; Richelson & Nelson, 1984). Similarly, selective or preferential D_2 antagonists such as the substituted benzamide sulpiride or the butyrophenone haloperidol, respectively, reproduced the essential clinical activity of less selective neuroleptics which antagonize both D_1 and D_2 receptors, such as the phenothiazines (e.g. fluphenazine) and the thioxanthenes (e.g. flupenthixol) (Seeman, 1980; Ehmann *et al.*, 1987); on this basis, D_2 receptor blockade was ascribed a prepotent or even exclusive role in mediating the antipsychotic activity of neuroleptics.

It should be emphasized here that the apparent strength of this hypothesis need not in itself indicate that hyperfunction of dopaminergic neurotransmission is fundamental to the pathophysiology of schizophrenia (Carlsson, 1988; Reynolds, 1989; Waddington, 1993b; see also Chapters 19 & 20), and alternative perspectives thereon have been presented (Davis *et al.*, 1991; Jaskiw & Weinberger, 1992; Waddington, 1993b). Equally, that strength should not blind us to the sometimes prominent action of many neuroleptics to variously block receptors for noradrenaline (α_1 and α_2), histamine (H_1), acetylcholine (muscarinic ACh) and 5-hydroxytryptamine (5-HT_{1A} and 5-HT_2) in human postmortem brain, though their affinities for these receptors fail to show the same correlation with clinical antipsychotic potency that is evident in relation to their D_2 receptor affinities (Richelson & Nelson, 1984; Wander *et al.*, 1987). Furthermore, it should not be overlooked that many neuroleptics can disrupt a variety of more basic, neuronal cellular functions, though often only at concentrations above those necessary to block

D_2 receptors (Waddington, 1989a; Nimgaonkar & Whatley, 1990).

Impact of PET on the D_2 blockade hypothesis

Positron emission tomography (PET) is an *in vivo* functional imaging technique that allows visualization of DA (and numerous other) receptor-binding sites in the living human brain and quantification of the extent of occupancy thereof in relation to dosage of neuroleptic administered; its application to schizophrenia has had a profound impact on how we 'view' the mechanism(s) of action of neuroleptic drugs (Waddington, 1989b).

Extent of D_2 vs. D_1 receptor occupancy during neuroleptic treatment

In the largest series of schizophrenic patients investigated in a systematic manner to date, it is apparent that near-maximal occupancy (70−89%) of available basal ganglia D_2 receptors is achieved in patients responding to treatment with relatively modest daily doses of various typical and newer neuroleptics from essentially all major chemical classes, e.g. chlorpromazine 200 mg daily; thioridazine 300−400 mg daily; trifluoperazine 10 mg daily; haloperidol 4−12 mg daily; haloperidol decanoate 50−70 mg monthly; flupenthixol 6 mg daily; flupenthixol decanoate 40 mg weekly; pimozide 8 mg daily; sulpiride 800 mg daily; and remoxipride 400 mg daily. At these doses, there is considerably less occupancy (0−44%) of D_1 receptors, with sulpiride demonstrating essentially complete D_2 selectivity, haloperidol a substantial preference for D_2 receptors, and thioridazine, flupenthixol and zuclopenthixol a lesser degree of preference for D_2 receptors (Farde *et al.*, 1992). These occupancies of D_2 vs. D_1 receptors in living patients by PET are in general accordance with results from receptor-binding studies *in vitro* subject to some greater preference for D_2 over D_1 receptors *in vivo* than might otherwise have been expected for putative 'non-selective' agents such as the phenothiazines and thioxanthenes. Investigation of the relationship between dose of typical neuroleptic administered and extent of D_2 receptor occupancy in a heterogeneous patient population indicated 150 mg of chlorpromazine equivalents daily to occupy approximately 50% of available receptors (Cambon *et al.*, 1987; Baron *et al.*, 1989); estimations of the dose of typical neuroleptic for essentially maximal (>75%) occupancy of D_2 receptors are approximately 400−500 mg of chlorpromazine equivalents daily using both PET (Baron *et al.*, 1989) and the related but less precise technique of single photon emission computerized tomography (SPECT) (Brucke *et al.*, 1992).

The above findings suggest that high doses of typical neuroleptics do not exert any greater putative primary mechanistic activity (i.e. D_2 receptor occupancy/blockade) than do considerably more modest doses; any additional therapeutic benefit of high-dose therapy with typical neuroleptics, which itself remains controversial, would seem to involve the recruitment only of actions at non-dopaminergic receptors, for which several such drugs show appreciable affinity, and/or reflect non-specific effects on brain function. Though pharmacokinetic-plasma level parameters will be considered in greater detail below, it should be noted here that occupancy of D_2 receptors by haloperidol appears to approach a maximum of 80−90% at plasma concentrations as low as 5−10 ng/ml, with concentrations as high as 90 ng/ml producing little or no further increase in occupancy (Wolkin *et al.*, 1989b); this might be in some accordance with recent clinical evidence that neither 30 nor 80 mg haloperidol daily showed any additional therapeutic benefit over 10 mg daily in the treatment of patients experiencing an acute episode or relapse of schizophrenia (Rifkin *et al.*, 1991), and that doses of haloperidol two- to 10-fold higher than its neuroleptic threshold did not lead to any greater alleviation of acute psychosis (McEvoy *et al.*, 1991).

Relationship to extrapyramidal side effects and therapeutic response

In the only series of schizophrenic patients investigated to date both for D_2 receptor occupancy by PET *and* for extrapyramidal side effects, those who experienced parkinsonism and/or akathisia while deriving benefit from treatment with modest doses of typical neuroleptics showed higher D_2 occupancies (76–89% vs. 70–81%) than did those who remained free of such side effects (Farde *et al.*, 1992). Thus, at least at such modest doses, it may be possible to titrate on an individual patient basis for a slightly lower dose that might induce fewer or less prominent extrapyramidal side effects without loss of antipsychotic effect (see also McEvoy *et al.*, 1991).

Regarding treatment failure, PET and SPECT studies have indicated that patients who do not respond even to substantial doses of haloperidol or other typical neuroleptics still demonstrate high (>85%) occupancy of D_2 receptors, to an extent indistinguishable from that evident in their responding counterparts (Wolkin *et al.*, 1989a; Coppens *et al.*, 1991; Pilowsky *et al.*, 1992). Thus, such lack of therapeutic response does not appear in the main to reflect any failure to attain adequate brain concentrations of neuroleptic or presumed primary mechanistic activity (i.e. D_2 receptor occupancy/blockade) and may rather reflect certain particular neuronal abnormalities in non-responding patients, the consequences of which cannot be ameliorated by D_2 receptor blockade. Such findings would not support the use of very high or megadoses of typical neuroleptics in the majority of those patients whose psychosis does not respond to more modest doses thereof.

Time course of D_2 occupancy in relation to therapeutic and adverse effects

It is widely held that the full antipsychotic effect of typical neuroleptic drugs may not be seen until 2–3 weeks following initiation of such treatment, though evidence for this proposition from controlled clinical trials is not substantial (Keck *et al.*, 1989). PET now indicates (Nordstrom *et al.*, 1992) that essentially maximal (73–91%) occupancy of D_2 receptors is obtained within a few hours of acute ingestion of modest doses (4–7.5 mg) of haloperidol, at least by volunteers. Such rapid

establishment thereof would be consistent with arguments that primary D_2 receptor blockade by typical neuroleptics is not in itself 'antipsychotic' but, rather, might initiate a critical series of slow, adaptive changes in presynaptic dopaminergic (and, subsequently, perhaps in other postsynaptic) neurones that show greater temporal contiguity with, and may ultimately underlie, alleviation of psychotic symptoms (see Pickar, 1988).

In normal volunteers, acute oral administration of 4–7.5 mg haloperidol induced akathisia over 3.5–24 h thereafter in several subjects at periods which coincided with maximal occupancy of basal ganglia D_2 receptors (Nordstrom *et al.*, 1992). Similarly, intravenous injection of 0.2–0.5 mg of the selective D_2 antagonist raclopride (as the ^{11}C-PET ligand) both to volunteers and to neuroleptic-naive schizophrenic patients induced akathisia over 10–25 min thereafter in the majority of subjects, at periods which again coincided with maximal ^{11}C-raclopride binding to D_2 receptors in the basal ganglia (Farde, 1992). These data have constituted the first demonstrations of a direct relationship between the time course of D_2 receptor occupancy by neuroleptics and induced pharmacological effects.

The search for visualization of extrastriatal DA receptors

Much of the above has concerned occupancy by neuroleptics of D_2 receptors in the basal ganglia, when the known dopaminergic innervations of extrastriatal areas may be of equal (or greater) relevance. This stems from limitations inherent to the PET technique which preclude spatial resolution of, for example, the nucleus accumbens from the caudate nucleus/putamen, and have not yet allowed ready visualization of such receptors in more distant regions because of the low density of their dopaminergic innervation and associated postsynaptic receptors (Farde *et al.*, 1988a). Evidence from *in vitro* receptor-binding studies in human postmortem brain indicates that D_2 receptors in the nucleus accumbens, while of somewhat lower density, show pharmacological characteristics indistinguishable from those in the basal ganglia in terms of affinity for neuroleptics (Reynolds *et al.*, 1982; Seeman & Ulpian, 1983; Richelson & Nelson, 1984), though it would be important and reassuring to have such characteristics of extrastriatal D_2 receptors confirmed *in vivo*.

Very recently, Kessler *et al.* (1992) have reported the visualization by SPECT of D_2 receptors in the thalamus, pituitary, hypothalamus and (medial) temporal lobe, as well as the basal ganglia, of a human volunteer using the selective D_2 antagonist ^{125}I-epidepride; the latter finding may be of particular importance, given the extent of current interest in putative developmental dysplasia and pathophysiology of medial temporal lobe structures in schizophrenia (Waddington, 1993b,c; see also Chapters 15 & 20, this volume).

Pharmacokinetics of neuroleptics in relation to PET indices of D_2 receptor occupancy

The pharmacokinetics of neuroleptic drugs are complex, due to a number of technical and procedural difficulties that have been reviewed previously in juxtaposition with classical pharmacokinetic principles, processes and parameters for such agents (Curry, 1986). Regarding the fundamental issue of whether there exist reliable relationships between neuroleptic dosage, plasma level and therapeutic/adverse effect, one authoritative review towards the end of the pre-PET era indicated that: (i) *moderate* doses are adequate for *most* patients; (ii) there exists little support for the general utility of unusually high doses; and (iii) antipsychotic efficacy might be related in a biphasic manner both to neuroleptic dosage and, possibly, to plasma concentration thereof (the 'therapeutic window' phenomenon) (Baldessarini *et al.*, 1988). Subsequent reviews (Van Putten *et al.*, 1991; Verghese *et al.*, 1991) have elaborated on these complexities, and have begun to note the potential significance of PET for clarification thereof by holding out the prospect of quantification of putative, primary mechanistic activity in relation to dose and plasma level.

Though there is evidence for a close curvilinear, hyperbolic relationship between total plasma haloperidol concentration and extent of D_2 receptor occupancy *in vivo* by PET (Wolkin *et al.*, 1989b), it has been argued that the free concentration of haloperidol may be the more relevant measure. The ultimate utility of this approach depends upon being able to demonstrate a relationship between extent of D_2 receptor occupancy and antipsychotic effect (Farde *et al.*, 1989). There is important preliminary evidence for a significant, positive relationship between the extent of reduction in the brief psychiatric rating scale scores during treatment with the new selective D_2 antagonist raclopride and the extent of D_2 receptor occupancy (Nordstrom *et al.*, 1993b). This complements the recent demonstration of a similar relationship between free neuroleptic concentration in patient plasma and the affinity for cloned D_2 receptors *in vitro* for all neuroleptics studied, except clozapine (Seeman, 1992). A long-standing controversy endures over whether there exists a 'therapeutic window' for neuroleptics in general, and for haloperidol in particular. While the two most recent, fixed dose/concentration studies are not entirely consistent as to whether the clinical improvement evident at lower plasma levels of haloperidol diminishes at higher levels, they are in some agreement that optimal therapeutic response is seen at modest levels thereof (5−12 ng/ml, Van Putten *et al.*, 1992; 2−13 ng/ml, Volavka *et al.*, 1992). These findings are in striking accordance with PET data indicating that essentially maximal occupancy of D_2 receptors is attained over plasma haloperidol levels of 5−15 ng/ml (Wolkin *et al.*, 1989b).

In terms of initiating neuroleptic treatment, the administration to normal volunteers of 2 and 4 mg haloperidol in PET studies produced D_2 receptor occupancies some 3−6 h later of 52 and 75%, respectively, at plasma levels below the limit of detection for the high-performance liquid chromatographic assay technique adopted (2 ng/ml); however, 7.5 mg haloperidol produced D_2 receptor occupancies of 83−92% at plasma levels of 5−6 ng/ml, and these measures appeared to endure for up to 30 h after acute oral administration (Nordstrom *et al.*, 1992). Regarding cessation of established neuroleptic treatment, when schizophrenic patients who had been receiving 15–20 mg haloperidol daily were followed after medication had been stopped, the decline in plasma level preceded by several days the decline in D_2 receptor occupancy measured by PET. By 1 week, both indices fell to control values (Smith *et al.*, 1988; see also Baron *et al.*, 1989). In a similar PET study, discontinuation of established treatment with 1200 mg sulpiride or 12 mg haloperidol daily was associated with a progressive decline in plasma levels over the subsequent 30–54 h, but occupancy of D_2 receptors endured at 65–85% (Farde *et al.*, 1988b). Such data would suggest some dissociation between plasma level and the extent of persistence of neuroleptic drugs in the brain, at least for sulpiride and haloperidol. There are limited clinical data that D_2 receptor occupancy may decline faster with chlorpromazine than haloperidol, as measured at 24 h following neuroleptic withdrawal (Smith *et al.*, 1988). This is supported by more robust data that butyrophenones may persist in the brain longer than phenothiazines (Cohen *et al.*, 1992).

The pharmacokinetics of the depot neuroleptics are recognized to be yet more complex than those of their orally administered counterparts, and following putative discontinuation they may persist for periods considerably beyond those recognized previously (Marder *et al.*, 1989; Simpson *et al.*, 1990). In the most relevant PET study, D_2 receptor occupancy remained high (53–80%) at up to 34 days following the last injection in patients on haloperidol decanoate 50–250 mg or fluphenazine decanoate 200 mg monthly for over 8 months (Baron *et al.*, 1989). In one patient evaluated at 4 months following the last of at least six monthly injections of 150 mg haloperidol decanoate, D_2 receptor occupancy at 17% was not evidently different from control values.

It is clear that PET is providing new insights into the pharmacokinetics of neuroleptic drugs by virtue of its ability to quantitate directly the extent of D_2 receptor occupancy in brain *vis-à-vis* dose administered and plasma level attained. In the face of evidence that brain-to-blood distribution may vary considerably between neuroleptic drugs, and may be particularly large for high- as opposed to low-potency agents (Tsuneizumi *et al.*, 1992), it is important to have available a technique with the potential to further disentangle these potentially serious pharmacokinetic confounds.

New strata of DA receptor subtypes and neuroleptic drug action

Over the past few years, hypotheses of neuroleptic drug action have had to accommodate new evidence from the application of molecular biological and gene cloning techniques that the number of DA receptor subtypes appears much larger than originally envisaged; the current situation encompasses at least six DA receptor sequences and, on the basis of their known pharmacological characteristics, these might best be subsumed under the umbrella of two *families* of 'D$_1$-like' (D_{1A}, D_{1B}/D_5) and 'D$_2$-like' ($D_{2long/short}$, D_3, D_4) receptors. Within the 'D$_1$-like' family, the classical D_1 receptor, with its general mesostriatal–mesocorticolimbic localization, has been designated D_{1A}, while its counterpart has been designated D_{1B} or D_5 and demonstrates a characteristic low-density and primarily corticolimbic localization. Of greater interest here are members of the 'D$_2$-like' family: the classical D_2 receptor, with its general mesostriatal–mesocorticolimbic localization, has been shown to exist in both 'long' and 'short' isoforms that appear to be generated via alternative splicing, with any functional distinction(s) between them being as yet obscure; the D_3 receptor shows a characteristic low-density localization primarily within corticolimbic regions, as does its D_4 counterpart (see Seeman, 1992; Sibley & Monsma, 1992).

There appears to be a good correlation between the affinities of typical neuroleptics and atypical antipsychotics for the cloned rat/human D_2 receptor and their free concentrations in patient plasma, subject to the exception of clozapine (see below) (Seeman, 1992). It has been reported recently that among an extensive range of chemically diverse typical neuroleptics and atypical antipsychotics, none were able to distinguish between either the cloned 'long' and 'short' splice variants of the human D_2 receptor or D_2 receptors in the rat striatum, nucleus accumbens and olfactory tubercle (Leysen *et al.*, 1993).

The properties of the cloned rat/human D_3 receptor have generated much interest as a potential novel target for antipsychotics, in terms of its high affinity for both typical neuroleptic and atypical antipsychotic drugs, and of its predominant 'peristriatal' limbic localization (Sokoloff *et al.*, 1990, 1992; Murray *et al.*, 1992). Though no known neuroleptics or atypical antipsychotics show any selectivity for D_3 over D_2 receptors, the extent of their preference for D_2 over D_3 receptors can vary within a modest 10-fold range, which may contribute to putative differences between individual agents; however, the correlation between the free concentrations of such drugs in patient plasma and K_i values (affinities) for the cloned D_3 receptor does not appear to be so strong as that for the cloned D_2 receptor (Seeman, 1992). Nevertheless, were selective D_3 antagonists to be identified, it would be important to investigate them for antipsychotic efficacy vs. side-effects liability, though it has been suggested that D_3 receptors may be normally occluded by endogenous DA to such an extent that they might not be occupied readily by such antagonists (Schotte *et al.*, 1992).

Similarly, the cloned D_4 receptor has also been offered as a potential novel target for antipsychotics on the basis of its high affinity for both typical neuroleptics and atypical antipsychotics, and a predominant corticolimbic localization. Most such drugs demonstrate some preferential affinity for D_2 over D_4 receptors within a modest 1- to 100-fold range, though clozapine is an exception in exhibiting approximately 10-fold selectivity for D_4 over D_2 receptors (Van Tol *et al.*, 1991). The correlation between the free concentration of such drugs in patient plasma and their affinities for the cloned D_4 receptor may not be so strong as that for the cloned D_2 receptor (Seeman, 1992). These findings will be discussed further below in the context of atypical antipsychotic drug action, together with any possible involvement of the family of 'D_1-like' receptors therein.

Clozapine and the enigma of atypical antipsychotic drug action

Over the past several years, there has been a resurgence of interest in atypical antipsychotic drug action following the *re*discovery in new, controlled trials that clozapine is an effective antipsychotic capable of reducing psychotic symptoms in a significant minority of those patients with schizophrenia who fail to respond to typical neuroleptics, while inducing markedly fewer (as distinct from no) extrapyramidal side effects (Claghorn *et al.*, 1987; Kane *et al.*, 1988; Pickar *et al.*, 1992). The increased risk for potentially fatal agranulocytosis inherent to clozapine and the necessity for a mandatory blood-count-monitoring programme, together with its liability to induce seizures, sedation, hypotension and hypersalivation (Baldessarini & Frankenburg, 1991) means that this important agent will not attain widespread use as a 'front-line' antipsychotic but, rather, remain a critical 'reserve' drug for patients who are unresponsive to or intolerant of conventional neuroleptics; nevertheless, it must contain important clues to the mechanism(s) of atypical antipsychotic drug action (Deutch *et al.*, 1991; Meltzer, 1991; Reynolds, 1992). However, clozapine is a highly non-selective compound which demonstrates an extensive range of actions at multiple levels of neuronal function associated with numerous neurotransmitter systems (Baldessarini & Frankenburg, 1991), and this seriously confounds the search for the basis of its greater therapeutic efficacy and reduced extrapyramidal side-effects liability.

Variants of the DA receptor blockade hypothesis

In preclinical studies, clozapine demonstrates at best modest pharmacological activity *in vivo* as a DA receptor antagonist (Niemegeers & Janssen, 1978; Baldessarini & Frankenburg, 1991; see also Chapter 21, this volume), and exhibits similarly modest affinity for both classical D_1 and D_2 receptors *in vitro* (Seeman, 1980, 1992). This modest affinity for D_2 receptors appears to show no evidence of regional (i.e. mesocorticolimbic) selectivity *in vitro* (Leysen *et al.*, 1993), while *ex vivo* studies suggest only limited preferential occupancy of limbic vs. striatal D_2 receptors (Meltzer & Stockmeier, 1992). There may, however, be more preferential effects on low-density cortical D_2 receptors in the course of chronic treatment (Janowsky *et al.*, 1992). Similarly, clozapine shows indistinguishably modest affinity for D_2 receptors in both the putamen and nucleus accumbens of human postmortem brain (Seeman & Ulpian, 1983; Richelson & Nelson, 1984).

Using PET or SPECT, clozapine occupies 0–63% of basal ganglia D_2 receptors in patients receiving from low to conventional doses (50–600 mg daily) relative to occupancies of 70% or more in those receiving from modest to conventional doses of typical neuroleptics (Brucke *et al.*, 1992; Farde *et al.*, 1992). This apparent difference held when patients responding to clozapine 150–600 mg daily were compared with patients showing a poor therapeutic response to typical neuroleptics (Pilowsky *et al.*, 1992); although one PET study has noted that clozapine 500 mg daily does not exhibit any occupancy of basal ganglia D_2 receptors, the failure to demonstrate more than 40% occupancy thereof by haloperidol 10 mg daily questions the representativeness of such findings (Karbe *et al.*, 1991). Using ^{11}C-clozapine as a PET ligand, basal ganglia binding was only partially displaced by haloperidol 2 mg daily or 1 mg i.v., suggesting that clozapine might bind to a site or sites additional to the D_2 receptor (Lundberg *et al.*, 1989).

In the only comparative PET study to date, clozapine 300–600 mg daily occupied 38–63% of D_2 *and* 35–52% of D_1 receptors in the basal ganglia (Farde *et al.*, 1992). This modest but very similar occupancy of both D_2 *and* D_1 receptors *in vivo* appears unique to clozapine (see above); it should be noted that the putative atypical antipsychotics sulpiride and remoxipride, which can also induce fewer extrapyramidal side effects than typical neuroleptics but have yet to be shown in controlled trials to share clozapine's efficacy in some otherwise neuroleptic-refractory patients,

are selective D_2 antagonists that occupy 71–78% of basal ganglia D_2 receptors (Farde *et al.*, 1992). In this regard, there is recent preclinical evidence that, despite its at best modest affinity for both classical DA receptor subtypes, clozapine appears to readily and preferentially attenuate D_1-mediated function (Murray & Waddington, 1990; Ellenbroek *et al.*, 1991; Waddington & Daly, 1992). The antipsychotic potential vs. side-effects liability of D_1 antagonism has been generally overlooked (see Waddington, 1988, 1992, 1993d) and will be considered further below.

Subsequent identification within the 'D_2-like' family of a D_4 receptor having a primarily corticolimbic localization and for which clozapine demonstrates some 10-fold higher affinity relative to the D_2 receptor, has generated some interest as a putative substrate of its atypical antipsychotic profile (Van Tol *et al.*, 1991); indeed, the discordance between the free concentration of clozapine in patient plasma and its K_i value for the cloned D_2 receptor may be reconciled when its K_i for the cloned D_4 receptor is substituted (Seeman, 1992). The D_4 receptor has recently been shown to exist as at least three, and perhaps seven, polymorphic variants in the human population, and it has been suggested that these might underlie individual differences in susceptibility to neuropsychiatric disease(s) and in responsiveness to antipsychotic medication (Van Tol *et al.*, 1992). However, a preliminary study of D_4 polymorphic allele frequencies between responders and nonresponders to clozapine has failed to reveal any significant differences (Shaikh *et al.*, 1993). As yet, there has been no evidence that clozapine, which shows more modest affinity for D_1 receptors, can distinguish between new members (D_{1A}, D_{1B}/D_5) of the 'D_1-like' family (Sunahara *et al.*, 1991), though it may preferentially attenuate dopaminergic function mediated via an as yet unidentified subtype of D_1 receptor (Daly & Waddington, 1994).

It should not be overlooked that clozapine might reduce dopaminergic function at levels other than or additional to the postsynaptic DA receptor, and there is a substantial and still evolving literature on its possible presynaptic effects. Some preclinical electrophysiological evidence has indicated that clozapine may induce 'depolarization block' of mesocorticolimbic, but not of mesostriatal, DA neurones over chronic treatment, but this leaves open the important question of any concomitant effects on DA release in presynaptic terminal areas. The literature here, in terms of *in vivo* dopaminergic cell body electrophysiology vs. various indices of presynaptic DA release (*ex vivo* neurochemistry, *in vivo* voltammetry, *in vivo* microdialysis) is large, often contradictory and extends to diverse (sometimes regionally specific) effects of clozapine on multiple neurochemical processes that include early gene expression (Baldessarini & Frankenburg, 1991; Deutch *et al.*, 1991, 1992; Meltzer, 1991; Chai & Meltzer, 1992). One recent study of sensory field potentials suggests that the non-dopaminergic actions of clozapine may be more important than anatomical selectivity (Lidsky & Banerjee, 1992).

The involvement of non-dopaminergic mechanisms

One influential hypothesis (Meltzer *et al.*, 1989) proposes that the higher affinity of clozapine for widely distributed 5-hydroxytryptamine (5-HT$_2$) than for D$_2$ receptors, which is also evident (by approximately 100-fold) in human postmortem brain (Richelson & Nelson, 1984; Wander *et al.*, 1987), underlies its atypical properties. Indeed, this combination of effects has been offered as a general mechanism for atypical antipsychotic drug action in terms of amelioration of the acute extrapyramidal side effects and, possibly, for augmenting the sometimes limited level of therapeutic efficacy associated with D$_2$ antagonist neuroleptics (Deutch *et al.*, 1991; Meltzer, 1991). As typical neuroleptics such as chlorpromazine can also show higher affinity for 5-HT$_2$ than for D$_2$ receptors (by approximately 10-fold) in human postmortem brain (Richelson & Nelson, 1984; Wander *et al.*, 1987), the hypothesis can accommodate such data only if the critical factor is the extent to which the former exceeds the latter, or if other actions are additionally involved.

PET studies with ^{11}C-clozapine have indicated that it appears to bind to a population of receptors in the frontal cortex that does not show a D$_2$ (i.e. haloperidoldisplaceable) profile (Lundberg *et al.*, 1989), and this might be consistent with the high affinity of clozapine for frontal cortex 5-HT$_2$ receptors in human postmortem brain (Wander *et al.*, 1987); however, this putative site was not characterized further. Recent PET studies indicate that patients receiving relatively low doses of clozapine (125–175 mg daily) show 84–87% occupancy of cortical 5-HT$_2$ receptors in association with 20% occupancy of basal ganglia D$_2$ receptors (Nordstrom *et al.*, 1993a).

In accordance with some preclinical studies and initially encouraging clinical findings with 5-HT$_3$ antagonists (see Meltzer, 1992), others have proposed that the moderate affinity of clozapine for 5-HT$_3$ receptors may be relevant to its atypical antipsychotic profile, in a manner either adjunctive to or independent of modest affinity for D$_2$ receptors (Watling *et al.*, 1990). While subsequent clinical studies with 5-HT$_3$ antagonists in schizophrenia have not proved encouraging (Newcomer *et al.*, 1992; but see Richmond *et al.*, 1993), it cannot be excluded that an optimal combination of D$_2$ and 5-HT$_3$ blockade may be of some relevance thereto.

Speculation (Pickar *et al.*, 1992) that the significant α_2 antagonist affinity of clozapine in human postmortem brain (Richelson & Nelson, 1984) may contribute to its enigmatic clinical profile might be clarified by studies in which α_2 antagonists are given as an adjunct to or a substitute for treatment with typical neuroleptics (Litman *et al.*, 1993).

Evidence for interactions between dopaminergic and glutamatergic systems in the brain and for glutamatergic dysfunction in schizophrenia has resulted in proposals that drugs which enhance glutamatergic tone may show or contribute to antipsychotic activity (Wachtel & Turski, 1990; Meltzer, 1991; Reynolds, 1992). Curiously, clozapine has recently been shown to have the highest affinity for hippocampal 5-HT$_{1A}$ receptors in human postmortem brain relative to several more typical neuroleptics and, as 5-HT$_{1A}$ receptors are enriched on cortical glutamatergic neurones, might conceivably influence these neurones via such receptors (Mason & Reynolds, 1992); however, any relative prepotence of clozapine at the 5-HT_{1A} receptor may be less evident in human postmortem frontal cortex (Wander *et al.*, 1987). Any significance for clozapine's atypical antipsychotic profile of its apparent action in preclinical studies to down-regulate 5-HT_{1C} receptors during chronic treatment (Hietala *et al.*, 1992) is entirely unknown.

There has been some speculation that 'sigma receptors', for which haloperidol and remoxipride demonstrate some affinity in addition to their D_2 antagonist activities, might play a role in anti-psychotic activity; however, clozapine does not have appreciable affinity for the sigma site, and there is as yet no consistent body of evidence for any particular role either in atypical antipsychotic activity specifically or in neuroleptic drug action in general (Deutsch *et al.*, 1988; Meltzer, 1991; Reynolds, 1992).

New putative atypical antipsychotic drugs

On the basis of these and other hypotheses, a number of new, putative atypical antipsychotics are currently in development. They either combine somewhat more restricted permutations of prop-erties from among the extensive range of those shown by clozapine or adopt alternative/additional therapeutic approaches, and some of these agents are considered below in approximate order of extent to which clinical information is available.

Risperidone

This agent is an extremely potent 5-HT_2 antag-onist with prominent (though approximately 25-fold less) D_2 antagonist and some α_1, α_2 and H_1 antagonist activity (Janssen *et al.*, 1988; Leysen *et al.*, 1992). Its preclinical psychopharmacological profile is predictive of antipsychotic efficacy but reduced extrapyramidal side-effects liability (Megens *et al.*, 1992b), and this has been sustained

by controlled clinical trials in relation both to positive and (as yet less certainly) to negative symptoms (Claus *et al.*, 1992; Chouinard *et al.*, 1993). A recent PET study in normal volunteers (Nyberg *et al.*, 1993) has indicated risperidone to occupy 45–68% of cortical 5-HT_2 vs. 40–55% of basal ganglia D_2 receptors at a dose (1 mg) somewhat lower than that (6 mg) which appears most effective clinically. It will be important to clarify such occupancy indices at more thera-peutically relevant doses of risperidone, in comparison with a typical neuroleptic such as chlorpromazine, which also shows appreciable 5-HT_2 as well as D_2 antagonist activity. Ocaperi-done is a more recent stable-mate, having an affinity for 5-HT_2 receptors similar to that of risperidone but almost equally high D_2 affinity, together with some affinity for α_1, α_2 and H_1 receptors (Leysen *et al.*, 1992; Megens *et al.*, 1992a). It has been suggested that risperidone might be preferable for maintenance treatment of chronic schizophrenic illness characterized by milder positive symptoms and a prominence of negative features, while ocaperidone might be particularly useful for treating the prominent positive symptoms of acute schizophrenic illness and/or florid exacerbations in the course of chronic illness (Megens *et al.*, 1992b), but it will require very carefully designed and executed clinical trials to substantiate this notion.

Zotepine

In contrast, this agent is a high-affinity antagonist of 5-HT_2, D_2, D_1 and α_1 receptors (Meltzer *et al.*, 1989). Despite a less striking preclinical psychopharmacological profile, it appears in con-trolled trials to show antipsychotic activity in patients with prominent negative symptoms while inducing relatively few extrapyramidal side effects (Barnas *et al.*, 1992).

Sertindole

Similarly, this agent is also a high-affinity antag-onist of 5-HT_2, D_2 and α_1 receptors with a preclinical psychopharmacological profile that suggests antipsychotic activity but reduced liability to induce extrapyramidal side effects (Sanchez *et al.*, 1991). Initial controlled clinical studies (Martin *et al.*, 1994) have suggested antipsychotic efficacy with relatively few extrapyramidal side effects in most patients.

Amperozide

By further contrast, amperozide is a moderately high-affinity $5-HT_2$ antagonist with little affinity for D_2 or D_1 receptors (Christensson & Bjork, 1990), though it may influence presynaptic dopaminergic function (Ichikawa & Meltzer, 1992). Its preclinical psychopharmacological profile is also predictive of antipsychotic activity but low extrapyramidal side-effects liability (Christensson & Bjork, 1990). Preliminary, open clinical studies appear to suggest efficacy that may encompass negative symptoms, in the face of modest extrapyramidal side effects in some patients (Axelsson *et al.*, 1991).

Olanzapine

There has been an extensive search for analogues of clozapine with comparable pharmacological actions but without its raised propensity to induce agranulocytosis, and olanzapine has evolved from such a programme. It is both a $5-HT_2$ and a D_2 antagonist whose preclinical psychopharmacological profile (Moore *et al.*, 1992) suggests antipsychotic activity but low liability to induce extrapyramidal side effects. Initial feedback from clinical studies indicates therapeutic activity that may encompass negative symptoms, in the face of relatively few extrapyramidal side effects (Wood *et al.*, 1994).

ICI 204,636

Similarly, this agent is a clozapine analogue with $5-HT_2$, D_2 and α_1 antagonist actions whose preclinical psychopharmacological profile would again predict antipsychotic activity but low extra-pyramidal side-effects liability. Initial trials indicate antipsychotic efficacy with little propensity to induce extrapyramidal reactions (Hirsh *et al.*, 1994).

D_2 autoreceptor agonists/postsynaptic partial agonists

One theoretical alternative to postsynaptic D_2 antagonism has been the 'selective' stimulation of so-called (D_2-like) autoreceptors on neuronal cell bodies/dendrites or presynaptic terminals of DA neurones which mediate inhibition of dopaminergic function. It was believed that such autoreceptors might be stimulated preferentially by low doses of DA agonists, such as apomorphine, or by selective agents, such as 3-(3-hydroxy-phenyl)-N-(l-propyl)piperidine (3-PPP), to result in antipsychotic activity but few extrapyramidal side effects (see Waddington, 1993a). Some initial, acute clinical investigations were encouraging (Tamminga *et al.*, 1986), but many subsequent studies with newer agents, such as talipexole, roxindole and pramipexole, have failed to indicate any consistent efficacy against positive, as opposed to negative, symptoms in schizophrenia (see Benkert *et al.*, 1992; Kasper *et al.*, 1992). Though there is evidence that pre- and postsynaptic D_2 receptors are actually similar, if not identical, entities, drugs such as U-68553B and PD 128483 continue to emerge as therapeutic candidates based on the fundamental premise, and their preclinical profiles appear worthy of clinical investigation (see Waddington, 1993a).

The concept of partial agonists having low intrinsic activity at D_2 receptors suggests that such agents would act as D_2 antagonists when tonic dopaminergic activity is high, or as limited D_2 agonists in the face of low tonic dopaminergic activity, and thus might exert therapeutic effects on both the positive and negative symptoms of schizophrenia with little induction of extrapyramidal side effects (Coward *et al.*, 1989). Initial clinical studies with agents such as terguride, SDZ 208-911 and -912 have not proved wholly convincing, with only limited efficacy and some extrapyramidal side effects being evident (Olbrich & Schanz, 1991; Waddington, 1993a; but see Potkin *et al.*, 1993). While there is evidence that D_2 autoreceptor agonism and postsynaptic D_2 receptor partial agonism may be variants of the same basic pharmacological property (see Waddington, 1993a), there may be scope for further trials with such agents.

D_1 receptor antagonists

In view of the weight of evidence for the primacy of D_2 blockade in the therapeutic actions of typical neuroleptic drugs, it came as some considerable surprise that initial preclinical studies with the first selective D_1 antagonist, SCH 23390, indicated it to be active in essentially all functional models predictive of antipsychotic activity (see Waddington, 1988; Ellenbroek *et al.*, 1989). This profile appears to have its basis in D_1:D_2 interactions that regulate critically the totality of dopaminergic neurotransmission (see Waddington, 1993a,d; Waddington & Daly, 1993). Newer, selective D_1 antagonists with more appropriate pharmacokinetics show a similarly provocative preclinical profile *vis-à-vis* putative therapeutic efficacy in schizophrenia (see Waddington & Daly, 1992), though there endures inconsistent evidence as to the liability of such agents to induce at least acute extrapyramidal side effects, both in non-human primates (Chipkin *et al.*, 1988; Casey, 1992) and in humans (Gessa *et al.*, 1991; Farde, 1992).

Two new selective D_1 antagonists, SCH 39166 (Chipkin *et al.*, 1988) and NNC-687 (together with its close congener NNC-756) (Andersen *et al.*, 1992), have entered clinical trials in schizophrenia, though those with SCH39166 have recently been discontinued; such studies will answer directly many important questions regarding the exclusivity or otherwise of D_2 antagonism as a fundamental basis of at least typical neuroleptic activity (see Waddington, 1993a).

Caveat

As new concepts of atypical antipsychotic drug action are explored clinically, the preclinical studies from which they derive come under intense scrutiny. Cautionary observations have emerged from studies with savoxepine which, despite an encouraging atypical preclinical profile ascribed to apparent selectivity for limbic (hippocampal) D_2 receptors (Bischoff *et al.*, 1988), has been reported to induce typical extrapyramidal side effects in the majority of patients (Wetzel *et al.*, 1991). Recent PET studies in normal volunteers indicate savoxepine to occupy up to 75% of basal ganglia D_2 receptors, even at low daily doses (Leenders *et al.*, 1993), and the compound has now been withdrawn from clinical development at some cost to the originating pharmaceutical company.

Conclusion

The basis of atypical antipsychotic drug action remains elusive, and this stems in no small measure from the prototype member of this category, clozapine, having so extensive a range of pharmacological actions as to seriously confound identification of its essential property(ies). Thus, the breadth of this range of actions of clozapine can be considered either as a rich reservoir for theorizing on or, alternatively, extremely muddy waters in which to fish for the substrate of atypical antipsychotic activity. Indeed, it cannot be excluded that the atypicality of clozapine is in fact related to so broad a range of effects on multiple levels of neuronal function, such that reproducing one or more individual properties in a new molecule may fail to reproduce the complete clinical profile of the progenitor compound. However, a number of those new, putative atypical antipsychotics that possess the more restricted combinations of properties from among the totality shown by clozapine will, if evaluated rigorously in a manner similar to clozapine, throw important light on these issues. It remains a chastening paradox that the only antipsychotic demonstrated so far to have greater therapeutic efficacy in otherwise neuroleptic-refractory patients should be more liable to induce a potentially fatal adverse reaction. Both arms of this paradox synergize in promoting the continuing search for new antipsychotic drugs.

Acknowledgement

The author is supported by the Health Research Board of Ireland.

References

Andersen, P.H., Gronvald, F.C. Hohlweg, R. *et al.* (1992) NNC-112, NNC-687 and NNC-756, new selective and highly potent dopamine D_1 receptor antagonists. *European Journal of Pharmacology*, **219**, 45−52.

Axelsson, R., Nilsson, A., Christensson, E. & Bjork, A. (1991) Effects of amperozide in schizophrenia: an open study of a potent 5-HT_2 receptor antagonist. *Psychopharmacology*, **104**, 287−292.

Baldessarini, R.J. & Frankenburg, F.R. (1991) Clozapine: a novel antipsychotic agent. *New England Journal of Medicine*, **324**, 746−754.

Baldessarini, R.J., Cohen, B.M. & Teicher, M.H. (1988) Significance of neuroleptic dose and plasma level in the pharmacological treatment of psychoses. *Archives of General Psychiatry*, **45**, 79−91.

Barnas, C., Stuppack, C.H., Miller, C., Haring, C., Sperner-Unterweger, B. & Fleischhacker, W.W. (1992) Zotepine in the treatment of schizophrenic patients with prevailingly negative symptoms. A double-blind trial vs. haloperidol. *International Clinical Psychopharmacology*, **7**, 23−27.

Baron, J.C., Martinot, J.L., Cambon, H. *et al.* (1989) Striatal dopamine receptor occupancy during and following withdrawal from neuroleptic treatment: correlative evaluation by positron emission tomography and plasma prolactin levels. *Psychopharmacology*, **99**, 463−472.

Benkert, O., Gründer, G. & Wetzel, H. (1992) Dopamine autoreceptor agonists in the treatment of schizophrenia and major depression. *Pharmacopsychiatry*, **25**, 254−260.

Bischoff, S., Christen, P. & Vassout, A. (1988) Blockade of hippocampal dopamine (DA) receptors: a tool for antipsychotics with low extrapyramidal side effects. *Progress in Neuro-Psychopharmacology and Biological Psychiatry*, **12**, 455−467.

Brucke, T., Roth, J., Podreka, I., Strobl, R., Wenger, S. & Asenbaum, S. (1992) Striatal dopamine D_2-receptor blockade by typical and atypical neuroleptics. *Lancet*, **339**, 497.

Cambon, H., Baron, J.C., Boulenger, J.P., Loc'h, C., Zarifian, E. & Maziere, B. (1987) *In vivo* assay for neuroleptic receptor binding in the striatum: positron tomography in humans. *British Journal of Psychiatry*, **151**, 824−830.

Carlsson, A. (1988) The current status of the dopamine hypothesis of schizophrenia. *Neuropsychopharmacology*, **1**, 179−186.

Carlsson, A. & Lindqvist, A. (1963) Effect of chlorpromazine or haloperidol on formation of 3-methoxytyramine in mouse brain. *Acta Pharmacologica et Toxicologica*, **20**, 140−144.

Casey, D.E. (1992) Dopamine D_1 (SCH 23390) and D_2 (haloperidol) antagonists in drug-naive monkeys. *Psychopharmacology*, **107**, 18−22.

Chai, B. & Meltzer, H.Y. (1992) The effect of chronic clozapine on basal dopamine release and apomorphine-induced DA release in the striatum and nucleus accumbens as measured by *in vivo* brain microdialysis. *Neuroscience Letters*, **136**, 47−50.

Chipkin, R.E., Iorio, L.C., Coffin, V.L., McQuade, R.D., Berger, J.G. & Barnett, A. (1988) Pharmacological profile of SCH 39166: a dopamine D_1 selective benzonaphthazepine with potential antipsychotic activity. *Journal of Pharmacology and Experimental Therapeutics*, **247**, 1093−1102.

Chouinard, G., Jones, B., Remington, G. *et al.* (1993) A Canadian multicenter placebo-controlled study of fixed doses of risperidone and haloperidol in the treatment of chronic schizophrenia patients. *Journal of Clinical Psychopharmacology*, **13**, 25−40.

Christensson, E. & Bjork, A. (1990) Amperozide: a new pharmacological approach in the treatment of schizophrenia. *Pharmacology and Toxicology*, Suppl. **1**, 5−7.

Claghorn, J., Honigfeld, G., Abuzzahab, F.S. *et al.* (1987) The risks and benefits of clozapine versus chlorpromazine. *Journal of Clinical Psychopharmacology*, **7**, 377−384.

Claus, A., Bollen, J., De Cuyper, H. *et al.* (1992) Risperidone versus haloperidol in the treatment of chronic schizophrenic inpatients: a multicentre double-blind comparative study. *Acta Psychiatrica Scandinavica*, **85**, 295−305.

Cohen, B.M., Tsuneizumi, T., Baldessarini, R.J., Campbell, A. & Babb, S.M. (1992) Differences between antipsychotic drugs in persistence of brain levels and behavioural effects. *Psychopharmacology*, **108**, 338−344.

Coppens, H.J., Sloof, C.J., Paans, A.M.J., Wiegman, T., Vaalburg, W. & Korf, J. (1991) High central D_2-dopamine receptor occupancy as assessed with positron emission tomography in medicated but therapy-resistant schizophrenic patients. *Biological Psychiatry*, **29**, 629−634.

Coward, D., Dixon, K., Enz, A. *et al.* (1989) Partial brain dopamine D_2 receptor agonists in the treatment of schizophrenia. *Psychopharmacology Bulletin*, **25**, 393−397.

Curry, S.H. (1986) Applied clinical psychopharmacology of schizophrenia. In Bradley, P.B. & Hirsch, S.R. (eds) *The Psychopharmacology and Treatment of Schizophrenia*, pp. 103−131. Oxford University Press, Oxford.

Daly, S.A. & Waddington, J.L. (1994) The effects of clozapine on behavioural responses to the selective 'D₁-like' agonist, RU24213, *British Journal of Pharmacology*, **113**, 839−844.

Davis, K.L., Kahn, R.S., Ko, G. & Davidson, M. (1991) Dopamine in schizophrenia: a review and reconceptualization. *American Journal of Psychiatry*, **148**, 1474−1486.

Deniker, P. (1983) Discovery of the clinical use of neuroleptics. In Parnham, M.J. & Bruinvels, J. (eds) *Discoveries in Pharmacology*, Vol. 1, *Psycho- and Neuro-pharmacology*, pp. 163−180. Elsevier, Amsterdam.

Deutch, A.Y., Lee, M.C. & Iadarola, M.J. (1992) Regionally specific effects of atypical antipsychotic drugs on striatal fos expression: the nucleus accumbens shell as a locus of antipsychotic action. *Molecular and Cellular Neurosciences*, **3**, 332−341.

Deutch, A.Y., Moghaddam, B., Innis, R.B. *et al.* (1991) Mechanisms of action of atypical antipsychotic drugs: implications for novel therapeutic strategies for schizophrenia. *Schizophrenia Research*, **4**, 121−156.

Deutsch, S.I., Weizman, A., Goldman, M.E. & Morihisa, J.M. (1988) The sigma receptor: a novel site implicated in psychosis and antipsychotic drug efficacy. *Clinical Neuropharmacology*, **2**, 105–119.

Ehmann, T.S., Delva, N.J. & Beninger, R.J. (1987) Flupenthixol in chronic schizophrenic inpatients: a controlled comparison with haloperidol. *Journal of Clinical Psychopharmacology*, **3**, 173–175.

Ellenbroek, B.A., Artz, M.T. & Cools, A. (1991) The involvement of dopamine D_1 and D_2 receptors in the effects of the classical neuroleptic haloperidol and the atypical neuroleptic clozapine. *European Journal of Pharmacology*, **196**, 103–108.

Ellenbroek, B.A., Willemen, A.P.M. & Cools, A.R. (1989) Are antagonists of dopamine D_1 receptors drugs that attenuate both positive and negative symptoms of schizophrenia? *Neuropsychopharmacology*, **2**, 191–199.

Farde, L. (1992) Selective D_1- and D_2-dopamine receptor blockade both induces akathisia in humans — a PET study with [^{11}C]SCH 23390 and [^{11}C]raclopride. *Psychopharmacology*, **107**, 23–29.

Farde, L., Wiesel, F.A., Halldin, C. & Sedvall, G. (1988b) Central D2- dopamine receptor occupancy in schizophrenic patients treated with antipsychotic drugs. *Archives of General Psychiatry*, **45**, 71–76.

Farde, L., Wiesel, F.A., Halldin, C., Sedvall, G. & Nilsson, L. (1989) Dopamine receptor occupancy and plasma haloperidol levels. *Archives of General Psychiatry*, **46**, 483–484.

Farde, L., Nordstrom, A.L., Wiesel, F.A., Pauli, S., Halidin, C. & Sedvall, G. (1992) Positron emission tomographic analysis of central D_1 and D_2 dopamine receptor occupancy in patients treated with classical neuroleptics and clozapine. *Archives of General Psychiatry*, **49**, 538–544.

Farde, L., Pauli, S., Hall, H. *et al.* (1988a) Stereoselective binding for ^{11}C-raclopride in living human brain — a search for extrastriatal central D2-dopamine receptors by PET. *Psychopharmacology*, **94**, 471–478.

Gessa, G.L., Canu, A., Del Zompo, M., Burrai, C. & Serra, G. (1991) Lack of acute antipsychotic effect of SCH 23390, a selective dopamine D_1 receptor antagonist. *Lancet*, **337**, 854–855.

Hietala, J., Koulu, M., Kuoppamäki, M., Lappalainen, J. & Syvälahti, E. (1992) Chronic clozapine treatment downregulates serotonin 5-HT-1c receptors in rat brain. *Progress in Neuro-Psychopharmacology and Biological Psychiatry*, **16**, 727–732.

Hirsch, S., Arvanitis, L., Miller, B. *et al.* (1994) A multicentre, double-blind placebo-controlled comparison of low and high dosage regimens of seroquel^{TM} in the treatment of hospitalised patients with acute exacerbation of subchronic or chronic schizophrenia. *European Neuropsychopharmacology*, **4**, 384–385.

Ichikawa, J. & Meltzer, H.Y. (1992) Amperozide, a novel antipsychotic drug, inhibits the ability of D-amphetamine to increase dopamine release *in vivo* in rat striatum and nucleus accumbens. *Journal of Neurochemistry*, **58**, 2285–2291.

Janowsky, A., Neve, K.A., Kinzie, J.M., Taylor, B., de Paulis, T. & Belknap, J.K. (1992) Extrastriatal dopamine D2 receptors: distribution, pharmacological characterization and region-specific regulation by clozapine. *Journal of Pharmacology and Experimental Therapeutics*, **261**, 1282–1290.

Janssen, P.A.J., Niemegeers, C.J.E., Awouters, F., Schellekens, K.H.L., Megens, A.A.H.P. & Meert, T.F. (1988) Pharmacology of risperidone (R 64 766), a new antipsychotic with serotonin-S_2 and dopamine-D_2 antagonistic properties. *Journal of Pharmacology and Experimental Therapeutics*, **244**, 685–693.

Jaskiw, G.E. & Weinberger, D.R. (1992) Dopamine and schizophrenia: a cortically correct perspective. *Seminars in the Neurosciences*, **4**, 179–188.

Johnstone, E.C. (1993) Schizophrenia: problems in clinical practice. *Lancet*, **341**, 536–538.

Johnstone, E.C., Crow, T.J., Frith, C.D., Carney, M.W.P. & Price, J.S. (1978) Mechanism of the antipsychotic effect in the treatment of acute schizophrenia. *Lancet*, **i**, 848–851.

Johnstone, E.C., Crow, T.J., Frith, C.D. & Owens, D.G.C. (1988) The Northwick Park 'functional' psychosis study: diagnosis and treatment response. *Lancet*, **ii**, 119–125.

Kane, J., Honigfeld, G., Singer, J., Meltzer, H. & Clozaril Collaborative Study Group (1988) Clozapine for the treatment-resistant schizophrenic. *Archives of General Psychiatry*, **45**, 789–796.

Karbe, H., Wienhard, K., Hamacher, K. *et al.* (1991) Positron emission tomography with (^{18}F)methylspiperone demonstrates D_2 dopamine receptor-binding differences of clozapine and haloperidol. *Journal of Neural Transmission (General Section)*, **86**, 163–173.

Kasper, S., Fuger, J., Zinner, H.-J., Bäuml, J. & Moller, H.-J. (1992) Early clinical results with the neuroleptic roxindole (EMD 49 980) in the treatment of schizophrenia — an open study. *European Neuropsychopharmacology*, **2**, 91–95.

Kebabian, J.W. & Calne, D.B. (1979) Multiple receptors for dopamine. *Nature*, **277**, 93–96.

Keck, P.E., Cohen, B.M., Baldessarini, R.J. & McElroy, S.L. (1989) Time course of antipsychotic effects of neuroleptic drugs. *American Journal of Psychiatry*, **146**, 1289–1292.

Kessler, R.M., Mason, N.S., Votaw, J.R. *et al.* (1992) Visualization of extrastriatal dopamine D_2 receptors in the human brain. *European Journal of Pharmacology*, **223**, 105–107.

Leenders, K.L., Antonini, A., Thomann, R. *et al.* (1993) *European Journal of Clinical Pharmacology*, **44**, 135–140.

Leysen, J.E., Gommeren, W., Mertens, J. *et al.* (1993) Comparison of *in vitro* binding properties of a series of dopamine antagonists and agonists for cloned human dopamine D_{2S} and D_{2L} receptors and for D_2 receptors in rat striatal and mesolimbic tissues, using [^{125}I] 2'-iodospiperone. *Psychopharmacology*, **110**, 27–36.

Leysen, J.E., Janssen, P.M.F., Gommeren, W., Wynants, J., Pauwels, P.J. & Janssen, P.A.J. (1992) *In vitro* and *in vivo* receptor binding and effects on monoamine turnover in rat brain regions of the novel antipsychotics risperidone and ocaperidone. *Molecular Pharmacology*, **41**, 494–508.

Lidsky, T.I. & Banerjee, S.P. (1992) Clozapine's mechanisms of action: non-dopaminergic activity rather than anatomical selectivity. *Neuroscience Letters*, **136**, 100–103.

Litman, R.E., Hong, W., Weissman, E., Su, T.P., Potter, W.Z. & Pickar, D. (1993) Augmentation of neuroleptics with idazoxan: focus on noradrenergic function in schizophrenia. *Schizophrenia Research*, **9**, 242.

Lundberg, T., Lindström, L.H., Hartvig, P. *et al.* (1989) Striatal and frontal cortex binding of 11-C-labelled clozapine visualized by positron emission tomography (PET) in drug-free schizophrenics and healthy volunteers.

Psychopharmacology, **99**, 8–12.

McEvoy, J.P., Hogarty, G.E. & Steingard, S. (1991) Optimal dose of neuroleptic in acute schizophrenia: a controlled study of the neuroleptic threshold and higher haloperidol dose. *Archives of General Psychiatry*, **48**, 739–745.

Marder, S.R., Hubbard, J.W., Van Putten, T. & Midha, K.K. (1989) Pharmacokinetics of long-acting injectable neuroleptic drugs: clinical implications. *Psychopharmacology*, **98**, 433–439.

Martin, P.T., Grebb, J.A., Schmitz, T.B. *et al.* (1994) Eficacy and safety of sertindole in double-blind, placebo-controlled trials of schizophrenic patients. *Schizophrenia Research*, **11**, 107.

Mason, S.L. & Reynolds, G.P. (1992) Clozapine has submicromolar affinity for $5-HT_{1A}$ receptors in human brain tissue. *European Journal of Pharmacology*, **22**, 397–398.

Megens, A.A.H.P., Niemegeers, C.J.E. & Awouters, F.H.L. (1992b) Antipsychotic profile and side-effect liability of haloperidol, risperidone, and ocaperidone as predicted from their differential interactions with amphetamine in rats. *Drug Development Research*, **26**, 129–145.

Megens, A.A.H.P., Awouters, F.H.L., Meert, T.F., Schellekens, K.H.L., Niemegeers, C.J.E. & Janssen, P.A.J. (1992a) Pharmacological profile of the new potent neuroleptic ocaperidone (R 79 598). *Journal of Pharmacology and Experimental Therapeutics*, **260**, 146–159.

Meltzer, H.Y. (1991) The mechanism of action of novel antipsychotic drugs. *Schizophrenia Bulletin*, **17**, 263–287.

Meltzer, H.Y. (1992) *Novel Antipsychotic Drugs*. Raven Press, New York.

Meltzer, H.Y. & Stockmeier, C.A. (1992) *In vivo* occupancy of dopamine receptors by antipsychotic drugs. *Archives of General Psychiatry*, **49**, 588–589.

Meltzer, H.Y., Matsubara, S. & Lee, J.C. (1989) Classification of typical and atypical antipsychotic drugs on the basis of dopamine D-1, D-2 and serotonin$_2$ pK_i values. *Journal of Pharmacology and Experimental Therapeutics*, **25**, 238–246.

Moore, N.A., Tye, N.C., Axton, M.S. & Risius, F.C. (1992) The behavioral pharmacology of olanzapine, a novel 'atypical' antipsychotic agent. *Journal of Pharmacology and Experimental Therapeutics*, **262**, 545–551.

Murray, A.M. & Waddington, J.L. (1990) The interaction of clozapine with dopamine D-1 versus dopamine D-2 receptor-mediated function: behavioural indices. *European Journal of Pharmacology*, **186**, 79–86.

Murray, A.M., Ryoo, H. & Joyce, J.N. (1992) Visualization of dopamine D$_3$-like receptors in human brain with [^{125}I] epidepride. *European Journal of Pharmacology* (Molecular Pharmacology Section), **227**, 443–445.

Newcomer, J.W., Faustman, W.O., Zipursky, R.B. & Csernansky, J.G. (1992) Zacopride in schizophrenia: a single-blind serotonin type 3 antagonist trial. *Archives of General Psychiatry*, **49**, 751–752.

Niemegeers, C.J.E. & Janssen, P.A.J. (1978) A systematic study of the pharmacological activities of dopamine antagonists. *Life Sciences*, **24**, 2201–2216.

Nimgaonkar, V.L. & Whatley, S.A. (1990) Specific effect of antipsychotic drugs on protein synthesis in human lymphomononuclear cells. *Journal of Neurochemistry*, **54**, 1934–1940.

Nordstrom, A.L., Farde, L. & Halldin, C. (1992) Time course of D$_2$-dopamine receptor occupancy examined by PET after single oral doses of haloperidol. *Psychopharmacology*, **106**, 433–438.

Nordstrom, A.L., Farde, L. & Halldin, C. (1993a) High 5-HT$_2$ receptor occupancy in clozapine-treated patients demonstrated by PET. *Psychopharmacology*, **110**, 365–367.

Nordstrom, A.L., Farde, L., Wiesel, F-A. (1993b) Central D2-dopamine receptor occupancy in relation to antipsychotic drug effects: a double-blind PET study of schizophrenic patients. *Biological Psychiatry*, **33**, 227–235.

Nyberg, S., Farde, L., Eriksson, L., Halldin, C. & Eriksson, B. (1993) 5-HT$_2$ and D$_2$ dopamine receptor occupancy in the living human brain: a PET study with risperidone. *Psychopharmacology*, **110**, 265–272.

Olbrich, R. & Schanz, H. (1991) An evaluation of the partial dopamine agonist terguride regarding positive symptoms reduction in schizophrenics. *Journal of Neural Transmission* (General Section), **84**, 233–236.

Pickar, D. (1988) Perspectives on a time-dependent model of neuroleptic action. *Schizophrenia Bulletin*, **14**, 255–268.

Pickar, D., Owen, R.R., Litman, R.E., Konicki, E., Gutierrez, R. & Rapaport, M.H. (1992) Clinical and biologic response to clozapine in patients with schizophrenia. *Archives of General Psychiatry*, **49**, 345–353.

Pilowsky, L.S., Costa, D.C., Ell, P.J., Murray, R.M., Verhoeff, N.P.L.G. & Kerwin, R.W. (1992) Clozapine, single photon emission tomography, and the D2 dopamine receptor blockade hypothesis of schizophrenia. *Lancet*, **340**, 199–202.

Potkin, S.G., Arnand, R. & Sandoz Collaborating Centres (1993) A partial dopamine agonist SDZ HDC 912 has antipsychotic efficacy. *Schizophrenia Research*, **9**, 247.

Reynolds, G.P. (1989) Beyond the dopamine hypothesis: the neurochemical pathology of schizophrenia. *British Journal of Psychiatry*, **155**, 305–316.

Reynolds, G.P. (1992) Developments in the drug treatment of schizophrenia. *Trends in Pharmacological Sciences*, **13**, 116–121.

Reynolds, G.P., Cowey, L., Rossor, M.N. & Iversen, L.L. (1982) Thioridazine is not specific for limbic dopamine receptors. *Lancet*, **ii**, 499–500.

Richelson, E. & Nelson, A. (1984) Antagonism by neuroleptics of neurotransmitter receptors of normal human brain *in vitro*. *European Journal of Pharmacology*, **103**, 197–204.

Richmond, G., Potkin, S.G., Plon, L., McElroy, T. & Jin, Y. (1993) Zacopride, a 5-HT3 receptor antagonist, may be an effective antipsychotic in schizophrenia. *Schizophrenia Research*, **9**, 247–248.

Rifkin, A., Doddi, S., Karajgi, B., Borenstein, M. & Wachspress, M. (1991) Dosage of haloperidol for schizophrenia. *Archives of General Psychiatry*, **48**, 166–170.

Sanchez, C., Arnt, J., Dragsted, N. *et al.* (1991) Neurochemical and *in vivo* pharmacological profile of sertindole, a limbic-selective neuroleptic compound. *Drug Development Research*, **22**, 239–250.

Schotte, A., Janssen, P.F.M., Gommeren, W., Luyten, W.H.L.M. & Leysen, J.E. (1992) Autoradiographic evidence for the occlusion of rat brain dopamine D$_3$ receptors *in vivo*. *European Journal of Pharmacology*, **218**, 373–375.

Seeman, P. (1980) Brain dopamine receptors. *Pharmacological*

Reviews, **32**, 229–313.

Seeman, P. (1992) Dopamine receptor sequences: therapeutic levels of neuroleptics occupy D$_2$ receptors, clozapine occupies D$_4$. *Neuropsychopharmacology*, **7**, 261–284.

Seeman, P. & Ulpian, C. (1983) Neuroleptics have identical potencies in human brain limbic and putamen regions. *European Journal of Pharmacology*, **94**, 145–148.

Shaikh, S., Collier, D., Kerwin, R.W. *et al.* (1993) Dopamine D4 receptor subtypes and response to clozapine. *Lancet*, **341**, 116.

Sibley, D.R. & Monsma, F.J. (1992) Molecular biology of dopamine receptors. *Trends in Pharmacological Sciences*, **13**, 61–69.

Simpson, G.M., Yadalam, K.G., Levinson, D.F., Stephanos, M.J., Lo, E.S. & Cooper, T.B. (1990) Single-dose pharmacokinetics of fluphenazine after fluphenazine decanoate administration. *Journal of Clinical Psychopharmacology*, **10**, 417–421.

Smith, M., Wolf, A.P., Brodie, J.D. *et al.* (1988) Serial [^{18}F]N-methylspiroperidol PET studies to measure changes in antipsychotic drug D-2 receptor occupancy in schizophrenic patients. *Biological Psychiatry*, **23**, 653–663.

Sokoloff, P., Giros, B., Martres, M.-P., Bouthenet, M.-L. & Schwartz, J.-C. (1990) Molecular cloning and characterization of a novel dopamine receptor (D3) as a target for neuroleptics. *Nature*, **347**, 146–151.

Sokoloff, P., Martres, M.-P., Giros, B., Bouthenet, J.-L. & Schwartz, J.-C. (1992) The third dopamine receptor (D$_3$) as a novel target for antipsychotics. *Biochemical Pharmacology*, **43**, 659–666.

Sunahara, R.K., Guan, H.-C., O'Down, B.F. *et al.* (1991) Cloning of the gene for a human dopamine D-5 receptor with higher affinity for dopamine than D-1. *Nature*, **350**, 614–619.

Tamminga, C.A., Gotts, M.D., Thaker, G.K., Alphs, L.D. & Foster, N.L. (1986) Dopamine agonist treatment of schizophrenia with N-propylnorapomorphine. *Archives of General Psychiatry*, **43**, 398–402.

Tsuneizumi, T., Babb, S.M. & Cohen, B.M. (1992) Drug distribution between blood and brain as a determinant of antipsychotic drug effects. *Biological Psychiatry*, **32**, 817–824.

Van Putten, T., Marder, S.R., Wirshing, W.C., Aravgirl, M. & Chabert, N. (1991) Neuroleptic plasma levels. *Schizophrenia Bulletin*, **17**, 197–216.

Van Putten, T., Marder, S.R., Mintz, J. & Poland, R.E. (1992) Haloperidol plasma levels and clinical response: a therapeutic window relationship. *American Journal of Psychiatry*, **149**, 500–505.

Van Tol, H.H.M., Bunzow, J.R., Guan, H.-C. *et al.* (1991) Cloning of the gene for a human dopamine D$_4$ receptor with high affinity for the antipsychotic clozapine. *Nature*, **350**, 610–614.

Van Tol, H.H.M., Wu, C.M., Guan, H.-C. *et al.* (1992) Multiple dopamine D4 receptor variants in the human population. *Nature*, **358**, 149–152.

Verghese, C., Kessel, J.B. & Simpson, G.M. (1991) Pharmacokinetics of neuroleptics. *Psychopharmacology Bulletin*, **27**, 551–563.

Volavka, J., Cooper, T., Czobor, P. *et al.* (1992) Haloperidol blood levels and clinical effects. *Archives of General Psychiatry*, **49**, 354–361.

Wachtel, H. & Turski, L. (1990) Glutamate: a new target in schizophrenia? *Trends in Pharmacological Sciences*, **11**, 219–220.

Waddington, J.L. (1988) Therapeutic potential of selective D-1 dopamine receptor agonists and antagonists in psychiatry and neurology. *General Pharmacology*, **19**, 55–60.

Waddington, J.L. (1989a) Schizophrenia, affective psychoses and other disorders treated with neuroleptic drugs: the enigma of tardive dyskinesia, its neurobiological determinants, and the conflict of paradigms. *International Review of Neurobiology*, **31**, 297–353.

Waddington, J.L. (1989b) Sight and insight; brain dopamine receptor occupancy by neuroleptics visualised in living schizophrenic patients by positron emission tomography. *British Journal of Psychiatry*, **154**, 433–436.

Waddington, J.L. (1992) Mechanisms of neuroleptic-induced extrapyramidal side effects. In Kane, J.M. & Lieberman, J.A. (eds) *Adverse Effects of Psychotropic Drugs*, pp. 246–265. Guilford Press, New York.

Waddington, J.L. (1993a) Pre- and postsynaptic D-1 to D-5 dopamine receptor mechanisms in relation to antipsychotic activity. In Barnes, T.R.E. (ed.) *Antipsychotic Drugs and their Side Effects*, pp. 65–85. Academic Press, London.

Waddington, J.L. (1993b) Schizophrenia: developmental neuroscience and pathobiology. *Lancet*, **341**, 531–536.

Waddington, J.L. (1993c) Neurodynamics of abnormalities in cerebral structure and metabolism in schizophrenia. *Schizophrenia Bulletin*, **19**, 55–69.

Waddington, J.L. (1993d) Future directions: the clinical significance and therapeutic potential of D-1:D-2 interactions in Parkinson's disease, schizophrenia and other disorders. In Waddington, J.L. (ed.) *D-1:D-2 Dopamine Receptor Interactions: Neuroscience and Psychopharmacology*, pp. 271–290. Academic Press, London.

Waddington, J.L. & Daly, S.A. (1992) The status of 'second generation' selective D$_1$ dopamine receptor antagonists as putative atypical antipsychotic agents. In Meltzer, H.Y. (ed.) *Novel Antipsychotic Drugs*, pp. 109–115. Raven Press, New York.

Waddington, J.L. & Daly, S.A. (1993) Regulation of unconditioned motor behaviour by D-1:D-2 interactions. In Waddington, J.L. (ed.) *D-1:D-2 Dopamine Receptor Interactions: Neuroscience and Psychopharmacology*, pp. 51–78. Academic Press, London.

Wander, T.J., Nelson, A., Okazaki, H. & Richelson, E. (1987) Antagonism by neuroleptics of serotonin 5-HT$_{1A}$ and 5-HT$_2$ receptors of normal human brain *in vitro*. *European Journal of Pharmacology*, **143**, 279–282.

Watling, K.J., Beer, M.S., Stanton, J.A. & Newberry, N.R. (1990) Interaction of the atypical neuroleptic clozapine with 5-HT$_3$ receptors in the cerebral cortex and superior cervical ganglion of the rat. *European Journal of Pharmacology*, **182**, 465–472.

Wetzel, H., Wiedmann, K., Holsboer, F. & Benkert, O. (1991) Savoxepine: invalidation of an 'atypical' neuroleptic response pattern predicted by animal models in an open clinical trial with schizophrenic patients. *Psychopharmacology*, **103**, 280–283.

Wolkin, A., Barouche, F., Wolf, A.P. *et al.* (1989a) Dopamine blockade and clinical response: evidence for two biological subgroups of schizophrenia. *American Journal of Psychiatry*, **146**, 905–908.

Wolkin, A., Brodie, J.D., Barouche, F. *et al.* (1989b) Dopamine receptor occupancy and plasma haloperidol levels. *Archives of General Psychiatry*, **46**, 482–483.

Wood, A.J., Beasley, C.M., Tollefson, G.D. & Tran, P.V. (1994) Efficacy of olanzapine in the positive and negative symptoms of schizophrenia. *European Neuropsychopharmacology*, **4**, 224–225.

Wysowski, D.K. & Baum, C. (1989) Antipsychotic drug use in the United States, 1976–1985. *Archives of General Psychiatry*, **46**, 929–932.

Chapter 19
The Neurochemistry
of Schizophrenia

F. OWEN AND M. D. C. SIMPSON

Introduction

It is generally accepted that genetic factors play a significant role in the aetiology of schizophrenia although the precise mode of inheritance of the disease remains obscure. If a component of schizophrenia is genetically determined, then it follows that a biochemical basis for the disease should be identifiable. The notion that the primary disturbance in schizophrenia has a neurochemical basis is plausible because the symptoms of the disease can be exacerbated or ameliorated by the administration of relatively simple chemical compounds and there is overwhelming evidence to suggest that these chemicals exert their effects by interactions with specific neurotransmitter mechanisms. Early investigations attempted to assess, indirectly, aspects of brain function using peripheral body fluids and tissues such as urine, blood, platelets or lymphocytes. More recently, neurotransmitter mechanisms have been studied directly in postmortem brain tissue from schizophrenics or *in vivo* using neuroimaging techniques. The advances that these recent studies have made to our understanding of the neurochemical basis of schizophrenia are presented in this chapter.

There have been many biochemical hypotheses of schizophrenia but the majority of investigations have attempted to demonstrate an association between schizophrenia and aberrant brain function of:

1 monoamine mechanisms;
2 amino acid neurotransmitters;
3 neuropeptides.

Monoamine mechanisms and schizophrenia

The monoamines of interest in relation to schizophrenia are dopamine, noradrenaline and 5-hydroxytryptamine (serotonin, 5-HT). Hypotheses suggesting the involvement of each of the amines and also their common degradative enzyme, monoamine oxidase (MAO), in the aetiology of schizophrenia have been proposed.

Dopamine

The dopamine 'hypothesis' of schizophrenia, which in its simplest form states that schizophrenia is associated with excessive dopaminergic function in the central nervous system (CNS), has persisted as the predominant neurochemical hypothesis of schizophrenia for three decades, although the presence of aberrant dopaminergic mechanisms in the brains of schizophrenic patients has yet to be established. The dopamine hypothesis arose from two lines of evidence. First, it has been well established that amphetamine and other dopamine-releasing drugs can induce a state closely resembling paranoid schizophrenia in mentally normal individuals (Connell, 1958; Griffiths *et al.*, 1972; Angrist *et al.*, 1974). The second line of evidence arose from studies on the mode of action of neuroleptic drugs that are effective in the treatment of schizophrenia. They comprise a wide variety of drugs that belong to several different chemical classes but have in common the ability to inhibit the dopamine-induced stimulation of adenylate cyclase *in vitro* (Clement-Cormier *et al.*, 1974; Miller *et al.*, 1974), and to displace the high-affinity binding of ligands to the dopamine receptor (Seeman *et al.*, 1975).

Strong support for the dopamine hypothesis was provided by the results of a clinical trial of the therapeutic efficacy of the optical isomers of the thioxanthene neuroleptic, flupenthixol (Johnstone *et al.*, 1978). Flupenthixol exists in a *cis* (or α) and a *trans* (or β) form which have many chemical and pharmacological features in common, except that α-flupenthixol is far more potent than β-flupenthixol in inhibiting dopamine-sensitive adenylate cyclase and also in displacing the high-affinity binding of ligands to the dopamine receptor. When the isomers were administered separately to a group of acute schizophrenics over a 4-week trial period, α-flupenthixol produced a significant improvement in the symptomatology, whereas β-flupenthixol was no more effective than a placebo.

However, investigations of the concentration of homovanillic acid (HVA — the major end product of dopamine metabolism) in the cerebrospinal fluid (CSF) have produced no evidence to suggest increased turnover of brain dopamine in schizophrenia (Bowers, 1974; Post *et al.*, 1975; Berger *et al.*, 1980a). Studies of the concentration of dopamine itself in postmortem brain tissue from schizophrenics have yielded equivocal results. Bird *et al.* (1977) reported significant increases in dopamine levels in samples of nucleus accumbens from schizophrenics but with similar levels to controls in the putamen, whereas Owen *et al.* (1978) reported increased dopamine levels in the caudate nucleus of schizophrenics and levels

similar to controls in the putamen and nucleus accumbens. Both groups found the brain concentrations of HVA to be similar in controls and schizophrenics, indicating no increase in brain dopamine turnover in the latter group (Owen *et al.*, 1978; Bird *et al.*, 1979). Moreover, Crow *et al.* (1979) reported that the activity of tyrosine hydroxylase, the rate-limiting enzyme in dopamine metabolism, was not increased in brain samples from schizophrenics.

However, a more recent report (Toru *et al*, 1988) describes increased brain concentrations of HVA as well as increased activity of tyrosine hydroxylase in postmortem samples from chronic schizophrenics. It is difficult to reconcile these conflicting results but it is known that neuroleptic drugs have profound effects on dopaminergic mechanisms. It is noteworthy that Bacopoulos *et al.* (1979) reported significant increases in HVA levels in several regions of postmortem brains from schizophrenics, but in the small number of neuroleptic-free patients included in the study HVA levels were no different from control values.

A finding that generated considerable interest was that of Reynolds (1983), who reported an increased concentration of dopamine in the left amygdala compared with the right amygdala of schizophrenics, but not in control samples. The asymmetry in dopamine concentrations in the amygdala was not shared by noradrenaline. Reynolds suggested that his finding supported the hypothesis that schizophrenia was associated with a dysfunction of the left temporal lobe (Flor-Henry, 1983).

Apart from the report by Reynolds (1983), which has remained unchallenged, the postmortem studies failed to provide unequivocal, verifiable evidence for increased dopamine turnover in the brains of schizophrenics.

Bowers (1974) and Crow *et al.* (1976) suggested that the postulated increased central dopaminergic function in schizophrenia might not result from increased dopamine turnover but from an increase in dopamine receptor sensitivity. The development of high-affinity ligand-binding techniques for assessing dopamine receptors (Seeman *et al.*, 1975) enabled this suggestion to be investigated.

Kebabian and Calne (1979) categorized dopamine receptors as D_1 or D_2. At that time, it was believed that D_1 receptors were linked to adenylate cyclase and did not bind with high affinity the butyrophenone class of neuroleptics, such as haloperidol or spiperone, whereas D_2 receptors were not linked to adenylate cyclase but bound to butyrophenones with high affinity. It has become clear that dopamine-receptor subtypes are considerably more complicated, but the initial distinction of D_1-like and D_2-like receptors persists.

The butyrophenones, particularly spiperone, proved to be useful ligands for binding studies. Therefore, the initial postmortem brain studies of dopamine receptors in schizophrenia involved the assessment of the D_2 receptor. Owen *et al.* (1978) reported significant increases in dopamine receptor numbers in samples of caudate, putamen and nucleus accumbens from schizophrenics. Similar findings were reported by other groups (Lee *et al.*, 1978; Lee & Seeman, 1980; Mackay *et al.*, 1980; Reynolds *et al.*, 1980; Hess *et al.*, 1987; Joyce *et al.*, 1988; Toru *et al.*, 1988).

Cross *et al.* (1981) used [^{3}H]flupenthixol (which binds with high affinity to both D_1 and D_2 receptors) as the primary ligand and the highly selective D_2 antagonist, domperidone, to resolve the binding into its D_1 and D_2 components; they reported a significant increase in binding to D_2 receptors but no elevation in binding to D_1 receptors in the schizophrenic group. Other workers have confirmed that unlike D_2 receptors there is no increase in high-affinity binding to D_1 receptors in brain samples from schizophrenics (Hess *et al.*, 1987; Czudek & Reynolds, 1988).

It has been well established that chronic neuroleptic administration to laboratory animals results in increased D_2 receptor numbers in the brain (Burt *et al.*, 1982). Therefore, although there is general agreement that dopamine D_2 receptors are increased in postmortem brains of schizophrenics, there remains a controversy over whether or not this increase is entirely due to neuroleptic medication and unrelated to the disease process.

Techniques based on position emission tomography (PET) and single photon emission tomography (SPET) for assessing neurotransmitter receptors in living human subjects have recently been developed (for review, see Sedvall *et al.*, 1986). However, the application of the techniques to studies of the dopamine receptor has failed to resolve the controversy over the state of the D_2 receptor in schizophrenia. Crawley *et al.* (1986), using a SPET technique with [^{77}Br]bromospiperone as ligand, demonstrated a small but just significant increase in striatum: cerebellum ratios of radioactivity (an index of D_2 receptor numbers) in neuroleptic-free schizophrenic patients. Using a PET technique with [^{11}C]methylspiperone as ligand, Wong *et al.* (1986) reported large, significant increases in D_2 receptors in neuroleptic-naive and also in neuroleptic-treated schizoprenics. Using the same ligand, Pearlson *et al.* (1993) reported similar increases in D_2 receptors in late-onset schizophrenia. On the other hand, the PET studies of Farde *et al.* (1990) using [^{11}C]raclopride as ligand and of Martinot *et al.* (1990) using [^{76}Br]bromospiperone as ligand revealed no significant differences in D_2 receptor numbers between controls and neuroleptic-free schizophrenic patients.

However, the application of molecular biological techniques to investigations of dopamine receptor subtypes has revealed that the topic is far more complicated than previously thought. At the present time five dopamine receptor subtypes (D_1–D_5) have been cloned and sequenced (Civelli *et al.*, 1991; Sunahara *et al.*, 1991). Of these, on the basis of similarities in gene structure and pharmacological profiles, D_1 and D_5 are said to be D_1-like and D_2, D_3 and D_4 are said to be D_2-like. A recent study of the D_4 receptor in postmortem brain samples from schizophrenics may help to resolve the apparent discrepancy between the reports on D_2 receptor levels observed in the *in vivo* PET studies (Seeman *et al.*, 1993). In this study, Seeman *et al.* used [^{3}H]emanopride to bind to D_2, D_3 and D_4 receptors and [^{3}H]raclopride to bind to D_2 and D_3 receptors, since raclopride has a relatively low affinity for the D_4 receptor. By subtracting the [^{3}H]raclopride binding from the [^{3}H]emanopride binding, it was deduced that the density of D_4 receptors was increased sixfold in schizophrenics, whereas the [^{3}H]raclopride binding itself was only marginally increased, in agreement with the findings of the PET study by Farde *et al.* (1990). Perhaps more importantly, Seeman *et al.* also reported that the [^{3}H]raclopride binding in tissue from schizophrenics, but not that from controls or from patients dying with Huntington's chorea or Parkinson's disease was unresponsive to guanine nucleotides, which normally cause an increase in the binding of the ligand. Seeman's observation suggests some functional alteration in the G-protein coupling of the dopamine receptor in schizophrenia, implicating the importance of the function of second messenger systems in schizophrenia. Second messenger systems are triggered by neurotransmitter receptor stimulation (Nahorski *et al.*, 1986). The transmitter–receptor complex then interacts with a guanine triphosphate (GTP)-binding protein, usually designated G-protein. Recent experimental advances have greatly clarified the second messenger systems underlying neurotransmitter actions, suggesting novel sites of action for psychotropic agents (Baraban *et al.*, 1989).

Dopamine receptors are thought to be functionally coupled to the cyclic adenosine monophosphate (AMP) and phosphoinositide (PI) second messenger system. The PI signalling system provides a link between receptors and intracellular calcium. Work on the PI transduction system in platelets from schizophrenic patients showed that the neurotransmitter hypotheses of neuroleptic action and schizophrenia could be extended beyond cell-surface receptors, providing a link between receptors and intracellular calcium (Essali *et al.*, 1992). The importance of such a mechanism is emphasized by the possible involvement of the PI transduction system in the therapeutic mode of action of both lithium and neuroleptics (Baraban *et al.*, 1989; Das *et al.*, 1992).

Since the dopamine-receptor subtypes have been cloned and sequenced, brain messenger ribonucleic acid (mRNA) expression for the subtypes can be investigated with absolute specificity using molecular biological techniques. Roberts *et al.* (1993) have reported the results of such a study on the isomers of the dopamine D_2 receptor. The isomers are generated by alternative splicing of one of the three exons, encoding the putative third intracellular loop of the receptor, thought to be involved in G-protein interaction. Roberts *et al.* reported an increased abundance of mRNA for the long and short isoforms in the schizophrenic group in some but not all brain regions studied, but with no differential distribution of the isoforms in the patient group. This result may prove of particular interest since although it is clear that chronic neuroleptic administration to laboratory animals results in increased D_2 receptor numbers in the brain, it is not clear that there is also a corresponding increase in receptor mRNA (Srivastava *et al.*, 1990; Van Tol *et al.*, 1990; Angulo *et al.*, 1991; Goss *et al.*, 1991).

Schmauss *et al.* (1993) investigated the expression of mRNA for dopamine D_3 receptors in samples from 12 brain regions of chronic schizophrenics and reported a selective loss of expression in parietal and motor cortices. Schmauss *et al.* cautiously suggested that many variables associated with either the course or therapeutic management of the disease may account for the selective loss of D_3 mRNA.

If the postulated aberrant central dopaminergic function in schizophrenia does indeed result from defective dopamine receptor function, then there is scope for considerably more research on the receptor subtypes (see also Chapter 20).

Noradrenaline

Stein and Wise (1971) suggested that the lack of goal-directed behaviour observed in schizophrenics might result from a deficit in the cortical noradrenergic reward system. They supported their hypothesis by reporting significant reductions in the activity of dopamine-β-hydroxylase (DBH) activity in postmortem brain samples from schizophrenics compared with controls (Wise & Stein, 1973). DBH catalyses the conversion of dopamine to noradrenaline and is a marker enzyme for noradrenergic neurones. Reduction in DBH activity could therefore be interpreted as a loss of noradrenergic neurones. Subsequently, however,

Wyatt *et al.* (1975) failed to find a reduction in DBH activity in brain samples from schizophrenics, but did observe that if patients with paranoid symptoms were omitted from the study the DBH activity of the remaining patients tended to be lower than that of controls.

Hartmann (1976) suggested that decreased brain DBH activity might lead to an accumulation of dopamine as well as a decrease in noradrenaline concentration, and that a change in the balance between the two monoamines might form the neurochemical basis of schizophrenia. However, Cross *et al.* (1978) reported no significant difference in DBH activity between controls and schizophrenics in all six regions of postmortem brain tissue examined. Moreover, Cross *et al.* found a significant inverse correlation between DBH activity and the time between death and autopsy. This group also reported that DBH activity was significant lower in neuroleptic-treated compared with neuroleptic-free patients.

The hypothesis by Stein and Wise (1971) of a central noradrenergic deficit in schizophrenia was particularly pertinent to patients with negative symptoms, but Crow *et al.* (1979) reported that patients with a preponderance of such symptoms did not represent a subgroup of schizophrenics with low DBH activity. It seems likely therefore that the postmortem lability of DBH and the effect of neuroleptic treatment on the activity of the enzyme are sufficient to explain the conflicting reports.

Maas and Landis (1968) and Maas *et al.* (1973) reported that a substantial proportion of 3-methoxy-4-hydroxyphenylglycol (MHPG) excreted in the urine was derived from the metabolism of noradrenaline in the brain. MHPG is the major end product of central noradrenaline metabolism and is present in urine either free or conjugated as MHPG-sulphate or MHPG-glucuronide.

Bond and Howlett (1974) and Bond *et al.* (1975) suggested that urinary MHPG-sulphate was specifically derived from the metabolism of noradrenaline in the brain, and that the glucuronide conjugate was derived from the peripheral metabolism of the amine. Joseph *et al.* (1976) therefore

exploited this suggestion in an attempt to assess brain noradrenaline turnover in living schizophrenic patients. Joseph *et al.* reported that although there was no difference between controls and neuroleptic-free chronic schizophrenics in the overall urinary excretion of MHPG-sulphate, there was a significant inverse correlation between MHPG-sulphate excretion and the severity of schizophrenic symptoms. This might suggest that severe forms of the illness are associated with a deficit in central noradrenergic function. However, in a subsequent study, Joseph *et al.* (1979b) failed to replicate their earlier finding of an inverse correlation between MHPG excretion and severity of schizophrenic symptoms and concluded that reduced brain noradrenaline turnover was neither necessary nor sufficient for schizophrenia to occur.

Noradrenergic receptors have been assessed in postmortem brain tissue using ligands for α and β receptor subtypes. No consistent differences between controls and schizophrenics were observed in early studies (Bennett *et al.*, 1979; Owen *et al.*, 1981b), although a more recent study reported alterations in the distribution of β_1 and β_2 receptors in the limbic structures of schizophrenics (Joyce *et al.*, 1992).

Serotonin

Wooley and Shaw (1954) were the first to hypothesize that schizophrenia might result from a deficiency in serotonergic function in the CNS. They based their postulate on the observation that drugs such as yohimbine, bufotenin and lysergic acid diethylamide (LSD), which have structural similarities to 5-HT, caused behavioural changes in animals and mental disturbances in humans. However, early reports of decreased concentrations of 5-hydroxyindoleacetic acid (5-HIAA — the major end product of 5-HT metabolism) were not confirmed by subsequent studies (Ashcroft *et al.*, 1966; Bowers *et al.*, 1969; Post *et al.*, 1975; Nyback *et al.*, 1983; Potkin *et al.*, 1983). Although plasma concentrations of tryptophan (the precursor of 5-HT) have been reported to be decreased in schizophrenic patients (Manowitz *et al.*, 1973; Domino & Krause, 1974), the administration of large oral doses has failed to produce consistent improvements in schizophrenic symptoms (Bowers, 1970; Wyatt *et al.*, 1972; Gillin *et al.*, 1976). Moreover, Pollin *et al.* (1961) reported that oral doses of tryptophan in conjunction with a monoamine oxidase inhibitor (MAOI), which would help to prevent the metabolic inactivation of brain 5-HT, markedly worsened the symptoms of some schizophrenics, suggesting that in some patients the disease may be associated with increased rather than decreased brain serotonergic function. It is interesting to note that several neuroleptic drugs are potent 5-HT antagonists as well as potent dopamine antagonists (Leyson *et al.*, 1978). However, clinical trials of the 5-HT antagonist, cinanserin, have clearly shown that the drug is ineffective in the treatment of schizophrenia (Gallant & Bishop, 1968; Holden *et al.*, 1971).

Direct investigation of brain serotonergic mechanisms in schizophrenia have also been carried out on postmortem tissue. Joseph *et al.* (1979a) measured the brain concentrations of tryptophan, 5-HT and 5-HIAA and found no evidence of changes in 5-HT metabolism associated with schizophrenia. In addition, Toru *et al.* (1988) reported that brain 5-HIAA levels were similar in controls and schizophrenics.

Early ligand-binding studies of 5-HT receptors in schizophrenia produced conflicting results. Thus, the report by Bennett *et al.* (1979) of reduced [^{3}H)LSD binding in frontal cortex samples from schizophrenics was not confirmed by Whitaker *et al.* (1981). However, it has now become clear that there are many subtypes of 5-HT receptors. Molecular biological studies have so far provided evidence for four main categories of human 5-HT receptors, namely 5-HT$_1$, 5-HT$_2$, 5-HT$_3$ and 5-HT$_4$. Five subtypes of the 5-HT$_1$ receptor (5-HT$_{1a}$, 5-HT$_{1b}$, 5-HT$_{1c}$, 5-HT$_{1d}$ and 5-HT$_{1e}$) have been identified (Heuring & Peroutka, 1987; Peroutka, 1988; Leonhardt *et al.*, 1989) and several selective ligands for binding studies of the 5-HT$_1$ receptor subtypes are available. Subtypes of 5-HT$_2$ receptors (5-HT$_{2a}$, 5-HT$_{2b}$) and 5-HT$_3$ receptors (5-HT$_{3a}$, 5-HT$_{3b}$, 5-HT$_{3c}$ and 5-HT$_{1d}$) have been reported (Richardson *et al.*,

1985; Pierce & Peroutka, 1989). Obviously, the early studies of 5-HT receptors in postmortem brain tissue from schizophrenics were insufficiently selective or comprehensive to provide meaningful results. Hashimoto *et al.* (1991) assessed 5-HT$_{1a}$ receptors using the specific ligand [^{3}H]8-hydroxy-2 (di-*n*-propyl-amino) tetralin ([^{3}H]8-OH-DPAT) and reported significant increases in receptor numbers in prefrontal and temporal cortex samples from schizophrenics compared with controls. Mita *et al.* (1986) reported a significant reduction in 5-HT$_2$ receptors in prefrontal cortex samples from schizophrenics. This finding was subsequently confirmed by Arora and Meltzer (1991) and Laruelle *et al.* (1993). The latter group also measured 5-HT reuptake sites using [^{3}H]paroxetine as ligand and reported decreases in several brain regions of schizophrenics; they concluded that prefrontal alterations in both presynaptic and postsynaptic serotonin receptors were present in at least some schizophrenic patients. In an autoradiographic study, Joyce *et al.* (1993) reported increased 5-HT reuptake sites in the dorsal putamen and caudate nucleus of schizophrenics and, consistent with the findings of Laruelle *et al.* (1993), observed a marked reduction in reuptake sites in the frontal cortex. Ohoha *et al.* (1993) recently reviewed the role of serotonin in schizophrenia and suggested that the alterations in serotonergic mechanisms in the prefrontal cortex of schizophrenics represented a cerebral cortex incapable of proper subcortical inhibition, resulting in increased dopaminergic function. Clearly, there is a need for additional investigations of the serotonergic system in schizophrenia.

MAO

Monoamine oxidase inactivates dopamine, noradrenaline and 5-HT in the brain by oxidative deamination. On the basis of the sensitivity of the enzyme to specific inhibitors and its selectivity for substrates, MAO has been classified as MAO-A and MAO-B. Serotonin is a preferred substrate for MAO-A and benzylamine or phenylethylamine for MAO-B (Johnston, 1968; Christmas *et al.*,

1972; Knoll & Magyar, 1972). Recently, the genes encoding MAO-A and MAO-B have been cloned and sequenced (Bach *et al.*, 1988).

Over 30 years ago, Lauer *et al.* (1958) and Pollin *et al.* (1961) reported that the administration of MAOIs to schizophrenics exacerbated their symptoms. The report by Murphy and Wyatt (1972) of a significant reduction in the activity of platelet MAO in chronic schizophrenics aroused considerable interest. Wyatt *et al.* (1973) then reported that not only was platelet MAO activity reduced in monozygotic twins discordant for schizophrenia but the enzyme activity was highly correlated between twins. In addition, there was a significant inverse correlation between MAO activity and the severity of the symptoms. Wyatt *et al.* suggested that reduced platelet MAO activity might prove to be a genetic marker for vulnerability to schizophrenia. Several groups replicated the finding of reduced platelet MAO activity in schizophrenics (Domino & Khanna, 1976; Murphy *et al.*, 1976; Berrettini *et al.*, 1978; Gruen *et al.*, 1982), while others reported platelet MAO activity in schizophrenics to be similar to control values (Murphy *et al.*, 1974; Owen *et al.*, 1976; Mann *et al.*, 1981). Platelet MAO activity has been reported to decrease with time on neuroleptic medication (Takahashi *et al.*, 1975; Friedhoff *et al.*, 1978; Delisi *et al.*, 1981; Owen *et al.*, 1981a), so it seems likely that the reduced platelet MAO activity reported in schizophrenia in some studies is a consequence of neuroleptic treatment.

Robinson *et al.* (1968) reported that MAO in platelets (which is exclusively MAO-B) had similar characteristics to the enzyme in liver and brain. The implication from the apparent reduction in platelet MAO of schizophrenic patients was that it might be reflecting a reduction in the activity of the enzyme in the brain. However, studies on postmortem brain tissue from schizophrenics lend little support to this notion.

Vogel *et al.* (1969), Domino *et al.* (1973), Schwartz *et al.* (1974), Wise *et al.* (1974), Cross *et al.* (1977) and Revely *et al.* (1981) all reported that MAO activity was similar in brain tissue from controls and schizophrenics. Fowler *et al.* (1981) reported a significant increase in the MAO-B:

MAO-A ratio in the pons of schizophrenics; they suggested that this was indicative of glial proliferation. This suggestion is consistent with the increase in MAO-B but not MAO-A reported in brain samples from patients dying with Alzheimer's disease where glial proliferation was present (Adolfsson *et al.*, 1980). Owen *et al.* (1987) reported significant reductions in MAO-B in frontal and temporal cortex and amygdala of schizophrenics in a subgroup with negative symptoms fulfilling the requirements of the type II syndrome described by Crow (1980). Most importantly, however, Green and Grahame-Smith (1978) demonstrated in the rat that reductions of greater than 70% in brain MAO activity are required to significantly affect mono-aminergic function in the brain. Reductions of such magnitude have never been reported in brain samples from schizophrenics, so it seems unlikely that MAO activity plays a significant role in the aetiology of schizophrenia.

Amino acid neurotransmitters and schizophrenia

The inhibitory amino acid neurotransmitter systems of gamma-aminobutyric acid (GABA) and the excitatory neurotransmitter, glutamate, have been extensively studied in relation to schizophrenia.

GABA

Roberts (1972) was the first to propose that GABA systems were defective in schizophrenia. Interactions between GABA (the major inhibitory neurotransmitter in the brain) and dopamine in striatal and limbic systems have been well established (Fuxe *et al.*, 1975; Santiago *et al.*, 1993), and it is plausible that a deficiency in GABAergic function in schizophrenia could result in excessive dopaminergic activity. Roberts suggested that his hypothesis could be readily tested by measuring the activity of glutamate decarboxylase (GAD), the enzyme responsible for decarboxylating glutamate to form GABA and a marker enzyme for GABAergic neurones. Bird *et al.* (1977)

measured GAD activity in samples from nucleus accumbens, putamen, amygdala and hippocampus from controls and schizophrenics and reported significant reductions in enzyme activity in all brain regions investigated in the schizophrenic group. Other workers, however, found GAD activity in postmortem brain samples from controls and schizophrenics to be similar (McGeer & McGeer, 1977; Roberts, 1977; Cross & Owen, 1979).

Subsequently, Bird *et al.* (1978) reported that a closer examination of necropsy reports revealed that death with bronchopneumonia was over-represented in the schizophrenic group and it was likely that terminal hypoxia adversely affected GAD activity.

The concentration of GABA itself in postmortem brain samples has also been assessed. Perry *et al.* (1979) reported significant reductions in GABA concentrations in samples of nucleus accumbens and thalamus from schizophrenics with the reductions being of similar magnitude to those previously reported in Huntington's chorea (Perry *et al.*, 1973; Bird & Iversen, 1974). However, Cross *et al.* (1979) were unable to confirm these findings and reported that there was no difference in the concentration of GABA in brain samples from schizophrenics compared with controls.

Reynolds *et al.* (1990) employed the binding of nipecotic acid to GABA uptake sites to assess the integrity of presynaptic GABAergic neurones. They observed a bilateral loss of [^{3}H]nipecotic binding in samples of hippocampus from schizophrenics. The results also showed a greater deficit of uptake sites in the left hemisphere, providing evidence for a lateralized loss of hippocampal neurones. Reynolds *et al.* suggested that this loss of hippocampal neurones could conceivably result in disinhibition of limbic dopamine systems and provide an explanation whereby neuroleptic treatment ameliorates the symptoms of schizophrenia.

Earlier ligand-binding studies of the GABA receptor in postmortem brain samples did not reveal significant differences between controls and schizophrenics (Bennett *et al.*, 1979; Owen *et al.*, 1981b), although more recent studies have reported increased binding to receptors in prefrontal cortex and the caudate nucleus (Hanada *et al.*, 1987) and cingulate gyrus (Benes *et al.*, 1992) of schizophrenics.

Pharmacological evidence does not support a significant role for GABAergic deficiency in the aetiology of schizophrenia. Thus, the GABA agonist baclofen has been demonstrated to be ineffective, or even detrimental, in the treatment of schizophrenia (Simpson *et al.*, 1975). In addition, Tamminga *et al.* (1978) reported that the administration of muscimol, another powerful GABA agonist, had no therapeutic efficacy in schizophrenia.

Glutamate

Glutamate is the most important excitatory neurotransmitter in the CNS (Fonnum, 1984). Within the cerebral cortex, glutamate is the primary transmitter of pyramidal neurones, the principal excitatory neurones of the cortex, which give rise to the corticocortical association fibres. Other glutamate fibres constitute cortical projections to the basal ganglia and limbic structures and also circuits within the hippocampus. These and other glutamate-operated neuronal pathways are of interest in the context of the aetiology of schizophrenia. The cortical association fibres converge in areas of cortex which integrate information from primary sensory cortex and other cortical association areas (Peinado & Mora, 1986). Many of the symptoms of schizophrenia may result from a breakdown in integration of cortical function.

The discovery and characterization of multiple glutamate receptors has stimulated new assessments of the relationship of glutamate function to the aetiology and treatment of schizophrenia. Responses to glutamate are mediated by several receptor subtypes, each with a unique distribution, with the highest levels in the cortex, basal ganglia and hippocampus (Greenamyre *et al.*, 1985). At the behavioural level, the function of glutamatergic pathways is not established, but evidence suggests that the *N*-methyl-D-aspartate (NMDA) glutamate-receptor subtype plays a role in memory processes. Schizophrenia may involve disorders of memory which are presented clinically in the form of delusions. Investigation of the NMDA glutamate-receptor complex in schizophrenia is of particular interest in view of reports that a single dose of phencyclidine (PCP), an NMDA-specific ligand, can precipitate a schizophrenia-like psychosis in susceptible subjects (Aniline & Pitts, 1982), and exacerbate symptoms in previously stabilized patients (Luby *et al.*, 1959). The clinical picture of PCP psychosis includes both positive and negative schizophrenic symptoms and thus more closely resembles the illness than does the psychosis induced by amphetamine (Peterson & Stillman, 1978). The site of action of the PCP-like drugs appears to be associated with the ion channel gated by the NMDA receptor.

An early interest in glutamate function in schizophrenia followed the finding of reduced CSF glutamate levels in chronic schizophrenic subjects (Kim *et al.*, 1980). The authors drew attention to the putative relationship between dopamine and glutamate neurones, and suggested that a primary deficit in corticostriatal glutamate neurones could result in a reduction in glutamatergic inhibition of dopamine release, with a consequential increase in dopaminergic tone. However, using a different method, Perry (1982) failed to find evidence for a decrease in CSF glutamate. Other studies have failed to demonstrate abnormalities in glutamate concentrations in CSF (Gattaz *et al.*, 1985) and striatal or extrastriatal regions of postmortem brain tissue (Korpi *et al.*, 1987; Toru *et al.*, 1988; Perry *et al.*, 1989) of schizophrenic subjects. In a study of 33 schizophrenic and 25 control subjects, Korpi *et al.* (1987) examined tissue glutamate concentrations in a number of brain regions with no positive findings. In contrast, Kutay *et al.* (1989) reported increases in glutamate content in a wide range of brain regions. Sherman *et al.* (1991) recently reported a reduction in glutamate release in cortical synaptosomes, compatible with a reduced number of glutamate terminals in schizophrenic cerebral cortex. However, the main disadvantage of measurements of tissue glutamate concentration is that the results reflect both the metabolic and

neurotransmitter pools of glutamate, the latter being the smaller of the two. A more positive outcome has been achieved by examination of the receptors and reuptake sites associated with the glutamate system.

Whereas most neurochemical studies in schizophrenia have aspired to develop a hypothesis based on the deficit or excess of a single neurotransmitter, the structural pathology appears to involve abnormalities in the development of cortical neurones (Lyon *et al.*, 1989), particularly affecting the hippocampus and parahippocampal gyrus (Roberts & Crow, 1987). Since the pathology does not involve a neurodegenerative process, profound deficits in neurochemical markers are not to be expected. However, the neurochemical correlates of abnormal patterns of neuronal circuitry may be regionally and neurochemically diverse. In view of the importance of glutamatergic neurones within cortical pathways, the details of abnormalities in glutamatergic connectivity have recently been examined at the level of the glutamate receptors. Studies have focused on temporal lobe structures, including the limbic components (Kerwin *et al.*, 1988; Deakin *et al.*, 1989) and the frontal cortex (Nishikawa *et al.*, 1983; Deakin *et al.*, 1989). The general impression from these studies is that in medial temporal structures there are deficits in glutamatergic markers, whereas in frontal cortex there are increases in these sites. In a study of 14 schizophrenic and matched control subjects, Deakin *et al.* (1989) observed marginal left lateralized reductions in glutamate uptake sites, labelled by [^{3}H]D-aspartate, in polar temporal cortex and amygdala. In drug-free patients there were marked deficits on the left in polar temporal cortex and amygdala and bilaterally in the hippocampus (Deakin *et al.*, 1990). The deficits were proposed to be related to temporal lobe atrophy, and it was suggested that schizophrenia involves abnormal glutamatergic innervation within the temporal lobe. That the deficits were asymmetrical implies that the pathological process may be left lateralized. The demonstration of lateralized deficits could provide a clue to the pathological substrate for theories of abnormal lateralization of cerebral function in schizophrenia

(Flor-Henry, 1983). While there was no evidence of an abnormality in [³H]kainate binding in the temporal lobe (Deakin *et al.*, 1989), a comparable study reported a reduction in the number of kainate receptors in the left hippocampus (Kerwin *et al.*, 1988). This finding was supported by autoradiographic evidence of left-sided reductions in kainate receptors in the hippocampal CA3/CA4 region, with bilateral reductions in the denatate gyrus and parahippocampal gyrus (Kerwin *et al.*, 1990). In contrast, NMDA sites were unchanged, while quisqualate sites were marginally reduced in CA3/CA4. A loss of mRNA encoding a non-NMDA glutamate receptor in the CA3 hippocampal subfield (Harrison *et al.*, 1991) is further evidence of a glutamate deficit in the hippocampus.

It has been suggested that dysfunction of frontal areas may be critical to the development of negative symptoms in schizophrenia (Fuster, 1980). This has been inferred from the observation that damage to the frontal cortex can induce a 'deficit state'. Frontal cortex lesions may produce symptoms which are similar to the type-II symptoms of schizophrenia. Evidence of structural pathology of the frontal cortex in schizophrenia is limited, although some computerized tomography (CT) studies report dilatation of frontal sulci (Shelton & Weinberger, 1986). However, imaging studies have indicated that frontal lobe functioning may be abnormal in schizophrenia. In particular, Szechtman *et al.* (1988) demonstrated in nevermedicated schizophrenic subjects a resting hyperfrontality which they suggested might result from a hyperinnervation of frontal areas. Several studies have now provided direct evidence compatible with an excessive glutamatergic innervation of orbital frontal cortex in schizophrenia. In an early study, Nishikawa *et al.* (1983) investigated [³H]kainate binding sites in four prefrontal cortical areas; they reported an increase in the density (B_{max}) of [³H]kainate binding in the medial frontal and eye-movement areas, a finding that has since been replicated (Toru *et al.*, 1988). In a study of 14 schizophrenic and matched control subjects there were regionally specific, highly significant bilateral increases in glutamate-uptake sites in the

orbitofrontal cortex (Deakin *et al.*, 1989). Kainate receptors were similarly increased in the same brain area (Deakin *et al.*, 1989), as was the NMDA receptor complex, labelled using [³H]thienylcyclohexylpiperidine ([³H]TCP) (Simpson *et al.*, 1992a). These results are convincing testimony to an increase in the number of glutamate synapses in orbital frontal cortex, a conclusion sustained by the finding of an increase in the density of layer V pyramidal neurones in the prefrontal area (Benes *et al.*, 1991).

Evidence from lesion studies in rodents suggests that the 5-HT$_{1A}$ receptor subtype may also be associated with the cell bodies of pyramidal neurones of the corticostriatal pathway (Francis *et al.*, 1992). It was suggested that the 5-HT$_{1A}$ site in the superficial layers of the human cortex may be a component of glutamatergic pyramidal neurones projecting to other ipsilateral cortical areas. These neurones appear to possess a particularly high complement of 5-HT$_{1A}$ sites, which may be especially important in the human cortex for regulating the activity of association fibres (Francis *et al.*, 1992). A recent autoradiographic study has demonstrated a bilateral increase in 5-HT$_{1A}$ receptors in superficial laminae of three medial orbital gyri of male schizophrenic subjects (Simpson *et al.*, 1993). An increase in 5-HT$_{1A}$ receptor message has also recently been observed in the orbital frontal cortex of the same brains (Balderson *et al.*, 1993). These increases are compatible with the reports of bilateral increases in glutamate markers in the orbital frontal cortex (Deakin *et al.*, 1989; Simpson *et al.*, 1992a) and with the suggestion that binding to the 5-HT$_{1A}$ receptor in the cerebral cortex is intimately associated with glutamatergic pyramidal neurones. It was suggested that the excess of glutamate markers in frontal cortical areas could signify the presence of a profusion of glutamate synapses, resulting from an abnormally dense afferent innervation, owing to a failure in the developmental 'pruning' processes which remodel the immature callosal/temporal projections during development (Deakin *et al.*, 1989). Benes *et al.* (1992) recently reported that glutamate-immunoreactive vertical fibres were increased in the anterior cingulate cortex of schizophrenic brains, although not in the prefrontal cortex. On the basis of these findings they suggested that altered patterns of gluta-matergic association fibre connectivity may con-tribute to the pathophysiology of schizophrenic psychosis. This finding is consistent with the interpretation of changes in glutamate markers as being due to an overabundant glutamatergic innervation of the frontal cortex.

Although there is little evidence of gross struc-tural abnormalities within the basal ganglia (Bogerts *et al.*, 1985; Brown *et al.*, 1986), imaging studies have demonstrated reduced metabolic activity of the basal ganglia in unmedicated schizophrenic subjects (Buchsbaum *et al.*, 1982; Sedvall *et al.*, 1984; Gur *et al.*, 1987). Hypo-metabolism could indicate an abnormal pattern of neuronal connectivity within the basal ganglia, or it may be a secondary functional consequence of pathology in other brain regions. Thus, functional, cytoarchitectural or neurochemical abnormalities could occur in the absence of gross anatomical change. In particular, the reciprocal control mechanisms governing glutamatergic and dopa-minergic neurotransmission in the striatal complex have been regarded as a possible substrate for schizophrenic pathology. While the details of the organization of glutamatergic and dopaminergic inputs to the striatum are under review (Carlsson & Carlsson, 1990), the functional relationship between glutamate and dopamine continues to create interest (see Chapter 20, this volume). Kornhuber *et al.* (1989) reported a 44% increase in the binding of [^{3}H]methyl-10.11-dihydro-5-H-dibenzocyclohepten-5, 10,-imine ([^{3}H] MK801), a marker of NMDA-type glutamate receptors, in the putamen of schizophrenic subjects. They suggested that this increase could be due to an upregulation of the PCP−NMDA receptor complex in response to a putative presynaptic glutamate deficit. However, chronic neuroleptic treatment itself induces an upregulation of the NMDA-associated PCP binding site (Byrd *et al.*, 1987) and cannot be discounted as a mechanism underlying the increase in [^{3}H]MK801 binding in the putamen. Nevertheless, substantial (40%) deficits in glutamate-uptake sites in the putamen

and globus pallidus have recently been reported (Simpson *et al.*, 1992b). Abnormalities within the pallidum are of interest in view of the report of unilaterally elevated blood flow in the left globus pallidus of unmedicated schizophrenic subjects (Early *et al.*, 1987). Bogerts *et al.* (1985) reported that the medial pallidal segment was reduced in size in schizophrenic brain, suggesting that this area is involved in the pathological process. A disruption of the cortical glutamatergic input to the basal ganglia could be relevant to the develop-ment of psychosis but could also relate to the spectrum of mild motor disturbances often de-scribed in the disease (Manschrek, 1986). Auto-radiographic studies will be required to address the question of the topographic distribution of the neurochemical abnormalities.

Neuropeptides and schizophrenia

In recent years considerable research effort has focused on neuroactive peptides and at least 40 such peptides have been identified in mammalian brain. The possible role of certain neuropeptides, in particular the opioids, in the aetiology of schizophrenia has received much attention. The effects of administering opioids to rats led to opposing views on the possible relationships between brain opioid function and schizophrenia. Bloom *et al.* (1976) observed a marked catatonia in rats after intraventricular injections of endor-phins and postulated that schizophrenia was associated with increased brain opioid production. In the same year, Jacquet and Marks (1976) reported that injection of endorphins into the periaqueductal grey of the rat brain produced effects similar to those produced by neuroleptic drugs, and hence suggested that schizophrenia may result from an underactivity of an endogenous antipsychotic system, i.e. a deficit in central opioid function.

Neither of these hypotheses received consistent support from the research that followed. Terenius *et al.* (1976) reported that opioid fractions in CSF from schizophrenics were elevated compared with those in controls and that the concentrations decreased after neuroleptic medication. This was confirmed by some groups (Lindström *et al.*, 1978; Domschke *et al.*, 1979; Rimon *et al.*, 1980) but not by others (Naber *et al.*, 1981). There have also been conflicting reports of the effects of opioid antagonists on schizophrenic symptoms. Thus, naloxone was reported by some groups to have beneficial effects in schizophrenia (Davis *et al.*, 1977; Emrich *et al.*, 1977; Gunne *et al.*, 1977) but was reported to be ineffective by others (Janowsky *et al.*, 1977; Volovka *et al.*, 1977). The effect of naloxone administration on schizophrenic symptomatology was reviewed by Mackay (1979), who concluded that whether or not naloxone was beneficial in the treatment of schizophrenia remained an unanswered question. Nevertheless, Pickar *et al.* (1982) reported the results of a World Health Organization collaborative study which concluded that short-term administration of naloxone to schizophrenics produced a significant selective reduction in auditory hallucinations, thus providing some, but hardly impressive, evidence for overactivity of brain opioid mechanisms in schizophrenia.

An apparently promising report that renal dialysis produced a significant amelioration of the severity of schizophrenic symptoms, possibly through the removal of aberrant or excess opioids (Wagemaker & Cade, 1977), was not confirmed in subsequent studies (Ferris, 1977; Levy, 1977; Weddington, 1977; Begleiter *et al.*, 1981; Hariprasad *et al.*, 1981).

The administration of opioids to schizophrenic patients has also produced results that have not provided conclusive support for the hypothesis that schizophrenia is associated with a deficit in brain opioid function. Administration of β-endorphin has produced little or no effect on the severity of psychotic symptoms (Kline *et al.*, 1977; Berger *et al.*, 1980b; Gerner *et al.*, 1980; Pickar *et al.*, 1981). However, administration of des-tyrosine-gamma-endorphin (DTγE) has been reported to have therapeutic efficacy in some schizophrenic patients (Verhoeven *et al.*, 1979; Emrich *et al.*, 1980; Van Ree *et al.*, 1980; Van Praag *et al.*, 1982). A possible basis for the therapeutic effect of this opioid may be aberrant cleavage of the β-endorphin fragment

from its polypeptide precursor (Van Ree & DeWied, 1981). Studies on postmortem brain material have also produced inconclusive results. Kleinman *et al.* (1983) reported decreased met-encephalin levels in the caudate nucleus of paranoid schizophrenics, whereas Lightman *et al.* (1979) found no differences between controls and schizophrenics in the brain concentrations of β-endorphin.

Iadarola *et al.* (1991) reported elevated levels of the opiod met-5-encephalin-org 6-gly 7-leu 8 (MERL) in samples of substantia nigra from schizophrenics, and suggested that their results indicated a selective alteration in the encephalin innervation of this brain region in schizophrenia. Iadarola *et al.* pointed out, however, that they could not rule out the possibility that the increase in MERL levels resulted from neuroleptic treatment.

Opioid receptors have also been assessed in postmortem brain tissue by high-affinity ligand binding, although these studies too have been inconclusive. Thus, Reisine *et al.* (1980) reported that [^{3}H]naloxone binding was significantly reduced in basal ganglia samples from schizophrenics. Since naloxone binds with equal affinity to μ, δ and κ opiate subtypes, Owen *et al.* (1985) used [^{3}H]etorphine as the ligand and resolved the binding into its μ and δ plus κ components but found no difference in the high-affinity binding to opioid receptors in the basal ganglia of schizophrenics.

Investigations of neuroactive peptides other than opioids in schizophrenia have also produced inconclusive results. Ferrier *et al.* (1983) reported that cholecystokinin-like immunoreactivity (CCK-LI) was significantly decreased in postmortem samples of temporal cortex from chronic schizophrenics, and that there were also decreases in CCK-LI in the hippocampus and amygdala that was selective to patients with negative symptoms. However, Kleinman *et al.* (1983) assessed CCK-LI in several brain regions, including those studied by Ferrier *et al*, and found no differences between controls and schizophrenics in any of the brain regions. Farmery *et al.* (1985) reported reduced high-affinity binding of CCK[33] in samples of hippocampus and frontal cortex from chronic schizophrenics. Virgo *et al.* (1994) have recently reported large decreases in mRNA for CCK in frontal and temporal cortices of schizophrenics with no significant correlation between mRNA loss and neuroleptic medication. This novel finding obviously warrants verification.

It has been established that CCK coexists with dopamine in mesolimbic neurones (Hökfelt *et al.*, 1980) and it has been suggested that after intracerebral injection of CCK-related peptides in the rat, CCK inhibits limbic dopaminergic activity with behaviourial effects that resemble those of antipsychotic drugs (Van Ree *et al.*, 1983). However, there have been conflicting reports (reviewed by Nair *et al.*, 1985) of the effects of CCK administration to schizophrenic patients.

The concentration of vasoactive intestinal polypeptide-like immunoreactivity (VIP-LI) has been reported to be similar to control values in CSF samples from chronic schizophrenics (Gjerris *et al.*, 1981). Perry *et al.* (1981) also found VIP-LI in entorhinal cortex samples from schizophrenics to be no different from that in controls. Other postmortem brain studies, however, have produced equivocal results. Thus, Roberts *et al.* (1983) reported significant increases in VIP-LI in the amygdala of schizophrenics, whereas Carruthers *et al.* (1984) found VIP-LI in this brain region of schizophrenics to be no different from that in controls.

Somatostatin-like immunoreactivity (SRIF-LI) in CSF samples from schizophrenics has been reported to be similar to control values. In an investigation of SRIF-LI levels in postmortem brain tissue, Ferrier *et al.* (1983) reported that the concentrations of the peptide in several cortical regions were no different from control values. In the same study, Ferrier *et al.* reported increased SRIF-LI in the thalamus of schizophrenics and reduced levels in the hippocampus of patients with negative symptoms. Nemeroff *et al.* (1983), on the other hand, found reduced SRIF-LI in the frontal cortex of schizophrenics.

Measurements of neurotensin-like immunoreactivity (NT-LI) in postmortem brain samples have also yielded conflicting results. Thus,

Nemeroff *et al.* (1983) found reductions of NT-LI in frontal cortex samples from schizophrenics, whereas Biggins *et al.* (1983) and Roberts *et al.* (1983) found NT-LI levels in several brain regions from schizophrenics to be similar to those in controls. There is general agreement that neurotensin binding sites are increased specifically in the substantia nigra of schizophrenic patients (Uhl & Kuhar, 1984; Farmery *et al.*, 1986). It also seems clear that this increase is the result of neuroleptic medication.

More recently, Frederiksen *et al.* (1991) reported reductions in the levels of galanin, arginine, vasopressin, neuropeptide Y and peptide YY in temporal cortex samples, but not hypothalamus samples, from chronic schizophrenics. They presented some evidence to suggest that the reduction in peptide levels was not the result of neuroleptic medications.

It has been well established that some peptides interact with dopamine in the brain and also coexist in some neurones. It seems likely, therefore, that research into neuroactive peptides in relation to schizophrenia will continue.

Concluding remarks

The dopamine hypothesis remains the predominant theory of schizophrenia and is the rationale behind most neurochemical investigations of the disease. However, despite considerable effort, direct, unequivocal neurochemical evidence to support the hypothesis has yet to be produced. Thus, early reports of increased dopamine D_2 receptors in postmortem brain samples from schizophrenics continue to be confirmed by some, but not all, groups and the effect of neuroleptic medication on the findings has still not been satisfactorily determined. The application of sophisticated neuroimaging techniques to assess neurotransmitter receptors *in vivo* has, unexpectedly, failed to resolve the controversy over the state of the dopamine D_2 receptor in schizophrenia. Impetus for further work on dopamine receptors has come from the demonstration of five receptor subtypes (D_1-D_2) in human brain. Although no specific ligand is presently available for the D_4 receptor, Seeman *et al.* (1993), using an indirect technique, have recently reported a sixfold increase in the receptor subtype in postmortem brain samples from schizophrenics. Such a technique is inherently inaccurate and this result requires the development of a specific D_4 ligand for a realistic verification. Research on brain serotonergic, and to a lesser extent noradrenergic, systems continues apace. Direct evidence, from studies of postmortem brain tissue, for alterations in serotonergic or noradrenergic mechanisms in schizophrenia has been limited. However, there is currently a general movement away from single-system theories of schizophrenia with more emphasis being placed on theories based on neural systems. There is much evidence to suggest extensive interactions between brain monoaminergic systems, whereby they can effectively alter dopaminergic activity. Clearly, there is plenty of scope for more research on this aspect of brain function in relation to schizophrenia.

Amino acid neurotransmitters, particularly glutamate, are also currently receiving much attention. Although some changes in ligand binding to GABA receptors have been reported, it is the research on glutamate systems that appears to be more rewarding. The reciprocal control mechanisms governing brain dopaminergic and glutamatergic mechanisms has often been suggested as a substrate for neurochemical theories of schizophrenia and there is now a degree of agreement that glutamatergic systems are altered in the brains of schizophrenics. Deakin *et al.*, (1989) have suggested that findings indicating increased numbers of glutamate synapses in orbital frontal cortex of schizophrenics result from a failure in the normal developmental 'pruning' process that remodels immature projections to the frontal cortex during development. Modulation of glutamate systems has been recognized as being of potential therapeutic importance in schizophrenia, so brain glutamatergic mechanisms are likely to receive considerable attention in future investigations.

Research on neuropeptides in schizophrenia has produced many equivocal results. However, since it has been well established that some peptides interact with dopamine in the brain and coexist with the amine in some neurones, so it seems likely that research on neuropeptides in relation to schizophrenia will also continue.

References

Adolfsson, R., Gottfries, C.G., Oreland, L., Wiberg, A. & Winblad, B. (1980) Increased activity of brain and platelet monoamine oxidase in dementia of Alzheimer type. *Life Sciences*, 27, 1029–1034.

Angrist, B., Sathanathan, G., Wilk, S. & Gershon, S. (1974) Amphetamine psychosis: behavioural and biochemical aspects. *Journal of Psychiatry Research*, 11, 13–23.

Angulo, J.A., Coirini, H., Ledoux, M. & Schumacher, M. (1991) Regulation by dopaminergic neurotransmission of dopamine D_2 mRNA and receptor levels in the striatum and nucleus accumbens of the rat. *Molecular Brain Research*, 11, 161–166.

Aniline, O. & Pitts, F.N. (1982) Phencyclidine: a review and perspectives. *Critical Reviews in Toxicology*, 10, 145–177.

Arora, R.C. & Meltzer, H.Y. (1991) Serotonin$_2$ (5-HT$_2$) receptor binding in the frontal cortex of schizophrenic patients. *Journal of Neural Transmission*, 85, 19–29.

Ashcroft, G.W., Crawford, T.B.B., Eccleston, D. *et al.* (1966) 5-hydroxyindole compounds in the cerebrospinal fluid of patients with psychiatric or neurological disease. *Lancet*, ii, 1049–1052.

Bach, A.W.J., Lau, N.C., Johnson, D.L. & Roth, R.H. (1988) Cloning of human liver monoamine oxidase A and B: molecular basis of differences in enzymatic properties. *Proceedings of the National Academy of Sciences USA*, 85, 4934–4938.

Bacopoulos, N.G., Spokes, E.G., Bird, E.D. *et al.* (1979) Antipsychotic drug action in schizophrenic patients: effects on cortical dopamine metabolism after long-term treatment. *Science*, 205, 1405–1407.

Balderson, D.J., Roberts, D.A., Deakin, J.F.W. & Owen, F. (1993) The abundance of serotonin 5HT$_{1A}$ receptor mRNA in post-mortem brain samples from controls and schizophrenics. *British Journal of Clinical Pharmacology*, 36, 490P.

Baraban, J.M., Worley, P.F. & Snyder, S.H. (1989) Second messenger systems and psychoactive drug action: focus on the phosphoinositide system and lithium. *American Journal Psychiatry*, 146, 1251–1260.

Begleiter, H., Porjesz, B. & Chou, C.L. (1981) Dialysis in schizophrenia: a double-blind evaluation. *Science*, 211, 1066–1068.

Benes, F.M., McSparren, J., Bird, E.D., San Giovanni, J.P. & Vincent, S.L. (1991) Deficits in small interneurones in prefrontal and cingulate cortices of schizophrenic and schizoaffective patients. *Archives of General Psychiatry*, 48, 996–1001.

Benes, F.M., Sorensen, I., Vincent, S.L., Bird, E.D. & Sathi, M. (1992) Increased density of glutamate-immunoreactive vertical processes in superficial laminae in cingulate cortex of schizophrenic brain. *Cerebral Cortex*, **2**, 503–512.

Bennett, J.P., Enna, S.J., Bylund, D.B., Gillin, J.C. & Wyatt, R.J. (1979) Neurotransmitter receptors in frontal cortex of schizophrenics. *Archives of General Psychiatry*, **36**, 927–934.

Berger, P.A., Faull, K.F., Killowski, J. *et al.* (1980a) Cerebrospinal fluid monoamine metabolites in depression and schizophrenia. *American Journal of Psychiatry*, **137**, 174–180.

Berger, P.A., Watson, S.J., Akil, H. *et al.* (1980b) Beta-endorphin and schizophrenia. *Archives of General Psychiatry*, **37**, 635–640.

Berrettini, W.H., Proxiałeck, W. & Vogel, W.H. (1978) Decreased platelet monoamine oxidase activity in chronic schizophrenia shown with novel substrates. *Archives of General Psychiatry*, **35**, 600–605.

Biggins, J.A., Perry, E.K., McDermott, J.R., Smith, A.I., Perry, R.H. & Edwardson, J.A. (1983) Post-mortem levels of thyrotropin-releasing hormone and neurotensin in the amygdala in Alzheimer's disease, schizophrenia and depression. *Journal of the Neurological Sciences*, **58**, 117–122.

Bird, E.D. & Iversen, L.L. (1974) Huntington's chorea: post-mortem measurement of glutamic acid decarboxylase, choline acetyltransferase and dopamine in basal ganglia. *Brain*, **97**, 457–472.

Bird, E.D., Crow, T.J., Iversen, L.L. *et al.* (1979) Dopamine and homovanillic acid concentration in the post-mortem brain in schizophrenia. *Journal of Physiology*, **293**, 36–37.

Bird, E.D., Spokes, E.G., Barnes, J., MacKay, A.V., Iversen, L.L. & Shepherd, M. (1977) Increased brain dopamine and reduced glutamic acid decarboxylase and choline acetyltransferase activity in schizophrenia and related psychoses. *Lancet*, **ii**, 1157–1159.

Bird, E.D., Spokes, E.G., Barnes, J., MacKay, A.V., Iversen, L.L. & Shepherd, M. (1978) Glutamic-acid decarboxylase in schizophrenia. *Lancet*, **i**, 156.

Bloom, F.E., Segal, D., Ling, N. & Guillemin, R. (1976) Endorphins: profound behavioural effects in rats suggest new etiological factors in mental illness. *Science*, **194**, 630–632.

Bogerts, B., Meertz, E. & Schonfeldt-Bausch, R. (1985) Basal ganglia and limbic system pathology in schizophrenia: a morphometric study of brain volume and shrinkage. *Archives of General Psychiatry*, **42**, 784–791.

Bond, P.A. & Howlett, D.R. (1974) Measurements of the two conjugates of 3-methoxy-4-hydroxyphenylglycol in urine. *Biochemical Medicine*, **10**, 219–228.

Bond, P.A., Dimitrakoudi, M., Howlett, D.R. & Jenner, F.A. (1975) Urinary excretion of the sulphate and glucorunide of 3-methoxy-4-hydroxyphenylglycol in a manic-depressive patient. *Psychological Medicine*, **5**, 279–285.

Bowers, M.B. Jr (1970) Cerebrospinal fluid 5-hydroxyindoles and behaviour after L-tryptophan and pyridoxine administration to psychiatric patients. *Neuropharmacology*, **9**, 599–604.

Bowers, M.B. Jr (1974) Central dopamine turnover in schizophrenic syndromes. *Archives of General Psychiatry*, **31**, 50–57.

Bowers, M.B., Heninger, G.R. & Gerbode, F.A. (1969) Cerebrospinal fluid 5-hydroxyindole acetic acid and homo-

vanillic acid in psychiatric patients. *International Journal of Neuropharmacology*, **8**, 225–262.

Brown, R., Colter, N., Corsellis, J.A.N. *et al.* (1986) Postmortem evidence of structural brain changes in schizophrenia. Differences in brain weight, temporal horn area and parahippocampal gyrus compared with affective disorder. *Archives of General Psychiatry*, **43**, 36–42.

Buchsbaum, M.S., Ingvar, D.H., Kessler, R. *et al.* (1982) Cerebral glucography with positron tomography: use in normal subjects and patients with schizophrenia. *Archives of General Psychiatry*, **39**, 251–259.

Burt, D.R., Creese, I. & Snyder, S.M. (1982) Antischizophrenic drugs: chronic treatment elevates dopamine receptor binding in brain. *Science*, **196**, 326–328.

Byrd, J.C., Bykov, V. & Rothman, R. (1987) Chronic haloperidol treatment upregulates rat brain PCP receptors. *European Journal of Pharmacology*, **149**, 121–122.

Carlsson, M. & Carlsson, A. (1990) Interactions between glutamatergic and monoaminergic systems within the basal ganglia – implications for schizophrenia and Parkinson's disease. *Trends in Neurosciences*, **13**, 272–276.

Carruthers, B. Dawbarn, B., De Quidt, M. *et al.* (1984) Changes of the neuropeptide content of the amygdala in schizophrenia. *British Journal of Pharmacology*, **81**, 19OP.

Christmas, A.J., Coulson, C.J., Maxwell, D.R. & Riddell, D. (1972) A comparison of the pharmacological and biochemical properties of substrate-selective monoamine oxidase inhibitors. *British Journal of Pharmacology*, **45**, 490–503.

Civelli, O., Bunzow, J.R., Grawdy, D.K., Zhou, Q.Y. & Van Tol, H.H.M. (1991) Molecular biology of the dopamine receptors. *European Journal of Pharmacology*, **207**, 277–286.

Clement-Cormier, Y.C., Kebabian, J.W., Petzgold, G.L. & Greengard, P. (1974) Dopamine-sensitive adenylate cyclase in mammalian brains: a possible site of action of antipsychotic drugs. *Proceedings of the National Academy of Sciences USA*, **71**, 1113–1117.

Connell, P.H. (1958) *Amphetamine Psychosis*. Maudsley Monograph No. 5. Chapman & Hall, London.

Crawley, J.C.W., Crow, T.J., Johnstone, E.C. *et al.* (1986) Dopamine D_2 receptors in schizophrenia studied *in vivo*. *Lancet*, **ii**, 224–225.

Cross, A.J. & Owen, F. (1979) The activities of glutamic acid decarboxylase and choline acetyltransferase in post-mortem brains of schizophrenics and controls. *Biochemical Society Transactions*, **7**, 145–146.

Cross, A.J., Crow, T.J. & Owen, F. (1981) ^{3}H-Flupenthixol binding in post-mortem brains of schizophrenics; evidence for a selective increase in dopamine D_2 receptors. *Biochemical Society Transactions*, **7**, 145–146.

Cross, A.J., Owen, F. & Crow, T.J. (1979) Gamma-aminobutyric acid in the brain in schizophrenia. *Lancet*, **i**, 560–561.

Cross, A.J., Crow, T.J., Glover, V., Lofthouse, R., Owen, F. & Riley, G.J. (1977) Monoamine oxidase activity in post-mortem brains of schizophrenics and controls. *British Journal of Clinical Pharmacology*, **4**, 719P.

Cross, A.J., Crow, T.J., Killpack, W.S., Longden, A., Owen, F. & Riley, G.J. (1978) The activities of brain dopamine-β-hydroxylase and catechol-*o*-methyltransferase in schizophrenics and controls. *Psychopharmacology*, **59**, 117–121.

Crow, T.J. (1980) Molecular pathology of schizophrenia: more than one disease process? *British Medical Journal*, **280**, 66–68.

Crow, T.J., Baker, H.F., Cross, A.J. *et al.* (1979) Monoamine mechanisms in chronic schizophrenia:post-mortem neurochemical findings. *British Journal of Psychiatry*, **134**, 249–256.

Crow, T.J., Deakin, J.F.W., Johnstone, E.C. & Longden, A. (1976) Dopamine and schizophrenia. *Lancet*, **ii**, 563–566.

Czudek, C. & Reynolds, G.P. (1988) Binding of ^{3}H-SCH 23 390 to post-mortem brain tissue in schizophrenia. *British Journal of Pharmacology*, **95**, 282.

Das, I., Essali, M.A., de Belleroche, J. & Hirsch, S.R. (1992) Inositol phospholipid turnover in platelets of schizophrenic patients. *Prostaglandins Leukotrienes and Essential Fatty Acids*, **46**, 65–66.

Davis, G.C., Bunney, W.E. Jr, DeFraites, E.G. *et al.* (1977) Intravenous naloxone administration in schizophrenic and affective illness. *Science*, **197**, 74–77.

Deakin, J.F.W., Slater, P., Simpson, M.D.C. *et al.* (1989) Frontal cortical and left temporal glutamatergic dysfunction in schizophrenia. *Journal of Neurochemistry*, **52**, 1781–1786.

Deakin, J.F.W., Slater, P., Simpson, M.D.C. & Royston, M.C. (1990) Disturbed brain glutamate and GABA mechanisms in schizophrenia. *Schizophrenia Research*, **3(1)**, 33.

DeLisi, L.E., Wise, C.D., Bridge, T.P., Potkin, S.G. & Wyatt, R.J. (1981) A probable effect of neuroleptic medication on platelet monoamine oxidase activity. *Psychiatry Research*, **2**, 179–186.

Domino, E.F. & Khanna, S.S. (1976) Decreased blood platelet MAO activity in unmedicated chronic schizophrenic patients. *American Journal of Psychiatry*, **133**, 323–326.

Domino, E.F. & Krause, R.R. (1974) Free and bound serum tryptophan in drug-free normal controls and chronic schizophrenic patients. *Biological Psychiatry*, **8**, 265–279.

Domino, E.F., Krause, R.R. & Bowers, J. (1973) Various enzymes involved with putative neurotransmitters. *Archives of General Psychiatry*, **29**, 195–201.

Domschke, W., Dickschas, A. & Mitznegg, P. (1979) CSF β-endorphin in schizophrenia. *Lancet*, **i**, 1024.

Early, T.S., Reiman, E.M., Raichle, M.E. & Spitznagel, E.L. (1987) Left globus pallidus abnormality in never-medicated patients with schizophrenia. *Proceedings of the National Academy of Sciences USA*, **84**, 561–563.

Emrich, H.M., Cording, C., Piree, S., Kolling, A., von Zerssen, D. & Herz, A. (1977) Indication of antipsychotic action of the opiate antagonist naloxone. *Pharmakopsychiatria*, **10**, 265–270.

Emrich, H.M., Zaudig, M., Zerssen, D.V., Herz, A. & Kissling, W. (1980) Des-tyr-gamma-endorphin in schizophrenia. *Lancet*, **ii**, 1364–1365.

Essali, M.A., Das, I., de Belleroche, J. & Hirsch, S.R. (1992) Calcium mobilization in platelets from schizophrenic and healthy subjects. Regulation by lithium and neuroleptics. *Journal of Psychopharmacology*, **6**, 389–394.

Farde, L, Wiesel, F.A., Stone-Elander, S. *et al.* (1990) D$_2$ dopamine receptors in neuroleptic-naive schizophrenic patients. *Archives of General Psychiatry*, **47**, 213–219.

Farmery, S.M., Crow, T.J. & Owen, F. (1986) ^{125}I-Iodotyrosyl-neurotensin binding in post-mortem brain: comparison of controls and schizophrenics patients. *British Journal of Pharmacology*, **88**, 380P.

Farmery, S.M., Owen, F., Poulter, M. & Crow, T.J. (1985) Reduced high-affinity cholecystokinin binding in hippocampus and frontal cortex of schizophrenic patients. *Life Sciences*, **36**, 473–477.

Ferrier, I.N., Roberts, G.W., Crow, T.J. *et al.* (1983) Reduced CCK-LI and SST-LI in the limbic lobe is associated with negative symptoms in schizophrenia. *Life Sciences*, **33**, 475–482.

Ferris, G.N. (1977) Can dialysis help the chronic schizophrenic? *American Journal of Psychiatry*, **134**, 1310.

Flor-Henry, P. (1983) Commentary and synthesis. In Flor-Henry, P. & Gruzelier, J. (eds) *Laterality and Psychopathology*, pp. 1–18. Elsevier, Amsterdam.

Fonnum, F. (1984) Glutamate: a neurotransmitter in mammalian brain. *Journal of Neurochemistry*, **42**, 1–11.

Fowler, C.J., Carlsson, A. & Winblad, B. (1981) Monoamine oxidase-A and -B activities in the brain stem of schizophrenics and non-schizophrenic psychotics. *Journal of Neural Transmission*, **52**, 23–32.

Francis, P.T., Pangalos, M.N., Pearson, R.C.A., Middleriss, D.N., Stratmann, G.C. & Bowen, D.M. (1992) 5-Hydroxytryptamine-1A but not 5-hydroxytryptamine-2 receptors are enriched on neocortical pyramidal neurones destroyed by intrastriatal volkensin. *Journal of Pharmacology and Experimental Therapeutics*, **261**, 1273–1281.

Frederiksen, S.I., Ekman, R., Gottfries, C.G., Widerlöv, E. & Jonsson, S. (1991) Reduced concentrations of galanin, arginine vasopressin, neuropeptide Y and peptide YY in the temporal cortex but not in hypothalamus of brains from schizophrenics. *Acta Psychiatrica Scandinavica*, **83**, 273–277.

Friedhoff, A.J., Miller, J.C. & Weissefeund, J. (1978) Human platelet MAO in drug-free and medicated schizophrenic patients. *American Journal of Psychiatry*, **135**, 952–955.

Fuster, J. (1980) *The Prefrontal Cortex*. Raven Press, New York.

Fuxe, K., Hökfelt, T., Ljungdahl, A., Agnati, L., Johansson, O. & Perez de la Mora, M. (1975) Evidence for an inhibitory GABAergic control of the mesolimbic dopamine neurons: possibility of improving treatment of schizophrenia by combined treatment with neuroleptics and GABAergic drugs. *Medical Biology*, **53**, 177–183.

Gallant, D.M. & Bishop, M.P. (1968) Cinanserin (SQ 10,643): a preliminary evaluation in chronic schizophrenic patients. *Current Therapy Research*, **10**, 461–463.

Gattaz, W.F., Gasser, T. & Beckmann, H. (1985) Multidimensional analysis of the concentrations of 17 substances in the CSF of schizophrenics and controls. *Biological Psychiatry*, **20**, 360–365.

Gerner, R.H., Catlin, D.H., Gorelick, D.A., Hui, K.K. & Li, C.H. (1980) Beta-endorphin: intravenous infusion causes behavioural changes in psychiatric inpatients. *Archives of General Psychiatry*, **37**, 642–647.

Gillin, J.C., Kaplan, J.A. & Wyatt, R.J. (1976) Clinical effects of tryptophan in chronic schizophrenia. *Biological Psychiatry*, **11**, 635–639.

Gjerris, A., Fahrenkrug, J., Bujholm, S. & Rafaelson, O.J. (1981) Vasoactive intestinal polypeptide (VIP) in cerebrospinal fluid in psychiatric disorders. *Biological Psychiatry*, **16**, 359–362.

Goss, J.R., Kelly, A.B., Johnson, S.A. & Morgan, G. (1991) Haloperidol treatment increases D_2 dopamine receptor protein independently of RNA levels in mice. *Life Sciences*, **48**, 1015–1022.

Green, A.R. & Grahame-Smith, D.G. (1978) Process regulating the functional activity of brain 5-hydroxytryptamine: results of animal experiments and their relevance to the understanding and treatment of depression. *Pharmacopsychiatrica*, **11**, 3–16.

Greenamyre, J.T., Olsen, J.M.M., Penney, J.B. Jr & Young, A.B. (1985) Autoradiographic characterisation of *N*-methyl-D-aspartate, quisqualate- and kainate-sensitive glutamate binding sites. *Journal of Pharmacology and Experimental Therapeutics*, **33**, 254–263.

Griffiths, J.D., Cavanaugh, J., Held, J. & Oates, J.A. (1972) Dextramphetamine: evaluation of psychomimetic properties in man. *Archives of General Psychiatry*, **26**, 97–100.

Gruen, R., Baron, M., Levitt, M. & Asnis, L. (1982) Platelet MAO activity and schizophrenic prognosis. *American Journal of Psychiatry*, **139**, 240–241.

Gunne, L., Lindström, L. & Terenius, L.M. (1977) Naloxone-induced reversal of schizophrenic hallucinations. *Journal of Neural Transmission*, **40**, 13–19.

Gur, R.E., Resnick, S.M., Alavi, A. *et al.* (1987) Regional brain function in schizophrenia. I. A positron emission tomography study. *Archives of General Psychiatry*, **44**, 119–125.

Hanada, S., Mita, T., Nishimo, N. & Tanaka, C. (1987) [^{3}H]-Muscimol binding sites increased in autopsied brains of chronic schizophrenics. *Life Sciences*, **40**, 259–266.

Hariprasad, M.K., Nadler, I.M. & Eisinger, R.P. (1981) Hemodialysis for manic schizophrenics: no psychiatric improvement. *Journal of Clinical Psychiatry*, **42**, 215–216.

Harrison, P.J., Mclaughlin, D. & Kerwin, R.W. (1991) Decreased hippocampal expression of a glutamate receptor gene in schizophrenia. *Lancet*, i, 450–452.

Hartmann, E. (1976) Schizophrenia: a theory. *Psychopharmacology*, **49**, 1–15.

Hashimoto, S., Nishino, N., Nakai, H. & Tanaka, C. (1991) Increase in serotonin $5HT1_A$ receptors in prefrontal and temporal cortices of brains from patients with chronic schizophrenia. *Life Sciences*, **48**, 355–363.

Hess, E.J., Bracma, M.S., Kleinman, J.E. & Creese, I. (1987) Dopamine receptor subtype imbalance in schizophrenia. *Life Sciences*, **40**, 1487–1497.

Heuring, R.E. & Peroutka, S.J. (1987) Characterization of a novel [^{3}H]-5-hydroxytryptamine binding site subtype in bovine brain membranes. *Journal of Neuroscience*, **7**, 894–903.

Hökfelt, T., Rehfeld, J.F., Skirboll, L., Ivemark, B., Goldstein, M. & Markey, K. (1980) Evidence for coexistence of dopamine and CCK in mesolimbic neurons. *Nature*, **285**, 476–478.

Holden, J.M.C., Keskiner, A. & Gannon, P. (1971) A clinical trial of an antiserotonin compound, cinanserin, in chronic schizophrenia. *Journal of Clinical Pharmacology*, **11**, 220–226.

Iadarola, M.J., Ofri, D. & Kleinman, J.E. (1991) Enkephalin, dynorphin and substance P in post-mortem substantia nigra from normals and schizophrenic patients. *Life Sciences*, **48**, 1919–1930.

Jacquet, Y.F. & Marks, N. (1976) The C-fragment of β-lipoprotein: an endogenous neuroleptic or antipsychotic. *Science*, **194**, 632–635.

Janowsky, D.S., Segal, D.S., Bloom, F. *et al.* (1977) Lack of effect of naloxone on schizophrenic symptoms. *American Journal of Psychiatry*, **134**, 926–927.

Johnston, J.P. (1968) Some observations on a new inhibitor of monoamine oxidase in brain tissue. *Biochemical Pharmacology*, **17**, 1285–1297.

Johnstone, E.C., Crow, T.J., Frith, C.D., Carney, M.W. & Price, J.S. (1978) Mechanism of the antipsychotic effect in the treatment of acute schizophrenia. *Lancet*, i, 848–851.

Joseph, M.H., Baker, H.F., Crow, T.J., Riley, G.J. & Risby, D. (1979a) Brain tryptophan metabolism in schizophrenia: a post-mortem study of metabolites of the serotonin and kynurenine pathways in schizophrenic and control subjects. *Psychopharmacology*, **62**, 279–285.

Joseph, M.H., Baker, H.F., Johnstone, E.C. *et al.* (1976) Determination of 3-methoxy-4-hydroxyphenylglycol conjugates in urine. Application to the study of central noradrenaline metabolism in unmedicated chronic schizophrenic patients. *Psychopharmacology*, **51**, 47–51.

Joseph, M.H., Baker, H.F., Johnstone, E.C. & Crow, T.J. (1979b) 3-Methoxy-4-hydroxyphenylglycol excretion in acutely schizophrenic patients during a controlled clinical trial of the isomers of flupenthixol. *Psychopharmacology*, **64**, 35–40.

Joyce, J.N., Lexow, N., Bird, E. & Winokur, A. (1988) Organisation of dopamine D_1 and D_2 receptors in human striatum: receptor autoradiographic studies in Huntingtons's disease and schizophrenia. *Synapse*, **2**, 546–577.

Joyce, J.N., Lexow, N., Kim, S.J. *et al.* (1992) Distribution of beta-adrenergic receptor subtypes in human post-mortem brain: alterations in limbic regions of schizophrenics. *Synapse*, **10**, 228–246.

Joyce, J.N., Shane, A., Lexow, N., Winokur, A., Casanova, M.F. & Kleinman, J.E. (1993) Serotonin uptake sites and serotonin receptors are altered in limbic systems of schizophrenics. *Neuropharmacology*, **8**, 315–316.

Kebabian, J.W. & Calne, D.B. (1979) Multiple receptors for dopamine. *Nature*, **271**, 93–96.

Kerwin, R.W., Patel, S. & Meldrum, B.S. (1990) Quantitative autoradiographic analysis of glutamate binding sites in the hippocampal formation in normal and schizophrenic brain post mortem. *Neuroscience*, **39**, 25–32.

Kerwin, R.W., Patel, S., Meldrum, B.S., Czudek, C. & Reynolds, G.P. (1988) Asymmetrical loss of glutamate receptor sub-type in left hippocampus in schizophrenia. *Lancet*, i, 583–584.

Kim, J.S., Kornhuber, H.H., Schmid-Burgk, W. & Holzmuller, B. (1980) Low cerebrospinal fluid glutamate in schizophrenic patients and a new hypothesis on schizophrenia. *Neuroscience Letters*, **20**, 379–383.

Kleinman, J.E., Iadorola, M., Govoni, S. *et al.* (1983) Post-mortem measurements of neuropeptides in human brain. *Psychopharmacology Bulletin*, **8**, 375–377.

Kline, N.S., Li, C.H., Lehmann, H.E., Lajtha, A., Laski, E. & Cooper, T. (1977) Beta-endorphin-induced changes in schizophrenia and depressed patients. *Archives of General Psychiatry*, **34**, 111–113.

Knoll, J. & Magyar, K. (1972) Some puzzling pharmacological effects of monoamine oxidase inhibitors. *Advances in Biochemical Psychopharmacology*, **5**, 393–408.

Kornhuber, J., Mack-Burkhardt, F., Riederer, P. *et al.* (1989) 3H-MK-801 binding sites in post-mortem brain regions of schizophrenic patients. *Journal of Neural Transmission*, **77**, 231–236.

Korpi, E.R., Kleinman, J.E., Goodman, S.I. & Wyatt, R.J. (1987) Neurotransmitter amino acids in post-mortem brains of chronic schizophrenic patients. *Psychiatry Research*, **22**, 291–301.

Kutay, F.Z., Pogun, S., Hariri, N., Peker, G. & Erlacin, S. (1989) Free amino acid level determinations in normal and schizophrenic brain. *Progress in Neuropsychopharmacology and Biological Psychiatry*, **13**, 119–126.

Laruelle, M., Abi-Dargham, A., Casanova, M., Toti, R., Weinberger, D.R. & Kleinman, J.E. (1993) Selective abnormality of prefrontal serotonergic receptors in schizophrenia: a post-mortem study. *Archives of General Psychiatry*, **50**, 810–818.

Lauer, J.W., Inskip, W.M., Bernsohn, J. & Zeller, E.A. (1958) Observations on schizophrenic patients after iproniazid and tryptophan. *Archives of Neurology and Psychiatry*, **80**, 122–130.

Lee, T. & Seeman, P. (1980) Elevation of brain neuroleptic-dopamine receptors in schizophrenia. *American Journal of Psychiatry*, **137**, 191–197.

Lee, T., Seeman, P., Tourtellotte, W.W., Farley, I.J. & Hornykiewicz, O. (1978) Binding of ³H-neuroleptics and ³H-apomorphine in schizophrenic brains. *Nature*, **274**, 897–900.

Leonhardt, S., Herrick-Davis, K. & Titeler, M. (1989) Detection of a novel serotonin receptor subtype (5-HT$_{1e}$) in human brain: interaction with a GTP-binding protein. *Journal of Neurochemistry*, **53**, 465–471.

Levy, N.B. (1977) Can dialysis help the chronic schizophrenic? *American Journal of Psychiatry*, **134**, 1311.

Leyson, J.E., Niemegeers, C.J.E., Tollenwaere, J.P. *et al.* (1978) Serotonergic component of neuroleptic receptors. *Nature*, **272**, 168–171.

Lightman, S.L., Spokes, E.G., Sagnella, G.A., Gordon, D. & Bird, E.D. (1979) Distribution of β-endorphin in normal and schizophrenic human brains. *European Journal of Clinical Investigation*, **9**, 377–379.

Lindström, L.H., Widerlöv, E., Gunne, L.M., Wahlström, A. & Terenius, L. (1978) Endorphins in human cerebrospinal fluid: clinical correlations to some psychotic states. *Acta Psychiatrica Scandinavica*, **57**, 152–164.

Luby, E.D., Cohen, B.D., Rosenbaum, G., Gottlieb, J.S. & Kelley, R. (1959) Study of a new schizophrenomimetic drug, Sernyl. *Archives of Neurology and Psychiatry*, **81**, 363–369.

Lyon, M., Barr, C.E., Cannon, T.D., Mednick, S.A. & Shore, D. (1989) Fetal neural development and schizophrenia. *Schizophrenia Bulletin*, **15**, 149–161.

Maas, J.W. & Landis, D.H. (1968) *In vivo* studies of the metabolism of norepinephrine in the central nervous system. *Journal of Pharmacology and Experimental Therapeutics*, **163**, 147–162.

Maas, J.W., Dekirmenjian, H., Garver, D., Redmond, D.E. Jr & Landis, D.H. (1973) Excretion of catecholamine metabolites following intraventricular injection of 6-hydroxydopamine in the macaca speciosa. *European Journal of Pharmacology*, **23**, 121–130.

McGeer, P.L. & McGeer, E.G. (1977) Possible changes in stiatal and limbic cholinergic systems in schizophrenia. *Archives of General Psychiatry*, **34**, 1319–1323.

Mackay, A.V.P. (1979) Psychiatric implications of endorphin research. *British Journal of Psychiatry*, **135**, 470–473.

Mackay, A.V.P., Bird, E.D., Spokes, E.G. *et al.* (1980) Dopamine receptors and schizophrenia: drug effect or illness? *Lancet*, **ii**, 915–916.

Mann, J.J., Kaplan, R.D., Georgotas, A., Friedman, E., Branchey, M. & Gershon, S. (1981) Monoamine oxidase activity and enzyme kinetics in three sub-populations of density-fractionated platelets in chronic paranoid schizophrenics. *Psychopharmacology*, **74**, 344–348.

Manowitz, P., Gilmour, D.G. & Racevskis, J. (1973) Low plasma tryptophan levels in recently hospitalized schizophrenics. *Biological Psychiatry*, **6**, 109–118.

Manschrek, T.C. (1986) Motor abnormalities in schizophrenia. In Nasrallah, H.A. & Weinberger, D.R. (eds) *Handbook of Schizophrenia*, Vol. 1, *The Neurology of Schizophrenia*, pp. 65–96. Elsevier, Amsterdam.

Martinot, J.L., Peron-Magnan, P., Huret, J.D. *et al.* (1990) Striata D$_2$ dopaminergic receptors assessed with positron emission tomography and [⁷⁶Br] bromospiperone in untreated schizophrenic patients. *American Journal of Psychiatry*, **147**, 44–50.

Miller, R.J., Horn, A.S. & Iversen, L.L. (1974) The action of neuroleptic drugs on dopamine stimulated-3′–5′-monophosphate production in neostriatum and limbic forebrain. *Molecular Pharmacology*, **10**, 759–766.

Mita, T., Hanada, S., Nishino, N. *et al.* (1986) Decreased serotonin S$_2$ and increased dopamine D$_2$ in chronic schizophrenics. *Biological Psychiatry*, **21**, 1407–1414.

Murphy, D.L. & Wyatt, R.J. (1972) Reduced platelet monoamine oxidase activity in chronic schizophrenia. *Nature*, **238**, 225–226.

Murphy, D.L., Belmaker, R. & Wyatt, R.J. (1974) Monoamine oxidase in schizophrenia and other behaviour disorders. *Journal of Psychiatry Research*, **11**, 221–247.

Murphy, D.L., Donelly, C.H., Miller, L. & Wyatt, R.J. (1976) Platelet monoamine oxidase in chronic schizophrenia: some enzyme characteristics relevant to reduced activity. *Archives of General Psychiatry*, **33**, 1377–1381.

Naber, D., Pickar, D., Post, R.M. *et al.* (1981) Endogenous opioid activity and β-endorphin immunoreactivity in csf of psychiatric patients and normal volunteers. *American Journal of Psychiatry*, **138**, 1457–1462.

Nahorski, R.N., Kendall, D.A. & Batty, I. (1986) Receptors

and phosphoinositide metabolism in the central nervous system. *Biochemical Pharmacology*, **35**, 2447–2453.

Nair, N.P.V., Lal, S. & Bloom, D.M. (1985) Cholecystokinin peptides, dopamine and schizophrenia — a review. *Progress in Neuropsychopharmacology and Biological Psychiatry*, **9**, 515–524.

Nemeroff, C.B., Mawberg, P.J., Widerlöv, E. *et al.* (1983) Neuropeptides in cerebrospinal fluid and post-mortem brain tissue of schizophrenics, Huntington's choreics and normal controls. *Psychopharmacology Bulletin*, **19**, 369–374.

Nishikawa, T., Takasima, M. & Toru, M. (1983) Increased ^{3}H-kainic acid binding in the pre-frontal cortex in schizophrenia. *Neuroscience Letters*, **40**, 245–250.

Nyback, H., Berggren, B.M., Hindmarsh, T., Sedvall, G. & Wiesel, F.A. (1983) Cerebroventricular size and cerebrospinal fluid monoamine metabolites in schizophrenic patients and healthy volunteers. *Psychiatry Research*, **9**, 301–308.

Ohouha, D.C., Hyde, T.M. & Kleinman, J.E. (1993) The role of serotonin in schizophrenia: an overview of the nomenclature, distribution and alterations of serotonin receptors in the central nervous system. *Psychopharmacology*, **112**, S5–S15.

Owen, F., Bourne, R.C., Crow, T.J., Fadhli, A.A. & Johnstone, E.C. (1981a) Platelet monoamine oxidase activity in acute shizophrenia: relationship to symptomatology and neuroleptic mediation. *British Journal of Psychiatry*, **139**, 16–22.

Owen, F., Bourne, R.C., Crow, T.J., Johnstone, E.C., Bailey, A.R. & Hershon, H.I. (1976) Platelet monoamine oxidase in schizophrenia: an investigation in drug-free chronic hospitalized patients. *Archives of General Psychiatry*, **33**, 1370–1373.

Owen, F. Bourne, R.C., Poulter, M., Crow, T.J., Paterson, S.J. & Kosterlitz, H.W. (1985) Tritiated etorphine and naloxone binding to opioid receptors in caudate nucleus in schizophrenics. *British Journal of Psychiatry*, **21**, 507–509.

Owen, F., Cross, A.J., Crow, T.J., Longden, A., Poulter, M. & Riley, G.J. (1978) Increased dopamine receptor sensitivity in schizophrenia. *Lancet*, **ii**, 223–226.

Owen, F., Cross, A.J., Crow, T.J., Lofthouse, R. & Poulter, M. (1981b) Neurotransmitter receptors in brain in schizophrenia. *Acta Psychiatrica Scandinavica*, **63**, (Suppl. 291), 20–28.

Owen, F., Crow, T.J., Frith, C.D. *et al.* (1987) Selective decreases in MAO-B activity in post-mortem brains from schizophrenic patients with type II syndrome. *British Journal of Psychiatry*, **151**, 514–519.

Pearlson, G.D., Tune, L.E., Wong, D.F. *et al.* (1993) Quantitative D_2 dopamine receptor PET and structural MRI changes in late-onset schizophrenia. *Schizophrenia Bulletin*, **19**, 783–795.

Peinado, J.M. & Mora, F. (1986) Glutamic acid as a putative transmitter of the interhemispheric corticocortical connections in the rat. *Journal of Neurochemistry*, **47**, 1598–6030.

Peroutka, S.J. (1988) 5-Hydroxytryptamine receptor subtypes: molecular biochemical and physiological characterization. *Trends in Neurosciences*, **11**, 496–500.

Perry, R.H., Dockray, G.J., Dimaline, R. *et al.* (1981) Neuropeptides in Alzheimer's disease, depression and schizophrenia. *Journal of Neurological Science*, **51**, 465–472.

Perry, T.L. (1982) Normal cerebrospinal fluid and glutamate levels do not support the hypothesis of abnormal gluataminergic neuronal dysfunction. *Neuroscience Letters*, **28**, 81–85.

Perry, T.L., Hansen, S. & Jones, K. (1989) Schizophrenia, tardive dyskinesia and brain GABA. *Biological Psychiatry*, **25**, 200–206.

Perry, T.L., Hansen, S. & Kloster, M. (1973) Huntington's chorea: deficiency of γ-aminobutyric acid in brain. *New England Journal of Medicine*, **288**, 337–342.

Perry, T.L., Kish, S.J., Buchanan, J. & Hansen, S. (1979) γ-Aminobutyric-acid deficiency in brain of schizophrenic patients. *Lancet*, **i**, 237–239.

Peterson, R.C. & Stillman, R.C. (1978) Phencyclidine: an overview. In *Phencyclidine Abuse: An Appraisal. National Institute of Drug Abuse Research Monograph*, **21**, 1–7.

Pickar, D., David, G.C., Schulz, S.C. *et al.* (1981) Behavioural and biological effects of acute beta-endorphin injection in schizophrenic and depressed patients. *American Journal of Psychiatry*, **138**, 160–166.

Pickar, D., Vartanian, F., Bunney, W.E. Jr *et al.* (1982) Short-term naloxone administration in schizophrenic and manic patients. *Archives of General Psychiatry*, **39**, 313–319.

Pierce, P.A. & Peroutka, S.J. (1989) Evidence for distinct 5-hydroxytryptamine binding site subtypes in cortical brain preparations. *Journal of Neurochemistry*, **52**, 656–658.

Pollin, W., Cardin, P.V. & Kety, S.S. (1961) Effects of amino acid feedings in schizophrenic patients treated with isoniazid. *Science*, **133**, 104–105.

Post, R.M., Fink, E. & Carpenter, W.T. (1975) Cerebrospinal fluid amine metabolites in acute schizophrenia. *Archives of General Psychiatry*, **32**, 1063–1069.

Potkin, S.G., Weinberger, D.R., Linnoila, M. & Wyatt, R.J. (1983) Low CSF 5-hydroxyindoleacetic acid in schizophrenic patients with enlarged ventricles. *American Journal of Psychiatry*, **140**, 21–25.

Reisine, T.D., Rossor, M., Spokes, E., Iversen, L.L. & Yamamura, H.I. (1980) Opiate and neuroleptic receptor alterations in human schizophrenic brain tissue. *Advances in Biochemical Psychopharmacology*, **21**, 443–450.

Revely, M.A., Glover, V., Sandler, M. & Spokes, E.G. (1981) Brain monoamine oxidase activity in schizophrenics and controls. *Archives of General Psychiatry*, **38**, 663–665.

Reynolds, G.P. (1983) Increased concentrations and lateral asymmetry of amygdala dopamine in schizophrenia. *Nature*, **305**, 527–528.

Reynolds, G.P., Czudek, C. & Andrews, H.B. (1990) Deficit and hemisphere asymmetry of GABA uptake sites in hippocampus in schizophrenia. *Biological Psychiatry*, **27**, 1038–1044.

Reynolds, G.P., Reynolds, L.M., Riederer, P., Jellinger, K. & Gabriel, E. (1980) Dopamine receptors and schizophrenia: drug effect or illness. *Lancet*, **ii**, 1251.

Richardson, B.P., Engel, G., Donatsch, P. & Stadler, P.A. (1985) Identification of serotonin M-receptor subtypes and their specific blockade by a new class of drugs. *Nature*, **316**, 126–131.

Rimon, R., Terenius, L. & Kampman, R. (1980) Cerebrospinal fluid endorphins in schizophrenia. *Acta Psychiatrica*

Scandinavica, **61**, 395−403.

Roberts, D.A., Balderson, D.J., Deakin, J.W.F. & Owen, F. (1993) The abundance of D_2 receptor mRNA isoforms in brain samples from controls and schizophrenics. *British Journal of Clinical Pharmacology*, **36**, 491P.

Roberts, E. (1972) An hypothesis suggesting that there is a defect in the GABA system in schizophrenia. *Neuroscience Research Program Bulletin*, **10**, 468−482.

Roberts, E. (1977) The γ-aminobutyric acid system and schizophrenia. In Usdin, E. & Barchas, J.D. (eds) *Neuroregulators and Psychiatric Disorders*, pp. 347−357. Oxford University Press, Oxford.

Roberts, G.W. & Crow, T.J. (1987) The neuropathology of schizophrenia: a progress report. *British Medical Bulletin*, **43**, 599−615.

Roberts, G.W., Ferrier, I.N., Lee, Y. *et al.* (1983) Peptides, the limbic lobe and schizophrenia. *Brain Research*, **288**, 199−211.

Robinson, D.S., Lovenberg, W., Keiser, H. & Sjoerdsma, A. (1968) Effects of drugs on human blood platelet and plasma amine oxidase activity *in vitro* and *in vivo*. *Biochemical Pharmacology*, **17**, 109−119.

Santiago, M., Machado, A. & Cano, J. (1993) Regulation of the prefrontal cortical dopamine released by $GABA_A$ and $GABA_B$ receptor agonists and antagonists. *Brain Research*, **630**, 28−31.

Schmauss, C., Haroutunian, V., Davis, K.L. & Davidson, M. (1993) Selective loss of dopamine D_3-type receptor mRNA expression in parietal and motor cortices of patients with chronic schizophrenia. *Proceedings of the National Academy of Sciences USA*, **90**, 8942−8946.

Schwartz, M.A., Aikens, A.N. & Wyatt, R.J. (1974) Monoamine oxidase activity in brains from schizophrenics and mentally normal individuals. *Psychopharmacologia*, **38**, 319−328.

Sedvall, G., Blomqvist, G., DePaulis, E. *et al.* (1984) PET studies on brain energy metabolism and dopamine receptors in schizophrenic patients and monkeys. In *Psychiatry; The State of the Art*, Vol. 2, pp. 305−312. Plenum Press, New York.

Sedvall, G., Farde, L., Persson, A. & Wiese, F.A. (1986) Imaging of neurotransmitter receptors in the living human brain. *Archives of General Psychiatry*, **43**, 995−1005.

Seeman, P., Hong-Chang, G. & Van Tol, H.H.M. (1993) Dopamine D4 receptors elevated in schizophrenia. *Nature*, **365**, 441−445.

Seeman, P., Chau-Wong, M., Tedesco, J. & Wong, K. (1975) Brain receptors for antipsychotic drugs and dopamine: direct binding assays. *Proceedings of the National Academy of Sciences USA*, **72**, 4376−4380.

Seeman, P., Hong-Chang & Van Tol, H.M.M. (1993) Dopamine D_4 receptors elevated in schizophrenia. *Nature*, **336**, 441−445.

Shelton, R.C. & Weinberger, D.R. (1986) X-ray computerised tomography studies of schizophrenia: a review and synthesis. In Nasrallah, H.A. & Weinberger, D.R. (eds) *The Neurology of Schizophrenia*, pp. 537−583. Elsevier, Amsterdam.

Sherman, A.D., Davidson, A.T., Baruah, S., Hegwood, T.S. & Waziri, R. (1991) Evidence of glutamatergic deficiency in

schizophrenia. *Neuroscience Letters*, **121**, 77−80.

Simpson, G.M., Lee, J.H., Shrivastva, R.K. & Branchy, M.M. (1975) Baclofen in schizophrenia. *Lancet*, **i**, 966−967.

Simpson, M.D.C., Slater, P. & Deakin, J.F.W. (1993) The autoradiographic distribution of abnormalities in $5HT_{1a}$ receptors in ventromedial prefrontal cortex in schizophrenia. *British Journal of Clinical Pharmacology*, **36**, 505.

Simpson, M.D.C., Slater, P., Royston, M.C. & Deakin, J.F.W. (1992a) Alterations in phencyclidine and sigma binding sites in schizophrenic brains: effects of disease process and neuroleptic medication. *Schizophrenia Research*, **6**, 41−48.

Simpson, M.D.C., Slater, P., Royston, M.C. & Deakin, J.F.W. (1992b) Regionally selective deficits in uptake sites for glutamate and gamma-aminobutyric acid in the basal ganglia in schizophrenia. *Psychiatry Research*, **42**, 273−282.

Srivastava, L.K., Morency, M.A., Bajwa, S.B. & Mishra, R.K. (1990) Effect of haloperidol on expression of dopamine D_2 receptor mRNAs in rat brain. *Journal of Molecular Neuroscience*, **2**, 155−161.

Stein, L. & Wise, C.D. (1971) Possible etiology of schizophrenia: progressive damage to the nonadrenergic reward system by 6-hydroxydopamine. *Science*, **171**, 1032−1036.

Sunahara, R.K., Guan, H.C., O'Dowd, B.F. *et al.* (1991) Cloning a human dopamine D5 gene with higher affinity for dopamine than D1. *Nature*, **350**, 614−617.

Szechtman, H., Nahmias, C., Garnett, S. *et al.* (1988) Effect of neuroleptics on altered cerebral glucose metabolism in schizophrenia. *Archives of General Psychiatry*, **45**, 523−532.

Takahashi, S., Yamane, H. & Naosuke, T. (1975) Reduction in blood platelet monoamine oxidase in schizophrenic patients on phenothiazines. *Folia Psychiatrica Neurologic Japonica*, **29**, 207−214.

Tamminga, C.A., Crayton, J.W. & Chase, T.N. (1978) Muscimol: GABA agonist therapy in schizophrenia. *American Journal of Psychiatry*, **135**, 746−747.

Terenius, L., Wahlström, A., Lindström, C. & Widerlöv, E. (1976) Increased CSF levels of endorphins in chronic psychosis. *Neuroscience Letters*, **3**, 157−162.

Toru, R.W., Watanabe, S., Shibuia. H. *et al.* (1988) Neurotransmitters, receptors and neuropeptides in post-mortem brains of schizophrenic patients. *Acta Psychiatrica Scandinavica*, **78**, 121−137.

Uhl, G.R. & Kuhar, M.J. (1984) Chronic neuroleptic treatment enhances neurotensin receptor binding in human and rat substantia nigra. *Nature*, **309**, 350−352.

Van Praag, H.M., Verhoeven, W.M.A., Van Ree, J.M. & De Wied, D. (1982) The treatment of schizophrenic psychoses with gamma-tyr-endorphins. *Biological Psychiatry*, **17**, 83−98.

Van Ree, J.M. & De Wied, D. (1981) Endorphins in schizophrenia. *Neuropharmacology*, **20**, 1271−1277.

Van Ree, J.M., De Wied, D., Verhoeven, W.M.A. & Van Praag, J. (1980) Antipsychotic effect of gamma-tyr endorphins in schizophrenia. *Lancet*, **ii**, 1363−1364.

Van Ree, J.M., Gaffori, O. & De Wied, D. (1983) In rats the behavioural profile of CCK-8 related peptides resembles that of antipsychotic agents. *European Journal of Pharmacology*, **93**, 63−78.

Van Tol, H.M.M., Riva, M., Civelli, O. & Crease, I. (1990)

Lack of effect of chronic dopamine receptor blockade on dopamine receptor mRNA level. *Neuroscience Letters*, **III**, 303–308.

Verhoeven, W.M.A., Van Praag, H.M., Van Ree, J.M. & De Wied, D. (1979) Improvement of schizophrenic patients treated with (des-tyr' -gamma-endorphin (DTγE). *Archives of General Psychiatry*, **36**, 294–298.

Virgo, L., De Belleroche, J., Barnes, T., Mortimer, A. & Hirsch, S. (1994) Differential changes in gene expression in cortical areas give insight into functional abnormalities occurring in schizophrenia. *Schizophrenia Research*, **11**, 126.

Vogel, W.H., Orfei, V. & Century, B. (1969) Activities of enzymes involved in the formation and destruction of biogenic amines in various areas of human brain. *Journal of Pharmacology and Experimental Therapeutics*, **165**, 196–203.

Volovka, J., Mallya, A., Baig, S. & Perez-Cruet, J. (1977) Naloxone in chronic schizophrenia. *Science*, **196**, 1227–1228.

Wagemaker, H.J. & Cade, R. (1977) The use of hemodialysis in chronic schizophrenia. *American Journal of Psychiatry*, **134**, 684–685.

Weddington, W.W. Jr (1977) Can dialysis help the chronic schizophrenic. *American Journal of Psychiatry*, **134**, 1310.

Whitaker, P.M., Crow, T.J. & Ferrier, I.N. (1981) Tritiated LSD binding in frontal cortex in schizophrenia. *Archives of General Psychiatry*, **38**, 278–280.

Wise, C.D. & Stein, L. (1973) Dopamine-β-hydroxylase deficits in the brains of schizophrenic patients. *Science*, **181**, 344–347.

Wise, C.D., Baden, M.M. & Stein, L. (1974) Post-mortem measurement of enzymes in human brain: evidence of a central noradrenergic deficit in schizophrenia. *Journal of Psychiatry Research*, **11**, 185–198.

Wong, D.F., Wagner, H.N. Jr, Tune, L.E. *et al.* (1986) Positron emission tomography reveals elevated D_2 dopamine receptors in drug-naive schizophrenics. *Science*, **234**, 1558–1562.

Wooley, D.W. & Shaw, E. (1954) A biochemical and pharmacological suggestion about certain mental disorders. *Proceedings of the National Academy of Sciences USA*, **40**, 228–231.

Wyatt, R.J., Murphy, D.L., Belmaker, R., Cohen, S., Donnelly, C.H. & Pollin, W. (1973) Reduced monoamine oxidase activity in platelets. A possible genetic marker for vulnerability to schizophrenia. *Science*, **179**, 916–918.

Wyatt, R.J., Schwarz, M.A., Erdelyi, E. & Barchas, J.D. (1975) Dopamine-β-hydroxylase activity in brains of chronic schizophrenic patients. *Science*, **187**, 368–370.

Wyatt, R.J., Vaughan, T., Calanter, M., Kaplan, J. & Green, R. (1972) Behavioural changes of chronic schizophrenic patients given L-5-hydroxytryptophan. *Science*, **177**, 1124–1126.

Chapter 20
The Dopamine Theory Revisited

A. CARLSSON

Introduction

In 1958, dopamine was identified and quantified as a normal brain constituent and was proposed to serve as an agonist in its own right in the control of psychomotor activity, in addition to its previously recognized role as a precursor to noradrenaline and adrenaline (Carlsson *et al.*, 1958). Reserpine was found to induce depletion of dopamine, and its psychomotor inhibitory action could be restored by the dopamine precursor L-dopa. In 1963, a specific stimulating action on dopamine (and noradrenaline) turnover of the major neuroleptics chlorpromazine and haloperidol was discovered and proposed to be due to blockade of dopamine (and noradrenaline) receptors (Carlsson & Lindqvist, 1963). When these studies were extended to a large number of antipsychotic agents, blockade of dopamine receptors, rather than of adrenergic receptors, appeared to be the common denominator (Andén *et al.*, 1970; Nybäck & Sedvall, 1970; Carlsson, 1978). This led to the notion that blockade of dopamine receptors is the most essential component in the action of the major antipsychotic agents. Similar views had been expressed by van Rossum (1966).

Abbreviations

7-OHDPAT: 7-hydroxy-2-(dipropylamino)tetraline

AP-5: DL--2-amino-5-phosphonopentanoic acid

MPTP: 1-methyl-4-phenyl-1,2,5,6-tetrahydropyridine

CPPene: 3-(2-carboxypiperazine-4-yl)-1-propenyl-1-phosphonic acid

DARPP-32: dopamine and cyclic AMP-regulated phosphoprotein-32

Today, there is overwhelming evidence that the major antipsychotic agents are capable of blocking dopamine receptors. Thus, they have been shown to antagonize the central actions of dopamine (formed from L-dopa or administered locally) and other dopaminergic agonists, actions such as stimulation of locomotor activity and stereotyped behaviour, and disruption of a discriminative task (for references, see Carlsson, 1983), inhibition of firing by dopaminergic neurones (Aghajanian & Bunney, 1974, 1977) and of dopamine synthesis and turnover (Carlsson *et al.*, 1977), hypothermia and decrease in prolactin secretion. The activation of adenyl cyclase, induced by dopaminergic receptor agonists *in vitro*, is antagonized, though not equally well by all neuroleptics (Kebabian & Greengard, 1971; Greengard, 1975), and the binding of dopaminergic receptor agonists to, for example, striatal membranes is counteracted (Seeman *et al.*, 1976; Creese *et al.*, 1976). The latter effect is closely correlated with the clinical dosage of a large number of neuroleptic agents.

The fact that dopaminergic agonists are capable of faithfully mimicking certain schizophrenic disease states led Randrup and Munkvad (1965) to propose that dopamine may be involved in schizophrenia. All the above observations form the basis for the 'dopamine hypothesis of schizophrenia'.

This theory has played a prominent role in schizophrenia research for almost three decades. However, some important caveats must be considered. First, the hypothesis rests almost entirely on indirect pharmacological evidence. A disturbance in dopaminergic functions in the brains of schizophrenic patients remains to be demonstrated beyond doubt (see below). Second, a fair proportion of schizophrenic patients respond poorly, or not at all, to treatment with antidopaminergic drugs. Poor responses are seen especially in cases with predominantly 'negative' symptomatology (affective flattening, poverty of speech, etc.; Crow, 1987). Third, dopaminergic agonists can only mimic the paranoid form of schizophrenia. Non-paranoid schizophrenia, and especially negative symptomatology, can be mimicked more faithfully by phencyclidine (PCP, 'angel dust'; Domino & Luby, 1973; Angrist, 1987), which appears to act

predominantly as an antagonist on the glutamatergic N-methyl-D-aspartate (NMDA) receptors (Lodge *et al.*, 1987). A deficient glutamatergic function in schizophrenia was proposed by Kornhuber *et al.* 1984 and Kim *et al.*, 1985.

The dopamine theory can best explain the 'positive' symptoms (hyperarousal, hallucinations, etc.) Negative symptoms are rather suggestive of dopaminergic hypofunction. However, positive and negative symptoms can apparently occur simultaneously. A truly comprehensive hypothesis must be able to offer an explanation of this phenomenon. Possibly, dopaminergic hyper- and hypofunction can occur simultaneously in different parts of the system. Alternatively, a non-dopaminergic system may be deficient, leading to differential dysfunctions within the dopaminergic system.

Another weakness of the dopamine theory is that the therapeutic efficacy of the antidopaminergic agents is not limited to schizophrenia but includes a variety of other psychotic states. Perhaps the theory should rather be called the 'dopamine hypothesis of psychosis'.

At present, it appears that the dopamine theory can serve best by providing a platform for attempts to analyse the neurotransmitter imbalances in schizophrenia and other psychotic states in some greater depth. Careful studies of the interaction between dopamine and other neurotransmitters thus seem essential. The present chapter will emphasize this aspect. Another strong impact of recent research dealing with the discovery of new dopamine receptor subtypes will be commented upon. However, before that, some recent postmortem data bearing on possible monoaminergic dysfunctions in schizophrenia will be briefly reviewed.

Does a dopaminergic dysfunction exist in schizophrenia?

One of the major claims in this area has been that the brains of schizophrenics have an increased density of dopamine D_2 receptors. This was originally based on postmortem observations but was challenged by some workers who suggested that the issue concerned an artefact induced by antipsychotic medication. Later, receptor densities were measured by means of positron emission tomography (PET), and again the claim was put forward that schizophrenics had an increased dopamine D_2 density in their brains, now in drug-naive patients. However, careful PET studies by Sedvall, Farde and their colleagues at the Karolinska Institute showed no difference in D_2 density between drug-naive schizophrenics and age-matched controls (for review, see Nordström *et al.*, 1993; Nordström, 1993).

A claim that dopamine levels are elevated in the left amygdala of the brains of schizophrenics (Reynolds, 1987) is interesting and deserves further examination.

A difficulty encountered in the search for biochemical abnormalities in schizophrenia deals with the probable heterogeneity of this disorder. An abnormality in a given subgroup may thus not show up because of contamination with other subgroups. In case the aberrations between subgroups go in opposite directions, mean values for a given variable could even be equal to control, and thus conventional statistical group comparisons would fail to demonstrate any differences.

The author's research group, in collaboration with Dr C.-G. Gottfries at the University of Goteborg, has carried out two studies on post-mortem brains, in which different monoaminergic indices were measured in several brain regions of schizophrenic and age-matched control patients. Conventional group comparisons did not reveal any differences. However, when a multivariate analysis was applied, aberrations in the schizophrenic groups were disclosed (Hansson *et al.*, 1994). Both studies suggested the existence of at least two subgroups of schizophrenic patients. The results of the first study are shown in Fig. 20.1. Here, the schizophrenic cases appear in two different clusters, each of which is different from the control group. The measurements underlying this result consisted of dopamine, serotonin and noradrenaline levels as well as some of their metabolites and precursors in several brain regions. One of the schizophrenic groups consisted of patients with paranoid schizophrenia and a relatively low degree of family history of psychosis. The other group consisted mainly of hebephrenic and catatonic schizophrenics and a high degree of family history of psychosis. In the paranoid group dopamine levels tended to be low, whereas serotonin precursor and metabolite levels were high. In the other schizophrenic group dopamine levels were

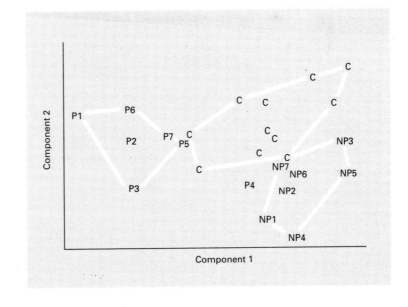

Fig. 20.1 Principal least squares discriminant analysis (PLSDA) of monoaminergic indices in several brain regions of chronic schizophrenic patients and age-matched controls. C, Controls; P, paranoid schizophrenics; NP, non-paranoid schizophrenics. The monoaminergic indices measured were: dopamine, 3-methoxy-tyramine, serotonin, 5-hydroxytryptophan, 5-hydroxyindoleacetic acid, noradrenaline, normetanephrine, tyrosine and tryptophan. (From Hansson *et al.*, 1994.)

almost normal, whereas serotonin as well as its precursor and metabolite levels were low. In the second study, a differentiation of schizophrenic patients into at least two groups showed up most strikingly in the caudate nucleus but was detectable also in the nucleus accumbens and a piece of limbic cortex. This study comprised the levels of dopamine, its deaminated metabolites and their cysteinyl adducts, as well as serotonin and 5-hydroxyindoleacetic acid. The larger subgroup tended to have lower monoaminergic indices, except for the cysteinyl adducts, which tended to be elevated, compared with controls; the reverse seemed to be true for the smaller subgroup. The deviations could not be accounted for by neuroleptic medication, because the unmedicated patients showed the strongest deviations from the controls.

Even though these observations are somewhat preliminary, it seems obvious that neither dopamine, serotonin nor noradrenaline can at present be dismissed as pathogenetic factors in schizophrenia. In any event, the data indicate that biochemical aberrations suggestive of neurotransmitter dysfunctions in the brain exist in schizophrenia and that this disorder does not seem to represent a single entity.

The role of dopamine-receptor subtypes in schizophrenia

Even though dopamine antagonists have been available for the treatment of schizophrenia for about 40 years, the therapeutic potential of this pharmacological principle still remains partly unexplored. This is true, for example, of the role of the various dopamine-receptor subtypes.

For a number of years dopamine receptors were assumed to consist of two subtypes, D_1 and D_2 (see Spano *et al.*, 1978; Kebabian & Calne, 1979). Thanks to molecular biology we now know that D_1 and D_2 actually represent two different receptor families (Sibley & Monsma, 1992). The D_1 family consists of D_1 and D_5, also called D_{1A} and D_{1B}, respectively, and the D_2 family consists of D_2 (D_{2A}, long, and D_{2B}, short), D_3 and D_4. At this time especially, the D_3 and D_4 subtypes are in focus.

One reason for the interest in the D_3 subtype is its regional distribution, with a strong localization to the ventral, 'limbic' parts of the basal ganglia, which are believed to be largely involved in mental functions, and are thus of considerable interest for the role of dopamine in schizophrenia (Sokoloff *et al.*, 1990). At present, little is known, however, about its function. To obtain conclusive information about the functional role of a given receptor subtype one needs to have access to sufficiently selective agonists, and especially antagonists. Until recently, no such compounds have been available in this case. The most selective antagonist, i.e. (+)-UH232, has only a three- to fivefold preference for D_3 vs. D_2 (Schwartz *et al.*, 1993). This agent has been described as a preferential dopamine-autoreceptor antagonist and is a mild behavioural stimulant (Svensson *et al.*, 1986); it is not known to what extent its pharmacological profile is related to its D_3 preference.

The currently used antipsychotic agents are either D_2 preferring or equally active on D_2 and D_3. Similarly, most of the agonists are poor discriminators in this respect; one exception is 7-OHDPAT, which has a relatively strong preference for the D_3 subtype (see Schwartz *et al.*, 1993). The difficulty in obtaining selectivity is not surprising, given the close structural similarity between the subtypes.

A number of antagonists with a sufficiently high selectivity for D_3 have recently been synthesized and tested in the author's laboratory in collaboration with Upjohn scientists. One of these agents, U99194A, shows a 20-fold preference for D_3 vs. D_2 and behaves as an antagonist *in vitro* as well as *in vivo* (Waters *et al.*, 1993b). Figure 20.2 summarizes the most salient findings. This agent is a behavioural stimulant with a characteristic dopaminergic profile but does not increase dopamine release, as measured by microdialysis. Its activity must then be assumed to be postsynaptic. It would thus appear that the D_3 subtype, in contrast to D_2, is behaviourally inhibitory. Analogous findings with D_3-preferring agonists support this view, i.e. they are inhibitory on behaviour in doses which do not change dopamine release (Svensson *et al.*, 1994). These investigations are in an early phase, and thus the con-

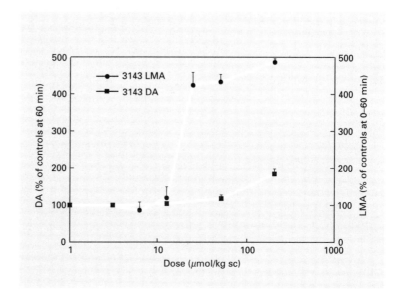

Fig. 20.2 Effect of U99194A on locomotor activity (LMA) and dopamine (DA) release, as measured by microdialysis in rat nucleus accumbens. (From Waters *et al.*, 1993b.)

clusions are still somewhat tentative.

Needless to say, the existence of a behaviourally inhibitory dopamine-receptor subtype, which has earlier been proposed from time to time, based on more indirect evidence (see Ståhle, 1992), can have important implications. For example, positive and negative symptoms in schizophrenia might arise from hypo- and hyperdopaminergia, respectively, mediated via dopamine D_3 receptors.

Perhaps clozapine's relatively broad blockade of dopamine receptors, encompassing the D_1 as well as the D_2 family, with some preference for D_4, can partly explain the favourable profile of this agent.

The main reason for the current interest in the D_4 dopamine-receptor subtype is clozapine's albeit limited preference for this subtype. [Whereas this preference has been claimed to reach one order of magnitude, recent data of Malmberg *et al.* (1993) suggest that it may be modest compared with the D_{2B} subtype.] Recently, Seeman *et al.* (1993) have presented data from postmortem schizophrenic patients suggesting a several-fold elevation of D_4 receptor density in the brains of these patients compared with age-matched controls. These results must await confirmation, using more D_4-selective ligands than those available today. Moreover, the possible influence of neuroleptic treatment must be carefully examined (see also Chapter 21).

Agents with preferential action on dopamine autoreceptors: partial dopamine-receptor agonists

Could dopaminergic drugs be used to counteract negative symptoms? Even though the amphetamines seem to possess the properties required for this purpose, they seem to be difficult to use in practice, in view of their too strong stimulant and addictive properties. Preferential dopamine-autoreceptor antagonists may turn out to be useful for this purpose. These are mild stimulants in rodents, and excessive stimulation and addiction will presumably be avoided by the postsynaptic receptor blockade that shows up after administration of higher doses. Examples of agents belonging to this class are the substituted aminotetralins (+)-UH232 and (+)-AJ76 (Svensson *et al.*, 1986). These agents are capable of blocking dopamine autoreceptors (D_2 and D_3), resulting in increased release of dopamine (Waters *et al.*, 1993a). They also block postsynaptic dopamine receptors, with a somewhat stronger action on the behaviourally inhibitory D_3 receptors than on the stimulant D_2 receptors. The net outcome of these actions is a mild stimulation of behaviour. A recently completed study of (+)-UH232 in healthy volunteers demonstrates psychotropic activity with predominantly stimulant properties (unpublished data of the present author's research group).

Agonists acting preferentially on dopamine autoreceptors may also turn out to be of therapeutic interest in schizophrenia (see Carlsson, 1975). In general, such agents seem to be partial dopamine-receptor agonists acting on the dopamine D_2 family. The apparent intrinsic activity of partial dopamine-receptor agonists appears to be more marked on the autoreceptors than on the postsynaptic receptors, owing to a higher responsiveness of the former (often ascribed to a higher 'receptor reserve'). This will result in behavioural inhibition which, however, will not reach the same high degree, e.g. with catalepsy, as that caused by classical neuroleptics. In fact, neuroleptic-induced catalepsy can be antagonized by partial dopamine-receptor agonists (Svensson et al., 1993). A partial dopamine D_2-receptor agonist with a suitable degree of intrinsic activity may thus turn out to possess antipsychotic properties without concomitant extrapyramidal side effects. Several such agents, which seem to share the properties of partial dopamine-receptor agonists, though with varying intrinsic activity, are now being used in clinical trials (Gründer et al., 1991; Klinke & Klieser, 1991; Naber, 1991; Wiedemann et al., 1991; Tamminga et al., 1992b).

Functional anatomy of the major dopaminergic pathways and their connections with other systems

Figure 20.3 shows the major neuronal circuitries connecting the basal ganglia with other brain regions. One major input to the striatum comes from the cerebral cortex. From the neocortex the input goes to the dorsal striatum, and from the allocortex (and the prefrontal cortex) to the ventral (limbic) striatum. Major projections from the dorsal and ventral striatum go to different thalamic nuclei via the dorsal and ventral pallidum, respectively. Finally, the loops are closed by projections from the thalamus back to the cortex (see also Chapter 21).

Inhibitory functions of the striatum

Carlsson and Carlsson (1990) have emphasized the inhibitory influence of the striatum on the thalamus and thus interpreted the cortico-striato-thalamo-cortical pathways as negative feedback loops. Originally, their conclusion was based on the fact that the mesostriatal dopaminergic pathways are behaviourally stimulating and that most neurophysiologists seem to agree that the dopaminergic input to the striatum has a mainly inhibitory action on striatal projection neurones. An inhibition of striatal function should thus result in behavioural stimulation. Further support was obtained when it was found that the behavioural stimulation induced by blockade of striatal NMDA receptors persisted in animals depleted of dopamine and other monoamines by means of reserpine and α-methyl-tyrosine. Thus, removal of the excitatory glutamatergic tone, acting on striatal cells, causes behavioural stimulation, and glutamate and dopamine can antagonize each other in the striatum (Carlsson & Carlsson, 1989a,b, 1990; Svensson & Carlsson, 1992; Fig. 20.4).

To account for the inhibitory influence of the striatum on the thalamus, Carlsson and Carlsson (1990) focused on the so-called indirect striato-pallido-thalamic pathways, which contain chains of three gamma-aminobutyric acidergic (GABAergic) neurones (and in addition one glutamatergic neurone originating in the subthalamic nucleus (STN) and projecting to the medial segment of the globus pallidus; see Fig. 20.3). More recently, they became aware of another GABAergic, indirect pathway, consisting of a three-neurone chain from the striatum to the thalamus, with the third GABAergic neurone located in the reticular nucleus of thalamus (Alheid et al., 1990; Parent et al., 1988, 1991). The latter nucleus is known to control most of the other thalamic nuclei. Taken together, these indirect three-neurone GABAergic pathways should be able to mediate an inhibitory impact on the thalamus, resulting in inhibition via the motor feedback loops as well as a reduced thalamic relaying of the sensory input to the cortex.

The neuroanatomy of the dorsal striatum is, generally speaking, more accurately mapped than

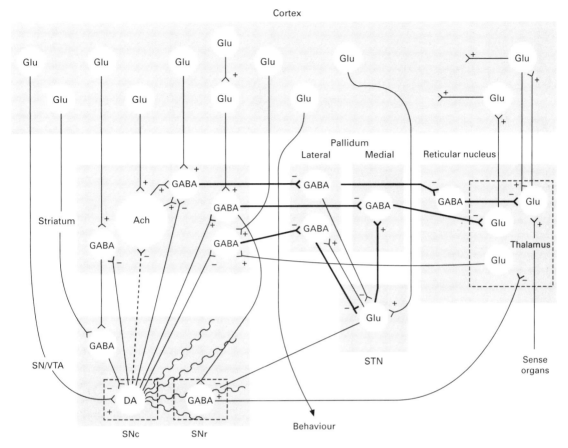

Fig. 20.3 Neurocircuitries of the basal ganglia. The pathways drawn with thick lines indicate some connections between the striatum and the thalamus, which are discussed in some detail in this chapter. The top and bottom pathways drawn with thick lines contain three GABAergic neurones and are referred to as 'indirect' pathways. The pathway in between contains two GABAergic neurones and is referred to as 'direct'. SN, Substantia nigra; VTA, ventral tegmental area; STN, subthalamic nucleus; Glu, glutamate; Ach, acetylcholine; DA, dopamine. (After Carlsson & Carlsson, 1990.)

that of the ventral striatum, but the principal organization and connections seem to be analogous (Heimer *et al.*, 1985). Among the least well-mapped areas of the basal forebrain is the so-called extended amygdala (Heimer *et al.*, 1991). However, this area seems to have an organization somewhat similar to that of the ventral striatum. For example, it receives glutamatergic and dopaminergic inputs from the (limbic) cortex and mesencephalon, respectively, and has strong projections, which are partly GABAergic, to the thalamus; in particular, projections to the reticular nucleus of the thalamus are of interest in this context (Steriade *et al.*, 1987; for further refer-

ences, see Heimer *et al.*, 1991). Heimer has emphasized the potential importance of the ventral striatum as well as the extended amygdala for mental functions. For the purpose of the present discussion it seems justified to include the extended amygdala in the total basal ganglia complex.

Although the dorsal and ventral striatum are often said to be involved in motor and mental functions, respectively, a strict functional distinction between the two portions is not well founded. For example, cognitive functions are probably regulated in part via certain regions within the dorsal striatum (Selemon & Goldman-Rakic,

Chapter 20

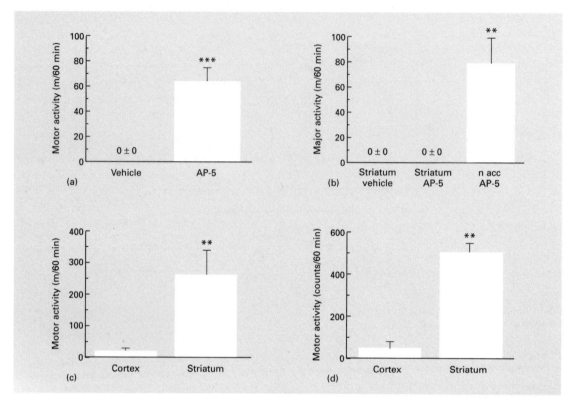

Fig. 20.4 Mice were monoamine depleted by means of pretreatment with reserpine (10 mg/kg) at 18 h and with α-methyl-tyrosine (500 mg/kg) at 2 h before the registration of locomotor activity commenced. (a) Effects of AP-5 injected into the nucleus accumbens: 10 min after the injection of AP-5 (5 μg) or vehicle the animals were placed in the circular tracks and locomotor activity was registered over 60 min. Shown are the means ± SEM, $n = 6-8$, *** $P = 0.0006$ vs. vehicle.
(b) Effects of AP-5 injected into the nucleus accumbens or dorsal striatum: 10 min after the injection of AP-5 (5 μg) or vehicle the animals were placed in the circular tracks and locomotor activity was registered over 60 min. Shown are the means ± SEM, $n = 4-6$, ** $P = 0.0039$ vs. AP-5 injected into the dorsal striatum. (c) Effects of AP-5 injected into the dorsal striatum or prefrontal cortex in combination with intraperitoneally administered clonidine: 10 min after the injection of AP-5 (10 μg) and immediately following the administration of clonidine (1 mg/kg) the animals were placed in the circular tracks and locomotor activity was measured over 60 min. Shown are the means ± SEM, $n = 6-8$, ** $P = 0.002$ vs. the prefrontal cortex. Note that the scale differs from that in (a) and (b). (From Svensson & Carlsson, 1992.) (d) Effects of methscopolamine injected into the dorsal striatum or prefrontal cortex in combination with intraperitoneally administered clonidine: immediately following the administration of methscopolamine (62 μg) and clonidine (1 mg/kg) the animals were placed in motility meters and locomotor activity was measured over 60 min. Shown are the means ± SEM, $n = 5-6$, ** $P = 0.0062$ vs. the prefrontal cortex. (From Carlsson *et al.*, 1992.)

1985; Goldman-Rakic & Selemon, 1986; Nauta, 1989). Even though a strict somatotropic organization appears to exist in the basal ganglia and its connections, the circuitries involved in various functions appear to be intimately intertwined, and this seems to be true of motor and mental functions alike. Pharmacologically, this close relation-ship shows up quite strikingly in the manipulation of various neurotransmitter functions, and this has given rise to the expression 'psychomotor activity'. From an evolutionary point of view, this close relation is not surprising, since motor and mental functions have probably evolved as a closely integrated unit.

In support of the functional importance of the indirect loop involving the STN, an increased firing rate has been recorded in this nucleus in MPTP-treated parkinsonian monkeys, and their defective motor functions have been dramatically improved by lesioning this nucleus (Bergman *et al.*, 1990) or by applying an NMDA-receptor antagonist locally in the medial pallidal segment (Graham *et al.*, 1990). The STN has connections with both the dorsal and ventral striatopallidal systems, but its role in mental functions is so far unknown. Vascular lesions damaging this nucleus typically induce a hyperkinetic syndrome called 'hemiballismus', which does not seem to involve any mental disturbances, if the lesion is distinctly localized to this nucleus (Meyers, 1968). This is in contrast to lesions in the pallidum and thalamus produced in antiparkinsonian surgery, where the risk of mental disturbances is considerable. Possibly, the GABAergic three-neurone chain projecting to the reticular nucleus, or a corresponding pathway from the extended amygdala, is especially important for mental functions.

Disinhibitory functions of the striatum

An essential part of the present working hypothesis is the postulate that a reduced striatal inhibition on the thalamus, brought about by either an increased dopaminergic or a reduced glutamatergic tone, should lead to an increase in arousal and psychomotor activity and to an increased sensory input relayed to the cortex (Carlsson, 1988; Carlsson & Carlsson, 1990; see also Carlsson, 1994, with references to literature on a filter defect in schizophrenia). If these changes go beyond a certain level the integrative capacity of the cortex will become insufficient and this will lead to psychosis with predominantly positive symptomatology. An excessive dopaminergic function may also lead to a disintegration of motor functions, as indicated by purposeless stereotyped behaviour.

This inhibitory function of the striatum appears to be exerted via the indirect pathways. However, the direct striato-pallido-thalamic pathways, which contain only two GABAergic neurones

(Penney & Young, 1986; Alexander & Crutcher, 1990), appear to serve an opposite function. The direct pathways should be able to mediate the excitatory glutamatergic input from the cortex to the thalamus via the striatum and the medial section of the pallidum — the pars reticulata of the substantia nigra (see Fig. 20.3). This should result in thalamic and behavioural stimulation, and the loops involved in this case should mediate positive feedback. The dopaminergic input to those striatal neurones which are involved in the direct pathways appears to be excitatory on these neurones (Pan *et al.*, 1985; see also Penney & Young, 1986), and dopamine should thus be behaviourally stimulating also via the direct pathways. In support of the behaviourally stimulating function of the direct pathways are, for example, experiments by Heim *et al.* (1986), who have demonstrated freezing and an inability to switch motor patterns in cats following local application of the GABA-receptor antagonist picrotoxin in the pars reticulata of the substantia nigra (regarded as part of the medial pallidum; Heimer *et al.*, 1985, 1991).

An important implication of an excitatory and inhibitory influence of dopamine on the direct and indirect pathways, respectively, will be that dopamine serves as a regulator of the balance between positive and negative feedback in the striatum. A low dopaminergic tone would favour negative feedback and a high tone, positive feedback. This will be apparent from the schematic diagrams depicted in Fig. 20.5.

Glutamatergic agonists applied locally in the nucleus accumbens have been found to induce behavioural stimulation (Donzanti & Uretsky, 1984; Boldry & Uretsky, 1988), perhaps by stimulating GABAergic projection neurones belonging to the direct pathways. Indeed, the direct pathways appear to be specifically involved in the initiation of movement by arousing executive centres via a disinhibitory mechanism, which in the case of eye movements involves the superior colliculi (Chevalier & Deniau, 1990).

It should be pointed out that the current description of direct and indirect pathways, as outlined above, is partly hypothetical. In actual

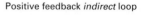

Positive feedback *direct* loop

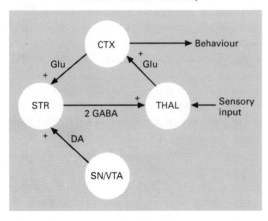

Positive feedback *indirect* loop

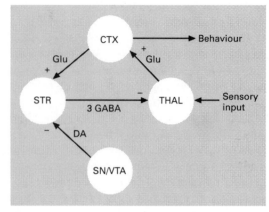

Fig. 20.5 Schematic diagram illustrating positive and negative feedback loops in the striatum, mediated via 'direct' and 'indirect' pathways, respectively. *Note* in this somewhat hypothetical scheme dopamine is excitatory on the direct and inhibitory on the indirect pathways, as first suggested by Penney and Young (1986). CTX, Cerebral cortex; STR, striatum; THAL, thalamus; SN, substantia nigra; VTA, ventral tegmental area; Glu, glutamic acid; DA, dopamine.

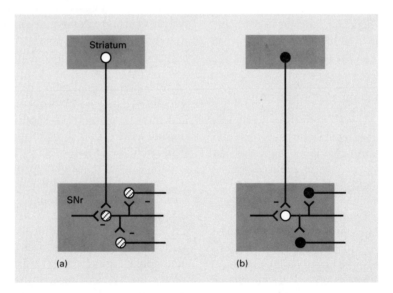

Fig. 20.6 The complex action of a striatal GABAergic neurone on neurones of the pars reticulata of the substantia nigra (SNr). Open circles represent silent neurones, hatched circles neurones of intermediate activity and filled circles neurones with high activity. In (a) the striatal neurone is silent and the SNr neurones show intermediate activity. In (b) the striatal neurone has started to fire, resulting in inhibition of the directly innervated SNr neurones, whereas the SNr neurones controlled via collaterals are released from inhibition and thus start to fire. (Reproduced with permission from Chevalier & Deniau, 1990.)

practice it may prove difficult to establish the number of inhibitory GABAergic neurones taking part in a given functional chain. As pointed out by Chevalier and Deniau (1990), stimulation of striatal neurones is not entirely inhibitory on nigral and pallidal neurones but actually causes increased firing of a fair proportion of neurones in these structures. The explanation offered to this phenomenon by Chevalier and Deniau is illustrated in Fig. 20.6. It is assumed that under baseline conditions striatal neurones may be silent (Fig. 20.6a). Neurones in substantia nigra, pars reticulata (SNr) may then show intermediate activity. If striatal neurones then start to fire, this will cause inhibition of nigral neurones directly innervated by the striatal neurones in question (Fig. 20.6b). However, nigral neurones communicate with other nigral neurones via axone collaterals. This will lead to increased firing of the latter neurones, owing to disinhibition. From a biochemical point of view, this will have important consequences. If GABAergic turnover is measured in the projection areas of SNr neurones, e.g. in the thalamus, the result of an increased striatal activity is hard to predict. The overall change could be either a decrease or an increase, or no change at all, depending on the proportion of the directly to the indirectly innervated neurones. No simple correlation to the behavioural outcome would be expected. By the same token, the consequences with regard to metabolism, measured, for example, by the deoxyglucose technique, would also be unpredictable. Despite this complication one should, of course, not feel discouraged to carry out these measurements of, for example, GABAergic activity and tissue metabolism.

When the behavioural interaction between glutamate and dopamine was examined at the postsynaptic level (in monoamine-depleted mice), it was observed that D_1 and D_2 agonists behaved differently. Whereas the behavioural actions of the D_1 agonist SKF 38393 and the mixed D_1/D_2 agonist apomorphine, given in threshold doses, were potentiated by the NMDA antagonist MK-801 (Carlsson & Carlsson, 1989b, 1990), the actions of D_2 agonists were antagonized by this agent (Svensson *et al.*, 1992b; Fig. 20.7). Similar results have been obtained by Morelli and Di Chiara (1990) and by Goodwin *et al.* (1992), using somewhat different experimental models. Thus, the responsiveness of the D_1 receptors is apparently suppressed by the glutamatergic tone. D_2 receptors, on the other hand, seem to operate in concert with the glutamatergic system to enhance behavioural stimulation. In other words, it seems as though glutamate can either inhibit or stimulate behaviour, and the outcome seems to depend to some extent on whether it interacts with D_1 or D_2 receptors. Another factor of importance in this context was found to be the behavioural baseline level of activity. Thus, with a low baseline activity, the ability of an NMDA-receptor antagonist to enhance locomotor activity is especially strong and may show up, though only weakly, even in conjunction with a D_2-receptor agonist. With a high baseline activity, an NMDA antagonist tends to be inhibitory, even in conjunction with a D_1-receptor agonist. Especially striking

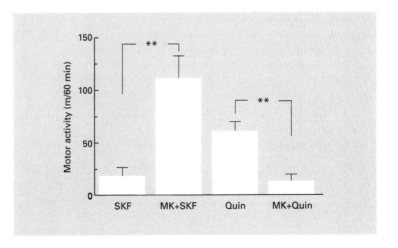

Fig. 20.7 Effects of dizocilpine (MK-801) in combination with either SKF 38393 or quinpirole on locomotor activity in monoamine-depleted mice. Dizocilpine (1 mg/kg) was given 60 min, and quinpirole (1 mg/kg) and SKF 38393 (8 mg/kg) were given immediately before the locomotor registration commenced. Locomotor activity was registered in the circular tracks over 60 min. Shown are the means ± SEM, $n = 5–6$, ** $P < 0.01$. (From Svensson *et al.*, 1992b.)

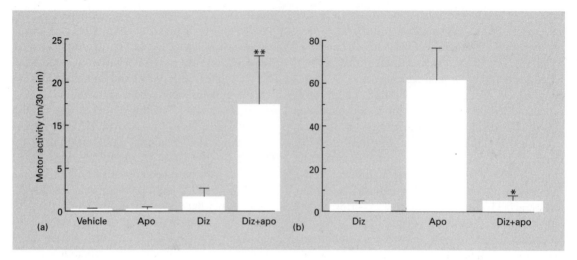

Fig. 20.8 (a) Effects of dizocilpine (diz) in combination with a subthreshold dose of apomorphine (apo) on locomotor activity in monoamine-depleted mice. Sixty minutes after the administration of dizocilpine (1.5 mg/kg) and immediately following the administration of apomorphine (0.1 mg/kg i.p.) the animals were placed in the circular tracks and locomotor activity was registered over 30 min. Shown are the means ± SEM, $n = 9–11$, ** $P < 0.01$ vs. dizocilpine. (From Carlsson & Carlsson, 1989.) (b) Effects of dizocilpine (diz) in combination with an effective *per se* dose of apomorphine (apo) on locomotor activity in monoamine-depleted mice. Sixty minutes after administration of dizocilpine (0.5 mg/kg) and immediately following administration of apomorphine (0.2 mg/kg s.c.) the animals were placed in circular tracks and locomotor activity was registered over 30 min. Shown are the means ± SEM, $n = 5–8$, * $P < 0.025$ vs. apomorphine given as the only treatment. (From Svensson *et al.*, 1992b.)

was the dependence on baseline activity in experiments with apomorphine, where MK-801 potentiated the behavioural stimulation induced by a threshold dose of apomorphine but antagonized the overt stimulation caused by a higher dose of this drug (Svensson *et al.*, 1992b; Fig. 20.8).

Perhaps even more striking are some more recent observations (Svensson *et al.*, 1992a, 1994) dealing with the effects of unilateral administration of the competitive NMDA antagonist AP-5 into the nucleus accumbens of the mouse. In the monoamine-depleted mouse this results in behavioural activation and contralateral rotation (Fig. 20.9). In mice with intact monoaminergic systems, this treatment induces predominantly ipsilateral rotation. These observations are in agreement with the model, because the indirect pathways and negative feedback should predominate in monoamine-depleted animals. Here, the unilateral loss of glutamatergic tone in the nucleus accumbens should reduce the parkinsonian inhibition ipsilaterally, leading to contralateral

rotation. In mice with an intact dopaminergic system the direct pathways and positive feedback should predominate, and thus unilateral inhibition of glutamatergic tone should cause loss of positive feedback ipsilaterally and ipsilateral rotation. The systemic administration of the dopamine D_2-receptor agonist quinpirole or the mixed D_1/D_2 agonist apomorphine to monoamine-depleted mice with unilateral reduction of glutamatergic tone, induced by AP-5, caused a switch of rotation from contralateral to ipsilateral. Thus, an increased D_2-receptor-mediated dopaminergic tone appears to switch the system from predominantly negative to positive feedback. On the other hand, the dopamine D_1-receptor agonist SKF 38393, injected systematically to monoamine-depleted mice with AP-5 given unilaterally into nucleus accumbens, caused increased contralateral rotation. These experiments strongly support the view that glutamate serves a dual function in the nucleus accumbens and that dopamine D_1 and D_2 receptors are differentially involved in this dual function.

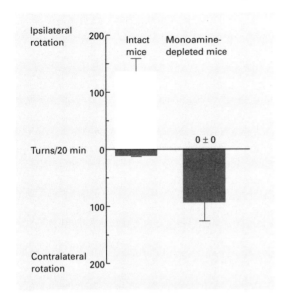

Fig. 20.9 Rotatory behaviour of mice following unilateral injection of the competitive *N*-methyl-D-aspartate (NMDA)-receptor antagonist AP-5 (5 µg) into the nucleus accumbens of mice. Shown are the number of rotations per 20 min following the injection of AP-5 (means ± SEM).

Thus, there are different pieces of evidence which independently indicate the occurrence of two mutually opposite behavioural functions of the corticostriatal glutamatergic system with respect to behaviour. It is tempting to link the pieces together and suggest that the behavioural stimulation observed after combined treatment with a D_1 agonist and an NMDA antagonist under conditions of a low baseline activity is mediated via the indirect pathways, whereas the inhibition seen after treatment with an NMDA antagonist in combination with a D_2 agonist under conditions of a high baseline level of activity is mediated via the direct pathways. A corollary would be that the striatal projection neurones of the direct and indirect pathways would be equipped with D_2 and D_1 receptors, respectively, but in view of some literature data arguing in a different direction (Gerfen *et al.*, 1990), as well as the complex D_1/D_2 interactions (Clark & White, 1987), it seems premature to claim such a strict anatomical distinction between the two receptor

subtypes. Moreover, the complication arising from the collateral inhibition mentioned above should be considered. Finally, it should be pointed out that in this context the behavioural D_1/D_2 interactions refer to the D_1/D_2 families rather than to individual receptor subtypes.

Although it is admittedly speculative, and despite the reservations mentioned above, it is tempting to propose that the direct pathways are critically involved in the negative symptomatology of schizophrenia. These pathways, which in contrast to the indirect pathways may tend to be phasic rather than tonic (Côté & Crutcher, 1991), appear to be crucial for the initiation of various types of motor and mental activity. If the glutamatergic input to these pathways becomes insufficient, it will result in negative symptomatology.

To summarize this speculative view, the glutamatergic input from the cortex to the striatum appears to have two mutually antagonistic behavioural functions, i.e. one mediating inhibition, tentatively via the indirect pathways, and the other mediating stimulation, via the direct pathways. Failure of either of the two would lead to positive and negative symptoms, respectively. Since these two components can be partly independent, it would explain why both positive and negative symptoms can exist side by side in varying proportions. Failure of glutamatergic pathways may lead to such mixed symptomatology. Such failure may, for example, be due to a genetically based defect of the NMDA receptor. Needless to say, a corticostriatal hypoglutamatergia would not necessarily be primary. It might be secondary to changes further upstream and related to the various structural and metabolic changes that have been repeatedly observed in the cerebral cortex and limbic−diencephalic system of schizophrenic patients (DeLisi, 1986; Kirch & Weinberger, 1986; Buchsbaum, 1990; Bogerts, 1991; Tamminga *et al.*, 1991, 1992c). Schizophrenic symptomatology can apparently also be induced by a downstream failure of striatal neurones, because such symptomatology may occur, and in fact precede motor disturbances, in cases of Huntington's chorea (Mattsson, 1974) (see also Chapter 20).

The role of cholinergic, noradrenergic and serotonergic mechanisms

Thus far we have argued that a neurotransmitter imbalance involving dopamine, glutamate and GABA in the cortico-striato-thalamic complex may play an important role in the pathogenesis of schizophrenia. Presumably, a number of other neurotransmitters also take part in this disturbance. This brief discussion will be limited to those small neurotransmitter molecules which occur abundantly within this complex, i.e. acetylcholine, noradrenaline and serotonin. Anticholinergic drugs can be psychotomimetic, and this neurotransmitter has long been discussed as a counterbalance to dopamine in the striatum. A behavioural synergism between dopamine and an α_2-adrenergic agonist has been known for a long time (Andén *et al.*, 1973), and several neuroleptic agents have antiadrenergic properties, which possibly contribute to the therapeutic response. Among these agents, clozapine has a particularly strong adrenolytic action. As to serotonin, 5-hydroxytryptamine (5-HT_2)-receptor agonists like lysergic acid diethylamide (LSD) are psychotomimetic. Recently, the 5-HT_2-receptor antagonist ritanserin has been reported to enhance the antipsychotic action of neuroleptics (Duinkerke *et al.*, 1993). Risperidone, a compound with combined dopamine- and 5-HT_2-receptor blocking activity, has been claimed to be a more efficacious antipsychotic than the conventional neuroleptics (Heylen & Gelders, 1990). Work in this area has been stimulated by the fact that clozapine is a fairly potent 5-HT_2-receptor antagonist (Nordström *et al.*, 1993; see Chapters 18, 21 and 25).

Recently, Gellman and Aghajanian (1991) reported that cortical 5-HT_2 receptors are located on GABAergic interneurones, on which they exert an excitatory influence; these can be blocked by 5-HT_2-receptor antagonists such as clozapine and risperidone. The excitation of the GABAergic interneurones causes inhibition of downstream pyramidal cell activity (cf. the psychotogenic action of glutamatergic antagonists). Muscimol, which is a GABA-A-receptor agonist and has been reported to be psychotogenic (Tamminga *et al.*, 1978), might also act by inhibiting glutamatergic neurones.

In experiments with monoamine-depleted mice, it has been found that in addition to glutamate the cholinergic system is apparently also involved in the regulation of postsynaptic monoaminergic receptor responsiveness. Thus, in monoamine-depleted mice, movements can be induced by the combined treatment with, on the one hand, a muscarinic receptor antagonist and, on the other hand, a subthreshold dose of an NMDA-receptor antagonist (Carlsson & Carlsson, 1989c). A similar interaction was found between a muscarinic receptor antagonist and an α_2-receptor agonist (Carlsson *et al.*, 1991). The striatum appears to play a crucial role in these interactions, as demonstrated by local applications of methylscopolamine and an α_2-receptor agonist in this structure (Carlsson *et al.*, 1992; see Fig. 20.4d, and unpublished data). The intrinsic cholinergic neurones in the ventral striatum thus seem to be involved in this interaction.

The potentiation of the D_1 agonist-induced behavioural stimulation by an NMDA-receptor antagonist, which was observed in monoamine-depleted mice, indicates an increased responsiveness of postsynaptic D_1 receptors following treatment with an NMDA-receptor antagonist. Moreover, NMDA antagonists are capable of increasing even more dramatically the responses to α_2-receptor agonists, again at the postsynaptic level (Carlsson & Carlsson, 1989b, 1990; Carlsson & Svensson, 1990a,b). The mechanism for the apparently strong suppressing action of NMDA receptors on dopamine D_1 and α_2-adrenergic receptors is not known. In the case of D_1 receptors, an interaction with NMDA receptors has been demonstrated at the level of DARPP-32 phosphorylation in striatal slices (Halpain *et al.*, 1990). Evidence for a change in D_1-receptor binding induced by dizocilpine has also been presented (Kobayashi & Inoue, 1993).

In Fig. 20.10 these interactions, leading to psychotogenic responses, are summarized in schematic form. Needless to say, this scheme is partly hypothetical.

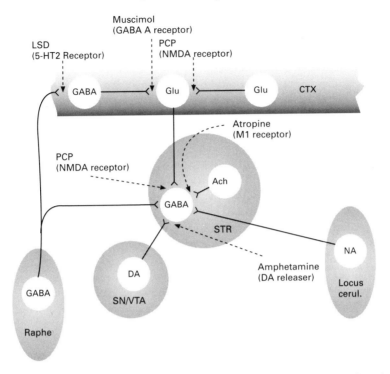

Fig. 20.10 Schematic diagram illustrating potential psychotogenic pathways and sites of action of psychotogenic and antipsychotic agents. Amphetamine and phencyclidine (PCP) are supposed to be psychotogenic by acting at least partly on striatal dopamine release and *N*-methyl-D-aspartate (NMDA) receptors, respectively, in the (limbic) striatum, although other sites may contribute. For example, PCP may act by blocking cortical NMDA receptors as well, for example, in the hippocampus, as indicated, leading to reduced tone in corticostriatal glutamatergic pathways. The 5-hydroxytryptamine (5-HT$_2$) agonist lysergic acid diethylamide (LSD) may act by stimulating cortical GABAergic interneurones, thereby reducing corticostriatal glutamatergic tone. LSD also seems to act on neurones in the striatum. The GABA-A-receptor agonist muscimol, which also appears to be psychotogenic (Tamminga *et al.*, 1978), may likewise act by reducing corticostriatal glutamatergic tone. Anticholinergic agents appear to act by blocking predominantly muscarinic M$_1$ receptors.

Is the neurotoxicity of amphetamines due to uncontrolled positive feedback? Possible implications for 'schizophrenic burnout'

It has been known for more than a decade that repeated excessive doses of methamphetamine can lead to degeneration of dopaminergic and serotonergic neurones, and that this neurotoxicity can be prevented by dopamine-receptor-blocking agents (see Gibb & Hotchkiss, 1979; Seiden *et al.*, 1988). Sonsalla *et al.* (1989) observed that NMDA-receptor antagonists, such as dizocilpine, PCP or ketamine, could also prevent this neuro-

toxicity. Marshall and colleagues (see O'Dell *et al.*, 1991a,b; Marshall *et al.*, 1993) discovered that following repeated methamphetamine injections, the release of dopamine in the striatum started to rise dramatically, as detected by means of microdialysis. This rise could be prevented by NMDA-receptor antagonists and by a dopamine D$_1$- or D$_2$-receptor-blocking agent.

Various mechanisms have been proposed to explain this neurotoxicity (see O'Dell *et al.*, 1991a,b; Marshall *et al.*, 1993). An alternative explanation, or at least a contributory factor, would be to postulate that excessive release of dopamine and stimulation of dopamine receptors disturbs the balance between the positive and negative feedback loops described above, leading to an uncontrolled positive feedback via the direct loop and excessive release of glutamate. Since glutamatergic neurotoxicity seems to act preferentially on cell bodies rather than axons, it seems reasonable to assume that the excessive glutamate release leading to neurotoxicity is mediated via corticofugal glutamatergic fibres impinging directly on the mesencephalic dopaminergic neurones (cf. Heimer *et al.*, 1991). We would therefore have to extend the positive feedback system to include not only corticostriatal but also corticonigral glutamatergic neurones. The advantage with this hypothesis is that it readily explains the excessive dopamine release following repeated dosage of methamphetamine and the protective action of both dopamine-receptor-blocking agents and NMDA-receptor antagonists. The neurotoxic action on serotonergic neurones might be explained by the existence of corticofugal glutamatergic neurones impinging also upon the serotonergic raphe neurones, which might thus be under the influence of the same positive feedback system as the dopaminergic neurones.

Observations following local application of glutamatergic antagonists in the substantia nigra suggest that GABAergic interneurones exist between glutamatergic and dopaminergic neurones in this nucleus (Dawbarn & Pycock, 1981). Since glutamatergic neurones have also been reported to impinge upon dopaminergic neurones directly (see Heimer *et al.*, 1991), it is tempting to propose that the cerebral cortex via two glutamatergic pathways can either stimulate nigral dopaminergic neurones directly or inhibit them (via GABAergic interneurones). Such a dual system exerted by the cerebral cortex via glutamatergic fibres in the striatum may be an example of a general principle of cortical control, which includes, for example, brain-stem dopaminergic, serotonergic and noradrenergic neurones. Such a dual system could tentatively explain why glutamatergic receptor antagonists can increase the firing of dopaminergic neurones in the ventrotegmental area of the mesencephalon, while at the same time inhibiting burst firing (Pawlowski *et al.*, 1990; Zhang *et al.*,

1992). The latter action could be due to reduced glutamatergic tone in the directly stimulating pathway, and the former to reduced glutamatergic tone in the indirect system, acting via GABAergic interneurones.

In this context the concept of 'schizophrenic burnout' seems worth considering. Cadet *et al.* (1987) proposed that this condition, where positive symptoms dominate initially but later yield to negative symptoms, may be due to the formation of free radicals during an initial hyperdopaminergic state, leading to degeneration of dopaminergic neurones with resultant negative symptomatology. Cadet *et al.* suggested that the use of neuroleptic drugs could induce an increased formation of free radicals and a defect state, due to neuronal degeneration. However, if a positive feedback, analogous to that suggested above to operate during methamphetamine intoxication, is the mechanism by which the assumed hyperdopaminergia during the active psychotic state causes neuronal degeneration, neuroleptics should rather improve the natural course of schizophrenia. In fact, the review of a large number of clinical studies reported by Wyatt (1991) supports the latter alternative.

Excitotoxicity may be also considered in synapses located within the cortex and forming part of positive feedback loops. These loops may also be involved in excitotoxicity occurring earlier in the individual's lifetime and may thus be involved in developmental pathogenetic mechanisms (cf. Weinberger, 1986).

Therapeutic potential of glutamatergic agents

Against the background of the hypothesis presented above, a most burning question deals with the glutamatergic system. It is reasonable to assume that PCP owes its psychotomimetic properties largely to its non-competitive interference with NMDA-receptor function. Much less is known about other glutamatergic antagonists. Ketamine is undoubtedly psychotomimetic and is also an NMDA-receptor antagonist by binding the PCP site, but it is less specific.

Amantadine and memantine, which are now believed to act at least in part as NMDA-receptor antagonists by binding to the PCP site (Kornhuber *et al.*, 1989), possess psychotomimetic properties. The most specific NMDA-receptor antagonist binding to the PCP site is dizocilpine (MK-801; Wong *et al.*, 1986). Unfortunately, the published data on the clinical profile of this agent are still sparse. Hopefully, some information on this matter will be released in the not too distant future. Another issue deals with the action of *competitive* NMDA antagonists on mental functions. At least one such agent (CPPene) has been found to be psychotomimetic (R. Markstein, personal communication).

Can glutamatergic agonists with antipsychotic properties be developed? A serious problem here is the potentially excitotoxic and convulsant properties of glutamatergic agonists. Can such effects be avoided, either by developing agonists acting as subtypes of glutamatergic receptors, which are not involved in excitotoxicity or cause convulsions, or by developing partial agonists, whose intrinsic activity is sufficient for antipsychotic activity but insufficient for inducing excitotoxicity or convulsions? Perhaps the development of agonists acting on allosteric sites of the NMDA receptors, such as the glycine and polyamine sites, might prove useful. Preliminary clinical trials with glycine and a glycine precursor have given somewhat contradictory results (Costa *et al.*, 1990; Tamminga *et al.*, 1992a).

The most important advantage of a glutamatergic agonist might be the ability to alleviate negative schizophrenic symptoms. As mentioned, glutamatergic agonists applied locally in the nucleus accumbens have been found to induce behavioural stimulation (Donzanti & Uretsky, 1984; Boldry & Uretsky, 1988), perhaps by stimulating GABAergic projection neurones belonging to the direct pathways.

Future outlook

In light of the knowledge accumulated during the past couple of decades, it seems clear that the hypothesis of hyperdopaminergia as the cause of schizophrenia is too simplistic. Admittedly, however, its heuristic value cannot be denied.

Schizophrenia is probably heterogeneous. This has been assumed for a long time and is supported by the recent postmortem data referred to at the beginning of this chapter. Paradoxically, this heterogeneity, though generally recognized, has been largely overlooked in the search for biochemical and other aberrations in schizophrenia; in many cases, a group of schizophrenics of mixed symptomatology has been compared with a control group, using conventional statistics. In light of the recent findings referred to above, it may prove worthwhile to re-examine some earlier data, using multivariate analysis and taking heterogeneity into account.

In Fig. 20.10, several neurotransmitters involved in psychotogenic mechanisms and some of their neuronal pathways were tentatively mapped. At present, it would seem unwise to disregard any of these neurotransmitters when discussing the pathogenesis of schizophrenia. Actually, more neurotransmitters may well have to be added to the list.

Perhaps the most fruitful approach would be to consider schizophrenia as a neurotransmitter imbalance syndrome with mixed aetiology. Intuitively, glutamate and dopamine may be looked upon as potential major players in this imbalance syndrome. This does not necessarily mean that they are aetiologically involved, however, in the sense that the ultimate cause resides in a glutamatergic or dopaminergic mechanism. It should also be noted that a disturbance in a given neurotransmitter system could just as well be pre- as postsynaptic. At present, focus has been largely on postsynaptic mechanisms, perhaps mainly because of recent advances in the study of receptors and their subtypes. This is not necessarily a bad strategy; even if the lesion should be located presynaptically, it is likely to have a secondary influence on postsynaptic receptors.

Regardless of whether schizophrenia researchers choose to study a special neurotransmitter or the interaction between different neurotransmitters, or wish to focus on pre- or postsynaptic mechanisms, they should not disregard the heterogeneity aspect. Whenever possible, they should try to apply multivariate analysis methods to the data. Perhaps they should try to look initially for aberrations in biochemical *patterns* rather than in individual components. If such aberrations are found, the next step would be to formulate a hypothesis to account for the aberration. For example, in one of the postmortem studies referred to above, paranoid schizophrenia seemed to be characterized by a pattern of changes involving, for example, a decrease in dopamine and an increase in serotonin precursor and metabolite levels. Since paranoid schizophrenic patients tend to respond well to antidopaminergic agents, it seems likely that they suffer from a *relative* hyperdopaminergia, despite their apparent *absolute* hypodopaminergia. In that case, it seems reasonable to suggest that the primary disturbance resides outside the dopaminergic system, at least at the presynaptic level. One possibility could be a postsynaptic dopaminergic receptor (D_2 or D_4) supersensitivity, which would or would not be accompanied by an increased dopamine-receptor density. Another possibility could be a subsensitivity of behaviourally inhibitory dopamine receptors (D_3). A third possibility could be that another neurotransmitter was primarily involved; for example, glutamate could be functioning at a subnormal level, causing increased dopamine-receptor sensitivity. These various alternatives may prove possible to investigate in postmortem as well as *in vivo* studies.

Not only dopamine but also serotonin might be secondarily changed in paranoid schizophrenia: the signs of increased serotonergic activity could be compensatory, for example, to the relative hyperdopaminergia. However, hyperserotonergia may also be considered a pathogenetic factor in paranoid schizophrenia.

In any event, it seems clear that the discovery of truly disease-related biochemical aberrations in the brains of schizophrenic patients will open up fruitful paths for further enquiry. The equipment and research tools now available, and soon forthcoming, for the study of schizophrenia are impressive. They extend from molecular biology to the highest levels of integration, including brain imaging in humans and sophisticated studies of animal and human behaviour. Further mapping of neuronal pathways in the brain, not least in the ventral forebrain with its cortical and subcortical connections, will probably add a great deal of useful knowledge, and help our understanding of the schizophrenic disturbances. Postmortem studies, *in vivo* imaging and cerebrospinal fluid analyses have already contributed considerably and will certainly continue to elucidate structural and metabolic changes, receptor aberrations, etc. in schizophrenia.

References

Aghajanian, G.K. & Bunney, B.S. (1974) Pre- and postsynaptic feedback mechanisms in central dopaminergic neurons. In Seeman, P. & Brown, G.M. (eds) *Frontiers of Neurology and Neuroscience Research*, pp. 4–11. University of Toronto Press, Toronto.

Aghajanian, G.K. & Bunney, B.S. (1977) Dopamine autoreceptors: pharmacological characterization by microiontophoretic single cell recording studies. *Naunyn-Schmiedebergs Archives of Pharmacology*, 297, 1–8.

Alexander, G.E. & Crutcher, M.D. (1990) Functional architecture of basal ganglia circuits: neural substrates of parallel processing. *Trends in Neurosciences*, 13, 266–271.

Alheid, G., Heimer, L. & Switzer, R.C. (1990) The basal ganglia. In Paxinos, G. (ed.) *The Human Nervous System*, pp. 483–582. Academic Press, San Diego.

Andén, N.-E., Butcher, S.G., Corrodi, H., Fuxe, K. & Ungerstedt, U. (1970) Receptor activity and turnover of dopamine and noradrenaline after neuroleptics. *European Journal of Pharmacology*, 11, 303–314.

Andén, N.-E., Strömbom, U. & Svensson, T.H. (1973) Dopamine and noradrenaline receptor stimulation: reversal of reserpine-induced suppression of motor activity. *Psychopharmacologia* (Berlin), 29, 289–298.

Angrist, B. (1987) Pharmacological models of schizophrenia. In Henn, F.A. & DeLisi, L.E. (eds) *Handbook of Schizophrenia*, Vol. 2, *Neurochemistry and Neuropharmacology of Schizophrenia*, pp. 391–424. Elsevier, Amsterdam.

Bergman, H., Wichmann, T. & DeLong, M.R. (1990) Reversal of experimental Parkinsonism by lesions of the subthalamic nucleus. *Science*, 249, 1436–1437.

Bogerts, B. (1991) The neuropathology of schizophrenia. In Häfner, H. & Gattaz, W.F. (eds) *Search for the Causes of Schizophrenia*, pp. 229–241. Springer-Verlag, Berlin.

Boldry, R.C. & Uretsky, N.J. (1988) The importance of dopaminergic neurotransmission in the hypermotility response produced by the administration of *N*-methyl-D-aspartic acid into the nucleus accumbens. *Neuropharmacology*, 27, 569–577.

Buchsbaum, M. (1990) The frontal lobes, basal ganglia, and temporal lobes as sites for schizophrenia. *Schizophrenia Bulletin*, **16**, 379–390.

Cadet, J.L., Lohr, J.B. & Jeste, D.V. (1987) Tardive dyskinesia and schizophrenic burnout: the possible involvement of cytotoxic free radicals. In Henn, F.A. & DeLisi, L.E. (eds) *Handbook of Schizophrenia*, Vol. 2, *The Neurochemistry and Neuropharmacology of Schizophrenia*, pp. 425–438. Elsevier, Amsterdam.

Carlsson, A. (1975) Dopaminergic autoreceptors. In Almgren, O., Carlsson, A. & Engel, J. (eds) *Chemical Tools in Catecholamine Research*, Vol. II, pp. 219–226. North Holland, Amsterdam.

Carlsson, A. (1978) Mechanism of action of neuroleptic drugs. In Lipton, M.A., DiMascio, A. & Killam, K.F. (eds) *Psychopharmacology. A Generation of Progress*, pp. 1057–1070. Raven Press, New York.

Carlsson, A. (1983) Antipsychotic agents: elucidation of their mode of action. In Parnham, M.J. & Bruinvels, J. (eds) *Discoveries in Pharmacology*, Vol. 1, *Psycho- and Neuro-Pharmacology*, pp. 197–206. Elsevier, Amsterdam.

Carlsson, A. (1988) The current status of the dopamine hypothesis of schizophrenia (with commentaries and the author's reply). *Neuropsychopharmacology*, **1**, 179–203.

Carlsson, A. (1994) Search for the neuronal circuitries and neurotransmitters involved in 'positive' and 'negative' schizophrenic symptomatology. *Fidia Research Foundation Neuroscience Award Lectures*, Vol. 5. Raven Press, New York. (In press.)

Carlsson, A. & Lindqvist, M. (1963) Effect of chlorpromazine and haloperidol on the formation of 3-methoxytyramine and normetanephrine in mouse brain. *Acta Pharmacologica et Torticologica*, **20**, 140–144.

Carlsson, A., Kehr, W. & Lindqvist, M. (1977) Agonist–antagonist interaction on dopamine receptors in brain, as reflected in the rates of tyrosine and tryptophan hydroxylation. *Journal of Neural Transmission*, **40**, 99–113.

Carlsson, A., Lindqvist, M., Magnusson, T. & Waldeck, B. (1958) On the presence of 3-hydroxytyramine in brain. *Science*, **127**, 471.

Carlsson, M. & Carlsson, A. (1989a) The NMDA antagonist MK-801 causes marked locomotor stimulation in monoamine-depleted mice. *Journal of Neural Transmission*, **75**, 221–226.

Carlsson, M. & Carlsson, A. (1989b) Dramatic synergism between MK-801 and clonidine with respect to locomotor stimulatory effect in monoamine-depleted mice. *Journal of Neural Transmission*, **77**, 65–71.

Carlsson, M. & Carlsson, A. (1989c) Marked locomotor stimulation in monoamine-depleted mice following treatment with atropine in combination with clonidine. *Journal of Neural Transmission*, **1**, 317–322.

Carlsson, M. & Carlsson, A. (1990) Interactions between glutamatergic and monoaminergic systems within the basal ganglia — implications for schizophrenia and Parkinson's disease. *Trends in Neurosciences*, **13**, 272–276.

Carlsson, M. & Svensson, A. (1990a) Interfering with glutamatergic neurotransmission by means of NMDA antagonist administration discloses the stimulatory potential of other transmitter systems. *Pharmacology, Biochemistry and Behavior*, **36**, 45–50.

Carlsson, M. & Svensson, A. (1990b) The non-competitive NMDA antagonists MK-801 and PCP, as well as the competitive NMDA antagonist SDZ EAA494 (D-CPPene), interact synergistically with clonidine to promote locomotion in monoamine-depleted mice. *Life Sciences*, **47**, 1729–1736.

Carlsson, M., Svensson, A. & Carlsson, A. (1991) Synergistic interactions between muscarinic antagonists, adrenergic agonists and NMDA antagonists with respect to locomotor stimulatory effects in monoamine-depleted mice. *Naunyn-Schmiedebergs Archives of Pharmacology*, **343**, 568–573.

Carlsson, M., Svensson, A. & Carlsson, A. (1992) Interactions between excitatory amino acids, catecholamines and acetylcholine in the basal ganglia. In Simon, R.P. (ed.) *Excitatory Amino Acids. Fidia Research Foundation Symposium Series*, Vol. 9, pp. 189–194. Thieme Medical Publishers, New York.

Chevalier, G. & Deniau, J.M. (1990) Disinhibition as a basic process in the expression of striatal functions. *Trends in Neurosciences*, **13**, 277–280.

Clark, D. & White, F.J. (1987) D_1 dopamine receptor — the search for a function: a critical evaluation of the D_1/D_2 dopamine receptor classification and its functional implications. *Synapse*, **1**, 347–388.

Costa, J., Khaled, E., Sramek, J., Bunney, W. Jr, & Potkin, S.G. (1990) An open trial of glycine as an adjunct to neuroleptics in chronic treatment-refractory schizophrenics. *Journal of Clinical Psychopharmacology*, **10**, 71–72.

Côté, L. & Crutcher, M.D. (1991) The basal ganglia. In Kandel, E.R., Schwartz, J.H. & Jessel, T.M. (eds) *Principles of Neural Science*, 3rd edn, pp. 647–659. Elsevier, Amsterdam.

Creese, I., Burt, D.R. & Snyder, S.H. (1976) Dopamine receptor binding predicts clinical and pharmacological potencies of antischizophrenic drugs. *Science*, **192**, 481–483.

Crow, T.J. (1987) Two syndromes of schizophrenia as one pole of the continuum of psychosis: a concept of the nature of the pathogen and its genomic locus. In Henn, F.A. & DeLisi, L.E. (eds) *Handbook of Schizophrenia*, Vol. 2, *The Neurochemistry and Neuropharmacology of Schizophrenia*, pp. 17–48. Elsevier, Amsterdam.

Dawbarn, D. & Pycock, C.J. (1981) Motor effects following application of putative excitatory amino acid antagonists to the region of the mesencephalic dopamine cell bodies in the rat. *Naunyn-Schmiedebergs Archives of Pharmacology*, **318**, 100–104.

DeLisi, L.E. (1986) The use of positron emission tomography to image regional brain metabolism in schizophrenia and other psychiatric disorders: a review. In Nasrallah, H.A. & Weinberger, D.R. (eds) *Handbook of Schizophrenia*, Vol. 1, *The Neurology of Schizophrenia*, pp. 309–324. Elsevier, Amsterdam.

Domino, E. & Luby, E.D. (1973) Abnormal mental states induced by phencyclidine as a model of schizophrenia. In Cole, J.O., Freedman, A.M. & Friedhoff, A.J. (eds) *Psychopathology and Psychopharmacology*, pp. 37–50. Johns Hopkins

University Press, Baltimore.

Donzanti, B.A. & Uretsky, N.J. (1984) Antagonism of the hypermotility response induced by excitatory amino acids in the rat nucleus accumbens. *Naunyn-Schmiedebergs Archives of Pharmacology*, **325**, 1−7.

Duinkerke, S.J., Botter, P.A., Jansen, A.A.I. *et al.* (1993) Ritanserin, a selective 5-HT$_{1C/2}$-antagonist, and negative symptoms in schizophrenia. A placebo-controlled double-blind trial. *British Journal of Psychiatry*, **163**, 451−455.

Gellman, R.L. & Aghajanian, G.K. (1991) IPSPs in pyramidal cells in piriform cortex evoked by monoamine excitation of interneurons demonstrate a convergence of inputs. *Society for Neuroscience Abstracts*, **17**(1), 989.

Gerfen, C.R., Engber, T.M., Mahan, L.C. *et al.* (1990) D$_1$ and D$_2$ dopamine receptor-regulated gene expression of striatonigral and striatopallidal neurons. *Science*, **250**, 1429−1432.

Gibb, J.W. & Hotchkiss, A.J. (1979) Role of striatonigral pathway and GABA systems in methamphetamine-induced depression of striatal tyrosine hydroxylase activity. In Usdin, E., Kopin, I.J. & Barchas, J. (eds) *Catecholamines. Basic and Clinical Frontiers*, Vol. 2, pp. 1125−1127. Pergamon Press, New York.

Goldman-Rakic, P.S. & Selemon, L.D. (1986) Topography of corticostriatal projections in nonhuman primates and implications for functional parcellation of the neostriatum. In Jones, E.G. & Peters, A. (eds) *Cerebral Cortex*, Vol. 5, pp. 447−466. Plenum Press, New York.

Goodwin, P., Starr, B.S. & Starr, M.S. (1992) Motor responses to dopamine D$_1$ and D$_2$ agonists in the reserpine-treated mouse are affected differentially by the NMDA receptor antagonist MK 801. *Journal of Neural Transmission*, **4**, 15−26.

Graham, W.C., Robertson, R.G., Sambrook, M.A. & Crossman, A.R. (1990) Injection of excitatory amino acid antagonists into the medial pallidal segment of a 1-methyl-4-phenyl-1,2,3,6-tetrahydropyridine (MPTP) treated primate reverses motor symptoms of parkinsonism. *Life Sciences*, **47**, PL91−97.

Greengard, P. (1975) Presynaptic and postsynaptic roles of cyclic AMP and protein phosphorylation at catechol-aminergic synapses. In Almgren, O., Carlsson, A. & Engel, J. (eds) *Chemical Tools in Catecholamine Research*, Vol. II, pp. 249−256. North Holland, Amsterdam.

Gründer, G., Wetzel, H., Hillert, A. & Benkert, O. (1991) Roxindole, a dopamine autoreceptor agonist, in the treatment of negative symptoms of schizophrenia. *Biological Psychiatry*, **29**, 390S.

Halpain, S., Girault, J.-A. & Greengard, P. (1990) Activation of NMDA receptors induces dephosphorylation of DARPP-32 in rat striatal slices. *Nature*, **343**, 369−371.

Hansson, L.O., Waters, N., Winblad, B., Gottfries, C.G. & Carlsson, A. (1994) Evidence for biomedical heterogeneity in schizophrenia: a multivariate study of monoaminergic indices in human post-mortal brain tissue. *Journal of Neural Transmission* (in press).

Heim, C., Schwarz, M., Klockgether, T., Jaspers, R., Cools, A.R. & Sontag, K.-H. (1986) GABAergic neurotransmission within the reticular part of the substantia nigra

(SNR); role for switching motor patterns and performance of movements. *Experimental Brain Research*, **63**, 375−381.

Heimer, L., Alheid, G.F. & Zaborszky, L. (1985) Basal ganglia. In Paxinos, G. (ed.) *The Rat Nervous System*, Vol. 1, *Forebrain and Midbrain*, pp. 37−86. Academic Press, New York.

Heimer, L., de Olmos, J., Alheid, G.F. & Zaborszky, L. (1991) 'Perestroika' in the basal forebrain: opening the border between neurology and psychiatry. *Progress in Brain Research*, **87**, 109−165.

Heylen, S.L.E. & Gelders, Y.G. (1990) *Risperidone: A Clinical Overview*. Paper presented at Satellite Symposium on Risperidone at the 17th congress of Collegium Internationale Neuro-Psychopharmacologicum, Kyoto, Japan.

Kebabian, J.W. & Calne, D.B. (1979) Multiple receptors for dopamine. *Nature*, **277**, 93−96.

Kebabian, J.W. & Greengard, P. (1971) Dopamine-sensitive adenyl cyclase: possible role in synaptic transmission. *Science*, **174**, 1346−1349.

Kim, J.S., Kornhuber, H.H., Kornhuber, J. & Kornhuber, M.E. (1985) Glutamic acid and the dopamine hypothesis of schizophrenia. In Shagass, C. (ed.) *Biological Psychiatry*, pp. 1109−1111. Elsevier, Amsterdam.

Kirch, D.G. & Weinberger, D.R. (1986) Anatomical neuropathology in schizophrenia: postmortem findings. In Nasrallah, H.A. & Weinberger, D.R. (eds) *Handbook of Schizophrenia*, Vol. 1, *The Neurology of Schizophrenia*, pp. 325−348. Elsevier, Amsterdam.

Klinke, A. & Klieser, E. (1991) Antidepressant effects of the new dopamine autoreceptor agonist EMD 49980 (Roxindol) in acute schizophrenia. *Biological Psychiatry*, **29**, 410S.

Kobayashi, K. & Inoue, O. (1993) An increase in the *in vivo* binding of [^{3}H]SCH 23390 induced by MK-801 in the mouse striatum. *Neuropharmacology*, **32**, 341−348.

Kornhuber, H.H., Kornhuber, J., Kim, J.S. & Kornhuber, M.E. (1984) Zur biochemischen Theorie der Schizophrenie. *Nervenarzt*, **55**, 602−606.

Kornhuber, J., Bormann, J., Retz, W., Hubers, M. & Riederer, P. (1989) Memantine displaces [^{3}H]MK-801 at therapeutic concentrations in postmortem human frontal cortex. *European Journal of Pharmacology*, **166**, 589−590.

Lodge, D., Aran, J.A., Church, J., Davies, S.N., Martin, D. & Zeman, S. (1987) Excitatory amino acids and phencyclidine drugs. In Hicks, T.P., Lodge, D. & McLennan, H. (eds) *Excitatory Amino Acid Transmission*, pp. 83−90. Alan Liss, New York.

Malmberg, Å.H., Jackson, D.M., Eriksson, A. & Mohell, N.A. (1993) Unique binding characteristics of antipsychotic agents interacting with human dopamine D$_{2A}$, D$_{2B}$ and D$_3$ receptors. *Molecular Pharmacology*, **43**, 749−754.

Marshall, J.F., O'Dell, S.J. & Weihmuller, F.B. (1993) Dopamine-glutamate interactions in methamphetamine-induced neurotoxicity. *Journal of Neural Transmission*, **91**, 241−254.

Mattsson, B. (1974) Huntington's chorea in Sweden. II. Social and clinical data. *Acta Psychiatrica Scandinavica*, Suppl. **255**, 221−235.

Meyers, R. (1968) Ballismus. In Vinken, P.J. & Bruyn, G.W. (eds) *Handbook of Clinical Neurology*, Vol. 6, *Diseases of the*

Basal Ganglia, pp. 476–490. North Holland, Amsterdam.

Morelli, M. & Di Chiara, G. (1990) MK-801 potentiates dopaminergic D_1 but reduces D_2 responses in the 6-hydroxydopamine model of Parkinson's disease. *European Journal of Pharmacology*, **182**, 611–612.

Naber, D. (1991) Efficacy and tolerability of the partial dopamine agonist SDZ HDC 912 in the treatment of schizophrenia. *Biological Psychiatry*, **29**, 409S.

Nauta, W.J.F. (1989) Reciprocal links of the corpus striatum with the cerebral cortex and limbic system: a common substrate for movement and thought? In Mueller, J. (ed.) *Neurology and Psychiatry: A Meeting of Minds*, pp. 43–63. Karger, Basel.

Nordström, A.-L. (1993) *PET Evaluation of Dopamine Hypotheses for Antipsychotic Drugs and Schizophrenia*. Thesis, Stockholm.

Nordström, A.-L., Farde, L. & Halldin, C. (1993) High 5-HT$_2$ receptor occupancy in clozapine treated patients. *Psychopharmacology*, **110**, 365–367.

Nybäck, H. & Sedvall, G. (1970) Further studies on the accumulation and disappearance of catecholamines formed from tyrosine 14-C in mouse brain. *European Journal of Pharmacology*, **10**, 193–205.

O'Dell, S.J., Wiehmuller, F.B. & Marshall, J.F. (1991a) Multiple methamphetamine injections induce marked increases in extracellular striatal dopamine which correlate with subsequent neurotoxicity. *Brain Research*, **564**, 256–260.

O'Dell, S.J., Wiehmuller, F.B. & Marshall, J.F. (1991b) Dopamine receptor antagonists attenuate methamphetamine-induced striatal dopamine overflow and terminal damage. *Society for Neuroscience Abstracts*, **17**, 1278.

Pan, H.S., Penney, J.B. & Young, A.B. (1985) Gamma-aminobutyric acid and benzodiazepine receptor changes induced by unilateral 6-hydroxydopamine lesions of the median forebrain bundle. *Journal of Neurochemistry*, **45**, 1396–1404.

Parent, A., Lavoie, B., Hazrati, L.-N. & Côté, P.-Y. (1991) Chemical anatomy of the basal ganglia in normal and parkinsonian monkeys. In *Abstracts of the 10th International Symposium on Parkinson's Disease*, Tokyo, p. 6.

Parent, A., Paré, D., Smith, Y. & Steriade, M. (1988) Basal forebrain cholinergic and noncholinergic projections to the thalamus and brainstem in cats and monkeys. *Journal of Comparative Neurology*, **277**, 281–301.

Pawlowski, L., Mathé, J.M. & Svensson, T.H. (1990) Phencyclidine activates rat A10 dopamine neurons but reduces burst activity and causes regularization of firing. *Acta Physiologica Scandinavica*, **139**, 529–530.

Penney, J.B. & Young, A.B. (1986) Striatal inhomogeneities and basal ganglia function. *Movement Disorders*, **1**, 3–15.

Randrup, A. & Munkvad, I (1965) Special antagonism of amphetamine-induced abnormal behaviour. Inhibition of stereotyped activity with increase of some normal activities. *Psychopharmacologia*, **7**, 416–422.

Reynolds, G.P. (1987) Postmortem neurochemical studies in schizophrenia. In Häfner, H., Gattaz, W.F. & Janzanik, W. (eds) *Search for the Causes of Schizophrenia*, pp. 236–240. Springer-Verlag, Heidelberg.

van Rossum, J.M. (1966) The significance of dopamine receptor blockade for the mechanism of action of neuroleptic drugs. *Archives Internationales de Pharmacodynamie et de Therapie*, **160**, 492–494.

Schwartz, J.-C., Levesque, D., Martres, M.-P. & Sokoloff, P. (1993) Dopamine D_3 receptor: basic and clinical aspects. *Clinical Neuropharmacology*, **16**, 295–314.

Seeman, P., Guan, H.-C. & Van Tol, H.H.M. (1993) Dopamine D_4 receptors elevated in schizophrenia. *Nature*, **365**, 441–445.

Seeman, P., Lee, M., Chau-Wong, M. & Wong, K. (1976) Antipsychotic drug doses and neuroleptic/dopamine receptors. *Nature*, **261**, 717–719.

Seiden, L., Commins, D., Vosmer, G., Axt, K. & Marek, G. (1988) Neurotoxicity in dopamine and 5-hydroxytryptamine terminal fields: a regional analysis in nigrostriatal and mesolimbic projections. *Annals of the New York Academy of Sciences*, **537**, 161–172.

Selemon, L.D. & Goldman-Rakic, P.S. (1985) Longitudinal topography and interdigitation of corticostriatal projections in the Rhesus monkey. *Journal of Neuroscience*, **5**, 776–794.

Sibley, D.R. & Monsma, F.J. Jr (1992) Molecular biology of dopamine receptors. *Trends in Pharmacological Science*, **13**, 61–69.

Sokoloff, P.B., Giros, B., Martres, M.-P., Bouthenet, M.-L. & Schwartz, J.-C. (1990) Molecular cloning and characterization of a novel dopamine receptor (D_3) as a target for neuroleptics. *Nature*, **347**, 146–151.

Sonsalla, P., Nicklas, W. & Heikkila, R. (1989) Role for excitatory amino acids in methamphetamine-induced nigrostriatal dopaminergic toxicity. *Science*, **243**, 398–400.

Spano, P.F., Govoni, S. & Trabucchi, M. (1978) Studies on the pharmacological properties of dopamine receptors in various areas of the central nervous system. *Advances in Biochemical Psychopharmacology*, **19**, 155–165.

Ståhle, L. (1992) Do autoreceptors mediate dopamine agonist-induced yawning and suppression of exploration? *Psychopharmacology*, **106**, 1–13.

Steriade, M. & Llinas, R.R. (1988) The functional states of the thalamus and the associated neuronal interplay. *Physiological Reviews*, **68**, 649–742.

Steriade, M., Parent, A. & Paré, D. & Smith, Y. (1987) Cholinergic and non-cholinergic neurons of cat basal forebrain project to reticular and mediodorsal thalamic nuclei. *Brain Research*, **408**, 372–376.

Svensson, A. & Carlsson, M.L. (1992) Injection of the competitive NMDA receptor antagonist AP-5 into the nucleus accumbens of monoamine-depleted mice induces pronounced locomotor stimulation. *Neuropharmacology*, **31**, 513–518.

Svensson, A., Carlsson, M.L. & Carlsson, A. (1992a) Interaction between glutamatergic and dopaminergic tone in the nucleus accumbens of mice: evidence for a dual glutamatergic function with respect to psychomotor control. *Journal of Neural Transmission*, **88**, 235–240.

Svensson, A., Carlsson, M.L. & Carlsson, A. (1992b) Differential locomotor interactions between dopamine D_1/D_2 receptor agonists and the NMDA antagonist dizocilpine in monoamine-depleted mice. *Journal of Neural Transmission*, **90**, 199–217.

Svensson, A., Carlsson, M.L. & Carlsson, A. (1994) Gluta-matergic neurons projecting to the nucleus accumbens can affect psychomotor functions in opposite directions depending on the dopaminergic tone. *Progress in Neuro-Psychopharmacology and Biological Psychiatry*, **18**, 1203–1218.

Svensson, K., Carlsson, A. & Waters, N. (1994) Locomotor inhibition by the D_3 ligand R-(+)-7-OH-DPAT is inde-pendent of changes in dopamine release. *Journal of Neural Transmission*, **95**, 71–74.

Svensson, K., Eriksson, E. & Carlsson, A. (1993) Partial dopamine receptor agonists reverse behavioral, biochemical and neuroendocrine effects of neuroleptics in the rat: potential treatment of extrapyramidal side effects. *Neuro-pharmacology*, **32**, 1017–1045.

Svensson, K., Johansson, A.M., Magnusson, T. & Carlsson, A. (1986) (+)-AJ 76 and (+)-UH 232: central stimulants acting as preferential dopamine autoreceptor antagonists. *Naunyn-Schmiedebergs Archives of Pharmacology*, **334**, 234–245.

Tamminga, C.A., Crayton, J.C. & Chase, T.N. (1978) Muscimol: GABA agonist therapy in schizophrenia. *American Journal of Psychiatry*, **135**, 746–748.

Tamminga, C.A., Cascella, N.G., Fakouhi, T.D. & Herting, R.L. (1992a) Enhancement of NMDA-mediated trans-mission in schizophrenia: effects of milacemide. In Meltzer, H.Y. (ed.) *Novel Antipsychotic Medications*, pp. 171–177. Raven Press, New York.

Tamminga, C.A., Cascella, N.G., Lahti, R.A., Lindberg, M. & Carlsson, A. (1992b) Pharmacological properties of (−)-3PPP (preclamol) in man. *Journal of Neural Transmission*, **88**, 165–175.

Tamminga, C.A., Kaneda, H., Buchanan, R. *et al.* (1991) The limbic system in schizophrenia. Pharmacologic and meta-bolic evidence. *Advances in Neuropsychiatry and Psycho-pharmacology*, **1**, 99–109.

Tamminga, C.A., Thaker, G.K., Gao, X.-M. *et al.* (1992c) Limbic system abnormalities in schizophrenia and neo-cortical alterations with deficit syndrome. *Archives of General Psychiatry*, **49**, 522–530.

Waters, N., Lagerkvist, S., Löfberg, L., Piercey, M. & Carlsson, A. (1993a) The dopamine D_3 receptor and auto-receptor preferring antagonists (+)-AJ76 and (+)-UH232; a microdialysis study. *European Journal of Pharmacology*, **242**, 151–163.

Waters, N., Svensson, K., Haadsma-Svensson, S.R., Smith, M.W. & Carlsson, A. (1993b) The dopamine D_3-receptor: a postsynaptic receptor inhibitory on rat locomotor activity. *Journal of Neural Transmission*, **94**, 11–19.

Weinberger, D.R. (1986) The pathogenesis of schizo-phrenia: a neurodevelopmental theory. In Nasrallah, H.A. & Weinberger, D.R. (eds) *Handbook of Schizophrenia*, Vol. 1, *The Neurology of Schizophrenia*, pp. 397–406. Elsevier, Amsterdam.

Wiedemann, K., Loycke, A., Krieg, J.C. & Holsboer, F. (1991) EMD 49980 – a novel dopamine autoreceptor agonist in the treatment of schizophrenic patients with negative symptoms. *Biological Psychiatry*, **29**, 422S.

Wong, E.H.F., Kemp, J.A., Priestley, T., Knight, A.R., Woodruff, G.N. & Iversen, L.L. (1986) The anticonvulsant MK-801 is a potent *N*-methyl-D-aspartate antagonist. *Proceedings of the National Academy of Sciences USA*, **83**, 7104–7108.

Wyatt, R.J. (1991) Neuroleptics and the natural course of schizophrenia. *Schizophrenia Bulletin*, **17**, 325–351.

Zhang, J., Chiodo, L.A. & Freeman, A.S. (1992) Electro-physiological effects of MK-801 on rat nigrostriatal and mesoaccumbal dopaminergic neurons. *Brain Research*, **590**, 153–163.

Chapter 21
Animal Neuropharmacology
and Its Prediction of Clinical Response

B. COSTALL AND R. J. NAYLOR

Introduction: the relevance of animal research to schizophrenia

Many neuropharmacologists who work with animals do so in the belief that their research may finally be relevant to an improved understanding of human physiology or pathology and its treatment. There may be direct attempts to model human illnesses in animal behavioural and biochemical tests, and the validity of the models must be subject to close scrutiny. The models can be designed to address the physiological basis of the systems underlying the disorder, its aetiology and/or its treatment. Assessing the validity of animal models in neuropsychopharmacological research is the subject of an excellent recent review (Willner, 1991) and is frequently one of judgement rather than detailed quantitative correlations. Willner (1991) suggests that the overall validity of any model is based on three aspects which allow a

synthesis of its overall validity; predictive validity, face validity and construct validity. Predictive validity means that performance in the test predicts performance in the condition being modelled; face validity means that there are phenomenological similarities between the two; and construct validity indicates that the model has a sound theoretical rationale. These are considered in relation to animal research and schizophrenia.

Construct validity

The design of an animal model of schizophrenia which has construct validity is a most daunting task. Indeed, it may be sensibly asked if this is possible at all in a single model. Thus, to establish construct validity would require that the aetiology of schizophrenia be known and could be simulated in animals. Given that the causation of schizophrenia is not known but is generally accepted to reflect a genetic predisposition with an environmental precipitant (Kendler, 1987), then clearly this is not possible. Even if it were known, there could be no guarantee that a given dysfunction would express itself in an identical manner in different species. Furthermore, given the breadth of dysfunction, the delusional thinking, hallucinations, incoherence or poverty of speech, inappropriate affect, social isolation, repetitive behaviour and others, the changing nature of schizophrenia over time and the virtual certainty that schizophrenia is more than one disease, then the modelling of schizophrenia in terms of construct validity remains to be achieved.

Face validity

Constructing animal models with face validity is an attempt to relate the symptoms of schizophrenia to similar behaviours in animals. Therefore, the first essential is to identify as precisely as possible the characteristic symptoms that define the profile of schizophrenia, accepting that there may be extreme variations in its presentations. If one is in aggreement with the criteria according to the *Diagnostic and Statistical Manual* DSM-III (APA, 1980), the initial phase may comprise both 'positive' and 'negative' behaviours. The positive behaviours with an 'active' quality are: (i) peculiar and bizarre behaviours; (ii) digressive speech or overelaboration, unnecessary repetitions or excessive purring; (iii) odd ideation, especially as bizarre or extremely unusual associations; and (iv) unusual perceptual experiences. The negative behaviours with a 'passive' quality are: (i) lack of personal hygiene or grooming; (ii) flat or inappropriate effect; and (iii) social isolation. In the final phase of the illness further positive behaviours: (i) delusional thinking; and (ii) hallucinations, especially of the auditory type, and negative behaviours: (i) incoherence or poverty of speech; and (ii) flat or inappropriate effect, are described. The difficulty, if not impossibility, of a direct measurement of many such behaviours in animals is obvious. But indirect measurement may afford an alternative approach.

It is hypothesized that the complex and changing presentation of the disease may reflect cardinal symptoms of an excessive response alternation or switching between a number of response alternatives, repetition or stereotype of a limited response type or constant shifting of response. This leads to an abnormal focusing and fragmentation of behaviour into non-adaptive and bizarre components (Lyon, 1991). The final consequence of this scenario is that fragmentation will prevent the completion of almost any complex behaviour, leading to the excessive repetition or stereotyped responding of a few and simple behavioural patterns. From this hypothesis, Lyon (1991) has compared human and animal symptoms that may be related to schizophrenia. For example, while digressive speech, overelaboration and repetitions in schizophrenia are not directly measurable in animals, indirect effects in animals could come from 'inappropriate switching or increased repetition of certain responses with exclusion of others, interfering with communicative, sexual or social behaviours; excessively repeated vocalization'. Unusual perceptions in humans might find indirect expression in animals as 'extremely concentrated examination of details, especially near objects, or body and hands; hyperstartle or sudden recoil to humanly undetectable stimuli; crouching, hiding and fearful responses to innocuous stimuli, or familiar individuals'. Hallucinations in humans might be indirectly measured in animals as 'behaviour directed at invisible objects, and having a sequential nature, with attention remaining concentrated on one spot during the activity, 'fly-catching' with co-ordinated eye, tongue and mouth movements (cats) or attack, flight or feeding behaviours associated with invisible stimuli (monkeys), excessive parasitotic-like grooming and biting at specific points on the skin (monkeys)'. The limiting factor for all such indirect measurements is the judgemental interpretation by the investigator of a verbal expression or body movement. For some behaviours it remains possible to directly measure analogous behaviour in the animal, e.g. increases in locomotor activity.

Predictive validity

The predictive value of behavioural and neuro-chemical models is based essentially on the clinical successes and failures of drug treatments. The model should discriminate between those compounds that relieve or exacerbate the symptoms of schizophrenia from those that do not. The models vary from behavioural paradigms where all drugs that are effective in the treatment of schizophrenia should be effective in the model, to simple or sophisticated neurochemical models or screens, which by definition will detect agents with an already defined mechanism of action.

It is preferable that drug potency in animal models should correlate with antipsychotic potency in humans, although species differences in the rate of drug metabolism may obscure the correlation. Discrepancies between the effect of a drug in animal models or screens and humans may also rise due to the study of acute drug effects in animals but chronic use in humans. It is rare for drugs to be administered chronically in screening tests in animals. Indeed, a single acute challenge is the norm. This must remain of concern when the antipsychotic action of drugs is not usually apparent until some 3−4 weeks of treatment. It also remains an interesting possibility that a false-negative result in a particular animal test may be revealing of the presence of differential drug activity in animal models and subgroups of clinical disorder. In other words, to expect an absolute correlation between data obtained from the acute use of drugs in animals and a serious and progressive human pathology is almost certainly naïve.

Animal tests in use for the prediction of antipsychotic activity

The chance detection of the antipsychotic actions of chlorpromazine prompted an intense search for other phenothiazines with similar actions, and other compounds from different chemical series. Many thousands of research papers and numerous reviews attest to the general consensus that the distinguishing mechanism of action of chlor-promazine, haloperidol, sulpiride and related antipsychotic agents is a dopamine-receptor blockade (see review by Costall & Naylor, 1980). Inevitably, this has dominated the design of animal tests and hypotheses as to the pathological disturbances in schizophrenia.

The dopamine hypothesis of schizophrenia

The evidence for an involvement of dopamine in schizophrenia is almost entirely based on pharmacological evidence using dopamine-receptor agonists and antagonists and has been exhaustively reviewed (see Costall & Naylor, 1985; Carlsson, 1988; and Chapter 20, this volume). Briefly, dopamine-receptor antagonists can attenuate the 'positive' symptoms of schizophrenia which can be exacerbated by amphetamine and dopamine agonists (Angrist *et al.*, 1974; Turner *et al.*, 1984). Indeed, the administration of amphetamine for a sufficient period of time in normal individuals can induce a paranoid psychotic-like behaviour. It has remained one of the most disquieting findings in schizophrenia research that for over 30 years there have been no consistent or marked biochemical changes in dopamine or its metabolism detected in the schizophrenic brain (Kleinman *et al.*, 1979). One of the few intriguing findings is by Reynolds (1983), who reported that levels of dopamine in the left amygdala were elevated in comparison to both levels in the right amygdala of schizophrenic brain and levels in either amygdala of control brain. The more recent evidence that the density of brain dopamine-receptor subtypes D_1 and D_2 may be differentially modified or involved in schizophrenia (Creese, 1988) is discussed elsewhere (Chapters 18 & 20, this volume). The lack of effect of the classical dopamine-receptor antagonists on the loss of functions in schizophrenia, i.e. the negative symptoms, has remained of continuing disappointment and concern. Brain-imaging techniques like computerized tomography (CT) and magnetic resonance imaging (MRI) have demonstrated ventricular enlargement and structural changes in the brains of schizophrenic patients, particularly in limbic structures and the temporal lobe (see

Shelton & Weinberger, 1987); these have been linked with the negative symptoms (Johnstone *et al.*, 1976; Crow, 1980). There are very important implications with respect to these studies in terms of an understanding of the pathogenesis of schizophrenia, the possibility of different patient subgroups, their treatment and outcome (see Crow, 1991). If the brain changes do reflect a progressive degeneration, then the treatment of many patients with chronic illness will require a fundamental revision. In turn, this will require new animal test procedures. This is beyond the scope of the present chapter but will undoubtedly be a critical issue in future studies.

Animal models that provide predictive validity of drug action in schizophrenia

The various models have been comprehensively reviewed (Ahlenius, 1991; Lyon, 1991) and are summarized below.

Stimulant drug models

Using many species, the administration of amphetamine as an acute injection or continuous treatment from implanted pellets causes highly consistent behavioural changes induced by the release of dopamine and/or the blockade of its uptake. Low doses cause increases in locomotor activity, which at higher doses are followed by peculiar or bizarre behaviour, abortive grooming and fragmentary movements, inappropriate or excessive switching and response stereotype (Ellinwood & Sudilovsky, 1973; Evenden & Robbins, 1983). The peripheral administration of other dopamine agonists can induce similar behaviours or components of this response. The injection or infusion of dopamine into the nucleus accumbens over a period of days again enhances locomotor activity and this is of a cyclical nature and dependent on basal responsiveness to dopamine agonist challenge (see Costall *et al.*, 1984). In any event, the effects of amphetamine and dopamine are inhibited by dopamine antagonists and there is an excellent correlation between the potency of traditional phenothiazine or butyro-

phenone compounds to inhibit a behaviour such as amphetamine-induced stereotypy and clinical antipsychotic potency (Costall & Naylor, 1980).

Drug-induced extrapyramidal side effects. The ability of drugs to block striatal dopamine receptors is revealed as a severe reduction in motor performance causing Parkinson-like side effects, dystonias, akathisia or dyskinesias in humans. Similar behaviours can be observed in primates and a 'catalepsy' or immobility is induced by neuroleptics in rodents. Again, for dopamine-receptor antagonists there is an excellent correlation between catalepsy induction, extrapyramidal side effects and antipsychotic/parkinsonism-inducing potential (Janssen *et al.*, 1965; Costall & Naylor, 1980).

Drug-induced endocrine effects. The tuberoinfundibular dopamine system moderates the release of hypothalamic/pituitary hormones. Dopamine inhibits the release of prolactin, and dopamine antagonists increase the release (Meltzer *et al.*, 1978). As would be expected, there is a good correlation between the ability of neuroleptics to increase prolactin and their antipsychotic potency.

Antagonism of emesis. Dopamine agonists such as apomorphine induce emesis in the dog, and its potent antagonism by dopamine antagonists has been used to evaluate potential antischizophrenic drugs (Niemegeers & Janssen, 1979). Again, there is a close correlation between the antiemetic potency of traditional neuroleptics and their antipsychotic potential (Costall & Naylor, 1980).

Sensorimotor gating models

Since the earliest studies of Kraepelin and Bleuler, abnormalities in attentional and information processing have been recorded in schizophrenia. McGhie and Chapman (1961) hypothesized that internal screening or gating mechanisms are impaired in schizophrenia, consciousness being flooded with an 'undifferentiated tide' of sensory data. Such deficits are thought to create a vulnerability to thought disorders (Gottschalk *et al.*, 1972). In normal subjects an event-related potential follows a novel stimulus; this is attenuated by a preliminary signal, i.e. 'prepulse inhibition'. In schizophrenic subjects an eye blink startle response shows less amplitude inhibition and less latency facilitation than does one in healthy subjects in response to prestimulus. This loss of prepulse inhibition was considered to lead to faulty information intake (Braff *et al.*, 1978). In animal models, apomorphine or amphetamine have been shown to attenuate prepulse inhibition via a neuroleptic-sensitive mechanism in the limbic system (Braff & Geyer, 1990). The finding indicates that an overactivity of limbic dopamine may cause a loss of sensorimotor gating with consequent disturbance of cognitive function.

The advantage of the startle reflex is its cross-species response to strong exteroceptive stimuli and a fine degree of experimental control (Geyer *et al.*, 1990). This is a newer model and it will be of particular interest to investigate a range of known antischizophrenic agents and other compounds to compare animal data with clinical results. It is worthy of serious investigation.

Thus, it is apparent that the animal models have a high ability for predicting the antipsychotic potency of dopamine-receptor antagonists. But to continue with such models to detect dopamine-receptor antagonists is merely to repeat the successes of the past, limiting future invention and innovation — and ultimately new therapies. Safer drugs without the extrapyramidal and endocrine side effects are urgently required to treat the positive symptoms, and the task of finding agents useful to treat the negative symptoms has barely begun. With this in mind, examples are taken and evidence is reviewed of recent neuropharmacological studies which may reveal future insights and treatments of schizophrenia.

5-Hydroxytryptamine$_2$ (5-HT$_2$) and 5-HT$_3$ receptors and schizophrenia

One of the earliest hypotheses of schizophrenia was focused around the role of 5-HT. This was founded on evidence that lysergic acid diethylamide (LSD) *N,N*-dimethyltryptamine and related agents induced hallucinations in humans and were known to interact with 5-HT receptors. It also gave rise to hypotheses as to a role for endogenous indolealkylamines in psychoses.

If agonist action on 5-HT receptors could have psychotomimetic effects, it was to be predicted that drugs acting to reduce 5-HT synthesis or release, or antagonize at 5-HT receptors would have antipsychotic effects. But fenfluramin or parachlorophenylalanine in disrupting 5-HT synthesis or release may also affect catecholamine function (see Barnes *et al.*, 1988). Also, of the 5-HT receptor antagonists that were available, methysergide or cypropeptadine lacked specificity for the 5-HT receptors. With these severe limitations in the choice of experimental probes, it is not surprising that no convincing evidence was obtained to support the hypothesis of an involvement of 5-HT or 5-HT-like compounds in schizophrenia. However, there has been a renaissance of interest in 5-HT and schizophrenia with the advent of compounds with highly selective effects on 5-HT receptor subtypes.

5-HT receptor subtypes

5-HT receptors are presently classified into four broad groups, 5-HT$_1$, 5-HT$_2$, 5-HT$_3$ and 5-HT$_4$, and the molecular, biochemical, physiological and pharmacological characterization of these receptors has been the subject of many reviews (see Bradley *et al.*, 1986; Humphrey, 1992; Weinshank *et al.*, 1992). With respect to 5-HT receptors and schizophrenia, this account focuses on the 5-HT$_2$ and 5-HT$_3$ receptors. It is emphasized that this is placed within the very important developments in the refinement of diagnostic criteria and the certainty of the heterogeneity of the syndrome (Andreasen, 1987; Brockington, 1986).

5-HT$_2$ receptors

The function, location and characteristics of 5-HT$_2$ receptors

Ketanserin was the first selective 5-HT$_2$ receptor antagonist (see review by Awouters *et al.*, 1988) and the use of this, and subsequently of other 5-HT$_2$ receptor antagonists, identified the receptor involvement in events as diverse as smooth muscle contraction, platelet aggregation and head twitches (see Bradley *et al.*, 1986). Such effects are induced by various 5-HT agonists, e.g. tryptamine, tryptophan, quipazine and LSD, and are blocked by 5-HT$_2$ antagonists. The use of 5-HT-receptor antagonists or reducing 5-HT function has also long been known to antagonize neuroleptic-induced catalepsy (Costall *et al.*, 1975) and this may assume particular importance with respect to the clinical studies using 5-HT$_2$ antagonists in the treatment of schizophrenia. Yet it remains clear that 5-HT$_2$ antagonists, when administered alone, fail to modify the motor, autonomic or cognitive performance of animals, or the turnover of 5-HT (Leysen & Pauwels, 1990; Leysen, 1992). This could indicate a very low or even absent endogenous stimulation of the 5-HT$_2$ receptor under normal physiological conditions.

The 5-HT neurones which originate in the raphe nuclei innervate the entire forebrain. It remains a most intriguing feature that within three terminal areas of the rat brain, the cerebral cortex, hippocampus and striatum, the majority of the ascending 5-HT pathways are non-junctional (Descarries *et al.*, 1990). It is also a pecularity that environmental stressors which reliably activate catecholamine neurones fail to activate 5-HT neurones (Jacobs *et al.*, 1990). But there remain others, not least the relative insensitivity of the 5-HT$_2$ receptor to 5-HT itself (Leysen, 1990) and its rapid desensitization to 5-HT agonists (see Leysen, 1992). High concentrations of 5-HT$_2$ receptors are found in the prefrontal cortex of all mammalian species, including humans (Leysen *et al.*, 1983; Schotte *et al.*, 1983). The 5-HT$_2$ receptors have been cloned and there is much similarity between the 5-HT$_{1C}$ and 5-HT$_2$ receptor.

5-HT$_2$ receptors, psychotomimetic drugs and schizophrenia

The possibility that phenylalkylamine, ergolene

and indolealkylamine hallucinogenic agents may exert their effects via the 5-HT$_2$ receptor has been investigated in animal behavioural and electrophysiological studies and in binding studies (see Aghajanian *et al.*, 1987). Many of the psychotomimetic agents have high affinity for the 5-HT$_2$/ 5-HT$_{1C}$ site (Hibert *et al.*, 1990) and facilitate the actions of 5-HT on the facial motor neurone (Aghajanian *et al.*, 1987). The latter observation would be particularly interesting if it could be extended to other neuronal systems.

If 5-HT$_2$ agonists can induce hallucinations, then 5-HT$_2$-receptor antagonists may have beneficial effects in schizophrenia, and the first evidence came from the use of pipamperone, but not in the direction anticipated from the animal studies. Pipamperone is a weak neuroleptic and considerably more potent as a 5-HT$_2$ antagonist. It was reported to be helpful in chronic schizophrenia, being anti-autistic, disinhibitory and facilitating resocialization (see Niemegeers, 1989). It was uncertain whether the clinical efficacy was due to the dopamine or 5-HT-receptor blockade or both. But in any event, the compound had no effect on the positive core symptoms. More selective 5-HT$_2$-receptor antagonists, such as ritan-

Table 21.1 Profile of 5-hydroxytryptamine (5-HT) and dopamine receptor ligands for the 5-HT$_{1C}$, 5-HT$_2$ and dopamine D$_2$ receptors. [From Leysen, 1992 (K$_i$ values, nM)]

Compound	Receptor subtype		
	5-HT$_2$	5-HT$_{1C}$	D$_2$
Ritanserin	0.24	0.6	–
Ketanserin	0.38	54	–
Pipamperone	1.0	100	130*
Methysergide	1.5	1.8	–
Risperidone	0.16	48	3.1
Flupenthixol	2.5	110	6.4
Chlorpromazine	2.7	25	2.8*
Clozapine	3.3	9.5	56*
Fluphenazine	3.5	300	1.9
Thioridazine	4.2	58	3.3*
Pimozide	6	380	1.2

* From Sokoloff *et al.* (1990) and Leysen *et al.* (1978).

serin, permitted a more precise investigation of the role of the 5-HT_2 receptor; clinical results indicated an improvement in mood, a notable increase in slow-wave sleep and a decrease in extrapyramidal side effects of concurrent neuroleptic therapy (Reyntjens *et al.*, 1986; Janssen, 1987; Awouters *et al.*, 1988; Pangalila-Ratu *et al.*, 1988).

Thus, from these preliminary studies the major effects of 5-HT_2-receptor blockade was not to alleviate the hallucinations and delusions but to improve the mood and sleep disorders with a valuable reduction in extrapyramidal side effects of concomitant neuroleptic therapy. Therefore, Janssen *et al.* synthesized agents with dopamine and 5-HT_2 receptor antagonism, and selected risperidone for clinical trial. It was reported to be efficacious in the treatment of psychotic and negative symptoms, with beneficial effects on mood and anxiety, and with little extrapyramidal disturbance (Janssen *et al.*, 1988; Castelao *et al.*, 1989; Meco *et al.*, 1989; Messoten *et al.*, 1989).

Such preliminary findings have given much encouragement to the development of a new class of antischizophrenic agents, and the preservation of 5-HT_2 and dopamine-receptor antagonism in a single drug can be seen in agents such as ORG5222 (Kelder *et al.*, 1984) and ICI 204,636 (Salama *et al.*, 1989). However, the best known agent is clozapine. This was developed over 20 years ago as an antipsychotic agent with a very low incidence of extrapyramidal disturbance (Angst *et al.*, 1971). In early studies we demonstrated its blockade of limbic dopamine function (Costall & Naylor, 1976) and this, together with its known affinity for the acetylcholine receptor, was believed to contribute to the antipsychotic potential and very low incidence of extrapyramidal disturbance (Coward *et al.*, 1989). The 5-HT-receptor antagonist effects of clozapine were considered important by only a few early investigators (Fink *et al.*, 1984). It was Meltzer (1989) who proposed that the 5-HT_2-receptor antagonism was important to its clinical effects and that schizophrenia may reflect a dysfunction in 5-HT and dopamine D_2 systems.

Clozapine affords one of the most important adjuncts to the treatment of schizophrenia, being the only known compound for the treatment of schizophrenic patients who do not respond to classical therapy. Indeed, given the regular haematological monitoring, this is the only clinical indication for its use, where some 50% of treatment-resistant patients demonstrate an improvement after 6 months of treatment. The possibility that the clinical profile of action of clozapine also reflects its more potent action on the D_4 receptor is beyond the present discussion (see Van Tol *et al.*, 1992).

There remain curious features to the hypotheses for the role of 5-HT_2 receptors in the drug treatment of schizophrenia. Many classical neuroleptic agents with high affinity for the dopamine receptor also have high affinity at low nanomolar concentrations for the 5-HT_2/5-HT_{1C} receptor (Table 21.1). Yet the presence of a 5-HT_2-receptor antagonism does not necessarily prevent the extrapyramidal side effects or relieve the negative symptoms. Further complexities are revealed in the actions of amperozide.

Amperozide is an atypical antipsychotic drug with an affinity for cortical 5-HT_2 receptors in *in vitro* binding assays 100-fold more potent than for striatal dopamine receptors (Meltzer *et al.*, 1989; Svartengren & Simonsson, 1990). Its ability to attenuate positive and negative schizophrenic symptoms could reflect a risperidone or clozapine-like profile. But, in *in vivo* binding assays, amperozide was found to be devoid of any ability to occupy striatal D_2 binding sites (Meltzer *et al.*, 1992) and was devoid of the ability to block dopamine D_2 sites in behavioural and biochemical tests (Waters *et al.*, 1989; Christensson, 1990). Its antipsychotic potency in a dose range of $5-20$ mg/day (Mertens *et al.*, 1989; Axelsson *et al.*, 1991) is therefore unlikely to be related to a dopamine-receptor blockade.

A further unusual pharmacological feature of amperozide is its surprisingly high potency in *in vivo* as compared with *in vitro* assays for the 5-HT_2 receptor; indeed, it is as potent as ritanserin (Meltzer *et al.*, 1989). These intriguing findings may raise many questions as to the mechanisms of action of amperozide as an antipsychotic agent and the relative roles of $5\text{-}HT_2$ and dopamine receptors in schizophrenia. Perhaps the answers may be partly found in a presynaptic action of amperozide, revealed by *in vivo* microdialysis, to inhibit the ability of amphetamine to stimulate dopamine release in the nucleus accumbens (Ichikawa & Meltzer, 1992). Confirmation of these findings may open a major new approach to the treatment of schizophrenia and indicate an important $5\text{-}HT_2$ control of dopamine release. In the immediate future, new therapies will be introduced to combine dopamine- and $5\text{-}HT_2$-receptor antagonist activities; a reduction in extrapyramidal side effects and improved treatment of the negative symptoms is predicted.

The $5\text{-}HT_3$ receptor

A neuronally located 5-HT receptor was first identified in the enteric nervous system (Gaddum & Picarelli, 1957). It was some 25 years before pharmacological tools were developed to characterize and locate the receptor, which was revealed to have an extensive distribution in the sensory and autonomic nervous systems and within the brain (see reviews by Fozard, 1989; Kilpatrick *et al.*, 1990).

Characterization, location and functional role of $5\text{-}HT_3$ receptors

$5\text{-}HT_3$ receptors show a susceptibility to antagonism by $5\text{-}HT_3$-receptor antagonists such as tropisetron and ondansetron, a resistance to the $5\text{-}HT_1$- and $5\text{-}HT_2$-receptor antagonists methysergide and ketanserin, and a responsiveness to the agonists 2-methyl-5-HT and phenylbiguanide. The $5\text{-}HT_3$ receptors are ligand-gated cation-selective ion channels mediating membrane depolarization and neuronal excitation; the response rapidly desensitizes (see review by Peters *et al.*, 1992). Evidence for interspecies variations in the pharmacological characteristics of the $5\text{-}HT_3$ receptor continues to grow (Peters *et al.*, 1992).

$5\text{-}HT_3$ receptors were first identified in the rat brain using the selective $5\text{-}HT_3$-receptor ligand

$[^3H]65630$ (Kilpatrick *et al.*, 1987). The density of $5\text{-}HT_3$ receptors was considerably lower than that of many other neurotransmitter receptors, but has been fully confirmed using homogenate and autoradiographic techniques in many studies involving many species, including humans (see Barnes *et al.*, 1989a; Kilpatrick *et al.*, 1989). The highest density of $5\text{-}HT_3$ receptors has been reported in the nucleus tractus solitarius and area postrema, with the limbic and cortical regions containing a significant density.

The development and use of the $5\text{-}HT_3$-receptor antagonists in the early 1980s indicated that in normal animals the compounds failed to effect behaviour or any other function. This has been amply confirmed and extended to humans, with the minor exception that $5\text{-}HT_3$-receptor antagonists cause constipation in some patients. This reflects a blockade of endogenous 5-HT function facilitating an enteric cholinergic drive.

This behavioural and biochemical inactivity to modify normal brain events has created considerable interest, within a perspective that the $5\text{-}HT_3$-receptor antagonists have an extraordinary breadth and potency of action to correct disturbed behaviour in animals. The behavioural and other effects of the $5\text{-}HT_3$-receptor antagonists have been extensively reviewed (Costall *et al.*, 1990) and are summarized below with respect to a potential role in the treatment of schizophrenia.

$5\text{-}HT_3$ receptors and animal behaviour

The control of limbic dopamine function. Evidence that the 5-HT innervation of the limbic system may moderate dopamine function was the starting point to investigate the possibility that $5\text{-}HT_3$ receptors were involved in mediating the effects of 5-HT (see review by Costall *et al.*, 1990). Ondansetron and other $5\text{-}HT_3$-receptor antagonists were shown to attenuate the behavioural hyperactivity caused by the injection of amphetamine or the infusion of dopamine into the nucleus accumbens or amygdala of the rat or marmoset (Costall *et al.*, 1987). The injection of a neurokinin agonist into the midbrain dopamine cell group increases both dopamine release in forebrain regions and locomotor activity. Both the behavioural and biochemical changes are prevented by ondansetron and tropisetron (Hagan *et al.*, 1990). Such effects induced by exogenous and endogenous dopamine challenge attest to the 5-HT$_3$-receptor antagonist role of 5-HT$_3$ receptors in limbic dopamine control. The inevitable comparison of the effectiveness of the 5-HT$_3$ antagonists and neuroleptics to inhibit the dopamine responses indicated that: (i) unlike the use of the neuroleptics, the 5-HT$_3$-receptor antagonists did not depress behaviour below normal, i.e. activity returned to normal levels; (ii) unlike the use of the neuroleptics, cessation of a dopamine/5-HT$_3$ antagonist administration was not followed by rebound hyperactivity; and indeed (iii) a single administration of ondansetron antagonized for many days the enhanced activity following a dopamine neuroleptic regimen. The additional effects of the 5-HT$_3$-receptor antagonists in failing to block drug-induced stereotyped behaviour or induce catalepsy further distinguished their effects from dopamine-receptor antagonists (Costall *et al.*, 1987).

5-HT$_3$ receptors and cognition. Ondansetron has been assessed in a habituation test in the mouse, a T-maze reinforced alternation task in rats and an object discrimination and reversal learning task in the marmoset. Ondansetron facilitated performance in: (i) aged mice and those impaired by scopolamine or lesions of the nucleus basalis magnocellularis; (ii) rats whose performance was impaired by scopolamine; and (iii) marmosets in the reversal learning task (Barnes *et al.*, 1990). The demonstration that 5-HT$_3$-receptor antagonists prevented the inhibitory effects of 5-HT$_3$ agonists to reduce acetylcholine release linked the behavioural data with a neurochemical correlate (Barnes *et al.*, 1989b). That is to say, the 5-HT-receptor antagonists may improve performance in cognitive tests by enhancing cholinergic function (see Bartus *et al.*, 1982). The studies provide the basis for a more detailed analysis of the potential to improve attention, reaction time, acquisition, memory, retrieval and other components of cognition.

5-HT$_3$ receptors and anxiety-related behaviours. 5-HT$_3$-receptor antagonists have an anxiolytic profile of action in the mouse black/white test, rat social interaction and other tests (see review by Costall *et al.*, 1990). Agents such as ondansetron are much more potent than the benzodiazepines, are not sedative and do not induce withdrawal phenomena after cessation of drug treatment. Indeed, the 5-HT$_3$-receptor antagonists can attenuate the 'anxiogenesis' following withdrawal from treatment with alcohol, cocaine, diazepam and nicotine (Costall *et al.*, 1990).

5-HT$_3$ receptors and schizophrenia

Measurement of 5-HT$_3$ recognition sites in autopsy material from the hippocampus of brains obtained from schizophrenic patients revealed no difference in density of [^{3}H]S(−)zacopride binding compared with that in control brains (Barnes, personal communication).

The animal experimentation showing that 5-HT$_3$-receptor antagonists attenuated a raised limbic dopamine function provided the rationale for the use of ondansetron in schizophrenia. In an open study in hospitalized patients with a DSM-III diagnosis of schizophrenia, ondansetron appeared to possess antipsychotic activity, the drug's efficacy appearing to be inversely related to dose. In a follow-up double-blind placebo-controlled study, the antipsychotic effects of ondansetron could not be definitely confirmed or rejected, the study being compromised by the inclusion of chlorpromazine. It was concluded that further studies are warranted (Meltzer, 1991).

The effect of ondansetron on cognition has been investigated clinically in age-associated memory impairment. In a double-blind placebo-controlled trial, it was concluded that there was a significant effect of ondansetron on two of the five primary outcome measures and that the drug merited further study (Crook & Lakin, 1991). The reader is referred elsewhere to the preliminary clinical investigations of the effect of ondansetron in anxiety and addictive disorders (Lader, 1991; Sellers *et al.*, 1991).

The ability of the 5-HT$_3$-receptor antagonists

to reduce limbic dopamine function and anxiety-related behaviours and improve cognitive performance in animals has ensured much interest in their continued testing in schizophrenia.

The *N*-methyl-D-aspartate (NMDA) receptor, glutamatergic systems and schizophrenia

The NMDA receptor and phencyclidine (PCP) psychosis

PCP, ketamine and related analogues were introduced as intravenous anaesthetics in the 1950s. They were described as 'dissociative anaesthetics' and produced pronounced changes in awareness (Domino *et al.*, 1965). Indeed, the severely dysphoric nature of the response limited their clinical usage. PCP was first used by Meyer *et al.* (1959) as a model of sensory deprivation and by Cohen *et al.* (1959) and Luby *et al.* (1962) as a model of schizophrenia. It has been described as the best drug-induced model of schizophrenia capable of mimicking both the positive and negative systems. This has provided the most important single stimulus for investigating the role of the NMDA receptor complex in schizophrenia.

However, in an important comparison of the symptoms of acute schizophrenia with those induced by PCP (Domino & Luby, 1981) (Table 21.2), it is clear that the intensity of the symptoms of acute schizophrenia does not entirely correlate with the effects of PCP. Furthermore, and most noticeably, the delusional thinking and auditory hallucinations observed in schizophrenia were virtually absent or not present with PCP. Indeed, it has been suggested that the behavioural changes induced by PCP more appropriately model an organic brain syndrome inducing delirium, including loss of memory and consciousness at higher doses (Domino, 1992). But in this event it would remain interesting to compare the effects of PCP with symptoms of chronic schizophrenia, particularly if the negative symptoms are the conse-

Table 21.2 Comparison of various symptoms of acute schizophrenia with those induced by phencyclidine (PCP) and lysergic acid ethylamide (LSD). (From Domino & Luby, 1981)

Symptom	Acute schizophrenia	PCP	LSD-25
Loosening of association	++++	++	++
Overinclusive thoughts	++++	++	++
Concreteness	++	++++	+
Ambivalence	+++	++	+++
Autistic dream states	+++	++++	++++
Affect disorder	++++	++	+++
Attention disorder	+++	+++	+++
Depersonalization	+++	++++	+++
Feelings of influence	+++	+	+
Delusional thinking	++++	+	++
Visual hallucinations		+	++++
Auditory hallucinations	++++		
Withdrawal	+++	+	+
Electroencephalogram changes		+++	++
Chlorpromazine response	+++	+	+++
Intensified by amphetamine	+++	+	+++
Catatonia	+	+	+
Clouding delirium	+	+++	++
Response to isolation	++	++	++

+ → ++++, minor to major

quence of organic brain disease. Also, and accepting that the effects of no drug precisely mirror the symptoms of schizophrenia, the past and probable future use of PCP may be profitable if its use allows a model that has predictive validity in the clinic. An understanding of the mechanism of action of PCP and the detection in animal models of novel antischizophrenic treatments requires an understanding of the NMDA receptor and glutaminergic systems within the brain.

The characteristics of the NMDA receptor

The structural requirements for the excitatory actions of amino acids such as L-glutamate were established by Curtis *et al.* in the 1960s (see Curtis & Watkins, 1960), and have led through an intensive series of investigations to an ever-growing number of receptors sensitive to NMDA, kainate and quisqualate and other agonist and antagonist ligands (see reviews by McLennan, 1988). The receptors activated by L-glutamate and related agents comprise the major class of receptors mediating fast excitatory neurotransmission (see review by Kelly & Crunelli, 1988). Through the activation of different receptor types, it would appear that a useful delineation of receptors can be made into those responses that are mediated via ligand-gated ion channels (i.e. ionotropic responses) and those that are mediated through G-proteins and second messenger systems (metabotropic responses) (Schoepp & Conn, 1993). With respect to the ionotropic responses, the receptors are differentiated into those specifically activated by NMDA receptors and a more diverse group of receptors activated by other ligands such as quisqualate/AMPA, kainate and L-AP4 (for non-NMDA receptors, see review by Watkins *et al.*, 1990). The latter group exhibits remarkable diversity but it is the NMDA receptor which is the major focus of interest in this chapter.

It must be stated that in its own right the NMDA receptor is a most unusual and complex receptor, clearly to be distinguished from other ligand-gated ion channels. There is abundant evidence that the NMDA receptor−channel complex appears sensitive to three endogenous signals,

two excitatory and one inhibitory (see review by Johnson & Ascher, 1987). The excitatory signals are glutamate and glycine, both of which are normally present in the cerebrospinal fluid (CSF) at concentrations capable of receptor activation. If such concentrations are actually achieved in the extracellular synaptic space, then the NMDA channels would be permanently activated. This is prevented by the entry of an inhibitory factor, magnesium ions (Mg^{2+}), into the channel associated with the NMDA receptor, preventing the current flow. This inhibitory effect is normally overcome by depolarization, which can come from a number of sources, including the release of glutamate onto non-NMDA as well as NMDA channels. In response to the three excitatory signals which will attenuate the Mg^{2+} blockade, the NMDA channel then moderates neuronal activity (Mayer *et al.*, 1984). The opening of the NMDA channel increases calcium ion (Ca^{2+}) permeability and the intracellular Ca^{2+} concentration, resulting in the activation of many Ca^{2+}-dependent enzymes, protein kinase C, proteases and others (MacDermott *et al.*, 1986). It has been hypothesized that the changes in Ca^{2+} might be relevant to the development of synaptic connections and learning and memory (Morris, 1988). Changes in Ca^{2+} permeability of the NMDA receptor might also contribute to cell death following damage to the nervous system (Olney, 1988).

Yet the receptor is also unique in other ways. It is distinguished from other known ligand-gated ion channels by its dependence on agonist binding at a closely located recognition site with high affinity for glycine. Other ligands for this strychnine-insensitive-glycine site are 7-chlorokynurenate, HA-966 and ACPC. The interaction of glycine with the NMDA receptor complex is essential for functioning of the NMDA receptor (Johnson & Ascher, 1987). There is a further potential site of action either within the ion channel or at a closely related site and with high affinity for PCP, dizocilpine (MK-801) and ketamine. The binding of these compounds attenuates current flow through the NMDA receptor, somewhat resembling the inhibitory action of Mg^{2+} (Honey *et al.*, 1985; Martin & Lodge, 1985). There are also further distinct sites of action for the poly-amines, ifenprodil, SL82.0715 and hydrogen ions (H^+) that can moderate the NMDA channel activity (Fig. 21.1).

The location of glutamatergic systems within the brain

Glutamate is the major excitatory transmitter candidate and the systems have been localized using immunocytochemical techniques and axonal transport of D-[^{3}H]aspartate and recording high-affinity uptake (Fagg & Foster, 1983; Fonnum, 1984; and review by Storm-Mathisen & Ottersen, 1988). Efferents from the neocortex, which include corticocortical as well as corticofugal connections, consistitute the most abundant glutamatergic pathways in the brain. Putative glutamatergic projections from the allocortex and from and within the hippocampus have also been detailed (Fig. 21.2). The complex arrangement of putative glutamatergic projections from sub-cortical structures is beyond the present discussion and can be found elsewhere (Storm-Mathisen & Ottersen, 1988). It remains clear that the gluta-matergic projections have a major distribution within the cortical and limbic brain regions with the potential for widespread influence on many central functions.

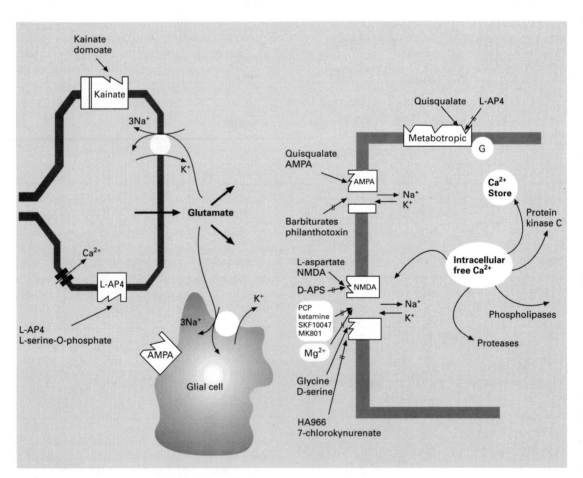

Fig. 21.1 A diagrammatic presentation of the *N*-methyl-D-aspartate (NMDA) receptor and its associated accoutrements and potential sites of drug action. After Lodge & Collinridge, 1990. For description, see text.

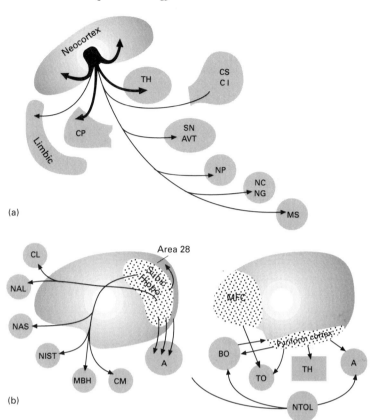

Fig. 21.2 Major efferent and intrinsic putative glutamatergic pathways from (a) the neocortex and (b) the allocortex. A, Amygdala; AVT, area ventralis tegmenti mesencephali; BO, bulbus olfactorius; CI and CS, colliculus inferior and superior; CL, contralateral hemisphere; CM, corpus mammillare; CP, caudatoputamen; MBH, mediobasal hypothalamus; MFC, medial frontal cortex; MS, medulla spinalis; NA, nucleus accumbens septi; NAS, nucleus accumbens; NC and NG, nucleus cuneatus and gracilis; NIST, nucleus interstitialis striae terminalis; NP, nuclei pontis; NR, nucleus ruber, NTOL, nucleus tractus olfactorii lateralis; SN, substantia nigra, TH, thalamus; TO, tuberculum olfactorium. After Storm-Mathisen & Ottersen, 1988.

Animal pharmacology

The NMDA receptor−channel complex has a number of sites at which different pharmacological agents may act: the NMDA transmitter recognition site, the associated ion channel, the glycine site and the polyamine site. Behavioural correlates have been reviewed by Willetts *et al.* (1990) and are summarized as follows.

Anticonvulsant activities

Seizures induced by a wide range of stimuli, electroshock, pentylenetetrazol, NMDA, kindling, sound in mice and light stimulation in baboons can be antagonized by compounds acting at all four sites. Thus, the NMDA antagonists have a broad spectrum of anticonvulsant activities and a detailed description of such activities has been reported elsewhere (Patel *et al.*, 1988).

Unconditioned behaviours

PCP, dizocilpine and other NMDA antagonists acting on the ion channel produce amphetamine-like effects in rodents. Increases in locomotor activity, stereotyped movements, circling behaviour and ataxia have been reported by many workers (see review by Snell & Johnson, 1986). In contrast, antagonists such as ifenprodil acting at the polyamine site induce muscle relaxation. The PCP-induced effects are attenuated by neuroleptics and 6-hydroxydopamine lesions of the mesolimbic dopamine system (French & Vatani, 1984) and are associated with increased limbic dopamine release (Bowers & Hoffman, 1984; Roa *et al.*, 1990). This is strongly supportive of an involvement of dopamine in the behavioural effects induced by NMDA ion channel blockers. This is not necessarily an exclusive role since 5-HT systems may also be involved (see Snell & Johnson,

1986). It also remains of interest that R(+)HA-966 (3-amino-1-hydro-xypyrrolid-2-one), an antagonist at the glycine modulatory site, blocks both the locomotor changes but not ataxia or the biochemical (dopamine release) effects of PCP and dizocilpine in mice and rats (Bristow *et al.*, 1993). Directly acting NMDA-receptor antagonists such as AP-5 also increase rodent motility (see Snell & Johnson, 1986), and in a potentially important finding MK-801 reversed the catalepsy induced by the dopamine antagonists raclopride and SCH23390 (Papa *et al.*, 1993).

Discriminative stimulus effects

NMDA antagonists acting at the ion channel produce a discriminate stimulus that is cross-generalized between species (rats, primates, pigeon) and drugs (Willetts *et al.*, 1990). This indicates that such agents produce a similar subjective effect, and provides substantial evidence that the PCP recognition site is a receptor that may play a physiologically relevant role. It remains interesting that compounds acting at the glycine site substitute for the non-competitive channel-blocking agents with variable efficacy (Willetts *et al.*, 1990) and ligands for the polyamine site not at all (Sanger & Jackson, 1988).

Learning and memory

The neurophysiological phenomena of long-term potentiation is hypothesized to be involved importantly in learning and memory and is disrupted by NMDA antagonists. Briefly, PCP-like drugs have been shown to disrupt rat performance in a swim-maze task, a two-level spatial alternation task and a Y-maze brightness discrimination task, and the acquisition of a new response sequence in monkeys (see review by Snell & Johnson, 1986).

Anti-anxiety effects

Non-competitive or competitive NMDA antagonists have variable effects to increase the rate of punished responding (Sanger & Jackson, 1989), whereas the polyamine site ligands are inactive (Snell & Johnson, 1986).

It becomes apparent from the animal work that compounds acting at different sites within the NMDA receptor complex have a commonality of effect, e.g. to reduce seizures, but differences elsewhere, e.g. anxiolytic-like potential, discriminatory properties. It is within such spectrums of effect and the different dose regimens required to produce such effects that investigators have sought a clinical relevance of drug action at the NMDA receptor complex to the treatment of schizophrenia.

The NMDA receptor and schizophrenia

Alterations in NMDA binding sites and glutamatergic function in schizophrenic brains

[^{3}H]TCP is a ligand for the PCP receptor and its use has revealed an increase, or a trend for an increase, in binding in the frontal cortex of schizophrenic brains as compared with controls (Simpson *et al.*, 1992; see also Toru *et al.*, 1988). Kornhuber *et al.* (1989) have also reported a small and non-significant increase in [^{3}H]MK-801 binding in the schizophrenic frontal cortex. However, Kerwin *et al.* (1988) report a decrease in [^{3}H]kainate binding in the left hippocampus (compared with the right) of schizophrenic brains, with [^{3}H]glutamate sites being relatively preserved. A decreased release of glutamate has been observed in the frontal and temporal cortex of schizophrenic patients (Sherman *et al.*, 1991). These preliminary observations are of interest, particularly if such findings can be confirmed in full saturation analysis studies and/or can be dissociated from the effects of antipsychotic medication. Also, significantly higher blood concentrations of glycine, glutamate and serine were found in schizophrenic patients (Macciardi *et al.*, 1990).

NMDA ligands in schizophrenia

Carlsson *et al.* (1991; Chapter 20, this volume) have developed the hypothesis that the excitatory effects of the excitatory amino acids may cause behavioural inhibition, mediated via the cortico-fugal glutamatergic/aspartatergic pathways. The authors have postulated a negative feedback loop from the cortex via the striatum and pallidum to an inhibition in the thalamus, attenuating the sensory information being relayed to the cortex. It is considered that the striatal dopaminergic pathways modulate via an inhibitory pathway this negative feedback loop, reducing striatal inhibition on the thalamus and increasing the sensory input. That is to say, the striatum is involved in sensorimotor gating, the pathogenesis of schizophrenia being broadened from a hyperdopaminergic to a hypoglutamatergic function. It follows that glutamatergic agonists may have antipsychotic potential.

A major challenge of a successful drug design based around the NMDA receptor is to eliminate the behavioural excitant potential. There are a number of possibilities and one point of attack is the glycine receptor. In a preliminary report, some 40% of chronic schizophrenic patients responded to the administration of high doses of glycine, in addition to the standard neuroleptic regimen, which was then reduced (Waziri, 1988). In a subsequent study in six chronically psychotic patients, there was a suggestion that glycine had a salutary effect in a few patients (Rosse *et al.*, 1989). It was considered that the limited actions of glycine might be related to a poor penetration through the blood–brain barrier. This prompted the use of milacemide (2-*n*-pentyl amino acetamide), an acylated prodrug of glycine, which readily crosses the blood–brain barrier (Christopher *et al.*, 1986). In this study involving five chronic schizophrenics, milacemide was associated with no improvement or a worsening in behaviour. Inappropriate dosing or adequate pools of endogenous glycine may have contributed to the lack of effect. But it remains of note that stereotypies induced by dizocilpine in rats are not counteracted by the glycine agonist D-cycloserine, indicating a failure of the glycine site to enhance NMDA receptor activity (see Kretschmer & Schmidt, 1992). But against this, milacemide has been shown to enhance the anticonvulsant actions of MK-801 in mice and to antagonize the behavioural and electrophysiological effects of PCP (Toth & Lajtha, 1986; Bertolino *et al.*, 1988).

Agonist action on the glycine receptor appears to be an absolute requirement for NMDA receptor activation, and the development of selective ligands is proceeding apace. HA966 was established as a low-efficacy partial agonist, and kynurenic acid as a full antagonist. From these structures a whole series of agonists, partial agonists and antagonists have been synthesized and are being extensively used to assess the functional role of the glycine receptor (see review by Kemp & Leeson, 1993). For example, (+)HA966 and its methyl derivative L687414 in contrast to PCP, fail to induce behavioural excitation in rodents (Singh *et al.*, 1990), and in neuroprotective doses fail to alter brain glucose utilization and have a better separation between anticonvulsant and sedative doses (Saywell *et al.*, 1991). It is these important differences which ensure that the glycine receptor remains an important target for potential therapeutic developments. Furthermore, cloning of the NMDA receptor introduces the distinct possibility of developing glycine subtype selective ligands.

In an area of intense pharmacological activity, it will be particularly interesting to record whether the animal neuropharmacology can finally be shown to produce a therapeutic benefit in schizophrenia.

The sigma site and psychoses

For many years the benzomorphan derivative (±)*N*-allylnormetazocine[(±)SKF10,047] was considered to be an antagonist at the μ opioid receptor subtype (Martin *et al.*, 1974). However, it was observed that the pattern of behavioural change induced by (±)SKF10,047 in the dog, a 'canine delirium', was different from that induced by the prototypical μ ligand morphine (Martin *et al.*, 1976), since the effects of (±)SKF10,047 could be antagonized by the opioid receptor antagonist naltrexone (Martin *et al.*, 1976). It was proposed that (±)SKF10,047 exerted its effects through the 'sigma opioid receptor'. A characterization of the sigma site and its establishment as a receptor relevant to schizophrenia research have proved to be an exceptionally challenging task. The potential relevance of sigma site ligands to schizophrenia is found in the biochemical effects of such agents and their behavioural actions to induce psychotic-like syndromes in animals or humans.

Characterization of the sigma site

In radioligand binding studies, the compounds which demonstrated the highest affinity for the sigma site were neuroleptic agents such as haloperidol and butaclomol (Su, 1982; Tam, 1983). But, in turn, it is most unlikely that the sigma site can be related to a dopamine receptor since dopamine and apomorphine displayed low affinity and, most importantly, the isomers of the neuroleptic butaclomol showed a reverse selectivity compared with the dopamine receptors (Seeman *et al.*, 1975). There are also theories for the existence of subtypes and/or different affinity states of the sigma binding site which are beyond the scope of the present discussion (Itzhak & Stein, 1990; Quirion *et al.*, 1992).

The sigma site and PCP

Interest in PCP relates to its ability to induce psychotic disorders in humans (see p. 410), to discriminate to (±)SKF10,047 and to induce a behavioural syndrome in animals similar to that induced by (+)SKF10,047 (Brady *et al.*, 1982). Early binding studies suggested a common site of action for (+)SKF10,047 and PCP, but the development of more selective ligands allowed a delineation of (+)SKF10,047 and PCP binding sites (Largent *et al.*, 1986).

The location of sigma and PCP binding sites

Sigma sites have been located mainly in the cerebellum, midbrain, hypothalamus and limbic brain areas, while PCP sites have been found mainly in the cortex, striatum and thalamus, with a heavy density of both binding sites in the hippocampus (see Largent *et al.*, 1986; Contreras *et al.*, 1988).

More recent studies indicate that the sigma binding site appears to have a subcellular location (Knight *et al.*, 1991a). This clearly has important implications for it is unlikely that such a site has a neurotransmitter role, such receptors being required on the cell membrane. There is one theory that the sigma site may be an enzyme related to cytochrome P-450 (Walther *et al.*, 1986).

But, against the hypothesis, known inducers of cytochrome P-450 activity fail to increase sigma ligand binding (Knight *et al.*, 1991b; see also Itzhak & Stein, 1990).

The functional role of the sigma binding site

The wealth of data from binding assays stands in contrast to our limited knowledge of the functional role of sigma binding sites. The first goal is to establish whether the binding site is a receptor, and there are numerous species in which this could be investigated. Thus, the sigma site has been identified in single aquatic life-forms through to humans (Vu *et al.*, 1990). However, notwithstanding the breadth of species available, there are very few indicators of a functional role for the sigma sites. This reflects the difficulty in use of many of the sigma site ligands: many have effects on other systems, e.g. the opiate or dopamine systems. It also reflects the preliminary nature of some of the pioneer studies.

In rats sensitized to (−)-*N*-allylnormetazocine, the administration of (+)butaclamol and (−)-*N*-allylnormetazocine induced a novel locomotor syndrome consisting of enhanced locomotion, retropulsion and sideways circling (Iwamoto, 1989). The behaviour was blocked by three agents with affinity for the sigma binding site: haloperidol, rimcazole and (±)BMY14802 (Ferris *et al.*, 1986). The model was taken to be a manifestation of the activation of the central sigma receptor system resulting in the release of an endogenous sigma ligand.

In a further rat study, (+)SKF10,047 increased dopamine metabolite levels in the striatum and olfactory tubercle; the effect of SKF10,047 was stereospecific and blocked not by naloxone but by the NMDA-receptor antagonist 3-[(±)-2-carboxypiperazin-4-yl]-propyl-1-phosphonic acid (Iyenger *et al.*, 1990a). Since the sigma receptor is not coupled to the NMDA receptor (Itzhak & Stein, 1990), the results are difficult to interpret, particularly in the absence of use of other sigma site antagonists. Similar comments would apply to the use of (+)SKF10,047 to stimulate ACTH release (Iyengar *et al.*, 1990b). Roles for the sigma site in the induction of emesis (Hudzik, 1991) and amnesia (Earley *et al.*, 1991) have also been claimed.

Evidence for a functional role of the sigma site has come from the links to the G-protein identified above and also to another second messenger system, the phosphoinositol system (Bowen *et al.*, 1988.

In a quite different system, cerebral glucose utilization is considered to reflect the energy-dependent activity of the brain. (+)Pentazocine and BMY14802 increased and rimcazole decreased glucose utilization in various brain areas with some correspondence to the sigma binding-site density (Della Puppa & London, 1989). The change in glucose utilization caused by the sigma ligands may reflect an unspecified functional activity. It is clear that more selective sigma-site ligands are required before the binding site can be characterized as a receptor, and for the binding data to be correlated to a functional change.

The sigma site and endogenous ligands

The possibility that there might exist endogenous ligands acting as agonists or antagonists at the sigma site has been investigated by a number of groups, with varying results. Claims have been made for the identification or isolation of putative endogenous sigma ligands, sigmaphin (Su *et al.*, 1986) or β-endopsychosis (DiMaggio *et al.*, 1988). Such substances have been found in both animal and human brain (Su *et al.*, 1986; Contreras *et al.*, 1987; DiMaggio *et al.*, 1988; Zhang *et al.*, 1988). The possibility that neuropeptide Y (NPY) and peptide YY (PYY) may be endogenous ligands comes from their demonstration of a high affinity for the sigma site (Roman *et al.*, 1991), but not in all studies (Tam & Mitchell, 1991). This is an area worthy of further study to substantiate the various claims and to identify the precise nature of any putative endogenous sigma site ligand.

The sigma/PCP binding site and psychoses

A major stimulus to investigations of the sigma/ PCP binding sites has been the possibility that it may be involved in psychoses. Thus, similarly to PCP (see p. 410), the benzomorphan derivatives such as (+)SKF10,047 can also induce dysphoria and a psychotomimetic syndrome of depersonalization and hallucinations. The subsequent realization that the sigma and PCP binding sites are not identical appears to exclude a common site of cellular interaction. But it remains an intriguing finding that haloperidol has a high affinity for the sigma site and that a number of novel potential antipsychotic compounds with different chemical structures and different pharmacologies have a common affinity for the sigma receptor, i.e. cinuperone (HR375), rimcazole (BW234u), tiospirone (BMY13859) and BMY14802 (Ferris *et al.*, 1986; Hall *et al.*, 1986; Su, 1986; Taylor *et al.*, 1991). It will be particularly interesting if the initial potential of such agents can be confirmed, since this would greatly enhance the hypothesis of the involvement of the sigma site in psychotic behaviour.

An additional approach would be to investigate the sigma/PCP binding sites in schizophrenic brains. Sigma and PCP recognition sites have been identified in the human brain in those areas implicated in schizophrenia (Sircar & Zukin, 1983; Weissman *et al.*, 1988). These sites have been investigated in postmortem assessments of tissue taken from both schizophrenic patients and PCP abusers (Weissman & De Souza, 1991). Using [³H]TCP, the results suggested that PCP recognition sites were not altered selectively in the brains of schizophrenics or PCP abusers. Using [³H]haloperidol at a single concentration of 1nmol/l, binding was significantly lower in the temporal cortex of the paranoid and undifferentiated schizophrenic groups when compared with normal controls. Using saturation studies, [³H]haloperidol B_{max} values were significantly lower in the temporal cortex of the paranoid schizophrenics. These findings may be important if the long-term effects of neuroleptic administration in influencing sigma binding can be eliminated from the effects of the disease itself.

Conclusion

A review of animal neuropharmacology and its prediction of clinical response allows certain broad conclusions. On the one hand, progress in the development of antischizophrenic drugs has been remarkable, given the almost total absence of knowledge as to the causes and biochemical pathology of schizophrenia. On the other hand, more effective treatments are urgently required, particularly for the negative symptoms in chronic schizophrenia.

From the examples drawn in this chapter, it becomes clear that once a group of compounds, such as the dopamine-receptor antagonists, have been shown to possess a clear benefit against the positive symptoms of schizophrenia, then biochemical tests which detect this particular pharmacological action will have a high predictive ability. But this is obvious and little more than an exercise in circuitry. Similar conclusions can be drawn from behavioural tests which can also detect the ability to reduce dopamine function. However, other biochemical and behavioural tests in animals have a clear advantage in allowing the detection of non-dopamine-receptor antagonists which nevertheless may affect other mechanisms moderating the dopamine system. The 5-HT_3-receptor antagonists are just one example. Even more importantly, the animal neuropharmacology described above may finally be shown to provide new therapies acting independently of the dopamine system.

The future use of animals to improve an understanding of schizophrenia and its treatment will require a pivotal and increasing synergy between the preclinical and clinical studies. Thus, it is to be regretted that the ability of 5-HT_2-receptor antagonists to prevent neuroleptic-induced extrapyramidal side effects in animals was shown 20 years ago, but is only now being introduced for clinical advantage. The 5-HT_3-receptor antagonists pose other challenges. Further clinical trials will be required to establish their potential and may require careful analysis in patient subgroups. It will be of interest to determine whether the ondansetron-induced improvements in cognitive performance in animals and age-associated memory disturbance in humans can be translated to a beneficial effect in schizophrenia. Similar comments may apply to the use of NMDA antagonists. Also, is it possible that the neuroprotective effects of NMDA antagonists could find benefit in chronic schizophrenia, with its known brain changes? Other data from animal tests may be more speculative and the potential value of sigma-site ligands would become more attractive if the sigma site could be shown to have a demonstrable and relevant receptor role. However, this does not necessarily exclude the possibility that the use of sigma ligands in humans may reveal new insights into schizophrenia and its treatment.

Yet, perhaps a real constraint to improvements in the drug treatment of schizoprenia is the self-imposed delineation of specific drug groups. For reasons of pharmacological convenience the present chapter has described separately the 5-HT_2, 5-HT_3, NMDA and sigma receptors. Yet, sigma ligands produce changes in serotonergic and noradrenergic brain function (Vander Maelan & Braselton, 1990), NMDA-receptor antagonists potentiate electrical responses elicited by 5-HT_3-receptor activation (Lovinger & White, 1991), 5-HT_2 receptors may interact with 5-HT_3 receptors to moderate transmitter release (Barnes *et al.*, 1989) and facilitate depolarization of neocortical neurones by NMDA (Rahman & Neuman, 1993), and 5-HT_3 receptors may moderate the release of a variety of neurotransmitters (Blandina *et al.*, 1988, 1991; Barnes *et al.*, 1989a; Paudice & Raiteri, 1991; Ropert & Guy, 1991).

From these few examples it is clear that a singular pharmacological manipulation may have a plurality of effects, whose consequences could be profound. They may even involve ultrastructural changes in axodendritic synapses (Vincent *et al.*, 1991). Perhaps future animal models will begin to address the extraordinarily complex nature of neurotransmitter interactions and herald a further progressive step towards the understanding and drug treatment of schizophrenia.

References

Aghajanian, G.K., Sprouse, J.S. & Rasmussen, K. (1987) Physiology of the midbrain serotonin system. In Meltzer, H.Y. (ed.) *Psychopharmacology: The Third Generation of Progress*, pp. 141–149. Raven Press, New York.

Ahlenius, S. (1991) Pharmacological evaluation of new antipsychotic drugs. In Willner, P. (ed.) *Behavioural Models in Psychopharmacology: Theoretical Industrial and Clinical Perspectives*, pp. 311–330. Cambridge University Press, Cambridge.

Andreasen, N.C. (1987) Schizophrenia: diagnosis and assessment. In Meltzer, H.Y. (ed.) *Psychopharmacology: The Third Generation of Progress*, pp. 1087–1094. Raven Press, New York.

Angrist, B., Lee, H.K. & Gershon, S. (1974) The antagonism of amphetamine-induced symptomatology by a neuroleptic. *American Journal of Psychiatry*, **131**, 817–819.

Angst, J., Berte, D., Berner, P., Heiman, H., Helrichen, H. & Hippius, H. (1971) Das klinische Wirkungsbird von Clozapin (Untersuchung mit dem AMP-System). *Pharmkopsychiatry*, **4**, 201–211.

APA (1980) *Diagnostic and Statistical Manual of Mental Disorders III*. Washington DC. American Psychiatric Association.

Awouters, F., Niemegeers, C.J.E., Megens, A.A.H.P., Meert, T.F. & Janssen, P.A.J. (1988) Pharmacological profile of ritanserin: a very specific central serotonin S_2-antagonist. *Drug Development Research*, **15**, 61–73.

Axelsson, R., Nilsson, A., Christensson, E. & Bjork, A. (1991) Effects of amperozide in schizophrenia. *Psychopharmacology*, **104**, 287–295.

Barnes, J.M., Barnes, N.M., Costall, B., Ironside, J.W. & Naylor, R.J. (1989a) Identification and characterisation of 5-hydroxytryptamine$_3$ recognition sites in human brain tissue. *Journal of Neurochemistry*, **53**, 1787–1793.

Barnes, J.M., Barnes, N.M., Costall, B., Naylor, R.J. & Tattersall, F.D. (1988) Reserpine, parachlorophenylalanine and fenfluramine antagonise cisplatin-induced emesis in the ferret. *Neuropharmacology*, **27**, 783–789.

Barnes, J.M., Barnes, N.M., Costall, B., Naylor, R.J. & Tyers, M.B. (1989b) 5-HT$_3$ receptors mediate inhibition of acetylcholine release in cortical tissue. *Nature*, **338**, 762–763.

Barnes, J.M., Costall, B., Coughlan, J. *et al.* (1990) The effects of ondansetron, a 5-HT$_3$ receptor antagonist, on cognition in rodents and primates. *Pharmacology, Biochemistry and Behaviour*, **35**, 955–962.

Bartus, R.T., Dean, R.L., Beer, B. & Lippa, A.S. (1982) The cholinergic hypothesis of geriatic memory dysfunction. *Science*, **217**, 408–417.

Bertolino, M., Vicini, S., Mazzetta, J. & Costa, E. (1988) Phencyclidine and glycine modulate NMDA-activated high conductance cationic channels by acting at different sites. *Neuroscience Letters*, **84**, 351–355.

Blandina, P., Goldfarb, J. & Green, J.P. (1988) Activation of a 5-HT$_3$ receptor releases dopamine from rat striatal slice. *European Journal of Pharmacology*, **155**, 349–350.

Blandina, P., Goldfarb, J. & Green, T.P. (1991) Stimulation of 5-HT$_3$ receptors inhibits release of endogenous noradrenaline from hypothalamus. In Fozard, J.R. & Saxena, P.R. (eds) *Serotonin: Molecular Biology, Receptors and Functional Effects*, pp. 322–329. Birkhauser Verlag, Basel.

Bowen, W.D., Kirshner, B.N., Newman, A.H. & Rice, K.C. (1988) Sigma receptors negatively modulate agonist-stimulated phosphoinositide metabolism in rat brain. *European Journal of Pharmacology*, **149**, 399–400.

Bowers, M.B. & Hoffman, F.J. (1984) Homovanillic acid in rat caudate and prefrontal cortex following phencyclidine and amphetamine. *Psychopharmacology* (Berlin) **84**, 136–137.

Bradley, P.B., Engel, S., Feniuk, W. *et al.* (1986) Proposals for the classification and nomenclature of functional receptors for 5-hydroxytryptamine. *Neuropharmacology*, **25**, 563–576.

Brady, K.T., Balster, R.L. & May, E.L. (1982) Stereoisomers of *N*-allyl normetazocine phencyclildine-like behavioural effects in squirrels, monkeys and rats. *Science*, **215**, 178–180.

Braff, D.L. & Geyer, M.A. (1990) Sensorimotor gating and the neurobiology of schizophrenia: human and animal model studies. *Archives of General Psychiatry*, **47**, 181–188.

Braff, D.L., Stone, C., Callaway, E., Geyer, M.A., Glick, I.D. & Bali, L. (1978) Prestimulus effects on human startle reflex in normals and schizophrenics. *Psychophysiology*, **15**, 339–343.

Bristow, L.J., Hutson, P.H., Thorn, L. & Tricklebank, M.D. (1993) The glycine/NMDA receptor antagonist, R-(+)-HA-966, blocks activation of the mesolimbic dopaminergic system induced by phencyclidine and dizocilpine (MK-801) in rodents. *British Journal of Pharmacology*, **108**, 1156–1163.

Brockington, I. (1986) Diagnosis of schizophrenia and schizoaffective psychoses. In Bradley, P.B. & Hirsch, S.R. (eds) *The Psychopharmacology and Treatment of Schizophrenia*, pp. 166–199. Oxford University Press, Oxford.

Carlsson, A. (1988) The current status of the dopamine hypothesis of schizophrenia. *Neuropsychopharmacology*, **1**, 179–186.

Carlsson, A., Carlsson, M. & Svensson, A. (1991) Glutamate receptor pharmacology: a novel approach to the treatment of schizophrenia. In Racagni, G., Brunello, N. & Fukuda, T. (eds) *Biological Psychiatry*, Vol. 2, pp. 751–753. Excerpta Medica, Amsterdam.

Castelao, J.F., Ferreira, L., Gelders, Y.G. & Heylen, S.L.E. (1989) The efficacy of the D$_2$ and 5-HT$_2$ antagonist risperidone (R64766) in the treatment of chronic psychosis: an open dose-finding study. *Schizophrenia Research*, **2**, 411–415.

Christensson, E. (1990) Effects of amperozide on induced turning behaviour in 6-OHDA lesioned rats. *Pharmacology and Toxicology*, Suppl. **1**, 22–28.

Christopher, J., Kutzner, T., Nguyen-Bui, N.D., Damien, C., Chatelain, P. & Gillet, L. (1986) Conversion of orally administered 2-*N*-pentylaminoacetamide into glycinamide and glycine in the rat brain. *Life Sciences*, **33**, 533–541.

Cohen, B.D., Rosenbaum, G., Luby, E.D., Gottlieb, J.S. & Yelen, D. (1959) Comparison of sernyl with other drugs. 1. Attention, motor function and proprioception. *Archives of General Psychiatry*, **1**, 651–656.

Contreras, P.C., Di Maggio, D.A. & O'Donohue, T.L. (1987)

An endogenous ligand for the sigma opioid binding site. *Synapse*, **1**, 57–61.

Contreras, P.C., Contreras, M.L., O'Donoghue, T.L. & Lair, C.C. (1988) Biochemical and behavioural effects of sigma and PCP ligands. *Synapse*, **2**, 240–243.

Costall, B. & Naylor, R.J. (1976) A comparison of the abilities of typical neuroleptic agents and of thioridazine, clozapine, sulpiride and metoclopramide to antagonise the hyperactivity induced by dopamine applied intracerebrally to areas of the extrapyramidal and mesolimbic systems. *European Journal of Pharmacology*, **40**, 9–19.

Costall, B. & Naylor, R.J. (1980) Assessment of the test procedures used to analyse neuroleptic action. *Review of Pure Applied Pharmaceutical Sciences*, **1**, 3–83.

Costall, B. & Naylor, R.J. (1985) Neurotransmitter hypothesis of schizophrenia. In Bradley, P.B. & Hirsch, S.R. (eds) *Psychopharmacology and Drug Treatment of Schizophrenia*, pp. 132–165. Oxford University Press, Oxford.

Costall, B., Domeney, A.M. & Naylor, R.J. (1984) Locomotor hyperactivity caused by dopamine infusion into the nucleus accumbens of rat brain: specificity of action. *Psychopharmacology*, **82**, 174–180.

Costall, B., Naylor, R.J. & Tyers, M.B. (1990) The psychopharmacology of 5-HT$_3$ receptors. *Pharmacology and Therapeutics*, **49**, 181–202.

Costall, B., Domeney, A.M., Naylor, R.J. & Tyers, M.B. (1987) Effects of the 5-HT$_3$ receptor antagonist GR38032F, on raised dopaminergic activity in the mesolimbic system of the rat and marmoset brain. *British Journal of Pharmacology*, **92**, 881–894.

Costall, B., Fortune, D.H., Naylor, R.J., Marsden, C.D. & Pycock, C.J. (1975) Serotonergic involvement with neuroleptic catalepsy. *Neuropharmacology*, **14**, 859–868.

Coward, D.M., Imperato, A., Urwyler, S. & White, T.G. (1989) Biochemical and behavioural properties of clozapine. *Psychopharmacology*, **99**, S6-S12.

Creese, I. (1988) Dopamine receptor subtypes differential regulatory characterisation and role in schizophrenia. *Neurochemistry International*, **13**, (SI) 24.

Crook, T. & Lakin, M. (1991) Effects of ondansetron in age-associated memory impairment. In Racagni, G., Brunello, N. & Fukuda, T. (eds) *Biological Psychiatry*, Vol. 2, pp. 888–890. Excerpta Medica, Amsterdam.

Crow, T.J. (1980) Molecular pathology of schizophrenia: more than one disease process? *British Medical Journal*, **200**, 66–68.

Crow, T.J. (1991) Brain changes in schizophrenia and their meaning. In Racagni, G., Brunello, N. & Fukuda, T. (eds) *Biological Psychiatry*, Vol. 1, pp. 511–514. Proceedings of the 5th World Congress of Biological Psychiatry, Florence, 9–14 June 1991. Excerpta Medica, Amsterdam.

Curtis, D.R. & Watkins, J.C. (1960) The excitation and depression of spinal neurones by structurally related amino acids. *Journal of Neurochemistry*, **61**, 117–141.

Della Puppa, A. & London, E.D. (1989) Cerebral metabolic effects of sigma ligands in the rat. *Brain Research*, **505**, 283–290.

Descarries, L., Audet, M.-A., Doucet, G. *et al.* (1990) Morphology of central serotonin neurones. Brief review of quantified aspects of their distribution and ultrastructure relationships. The neuropharmacology of serotonin. *Annals of the New York Academy of Sciences*, **600**, 81–92.

DiMaggio, D.A., Contreras, P.C. & O'Donohue, T.L. (1988) Biological and chemical characterisation of the endopsychosins: distinct ligands for PCP and sigma sites. In Domino, E.F. & Kamenka, J.M. (eds) *Sigma and Phencyclidine-like Compounds as Molecular Probes in Biology*, pp. 157–171. NPP Books, Ann Arbor.

Domino, E.F. (1992) Chemical dissociation of human awareness: focus on non-competitive NMDA receptor antagonists. *Journal of Psychopharmacology*, **6**, 418–424.

Domino, E.F. & Luby, E.D. (1981) Abnormal mental states induced by phencyclidine as a model of schizophrenia. In Domino, E.F. (ed.) *PCP (Phencyclidine): Historical and Current Perspectives*, pp. 401–418. NPP Books, Ann Arbor.

Domino, E.F., Chodoff, P. & Corssen, G. (1965) Pharmacologic effects of Cl–581, a new dissociative anaesthetic in man. *Clinical Pharmacology Therapeutics*, **6**, 279–291.

Earley, B., Burke, M., Leonard, B.E., Gouret, C.J. & Junien, J.L. (1991) Evidence for an antiamnesic effect of JO1784 in the rat: a potent and selective ligand for the sigma receptor. *Brain Research*, **546**, 282–286.

Ellinwood, E.H. & Sudilovsky, A. (1973) Chronic amphetamine intoxication. Behavioural model of psychoses. In Cole, J.O., Freedman, A.M. & Friedhoff, A.J. (eds) *Psychopathology and Psychopharmacology*, pp. 231–247. John Hopkins University Press, Baltimore.

Evenden, J.L. & Robbins, T.W. (1983) Increased response switching, perseveration and perseverative switching following d-amphetamine in the rat. *Psychopharmacology*, **80**, 67–73.

Fagg, G.E. & Foster, A.C. (1983) Amino acid neurotransmitters and their pathways in the mammalian central nervous system. *Neuroscience*, **9**, 701–719.

Ferris, R.M., Tang, F.L.M., Chang, K.-J. & Russell, A. (1986) Evidence that the potential antipsychotic agent rimcazole (BW234U) is a specific, competitive antagonist of sigma sites in brain. *Life Sciences*, **38**, 2329–2337.

Fink, H., Morgenstern, R. & Oesfssner, W. (1984) Clozapine — a serotonic antagonist? *Pharmacology, Biochemistry and Behaviour*, **20**, 513–517.

Fonnum, F. (1984) Glutamate: a neurotransmitter in mammalian brain. *Journal of Neurochemistry*, **42**, 1–11.

Fozard, J.R. (1989) The development and early clinical evaluation of selective 5-HT$_3$ receptor antagonists. In Fozard, J.R. (ed.) *The Peripheral Actions of 5-Hydroxytryptamine*, pp. 354–376. Oxford Medical Publications, Oxford.

French, A.D. & Vatani, G. (1984) Phencyclidine-induced locomotor activity in the rat is blocked by 6-hydroxydopamine lesion of the nucleus accumbens: comparisons to other psychomotor stimulants. *Psychopharmacology* (Berlin) **82**, 83–88.

Gaddum, J.H. & Picarelli, Z.P. (1957) Two kinds of tryptamine receptor. *British Journal of Pharmacology*, **12**, 323–328.

Geyer, M.A., Swerdlow, N.R., Mansbach, R.S. & Bratt, D.L. (1990) Startle response models of sensorimotor gating and habituation deficits in schizophrenia. *Brain Research Bulletin*, **25**, 485–498.

Gottschalk, L.A., Haer, J.L. & Bates, D.E. (1972) Effect of sensory overload on psychological state. *Archives of General Psychology*, **27**, 451–457.

Hagan, R.M., Jones, B.J., Jordan, C.C. & Tyers, M.B. (1990) Effect of 5-HT₃ receptor antagonists on responses to selective activation of mesolimbic dopaminergic pathways in the rat. *British Journal of Pharmacology*, **99**, 227–232.

Hall, H., Sallemack, M. & Jerning, E. (1986) Effects of remoxipride and some related new substituted salicylamides on rat brain receptors. *Acta Pharmacologia et Toxicologia*, **58**, 61–70.

Hibert, M.F., Mir, A.K. & Fozard, J.R. (1990) Serotonin (5-HT) receptors. In Emmot, J.C. (ed.) *Comprehensive Medicinal Chemistry*, Vol. 3, pp. 567–600. Pergamon Press, Oxford.

Honey, C.R., Miljkovic, Z. & McDonald, J.F. (1985) Ketamine and phencyclidine cause a voltage-dependent block of responses to L-aspartic acid. *Neuroscience Letters*, **61**, 135–139.

Hudzik, T.J. (1991) Sigma ligand-induced emesis in the pigeon. *Pharmacology, Biochemistry and Behaviour*, **41**, 215–217.

Humphrey, P.A.A. (1992) 5-Hydroxytryptamine receptors and drug discovery. In Langer, S.Z., Brunello, N., Racagni, G. & Mendlewicz, J. (eds) *Serotonin Receptor Subtypes: Pharmacological Significance and Clinical Implications*, Vol. 1, *International Academy of Biomedical Drug Research*, pp. 129–139. Karger, Basel.

Ichikawa, J. & Meltzer, H.Y. (1992) The effect of chronic atypical antipsychotic drugs and haloperidol in amphetamine-induced dopamine release *in vivo*. *Brain Research Bulletin*, **574**, 98–104.

Itzhak, Y. & Stein, I. (1990) Sigma binding sites in the brain: an emerging concept for multiple sites and their relevance for psychiatric disorders. *Life Sciences*, **47**, 1073–1081.

Iwamoto, E.T. (1989) Evidence for a model of activation of central sigma systems. *Life Sciences*, **44**, 1547–1554.

Iyengar, S., Dilworth, V.M., Mick, S.J. *et al.* (1990a) Sigma receptors modulate both A9 and A10 dopaminergic neurones in the rat brain: functional interaction with NMDA receptors. *Brain Research*, **524**, 322–326.

Iyengar, S., Mick, S., Dilworth, V. *et al.* (1990b) Sigma receptors modulate the hypothalamic-pituitary adrenal (HPA) axis centrally: evidence for a functional interaction with NMDA receptors, *in vivo*. *Neuropharmacology*, **29**, 299–303.

Jacobs, B.L., Wilkenson, L.O. & Fornal, C.A. (1990) The role of brain serotonin. A neurophysiological perspective. *Neuropsychopharmacology*, **3**, 473–479.

Janssen, P.A.J. (1987) Does ritanserin, a potent serotonin-S₂ antagonist, restore energetic functions during the night. *Journal of the Royal Society of Medicine*, **80**, 409–414.

Janssen, P.A.J., Niemegeers, C.J.E. & Schellekens, K.L.H. (1965) Is it possible to predict clinical effects of neuroleptic drugs (major tranquillizers) from animal data? *Arzneimittel-Forschung*, **15**, 104–117.

Janssen, P.A.J., Niemegeers, C.J.E., Awouters, F., Schellekens, K.H.L., Megens, A.A.H. & Meert, T.F. (1988) Pharmacology of risperidone (R64766), a new antipsychotic with serotonin-S₂ and dopamine-D₂ antagonistic properties. *Journal of Pharmacology and Experimental Therapeutics*, **244**, 685–693.

Johnson, J.W. & Ascher, P. (1987) Glycine potentiates the NMDA response in cultured mouse brain neurons. *Nature*, **325**, 529–531.

Johnstone, E.C., Crow, T.J., Frith, C.D., Husband, J. & Kreel, L. (1976) Cerebral ventricular size and cognitive impairment in chronic schizophrenia. *Lancet*, **2**, 924–926.

Kelder, J., de Boer, Th., Graals, J.S. & Wieringa, J.H. (1984) Tetracyclic neuroleptics related to mianserin: SAR and strategies in the design of bioactive compounds. In Segeberg, B. & Seydel, J.K. (eds) *Proceedings of the 5th European Symposium on QSAR*, Berlin, p. 162. VCH, Berlin.

Kelly, J.S. & Crunelli, V. (1988) Glutamate as a mediator of fast synaptic transmission. In Lodge, D. (ed.) *Excitatory Amino Acids in Health and Disease*, pp. 187–202. Wiley, Chichester.

Kemp. J.A. & Leeson, P.D. (1993) The glycine of the NMDA receptor — five years on. *Trends in Pharmacological Science*, **14**, 20–25.

Kendler, K.S. (1987) The genetics of schizophrenia. In Meltzer, H.Y. (ed.) *Psychopharmacology: The Third Generation of Progress*, pp. 705–713. Raven Press, New York.

Kerwin, R.W., Patel, S., Meldrum, B.S., Czudek, C. & Reynolds, G.P. (1988) Asymmetrical loss of glutamate receptor subtype in left hippocampus in schizophrenia. *Lancet*, **1**, 583–584.

Kilpatrick, G.J., Bunce, K.T. & Tyers, M.B. (1990) 5-HT₃ receptors. *Medical Research Review*, **10**, 441–475.

Kilpatrick, G.J., Jones, B.J. & Tyers, M.B. (1987) Identification and distribution of 5-HT₃ receptors in rat brain using radioligand binding. *Nature*, **330**, 746–748.

Kilpatrick, G.J., Jones, B.J. & Tyers, M.B. (1989) Binding of the 5-HT₃ ligand, [³H]GR65630, to rat area postrema, vagus nerve and the brains of several species. *European Journal of Pharmacology*, **159**, 157–164.

Kleinman, J.E., Bridge, P., Karoum, F. *et al.* (1979) Catecholamines and metabolites in the brains of psychotics and normals: post mortem studies. In Usdin, E., Kopin, I.J. & Barchas, J. (eds) *Catecholamines: Basic and Clinical Frontiers*, pp. 1845–1847. Pergamon Press, New York.

Knight, A.R., Noble, A., Wong, E.H.F. & Middlemiss, D.N. (1991a) The subcellular distribution and pharmacology of the sigma recognition site in the guinea pig brain and liver. *Molecular Pharmacology*, **1**, 71–75.

Knight, A.R., Wyatt, C. & Middlemiss, D.N. (1991b) Spironolactone causes a rapid down regulation of sigma recognition sites in guinea pig brain and liver. *Neuropharmacology*, **30**, 923–925.

Kornhuber, J., Mack-Burkhardt, F., Riederer, P., Hebenstreit G.F., Reynolds, G.P., Andrews, H.B. & Beckman, H. (1989) [³H]Mk-801 binding sites in postmortem brain regions of schizophrenic patients. *Journal of Neural. Transmission* **77**, 231–236.

Kretschmer, B.D. & Schmidt, N.W. (1992) Glycine agonists in the treatment of schizophrenia? *Clinical Neuropharmacology*, **15**, 157–161.

Lader, M.H. (1991) Ondansetron in the treatment of anxiety.

In Racagni, G., Brunello, N. & Fukuda, T. (eds) *Biological Psychiatry*, Vol. 2, pp. 885–887. Excerpta Medica, Amsterdam.

Largent, B.L., Gundlack, A.L. & Snyder, S.H. (1986) Pharmacological and autoradiographic discrimination of sigma and phencyclidine receptor binding sites in brain with (+)[^{3}H]SKF10,047, (+)[^{3}H]3-3-[3-hydroxyphenyl]- *N*-(1-propyl)piperidine and [^{3}H]-1-1-(2-thienyl cyclohexyl)piperidine. *Journal of Pharmacology and Experimental Therapeutics*, **238**, 739–748.

Leysen, J.E. (1990) Gaps and peculiarities in 5-HT$_2$ receptor studies. *Neuropsychopharmacology*, **3**, 361–369.

Leysen, J.E. (1992) 5-HT$_2$ receptors: location, pharmacological, pathological and physiological role. In Langer, S.Z., Brunello, N., Racagni, G. & Mendlewicz, J. (eds) *Serotonin Receptor Subtypes: Pharmacological Significance and Clinical Implications*, Vol. 1, *International Academy of Biomedical Drug Research*, pp. 31–43. Karger, Basel.

Leysen, J.E. & Pauwels, P. (1990) 5-HT$_2$ receptors, roles and regulation. The neuropharmacology of serotonin. *Annals of the New York Academy of Sciences*, **600**, 183–193.

Leysen, J.E., Gommeron, W. & Laduron, P.M. (1978) Spiperone: a ligand of choice for neuroleptic receptors. 1. Kinetic characteristics of 'in vitro' binding. *Biochemical Pharmacology*, **27**, 307–316.

Leysen, J.E., Van Gompel, P., Verwimp, M. & Niemegeers, C.J.E. (1983) Role and localisation of serotonin (S$_2$) receptor binding sites. Effects of neuronal lesions. In Mandel, P. & De Feudis, F.V. (eds) *CNS Receptors: From Molecular Pharmacology to Behaviour*, pp. 373–383. Raven Press, New York.

Lodge, D. & Collingridge, G. (1990) Pharmacology of excitatory amino acids. *Trends in Pharmacologic Science*.

Lovinger, D.M. & White, G. (1991) Ethanol potentiation of 5-hydroxytryptamine$_3$ receptor-mediated ion current in neuroblastoma cells and isolated adult mammalian neurons. *Molecular Pharmacology*, **40**, 263–270.

Luby, E.D., Gottlieb, J.S., Cohen, B.D., Rosenbaum, G. & Domino, E.F. (1962) Model psychoses and schizophrenia. *American Journal of Psychiatry*, **119**, 61–67.

Lyon, M. (1991) Animal models of mania and schizophrenia. In Willner, P. (ed.) *Behavioural Models in Psychopharmacology: Theoretical, Industrial and Clinical Perspectives*, pp. 253–310. Cambridge University Press, Cambridge.

Macciardi, F., Lucca, A., Catalano, M., Marino, C., Zanardi, R. & Smeraldi, E. (1990) Amino acid patterns in schizophrenia: some new findings. *Psychiatry Research*, **32**, 63–70.

MacDermott, A.B., Mayer, M.L., Westbrook, G.L., Smith, S.J. & Barker, J.L. (1986) NMDA-receptor activation increases cytoplasmic calcium concentration in cultured spinal cord neurones. *Nature*, **321**, 519–522.

McGhie, A. & Chapman, J. (1961) Disorders of attention and perception in early schizophrenia. *British Journal of Medicine and Psychology*, **34**, 103–116.

McLennan, H. (1988) The pharmacological characterisation of excitatory amino acid receptors. In Lodge, D. (ed.) *Excitatory Amino Acids in Health and Disease*, pp. 1–11. Wiley, Chichester.

Martin, D. & Lodge, D. (1985) Ketamine acts as a non-competitive *N*-methyl-D-aspartate antagonist in frog spinal cord *in vitro*. *Neuropharmacology*, **24**, 999–1003.

Martin, W.R., Eades, C.G., Fraser, H.F. & Wikler, A. (1974) Morphine physical dependence in the dog. *Journal of Pharmacology and Experimental Therapeutics*, **189**, 759–771.

Martin, W.R., Eades, C.G., Thompson, J.A., Huppler, R.E. & Gilbert, P.E. (1976) The effects of morphine- and nalorphine-like drugs in the non-dependent and morphine-dependent chronic spinal dog. *Journal of Pharmacology and Experimental Therapeutics*, **197**, 517–532.

Mayer, M., Westbrook, G.L. & Guthrie, P.B. (1984) Voltage dependent block by Mg^{2+} of NMDA responses. *Nature*, **309**, 261–263.

Meco, G., Bedini, L., Bonitati, V. & Sonsini, U. (1989) Risperidone in the treatment of chronic schizophrenia with tardive dyskinesia. *Current Therapy Research*, **46**, 876–883.

Meltzer, H.Y. (1989) Clinical studies on the mechanism of action of clozapine: the dopamine–serotonin hypothesis of schizophrenia. *Psychopharmacology*, **99**, S18–S27.

Meltzer, H.Y. (1991) Studies on ondansetron in schizophrenia. In Racagni, G., Brunello, N. & Fukuda, T. (eds) *Biological Psychiatry*, Vol. 2, pp. 891–893. Excerpta Medica, Amsterdam.

Meltzer, H.Y., Goode, D.J. & Fang, V.S. (1978) The effect of psychotropic drugs on endocrine function. 1. Neuroleptics, precursors and agonists. In Lipton, M.A., Di Mascio, A. & Killam, K.F. (eds) *Psychopharmacology: A Generation of Progress*, pp. 509–529. Raven Press, New York.

Meltzer, H.Y., Matsubara, S. & Lee, J.-C. (1989) Classification of typical and atypical antipsychotic drugs on the basis of dopamine D-1, D-2 and serotonin$_2$ pK_i values. *Journal of Pharmacology and Experimental Therapeutics*, **251**, 238–244.

Meltzer, H.Y., Zhang, Y. & Stockmeier, C.A. (1992) Effect of amperozide on rat cortical 5-HT$_2$ and striatal and limbic dopamine D$_2$ receptor occupancy: implications for antipsychotic action. *European Journal of Pharmacology*, **216**, 67–71.

Mertens, C., De Wilde, J., Dierick, M., Bergman, L. & Gustavsson, G. (1989) Clinical trials of amperozide on schizophrenia. In *VIIIth World Congress of Psychiatry*, p. 502. Medica International Congress Series 899. Excerpta, Amsterdam.

Messoten, F., Suy, E., Pietquin, M., Buton, P., Heylen, S. & Gelders, Y. (1989) Therapeutic effect and safety of increasing doses of risperidone (R64766) in psychotic patients. *Psychopharmacology*, **99**, 445–449.

Meyer, J.S., Greifstein, F. & De Vaults, M. (1959) A new drug causing symptoms of sensory deprivation: neurological electroencephalographic and pharmacologic effects of sernyl. *Journal of Nervous and Mental Disease*, **129**, 54–61.

Morris, R.G.M. (1988) Elements of hypothesis concerning the participation of hippocampal NMDA receptors in learning. In Lodge, D. (ed.) *Excitatory Amino Acids in Health and Disease*, pp. 297–320. Wiley, Chichester.

Niemegeers, C.J.E. (1989) 5-HT$_2$ antagonists — role in the treatment of psychosis. Paper presented at the International Conference *New Developments in the Understanding and Treatment of Schizophrenia*, The Royal College of Physicians, London, 6th December.

Niemegeers, C.J.E. & Janssen, P.A.J. (1979) A systemic study of the pharmacological activities of dopamine antagonists. *Life Sciences*, **24**, 2201–2216.

Olney, J.W. (1988) Endogenous excitotoxins and neuropathological disorders. In Lodge, D. (ed.) *Excitatory Amino Acids in Health and Disease*, pp. 337–352. Wiley, Chichester.

Pangalila-Ratu, Langi, E.A. & Janssen, A.A.I. (1988) Ritanserin in the treatment of generalised anxiety disorders: a placebo controlled trial. *Human Psychopharmacology*, **3**, 207–212.

Papa, S.M., Engber, T.M., Boldry, R.C. & Chase, T.N. (1993) Opposite effects of NMDA and AMPA receptor blockade on catalepsy induced by dopamine receptor antagonists. *European Journal of Pharmacology*, **232**, 247–253.

Patel, S., Chapman, A.G., Millan, M.H. & Meldrum, B.S. (1988) Epilepsy and excitatory amino acid antagonists. In Lodge, D. (ed.) *Excitatory Amino Acids in Health and Disease*, pp. 353–378. Wiley, Chichester.

Paudice, P. & Raiteri, M. (1991) Cholecystokinin release mediated by 5-HT$_3$ receptors in rat cerebral cortex and nucleus accumbens. *British Journal of Pharmacology*, **103**, 1790–1794.

Peters, J.A., Malone, H.M. & Lambert, J.J. (1992) Recent advances in the electrophysiological characterisation of 5-HT$_3$ receptors. *Trends in Pharmacological Sciences*, **13**, 391–397.

Quirion, R., Bowen, W.D., Itzhak, Y. *et al.* (1992) A proposal for the classification of sigma binding sites. *Trends in Pharmacological Sciences*, **13**, 85–86.

Rahman, S. & Neuman, R.S. (1993) Activation of 5-HT$_2$ receptors facilitate depolarization of neocortical neurons by *N*-methyl-D-aspartate. *European Journal of Pharmacology*, **231**, 347–354.

Rao, T.S., Kim, H.S., Lehmann, J., Martin, L.L. & Wood, P.L. (1990) Differential effects of phencyclidine (PCP) and ketamine on mesocortical and mesostriatal dopamine release *in vivo*. *Life Sciences* **45**, 1065–1072.

Reynolds, G.P. (1983) Increased concentrations and lateral asymmetry of amygdala dopamine in schizophrenia. *Nature*, **305**, 527–528.

Reyntjens, A., Gelders, Y.G., Hoppenbrouwers, M.-L.J.A. & Bussche, G.V. (1986) Thymosthenic effects of ritanserin (R55667), a centrally acting serotonin S$_2$-receptor blocker. *Drug Development Research*, **8**, 205–211.

Roman, F.J., Pascaud, X., Duffy, O., Vauche, D., Martin, B. & Junien, J.L. (1991) Neuropeptide Y and peptide YY interact with rat brain sigma and PCP binding sites. *European Journal of Pharmacology*, **174**, 301–302.

Ropert, N. & Guy, N. (1991) Serotonin facilitates GABAergic transmission in CA1 region of rat hippocampus *in vivo*. *Journal of Physiology*, **441**, 121–136.

Rosse, R.B., Thent, S.K., Banay-Schwartz, M., Leighton, M., Scarella, E., Cohen, C.G. & Deutsch, S.I. (1989) Glycine adjuvant therapy to conventional neuroleptic treatment in schizophrenia: an open-label, pilot study. *Clinical Neuropharmacology* **12**, 416–424.

Salama, A.I., Saller, C.F., Goldstein, J.M. *et al.* (1989) The preclinical pharmacology of ICI204636, a new atypical agent. *Proceedings of the 28th Annual Meeting of ACNP*, Maui, Hawaii, p. 124.

Sanger, D.J. & Jackson, A. (1988) Is the discriminative stimulus produced by phencyclidine due to an interaction with *N*-methyl-D-aspartate receptors. *Psychopharmacology*, **96**, 87–92.

Sanger, D.J. & Jackson, A. (1989) Effects of phencyclidine and other *N*-methyl-D-aspartate antagonists on the schedule-controlled behaviour of rats. *Journal of Pharmacology and Experimental Therapy*, **248**, 1215–1221.

Saywell, K., Singh, L., Oles, R.J. *et al.* (1991) The anticonvulsant properties in the mouse of the glycine/NMDA receptor antagonist L.687,414. *British Journal of Pharmacology*, **102**, 66P.

Schoepp, D.D. & Conn, P.J. (1993) Metabotropic glutamate receptors in brain function and pathology. *Trends in Pharmacological Sciences*, **14**, 13–20.

Schotte, A., Maloteaux, J.M. & Laduron, P.M. (1983) Characterisation and regional distribution of serotonin S$_2$-receptors in human brain. *Brain Research*, **276**, 231–235.

Seeman, P., Chau-Wong, M., Tedesco, J. & Wong, K. (1975) Brain receptors for antipsychotic drugs and dopamine: direct binding assays. *Proceedings of the National Academy of Sciences USA*, **72**, 4376–4380.

Sellers, E.M., Romach, M.K., Frecker, R.C. & Higgins, G.A. (1991) Efficacy of the 5-HT$_3$ antagonist ondansetron in addictive disorders. In Recagni, G., Brunello, N. & Fukuda, T. (eds) *Biological Psychiatry*, Vol. 2, 894–897. Excerpta Medica, Amsterdam.

Shelton, R.C. & Weinberger, D.R. (1987) Brain morphology in schizophrenia. In Meltzer, H.Y. (ed.) *The Third Generation of Progress*, pp. 773–781. Raven Press, New York.

Sherman, A.D., Davidson, A.T., Baruah, S., Hegwood, T.S. & Waziri, R. (1991) Evidence of glutamatergic deficiency in schizophrenia. *Neuroscience Letters*, **121**, 77–80.

Simpson, M.D.C., Slater, P., Royston, M.C. & Deakin, J.F.W. (1992) Alterations in phencyclidine and sigma binding sites in schizophrenic brains. *Schizophrenia Research*, **6**, 41–48.

Singh, L., Donald, A.E., Foster, A.C. *et al.* (1990) Enantiomers of HA-966 (3-amino-1-hydroxypyrrolid-2-one) exhibit distinct central nervous system effects: (+)HA-966 is a selective glycine/*N*-methyl-D-aspartate receptor antagonist, but (−)HA966 is a potent γ-butyrolactone-like sedative. *Proceedings of the National Academy of Sciences USA*, **87**, 347–351.

Sircar, R. & Zukin, S.R. (1983) Characterisation of specific sigma opiate/phencyclidine (PCP)-binding sites in the human brain. *Life Sciences* **33**, 259–262.

Snell, L.D. & Johnson, K.M. (1986) Characterisation of the inhibition of excitatory amino-acid-induced neurotransmitter release in the rat striatum by phencyclidine-like drugs. *Journal of Pharmacology and Experimental Therapeutics*, **238**, 938–946.

Sokoloff, P., Giros, B., Martres, M.-P., Bouthenet, M.-L. & Schwartz, J.C. (1990) Molecular cloning and characterisation of a novel dopamine receptor (D$_3$) as a target for neuroleptics. *Nature*, **347**, 146–151.

Storm-Mathisen, J. & Ottersen, O.P. (1988) Anatomy of putative glutamatergic neurons. In Alvoli, M., Reader, T.A., Dykes, R.M. & Gloor, P. (eds). *Neurotransmitters and*

Cortical Function, pp. 39–70. Plenum, New York.

Su, T.P. (1982) Evidence for sigma opioid receptor: binding of [^{3}H]SKF10,047 to etorphine-inaccesible sites in guinea pig brain. *Journal of Pharmacology and Experimental Therapeutics*, **223**, 284–290.

Su, T.P. (1986) HR 375A: a potential antipsychotic drug that interacts with dopamine D$_2$ receptors and sigma receptors in the brain. *Neuroscience Letters*, **71**, 224–228.

Su, T.P., Weissman, A.D. & Yeh, S.Y. (1986) Endogenous ligands for sigma opioid receptors in the brain ('sigma phin'): evidence from binding assays. *Life Sciences*, **38**, 2199–2210.

Svartengren, J. & Simonsson, P. (1990) Receptor binding properties of amperozide. *Pharmacology and Toxicology*, Suppl. **1**, 8–14.

Tam, S.W. (1983) Naloxone inaccessible sigma receptor in rat central nervous system. *Proceedings of the National Academy of Sciences USA*, **80**, 6703–6707.

Tam, S.W. & Mitchell, K.N. (1991) Neuropeptide Y and peptide YY do not bind to brain sigma and phencyclidine binding sites. *European Journal of Pharmacology*, **193**, 121–122.

Taylor, D.P., Eison, M.S., Moon, S.L. & Yocca, F.D. (1991) BMY 14802: a potential antipsychotic with selective affinity for sigma binding sites. In Tamminga, C.A. & Schultz, S.C. (eds) *Advances in Neuropsychiatry and Psychopharmacology*, Vol. 1, *Schizophrenia Research*. Raven Press, Australia.

Toru, M., Watanabe, S., Shibuya, H. *et al.* (1988) Neurotransmitters, receptors and neuropeptides in post-mortem brains of chronic schizophrenic patients. *Acta Psychiatrica Scandinavica*, **78**, 121–137.

Toth, E. & Lajtha, A. (1986) Antagonism of phencyclidine-induced hyperactivity by glycine in mice. *Neurochemistry Research*, **11**, 393–400.

Turner, T., Cookson, J.C., Wass, J.A.H., Drury, P.C., Price, P.A. & Besser, G.M. (1984) Psychotic reactions during treatment of pituitary tumours with dopamine agonists. *British Medical Journal*, **289**, 1101–1103.

Van der Maelan, C.P. & Braselton, J.P. (1990) Effects of a potential antipsychotic, BMY 14802, on firing of central serotonergic and noradrenergic neurons in rats. *European Journal of Pharmacology* **179**, 357–366.

Van Tol, H.H.M., Wu, C.M., Guan, H.-C. *et al.* (1992) Multiple dopamine D$_4$ receptor variants in the human population. *Nature*, **358**, 149–152.

Vincent, S.L., McSparren, J., Wang, R.Y. & Benes, F.M. (1991) Evidence four ultrastructural changes in cortical axodendritic synapses following long-term treatment with haloperidol or clozapine. *Neuropsychopharmacology*, **5**, 147–155.

Vu, T.H., Weissman, A.D. & London, E.D. (1990) Pharmacological characteristics and distributions of sigma and phencyclidine receptors in the animal kingdom. *Journal of Neurochemistry*, **54**, 598–603.

Walther, B., Ghersi-Egea, J.F., Minn, A. & Siest, G. (1986) Subcellular distribution of cytochrome P450 in the brain. *Brain Research*, **375**, 338–344.

Waters, N., Petersson, G., Carlsson, A. & Svensson, K. (1989) The putatively antipsychotic agent amperazide produces behavioural stimulation in the rat. *Naunyn-Schmiedebergs Archives of Pharmacology*, **340**, 161–169.

Watkins, J.C., Krogsgaard-Larsen, P. & Honor, T. (1990) Structure–activity relationships in the development of excitatory amino acid receptor agonists and competitive antagonists. *Trends in Pharmacological Science*, **11**, 25–33.

Waziri, R. (1988) Glycine therapy of schizophrenia. *Biological Psychiatry*, **23**, 210–211.

Weinshank, R.L., Adham, N., Zgombick, J., Bard, J., Branchek, T. & Hartig, P.R. (1992) Molecular analysis of serotonin receptor subtypes. In Langer, S.Z., Brunello, N., Racagni, G. & Mendlewicz, J. (eds) *Serotonin Receptor Subtypes: Pharmacological Significance and Clinical Implications*, pp. 1–12. Karger, Basel.

Weissman, A.D. & De Souza, E.B. (1991) Post mortem investigations of sigma and PCP receptors in psychosis. In Racagni, G., Brunello, N. & Fukuda, T. (eds) *Biological Psychiatry*, Vol. 1, pp. 498–500. Excerpta Medica, Amsterdam.

Weissman, A.D., Su, T.P., Hedreen, J.C. & London, E.D. (1988) Sigma receptors in postmortem human brains. *Journal of Pharmacology and Experimental Therapeutics* **247**, 29–33.

Willetts, J., Balster, R.L. & Leander, J.D. (1990) The behavioural pharmacology of NMDA receptor antagonists. *Trends in Pharmacological Science*, **11**, 423–428.

Willner, P. (1991) Behavioural models in psychopharmacology. In Willner, P. (ed.) *Behavioural Models in Psychopharmacology: Theoretical, Industrial and Clinical Perspectives*, pp. 3–18. Cambridge University Press, Cambridge.

Zhang, A.Z., Mitchell, K.N., Cook, L. & Tam, S.W. (1988) Human endogenous ligands for sigma and phencyclidine receptors. In Domino, E.F. & Kamenka, J.M. (eds) *Sigma and Phencyclidine-like Compounds as Molecular Probes in Biology*, pp. 238–352. NPP Books, Ann Arbor.

Chapter 22
Brain Imaging

P. F. LIDDLE

Introduction

Schizophrenia is a subtle, yet potentially devastating, disorder of the highest human faculties. A detailed understanding of the neuronal mechanisms associated with this subtle disorder remains an elusive goal, not only because the human brain is an extremely complex organ, but also because it is relatively inaccessible to investigation during life. In the past two decades, refinement of imaging techniques has provided access to the function and structure of the living brain. There are three main domains in which we might look for brain abnormality in schizophrenia. First, we might seek the location of the cerebral damage that creates a predisposition to schizophrenia by examining macroscopic brain structure using X-ray computerized tomography (CT) or magnetic resonance imaging (MRI). Second, to establish the relationship between disordered neural activity and the clinical features of schizophrenia, we might employ functional imaging techniques, such as positron emission tomography (PET), single photon emission tomography (SPET) or brain electrical activity mapping (BEAM), to generate images of regional neuronal activity. Third, we might seek an understanding of the nature of the pathological process that impairs neuronal function by imaging

the molecular components of brain tissue, including key functional elements such as neuroreceptors, which can be imaged using PET or SPET, or structural elements such as membrane phospholipids, which can be imaged using magnetic resonance spectroscopy (MRS).

Macroscopic brain structure

Enlargement of cerebral ventricles

Early studies of macroscopic brain structure employing pneumoencephalography revealed that at least some schizophrenic patients had enlarged cerebral ventricles. For example, in a pneumoencephalographic study of 212 schizophrenic patients, aged less than 50 but nonetheless long-term institutional residents, Huber (1964) found that 81.6% exhibited evidence of atrophy, most commonly enlargement of the third ventricle. In the mid-1970s, the advent of the relatively non-invasive technique of X-ray CT offered the prospect of further progress in the quest for evidence that schizophrenia is associated with demonstrable brain abnormality. The first X-ray CT study by Johnstone et al. (1976), performed in a group of 18 severely impaired patients in long-term institutional care, confirmed Huber's observation of ventricular enlargement, and subsequent studies, which have included less severely impaired subjects, have produced further confirmation despite some discordant findings. In a comprehensive review of X-ray CT studies, in which patients had been compared with prospectively ascertained volunteers scanned concurrently with the patient group, Lewis (1990) reported that 12 of 21 studies had found a significant increase in lateral ventricular size, seven of the nine studies that examined the third ventricle found a significant increase in width of that ventricle, and four of the eight studies which examined cortical sulci had found significant sulcal enlargement.

However, a simple count of the number of studies reporting significant differences between patients and normal controls, without considering the statistical power of each study, gives no indication of the magnitude of the increase in ventricular size. In an attempt to estimate the magnitude of the effect, Raz and Raz (1990) performed a meta-analysis of CT and MRI studies. They defined effect size as the ratio of difference between mean ventricular volume in patients and controls divided by the pooled standard deviation, for each study. They found that the effect size for the various studies was normally distributed with a mean value of approximately 0.6 standard deviations. Thus, there is convincing evidence that the mean ventricular volume in patients is larger than in normal individuals, but the magnitude of the effect is relatively small, and it is not surprising that some individual studies have failed to find a significant effect.

Reductions in cerebral tissue volume

Enlargement of cerebrospinal fluid (CSF) spaces, such as the cerebral ventricles and cortical sulci, imply that there is a deficit in the amount of brain tissue. The advent of MRI, which provides not only higher spatial resolution, but also the ability to distinguish between grey and white matter, offered the possibility of defining more clearly the locus of the implied deficit in amount of brain tissue. The majority of studies, such as those by Suddath *et al.* (1990) and by Zipursky *et al.* (1992),

indicate a defect in grey matter volume, although some studies (Breier *et al.*, 1992) also found deficits in white matter. In addition to diminished tissue volume, MRI scans reveal an excess of developmental abnormalities such as cavum septum pellucidum (Jurjus *et al.*, 1993) and grey matter heterotopias.

The question of whether structural abnormality is confined principally to a specific lobe of the brain remains controversial. There have been consistent reports of structural abnormality in temporal lobes, in both medial structures, such as hippocampal formation (Suddath *et al.*, 1989, 1990), and in lateral areas, such as superior temporal gyrus (Shenton *et al.*, 1992). Although abnormality is more pronounced on the left, there are also abnormalities in the right temporal lobe (Suddath *et al.*, 1990). While findings of overt structural abnormality in other lobes have been less consistent, the balance of evidence indicates that there are widespread deficits in brain tissue, especially in frontal, temporal and parietal lobes. Zipursky *et al.* (1992) measured grey matter volume in six regions that spanned the brain, and found that in schizophrenic patients the mean grey matter volume was significantly less than normal in five of the regions and exhibited a trend towards being significantly less in the sixth region.

Is cerebral tissue volume diminished in all cases?

In most quantitative studies of brain structure the measurements exhibit a unimodal distribution, suggesting that the patients belong to a single population in which mean brain tissue volume is diminished in comparison with normal, even though many individual patients have values lying within the normal range. For example, Zipursky *et al.* (1992) plotted regression curves defining the normal range for grey matter volume (as a proportion of intracranial volume) as a function of age in normal individuals, and found an excess of schizophrenic patients with grey matter volume within the lower half of the normal range for their age, as well as an excess of cases with values more than two standard deviations below the normal mean.

Suddath *et al.* (1990) compared the volumes of medial temporal lobe structures in 15 pairs of identical twins discordant for schizophrenia, and demonstrated that in 14 pairs the twin with schizophrenia had the smaller left hippocampal volume, while in 13 pairs the schizophrenic twin had the smaller right hippocampal volume. Measurements of ventricular volume showed that the affected twin tended to have larger third and lateral ventricles, consistent with the expectation of an inverse relationship between ventricular size and brain tissue volume. The findings of Suddath *et al.* are consistent with the observation by Reveley *et al.* (1982) that within a group of seven discordant identical twin pairs, the affected twin had a larger ventricular brain ratio (VBR) in six of the pairs. Thus, studies of discordant twins indicate that virtually all schizophrenic patients have a reduction in cerebral tissue compared with that expected if they had not been ill.

Is there progressive structural change?

Ventricular enlargement has been detected in the early stages of the illness (Schulz *et al.*, 1983; Turner *et al.*, 1986). The majority of studies which have examined the relationship between lateral ventricular size and duration of illness prior to scanning have not found a significant relationship. The available evidence from longitudinal studies, in which a follow-up scan was performed several years after the initial scan, suggests that ventricular enlargement is not progressive in the majority of cases (e.g. Nasrallah *et al.*, 1986; Illowsky *et al.*, 1988; Vita *et al.*, 1988), though there is evidence of progression in a minority.

Clinical correlates of structural abnormality

The finding of ventricular enlargement in at least some schizophrenic patients, together with the clinical evidence that florid schizophrenic symptoms tend to respond to treatment with dopamine-blocking drugs, led Crow (1980) to propose that there are two types of pathological process in schizophrenia. The proposed type I process involves biochemical imbalance and is reflected in positive symptoms, such as delusions, hallucinations and formal thought disorder, which tend to occur in acute episodes. The proposed type II process involves loss of cerebral tissue and is reflected in negative symptoms, such as poverty of speech and blunted affect, which tend to be persistent. This formulation implies that ventricular enlargement is associated with negative symptoms. However, of the 18 X-ray CT studies reviewed by Lewis (1990) which have examined the issue, only five revealed a significant association between negative symptoms and ventricular enlargement. Thus, the evidence provides only modest support for the cardinal hypothesis arising from the concept of the type-II disease process.

The most consistently reported clinical correlate of ventricular enlargement is impaired performance in cognitive tests. Johnstone *et al.* (1976) found that ventricular enlargement was associated with impaired performance in the Withers and Hinton battery, which consists of tests of various aspects of cognitive function, including concentration, verbal memory and reasoning. Golden *et al.* (1980) demonstrated an association between ventricular enlargement and impairment in the Luria–Nebraska battery, which embraces a wide range of aspects of neuropsychological function. Many other studies have reported similar findings. A few studies have sought to relate the locus of diminution of cerebral tissue to specific cognitive impairments. For example, Raine *et al.* (1992) found that reduced frontal tissue volume was correlated with impaired performance in neuropsychological tests of frontal lobe function.

The question of how brain structural abnormalities might relate to dopaminergic hyperactivity is of major importance in understanding schizophrenia. Employing the plasma homovanillic acid level as a measure of dopaminergic activity, Breier *et al.* (1993) demonstrated that schizophrenic patients exhibit an abnormally large increase in dopaminergic activity in response to pharmacologically induced stress. They found that the magnitude of this dopaminergic response is inversely related to frontal lobe volume.

Images of brain function

Regional cerebral blood flow (rCBF) and glucose metabolism (rCMRglu)

Imaging techniques

Simple motor tasks or sensory experiences are associated with increases in rCBF in the relevant primary motor or sensory areas, indicating that rCBF is an index of local neuronal activity. Typically, the rise in rCBF occurs over a time scale of several seconds after onset of the neuronal activity. rCBF is a more sensitive index of transient neuronal activity than is rCMRglu (Raichle *et al.*, 1987). However, it is probable that rCMRglu and rCBF provide similar indices of steady state cerebral activity.

The established techniques for imaging rCBF are the cortical probe technique using radioactive xenon (^{133}Xe), SPET using exametazime (HMPAO) labelled with the metastable technetium isotope ^{99m}Tc and PET using the positron-emitting oxygen isotope ^{15}O.

The cortical probe technique employs an array of detectors placed on the scalp to detect the spatial distribution of radioactivity in the lateral and superior aspects of the cerebral cortex during the inhalation of ^{133}Xe. Although the technique has access only to superficial brain regions, it is sensitive and entails exposure to a level of radiation low enough to allow multiple repeated scans. SPET employs tomographical reconstruction, and can therefore provide images of the entire brain, though sensitivity to regions deep within the brain is relatively poor because of absorption of photons in the brain tissue. The major limitation of the rCBF technique using SPET with ^{99m}Tc-HMPAO is high radiation exposure. Exposure in a single scan is approximately equivalent to a year's exposure to background radiation, restricting the possibilities for repeated scanning.

PET is a far more cumbersome technique because it entails the use of short-lived positron-emitting isotopes, and hence requires a nearby cyclotron, but offers the possibility of virtually uniform sampling of the entire brain. Images of rCBF can be obtained following administration of either water or carbon dioxide labelled with ^{15}O, which has a half-life of 2.1 min, allowing the recording of multiple images of rCBF in different states of brain activity within a single session. The cumulative radiation dose after 10 repeated images is approximately equal to the annual dose arising from exposure to background radiation. PET can also be used to obtain images of rCMRglu after infusion of deoxyglucose labelled with ^{18}F, which has a half-life of approximately 2 h. However, this technique provides images of brain activity averaged over approximately 30 min, and does not allow imaging of a multiplicity of brain states in one individual in a single session.

Recently developed techniques using MRI to detect changes in the local concentration of deoxyhaemoglobin when capillaries dilatate in response to neuronal activation, hold the promise of non-invasive imaging of brain function with higher spatial and temporal resolution than is possible with PET (Neil, 1993). These techniques have been used to image neuronal activity in normal subjects, but have yet to be used in schizophrenia.

Landmarks in the history of functional imaging in schizophrenia

The earliest studies of rCBF in schizophrenia using the cortical probe technique (Ingvar & Franzen, 1974) revealed relative underactivity of frontal cortex relative to postcentral cortical regions in chronic schizophrenic patients. However, subsequent studies provided conflicting results. Mathew *et al.* (1982) found global reduction in rCBF, but no relative hypofrontality in a group of 23 patients, most of whom were receiving medication. Ariel *et al.* (1983) found relative hypofrontality in the left hemisphere in a study of 29 patients, most of whom were receiving medication. In a study of 15 medicated patients, Gur *et al.* (1983) did not find relative hypofrontality, and in a subsequent study of 19 unmedicated patients, the same investigators (Gur *et al.*, 1985) again found no evidence of hypofrontality.

Some, but not all, of the early PET studies of

regional metabolism also reported evidence of hypofrontality. Buchsbaum *et al.* (1982) found a reduction in prefrontal rCMRglu relative to posterior rCMRglu in the resting state in a group of eight patients who were not receiving medication at the time of scanning, and Farkas *et al.* (1984) observed similar hypofrontality in a group of 13 subjects, of whom seven were unmedicated. Wolkin *et al.* (1985) found reduced absolute frontal and temporal lobe rCMRglu in 10 unmedicated chronic schizophrenic patients. After recommencement of medication, temporal metabolism returned towards normal, but hypofrontality persisted. DeLisi *et al.* (1985) found no significant change in anterior–posterior rCMRglu gradient between the medication-free and medicated states in nine chronic schizophrenic patients. In the first PET study of acutely ill patients with minimal prior antipsychotic medication, Sheppard *et al.* (1983) measured regional oxygen metabolism in 12 patients, six of whom were medication naive, and did not find hypofrontality.

In evaluating the discrepancies between the findings of different studies, it is necessary to consider not only differences between the patients' clinical state and medication, but the possibility that other factors which produce variance in observed patterns of rCBF (or metabolism) might conceal true differences in brain function between patients and controls. For example, it is necessary to take account of variations in brain size, shape and orientation that make it difficult to ensure that the same regions are being compared in all subjects. In light of subsequent evidence (reviewed below) that patterns of rCBF in schizophrenia can include local increases and local decreases in rCBF in nearby regions, imprecise location of relatively arbitrarily determined regions of interest is likely to obscure true differences. Another source of potentially confounding variance is variation in global cerebral blood flow (and metabolism) that is unrelated to local neuronal activity. These global variations have only a minor effect on ratios such as the ratio of anterior to posterior rCBF, but such ratios provide only a crude indication of the pattern of brain activity. If local values of rCBF or metabolism are to be interpreted in term of local neural activity, it is essential to take account of global variations.

Although debate about the best way of dealing with these potentially confounding sources of variance in rCBF (or metabolism) still continues, methods have been steadily refined by the PET group at Washington University, Missouri (Fox *et al.*, 1985; Perlmutter *et al.*, 1985) and later by the PET group at Hammersmith Hospital, England (Friston *et al.*, 1990, 1991). In the method developed at Washington University, regions of interest are defined from a stereotactic atlas of the brain and located on the PET image by reference to reliable anatomical landmarks. Whole-brain blood flow is measured, and regional flow is expressed as the ratio of regional to whole-brain blood flow. This approach makes the physiologically implausible assumption that rCBF changes due to local neuronal activity are proportional to concurrent global flow, but errors from such an assumption are likely to be small. In the Hammersmith method, the image of each subject is plastically transformed to match a standard template. Effects of variation in whole-brain blood flow are removed by analysis of covariance.

Using the approach developed at Washington University, Early *et al.* (1987) measured rCBF in two separate groups of five medication-naive acute schizophrenic patients, and in both groups found an increase in resting state rCBF in the left globus pallidus in comparison with controls, but there were no significant differences in frontal rCBF. Thus, by 1987, the balance of evidence indicated that schizophrenic patients exhibit abnormal rCBF or regional metabolism when in the resting state, but different schizophrenic patients exhibit different patterns of abnormality. In general, hypofrontality is more prevalent in chronic patients. In retrospect, this variability between patients is scarcely surprising as cerebral activity during a resting state is likely to be influenced by concurrent symptoms. Recent studies have explicitly utilized the fact that rCBF reflects current mental activity, and have either directly or indirectly measured the change in rCBF between a mental state of interest and a control mental state.

Two principal approaches have been used. One approach seeks to determine the pattern of cerebral activity associated with a specific type of symptom by comparing rCBF in the presence and the absence of that type of symptom. This type of approach is exemplified in the studies by Liddle *et al.* (1992) and McGuire *et al.* (1993). The other approach, developed in a series of seminal studies by Weinberger *et al.* (1986, 1988, 1992), compares cerebral activity during performance of a neuropsychological task which engages mental processes implicated in schizophrenia with that during an appropriate reference state. Such neuropsychological activation studies do not directly reveal the pattern of cerebral activity associated with the occurrence of a particular type of symptom, although the cerebral activity associated with the neuropsychological task might be influenced by the symptom profile.

Cerebral activity associated with specific types of symptoms

The most direct strategy for establishing the relationship between cerebral activity and a particular symptom is to compare rCBF when the symptom of interest is present with rCBF in the same subject when the symptom has resolved. This strategy was adopted by McGuire *et al.* (1993) in their SPET study of rCBF pattern associated with auditory hallucinations. They found that auditory hallucinations are associated with increased rCBF in Broca's area and, to a lesser extent, in medial frontal cortex and left medial temporal cortex.

The difficulty with this approach is that factors other than the expression of the relevant symptom might have changed between the two measurements. In particular, other symptoms or effects of medication might change. An alternative second strategy exploits the fact that schizophrenia is a multidimensional illness in which particular groups of symptoms vary independently of other groups of symptoms. The pattern of correlations between symptoms indicate that the illness can be described in terms of four virtually orthogonal dimensions (Liddle, 1994). One dimension is

bipolar, so there are five major groups of symptoms (or syndromes).
1 *Reality distortion* (delusions and hallucinations).
2 *Disorganization* (formal thought disorder, inappropriate affect).
3 *Psychomotor poverty* (poverty of speech, flat affect, decreased movement).
4 *Psychomotor excitation* (pressure of speech, labile or affect, increased movement).
5 *Depression* (depressed mood, hopelessness, low self-esteem).
Psychomotor poverty and excitation lie at opposite poles of a single dimension which is virtually orthogonal to the other three dimensions. Since the dimensions are virtually orthogonal, it is possible to examine the correlation between rCBF and each syndrome, with the expectation that the confounding effects of variation in symptoms from orthogonal dimensions will be trivial. Of the five syndromes, reality distortion, disorganization and psychomotor poverty are especially characteristic of schizophrenia, and these three syndromes have been subjected to detailed study.

In a PET study of medicated patients with stable symptoms, Liddle *et al.* (1992) found that each of the three cardinal syndromes is associated with a specific pattern of rCBF in multimodal association cortex and related subcortical nuclei. In particular, psychomotor poverty is associated with decreased rCBF in prefrontal cortex and left parietal cortex, and increased rCBF in the caudate nuclei; disorganization with increased rCBF in right anterior cingulate, and decreased rCBF in right ventral prefrontal cortex; while reality distortion is associated with increased rCBF in left medial temporal lobe and with decreased rCBF in posterior cingulate and left lateral temporal lobe. In a SPET study of unmedicated patients, Ebmeier *et al.* (1993) confirmed the negative correlation between psychomotor and prefrontal rCBF, the positive correlation between disorganization and rCBF in right anterior cingulate and the negative correlation between reality distortion and left lateral temporal rCBF. It is noteworthy that Ebmeier *et al.* did not observe a positive correlation between reality distortion and left medial temporal rCBF. However, the balance of evidence indicates that reality distortion can be associated with increases in left temporal rCBF. In particular, Kurachi *et al.* (1985), Musalek *et al.* (1989), Matsuda *et al.* (1989) and Suzuki *et al.* (1993) have all reported an association between hallucinations and increased rCBF in left temporal lobe.

The observation of an association between psychomotor poverty and decreased prefrontal rCBF is consistent not only with Ingvar and Franzen's (1974) original observation of hypofrontality in chronic patients who exhibited inactivity and autism, but also with most subsequent studies that have examined the relationship between regional cerebral activity and the core negative symptoms which make up the psychomotor poverty syndrome. For example, using SPET to measure rCBF, Suzuki *et al.* (1992) found an association between severity of negative symptoms and hypofrontality. Using PET studies to measure rCMRglu in unmedicated patients, Wolkin *et al.* (1992) and Tamminga *et al.* (1992) reported an association between negative symptoms and decreased frontal rCMRglu. Thus, the association between the core negative symptoms that make up the psychomotor poverty syndrome and decreased frontal activity is a very robust finding.

Evidence from neuropsychological studies indicates that psychomotor poverty, disorganization and reality distortion are associated with disorder of the supervisory processes responsible for initiation, selection and monitoring of self-generated mental activity, respectively. Consistent with this, in the case of each of these three syndromes, the pattern of rCBF associated with each of these three syndromes includes the cortical site that is most strongly activated in normal individuals during the performance of the type of supervisory mental process implicated in that syndrome (Liddle, 1993).

It might be predicted that the psychomotor excitation syndrome would be characterized by the opposite pattern of cerebral activity to that seen in psychomotor poverty, and in particular, that it would be associated with frontal hyperactivity. The available circumstantial evidence supports this hypothesis. For example, in the group of undedicated, acutely ill patients studied by Ebmeier *et al.* (1993), the patient group as a whole exhibited increased frontal rCBF when compared with normal control subjects, even though within the schizophrenic patient group there was a significant negative correlation between rCBF and severity of psychomotor poverty. It is likely that in these acute patients, the group mean score on the psychomotor dimension inclined towards psychomotor excitation, and the observed net frontal hyperactivity in the group reflects an association between psychomotor excitation and frontal hyperactivity.

In view of the multidimensional nature of schizophrenia, it is perhaps scarcely surprising that studies which have compared resting-state cerebral activity in schizophrenic patients with that in normal controls without taking account of the specific symptom profile of the patients, have produced conflicting findings. However, when the symptom profile is taken into account, a more consistent picture is obtained.

Neuropsychological activation in schizophrenia

Using the cortical probe technique, Weinberger *et al.* (1986) demonstrated that unmedicated schizophrenic patients produce a lesser degree of activation of the dorsolateral prefrontal cortex than do normal individuals during performance of the Wisconsin card sorting test (WCST), a task which demands flexibility in problem solving. This task is well established as a test of frontal lobe function. Furthermore, it is a task that many schizophrenic patients perform poorly. In their study, Weinberger *et al.* found that in the patients there was a strong correlation between frontal rCBF and WCST performance, indicating that the level of ability to activate frontal lobes was the limiting factor that determined performance. In a companion study, Berman *et al.* (1986) demonstrated that the impaired frontal function was independent of antipsychotic medication, and of factors such as attention, mental effort and severity of psychotic symptoms. Furthermore, in a subsequent study of monozygotic twins, Berman *et al.* (1992) demonstrated that in all discordant twin pairs studied, the affected twin showed evidence of lower frontal activity during the WCST, suggesting that a degree of environmentally determined frontal impairment occurs in virtually all cases of schizophrenia. In the majority of concordant affected twin pairs, the twin who had received more antipsychotic medication exhibited somewhat less impaired frontal activation, indicating that frontal impairment is not due to prior medication.

In a series of studies, Weinberger's group obtained evidence that the degree of diminished prefrontal activation during WCST performance is correlated with reduced hippocampal volume (Weinberger *et al.*, 1992), reduced dopaminergic activity (Weinberger *et al.*, 1988), and might be reversed by the dopamine agonist, amphetamine (Daniel *et al.*, 1991).

Using SPET, Andreasen *et al.* (1992) demonstrated that medication-naive schizophrenic patients produce less activation of medial prefrontal cortex than do normal individuals during the Tower of London test, a task which requires strategy planning. A similar finding was obtained in patients who had previously taken medication for long periods. This study confirms that frontal lobe impairment in schizophrenia is not merely a consequence of prior treatment. Warkentin *et al.* (1989) demonstrated that schizophrenic patients fail to exhibit normal activation of prefrontal cortex during verbal fluency tasks. Buchsbaum *et al.* (1992), using PET to measure rCMRglu, demonstrated that medication-naive schizophrenic patients exhibited less activity in frontal cortex when scanned during performance of the continuous performance test (CPT), a task expected to activate frontal cortex, although interpretation of this finding is confounded by the absence of comparison with metabolism in a baseline mental state. The observed deficit might reflect either frontal underactivity at rest or a failure to activate frontal cortex normally.

Studies that demonstrate lesser frontal activation in schizophrenic patients during 'frontal' tasks which the patients perform poorly do not address the question of whether or not patients activate frontal cortex as much as normal individuals do, when both groups perform a 'frontal' task at the same rate. This question can be addressed by imaging rCBF during the generation of words at a rate which is paced so that all subjects produce words at the same rate. In such a study, Liddle *et al.* (1994) demonstrated that the magnitude of the frontal activation associated with generation of words is as great in patients with substantial poverty of speech as it is in normal subjects generating words at the same rate. However, in the patients, the relationship between the frontal activation and activity in other cerebral areas, especially the temporal cortex, was quite different from that observed in normals (Fig. 22.1). This indicates that hypofrontality does not reflect a fixed loss of function, but rather a dynamic imbalance between cerebral regions consistent with the proposal that the essential abnormality lies in the pattern of correlation between activity in different parts of the brain, especially between frontal and temporal activity.

The overall pattern of correlation between neural activity in different brain areas during tasks such as word generation can be expressed in terms of principal components of the covariance matrix representing pairwise associations between activity in all relevant pairs of pixels in the image. In normal subjects generating words, a major fraction of the covariance between pixels is accounted for by the first principal component (Friston *et al.*, 1993). This principal component has positive loadings in lateral and medial frontal cortex and thalamus, and negative loadings in lateral temporal cortex, bilaterally. It is possible to determine the degree to which the normal pattern of cerebral activity represented by this principal component contributes to the covariance between cerebral areas in schizophrenic patients when generating words, by calculating the two-norm, which is the product of the covariance matrix (for patients) by the vector that represents the principal component (for normals). In three separate groups of patients differing in symptom profiles, the normal pattern of cerebral activity was found to contribute only a trivial amount to the covariance in the patients, consistent with the proposal that the cardinal difference between patients and

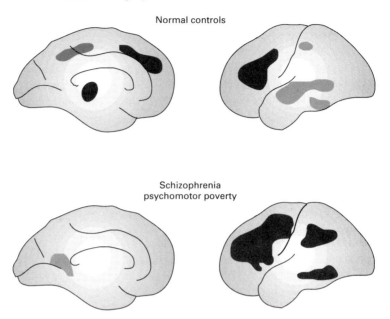

Normal controls

Schizophrenia
psychomotor poverty

Fig. 22.1 Areas of significant change in left-hemisphere regional cerebral blood flow (rCBF) in six normal subjects and in six schizophrenic patients with psychomotor poverty, when generating words paced at the rate of one word every 3 s (compared with repeating words at the same rate). In normal subjects, the major features include increased activity in lateral and medial frontal cortex and thalamus, and suppression of activity in the temporal lobe. In patients, frontal activation is accompanied by abnormal activation in temporal and parietal lobes, and an absence of thalamic activation.

normals lies not so much in the ability to activate a specific cerebral area as in the pattern of functional connectivity between areas.

Electrical activity

Electrical activity detected by scalp electrodes provides an indication of neuronal activity. Unfortunately, the spatial variation of scalp electrical potential provides a very diffuse image of the location of the underlying neuronal events. However, the temporal resolution of electrical measurements can match the time scale of neuronal events. There are two main approaches to displaying the electrical signals. The first approach is to map the spatial distribution of energy in the electroencephalographic (EEG) freuency bands, α, β, δ and θ, derived by spectral analysis of the signals detected by an array of electrodes distributed over the surface of the scalp. However, it is difficult to relate the distribution of energy in frequency bands to underlying neuronal or mental events. In view of the likelihood that functional connectivity between different brain regions is disordered in schizophrenia, potentially the most useful information that can be derived from

spatially distributed spectral data is the correlation between neural activity in different brain regions.

The second approach is to time-lock the electrical recording to a specific event such as the occurrence of a novel, task-relevant stimulus embedded in a train uniform stimuli, and to record the temporal variation of electrical potential following the target stimulus. The various peaks in these event-related potentials (ERPs) can be interpreted in terms of different components of information processing. Although the spatial variation in scalp potential provides a very imprecise indication of the location of the neural events generating the potentials, it is possible to enhance the anatomical information by relating variation (between subjects) in ERPs to variation in structure or function measured with a tomographical imaging technique, such as PET or MRI.

Schizophrenic patients exhibit a variety of abnormalities in the spatial distribution of energy in the various EEG frequency bands (Morihisa *et al.*, 1983), indicating disordered function in frontal, temporal and parietal lobes. Patients with differing symptom profiles exhibit differing patterns. In particular, Gruzelier *et al.* (1994) examined the spatial distribution of energy in the

α and β_1 EEG bands, associated, respectively, with a withdrawn syndrome and with an active syndrome; these correspond approximately to the psychomotor poverty and psychomotor excitation syndromes described above. They concluded that the withdrawn syndrome is characterized by relative underactivity of the left hemisphere compared with the right, while the active syndrome is characterized by relative overactivity of the left hemisphere. These findings are consistent with the observation that psychomotor poverty is associated with a decrease in cortical rCBF that is more extensive in the left hemisphere than in the right (Liddle *et al.*, 1992).

Morrison-Stewart *et al.* (1991) examined the relationship between EEG activity detected at different scalp sites and demonstrated that in normal individuals there is an increase in α wave coherence between left frontal and parietal regions and decreases in coherence between left frontal and temporal regions during a continuous calculation task, while in schizophrenic patients performing the same task, there was an increase in coherence between left frontal and temporal areas. As in the case of the PET measurements of functional connectivity during word generation (discussed above), these findings of altered coherence between regions indicate that schizophrenic patients have abnormal functional connectivity between cortical regions, especially between left frontal and temporal regions.

The most frequently replicated ERP abnormality in schizophrenia is a decrease in amplitude of the P3 peak (sometimes denoted P300) that occurs approximately 300 ms after a novel, task-relevant stimulus (Pfefferbaum *et al.*, 1989). The latency of the P3 peak also tends to be longer, but latency appears to be more sensitive to specific clinical features, with longer latency seen in patients having greater cognitive impairment. Romani *et al.* (1987) found that the latency was greatest in disorganized patients.

Abnormality of P3 is not specific to schizophrenia and occurs in various other cerebral conditions which impair the processing of information. The P3 peak appears to comprise separate components denoted P3a and P3b. P3a is sensitive to the novelty of the stimulus, while P3b is influenced by the degree of relevance of the stimulus to the response that the subject is required to make. Studies of the spatial variation in amplitude of P3 have reported a diminution over the left temporal lobe in schizophrenia (Morstyn *et al.*, 1983), although some studies have not replicated this observation (Pfefferbaum *et al.*, 1989). Combining the measurement of P3 with MRI imaging, McCarley *et al.* (1993) found a strong correlation between P3 amplitude reduction and reduction of the volume of tissue in the left superior temporal gyrus.

Molecular composition of brain tissue

PET studies of neuroreceptors

D_2 receptors in drug-naive patients

In view of the seminal role played by the dopamine hypothesis of schizophrenia, the question of dopamine D_2-receptor density in drug-naive patients was for several years one of the most tantalizing questions for schizophrenia researchers. In principle, D_2-receptor density in the basal ganglia can be estimated by using PET to obtain images of the accumulation of a D_2-receptor antagonist labelled with a positron-emitting isotope. In practice, the task is made difficult by a number of potentially confounding factors, including the fact that distribution of the labelled ligand is governed by many physiological processes in addition to specific receptor binding. Wong *et al.* at the John Hopkins Hospital, Baltimore, developed a technique for measuring D_2-receptor density using the ligand $[^{11}C]$-N-methyl-spiperone. Because the binding of N-methyl-spiperone does not reach equilibrium during the time course of a PET experiment, the mathematical model simulating the accumulation is complex and depends on several assumptions about the behaviour of the ligand. Using this technique in a study of drug-naive patients, Wong *et al.* (1986) found evidence of an increase in D_2-receptor number.

Meanwhile, Farde, Sedvall and colleagues at the Karolinska Institute in Stockholm developed a technique based on the D_2 ligand, [^{11}C]raclopride, which reaches equilibrium during the course of a PET experiment. Because equilibrium is achieved, a simpler mathematical model can be used to describe the accumulation of ligand. Farde *et al.* (1990) found no evidence of a generalized increase in D_2-receptor number in the basal ganglia of drug-naive patients, although they did find evidence of an increase in the left putamen compared with the right.

Initial attempts to explain the discrepancy between the findings of the John Hopkins and Karolinska groups centred on the validity of the different mathematical models used to simulate the accumulation of labelled ligand, and on issues such as whether or not differences between patients and controls in endogenous dopamine levels might generate a false-negative result when using the raclopride method. More recent studies by the John Hopkins group report that the finding of excess D_2 receptors appears to be confined to a subgroup of patients with a long history of illness prior to the study (Tune *et al.*, 1992). Thus, it is possible that a major factor in the differences between the findings of the two groups is subject selection. On balance, the evidence suggests that in drug-naive patients with illness of recent onset, there is no significant generalized increase in D_2-receptor number in the basal ganglia.

D_2 blockade by antipsychotic medication

In the presence of an unlabelled D_2 blocking drug, the number of receptors available for binding of a labelled ligand is reduced and measurement of the reduction in available D_2 receptors provides an estimate of the degree of receptor blockade by the unlabelled drug. By measuring the binding of [^{11}C]raclopride during treatment with anti-psychotic medication, Farde *et al.* (1988) demonstrated that typical antipsychotics such as haloperidol produce blockade of greater than 70% of D_2 receptors in the basal ganglia at therapeutic doses. On the other hand, atypical antipsychotic agents such as clozapine produce approximately 60% blockade of D_2 receptors at therapeutic doses. Using [^{18}F]N-methyl-spiperone as the labelled D_2 ligand, Wolkin *et al.* (1989) demonstrated that during treatment with haloperidol, patients who do not respond to treatment have a level of D_2 occupancy similar to that seen in treatment responders. Thus, PET studies using labelled D_2 ligands have demonstrated that typical antipsychotic drugs do in fact block central D_2 receptors, but in some patients symptoms can persist despite a high level of D_2 blockade. On the other hand, drugs such as clozapine apparently achieve their antipsychotic effect at moderate levels of D_2 blockade, implying that some other receptor type plays a role in mediating the therapeutic effect of this atypical antipsychotic agent.

MRS studies of membrane phospholipids

MRS is a technique capable of measuring the regional distribution of molecules containing atoms with a magnetic moment. The naturally occurring phosphorus isotope ^{31}P has magnetic moment and therefore exhibits resonant absorption and subsequent emission of radio frequency energy when in a strong magnetic field. The precise frequency of resonance is determined by the chemical environment of the ^{31}P atom. ^{31}P atoms in different molecular species, such as phosphomonoesters (PMEs) and phosphodiesters (PDEs), resonate at slightly different frequencies when subjected to a particular external magnetic field, and hence can be distinguished from each other and from ^{31}P atoms in other molecular species. Unfortunately, the spatial resolution of MRS is poor compared with either MRI or PET.

Pettigrew *et al.* (1991) measured the strength of the magnetic resonance signals from PMEs and PDEs in the frontal cortex of young, first-onset, medication-free schizophrenic patients and found evidence of a decrease in PMEs and an increase in PDEs compared with matched controls. PMEs and PDEs occur in brain cell membranes. A decrease in PMEs suggests a reduction in membrane synthesis, while an increase in PDEs suggests an increased rate of breakdown of cell membranes.

MRS studies of *N*-acetyl aspartate (NAA)

Hydrogen atoms (^{1}H) also have a strong magnetic moment, but in view of the abundance of water in tissue, it is necessary to use special techniques to suppress the magnetic resonance signal from H in water if the signals from H atoms in other molecular species are to be detected. When the water signal is suppressed, one of the species which can be detected is NAA, which occurs within neurones and is an index of neuronal density. Nasrallah *et al.* (1992) reported a reduction in the signal from NAA in the temporal lobe in schizophrenic patients.

Conclusion

Structural imaging studies have provided robust evidence for a deficit in amount of tissue in the temporal lobes, and the balance of evidence also indicates deficits in other areas, including the frontal lobes. The finding that deficits are detectable from the earliest phases of the illness, together with the observation that developmental anomalies are relatively common, is consistent with the hypothesis that the underlying pathological process has its origin early in the development of the nervous system.

Functional imaging techniques provide strong evidence for widespread disturbance of brain function, especially in the association cortex of frontal and temporal lobes. Different patterns of disturbed cerebral activity are associated with different symptom profiles. For example, frontal underactivity is associated with psychomotor poverty (core negative symptoms). However, latent hypofrontality occurs even in patients who do not exhibit marked negative symptoms, and can be made manifest by imaging during tasks which normally engage frontal cortex. The study of discordant twins suggests that at least a minor degree of frontal impairment occurs in most cases. The abnormalities of function appear to reflect a dynamic imbalance between different cerebral regions consistent with the hypothesis that the essential functional abnormality in schizophrenia is a disturbance of functional connectivity in the neural networks serving the supervisory mental functions responsible for the initiation, selection and monitoring of self-generated mental activity.

References

Andreasen, N.C., Rezai, K., Alliger, R. *et al.* (1992) Hypofrontality in neuroleptic-naive patients and in patients with chronic schizophrenia. Assessment with Xenon 133 single-photon emission computed tomography and the Tower of London. *Archives of General Psychiatry*, **49**, 943–958.

Ariel, R.N., Golden, C.J., Berg, R.A. *et al.* (1983) Regional cerebral blood flow in schizophrenics. *Archives of General Psychiatry*, **40**, 258–263.

Berman, K.F., Zec, R.F. & Weinberger, D.R. (1986) Physiologic dysfunction of dorsolateral prefrontal cortex in schizophrenia. II. Role of neuroleptic treatment, attention, and mental effort. *Archives of General Psychiatry*, **43**, 126–135.

Berman, K.F., Torrey, E.F., Daniel, D.G. & Weinberger, D.R. (1992) Regional cerebral blood flow in monozygotic twins discordant and concordant for schizophrenia. *Archives of General Psychiatry*, **49**, 927–935.

Breier, A., Buchanan, R.W., Elkashef, A., Manson, R.C., Fitzpatrick, B. & Gillad, F. (1992) Brain morphology and schizophrenia: a magnetic resonance imaging study of limbic, prefrontal cortex and caudate structures. *Archives of General Psychiatry*, **49**, 921–926.

Breier, A., Davis, O.R., Buchanan, R.W., Moricle, L.A. & Munson, R.C. (1993) Effects of metabolic perturbation on plasma homovanillic acid in schizophrenia: relationship to prefrontal cortex volume. *Archives of General Psychiatry*, **50**, 541–550.

Buchsbaum, M.S., Haier, R.J., Potkin, S.G. *et al.* (1992) Frontostriatal disorder in cerebral metabolism in never-medicated schizophrenics. *Archives of General Psychiatry*, **49**, 935–942.

Buchsbaum, M.S., Ingvar, D.H., Kessler, R. *et al.* (1982) Cerebral glucography with positron tomography. *Archives of General Psychiatry*, **39**, 251–259.

Crow, T.J. (1980) The molecular pathology of schizophrenia: more than one disease process. *British Medical Journal*, **280**, 66–68.

Daniel, D.G., Weinberger, D.R., Jones, D.W. *et al.* (1991) The effect of amphetamine on regional cerebral blood flow during cognitive activation in schizophrenia. *Journal of Neuroscience*, **11**, 1907–1917.

DeLisi, L.E., Holcomb, H.H., Cohen, R.M. *et al.* (1985) Positron emission tomography in schizophrenic patients with and without neuroleptic medication. *Journal of Cerebral Blood Flow and Metabolism*, **5**, 201–206.

Early, T.S., Reiman, E.R., Raichle, M.E. & Spitznagel, E.L. (1987) Left globus pallidus abnormality in never-medicated patients with schizophrenia. *Proceedings of the National Academy of Science*, **84**, 561–563.

Ebmeier, K.P., Blackwood, D.H.R., Murray, C. *et al.* (1993) Single photon emission tomography with 99mTc-exametazime in unmedicated schizophrenic patients. *Biological Psychiatry*, 33, 487–495.

Farde, L., Weisel, F.A., Halldin, C. & Sedvall, G. (1988) Central D2-dopamine receptor occupancy in schizophrenic patients treated with antipsychotic drugs. *Archives of General Psychiatry*, 45, 71–76.

Farde, L., Weisel, F.A., Stone-Elander, S. *et al.* (1990) D2 dopamine receptors in neuroleptic naive schizophrenic patients. *Archives of General Psychiatry*, 47, 213–219.

Farkas, T., Wolf, A., Jaeger, J. *et al.* (1984) Regional brain glucose metabolism in chronic schizophrenia: a positron emission transaxial tomographic study. *Archives of General Psychiatry*, 41, 293–300.

Fox, P., Perlmutter, J. & Raichle, M. (1985) A stereotactic method of anatomical localization for positron emission tomography. *Journal of Computer Assisted Tomography*, 9, 141–153.

Friston, K.J., Frith, C.D., Liddle, P.F. & Frackowiak, R.S.J. (1991) Plastic transformation of PET images. *Journal of Computer Assisted Tomography*, 15, 634–639.

Friston, K.J., Frith, C.D., Liddle, P.F. & Frackowiak, R.S.J. (1993) Functional connectivity: the principal component analysis of large (PET) data sets. *Journal of Cerebral Blood Flow and Metabolism*, 13, 5–14.

Friston, K.J., Frith, C.D., Liddle, P.F., Lammertsma, A.A., Dolan, R.D. & Frackowiak, R.S.J. (1990) The relationship between global and local changes in PET scans. *Journal of Cerebral Blood Flow and Metabolism*, 10, 458–466.

Golden, C.J., Moses, J.A., Zelazowski, R. *et al.* (1980) Cerebral ventricular size and neuropsychological impairment in young chronic schizophrenics. *Archives of General Psychiatry*, 37, 619–623.

Gruzelier, J.G., Laws, K., Liddiard, D. *et al.* (1994) Topographical EEG during words and faces memory tasks in syndromes of schizophrenia. *Schizophrenia Research*, 11, 199.

Gur, R.E., Gur, R.C., Skolnick, B.E. *et al.* (1985) Brain function in psychiatric disorders. III. Regional cerebral blood flow in unmedicated schizophrenics. *Archives of General Psychiatry*, 42, 329–334.

Gur, R.E., Skolnick, B.E., Gur, R.C. *et al.* (1985) Brain function in psychiatric disorders. I. Regional cerebral blood flow in medicated schizophrenics. *Archives of General Psychiatry*, 40, 1250–1254.

Huber, G. (1964) Neuroradiologie und Psychiatrie. In Gruhle, H.W., Jung, R., Mayer-Gross, W. & Muller, M. (eds) *Psychiatrie der Gegenwart, Forschung und Praxis*, Vol. 1, *Grundlagenforschung zur Psychiatrie*, Part B. Springer-Verlag, Berlin, pp. 253–290.

Illowsky, B., Juliano, D.M., Bigalow, L.B. & Weinberger, D.R. (1988) Stability of CT scan findings in schizophrenia. *Journal of Neurology, Neurosurgery and Psychiatry*, 51, 209–212.

Ingvar, D.H. & Franzen, G. (1974) Abnormalities of cerebral blood flow distribution in patients with chronic schizophrenia. *Acta Psychiatrica Scandinavica*, 50, 425–462.

Johnstone, E.C., Crow, T.J., Frith, C.D., Husband, J. & Kreel, L. (1976) Cerebral ventricular size and cognitive impairment in chronic schizophrenics. *Lancet*, 2, 924–926.

Jurjus, G.J., Nasrallah, H.A., Olson, S.C. & Schwarzkopf, S.B. (1993) Cavum septum pellucidum in schizophrenia, affective disorder and healthy controls: a magnetic resonance imaging study. *Psychological Medicine*, 23, 319–322.

Kurachi, M., Kobayashi, K., Matsubara, R. *et al.* (1985) Regional cerebral blood flow in schizophrenia disorders. *European Neurology*, 24, 176–181.

Lewis, S.W. (1990) Computerised tomography in schizophrenia 15 years on. *British Journal of Psychiatry*, 157, (Suppl. 9), 16–24.

Liddle, P.F. (1993) The psychomotor disorders: disorders of the supervisory mental processes. *Behavioural Neurology*, 6, 5–14.

Liddle, P.F. (in press) Inner connections within the domain of dementia praecox: the role of supervisory mental processes in schizophrenia. *European Archives of Psychiatry and Clinical Neuroscience*.

Liddle, P.F., Friston, K.J., Frith, C.D., Jones, T., Hirsch, S.R. & Frackowiak, R.S.J. (1992) Patterns of cerebral blood flow in schizophrenia. *British Journal of Psychiatry*, 160, 179–186.

Liddle, P.F., Herold, S., Fletcher, P., Friston, K.J., Silbersweig, D. & Frith, C.D. (1994) A PET study of word generation in schizophrenia. *Schizophrenia Research*, 11, 168.

McCarley, R.W., Shenton, M.E., O'Donnel, B.F. *et al.* (1993) Auditory P300 abnormalities and left superior temporal gyrus volume reduction in schizophrenia. *Archives of General Psychiatry*, 50, 190–197.

McGuire, P.K., Shah, G.M.S. & Murray, R.M. (1993) Increased blood flow in Broca's area during auditory hallucinations in schizophrenia. *Lancet*, 342, 703–706.

Mathew, R.J., Duncan, G.C., Weinman, M.L. & Barr, D.L. (1982) A study of regional cerebral blood flow in schizophrenia. *Archives of General Psychiatry*, 39, 1121–1124.

Matsuda, H., Gyobu, T., Hisada, K. & Ii, M. (1989) SPECT imaging of auditory hallucination using ^{123}I-IMP. *Advances in Functional Neuroimaging*, 2, 9–16.

Morihisa, J.M., Duffy, F.H. & Wyatt, R.J. (1983) Brain electrical activity mapping (BEAM) in schizophrenic patients. *Archives of General Psychiatry*, 40, 719–728.

Morrison-Stewart, S.L., Williamson, P.C., Corning, W.C., Kutcher, S.P. & Merskey, H. (1991) Coherence on electroencephalography and aberrant functional organization of the brain in schizophrenic patients during activation tasks. *British Journal of Psychiatry*, 159, 636–644.

Morstyn, R., Duffy, F.H. & McCarley, R.W. (1983) Altered P300 topography in schizophrenia. *Archives of General Psychiatry*, 40, 729–734.

Musalek, M., Podreka, I., Walter, H. *et al.* (1989) Regional brain function in hallucinations: a study of regional cerebral blood flow with 99m-Tc-HMPAO-SPECT in patients with auditory hallucinations, tactile hallucinations and normal controls. *Comprehensive Psychiatry*, 30, 99–108.

Nasrallah, H.A., Olsen, S.C., McCalley-Witters, M., Chapman, S. & Jacoby, C.G. (1986) Cerebral ventricular enlargement in schizophrenia; a preliminary follow-up study. *Archives of General Psychiatry*, **43**, 157–159.

Nasrallah, H.A., Skinner, T.E., Schmalbrock, P. & Robitaille, P.M. (1992) In vivo proton magnetic resonance spectroscopy (MRS) of the hippocampus/amygdala region in schizophrenia. Schizophrenia Research, 6, 150.

Neil, J.J. (1993) Functional imaging of the central nervous system using magnetic resonance imaging and positron emission tomography. *Current Opinion in Neurology*, **6**, 927–933.

Perlmutter, J.S., Herscovitch, P., Powers, W.S., Fox, P.T. & Raichle, M.E. (1985) Standardized mean regional method for calculating global positron emission tomographic measurements. *Journal of Cerebral Blood Flow and Metabolism*, **5**, 476–478.

Pettigrew, J.W., Keshaven, M.S., Panchalingram, K. *et al.* (1991) Alterations in brain high-energy phosphate and membrane phospholipid metabolism in first episode, drug-naive schizophrenics. A pilot study of dorsal prefrontal cortex by *in vivo* phosphorous-31 magnetic resonance spectroscopy. *Archives of General Psychiatry*, **48**, 563–568.

Pfefferbaum, A., Ford, J.M., White, P.M. & Roth W.T. (1989) P3 in schizophrenia is affected by stimulus modality, response requirements, medication status, and negative symptoms. *Archives of General Psychiatry*, **46**, 1035–1044.

Raichle, M.E., Fox, P.T., Mintun, M.A. & Dense, C. (1987) Cerebral blood flow and oxidative glycolysis are uncoupled by neuronal activity. *Journal of Cerebral Blood Flow and Metabolism*, **7** (Suppl. 1), S300.

Raine, A., Lencz, T., Reynolds, G.P. *et al.* (1992) An evaluation of structural and functional prefrontal deficits in schizophrenia: MRI and neuropsychological measures. *Psychiatry Research: Neuroimaging*, **45**, 123–137.

Raz, S. & Raz, N. (1990) Structural brain abnormalities in the major psychoses: a quantitative review of the evidence from computerized imaging. *Psychological Bulletin*, **108**, 93–108.

Reveley, A.M., Reveley, M.A., Clifford, C.A. & Murray, R.M. (1982) Cerebral ventricular size in twins discordant for schizophrenia. *Lancet*, **1**, 540–541.

Romani, A., Merello, S., Gozzoli, L., Zerbi, F., Grassi, M. & Cosi, V. (1987) P300 and CT scan in patients with chronic schizophrenia. *British Journal of Psychiatry*, **151**, 506–513.

Schulz, S.C., Koller, M., Kishore, P.R., Hamer, R.M., Gehl, J.J. & Friedel, R.O. (1983) Ventricular enlargement in teenage patients with schizophrenia spectrum disorder. *American Journal of Psychiatry*, **140**, 1592–1595.

Shenton, M.E., Kikinis, R., Jolesz, F.A. *et al.* (1992) Abnormalities of the left temporal lobe and thought disorder in schizophrenia: a quantitative magnetic resonance imaging study. *New England Journal of Medicine*, **327**, 604–612.

Sheppard, G., Gruzelier, J., Manchanda, R. *et al.* (1983) ^{15}O positron emission tomographic scanning of predominantly never-treated acute schizophrenic patients. *Lancet*, **ii**, 1448–1452.

Suddath, R.L., Casanova, M.F., Goldberg, T.E., Daniel, D.G., Kelsoe, J.R. & Weinberger, D.R. (1989) Temporal lobe pathology in schizophrenia. *American Journal of Psychiatry*, **146**, 464–472.

Suddath, R.L., Christison, G.W., Torrey, E.F., Casanova, M.F. & Weinberger, D.R. (1990) Anatomical abnormalities in the brains of monozygotic twins discordant for schizophrenia. *New England Journal of Medicine*, **322**, 789–794.

Suzuki, M., Kurachi, M., Kawasaki, Y., Kiba, K.B. & Yamaguchi, N. (1992) Left hypofrontality correlates with blunted affect in schizophrenia. *Japanese Journal of Psychiatry and Neurology*, **46**, 653–657.

Suzuki, M., Yuasa, S., Minabi, Y., Murata, M. & Kurachi, M. (1993) Left superior temporal blood flow increases in schizophrenic and schizophreniform patients with auditory hallucinations: a longitudinal case study using ^{123}I-IMP SPECT. *European Archives of Psychiatry and Clinical Neuroscience*, **242**, 257–261.

Tamminga, C.A., Thaker, G.K., Buchanan, R. *et al.* (1992) Limbic system abnormalities identified in schizophrenia using positron emission tomography with fluorodeoxyglucose and neocortical alterations with deficit syndrome. *Archives of General Psychiatry*, **49**, 522–530.

Tune, L.E., Wong, D.F. & Pearlson, G.D. (1992) Elevated dopamine D2 receptor density in 23 schizophrenic patients: a positron emission tomography study with $[^{11}C]N$-methyl-spiperone. *Schizophrenia Research*, **6**, 147.

Turner, S.W., Toone, B.K. & Brett-Jones, J.R. (1986) Computerized tomographic scan changes in early schizophrenia: preliminary findings. *Psychological Medicine*, **16**, 219–225.

Vita, A., Sacchetti, E., Valvassori, G. & Cazzullo, C.L. (1988) Brain morphology in schizophrenia: a 2- to 5-year CT scan follow-up study. *Acta Psychiatrica Scandinavica*, **78**, 618–621.

Warkentin, S., Nilsson, A., Risberg, J. & Karlson, S. (1989) Absence of frontal lobe activation in schizophrenia. *Journal of Cerebral Blood Flow and Metabolism*, **9**, S354.

Weinberger, D.R., Berman, K.F. & Illowsky, B.P. (1988) Physiological dysfunction of the dorsolateral prefrontal cortex in schizophrenia. III. A new cohort and evidence for a monoaminergic mechanism. *Archives of General Psychiatry*, **45**, 609–615.

Weinberger, D.R., Berman, K.F. & Zec, R.F. (1986) Physiologic dysfunction of dorsolateral prefrontal cortex in schizophrenia. 1. Regional cerebral blood flow evidence. *Archives of General Psychiatry*, **43**, 114–124.

Weinberger, D.R., Berman, K.F., Suddath, R. & Torrey, E.F. (1992) Evidence of dysfunction of a prefrontal-limbic network in schizophrenia: a magnetic resonance imaging and regional cerebral blood flow study of discordant monozygotic twins. *American Journal of Psychiatry*, **149**, 890–897.

Wolkin, A., Barouche, F., Wolf, A.P. *et al.* (1989) Dopamine blockade and clinical response: evidence for two biological subgroups of schizophrenia. *American Journal of Psychiatry*, **146**, 905–908.

Wolkin, A., Jaeger, J., Brodie, J.D. *et al.* (1985) Persistence of cerebral metabolic abnormalities in chronic schizophrenia as determined by positron emission tomography. *American Journal of Psychiatry*, **142**, 564–571.

Wolkin, A., Sanfilipo, M., Wolf, A.P., Angrist, B., Brodie, J.D. & Rotrosen, J. (1992) Negative symptoms and hypofrontality in chronic schizophrenia. *Archives of General Psychiatry*, **49**, 959–965.

Wong, D.F., Wagner, H.N., Tune, L.E. *et al.* (1986) Positron emission tomography reveals elevated D2 dopamine receptors in drug-naive schizophrenics. *Science*, **234**, 1558–1563.

Zipursky, R.B., Lim, K.O., Sullivan, E.V., Brown, B.W. & Pfefferbaum, A. (1992) Widespread cerebral grey matter volume deficits in schizophrenia. *Archives of General Psychiatry*, **49**, 195–205.

PART 3
PHYSICAL TREATMENTS

Chapter 23
The Clinical Treatment of Schizophrenia with Antipsychotic Medication

S. R. HIRSCH AND T. R. E. BARNES

Introduction

The discovery in the 1950s that chlorpromazine (Delay & Bernitzer, 1952) and reserpine (Kline, 1954) possessed tranquillizing properties that were especially effective in patients with schizophrenia led to the introduction of a series of antipsychotic drugs, many of which have been continually in use since that time. These agents are commonly referred to as conventional or classical neuroleptics, noteworthy because they cause extrapyramidal side effects, in contrast to the more recent, atypical compounds, such as clozapine, which have much less tendency to cause such problems. In addition to a beneficial effect on the cognitive and perceptual disturbances of the condition, the classical neuroleptics are able to control excitement and unpredictable behaviour. Furthermore, these drugs allow patients prolonged periods of remission which offer new opportunities for social management and care within the community. Nevertheless, these dramatic improvements in patient care have been at the expense of a wide range of side effects and adverse effects, and the impact of these drugs on the natural course of the illness may be limited. Evidence from 12 follow-up studies, each extending over 10 years, suggests that the number of patients who fully recover from the condition has not changed since 1908, when E. Bleuler first proposed the term 'schizophrenia' (Stephens, 1970; Tsuang, 1982). M. Bleuler's observations of over 2000 cases, 208 of which he personally followed up for more than 20 years, substantiate this view (Bleuler, 1974). Thus, while medication generally produces a more speedy remission of the illness, with a considerable decrease in the severity of positive symptoms, in the majority of cases it cannot be considered curative.

The improvements which have occurred in the quality of life and social functioning of patients in recent years can be ascribed partly to improved compliance with medication facilitated by the use of long-acting, depot medication and more intensive follow-up of patients who have been discharged from hospital, as well as improvements in the hospital milieu (Wing & Brown, 1970), rehabilitation (Chapter 30, this volume), psychosocial treatments (Leff, 1994; Chapter 31, this volume) and improved community care (Chapter 32, this volume). The use of adjunctive medication and the advent of clozapine and other 'atypical' neuroleptics have, as yet, had only a marginal effect in terms of the totality of the problem (Chapter 25, this volume), but new developments in treatment bring the prospect of real advances in efficacy of treatment and a reduction of unwanted side effects. In this chapter we review present knowledge on the use and effectiveness of conventional antipsychotic treatment.

Effects of medication

Effectiveness

The efficacy of neuroleptic medication for acute schizophrenia has been proved beyond doubt. Neuroleptics are drugs with pharmacological features similar to those of chlorpromazine, having relatively strong, antipsychotic, tranquillizing effects relative to their hypnotic effect but also causing extrapyramidal side effects which are relevant to their antipsychotic action in so far as they reflect activity at dopamine receptors.

Davis and Garver (1978) summarized the initial evidence of antipsychotic effect. Out of 207 double-blind comparative studies, 86% showed a significant advantage of neuroleptic antipsychotic medication over placebo in reducing the acute symptoms of schizophrenia; barbiturates had no antipsychotic effect and promazine and mepazine showed only weak antipsychotic activity. In a further analysis of 66 trials comparing chlorpromazine and placebo, 11 failed to demonstrate a significant treatment effect, perhaps because the numbers were small or the dosage inadequate: chlorpromazine proved superior to placebo in all studies using daily doses of 500 mg or more. The magnitude of the treatment effect was demonstrated in a large-scale trial of acutely ill patients (Cole et al., 1964). Of patients receiving active medication, 75% showed considerable improvement compared with 16% receiving placebo. Nearly 90% of patients treated with placebo showed no change or became worse. Similar rates of improvement for acutely admitted schizophrenics were observed in a sample of all admissions during 1 year to a psychiatric unit from a catchment area population of 90 000 (Knights & Platt, 1980).

Specific antipsychotic effects of neuroleptics

Positive symptoms

Neuroleptics have a specific effect on psychotic features such as delusions and paranoid thinking, hallucinations and thought disorder. The drugs are able to reduce the intensity of such features, shorten the acute episodes or exacerbations of the schizophrenic illness where such symptoms are prominent, and reduce the likelihood of their recurrence. Note that these effects are not specific to schizophrenia, but apply equally well to the positive psychotic symptoms of mania, depression and organic psychosis, although the preventive aspect has not been established in these conditions.

While there is no doubt that antipsychotic agents are the mainstay of treatment for florid episodes of schizophrenia, there is a marked heterogeneity of response. A substantial minority of patients, perhaps 10–20%, will derive little benefit from conventional antipsychotic drug therapy, although a smaller proportion would seem to be completely resistant (Davis et al., 1980; Kane, 1987). Even at an early stage of the illness, a small proportion of patients will show a lack of response. For example, in an early study of 92 first-episode patients, 4.4% could not be discharged from hospital within 6 months (May, 1968). In a similar study of 253 patients, 6.5% did not achieve discharge within the 2-year follow-up period, predominantly owing to persistence of positive symptoms (MacMillan et al., 1986). In a later study of 70 schizophrenic patients, Loebel et al. (1993) found that 16% 'did not recover' from their first episode. Furthermore, many of those patients who improve on drug treatment are nevertheless left with residual positive symptoms that compromise their social functioning and cause anxiety and distress.

Effect of delay in initiating treatment. A school of opinion has developed in recent years which argues that delay in initiating treatment causes a worse prognosis or an increased susceptibility to relapse. The question is whether the more recent observations of a higher relapse rate with a longer period of untreated illness have a causal explanation or are merely a consequence of the long-established clinical observation of a worse prognosis with gradual onset of illness, as well as the fact that chronic patients have a higher risk of relapse. Poor response to treatment in chronic, as opposed to acute, patients is axiomatic.

Thus, Angrist and Schulz (1990) reviewed 10 studies of psychiatric patients in the USA in the mid-1950s, when antipsychotic drugs were first introduced. In six of the studies, chronic patients showed 'less brisk therapeutic responses than acute/recently hospitalized patients'. This could reflect a gradual worsening of the illness or a loss of responsiveness to antipsychotic drugs over time, or could be interpreted as evidence that delay in starting treatment may predispose to a poorer outcome. Crow et al. (1986) studied 120 first-episode schizophrenic patients from Northwick Park Hospital who were randomly allocated to placebo or active antipsychotic drug. Within 2 years, 46% of the drug-treated group had relapsed compared with 62% of those on placebo. The duration of illness before starting medication was significantly related to the risk of relapse, regardless of treatment, in that relapse was greater for patients in whom this period was longer than 1 year. Another prospective study of first-episode schizophrenia in New York found a similar association between relapse and an illness duration of 1 year or more before antipsychotic medication was started (Loebel et al., 1992). These findings can be explained in terms of type of illness, that is, in illness with an inherently high risk of relapse, certain symptoms may lead to delay in hospital admission. Alternatively, the social and psychological disruption of a long period of untreated

psychotic illness might lead to a poor prognosis. Wyatt (1991) has argued that persistent, untreated psychosis might be biologically toxic and responsible for long-term morbidity, but the association between florid acute episodes and good response to treatment was well described prior to the introduction of neuroleptic medication or electroconvulsive therapy (ECT). Whether or not treating patients quickly after the onset of schizophrenia reduces susceptibility to relapse is an area that warrants further careful investigation.

Negative symptoms

A limitation of classical antipsychotic drug treatment is that it appears to have little effect on either the chronic course of the illness (Csernansky et al., 1985) or the negative symptoms (Crow, 1985), in that inactivity and isolation remain a serious problem for many. Moreover, it may be difficult to distinguish between the extrapyramidal side effects of medication, particularly bradykinesia, and the negative symptoms of schizophrenia (Johnson, 1981; Prosser et al., 1987; Barnes, 1994). However, a host of uncontrolled studies have examined the relationship between dose of antipsychotic drug and negative symptomatology, and the majority failed to find a significant correlation (Barnes & Liddle, 1990).

The negative symptoms characterizing the type-II syndrome were initially described by Crow (1985) as being unresponsive to drug treatment. While the consensus view at present is that negative symptoms are not appreciably aggravated by antipsychotic drugs, opinion is divided as to whether the drugs have no effect or may improve negative symptoms (Johnstone et al., 1978; Angrist et al., 1980; Goldberg, 1985). For example, a study by Breier et al. (1987) seemed to suggest a beneficial effect for antipsychotics on negative symptoms. They carried out a prospective, double-blind, placebo-controlled study to test the effects of antipsychotic withdrawal on ratings of negative and positive symptoms. In their small sample of young, chronic schizophrenic patients, scores for both positive and negative symptoms increased during a period of drug withdrawal and decreased with the reinstitution of drug treatment.

Some authors find it useful in this respect to distinguish between secondary negative symptoms which may be due to active avoidance and withdrawal secondary to delusional and paranoid thinking, from primary negative symptoms which represent a true absence of activity, drive and volition and a poverty of thought and flatness of affect (Carpenter *et al.*, 1988). It is reasoned that the former are more likely to respond to medication because they are secondary to treatment-responsive positive symptoms (Barnes, 1994).

Claims for a particular beneficial effect on negative symptoms have been made for some of the antipsychotic drugs more recently introduced, particularly pimozide (Van Kammen *et al.*, 1987; Feinberg *et al.*, 1988), low-dose sulpiride (Petit *et al.*, 1987), clozapine (Kane & Mayerhoff, 1989), amisulpride (Boyer *et al.*, 1990), risperidone (Claus *et al.*, 1992; Marder, 1992; Hoyberg *et al.*, 1993) and ritanserin (Duinkerke *et al.*, 1993). These results are intriguing and encouraging, and further controlled studies are warranted. One question regarding interpretation of these findings refers again to the difficulties of calculating equivalent dosages. The two drugs being compared may not be equivalent in their dosage for antipsychotic efficacy or ability to produce side effects. Thus, the apparent specific benefit on negative symptoms of one drug might reflect a superior effect on positive symptoms causing a reduction in secondary negative symptoms, or relatively less sedative or extrapyramidal effects.

Comparative effectiveness of classical neuroleptics

There is a lack of good data on the equivalent efficacy of the classical neuroleptics. Nevertheless, no consistent differences have been demonstrated in terms of antipsychotic potency or effects on individual symptoms, syndromes or schizophrenia subgroups, and the clinical choice is largely dependent upon the side-effects profile (Hollister, 1974). For example, when Davis and Garver (1978) evaluated the results from 134 double-blind comparisons between 21 different neuroleptics and chlorpromazine, none was superior to chlorpromazine in any of the trials. Mepazine, promazine and phenobarbitone were consistently inferior, except when chlorpromazine was used in insufficient dosage (usually below 400 mg a day).

Recent years have seen the introduction of a number of atypical neuroleptic compounds, the defining feature of which is a lower liability for motor side effects, and, in the case of clozapine, a demonstrable superiority to chlorpromazine in patients who have proved resistant to trials of various classes of classical neuroleptics (Kane *et al.*, 1988). These 'atypical' neuroleptics are considered in detail in Chapter 25.

Are there any differences in efficacy between the various depot preparations currently available? Comparative studies of depot drugs have generally failed to find any substantial differences between them in respect of relapse prevention (Kissling *et al.*, 1985; Eberhard & Hellbom, 1986). In one of the few studies reporting a significant difference, McKane *et al.* (1987) found that relapse was more frequent in schizophrenic patients treated for 60 weeks with haloperidol decanoate compared with a comparison group of patients treated with fluphenazine decanoate. However, the authors suggest that one explanation is that the dose of haloperidol was low relative to the dose of fluphenazine. As already mentioned, the problem of calculating equivalent doses (see Rey *et al.*, 1989) bedevils the comparative study of treatments for schizophrenia because the ratio of the dose causing side effects to the dose achieving an antipsychotic effect differs from one drug to another, so there is a tendency for the clinical effect to differ if the side effects are kept constant and vice versa.

Time course and mechanism of action

Sedative action

There are important differences in the time course of the specific antipsychotic effects. The sedative action is immediate as soon as adequate blood levels are reached, which is within 10 min using intravenous haloperidol. Agitation and excitement that have been controlled by treatment can re-emerge quickly when medication is omitted. Less potent barbiturates and benzodiazepines in high doses, as well as paraldehyde, have been used to quell excitement. However, barbiturates are rapidly hypnotic and suppress brain-stem functions, making medical examination more difficult. They also carry all the other potential dangers of unconsciousness and respiratory failure that can usually be avoided by neuroleptics if used judiciously but in sufficient dosage.

Antipsychotic action

Comparisons of neuroleptics with placebo in newly admitted patients show that the antipsychotic effect develops slowly over 2–3 weeks, by which time a significant advantage for the neuroleptics is evident (Davis & Garver, 1978). Nevertheless, most patients will improve to some extent following admission to hospital, even if receiving only placebo treatment, although the response is usually partial and temporary. The sedative action of neuroleptics may be useful in the early stages while the slower antipsychotic effect has a chance to develop. Keck *et al.* (1989) could find only a few studies that had systematically examined the onset of the antipsychotic effect; beneficial responses began over vastly different periods, from hours to weeks. Generally, the most rapid effect on psychotic symptoms is achieved between 2 and 6 weeks, after which further improvement takes place slowly over months. Some patients run an erratic course, slowly improving over 6 months or more, with further gradual improvements over the next few years. For such patients, it may be unclear whether all the recovery is attributable to medication. There is no evidence to suggest that tolerance develops to the antipsychotic effects of neuroleptics.

There is some suggestion from clinical trials that the use of anticholinergics in combination with neuroleptics delays the emergence of the antipsychotic effects (Singh & Kay, 1975, 1979; Johnstone *et al.*, 1983). Crow *et al.* (1981) found that patients randomly assigned not to receive anticholinergics improved more rapidly until the tenth day when they received anticholinergics. However, in practice, clinicians do not have the impression that anticholinergics significantly disadvantage patients in the course of their recovery.

Relapse prevention

New positive symptoms may be uncovered in the early stages of treatment, particularly if the initial presentation was characterized by inhibition, paranoid guarding or withdrawal, on the one hand, or gross excitement with disinhibition on the other. Whether such symptoms are genuinely new or only covert psychotic features revealed as the patient becomes less guarded and more articulate might be seen as a philosophical point, although it is of practical relevance when trying to establish a symptom baseline for treatment trials. Generally, psychotic symptoms do not continue to develop once treatment has begun.

Numerous well-controlled trials (Davis, 1975) have confirmed the observation of Leff and Wing (1971) that relapse can occur any time after discontinuing prophylaxis, but about 50% of patients will relapse between 3 and 10 months; the mode occurs at 3–5 months. This will be discussed further in the section on maintenance treatment.

Relative effects of antipsychotic drugs and their pharmacology

Beliefs about differences between drugs, for example that chlorpromazine is better for excited, disorientated or hostile patients or that fluphenazine is better for those whose illness is characterized by paranoid delusions or thought disorder, may be partly explained in terms of differences in their side effects when drugs are compared at doses necessary to achieve an equivalent antipsychotic effect.

Potency

If the effectiveness of neuroleptics is defined as their ability to achieve the desired antipsychotic effect, potency can be defined in terms of the minimum amount of drug in milligrams required to achieve this. On such a basis, chlorpromazine, thioridazine and clozapine are regarded as low-potency neuroleptics, that is they require high dosage as compared to fluphenazine, haloperidol, pimozide or risperidone, which are examples of high-potency drugs. However, none of the classical neuroleptic drugs has demonstrable superiority in antipsychotic efficacy in schizophrenia. Most of the reported differences between classical neuroleptics in their antipsychotic effect are probably due to a failure to ensure that drugs are used in equivalent dosage.

Davis (1976) produced a table of the relative potencies of standard neuroleptics, based on the average daily dose used in published double-blind trials which had allowed flexible adjustment of dosage to obtain an optimal clinical response compared with chlorpromazine. The clinical doses administered were higher than those generally prescribed today and studies of chronic patients were not separated from acute. Nevertheless, the relative clinical potency of different drugs is largely supported by the high correlation between clinical potency and *in vivo* binding affinity for D_2 dopamine receptors, but not other receptor types (Peroutka & Snyder, 1980). These binding affinities are a measure of the amount of drug necessary to displace 50% of a tritiated (radioactive) ligand

such as spiperone, a powerful D_2 dopamine-receptor binding agent, from striatal brain. However, this method cannot be used to calculate 'dose equivalence', as the dose–response curve for chlorpromazine is sigmoidal in shape, not a straight line, and the equivalence referred to applies only to the dopamine-binding properties of chlorpromazine, not its effect on other receptors. This ratio of a drug's potency compared to chlorpromazine has led to the concept of *chlorpromazine equivalents*, usually expressed in milligrams per day, calculated on the basis of the clinical studies referred to above and various biochemical measurements (Rey *et al.*, 1989).

Table 23.1 shows a summary review of the binding affinities of different neuroleptic drugs for several relevant different receptors. Note that while chlorpromazine is four times as potent as haloperidol on the α-noradrenergic receptor, in practice reference to the dopamine-receptor binding affinities shows that it is 1/50th as potent as haloperidol on dopamine receptors to achieve the same antipsychotic dose. Thus, chlorpromazine will have $50 \times \frac{1}{4}$ (12.5) times the effect on noradrenergic receptors compared to haloperidol. The correlation between the average dose determined by Davis and the relative potency determined by a drug's binding affinity to D_2 dopamine receptors

Table 23.1 Binding affinities of neuroleptic drugs at receptors for different neurotransmitters. (After Leysen, 1981)

Drug	Dopamine*	Serotonin†	Histamine‡	Noradrenaline§	Acetylcholine‖
Chlorpromazine	50	20	7	2	162
Thioridazine	15	36	40	3	77
Chlorprothixene	11	3.5	6	1	39
Haloperidol	1	48	4390	8	4370
Pimozide	1	33	>10 000	41	1022
Clozapine	156	16	4	7	31
Sulpiride	31	>10 000	>10 000	>1000	>10 000

Affinity expressed as equilibrium inhibition constant, K_i in nmol/l, for ligands indicated.
* Binding of [³H]haloperidol in striatum of rat (Leysen *et al.*, 1977).
† Binding of [³H]spiperone in frontal cortex of rat (Leysen *et al.*, 1978).
‡ Binding of [³H]pyrilamine, H_1 receptors, in guinea pig cerebellum (Chang *et al.*, 1978).
§ Binding of [³H]WB4101, α_1 receptors, in forebrain of rat (Greenberg *et al.*, 1976).
‖ Binding of [³H]dexetimide, muscarinic receptors, in striatum of rat (Laduron *et al.*, 1979).

is greater than, $r_p = 0.90$ (Pearson correlation coefficient), one of the strongest biological correlations observed in nature. This has led many to conclude that the clinical action of an antipsychotic is due solely to its actions on dopamine receptors; but the advent of atypical neuroleptics has challenged this notion and shown the pharmacology is more complicated and affected by other neurotransmitter systems such as the serotonin system. Furthermore, clozapine can be an effective antipsychotic at doses that are associated with significantly lower levels of *in vivo* binding of the D_2 receptors compared with that produced by the effective clinical doses of classical neuroleptics (Farde *et al.*, 1992).

Difference in clinical action based on pharmacology

The pharmacology of neuroleptic medication is explained in Chapters 18, 20 and 21. Briefly, the antipsychotic properties of classical or standard neuroleptics are normally explained by action on dopamine D_2 receptors in the mesolimbic and mesocortical systems, although selective effects on noradrenergic receptors, serotonin (5-hydroxytryptamine; $5\text{-}HT_2$) receptors and other dopamine-receptor subtypes may play a role. Molecular genetics has identified several new subtypes of dopamine receptors, which may be divided into at least two major families: the D_1-like group (D_{1A}, D_{1B} and D_5) and the D_2-like group (D_{2long}, D_{2short}, D_3 and D_4). The significance of these dopamine-receptor subtypes in the mediation of antipsychotic activity is uncertain at present (see Waddington, 1993). However, the D_4 dopamine receptor may be of particular interest, as clozapine binds to this receptor subtype with an affinity 10 times higher than that to the D_2 or D_3 receptors. Recent evidence of polymorphism in the D_4 receptor (Van Tol *et al.*, 1992) may be relevant to individual response to antipsychotic treatment (Kennedy *et al.*, 1994; Shaikh *et al.*, 1994).

The sedation caused by these drugs has been explained by effects on noradrenergic and histamine receptors, and the extrapyramidal side effects by the extent to which the action on nigrostriatal dopaminergic receptors is unopposed by simultaneous strong activity on muscarinic cholinergic receptors (for example, contrast haloperidol and thioridazine in Table 23.1) and possibly $5\text{-}HT_2$ and other receptors. Each drug has its own profile of receptor-binding affinities (see Table 23.1). This may partly explain why some so-called low-potency neuroleptics are more sedative, at least when initially administered, while the high-potency neuroleptics have a greater tendency to cause acute dystonic and parkinsonian reactions, due to unopposed dopaminergic blockade of the nigrostriatal systems. Some of the substituted benzamides are an exception because they are more selective for the D_2 family of receptors but have a low D_2 affinity. Furthermore, they are considered to have a more potent effect on the mesolimbic and mesocortical neurones than nigrostriatal neurones (Gerlach, 1993).

A psychiatrist's choice of medication for an individual patient will be influenced by factors such as the sedative properties of a drug and the tendency to cause extrapyramidal symptoms. The central α-adrenergic activity is also relevant, being responsible for not only sedation but also postural hypotension, via effects on the peripheral vasculature.

Those prescribing antipsychotic drugs should beware of claims by manufacturers and researchers about the specificity of antipsychotic action for any drug or the absence of particular side effects. Such claims are often based on a limited number of studies or a failure to appreciate that differences observed in a particular study may be due to differences in dosage rather than inherent activity or different effects on receptor sites. A competent appraisal of the benefits and unwanted side effects of different medication should always be based on repeated trials carried out by independent investigators and widespread clinical use. Occasionally, this process will be punctuated by the exceptional breakthrough in treatment which alters clinical practice.

Responses to individual drugs and serum levels

The clinical utility of measuring plasma levels of antipsychotic drugs remains uncertain. The steady-state plasma concentrations of antipsychotic drugs show considerable interindividual variation, and most early studies failed to find any clear association between blood levels and response. There are a number of methodological problems in this work. For example, an intrinsically poor responder to drugs may end up on high doses as a reflection of the therapeutic optimism of the clinician who admits defeat only after raising the dose to a high level. Nevertheless, in a dose—response study the data on such patients could be interpreted as showing that high blood levels were counter-therapeutic.

However, in the last decade there have been enormous advances in the laboratory techniques available for measuring antipsychotic drug levels. Relevant studies have been reviewed by Dahl (1986), who considered that plasma-level monitoring could help to reduce drug toxicity and increase the chances of a beneficial response for a small number of drugs. He concluded that dose reduction was a reasonable strategy for patients showing plasma drug concentrations above the upper limit of the therapeutic range. Dahl suggested that a therapeutic plasma concentration range existed for haloperidol. Perry *et al.* (1988) reviewed the evidence for such a 'therapeutic window' for haloperidol and concluded that a similar but narrower plasma-level range of around $12-17\,\mu g/l$ was associated with the best response with psychosis.

Chronic treatment with antipsychotic agents might be expected to cause tolerance but this does not seem to be the case clinically for the majority of patients. Addressing this issue, Cohen *et al.* (1987) studied a group of 76 schizophrenic outpatients who had been receiving depot fluphenazine for periods ranging from 3 to 23 years. They failed to find a correlation between the duration of treatment and dose, plasma level or serum prolactin. This suggests that there are no marked changes in the metabolism of fluphenazine and no

development of tolerance in the dopamine receptors which elevate prolactin even with extended administration.

Practical clinical issues

Who to treat?

Kane *et al.* (1982) carried out a randomized placebo-controlled trial on 28 schizophrenic patients with a duration of illness less than 3 months, and therefore classified as schizophreniform psychosis by the *Diagnostic and Statistical Manual* DSM-III. There were no relapses in the group receiving active fluphenazine decanoate, but 41% of the patients receiving placebo relapsed within 1 year. This study suggests that even first-illness patients, who as a group have a lower relapse rate, benefit if they are maintained on neuroleptic medication. However, it is worth noting that of the 14 patients given active medication in this study, three dropped out and three developed toxic reactions.

It may be worthwhile to consider offering schizophrenic patients a period off treatment at various stages of the illness. Contrary to traditional views, treated schizophrenics rarely show progressive deterioration after 5 years (Bleuler, 1974), unless it is due to harmful treatment or environmental influences such as poverty of stimulation or excessive arousal (see Chapter 29). Moreover, up to 25% of unselected schizophrenic patients admitted to hospital remit even without medication, hence the value of hospitalization before modern somatic treatment (Cole *et al.*, 1964). While spontaneous remission is more likely to occur among the group traditionally recognized to have a good prognosis (that is those patients characterized by features such as an acute, florid onset and good previous personality), it is not possible to identify reliably patients who will recover spontaneously unless they are first tried without medication. Moreover, patients improve at equal rates during the first $2-3$ weeks after admission, whether on active medication or placebo; after that period, those on drugs do better. Once treatment has begun, the patient is likely to remain on it for months, even after discharge. While there may be theoretical advantages to observing the patient for a period before starting medication, practical considerations in the treatment setting and the pressures for rapid management and discharge usually preclude this.

This rule applies equally to chronic patients stabilized in an unstressful environment. While some chronic patients require neuroleptics for sedation, and others need them to control or prevent the emergence of florid symptoms, a sizeable proportion of chronic patients, between 30 and 70%, are unchanged in the short term when medication is withdrawn (Prien & Klett, 1972). Given the risk of developing tardive dyskinesia and the fact that treatment can be rapidly restarted in patients under observation, consideration should be given to testing patients' needs for treatment by gradually weaning them off. A small proportion of patients will improve when medication is reduced, even if they are very disturbed — possibly due to the alleviation of side effects such as akathisia. At the same time, before deciding to withdraw or reduce the dose, the potential risks to the patient should be carefully considered, taking into account the nature and severity of previous relapses.

Acute psychiatric emergencies

A major clinical problem is the pharmacological management of the gross agitation, excitement and violent behaviour sometimes found in association with psychosis. Practice varies from country to country and has changed dramatically in recent years. Moderate doses of the more sedating, low-potency neuroleptics can be effective but may be too sedative or cause postural hypotension even in moderate doses, and there is also the risk of cardiotoxic side effects (Mehtonen *et al.*, 1991), particularly in high doses. Moderately high doses of high-potency neuroleptics, such as haloperidol (10–20 mg/day) or the more sedating but short-acting droperidol, can be effective, although cardiotoxic effects have also been reported with such drugs (see Edwards & Barnes, 1993). Sedation begins within 30 min of orally administered

haloperidol or fluphenazine and within 10 min or so of an intravenous injection.

A consensus statement from the Royal College of Psychiatrists (Thompson, 1994) warned of the dangers attendant upon the use of intravenous or intramuscular neuroleptics in emergency situations. These include the rapid increase in blood levels compared with oral administration and the particularly rapid absorption of an intramuscular injection in a patient who is very active. The relevance of such factors to the possible association between antipsychotic drugs and sudden unexpected death is unclear (see Edwards & Barnes, 1993), but Simpson *et al.* (1987) concluded that antipsychotic drugs may cause sudden death by interacting with the effects of stress and physical activity, increasing the vulnerability to cardiac arrhythmias and other autonomic complications.

For emergency use, many clinicians would now avoid very high doses of neuroleptic medication, and prescribe a combination of high-potency neuroleptic and benzodiazepine: the former for its eventual antipsychotic effect and the latter to achieve short-term sedation (Thompson, 1994). Haloperidol 10 mg orally plus 2–4 mg lorazepam, repeated if necessary after 1–2 h, is an example of such a regimen. Use of such a combination seems to result in lower overall dosage and less risk of acute dystonia (Barbee *et al.*, 1992; Hirsch & Barnes, 1994). If response to drug treatment is slow or inadequate, ECT can be a relatively safe and effective method of calming persistent psychotic excitement, and it carries a lower risk:benefit ratio than persistence with polypharmacy in high doses (Hirsch & Barnes, 1994; Thompson, 1994).

Patients chronically exposed to large doses of alcohol, sedative or neuroleptics may require higher doses because of tolerance. Curiously, large doses of intravenous haloperidol have been used safely in post-heart surgery patients with no effect on arterial pressure, pulse pressure, pulmonary atrial pressure, cardiac rhythm or respiratory rate (Ayd, 1978).

Dose–response relationships

Rapid neuroleptization strategy

With regard to the treatment of acute psychotic episodes, some clinicians hold the view that the early use of high doses of antipsychotic drugs, perhaps with intramuscular administration, will produce remission more rapidly and effectively. While the original, open studies of this 'rapid neuroleptization' approach were encouraging, subsequent controlled studies comparing high-dose strategies with standard dosage regimens revealed no significant superiority for high dosage in either degree or rapidity of response in acutely ill schizophrenic patients (see Kane, 1993). Thus, although the rapid neuroleptization technique has been widely adopted by clinicians, systematic investigation has not found it to possess any particular advantage over a more restrained oral regime.

Neuroleptic threshold hypothesis

Baldessarini *et al.* (1988) concluded that the appearance of parkinsonism and other acute, drug-induced movement disorders seemed to coincide with the upper limit of the therapeutic dose range in many cases. This is in line with the traditional strategy of titrating the dose, using the appearance of extrapyramidal side effects as an indicator of effective antidopaminergic dosage. A refined version of this approach, the neuroleptic threshold hypothesis, states that when antipsychotic drugs are initially administered the first appearance of a modest increase in muscle tone indicates that the optimum therapeutic dosage has been reached (Haase & Janssen, 1965; McEvoy, 1986).

A recent controlled study in patients with schizophrenic or schizoaffective disorder (McEvoy *et al.*, 1991a) found no therapeutic advantage for doses of haloperidol 2–10 times higher than the mean dose achieved using neuroleptic threshold approach. Nearly 75% of the patients on the neuroleptic threshold dose showed clinical recovery over 5 weeks. There was no greater improve-

ment in those patients receiving the higher doses, although they experienced significant increases in distressing extrapyramidal side effects. These findings suggest that the neuroleptic threshold hypothesis is worthy of exploration as a rational basis for prescribing antipsychotic drugs.

Optimum dose range

With regard to an optimum dose range for antipsychotic drugs, haloperidol has been the drug most commonly investigated. Several studies suggest the existence of an optimum dose range for oral haloperidol in acute psychosis (Van Putten *et al.*, 1990; McEvoy *et al.*, 1991a; Rifkin *et al.*, 1991). For example, Van Putten *et al.* (1990) assigned acute admissions to either 5, 10 or 20 mg haloperidol for 4 weeks. The 20-mg daily dose was more effective for psychotic symptoms in the first week or so, compared with 5 mg, and marginally superior to the 10-mg dose. However, by the second week of treatment, the higher dose seemed to be having 'psychotoxic' effects. An increased frequency and severity of side effects was observed with the 20-mg dose, particularly bradykinesia and akathisia, which were associated with non-compliance, anxiety, dysphoria, withdrawal and apathy. The authors concluded that for a proportion of newly admitted, severely psychotic patients, daily doses as low as 5 mg/day of haloperidol or its equivalent may be adequate, particularly after 1–2 weeks with doses of 10–20 mg. The higher initial dose may have been helpful in sedating excited behaviour.

Similarly, Rifkin *et al.* (1991) compared treatment with 10, 30 or 80 mg/day of oral haloperidol over 6 weeks in a double-blind trial with newly admitted patients with schizophrenia. The findings revealed no therapeutic advantage for patients treated with doses of haloperidol higher than 10 mg/day. However, the higher doses were not associated with more or worse side effects, a finding that may have been partly related to the prophylactic use of an anticholinergic, benztropine mesylate 6 mg/day.

The results of these studies provide little evidence for the efficacy of antipsychotic drug treatment outside the standard clinical dosage range, when considering schizophrenic patients as a group. Furthermore, the findings suggest that in both acute and long-term treatment, antipsychotic drugs have traditionally been prescribed at dosages greater than necessary for adequate clinical response. Baldessarini *et al.* (1988) reviewed 33 studies from 1959–85 involving random assignment of 2346 chronically psychotic patients to at least two doses of an antipsychotic. They concluded that increasing the daily dose above 600 mg chlorpromazine equivalents a day gives diminishing returns, conferring little additional therapeutic benefit but an increased risk of side effects: there was a consistently higher risk of motor side effects at higher daily doses (average 5200 mg chlorpromazine equivalents) compared with lower doses (average 400 mg chlorpromazine equivalents). Jain *et al.* (1988) carried out a meta-analysis of 12 studies comparing high and conventional doses of antipsychotics in chronic, hospitalized schizophrenic patients. They estimated that only a fraction of the patients treated with high doses showed a better response, and in these patients bioavailability issues and other pharmacodynamic factors may be relevant. Some of the patients receiving very high dosages were noted to have electrocardiogram (ECG) and electroencephalogram (EEG) abnormalities (Dencker *et al.*, 1981; Jain *et al.*, 1988).

High-dose/megadose studies

Over the last decades, the use of very high doses of antipsychotic drugs for behaviourally difficult patients refractory to standard doses has become fashionable, despite a lack of systematic evidence for any superior efficacy for such treatment either acutely or over a medium- to long-term basis (Baldessarini *et al.*, 1988). At three centres in the USA, Reardon *et al.* (1989) documented a significant increase in the dosage of antipsychotic drugs prescribed for acute in-patients with schizophrenia over the decade from 1973 to 1982. Overall, there was a doubling of the mean daily dose received, the peak dose reached and the dosage at discharge. One explanation for this

increase was that it represented a response from clinicians to the pressure to discharge patients, the underlying belief being that increased doses would lead to a more rapid remission.

High doses are particularly popular with forensic psychiatrists who tend to deal with patients characterized by disturbed behaviour and violence. Forensic psychiatrists are also under greater pressure to render their patients asymptomatic as a requisite for their return to the community. Although many clinicians in this area are committed to the concept that high doses or megadoses are beneficial and report that patients deteriorate when the doses are lowered, no clear accounts of appropriate dose levels or clinical indicators have been forthcoming.

One key question is whether increasing the dosage can improve outcome in those patients who have failed to respond to conventional dose levels. Many of the trials that have attempted to assess the response of treatment-resistant patients to high doses or megadoses have had methodological problems, such as small sample sizes and the lack of a consistent, valid definition of treatment resistance (Kane, 1993). There has also been a wide variation between studies in the definition of high and standard doses. For example, Quitkin *et al.* (1975) compared 1200 mg of oral fluphenazine a day (equivalent to at least 60 000 mg chlorpromazine; Rey *et al.*, 1989) with 30 mg/day of the same drug (equivalent to at least 1500 mg chlorpromazine), while McClelland *et al.* (1976) compared 250 mg of depot fluphenazine weekly with 12.5 mg/week.

These and other controlled studies comparing very high doses with standard dose treatment (Itil *et al.*, 1970; Quitkin *et al.*, 1975; McClelland *et al.*, 1976; McCreadie *et al.*, 1979; Bjorndal *et al.*, 1980) all failed to show a statistically significant advantage for the megadose regimen. These findings are not incompatible with the clinical observation that individual patients may occasionally show a dramatic response. However, specific characteristics of those patients responding to high doses have not been identified, although some studies hint that schizophrenic patients under 40 years of age and hospitalized for less than 10 years may tend to benefit from high doses, but not megadoses (Gardos *et al.*, 1973). Other reports suggest that pharmacokinetic variables may be relevant in some treatment-resistant patients who improve with high doses (McCreadie *et al.*, 1979). In the few studies where follow-up data were collected, there was tentative evidence that the benefit with high-dose treatment can be maintained with subsequent lower maintenance doses (McCreadie & MacDonald, 1977; Bjorndal *et al.*, 1980; Cookson *et al.*, 1983).

High doses of antipsychotic medication may be less safe than previously considered, being associated with pharyngeal and laryngeal dystonia that can prove fatal. An increased risk of the neuroleptic malignant syndrome has been reported, although a clear relationship between drug dose and neuroleptic malignant syndrome was not noted within the lower ranges (Keck *et al.*, 1991). Another possible hazard of high-dose treatment is an association with violent, disturbed behaviour (Barnes & Bridges, 1980). In a placebo-controlled study by Herrera *et al.* (1988), violence in treatment-resistant, schizophrenic in-patients showed a marked increase with high-dose haloperidol (increasing to 60 mg/day) over 6 weeks, but not with the low-potency antipsychotics chlorpromazine (1800 mg/day) and clozapine (900 mg/day). One possible explanation is that the violent behaviour is a response to the stressful subjective experience of akathisia.

New forms of treatment for those patients proving resistant to conventional antipsychotic drugs include clozapine and adjunctive medication, such as lithium, carbamazepine, sodium valproate and benzodiazepines. In the light of these advances, the argument for the prolonged use of very high doses of standard antipsychotic drugs becomes difficult to sustain.

Maintenance treatment

The prophylactic action of neuroleptics preventing the recurrence or recrudescence of schizophrenic symptoms has now been well established in over 35 double-blind trials dealing with over 3700 chronic in- and out-patients (Davis *et al.*, 1993).

Relapse rates on placebo ranged from 30 to 100% with a mean of 55%, and on active medication from 0 to 49% with a mean of 21%. Differences between studies mostly depend on the length of follow-up and selection of cases (Hirsch & McCrae, 1986). It is interesting to note that when medication is withdrawn, schizophrenic symptoms tend to return in the same order as in previous episodes (Hirsch *et al.*, 1973; Wistedt, 1981). Baldessarini *et al.* (1988) reviewed the literature on relapse prevention with antipsychotic medication and interpreted the data available as suggesting that doses between 50 and 150 mg chlorpromazine equivalents a day were sufficient to protect half of the patients evaluated.

Oral vs. depot preparations

Relapse prevention

Although the value of oral medication had been confirmed earlier (Leff & Wing, 1971), a strongly held view has developed among clinicians, especially in Britain, that depot injections are more successful in preventing relapse. This view was largely formed by the early 'mirror-image' studies (Denham & Adamson, 1971; Johnson, 1993) which demonstrated impressive reductions in the frequency and severity or relapse in patients following the introduction of depot maintenance treatment.

The development of special clinics and district psychiatric nurses for administering injections has improved patient care and follow-up, but the route of administration does not prove to be a critical factor when treatments are compared under similar conditions. Studies comparing oral and depot forms of a neuroleptic such as penfluridol (Quitkin *et al.*, 1978) or fluphenazine found relapse rates below 30% over 1 year for both oral and depot medication. About 65% of patients relapsed when switched to placebo, depending on the length of treatment (Davis, 1975). In two studies of selected patients, clinical differences between those treated with pimozide tablets and fluphenazine injections were not significant (Falloon *et al.*, 1978a; Barnes *et al.*, 1983), although in one of the studies there were differences in social functioning, ascribed to extrapyramidal side effects and possibly to differences between doses (Falloon *et al.*, 1978b).

Nevertheless, despite the apparent lack of difference in relapse rate during controlled trials, a meta-analysis based on six studies carried out by Davis *et al.* (1993) using the Mantel−Haenszel test revealed that significantly fewer patients on depot medication relapsed than with oral medication ($P < 0.0002$).

Compliance

In practice, one is likely to achieve better results with long-acting depot injections because schizophrenics are unreliable when left to administer their own medication. Poor compliance figures of 30−50% have been reported in some maintenance studies with oral medication (Kane, 1987), even though clinical trials are likely to recruit the more compliant patients. While the close nursing supervision associated with depot injection clinics seems to assure guaranteed medication delivery, 10−15% will still default from treatment over 2 years (Johnson, 1993). However, covert non-compliance is not possible with a depot regimen.

The problem associated with poor compliance and follow-up may not be reflected in clinical trials such as those quoted in which patients are highly selected and closely observed. This view is supported by the findings of a study by Johnson (1978) of 287 schizophrenics from a catchment area followed up for a year after discharge from hospital. Out of 187 patients receiving depot preparations, only 23% relapsed over the following period compared with 37% on oral medication and 63% of those stopping treatment. However, as the patients were self-selected or prescribed oral or depot medication by clinical choice, bias in selection may account for the different relapse rates of different groups. In a 7- to 8-year follow-up of patients on depot medication (Curson *et al.*, 1985), there were significant correlations between the number of illness episodes and simple measures of poor compliance, such as not turning up to the clinic for injections but having them at home, or refusing injections. From such data, it is difficult to unravel whether poor compliance is a cause or effect of clinical deterioration, or whether both may be relevant.

Bioavailability

Oral antipsychotic drugs are converted to inactive metabolites by non-specific enzymes in the gut wall and rapidly metabolized during the first pass through the liver. Thus, only a small proportion of the dose reaches the systemic circulation. Such problems are largely overcome by intramuscular or depot injections. Although, theoretically, the bioavailability difficulties associated with oral medication are largely obviated by depot preparations, there is a lack of studies demonstrating the value of this clinically. Any therapeutic superiority found for depot medication compared with oral drugs could be explained by the avoidance of compliance problems rather than bioavailability problems.

Risk of overdose

The risk of deliberate or inadvertent overdose with antipsychotic drugs is eliminated by depot injections. This may be important considering that suicide, often of an impulsive nature, is a relatively common cause of death in schizophrenia with a life-time prevalence of 10−15% (Cohen *et al.*, 1990). Dencker and May (1988) estimate a figure of 2 per 100 young schizophrenic patients a year.

Regular clinical contact

The arrangements for the administration of injections often involve the establishment of a special clinic where each patient is in regular contact with a trained community nurse, who can monitor a patient's response to medication and changing symptomatology (Gaind & Barnes, 1981) and liaise with relatives and other carers.

The disadvantages of such clinics are that they are often hospital based and inconveniently sited. Marriott (1978) found that 65% of the patients attending such a clinic depended on public transport. Clinic times tend to be limited so that a large number of patients are seen within a short time, allowing little individual attention to each patient. We may be moving now from a clinic-based service to a system of care delivered by nurses in the home or in community health centres or day centres.

Extrapyramidal side effects: drug differences and treatment during maintenance

Like oral medication, the claim that depot neuroleptics differ in their specific actions does not stand up to scrutiny. *cis*-Clopenthixol, haloperidol decanoate, penfluridol (an oral preparation given weekly) and pipothiazine palmitate have not shown any consistent pattern of superiority over fluphenazine decanoate, flupenthixol decanoate, or each other. Knights *et al.* (1979) were unable to find any meaningful differences in the course or outcome of 57 schizophrenic patients randomly assigned to fluphenazine decanoate or flupenthixol decanoate, and followed for 6 months after leaving hospital. However, frequent assessment revealed a high incidence of extrapyramidal side effects. At any point in time, about 20% of the patients exhibited parkinsonian symptoms, but there was a constant interchange between those affected and those not. After 6 months on maintenance medication, nearly 90% of the patient sample had been assessed as showing extrapyramidal symptoms on at least one occasion. These findings emphasize the high frequency of extrapyramidal side effects during the initial stage of treatment with depot neuroleptics.

When they occur, extrapyramidal symptoms can be tackled successfully in two-thirds of cases by reducing the dosage (Johnson, 1978). Anticholinergic medication is effective for extrapyramidal problems occurring with acute neuroleptic treatment, but the need for long-term administration after control of the acute symptoms is uncertain (Johnson, 1978; Barnes, 1990). This is partly because the studies of anticholinergic withdrawal in patients on maintenance antipsychotic drug

treatment show a wide variation in the proportion of patients experiencing a relapse of parkinsonism, from 68 (Manos *et al.*, 1981) to 4% (McClelland *et al.*, 1974). Investigators such as Caroli *et al.* (1975), Rifkin *et al.* (1978) and Manos *et al.* (1981), who found moderate to severe parkinsonism reappeared in a relatively high proportion of those patients withdrawn from anticholinergics, came to the conclusion that the risk:benefit ratio was balanced in favour of continuing anticholinergic treatment. However, investigators such as Orlov *et al.* (1971), Klett *et al.* (1972), McClelland *et al.* (1974) and Perenyi *et al.* (1983), who reported a relatively low recurrence of parkinsonian symptoms, were of the opinion that the long-term administration of these drugs was unnecessary for the majority of patients.

A consensus statement by the World Health Organization on the prophylactic use of anticholinergics in patients on long-term neuroleptic treatment (WHO, 1990) suggested that when antipsychotic treatment is started, the addition of anticholinergic agents was indicated only if parkinsonism developed. The anticholinergics should then be stopped later to allow the need for continued use to be assessed. These treatment recommendations are prudent. Without regular review, patients may receive antiparkinsonian drugs indefinitely, with the hazards of anticholinergic side effects in the long term (see Barnes & Edwards, 1993) and possibly an increase in the dose requirement of antipsychotic treatment as a result of enzyme induction and the more rapid metabolism of neuroleptics (Lader, 1979).

Effects of discontinuing maintenance treatment

Maintenance treatment can be withdrawn from a proportion of patients for many months without adverse effects. The mean time before relapse is about 4.5 months (Letemendia *et al.*, 1967; Hirsch *et al.*, 1973; Hogarty & Ulrich, 1977). After withdrawal, the number who relapse accumulates over time at a rate which decreases exponentially. Using life-table methods, Hogarty and Ulrich (1977) calculated survival rates for 374 patients treated with oral chlorpromazine or placebo. The longer patients survived without relapse, the lower the risk became. In the first months, the risk of relapse for those patients receiving placebo was 13%, while the risk for those on active drug was 4%. By the end of 2 years, the figures had declined to 3 and 1.5%, respectively. However, in their meta-analysis, Davis *et al.* (1993) noted that there was an exponential decline of 10% a month in the number of patients who survived without relapse after withdrawal from medication. The exponential relationship is accounted for by the decreasing number of patients who are at risk of relapse. Thus, for a sample of 100 patients, there would be 90 remaining after the first month, 81 after the second, 73 after the third, etc. Overall, medication lowered the risk of relapse by a factor of 3.

Extrapolating their results beyond 3 years, Hogarty and Ulrich estimated that eventually 65% of patients on active medication would relapse compared with 87% of those receiving placebo. This seems to suggest that medication will indefinitely prevent relapse in 22% of patients, but only postpone relapse in 65%. Furthermore, 13% of patients will survive without treatment. These predictions are supported to some extent by data from a 7-year follow-up study of 81 schizophrenic patients who had been well maintained in a depot phenothiazine clinic (Curson *et al.*, 1985). Excluding 12 patients who died and five for whom there were imcomplete data, 83% of the 63 patients followed up had suffered at least one relapse. In accord with the predictions of Hogarty and Ulrich, 68% had a relapse within 7 years while taking medication. This compares with a relapse rate of 63% within 13 months for 39 patients during periods when they were not receiving medication. This study again emphasizes that the main effect of maintenance medication is to reduce considerably the rate of relapse and prolong the interval between illness episodes, but only in a minority of cases are such illness episodes eliminated altogether.

Relationship of serum drug level to relapse

The peak relapse rate following discontinuation of depot phenothiazines occurs around 18 weeks. This coincides with the period when fluphenazine decanoate ceases to be detectable in most patients. However, Wiles and Wistedt (1981) were able to detect fluphenazine decanoate by radioimmunoassay in the serum of some patients for up to 6 months, although flupenthixol decanoate was not detectable after 9 weeks. This is in line with the observation that patients tend to relapse earlier after discontinuation of flupenthixol decanoate compared with fluphenazine decanoate. It has also been noticed that patients who relapse in the first 3 months after withdrawal have a fall in serum levels. Antipsychotic drugs tend to persist in the blood longer in elderly patients and relapse occurs more slowly after withdrawal (Wiles & Wistedt, 1981; Wistedt, 1981). Marder (personal communication) found that patients with low blood levels of fluphenazine, for example 0.4–0.5 mg/ml, could have their risk of relapse reduced by adding even a small dose of neuroleptic (Marder *et al.*, 1987).

When can medication be stopped?

While clinical studies have convincingly demonstrated the continuing benefit to patients of drug maintenance as compared to placebo, the findings do not answer the more practical question of what is the likelihood of relapsing if medication is withdrawn after several years of treatment. During the first year after discharge, if medication is withdrawn the relapse rate is particularly high (Hirsch *et al.*, 1973). Three groups report relapse rates in the order of 65% for patients withdrawn from treatment for a year after surviving 2, 3 and 5 years on medication (Hogarty *et al.*, 1976; Cheung, 1981). This is a similar rate to that reported by Curson *et al.* (1985) (see above).

Kane (1987) reviewed those studies of relapse in 'good-prospect' patients who had been specially selected to discontinue maintenance medication on the basis that they wished to stop, were in remission, and had good social control. Overall, the mean relapse rate over the follow-up period, which ranged from 6 months to 2 years, was around 75% (see Table 23.2). In three of the studies (Hirsch *et al.*, 1973; Dencker *et al.*, 1980; Wistedt, 1981), the relapse rates were over 90%. These studies provide no indication of recovery over time in patients, even if their illness has remained well controlled.

One explanation for these findings would be the development of neuroleptic dependence, which is consistent with the idea of postsynaptic receptor supersensitivity, induced by chronic blockade of dopamine receptors. Chouinard and Jones (1980) have proposed the existence of a supersensitivity psychosis, a syndrome of increasing tolerance to neuroleptics and the rapid emergence of psychosis and tardive dyskinesia when drugs are withdrawn. However, there is no evidence of tolerance development to maintenance neuroleptics. To the contrary, maintenance doses are usually much lower than the acute treatment dose and tend to remain relatively constant.

Strategies to reduce exposure to medication

Low-dose maintenance and drug holidays. The disadvantages of long-term antipsychotic treatment include weight gain, sexual dysfunction and motor disorders such as tardive dyskinesia, akathisia and bradykinesia; these alter a patient's social presentation and are associated with distress and depression (Rifkin *et al.*, 1975; Barnes & Edwards,

1993). There is much to commend reducing the dose of long-term neuroleptics.

Early experimental studies to test the effects of low dosage compared treatment for 3 days a week on alternate days with daily treatment. The patients on the low-dose regimen experienced significantly higher rates of relapse (Caffey *et al.*, 1964; Prien *et al.*, 1973). The effective dose reduction was up to 43% but the studies lasted only 4 months, an insufficient period to assess the longer term effect of reducing maintenance dosage.

Capstick (1980) withdrew patients from depot neuroleptic medication by gradually increasing the periods between injections by 1 week and slowly decreasing the dose over a 6-month period. When medication had been reduced to a dosage of 3 mg fluphenazine decanoate every 8 weeks, it was stopped. In the first 6 months after drug discontinuation, 40% of the patients relapsed, and a further 40% relapsed over the next 18 months. Thus, there was an overall relapse rate of 80% over a 2-year period. In 1979, Kane *et al.* reported an open study of 57 patients in which standard doses of fluphenazine decanoate (12.5–50 mg every 2–4 weeks) were reduced to one-tenth. Among the patient sample, 26% relapsed in the following 6 months. In both of these studies, symptoms quickly remitted when medication was reintroduced and admission to hospital was not usually necessary.

A subsequent double-blind controlled study (Kane *et al.*, 1983) randomly allocated 126 patients

Table 23.2 Relapse rate following drug discontinuation after long-term remission

Reference	Time in remission	Duration of follow-up	Relapse rate (%)
Wistedt (1981)	>6 months	1 year	100
Hirsch *et al.* (1973)	<1 year	9 months	92
Johnson (1976)	1–2 years	6 months	53
Dencker *et al.* (1980)	2 years	2 years	99
Johnson (1981)	1–4 years	18 months	80
Hogarty *et al.* (1976)	2–3 years	1 year	65
Hirsch *et al.* (1973)	1–5 years	9 months	66
Cheung *et al.* (1981)	3–5 years	18 months	62

to receive either 1.25–5 mg fluphenazine decanoate or 12.5–50 mg fluphenazine decanoate every 2 weeks. This 90% dosage reduction brought about a 56% relapse rate in the first year compared with a 7% relapse rate in patients maintained on standard doses. However, only 7% of the patients receiving the low dose required hospitalization and the social sequelae of relapse were minimal. Furthermore, on the lower dose regimen, patients appeared to have a better adjustment with less social withdrawal, blunting of affect and motor retardation. This study suggested that the value of a low dose turns on the degree to which advantages such as improved social functioning and a greater sense of well-being outweigh the higher rate of symptom recrudescence, which nonetheless responds quickly to a rapid augmentation of the medication.

In the UK, Johnson *et al.* (1987) reported a double-blind trial comparing flupenthixol decanoate in a standard dose of 40 mg every 2 weeks with half that dose. At the end of 1 year, the relapse rate in the lower dose group was 32%, significantly higher than the 10% relapse rate in the group receiving the full-dose regimen. In order to examine the long-term effects of neuroleptic dose reduction, Johnson *et al.* (1987) followed up the group of patients receiving 50% of their original neuroleptic dose for a total of 3 years. Patients who were on the standard dose were switched to the lower dose group, though these patients were then rated unblind. For patients completing 2 years, there was a 56% overall relapse rate, and for patients completing 3 years, a 70% relapse rate was observed. With respect to side effects, no differences were observed between the standard-dose group and the 50% neuroleptic dose reduction group during the first year of double-blind comparison. This finding indicates that a neuroleptic dose reduction of a half or more leads to a significantly higher rate of relapse, although the relapse can often be controlled at an early stage. Nevertheless, a considerable proportion of patients did not relapse, even at the end of 2 years, suggesting that this approach could be tried on a case-by-case basis where dose reduction is important.

Targeted brief intermittent treatment. The second strategy to reduce exposure to medication had its origin in the retrospective study of Herz and Melville (1980), who questioned 145 schizophrenics and their relatives about symptoms which appeared in the period leading up to relapse. Depressed mood, agitation, anger and social withdrawal were common in the 3-week prodromal period prior to the re-emergence of florid schizophrenic symptoms. These 'prodromal symptoms' were reported by 70% of patients, and by the patient and/or relatives in over 90% of cases. Symptoms experienced by more than 50% of patients included tension and nervousness; loss of sleep, appetite, interest and concentration; memory loss; thoughts of being laughed at or being noticed; and a feeling of being excited, depressed or worthless. Dencker *et al.* (1980), Wistedt (1981) and Capstick (1980) all reported similar findings.

Knights and Hirsch (1981) found that depressive and neurotic symptoms were prevalent in the acute phase of the illness and continued to come and go during the recovery phase (Knights *et al.*, 1979), again supporting the view that they are an integral part of schizophrenic pathology. Thus, the concept that one might be able to treat patients with neuroleptics for brief periods only when they are about to relapse using early neurotic and nonspecific prodromal symptoms as warnings of impending relapse suggested itself as a possible alternative strategy to continuous neuroleptic medication (Herz & Melville, 1980). The treatment intervention would be triggered by patients or relatives becoming aware of the emergence of neurotic and non-specific symptoms.

Such a strategy has now been tested in four randomized, controlled clinical trials comparing 'targeted' or 'brief intermittent' treatment (also called early intervention treatment) with standard continuous long-term prophylactic medication. The studies of Herz *et al.* (1991) and Jolley *et al.* (1990) were placebo controlled, and those of Carpenter *et al.* (1990) and the German multicentred trial (Pietzcker *et al.*, 1994) were open. In the studies of Herz *et al.* and Pietzcker *et al.*, patients were allowed to receive oral or depot medication. Carpenter *et al.* (1990) allowed only oral medication, while the patients in the trial of Jolley *et al.* were restricted to depot treatment. The study patients received regular, supportive psychotherapy in all the studies except the UK trial (Jolley *et al.*, 1990), although in that study patients were seen monthly for research assessment.

The German study tested an important additional hypothesis by including a third treatment group which received what they called 'crisis intervention treatment', that is adjunctive medication was prescribed only if there was frank evidence of psychotic deterioration. This study was the most ambitious and had the largest sample; 3481 patients were screened and 122 were allocated to receive continuous treatment, 127 brief intermittent treatment and 122 'crisis intervention'.

For all these studies, the clinical outcome at 2 years revealed a large and significant advantage for continuous treatment over brief intermittent treatment. Taking into account dropouts and admissions to hospital, over half did poorly on intermittent treatment. Prodromal symptoms were more frequently associated with brief intermittent treatment in the three studies in which they were systematically assessed. The dropout rate was significantly higher on brief intermittent treatment in all groups but was as high as 46% in the study by Herz *et al.*, which otherwise was the only one to find no difference in admission rate and symptom recurrence for those who remained in this study. It would appear that a difference in dropouts may have prejudiced this study, and may have accounted for the lower rate of relapse and symptom recurrence for those who remained in the study. Brief intermittent therapy was associated with higher rates of symptom recurrence and relapse in the other three studies but they had lower dropout rates.

Although less effective than continuous treatment, early brief treatment when prodromal symptoms occurred was associated with a significantly lower relapse rate (49%) in the German multicentre trial compared with the 63% relapse rate of the 'crisis intervention group', for whom medication was offered only when psychotic symptoms

or relapse occurred. The relapse rate on standard continuous maintenance treatment in this study was only 23%

A subsidiary hypothesis for this research was that with only intermittent treatment there might be a benefit in terms of improved well-being and long-term social functioning, and relapses would be milder, even if more frequent. In practice, relapses were more frequent and their severity was not studied, but social functioning was not improved on intermittent treatment in any of the four studies. Targeted, intermittent treatment showed no consistent superiority in terms of patients' sense of well-being or burden to unemployment or social stability (Jolley *et al.*, 1989). Finally, there were no significant differences between groups over time on measurements of extrapyramidal side effects or tardive dyskinesia, despite a 30 (Carpenter *et al.*, 1990) to 63% (Jolley *et al.*, 1990) relative decrease in the total amount of neuroleptic exposure for the brief intermittent treatment groups during the trial.

These findings clearly indicate that, at least on a group basis, reducing the exposure to neuroleptic dosage by low dose or intermittent targeted treatment is associated with an increased rate of symptom emergence, a higher relapse rate and more hospitalizations over 2 years, without a demonstrable gain in either improved social functioning or reduced neurological side effects. Yet, it must be noted that some 40% or more of patients survived 2 years on targeted intermittent treatment without relapse, so it may be a treatment worthy of trial when there are special indications to reduce dosage in alert and compliant patients.

A combined low-dose/augmentation strategy. In contrast to either a simple low-dose medication strategy or early brief, targeted intervention, there have been two published studies which combined these two approaches. In the first study, patients in the experimental group were given low doses but the clinician augmented the medication as soon as prodromal or early schizophrenic symptoms appeared. Marder *et al.* (1987) compared a standard dose of 25 mg fluphenazine decanoate every 2 weeks with 5 mg fluphenazine decanoate every 2 weeks. Approximately 30% of patients in both groups showed an exacerbation during the first year, while 69% of those in the low-dose group showed a significantly higher rate of early signs of relapse by the end of a 2-year follow-up period. If early signs of relapse emerged, including non-specific prodromal symptoms, clinicians were allowed to double the dose. Patients were considered survivors if this dose increase controlled the symptoms within a few days, otherwise they were considered to have relapsed. Symptom evaluation following dose augmentation showed similar relapse rates in both groups: 44% for the patients in the low-dose group with augmentation, and 31% for patients maintained on the standard neuroleptic dose. The difference was not significant.

Hogarty *et al.* (1988) carried out a study of similar design in which the average low-dose treatment with fluphenazine decanoate was 3.8 mg every 2 weeks and the average standard dose treatment was 25.7 mg every 2 weeks. This study did not show a significant difference in exacerbation rates between the two treatments prior to augmentation, but there was a significant reduction in relapse rates in both treatment groups when dosage was increased for patients who threatened relapse. Of patients in the low-dose treatment group, 49% showed an exacerbation, but only 28% were regarded as having relapsed after medication was increased. The respective figures for the standard dose group were 45 and 22%.

These findings suggest that a possible alternative to full-dose maintenance neuroleptic medication can be a low-dose medication regimen combined with a dose augmentation strategy when prodromal or early symptoms of relapse appear. A reasonable approach to reducing exposure to medication for a limited number of patients might be to slowly reduce the dose, for example by 50% over 3−6 months and then perhaps to 25% of the original dose, in combination with a dose augmentation programme in which the dose is at least doubled when prodromal or early symptoms of relapse appear. When the symptoms have been controlled for a period of 2 weeks, the dose could be reduced back to the original low dose. However, in this regard it is relevant to note that the value of prodromal symptoms in heralding relapse may be limited. In a prospective study over a year, Malla and Norman (1994) examined the relationship between non-psychotic prodromal symptoms and subsequent psychotic symptoms in 55 schizophrenic out-patients. Only in a relatively small proportion of patients did prodromal symptoms show a significant correlation with the subsequent level of psychotic symptoms, and a large proportion of psychotic episodes occurred without prodromal symptoms being identified.

Long-term effects of relapse and consequences of placebo-controlled trials

Good clinical practice involves deciding when treatment should be initiated, and when it should be stopped or continued, taking into account a reasoned response to a patient's desire to come off treatment. This requires an assessment of the benefits of treatment balanced against its risks. The same clinical judgement is involved when deciding whether a patient should enter a controlled clinical trial, especially a placebo-controlled trial. Some licensing authorities require such evidence for new antipsychotic compounds, and it is probably fair to say that proof of clinical efficacy is never complete without a placebo-controlled study.

Do placebo-controlled trials have long-term disadvantageous consequences for schizophrenics? The follow-up study by Curson *et al.* (1985) of patients who had originally entered a randomized, placebo-controlled trial on the basis of being well established and stable on depot fluphenazine decanoate provides useful evidence. In the initial placebo-controlled trial, 66% of the placebo group and 8% of those on active medication relapsed over 9 months (Hirsch *et al.*, 1973). Sixty-four patients were subsequently followed up with a repeat assessment of clinical, social and neurological functioning as well as a detailed examination of their clinical histories during the intervening 7−8 years. There were no differences between the original drug and placebo trial groups in terms of the number of subsequent deaths, the frequencies of relapse, companionship, marital status, employment status, number of admissions, number of episodes of illness, total time spent on depot medication, status of follow-up and mean time to relapse if medication had been discontinued. Similarly, comparing those 20 patients who received neuroleptics continuously during the follow-up with 22 who had relapsed within 13 months of discontinuing treatment, there were no significant differences on the same variables at follow-up.

Curson *et al.* (1985) reported a significant positive correlation between the number of relapses an individual had suffered and social outcome. This can be interpreted in two ways. The most economic explanation is that the worst patients have the worst outcome. This is consistent with conventional thinking about schizophrenia, that patients with more gradual onset, more insidious symptoms and slower deterioration prior to onset or relapse are likely to fare worse. Supportive evidence comes from a study of over 100 newly admitted, acute schizophrenic patients treated with haloperidol as part of an investigation of neuroleptic-threshold dosage (McEvoy *et al.*, 1991b). Rapid clinical response was most powerfully predicted by a short period of active illness, that is less than 1 month prior to admission. A more gradual clinical response was associated with a duration of illness of less than 6 months, while active illness of more than 6 months prior to admission was one of the factors associated with a lack of response.

The second explanation is that acute relapse has a deleterious effect on negative symptoms and social functioning, and there are lasting deficits in these areas following relapse (Davis *et al.*, 1993). Evidence in accord with this notion is available from the prospective follow-up study by Johnson *et al.* (1983) of 60 chronic schizophrenic patients withdrawn from drug treatment, compared with a control group continuing on medication. Those stopping drug treatment not only had significantly more acute psychotic episodes, but the relapses were more severe when rated on a number of

relevant criteria. In those patients suffering relapse, both work and social functioning were adversely affected, and the majority had not regained their pre-relapse level of functioning a year after recovery from the acute symptoms. Furthermore, in a 1-year follow-up study by Barnes *et al.* (1983), a sample of schizophrenic patients who had continued on medication and remained relatively free of relapse showed a specific improvement in social performance. These findings could mean that relapse can leave a residual impairment of social functioning, although with a period of illness stability, that is to say free of relapse, there is potential for recovery. If this were true, the prophylactic role of antipsychotic drugs would serve not only to reduce the mental distress and adverse personal and social consequences of psychotic relapse, but also to retard a decline in respect of some aspects of the defect state.

This work reinforces the value of studies that have adopted more refined criteria of outcome than simply the number of relapses suffered in treatment studies of schizophrenia. Long-term outcome is increasingly being judged on a range of relevant clinical variables such as the level and quality of social adjustment and functioning, the presence and severity of negative symptoms and side effects.

Treatments in the elderly

There has been little published research of differences in dosage requirements or dose–response relationships for the treatment of schizophrenia in patients over 65 years of age. However, the way drugs are handled by the body and their effect on body systems changes in the elderly in a predictable manner and must therefore be kept in mind when prescribing drugs. Most of our knowledge of changes in drug metabolites in the elderly is based on research with non-psychiatric drugs. However, although important, age is but one factor influencing the observed variation in the handling and response to psychotropic medication. Individual response to dosage is itself subject to considerable differences in the elderly.

Several factors are likely to cause an increased availability of drugs with advancing age, leading to a higher plasma concentration and more severe adverse and unwanted effects relative to the amount of drug prescribed. First-pass metabolism, particularly for lipid-soluble agents which have a high uptake by the liver, normally reduces the bioavailability of antipsychotic drugs by over 80%, but this can be greatly reduced in the elderly, in which case the dosage needs to be reduced accordingly. Renal clearance can also decline markedly with age and this is particularly relevant for lithium, which is excreted by the kidney, but again there is marked variation between individuals. Most antipsychotics are metabolized by the liver and this process may also be affected with ageing, due mostly to a decrease in liver size (reduced by 20–40% from the third to the ninth decades of life) and hepatic blood flow.

Sensitivity to drugs also changes with age and can interfere with the body's homeostatic processes. For example, postural hypotension is more common in the elderly, especially with drugs which affect vasomotor control, predisposing them to falls. Thermoregulatory reflexes may be blunted by neuroleptics, predisposing the elderly to accidental hypothermia; and animal data suggest that D_1 and D_2 receptor populations are reduced with age, which should indicate lower dose requirements for the same effect. These effects are reviewed in greater detail by Woodhouse (1992), who was able to find only five studies of the pharmacokinetics of antipsychotic drugs in relation to age. These suggest that drug plasma concentrations may increase by up to twofold in the elderly on thioridazine, and a similar tendency was observed for haloperidol.

Extrapyramidal side effects, tardive dyskinesia and neuroleptic malignant syndrome are all understood as a consequence of the central action of standard neuroleptic medication which blocks D_1 and D_2 dopamine receptors. But there are no systematic studies to show that the elderly have a higher incidence of these syndromes, as might be expected if afferent neurones are rendered either more sensitive or less sensitive by a decrease in the number of dopamine receptors with advancing

age. When treating the elderly, clinicians need to appreciate the increasing risk of developing tardive dyskinesia with age (see Chapter 27). This, and general experience borne out of practice, dictates that all psychotropic medication for the elderly should be started in very low doses compared with that for younger adults, and should be gradually increased as tolerated, the expectation being that the therapeutic aim will usually be achieved at relatively low doses. Examples of starting doses in the elderly are haloperidol 0.5 mg, chlorpromazine 25 mg and thioridazine 10 mg.

A general observation is that many of the unwanted side effects and complications of other medication may be exacerbated by concomitant neuroleptic treatment, complications such as agranulocytosis, a fall in blood platelets, cardiac arrhythmias and postural hypotension. Patients should always have a baseline blood pressure, full blood count and an ECG prior to starting treatment, and should be regularly monitored if abnormalities are observed. The general dictum is, when medicating the elderly start with low doses and increase slowly.

Relative contributions of experiential factors and drug treatment

The importance of antipsychotic medication in terms of its effect on the recurrence of acute and chronic symptoms and relapse rates may be less than psychiatrists generally appreciate. Davis (1976) calculated a correlation of $r_p = 0.60$ between medication–no medication and improvement–deterioration from a large series of placebo-controlled studies. This suggests that drugs account for only about 36% of the variance between improvement and no improvement in acute patients randomly assigned to either receive or not receive medication.

The results of a follow-up study by Vaughn and Leff (1976) reinforced previous findings regarding patients returning to live with relatives who had been rated high on expressed emotion (EE) (see Chapters 29 and 31). The correlation between continuation on maintenance medication and relapse was only $r_p = 0.39$, explaining 15% of the variance. Returning to live with a relative who was rated high on EE had a similar correlation with relapse ($r_p = 0.45$), but continuing to take medication appeared to be independent of EE in the social environment. Even the amount of time spent in contact with a high-EE relative had a significant effect on the relapse rate independent of medication; 69% of those spending more than 35 h a week with a high-EE relative relapsed compared with 35% of those spending less time in contact. Patients who returned to live with relatives rated low on EE had a low relapse rate regardless of whether they were on medication or not, about 13% in the first year, but an advantage emerged even in this group on medication when they were followed for 2 years (Leff & Vaughn, 1981). In contrast, patients living in the high-risk, high-EE environments experienced a significant protective effect from medication which was strongly evident even in the first year, decreasing their relapse rate by a third to a half. Thus, contact with a high-EE relative played as strong a role in determining whether a patient relapsed as whether or not the patient was on medication, and the two acted independently. These studies suggest that social experience is a strong factor in provoking relapse, but drugs can modify the influences remedially in the acutely ill, and prophylactically after patients have recovered. For further discussion of the role of psychosocial factors and the use of psychosocial treatments, see Chapters 29 and 31.

References

Angrist, B. & Schulz, S.C. (1990) Introduction. In Angrist, B. & Schulz, S.C. (eds) *The Neuroleptic-Nonresponsive Patient: Characterisation and Treatment*, pp, xvii–xxviii. American Psychiatric Press, Washington DC.

Angrist, B., Rotrosen, J. & Gershon, S. (1980) Response to apomorphine, amphetamine and neuroleptics in schizophrenic subjects. *Psychopharmacology*, **67**, 31–38.

Ayd, F.J. (1978) Intravenous haloperidol therapy. *International Drug Therapy Newsletter*, Baltimore.

Baldessarini, R.J., Cohen, B.M. & Teicher, M.H. (1988) Significance of neuroleptic dose and plasma level in the pharmacological treatment of psychosis. *Archives of General Psychiatry*, **45**, 79–91.

Barbee, J.G., Mancuso, D.M., Freed, C.R. & Todorov, A.A. (1992) Alprazolam as a neuroleptic adjunct in the emergency treatment of schizophrenia. *American Journal of Psychiatry*, **148**, 506–510.

Barnes, T.R.E. (1990) Comment on the WHO consensus statement. *British Journal of Psychiatry*, **156**, 413–414.

Barnes, T.R.E. (1994) Issues in the clinical assessment of negative symptoms: editorial review. *Current Opinion in Psychiatry*, **7**, 35–38.

Barnes, T.R.E. & Bridges, P.K. (1980) Disturbed behaviour induced with high-dose antipsychotic drugs. *British Medical Journal*, **281**, 274–275.

Barnes, T.R.E. & Edwards, J.G. (1993) The side-effects of antipsychotic drugs. I. CNS and neuromuscular effects. In Barnes, T.R.E. (ed.) *Antipsychotic Drugs and Their Side-Effects*, pp. 213–247. Academic Press, London.

Barnes, T.R.E. & Liddle, P.F. (1990) Evidence for the validity of negative symptoms. In Andreasen, N.C. (ed.) *Schizophrenia: Positive and Negative Symptoms and Syndromes*, Vol. 24, *Modern Problems in Pharmacopsychiatry*, pp. 43–72. Karger, Basel.

Barnes, T.R.E., Milavic, G., Curson, D.A. & Platt, S.D. (1983) Use of the Social Behaviour Assessment Schedule (SBAS) in a trial of maintenance antipsychotic therapy in schizophrenic outpatients: pimozide versus fluphenazine. *Social Psychiatry*, **18**, 193–199.

Bjorndal, N., Bjere, M., Gerlach, J. *et al.* (1980) High dosage haloperidol therapy in chronic schizophrenic patients: a double-blind study of clinical response, side-effects, serum haloperidol, and serum prolactin. *Psychopharmacology*, **67**, 17–23.

Bleuler, M. (1974) The long-term course of the schizophrenic psychoses. *Psychological Medicine*, **4**, 244–254.

Boyer, P., Lecrubier, Y. & Puech, A.J. (1990) Treatment of positive and negative symptoms: pharmacologic approaches. In Andreasen, N.C. (ed.) *Schizophrenia: Positive and Negative Symptoms and Syndromes*, Vol. 24, *Modern Problems in Pharmacopsychiatry*, pp. 152–174. Karger, Basel.

Breier, A., Wolkowitz, O.M., Doran, A.R. *et al.* (1987) Neuroleptic responsivity of negative and positive symptoms in schizophrenia. *American Journal of Psychiatry*, **144**, 1549–1555.

Caffey, E.M., Diamond, L.S., Frank, T.V. *et al.* (1964) Discontinuation or reduction of chemotherapy in chronic schizophrenics. *Journal of Chronic Disease*, **17**, 347–359.

Capstick, N. (1980) Long-term fluphenazine decanoate. Maintenance dosage requirements of chronic schizophrenic patients. *Acta Psychiatrica Scandinavica*, **61**, 256–262.

Caroli, F., Littre-Poirrier, M.-F., Ginestet, D. & Deniker, P. (1975) Essai d'interruption des antiparkinsoniens dans les traitements neuroleptiques au long cours. *Encephale*, **I**, 69–74.

Carpenter, W., Hanlon, T., Heinrichs, D., Kirkpatrick, B., Levine, J. & Buchanan, R. (1990) Continuous versus targeted medication in schizophrenic patients: outcome results. *American Journal of Psychiatry*, **147**, 1138–1148.

Carpenter, W.T., Heinrichs, D.W. & Wagman, A.M. (1988) Deficit and non-deficit forms of schizophrenia: the concept. *American Journal of Psychiatry*, **145**, 578–583.

Chang, R.S.L., Tran, V.T. & Synder, S.H. (1978) Histamine H_1 receptors in brain labelled with ^{3}H-mepyramine. *European Journal of Pharmacology*, **48**, 463–464.

Cheung, H.K. (1981) Schizophrenics fully remitted on neuroleptics for 3–5 years – to stop or continue drugs. *British Journal of Psychiatry*, **138**, 490–494.

Chouinard, G. & Jones, B. (1980) Neuroleptic-induced supersensitivity psychosis with clinical and pharmacological characteristics. *American Journal of Psychiatry*, **137**, 16–21.

Claus, A., Bollen, J., De Cuyper, H. *et al.* (1992) Risperidone versus haloperidol in the treatment of chronic schizophrenia in patients: a multicentre double-blind comparative study. *Acta Psychiatrica Scandinavica*, **85**, 295–305.

Cohen, B.M., Chouinard, G., Waternaux, C., Schachter, H., Jones, B. & Sommer, B. (1987) Plasma concentration of neuroleptic and serum prolactin in patients chronically receiving depot fluphenazine: no evidence of tolerance. *Human Psychopharmacology*, **2**, 171–176.

Cohen, L.J., Teat, M.A. & Brown, R.K. (1990) Suicide and schizophrenia – data from a prospective community treatment study. *American Journal of Psychiatry*, **147**, 602–607.

Cole, J., Kleberman, G.L. & Goldberg, S.C. (1964) Phenothiazine treatment of acute schizophrenia. *Archives of General Psychiatry*, **10**, 246–261.

Cookson, I.B., Muthu, M.S., George, A. & Dewey, M. (1983) High-dose neuroleptic treatment of chronic schizophrenic patients. *Research Communications in Psychology, Psychiatry and Behavior*, **8**, 1–8.

Crow, T.J. (1985) The two-syndrome concept: origins and current status. *Schizophrenia Bulletin*, **11**, 471–486.

Crow, T.J., Frith, C.D., Johnson, E.C. & Owens, D.T. (1981) The influence of anti-cholinergic medication on the extrapyramidal and anti-psychotic effects of neuroleptic drugs in the treatment of acute schizophrenia. *Biological Psychiatry*, **16**, 790–792.

Crow, T.J., MacMillan, J.F., Johnson, A.L. & Johnstone, E.C. (1986) The Northwick Park study of first-episode schizophrenia II. A randomised controlled trial of prophylactic neuroleptic treatment. *British Journal of Psychiatry*, **148**, 120–127.

Csernansky, J.G., Kaplan, J. & Hollister, L.E. (1985) Problems in classification of schizophrenics as neuroleptic responders and nonresponders, *Journal of Nervous and Mental Disease*, **173**, 325–331.

Curson, D.A., Barnes, T.R., Bamber, R.W., Platt, S.D., Hirsch, S.R. & Duffy, J.A. (1985) 7-year follow-up study of MRC 'Modecate' trial. *British Journal of Psychiatry*, **146**, 464–480.

Dahl, S.G. (1986) Plasma level monitoring of antipsychotic drugs: clinical utility. *Clinical Pharmacokinetics*, **11**, 36–61.

Davis, J.M. (1975) Overviews: maintenance therapy in psychiatry in schizophrenia. *American Journal of Psychiatry*, **132**, 1237–1245.

Davis, J.M. (1976) Comparative doses and costs of antipsychotic medication. *Archives of General Psychiatry*, **33**, 858–861.

Davis, J.M. & Garver, D.L. (1978) Neuroleptics: clinical use in psychiatry. In Iversen, L., Iversen, S. & Snyder, S. (eds) *Handbook of Psychopharmacology*, Plenum Press, New York.

Davis, J.M., Dysken, M., Haberman, S., Javaid, I., Chang, S. & Killian, G. (1980) Use of survival curves in analysis of antipsychotic relapse studies with long-term effects of neuroleptics. In Cattabeni, F., Spano, P.F., Racagni, G. &

Costa, E. (eds) *Advances in Biochemistry and Psychopharmacology*, Vol. 24, Raven Press, New York.

Davis, J.M., Janicak, P., Singla, A. & Sharma, R.P. (1993) Maintenance antipsychotic medication. In Barnes, T.R.E. (ed.) *Antipsychotic Drugs and Their Side-Effects*, pp. 183–203. Academic Press, London.

Delay, J. & Bernitzer, P. (1952) Le traitment des psychoses par une méthode neuroleptique dérivée de l'hibernothérapie. In Ossa, P.C. (ed.) *Congrès de Médecins Aliénistes et Neurologistes de France*, pp. 497–502. Masson, Paris.

Dencker, S.J. & May, P.R.A. (1988) From chronic mental hospital care to integration in society. In Dencker, S.J. & Kulhanek, F. (eds) *Treatment Resistance in Schizophrenia*, pp. 13–21. Vieweg, Wiesbaden.

Dencker, S.J., Lepp, M. & Malm, U. (1980) Do schizophrenics well adapted in the community need neuroleptics? A depot withdrawal study. *Acta Psychiatrica Scandinavica*, Suppl. **279**, 64–66.

Dencker, S.J., Enoksson, P., Johansson, L., Lundin, L. & Malm, U. (1981) Late (4–8 years) outcome of treatment with megadoses of fluphenazine enanthate in drug-refractory schizophrenics. *Acta Psychiatrica Scandinavica*, **63**, 1–12.

Denham, J. & Adamson, L. (1971) The contribution of fluphenazine enanthate and decanoate in the prevention of readmission of schizophrenic patients. *Acta Psychiatrica Scandinavica*, **47**, 420–430.

Duinkerke, S.J., Botter, P.A., Jansen, A.A. *et al.* (1993) Ritanserin, a selective 5HT2/1C antagonist reduced negative symptoms in schizophrenia: a placebo-controlled double-blind trial. *British Journal of Psychiatry*, **163**, 451–455.

Eberhard, G. & Hellbom, E. (1986) Haloperidol decanoate and flupenthixol decanoate in schizophrenia: a long-term double-blind cross-over comparison. *Acta Psychiatrica Scandinavica*, **4**, 255–262.

Edwards, J.G. & Barnes, T.R.E. (1993) The side-effects of antipsychotic drugs. II. Effects on other physiological systems. In Barnes, T.R.E. (ed) *Antipsychotic Drugs and Their Side-Effects*, pp. 249–275, Academic Press, London.

Falloon, I., Watt, D.C. & Shepherd, M. (1978a) A comparative controlled trial of pimozide and fluphenazine decanoate in continuation therapy of schizophrenia. *Psychological Medicine*, **8**, 59–70.

Falloon, I., Watt, D.C. & Shepherd, M. (1978b) The social outcome of patients in a trial of long-term continuation therapy in schizophrenia and pimozide vs fluphenazine. *Psychological Medicine*, **8**, 265–274.

Farde, L., Norstrom, A.-L., Wiesel, F.-A., Pauli, S., Halldin, C. & Sedvall, G. (1992) Positron emission tomographic analysis of central D_1 and D_2 dopamine receptor occupancy in patients treated with classical neuroleptics and clozapine: relation to extrapyramidal side-effects. *Archives of General Psychiatry*, **49**, 538–544.

Feinberg, S.S., Kay, S.R., Elijovich, L.R., Fiszbein, A. & Opler, L.A. (1988) Pimozide treatment of the negative schizophrenic syndrome: an open trial. *Journal of Clinical Psychiatry*, **49**, 235–238.

Gaind, R.N. & Barnes, T.R.E. (1981) Depot neuroleptic clinics. In Van Praag, H.M., Lader, M.H., Rafaelson, O.J. & Sachar, E.J. (eds) *Handbook of Biological Psychiatry*, Part

VI, *Practical Applications of Psychotropic Drugs and Other Biological Treatments*, pp. 149–179. Marcel Dekker, New York.

Gardos, G., Cole, J.O. & Orzack, M.H. (1973) The importance of dosage in antipsychotic drug administration — a review of dose — response studies. *Psychopharmacologia*, **29**, 221–230.

Gerlach, J. (1993) Pharmacology and clinical properties of selective dopamine antagonists with focus on substituted benzamides. In Barnes, T.R.E. (ed.) *Antipsychotic Drugs and Their Side-Effects*, pp. 45–63. Academic Press, London.

Goldberg. S.C. (1985) Negative and deficit symptoms in schizophrenia do respond to neuroleptics. *Schizophrenia Bulletin*, **11**, 453–456.

Greenberg, D.A., U'Pritchard, D.C. & Synder, S.H. (1976) α-Noradrenergic receptor binding in mammalian brain. *Life Sciences*, **19**, 69–76.

Haase, H.J. & Janssen, P.A.J. (1985) *The Action of Neuroleptic Drugs*, 2nd edn. Elsevier Science, New York.

Herrera, J.N., Sramek, J.J., Costa, J.F., Roy, S., Heh, C.W. & Nguyen, B.N. (1988) High potency neuroleptics and violence in schizophrenics. *Journal of Nervous and Mental Disease*, **176**, 558–561.

Herz, M. & Melville, C. (1980) Relapse in schizophrenia. *American Journal of Psychiatry*, **137**, 801–805.

Herz, M.I., Glazer, W.M., Mostert, M.A. *et al.* (1991) Intermittent versus maintenance medication in schizophrenia. Two year results. *Archives of General Psychiatry*, **48**, 333–339.

Hirsch, S.R. (1986) Clinical treatment of schizophrenia. In Bradley, R.B. & Hirsch, S.R. (eds) *The Psychopharmacology and Treatment of Schizophrenia*, pp. 286–339. Oxford University Press, Oxford.

Hirsch, S.R. & Barnes, T.R.E. (1994) Clinical use of high-dose neuroleptics. *British Journal of Psychiatry*, **164**, 94–96.

Hirsch, S.R. & Macrae, K.D. (1986) Essential elements in the design of clinical trials. In Bradley, P.B. & Hirsch, S.R. (eds) *The Psychopharmacology and Treatment of Schizophrenia*, pp. 212–233. Oxford Medical Publications, Oxford.

Hirsch, S.R., Gaind, R., Rohde, P.D., Stevens, B.C. & Wing, J.C. (1973) Outpatient maintenance of chronic schizophrenic patients with long-acting fluphenazine: double-blind placebo trial. *British Medical Journal*, **1**, 633–637.

Hogarty, G.E. & Ulrich, R.(1977) Temporal effects of drug and placebo in delaying relapse in schizophrenic outpatients. *Archives of General Psychiatry*, **34**, 297–301.

Hogarty, G.E., McEvoy, J.P., Munetz, M. *et al.* (1988) Dose of fluphenazine, familial expressed emotion and outcome in schizophrenia. *Archives of General Psychiatry*, **45**, 797–805.

Hogarty, G.E., Ulrich, R., Mussare, R. & Aristigueta, N. (1976) Drug discontinuation among long-term successfully maintained schizophrenic outpatients. *Diseases of the Nervous System*, **37**, 494–500.

Hollister, L.E. (1974) Clinical differences among phenothiazines in schizophrenia. In *Advances in Biomedical Psychopharmacology*. Vol. 9, pp. 617–73.

Hoyberg, O.J., Fensbo, C., Remvig, J., Lingjaerde, O., Sloth-Nielsen, M. & Salvesen, I. (1993) Risperidone versus perphenazine in the treatment of chronic schizophrenic patients with acute exacerbations. *Acta Psychiatrica Scandinavica*, **88**, 395–402.

Itil, T.M., Keskiner, A., Heinemann, L., Han, T., Gannen, P. & Hsu, W. (1970) Treatment of resistant schizophrenia with extreme high-dosage fluphenazine hydrochloride. *Psychosomatics*, **11**, 456–463.

Jain, A.K., Kelwala, S. & Gershon, S. (1988) Antipsychotic drugs in schizophrenia: current issues. *International Clinical Psychopharmacology*, **3**, 1–30.

Johnson, D.A.W. (1976) The duration of maintenance therapy in chronic schizophrenia. *Acta Psychiatrica Scandinavica*, **53**, 298–301.

Johnson, D.A.W. (1977) Practical considerations in the use of depot neuroleptics for the treatment of schizophrenia. *British Journal of Hospital Medicine*, **17**, 546–559.

Johnson, D.A.W. (1978) The prevalence and treatment of drug-induced extrapyramidal symptoms. *British Journal of Psychiatry*, **132**, 27–30.

Johnson, D.A.W. (1981) Studies of depressive symptoms in schizophrenia. *British Journal of Psychiatry*, **139**, 89–101.

Johnson, D.A.W. (1993) Depot neuroleptics. In Barnes, T.R.E. (ed.) *Antipsychotic Drugs and Their Side-Effects*, pp. 205–212. Academic Press, London.

Johnson, D.A.W., Ludlow, J.M., Street, K. & Taylor, R.D.W. (1987) Double-blind comparison of half-dose and standard-dose flupenthixol decanoate in the maintenance treatment of stabilised outpatients with schizophrenia. *British Journal of Psychiatry*, **151**, 634–638.

Johnson, D.A.W., Pasterski, G., Ludlow, J.M., Street, K. & Taylor, R.D.W. (1983) The discontinuance of maintenance neuroleptic therapy in chronic schizophrenic patients: drug and social consequences. *Acta Psychiatrica Scandinavica*, **6**, 339–352.

Johnstone, E., Crow, T., Ferrier, N. *et al.* (1983) Adverse effects of anticholinergic medication on positive schizophrenic symptoms. *Psychological Medicine*, **13**, 513–527.

Johnstone, E., Crow, T., Frith, C., Carney, M. & Price, J. (1978) The mechanism of the antipsychotic effect in the treatment of acute schizophrenia. *Lancet*, **i**, 848–851.

Jolley, A.G., Hirsch, S.R., McRink, A. & Manchanda, R. (1989) Trial of brief intermittent neuroleptic prophylaxis for selected schizophrenic outpatients: clinical outcome at one year. *British Journal of Psychiatry*, **298**, 985–990.

Jolley, A.G., Hirsch, S.R., Morrison, E., McRink, A. & Wilson, L. (1990) Trial of brief intermittent neuroleptic prophylaxis for selected schizophrenic outpatients: clinical and social outcome at two years. *British Medical Journal*, **301**, 837–842.

Kane, J.M. (1987) Treatment of schizophrenia. *Schizophrenia Bulletin*, **13**, 133–156.

Kane, J.M. (1993) Acute treatment. In Barnes, T.R.E. (ed.) *Antipsychotic Drugs and Their Side-Effects*, pp. 169–181. Academic Press, London.

Kane, J.M. & Mayerhoff, D. (1989) Do negative symptoms respond to pharmacological treatment? *British Journal of Psychiatry*, **155** (Suppl. 7), 115–118.

Kane, J., Rifkin, A., Quitkin, F. & Klein, D.F. (1982) Fluphenazine vs. placebo in patients who remitted, acute first-episode schizophrenia. *Archives of General Psychiatry*, **39**, 70–73.

Kane, J.M., Honigfeld, G., Singer, J. & Meltzer, H. (1988) Clozapine for the treatment-resistant schizophrenic. A double-blind comparison with chlorpromazine. *Archives of*

General Psychiatry, **45**, 789–796.

Kane, J., Rifkin, A., Quitkin, F. *et al.* (1979) How does fluphenazine decanoate aid in maintenance treatment of schizophrenia. *Psychiatry Research*, **1**, 341–348.

Kane, J., Rifkin, A., Woerner, M. *et al.* (1983) Low-dose neuroleptic treatment of outpatient schizophrenics. *Archives of General Psychiatry*, **40**, 893–896.

Keck, P.E., Cohen, B.M., Baldessarini, R.J. & McElroy, S.L. (1989) Time course of antipsychotic effects of neuroleptic drugs. *American Journal of Psychiatry*, **146**, 1289–1292.

Keck, P.E., Pope, H.G. & McElroy, S.L. (1991) Declining frequency of neuroleptic malignant syndrome in a hospital population. *American Journal of Psychiatry*, **148**, 880–882.

Kennedy, J.L., Petronis, A., Macciardi, F., Van Tol, H.M. & Seeman, P. (1994) The dopamine D4 receptor and schizophrenia. *Schizophrenia Reseaarch*, **11**, 145.

Kissling, W., Moller, H.J., Walter, K., Wittmann, B., Krueger, R. & Trenk, D. (1985) Double-blind comparison of haloperidol decanoate and fluphenazine decanoate effectiveness, side-effects, dosage and serum levels during a six-months treatment for relapse prevention. *Pharmacopsychiatry*, **18**, 240–245.

Klett, C.J., Point, P. & Caffey, E. (1972) Evaluating the long-term need for antiparkinson drugs by chronic schizophrenics. *Archives of General Psychiatry*, **26**, 375–379.

Kline, N.S. (1954) Use of Rauwolfia serpentinia bentyl in neuropsychiatric conditions. *Annals of the New York Academy of Science*, **59**, 107–132.

Knights, A. & Hirsch, S.R. (1981) Revealed depression and drug treatment for schizophrenia. *Archives of General Psychiatry*, **38**, 806–811.

Knights, A. & Platt, S. (1980) Clinical change as a function of brief admission to hospital in a controlled study using the PSE. *British Journal of Psychiatry*, **137**, 170–180.

Knights, A., Okasha, M.S., Salih, M. & Hirsch, S.R. (1979) Depressive and extra-pyramidal symptoms and clinical effects: a trial of fluphenazine versus flupenthixol in maintenance of schizophrenic outpatients. *British Journal of Psychiatry*, **135**, 515–524.

Lader, M. (1979) Monitoring plasma concentrations of neuroleptics. *Pharmacopsychology*, **9**, 170–177.

Laduron, P.M., Verwimp, M. & Leysen, J.E. (1979) Stereospecific *in vitro* binding of ^{3}H-dexetimide to brain muscarinic receptors. *Journal of Neurochemistry*, **32**, 421–427.

Leff, J.P. (1994) Working with the families of schizophrenic patients. *British Journal of Psychiatry*, **164** (Suppl. 23), 71–76,

Leff, J.P. & Vaughn, C. (1981) The role of maintenance therapy and relatives expressed emotion in relapse of schizophrenia: a two-year follow-up. *British Journal of Psychiatry*, **139**, 102–104.

Leff, J.P. & Wing, J.K. (1971) Trial of maintenance therapy in schizophrenia. *British Medical Journal*, **3**, 599–604.

Letemendia, F.J.J., Harris, A.D. & Williams, P.J.A. (1967) The clinical effects on a population of chronic schizophrenic patients of administrative changes in hospital. *British Journal of Psychiatry*, **113**, 959–971.

Leysen, J.E., Tollenaere, J.P., Koch, M.H.J. & Laduron, P.M. (1977) Differentiation of opiate and neuroleptic receptor binding in rat brain. *European Journal of Pharmacology*, **43**, 253–267.

Leysen, J.E., Niemegeers, C.J.E., Tollenaere, J.P. & Laduron, P.M. (1978) Serotonergic component of neuroleptic receptors. *Nature*, **272**, 168–171.

Leysen, J.E. (1981) Review on neuroleptic receptors: specificity and multiplicity of *in vitro* binding related to pharmacological activity. In Usdin, E., Dahl, S.G., Gram, L.F. & Lingjaerde, O. (eds) *Clinical Pharmacology in Psychiatry: Neuroleptic and Antidepressant Research*, pp. 35–62. Macmillan, London.

Loebel, A.D., Lieberman, J.A., Alvir, J.M., Mayerhoff, D.I., Geisler, S.H. & Szymanski, S.R. (1993) Duration of psychosis and outcome in first-episode schizophrenia. *American Journal of Psychiatry*, **149**, 1183–1188.

Loebel, A.D., Lieberman, J.A., Alvir, J.M.J. *et al.* (1993) Duration of psychosis and outcome in first-episode schizophrenia. *American Journal of Psychiatry*, **149**, 1183–1188.

McClelland, H.A., Blessed, G., Bhate, S., Ali, N. & Clarke, P.A. (1974) The abrupt withdrawal of antiparkinsonian drugs in schizophrenic patients. *British Journal of Psychiatry*, **124**, 151–159.

McClelland, H.A., Farquharson, R.G., Leyburn, P., Furness, J.A. & Schiff, A.A. (1976) Very high dose fluphenazine decanoate. *Archives of General Psychiatry*, **33**, 1435–1439.

McCreadie, R.G. & MacDonald, I.M. (1977) High dosage haloperidol in chronic schizophrenia. *British Journal of Psychiatry*, **131**, 310–316.

McCreadie, R.G., Flanagan, W.L., McKnight, J. & Jorgensen, A. (1979) High dose flupenthixol decanoate in chronic schizophrenia. *British Journal of Psychiatry*, **135**, 175–179.

McEvoy, J.P. (1986) The neuroleptic threshold as a marker of minimum effective neuroleptic dose. *Comprehensive Psychiatry*, **27**, 327–335.

McEvoy, J.P., Hogarty, G.E. & Steingard, S. (1991a) Optimal dose of neuroleptic in acute schizophrenia. *Archives of General Psychiatry*, **48**, 739–745.

McEvoy, J.P., Schooler, N.R. & Wilson, W.H. (1991b) Predictors of therapeutic response to haloperidol in acute schizophrenia. *Psychopharmacology Bulletin*, **27**, 97–101.

McKane, J.P., Robinson, A.D.T., Wiles, D.H., McCreadie, R.G. & Stirling, G.S. (1987) Haloperidol decanoate vs. fluphenazine decanoate as maintenance therapy in chronic schizophrenic in-patients. *British Journal of Psychiatry*, **151**, 333–336.

MacMillan, J.F., Gold, A., Crow, T.J. *et al.* (1986) The Northwick Park study of first episodes of schizophrenia. III. *British Journal of Psychiatry*, **148**, 128–133.

Malla, A.K. & Norman, R.M.G. (1994) Prodromal symptoms in schizophrenia. *British Journal of Psychiatry*, **164**, 487–493.

Manos, N., Gkiouzepas, J. & Logothetis, J. (1981) The need for continuous use of antiparkinsonian medication with chronic schizophrenic patients receiving long-term neuroleptic therapy. *American Journal of Psychiatry*, **138**, 184–188.

Marder, S.R. (1992) Risperidone: clinical development: North American results. *Clinical Neuropharmacology*, **15**, (Suppl. 1), 92–93.

Marder, S.R., Van Putten, T., Mintz, J., Lebell, M., McKenzie, J. & May, P.R. (1987) Low and conventional dose maintenance therapy with fluphenazine decanoate: two-year outcome. *Archives of General Psychiatry*, **44**, 518–521.

Marriott, P.A. (1978) A five-year follow-up at a depot phenothiazine clinic: patterns and problems. In Ayd, F.J. (ed) *Depot Fluphenazines: Twelve Years of Experience*, pp. 46–69. Ayd Medical Communications, Baltimore.

May, P.R.A. (1968) *Treatment of Schizophrenia: A Comparative Study of Five Treatment Methods*. Science House, New York.

Mehtonen, O.P., Aranko, K., Malkonen, L. & Vapaatalo, H. (1991) A study of sudden death associated with the use of antipsychotic or antidepressant drugs: 49 cases in Finland. *Acta Psychiatrica Scandinavica*, **84**, 58–64.

Orlov, P., Kasparian, G., DiMascio, A. & Cole, J.O. (1971) Withdrawal of antiparkinson drugs. *Archives of General Psychiatry*, **25**, 410–412.

Perenyi, A., Gardos, G., Samu, I., Kallos, M. & Cole, J.O. (1983) Changes in extrapyramidal symptoms following anticholinergic drug withdrawal. *Clinical Neuropharmacology*, **6**, 55–61.

Peroutka, S. & Snyder, S.H. (1980) Relationship of neuroleptic drug effects at brain dopamine, serotonin, alpha-adrenergic, and histamine receptors to clinical potency. *American Journal of Psychiatry*, **137**, 1518–1522.

Perry, P.J., Pfohl, B.M. & Kelly, M.W. (1988) The relationship of haloperidol concentrations to therapeutic response. *Journal of Clinical Psychopharmacology*, **8**, 38–42.

Petit, M., Zann, M., Lesieur, P. & Colonna, L. (1987) The effect of sulpiride on negative symptoms of schizophrenia (letter). *British Journal of Psychiatry*, **150**, 270–271.

Pietzcker, A., Gaebel, W., Kopcke, W. *et al.* (1994) Intermittent versus maintenance neuroleptic long-term treatment in schizophrenia – 2-year results of a German multicentre study. *Journal of Psychiatry Research*, **27**(4), 321–339.

Prien, R.F. & Klett, C.C. (1972) An appraisal of the long-term use of tranquillizing medication with hospitalized chronic schizophrenics. *Schizophrenia Bulletin*, **5**, 64–73.

Prien, R.F., Gillis, R.P. & Caffey, E.M. (1973) Intermittent pharmacotherapy in chronic schizophrenia. *Hospital and Community Psychiatry*, **24**, 317–322.

Quitkin, F., Rifkin, A., Kane, J., Ramos-Lorenzi, J. & Klein, D. (1978) Long-action oral vs injectable antipsychotic drugs in schizophrenics. *Archives of General Psychiatry*, **35**, 889–892.

Quitkin, F., Rifkin, A. & Klein, D.F. (1975) Very high dosage versus standard dosage fluphenazine in schizophrenia: a double-blind study of non-chronic treatment refractory patients. *Archives of General Psychiatry*, **32**, 1276–1281.

Reardon, G.T., Rifkin, A., Schwartz, A., Myerson, A. & Siris, S.G. (1989) Changing patterns of neuroleptic dosage over a decade. *American Journal of Psychiatry*, **146**, 726–729.

Rey, M.-J., Schulz, P., Costa, C., Dick, P. & Tissot, R. (1989) Guidelines for the dosage of neuroleptics. I. Chlorpromazine equivalents of orally administered neuroleptics. *International Clinical Psychopharmacology*, **4**, 95–104.

Rifkin, A., Quitkin, F. & Klein, D.F. (1975) Akinesia: a poorly recognised drug-induced extrapyramidal disorder. *Archives of General Psychiatry*, **32**, 672–674.

Rifkin, A., Quitkin, F., Kane, J.M., Struve, F. & Klein, D.F. (1978) Are prophylactic antiparkinson drugs necessary? *Archives of General Psychiatry*, **35**, 483–489.

Rifkin, A., Doddi, S., Karajgi, B. *et al.* (1991) Dosage of haloperidol for schizophrenia. *Archives of General Psychiatry*, **48**, 166–170.

Shaikh, S., Collier, D., Gill, M., Pilowsky, L., McMillan, A.M., Sham, P. & Kerwin, R. (1994) D4 polymorphism in schizophrenics treated with clozapine. *Schizophrenia Research*, **11**, 146.

Simpson, G.M., Davis, J., Jefferson, J.W. & Perez-Cruet, J.F. (1987) Sudden deaths in psychiatric patients: the role of neuroleptic drugs. *America Psychiatric Association Task Force Report*, No. 27.

Singh, M.M. & Kay, S.R. (1975) A comparative study of haloperidol and chlorpromazine in terms of clinical effects and therapeutic reversal with benztropine in schizophrenia. *Psychopharmacologia*, **43**, 103–113.

Singh, M.M. & Kay, S.R. (1979) Dysphoric response to neuroleptic treatment in schizophrenia: its relationship to autonomic arousal and prognosis. *Biological Psychiatry*, **14**, 277–294.

Stephens, J.H. (1970) Long-term course and prognosis in schizophrenia. *Seminars in Psychiatry*, **2**, 464–485.

Thompson, C. (1994) The Use of High-Dose Antipsychotic Medication. *British Journal of Psychiatry*, **164**, 448–458.

Tsuang, M.T. (1982) Long-term outcome in schizophrenia. *Trends in Neuroscience*, **June**, 203–207.

Van Kammen, D.P., Hommer, D.W. & Malas, K.L. (1987) Effect of pimozide on positive and negative symptoms in schizophrenic patients: are negative symptoms state dependent? *Neuropsychobiology*, **18**, 113–117.

Van Putten, T., Marder, S.R. & Mintz, J. (1990) A controlled dose comparison of haloperidol in newly admitted schizophrenic patients. *Archives of General Psychiatry*, **47**, 754–758.

Van Tol, H.M., Wu, C.M., Guan, H.-C. *et al.* (1992) Multiple dopamine D4 receptor variants in the human population. *Nature*, **358**, 149–152.

Vaughn, C. & Leff, J. (1976) The influence of family and social factors on the course of psychiatric illness. *British Journal of Psychiatry*, **129**, 125–137.

Waddington, J.L. (1993) Pre- and postsynaptic D_1 to D_5 dopamine receptor mechanisms in relation to antipsychotic activity. In Barnes, T.R.E. (ed.) *Antipsychotic Drugs and Their Side-Effects*, pp. 65–85. Academic Press, London.

WHO Heads of Centres (1990) Prophylactic use of anticholinergics in patients on long-term neuroleptic treatment: a consensus statement. *British Journal of Psychiatry*, **156**, 412.

Wiles, D. & Wistedt, B. (1981) *The Relationship of Serum Fluphenazine Decanoate Levels to Relapse Following Withdrawal of Medication*. Poster F522, Third World Congress of Biology and Psychiatry, Stockholm.

Wing, J.K. & Brown, G.W. (1970) *Institutionalism and Schizophrenia: A Comparative Study of Three Mental Hospitals 1966–1968*. Cambridge University Press, Cambridge.

Wistedt, B. (1981) A depot neuroleptic withdrawal study. *Acta Psychiatrica Scandinavica*, **64**, 65–84.

Woodhouse, K. (1992) The pharmacology of major tranquillisers in the elderly. In Katona, C. & Levy, R. (eds) *Delusions of Hallucinations in Old Age*, pp. 89–92. R.C. Psych, Gaskill, London.

Wyatt, R.J. (1991) Neuroleptics and the natural course of schizophrenia. *Schizophrenia Bulletin*, **17**, 325–351.

Chapter 24
Treatment-Resistant Schizophrenia

S. C. SCHULZ AND P. F. BUCKLEY

Chapter outline

The objectives of this chapter are to provide a timely and critical appraisal of current perspectives on the definition and concept of treatment resistance in schizophrenia, to explore its proposed clinical and neurobiological characteristics, and to evaluate the rationale and effectiveness of present-day pharmacological practice, in particular the use of antipsychotic augmentation strategies in the management of treatment-resistant patients.

Until the 1980s the concept of non-response to antipsychotic medication was very poorly defined and was usually synonymous with long-term hospital stay. With the initiation of the clozapine study of treatment of last resort in the USA, treatment resistance was defined by stringent research criteria which largely emphasized the severity and chronicity of psychotic symptoms. The basic tenets of this approach have come under sharp scrutiny and it is now acknowledged that this narrow focus underestimates both the clinical impact and the complexity of treatment resistance. The concept of persistent disability has broadened appropriately to encompass functional and psychosocial dimensions. The utility of such a multidimensional perspective and its research and clinical validity are emphasized.

Differences between treatment responders and non-responders have frequently emerged when subjects are compared along clinical parameters (e.g. age at onset), cognitive and neurological function, electroencephalogram (EEG) rhythms, neuroimaging of cerebral morphology and plasma metabolite patterns. While single variable comparisons have detected such abnormalities, subsequent research has yielded disparate and often contradictory results (e.g. computerized tomography (CT) findings in treatment resistance) and a more integrative, multivariable research evaluation of treatment-resistant patients is now advocated. This approach offers most promise in delineating a putative subgroup of poorly responsive patients.

The advent of clozapine as an effective treatment option has necessitated a reformulation of the pharmacological management of treatment resistance. This is addressed in Chapters 18 and 25. In particular, the role of antipsychotic augmentation strategies needs careful re-evaluation and this process would be aided by research comparing the efficacy of these approaches with clozapine therapy and other new agents. In this chapter, we review the relative merits of the most commonly used other strategies, including the addition of benzodiazepines, lithium, carbamazepine and serotonin agonists, as well as some more experimental agents such as the neurotransmitter cholecystokinin (CCK). Electroconvulsive therapy (ECT) is addressed in Chapter 26. We also describe an approach to the clinical assessment and care of the treatment-resistant patient. The close integration of pharmacological therapies with behavioural, cognitive and social skills management in the treatment plan is stressed.

Introduction

Some 20–40% of patients will prove resistant to standard antipsychotic treatments. If the definition of treatment resistance or persistent symptoms is broadened beyond psychopathology measures to include vocational, social and cognitive domains, then it is suggested that more patients could be classified as treatment resistant (Meltzer, 1992a). Moreover, present figures are largely based on stringent research criteria (Kane *et al.*, 1988) and thus may underestimate this problem by not including the many patients who manifest an incomplete response to antipsychotics (Osser & Albert, 1990). A recent report on the initial findings from a multicentre trial of treatment strategies involving 300 patients with schizophrenia supports this assertion (Keith *et al.*, 1991). This study, evaluating maintenance antipsychotic treatments and their interaction with family therapies, has demonstrated that just short of 40% of patients remained poorly stabilized at 6 months of treatment. Equally discouraging, a substantial number of those who showed initial treatment response were unable to sustain this through to the second year of observation. In addition, there is now evidence (Lieberman *et al.*, 1989, 1992, 1993; Kane *et al.*, 1992) to suggest that treatment resistance may emerge and persist even from the earliest phase of the illness. In a prospective study of the treatment outcome and psychobiology in a well-characterized sample of 70 patients with 'first-episode' schizophrenia (Lieberman *et al.*, 1989, 1992), eight patients were refractory to all phases of the treatment algorithm and subsequently received treatment with clozapine. These findings, in conjunction with earlier reports (Johnstone *et al.*, 1990), support the notion that treatment resistance is not merely the result of institutionalization or of acquired disabilities but, rather, represents a putative 'endogenous' trait which (regrettably) shows remarkable consistency over time. The seminal study of Kane *et al.* (1988)

further supports this viewpoint. Here, 305 patients with current evidence of a severe, symptomatic schizophrenic illness were carefully determined as having a prior history of treatment resistance using stringent historical criteria (see Table 24.1). These patients were then enrolled in a 6-week prospective trial of haloperidol (60 mg/day) to confirm their apparent treatment non-responsivity. At the conclusion of this phase, only five patients emerged as treatment responders.

Defining poor response to treatment

Historically, the concept of non-response to antipsychotic medication was ill defined and largely synonymous with chronic hospitalization. In refining this to ensure methodological rigour and clear characterization of study samples, many researchers have sought explicit definitions of treatment resistance (Table 24.1). Definitions have often been related to the purpose of the individual project, e.g. treatment of last resort (Kane *et al.*, 1988) or differences between groups (Schulz *et al.*, 1989). These definitions have not addressed clinical questions, such as when to change treatment. In general, the use of psychopathology rating scales has enhanced the reproducibility and consistency of the definition of poor response to neuroleptics. A cut-off point of 20% decrease in brief psychiatric rating scale (BPRS) total score has been widely adopted as a measure of response to antipsychotics (Kane *et al.*, 1988). However, in reality, this has been somewhat arbitrarily defined and emanated largely from earlier trials intended merely to indicate that antipsychotic medications were active. Thus, a 20% decrement in BPRS symptomatology *per se* is not an immutable benchmark and may, in some instances, confer the erroneous impression that substantial improvement or satisfactory clinical 'response' has been attained. A patient with an initial BPRS score of 48 may indeed achieve a 20% fall in BPRS with treatment (to a value $\leq$38) and yet still exhibit substantial impairment. Furthermore, if another patient at an initial BPRS rating of 38 fails to attain a similar 20% reduction in BPRS, then this subject will be designated a

Table 24.1 Representative criteria for treatment-resistant schizophrenia

Reference	Criteria
Hall *et al.* (1968)	Male phenothiazine-resistant schizophrenic in-patients (median current hospitalization 50 months, range 3 months–40 years; numerous previous hospitalizations)
McCreadie and McDonald (1977)	Drug-resistant male in-patients in long-stay unit (previous two to three courses of neuroleptics; persistent symptoms)
Kane *et al.* (1988)	Historical: no period of good functioning or significant symptomatic relief within preceding 5 years despite at least two courses of neuroleptics (doses ≥ 1000 mg/day chlorpromazine) for 6 weeks Cross-sectional: BPRS score ≥ 45, score of ≥ 4 on at least two of conceptual disorganization, suspiciousness, hallucinatory behaviour, unusual thought content; CGI score of ≥ 4 Prospective: 6-week trial of haloperidol (60 mg/day) fails to reduce BPRS by 20% or to below 35, or fails to reduce CGI to below 3
Schulz *et al.* (1989)	Prospective: after 4-week trial of haloperidol (dosage which achieves blood level of 8–25 ng/ml) patients score ≥ 40 on BPRS, or ≥ 4 on Bunney–Hamburg psychosis scale
Brenner *et al.* (1990)	Seven levels of treatment response incorporating evaluation of symptomatology, personal and social adjustment: level 1, clinical remission; level 2, partial remission; level 3, slight resistance; level 4, moderate resistance; level 5, severe resistance; level 6, refractory; level 7, severely refractory

BPRS, brief psychiatric rating scale; CGI, clinical global impression.

'non-responder' and, yet, will likely possess an end point BPRS score which is broadly similar to that of the 'responder'. Quite apart from the selection of a particular definition of responsiveness, the use of this cut-off point has other related implications. For example, the acutely psychotic patient (e.g. BPRS of 58) may attain this 20% decrement more readily with treatment than another patient who, while not as floridly psychotic (e.g. BPRS of 38), may nevertheless experience disabling symptoms. In such circumstances, there is a differential effect through the range of BPRS rating with greater improvement at the lower range being necessary to be considered a 'responder' than at higher baseline points on the scale. This differential effect may underrepresent the true estimate of treatment resistance (Thompson *et al.*, 1994). The approach of Kane *et al.* (1988) and Schulz *et al.* (1989) stressed a specific level of symptomatology as the guideline for response. In

both reports, a definite BPRS score was chosen as representing a mild level of symptoms. This is more like a medical approach to symptoms in that it aims at remission of symptoms or at least reduction to a low level. The criteria of Kane *et al.* also included historical criteria, which are important for studies of treatments of last resort, while Schulz *et al.* (1989) included requirements of adequate medication levels before labelling a person resistant.

A related issue concerns the relative effectiveness of standard antipsychotics to ameliorate positive and negative symptoms of schizophrenia (Goldberg, 1985; Meltzer *et al.* 1986) and the extent to which this effect ultimately impinges upon the characterization of treatment-resistant schizophrenia. The type I/type II model of schizophrenia (Crow, 1980) considered the importance of symptomatology in response to antipsychotics in schizophrenic patients and suggested that positive symptoms were remediated by these drugs, while negative symptoms were persistent and refractory to conventional treatments. However, observations with typical (Goldberg, 1985; Meltzer *et al.*, 1986) and atypical antipsychotic medications (Kane *et al.*, 1988) challenge this notion. The differential effect of antipsychotics (or lack thereof) on positive and negative symptoms *specifically* among treatment-resistant patients alone is less clear. Indeed, just as fundamental differences emerge between 'deficit' and 'non-deficit' forms of schizophrenia (Buchanan *et al.*, 1993), one could expect patients with persistent, treatment-resistant positive symptomatology to show neurobiological differences from those patients whose treatment-resistant illness is characterized by enduring negative symptomatology. This distinction has yet to be appropriately addressed strictly within the context of antipsychotic non-responsivity.

In addition, while psychopathology scales do attempt to take due account of the impact of symptomatology on overall functioning, they may fall short in appraising the qualitative nature and clinical ramifications of the disability which the persistently psychotic patient presents to the psychiatrist. Thus, it seems inappropriate to equate the treatment resistance of a patient with chronic delusions and hallucinations for which he/she retains (albeit partial) insight and functional capacity with that of the patient whose apathy and amotivation result in severe social withdrawal and secondary deficits. Similarly, the quality of the persistent psychotic experiences import different functional significance which will duly influence the extent of treatment responsiveness; this point is most readily observed with patients whose bizarre delusions are associated with marked social disruption and functional decline, in contrast with others, experiencing similar intensity of delusions but of a less bizarre nature and which impact less on overall social functioning.

A dichotomous view of treatment response, largely derived from the application of psychopathology rating scales, assumes that patients who are deemed poor responders to antipsychotic therapy constitute a homogeneous group. While therapeutic trials have largely focused on overall group effects between responders and non-responders, it is nevertheless apparent (and accords with clinical practice) that non-responders of themselves show considerable diversity in therapeutic response; thus, within a group of non-responders, some may show only modest response to an experimental treatment, others a minimal change in symptoms and a few show an actual deterioration with treatment (Elizur, 1979; Wolkowitz *et al.*, 1988). Such differences may impart fundamental implications for our understanding of treatment response but, largely because of inadequate sample sizes, this issue has yet to be subjected to appropriate scientific enquiry.

The alternative perspective posits that treatment resistance is not a marker for discrete response groups but, rather, is best conceptualized as a continuum (Brenner *et al.*, 1990). This notion lends credence to the clinical observation that the majority of patients do not fall within a strictly defined responder−non-responder distinction, but are in fact suboptimal responders who continue to exhibit persistent symptomatology and functional disability (Brenner *et al.*, 1990; Kane *et al.*, 1990; Osser & Albert, 1990). Such 'partial responders' have now become an important focus of interest, particularly as we struggle to establish a valid and clinically meaningful classification of treatment resistance. Furthermore, with the availability of clozapine as an effective treatment option for severely ill patients, the characterization and management strategies for the partial responder have come under sharp review.

In addition to addressing the potential confounding variables of poor compliance (Weiden *et al.*, 1991), drug bioavailability (Van Putten *et al.*, 1991) and a putative therapeutic window (Schulz *et al.*, 1984; Bitter *et al.*, 1991), there has been greater recognition of a multidimensional perspective to treatment resistance and of the complexity of interrelationships between positive and negative symptomatology, functional deficits and behavioural disturbance (Brenner *et al.*, 1990; Meltzer, 1990, 1992b). It has been acknowledged that improvement in cognitive function and psychopathology may, in some instances, occur independently of each other (Goldberg *et al.*, 1987, 1993) and that such measures may exert different, yet equally pertinent, influences on eventual treatment outcome (Goldberg *et al.*, 1987; Meltzer, 1992b). Recommendation that other facets of the illness receive particular attention in a manner similar to assessing symptomatology has led to the incorporation of such scales (quality of life scale, Heinrichs *et al.*, 1984; independent living skill survey, Wallace, 1986) into the routine evaluation of treatment response.

The potential significance of comorbid disorders in treatment-resistant schizophrenia has received insufficient attention in relation to poor response or persistent illness. While the presence of affective symptoms has traditionally been viewed as a favourable prognostic sign (Strauss & Carpenter, 1972), this may in part have been attributable to the diagnostic overlap between mood disorders and schizophrenia. Recent developments in the classification of psychiatric disorders have helped clarify the nosological relationships between affective disorders, schizoaffective disorder and schizophrenia, and this has facilitated a more direct enquiry of the relevance of depression in schizophrenia (Green *et al.*, 1990). However, it is presently unclear whether depressive symptoms are more prominent in treatment-resistant patients and the morbidity of affective symptoms has been underexplored. The efficacy of antidepressant medication in treating depression in schizophrenia has not been fully established; however, Siris (1991) has pointed the way to a more informed use of antidepressants. Recently, Siris *et al.* (1994) have shown that maintenance antidepressant therapy for secondary depression in schizophrenia is associated with less depressive *and* psychotic relapses. Unfortunately, some patients continue to exhibit prominent depressive features, despite adequate doses and trials of various antidepressants.

Similarly, obsessional symptoms were considered to import good prognostic outcome (Rosen, 1957), yet in clinical practice these patients appear to be less responsive to treatment and their obsessional symptoms do not seem to be readily amenable to treatment with antiobsessional drugs. There is, however, a marked paucity of research on this topic. In contrast, there has been a growing appreciation of the extent of comorbid substance abuse in schizophrenia (Seibyl & Lieberman, 1993; Buckley *et al.*, 1994). Patients who abuse illicit drugs or alcohol are more likely to have more prominent symptomatology, more frequent relapses and repeated hospitalizations (Seibyl & Lieberman, 1993). The potentially deleterious interaction of substance abuse and psychosis in such individuals may (quite apart from interrelated adverse factors such as social deprivation and treatment compliance) confer a relative resistance to neuroleptic treatment. The neurochemical basis for such an effect, possibly acting through alteration of dopamine-receptor sensitivity, merits further attention since it may suggest more effective, alternative treatment strategies for treatment-resistant schizophrenic patients who have comorbid substance abuse (Buckley *et al.*, 1994).

Finally, our understanding of the nature of treatment resistance in schizophrenia has been advanced by the recent upsurge of research on the earliest phases of schizophrenia (Lieberman *et al.*, 1992). This work has highlighted the severity of disability already evident in first-episode patients, including prominent cognitive impairment (Hoff *et al.*, 1992; Kenney & Schulz, 1993) and structural abnormalities of cerebral morphology (Lieberman *et al.*, 1993). Prospective evaluation of treatment responsivity in some of these samples (Lieberman *et al.*, 1989, 1992, 1993; Johnstone *et al.*, 1990) indicates the early emergence of treatment resistance. Moreover, detailed assessment of the onset of illness and duration of psychosis prior to the commencement of treatment with antipsychotic medication (Johnstone *et al.*, 1990; Loebel *et al.*, 1992) suggests that a prolonged interval of untreated psychosis may of itself be biologically toxic and thereby import subsequent treatment resistance. A recent review of the onset and treatment outcome of schizophrenia supports this assertion (Wyatt, 1991).

Aetiological implications of treatment resistance

The notion of aetiological heterogeneity within schizophrenia is an enduring hypothesis which has been tested from a variety of research stances, and posits that by studying distinct illness subgroups, we may ultimately elucidate further the pathophysiological basis of schizophrenia itself (Dalen & Hayes, 1990; but see Daniel & Weinberger, 1991). This approach has been applied to the study of responsivity to antipsychotic medication with mixed success (Csernansky *et al.*, 1985; Garver *et al.*, 1988; Brown & Herz, 1989; Schulz *et al.*, 1989). Differences between treatment responders and non-responders have been sought on clinical variables (Kolakowska *et al.*, 1985; Barkto *et al.*, 1990; Keefe *et al.*, 1990), biochemical variables (Kahn & Davidson, 1993), electrophysiological parameters (Itil & Shapiro, 1981) and neuroimaging abnormalities (Friedman *et al.*, 1992). These various lines of enquiry are highlighted in Tables 24.2 and 24.3. In broad outline, the results of these studies have been largely conflicting with positive findings often not being replicated or occasionally being contradicted subsequently. This may be because of previous poor methodology of classification or a combination of both. An explanation may lie in the observation that few studies have sought to characterize treatment-resistant patients along multiple variables, but rather through univariate comparisons. The single-variable approach appears too insensitive to determine discrete pathobiological differences and more integrative, multivariable research evaluation of treatment-resistant and responsive patients is more likely to delineate any putative subgroup of treatment-resistant patients.

Alternatively, a threshold model of treatment resistance may be relevant, where the cumulative effect of putative aetiological factors is associated with a greater likelihood of showing treatment resistance. Thus, patients might be evaluated at multiple levels; neuroimaging [functional — positron emission tomography (PET), single photon emission computerized tomography

(SPECT), magnetic resonance spectroscopy, computerized EEG; structural — magnetic resonance imaging (MRI)], biochemical [cerebrospinal fluid (CSF) and plasma dopaminergic and serotonergic metabolite studies; neuroendocrine challenge studies; methylphenidate challenge], electrophysiological (eye tracking, sensory gating), neuropsychological (including activation studies) and phenomenological characterization. Many of these data are now being accumulated in first-episode and early-phase schizophrenia treatment studies (Lieberman *et al.*, 1992). In the study of first-episode schizophrenia (Lieberman *et al.*, 1989, 1993), 12 out of 70 patients had not responded to the treatment algorithm after 1 year. Brain pathomorphology on MRI, eye tracking, basal growth hormone level and response to apomorphine challenge, and methylphenidate response were studied in relation to time and level of remission achieved. Abnormal brain morphology (specifically, ventricular enlargement but not cortical or medial temporal lobe abnormalities) and elevated basal growth hormone were associated with poor treatment response. Apomorphine or methylphenidate challenge, or eye tracking dysfunction were not associated with either time to or level of remission.

Treatment variables

Plasma antipsychotic levels have also been investigated as a potential factor in the expression of treatment resistance in schizophrenia (Davis *et al.*, 1978; Schulz *et al.*, 1984; Bitter *et al.*, 1991). The wide interindividual variations in reported antipsychotic plasma levels have been interpreted to indicate a possible therapeutic window (Bitter *et al.*, 1991; Van Putten *et al.*, 1991), with low levels being ineffective in treatment and high levels being associated with symptom exacerbation and/or treatment toxicity (especially neuroleptic intolerance) (Rifkin *et al.*, 1991). This hypothesis is supported clinically by the findings of Van Putten *et al.* (1988) who noted symptomatic improvement in patients after medication withdrawal. This therapeutic window has been invoked as a possible explanation for poor response to anti-

Table 24.2 Variables studied in relation to treatment resistance in schizophrenia

Variable	Key studies	Association	Comment
Age at onset	Kolakowska *et al.* (1985)	(+)	Some, but not all, studies report an earlier age at onset in TR patients
	Nimgaonkar *et al.* (1988)	(+)	
	Bartko *et al.* (1990)	(−)	
Family history of schizophrenia	Nimgaonkar *et al.* (1988)	(−)	A positive family history may predict poor response to treatment
	Silverman *et al.* (1987)	(+)	
Poor premorbid function	Kolakowska *et al.* (1985)	(+)	Poor premorbid adjustment associated with TR
	Bartko *et al.* (1990)	(+)	
	Keefe *et al.* (1990)	(+)	
Subtype of schizophrenia	Kolakowska *et al.* (1985)	(−)	Findings suggest no relationship with TR
	Losonczy *et al.* (1986)	(−)	
	Bartko *et al.* (1990)	(−)	
Symptoms at first presentation	Crow (1980)	(+)	More negative symptoms associated with TR, less clear relationship now
	Kolakowska *et al.* (1985)	(+)	
	Lieberman *et al.* (1993)	(−)	
NSS	Kolakowska *et al.* (1985)	(−)	NSS associated with poor treatment response?
	Bartko *et al.* (1989)	(−)	
	Schulz *et al.* (1989)	(+)	
	Johnstone *et al.* (1990)	(+)	
Neuropsychological impairment	Kolakowska *et al.* (1985)	(+)	Cognitive impairment appears to be associated with TR
	Bartko *et al.* (1989)	(−)	
	Schulz *et al.* (1989)	(+)	
EEG abnormalities	Itil and Shapiro (1981)	(+)	Idiopathic EEG abnormalities more common in TR patients
Structural brain imaging	See Table 24.3		
Functional brain imaging	Wolkin *et al.* (1989)	(−)	No differences in dopamine-receptor occupancy between good and poor responders; metabolic differences in glucose in basal ganglia metabolism on PET in striatum
	Buchsbaum *et al.* (1992)	(+)	
Prolactin response	Meltzer and Fang (1976)	(+)	Elevated prolactin correlated with improvement in treatment response
	Kolakowska *et al.* (1985)	(−)	
GH response	Beasley *et al.* (1984)	(+)	Blunted GH associated with poor response to neuroleptics
	Garver *et al.* (1988)	(+)	
Plasma HVA	Bowers *et al.* (1984); Bowers (1990)	(+)	High pretreatment HVA and decrease with neuroleptic treatment correlated with good response; poor responders show a lower baseline HVA and little alteration with neuroleptic treatment
	Chang *et al.* (1988)	(+)	
	Davidson *et al.* (1991)	(+)	
Noradrenergic activity	Sternberg *et al.* (1981, 1982)	(−)	Low CSF levels of dopamine β-hydroxylase in TR
Immunological activity	Van Kammen *et al.* (1994)	(+)	Reduced CSF interleukin-2 immunoreactivity in relapsing patients

TR, treatment resistant; NSS, neurological soft signs; EEG, electroencephalogram; PET, positron emission tomography; GH, growth hormone; HVA, homovanillic acid; CSF, cerebrospinal fluid.

Table 24.3 A representative sample of studies investigating structural brain-imaging parameters and treatment response in schizophrenia

Brain-imaging parameter	Positive association	No association	Comment
Pneumencephalography			
Lateral ventricular enlargement	Cazzullo (1963)		Ventricular enlargement associated with poor treatment response; addition of abnormal electroencephalogram findings increased predictive power
Computerized tomography			
Ventricular brain ratio	Weinberger *et al.* (1980) Schulz *et al.* (1983) Pandurangi *et al.* (1989)	Losonczy *et al.* (1986) Shelton *et al.* (1988) Schulz *et al.* (1989)	Computerized tomography findings have been inconsistent in results in relation to ventricular brain ratio, third ventricular enlargement or sulcal prominence
Third ventricular enlargement	Kaplan *et al.* (1990)	Shelton *et al.* (1988)	
Sulcal prominence	Kaiya *et al.* (1989) Friedman *et al.* (1991)	Nasrallah *et al.* (1983) Nimgaonkar *et al.* (1988)	
Magnetic resonance			
Qualitative/focal abnormalities	Lieberman *et al.* (1989)		Excess of focal findings in treatment-resistant patients
Ventricular volume	Lieberman *et al.* (1993)	Miller *et al.* (1991)	Lateral and third ventricular volume associated with poor treatment response
Cerebellar vermis: brain ratio	Uematsu and Kaiya (1988)		Smaller vermis:brain ratio in treatment-responsive patients

A more complete list of imaging studies is reviewed by Friedman *et al.* (1992).

psychotics (Baldessarini *et al.*, 1988).

PET studies (Smith *et al.*, 1988; Wolkin *et al.*, 1989; Wolkin, 1990) combining measurements of plasma antipsychotic levels with dopamine occupancy have indicated a close relationship between receptor occupancy and plasma values at blood levels of 5–15 ng/ml, levels which are essentially indistinguishable from those cited in clinical studies evaluating clinical response and blood levels of antipsychotics (Rifkin *et al.*, 1991); moreover, above serum values of 20 ng/ml, an asymptotic relationship exists between PET receptor occupancy and plasma level, consistent with the frequent clinical observation that further increases in antipsychotic dosage in most non-responsive patients do not result in any substantial symptomatic benefit (Wolkin, 1990).

At another level, the role of high expressed emotion (HEE) in the persistence of illness represents an alternative, but equally important, variable (see Chapter 29 for full discussion). While this relationship is complex, it does not appear to be mediated through the emergence of medication non-compliance in patients from HEE families, but rather, appears to act via a psychophysiological/ stress-diathesis mechanism (Kavanagh, 1992).

Treatment strategies

The advent of clozapine and other atypical antipsychotics (see Chapters 18 and 25) as effective treatment options for treatment-resistant patients has necessitated a re-evaluation of the guidelines for pharmacological management of treatment resistance. Treatment algorithms for the poorly responsive schizophrenic patient need to be clearly delineated, perhaps analogous to severe medical conditions such as treatment-resistant rheumatoid arthritis, for which there are recognized guidelines for the use of first-line, second-line and more aggressive treatment options (Kushner & Dawson, 1992). To date, issues concerning the definitions of treatment-resistant schizophrenia (see earlier) and the determination of which agents may be of use in such circumstances have dominated our research and clinical practice, and we have yet to incorporate these aspects within a coherent treatment algorithm. Such endeavours require consideration of the risk:benefit *and* cost:benefit ratios of each potential treatment option. For instance, although the efficacy of clozapine in the treatment of well-characterized treatment-resistant patients is clearly established (Kane *et al.*, 1988; Naber & Hippius, 1990; see also Chapter 25), the risks and side-effect profile of this drug have led to a disparity around the world in its use in partial responders or treatment-responsive patients. Furthermore, these issues are also intricately related to more complex fiscal and health-care provision concerns which continue to influence the wider implementation of clozapine treatment (Healy, 1993). Thus, indications for use of augmentation strategies as opposed to direct initiation of treatment with clozapine will vary widely from country to country, reflecting health-policy issues perhaps more than clinical requirements. In addition, other important research questions remain to be answered. For example, clozapine has to date been compared only in relation to standard antipsychotic medications alone, and it is unclear whether a particular augmentation treatment might achieve comparable results to those observed with clozapine. In the absence of such research, it seems appropriate to recommend clozapine as the treatment of choice for the clearly treatment-resistant patient and to use augmentation strategies in the partial responder or those

who do not wish to take this drug or who cannot tolerate clozapine treatment. However, such first-line and second-line treatment recommendations are presently dependent upon the issues discussed above and are likely to vary greatly in clinical application and to be subject to change as further research and treatments become available. Presently, the most frequently used augmentation strategies include the addition of lithium, carbamazepine, benzodiazepines, serotonin agonists or ECT (Table 24.4).

The introduction of lithium into the USA led to some earlier trials of its efficacy as a single agent in the treatment of schizophrenia, the results of which were disappointing [see Schulz *et al.* (1990) for review]. Small *et al.* (1975) initially investigated the response to lithium augmentation of neuroleptic treatment among 22 neuroleptic-resistant patients, and found a distinct benefit with the addition of lithium; this effect was not confined to improvement in agitation but also in psychotic symptoms. Subsequent studies (Biederman *et al.*, 1979; Growe *et al.*, 1979; Carmen *et al.*, 1981) have confirmed this benefit, pointing to a synergistic mechanism of effect, and have collectively demonstrated a low level of side effects. However, more recent research, as part of the National Institute of Mental Health (NIMH) treatment strategies in schizophrenia collaborative study, does not support the initial optimism for the efficacy of lithium as an augmenting agent (Schulz *et al.*, unpublished data), although all patients in this study were out-patients — a significant difference from the first four studies. Wilson (1993) has also not found lithium to be an effective augmenting agent in state hospital patients. When used in clinical practice, careful monitoring of lithium serum levels and use of lithium dosages within the range for treating bipolar disorder are recommended. Also, high doses of neuroleptic should be avoided during lithium augmentation, especially in light of more recent speculation concerning a causal effect of lithium in some cases of neuroleptic malignant syndrome (Buckley *et al.*, 1991).

The rationale for introducing trials of carbamazepine to augment the neuroleptic effect in

Table 24.4 Augmentation strategies in treatment-resistant schizophrenia

Agent	Comment
Lithium	Blood level of 0.6–0.8 mEq/l; monitor of lithium side effects and serum level; neurotoxicity
Carbamazepine	Blood level of 9–12 ng/ml; monitor for side effects and serum level ± neuroleptic blood level (due to enzyme induction); helpful in patients with aggressive/idiopathic electroencephalogram abnormalities
Benzodiazepines	May reduce delusions, thought disorder and anxiety; sedation, withdrawal symptoms and psychotic relapse may be problematic
Azopirones	Buspirone (15–40 mg/day) may reduce anxiety and negative symptoms
Reserpine	Rarely used now, as hypotension and depression limit tolerability; efficacy not clearly established
Propranolol	Rarely used now, as hypotension and depression limit tolerability; efficacy not clearly established
Endorphins, vasopressin, cholecystokinin, verapamil, GABAergic drugs	Efficacy not clearly established; GABAergic drugs may have role in concomitant tardive dyskinesia
L-dopa, bromocriptine, d-amphetamine	May ameliorate persistent negative symptoms; risk of precipitating relapse
Electroconvulsive therapy	Agitation, perplexity, depressed mood may favour good response; maintenance treatment required but risk of side effects (e.g. memory loss) may outweigh limited efficacy

GABA, gamma-aminobutyric acid.

treatment-resistant patients lies in its antiepileptic efficacy and in the observation that patients with schizophrenia who manifest violent behaviour frequently exhibit EEG abnormalities. In a double-blind study of chronically psychotic patients with temporal lobe abnormalities on EEG, observed in the absence of any overt seizures (Neppe, 1983), nine out of 11 patients benefited from concomitant carbamazepine treatment. The addition of carbamazepine has proved of benefit in aggressive, treatment-unresponsive patients [see Schulz *et al.* (1990) for review]. However, carbamazepine does not appear to be superior to lithium in its augmenting effect (Schulz *et al.* 1989, 1990), nor does it possess significant effect when administered independently of neuroleptics

(Carpenter *et al.*, 1991). Careful serial monitoring of carbamazepine serum levels is advisable; furthermore, plasma levels of antipsychotics may also require monitoring as carbamazepine is known to influence the metabolism of these drugs (Kahn *et al.*, 1990).

Although benzodiazepines have a longer history of use as an augmenting agent (Wolkowitz & Pickar, 1991), they share many characteristics with the other agents; namely, their effect is limited to combination treatment with neuroleptics alone, is seen in a minority of patients, reduces positive symptomatology (perhaps also negative symptoms) and (more critically) the persistence of effect over time is unclear (Wolkowitz *et al.*, 1990). Claims for superior efficacy of high-potency over low-potency agents are presently unsubstantiated (Csernansky *et al.*, 1988; Wolkowitz *et al.*, 1988). Since the dose required to be effective is relatively modest (mean dose of alprazolam of 2.8 mg — Wolkowitz *et al.*, 1988), concerns about rebound of psychotic symptoms may be minimized by using a gradual withdrawal regimen.

Interest in serotonergic interactions in schizophrenia and recognition that patients may show different pharmacological responsivity has prompted trials of 5-hydroxytryptamine (5-HT) agonists in treatment-resistant patients. A recent open trial of buspirone in 20 patients indicated a modest improvement in symptomatology, particularly in depressive and anxiety features (Goff *et al.*, 1991). However, since plasma haloperidol levels also rose by 26%, a direct clinical effect attributable to the addition of buspirone is speculative and must await further investigation. The efficacy of 5-HT reuptake inhibitors in treatment-resistant patients has also been examined (Goff *et al.*, 1990; Silver & Nasser, 1992). Fluoxetine added to antipsychotic medication produced substantial improvements in both positive and negative symptoms in a small open trial (Goff *et al.*, 1990), while fluvoxamine augmentation was shown to ameliorate negative symptoms in another study (Silver & Nasser, 1992).

Reserpine and propranolol have also been advocated as effective agents in treatment-resistant schizophrenia (Hayes & Schulz, 1983; Berlant, 1990; Christison *et al.*, 1991). However, the results of limited studies are conflicting, and at the dosages typically employed optimal treatment dosage may be constrained by the hypotensive effect of these agents. In addition, pharmacokinetic interactions with antipsychotic drugs may complicate the use of propranolol, other β-adrenergic drugs, or other potential augmentation agents (Goff & Baldessarini, 1993). A range of experimental agents (e.g. endorphins, vasopressin, CCK and gamma-aminobutyric acidergic agonists) and other agents (e.g. verapamil) have also been tried but, in general, study samples are small (Christison *et al.*, 1991) and results are not encouraging. Although dopaminergic drugs or stimulants (L-dopa, bromo-

criptine, d-amphetamine) may also induce psychotic exacerbations, the addition of these agents may be helpful in some patients with predominantly negative symptomatology.

The use of ECT in treatment-resistant schizophrenia is discussed in Chapter 26.

Managing the poorly responsive patient

Although there has been increased attention on persistently ill patients in the last 15 years, treatment strategies have followed trial and error practices, resulting in an insufficient trial of individual antipsychotics or inappropriate dosage regimens, such as high-dose therapy (Hirsch & Barnes, 1994). Greater appreciation of the complexity of treatment resistance confers the need to procure all available data on previous treatments, hospitalizations and subsequent care to determine the range and duration of treatments employed and their efficacy with regard to *both* symptomatology and level of sustained social functioning. Furthermore, this historical approach will provide a useful vantage point to carefully re-evaluate the diagnosis and detail the distinct pattern of symptomatology (e.g. comorbid depressive or anxiety symptoms) (Table 24.5). Presently, we lack sufficient research data on the differential treatment responsivity of treatment-resistant patients with persistent depressive, anxiety or obsessional symptoms, but it nevertheless seems intuitive that such patients may have different treatment needs. More evidence is available to suggest that substance abusers have specific treatment requirements and, possibly, a different pharmacological responsivity (Buckley *et al.*, 1994). In addition, a small minority of patients may have unforeseen physical illness which may contribute to poor treatment response and chronicity of illness. Appropriate evaluation for this is important. The determination of the presence and severity of tardive dyskinesia — objectively quantified using a rating scale — is a further facet of the assessment of these patients and will be important in the choice of subsequent pharmacological treatment.

If it appears that the patient has had an insuf-

Table 24.5 Important considerations in the evaluation and management of the treatment-resistant patient

Historical	Current	Prospective
Premorbid function	Clarity of diagnosis	Need for therapeutic trial to establish poor response
Persistence of symptoms	Secondary disabilities	Integration of psychosocial and rehabilitative measures
Psychosocial attainment	Current physical illness	Objective assessment of improvement and residual impairments, side effects, tardive dyskinesia
Neuroleptic treatment	Tardive dyskinesia	
Type		
Dosage	Substance abuse	
Duration		
Side effects	Compliance/motivation	
Compliance	Current strengths/level of support	
Level of social support	Level of insight	

ficient trial of a standard antipsychotic, then a prospective trial should be given. Reinstituting treatment with a conventional antipsychotic drug to affirm a suspected poor response necessitates a duration of at least 4–6 weeks of close observation of symptomatic and behavioural change. In some cases, estimating the blood level of the antipsychotic may be helpful. However, patients who have already experienced standard treatment and are on high-dose or polypharmacy treatment should be considered for a period of drug reduction or a no-medication holiday (Van Putten *et al.*, 1988). This should help determine whether continued symptoms are in part due to side effects of akathisia, parkinsonism or toxic effects of the current regime. Drug administration needs to be closely monitored to ensure compliance and to check for the emergence of side effects; intolerance to antipsychotics is a not infrequent attribute in such patients. This assessment should preferably incorporate rating scales to objectify treatment response or lack thereof. This process demands a good therapeutic relationship between the patient and clinician, and the patient should be given an understandable rationale for the treatment programme with emphasis on the need to comply so that the clinician can achieve at least a 6-week duration of specific treatment before the adequacy of therapeutic response is determined. Blood-level determinations may be helpful in

a small group of patients. Furthermore, such a programme should encompass the wider dimensions of multidisciplinary treatment, including behavioural, cognitive and social skills management. These approaches may prove beneficial even in those patients with marked disabilities and are discussed in Chapter 30. Finally, the issue of which augmentation strategy or, alternatively, whether to opt directly for clozapine treatment in these patients has been discussed earlier.

Concluding remarks

Patients who are poorly responsive to treatment with antipsychotic medication represent the most disadvantaged sector of our services and, accordingly, merit particular consideration for further research. Clear delineation of treatment resistance and of the range of symptomatic and functional disabilities are the cornerstones of devising an appropriate management plan in such cases. Effective treatment relies upon the close integration of behavioural, psychosocial and pharmacological components. Hopefully, future developments in our understanding of the neurobiological mechanism(s) underlying treatment resistance will result in more specific and efficacious treatment options than are presently available.

References

Baldessarini, R.J., Cohen, B.M. & Teicher, M.H. (1988) Significance of neuroleptic dose and plasma level in the pharmacological treatment of psychoses. *Archives of General Psychiatry*, **45**, 79–91.

Barkto, G., Frecska, E., Horvath, S., Zador, G. & Arato, M. (1990) Predicting neuroleptic response from a combination of multilevel variables in acute schizophrenic patients. *Acta Psychiatrica Scandinavica*, **82**, 408–412.

Barkto, G., Frecska, E., Zador, G. & Herczeg, I. (1989) Neurological features, cognitive impairment, and neuroleptic response in schizophrenic patients. *Schizophrenia Research*, **2**, 311–313.

Beasley, C.M., Magnusson, M. & Garver, D.L. (1984) TSH response to TRH and haloperidol response latency in psychosis. *Biological Psychiatry*, **52**, 714–716.

Berlant, J.L. (1990) Presynaptic modulators of dopamine synthesis in the treatment of chronic schizophrenia. In Angrist, B. & Schulz, S.C. (eds) *The Neuroleptic Nonresponsive Patient: Characterization and Treatment*, pp. 137–152. American Psychiatric Association, Washington DC.

Biederman, J., Lerner, Y. & Belmaker, R.H. (1979) Combination of lithium carbonate and haloperidol in schizoaffective disorder: a controlled study. *Archives of General Psychiatry*, **36**, 327–333.

Bitter, I., Volovka, J. & Scheurer, J. (1991) The concept of the neuroleptic threshold: an update. *Journal of Clinical Psychopharmacology*, **11**, 28–33.

Bowers, M.B. Jr (1990) Catecholamine metabolites in plasma as correlates of neuroleptic response. In Angrist, B. & Schulz, S.C. (eds) *The Neuroleptic Nonresponsive Patient: Characterization and Treatment*, pp. 23–33. American Psychiatric Association, Washington DC.

Bowers, M.B. Jr, Swigar, M.E. & Jatlow, P.I. (1984) Plasma catecholamine metabolites and early response to haloperidol. *Journal of Clinical Psychiatry*, **45**, 249–251.

Brenner, H.D., Dencker, S.J., Goldstein, M.J. *et al.* (1990) Defining treatment refractoriness in schizophrenia. *Schizophrenia Bulletin* **16(4)**, 551–561.

Brown, W.A. & Herz, L.R. (1989) Response to neuroleptic drugs as a device for classifying schizophrenia. *Schizophrenia Bulletin*, **15(1)**, 123–129.

Buchanan, R., Brier, A., Kirkpatrick, B. & Carpenter, W. Jr (1993) Structural differences between 'deficit' and 'non-deficit' forms of schizophrenia. *American Journal of Psychiatry*, **150**, 89–94.

Buchsbaum, M.S., Potkin, S.G., Siegel, B.V. *et al.* (1992) Striatal metabolic rate and clinical response to neuroleptics in schizophrenia. *Archives of General Psychiatry*, **49**, 966–974.

Buckley, P., Freyne, A., McCarthy, A. & Larkin, C. (1991) Neuroleptic malignant syndrome. *Irish Journal of Medical Science*, **6**, 125–130.

Buckley, P., Way, L., Thompson, P. & Meltzer, H.Y. (1994) Substance abuse in treatment-resistant schizophrenic patients: implications for clozapine therapy. *American Journal of Psychiatry*, **151**, 354–359.

Carmen, J., Bigelow, L.B. & Wyatt, R.H. (1981) Lithium combined with neuroleptics in chronic schizophrenic and schizoaffective patients. *Journal of Clinical Psychiatry*, **42**, 124–128.

Carpenter, W.T., Kurz, R., Kirkpatrick, B. *et al.* (1991) Carbamazepine maintenance treatment in outpatient schizophrenics. *Archives of General Psychiatry*, **48**, 69–72.

Cazzullo, C.L. (1963) Biological and clinical studies on schizophrenia related to pharmacological treatment. *Recent Advances in Biological Psychiatry*, **5**, 114–143.

Chang, W., Chen, T. & Lee, C. (1988) Plasma homovanillic acid levels and subtyping of schizophrenia. *Psychiatry Research*, **23**, 261–267.

Christison, G.W., Kirch, D.G. & Wyatt, R.J. (1991) When symptoms persist: choosing among alternative somatic treatments for schizophrenia. *Schizophrenia Bulletin*, **17**, 217–245.

Crow, T.J. (1980) Molecular pathology of schizophrenia. More than one disease process? *British Medical Journal*, **1**, 66–68.

Csernansky, J.G., Kaplan, J. & Hollister, L.E. (1985) Problems in classification of schizophrenics as neuroleptic responders and nonresponders. *Journal of Nervous Mental Disorders*, **173**, 325–331.

Csernansky, J.G., Riney, S.J., Lombroso, L., Overall, J.E. & Hollister, L.E. (1988) Double-blind comparison of alprazolam, diazepam, and placebo for the treatment of negative schizophrenic symptoms. *Archives of General Psychiatry*, **45**, 655–659.

Dalen, P. & Hayes, P. (1990) The aetiological heterogeneity of schizophrenia: the problem and the evidence. *British Journal of Psychiatry*, **157**, 119–122.

Daniel, D.G. & Weinberger, D.R. (1991) Ex multi uno: a case for neurobiological homogeneity in schizophrenia. In Tamminga, C.A. & Schulz, S.C. (eds) *Advances in Neuropsychiatry and Psychopharmacology, Schizophrenia Research*, Vol. 1, pp. 227–235. Raven Press, New York.

Davidson, M., Kahn, R.S., Knott, P. *et al.* (1991) The effect of neuroleptic treatment on plasma homovanillic acid concentrations and schizophrenic symptoms. *Archives of General Psychiatry*, **48**, 910–913.

Davis, J.M., Erickson, S. & Dekirmenjian, H. (1978) Plasma levels of antipsychotic drugs and clinical response. In Lipton, L.A., DiMascio, A. & Killam, K.F. (eds) *Psychopharmacology: A Generation of Progress*, pp. 905–916. Raven Press, New York.

Elizur, A., Segal, Z. & Yeret, A. (1979) Antipsychotic effect of propranolol on chronic schizophrenics: study of a gradual treatment regimen. *Psychopharmacology*, **60**, 189–194.

Friedman, L., Knutson, L., Shurell, M. & Meltzer, H.Y. (1991) Prefrontal sulcal prominence is inversely related to response to clozapine in schizophrenia. *Biological Psychiatry*, **29**, 865–877.

Friedman, L., Lys, C. & Schulz, S.C. (1992) The relationship of structural brain imaging parameters to antipsychotic treatment response: a review. *Journal of Psychiatry and Neuroscience*, **17**, 42–54.

Garver, D.L., Kelly, K., Fried, K.A., Magnusson, M. & Hirschowitz, J. (1988) Drug response patterns as a basis of nosology for the mood-incongruent psychoses (the schizophrenias). *Psychological Medicine*, **18**, 873–885.

Goff, D.C. & Baldessarini, R.J. (1993) Drug interactions with antipsychotic agents. *Journal of Clinical Psychopharmacology*, **13**, 57–67.

Goff, D.C., Brotman, A.W., Waites, M. & McCormick, S. (1990) Trial of fluoxetine added to neuroleptics for treatment-resistant schizophrenic patients. *American Journal of Psychiatry*, **47**, 492–494.

Goff, D.C., Midha, K.K., Brotman, A.W., McCormick, S., Waites, M. & Anies, E.T. (1991) An open trial of buspirone added to neuroleptics in schizophrenic patients. *Journal of Clinical Psychopharmacology*, **11**, 193–197.

Goldberg, S.C. (1985) Negative and deficit symptoms in schizophrenia do respond to neuroleptics. *Schizophrenia Bulletin*, **11**, 453–456.

Goldberg, T.E., Greenberg, R.D., Griffin, S.J. *et al.* (1993) The effect of clozapine on cognition and psychiatric symptoms in patients with schizophrenia. *British Journal of Psychiatry*, **162**, 43–48.

Goldberg, T.E., Weinberger, D.R., Berman, K.F., Pliskin, N.H. & Podd, M.H. (1987) Further evidence of dementia of the prefrontal type in schizophrenia? *Archives of General Psychiatry*, **44**, 1008–1014.

Green, M.F., Nuechterlein, K.H., Ventura, J. & Mintz, J. (1990) The temporal relationship between depressive and psychotic symptoms in recent-onset schizophrenia. *American Journal of Psychiatry*, **147**, 179–182.

Growe, G.A., Crayton, J.A. & Klass, D.B. (1979) Lithium in chronic schizophrenia. *American Journal of Psychiatry*, **136**, 454–455.

Hall, W.B., Vestre, N.D., Schiele, B.C. & Zimmerman, R. (1968) A controlled comparison of haloperidol and fluphenazine in chronic treatment-resistant schizophrenics. *Diseases of the Nervous System*, **29**, 405–408.

Hayes, P.E. & Schulz, S.C. (1983) The use of beta-adrenergic blocking agents in anxiety disorders and schizophrenia. *Psychopharmacology*, **3**, 101–117.

Healy, D. (1993) Psychopharmacology and the ethics of resource allocation. *British Journal of Psychiatry*, **162**, 23–28.

Heinrichs, D.W., Hanlon, E.T. & Carpenter, W.T. Jr (1984) The quality of life scale: an instrument for rating the deficit syndrome. *Schizophrenia Bulletin*, **10**, 388–398.

Hirsch, S.R. & Barnes, T.R.E. (1994) Clinical use of high-dose neuroleptics. *British Journal of Psychiatry*, **164**, 94–96.

Hoff, A.L., Riordan, M., O'Donnell, D.W., Morris, L. & DeLisi, L.E. (1992) Neuropsychological functioning of first-episode schizophrenic patients. *American Journal of Psychiatry*, **147**, 898–903.

Itil, T.M. & Shapiro, D. (1981) Computerized EEG as a predictor of response in treatment resistant schizophrenia. *Journal of Nervous Mental Disorders*, **169**, 629–634.

Johnstone, E.C., McMillan, F.J., Frith, C.D., Benn, D.K. & Crow, T.J. (1990) Further investigation of the predictors of outcome following first schizophrenic episodes. *British Journal of Psychiatry*, **157**, 182–189.

Kahn, E.M., Schulz, S.C., Perel, J.M. & Alexander, J.E. (1990) Change in haloperidol level due to carbamazepine: a complicating medication for schizophrenia. *Journal of*

Clinical Psychopharmacology, **10**, 54–57.

Kahn, R.S. & Davidson, M. (1993) On the value of measuring dopamine, norepinephrine and their metabolites in schizophrenia. *Neuropsychopharmacology*, **8**, 93–95.

Kaiya, H., Uematsu, M., Ofuji, M., Nishida, A., Morikiyo, M. & Adachi, S. (1989) Computerized tomography in schizophrenia. Familial versus non-familial forms of illness. *British Journal of Psychiatry*, **155**, 444–450.

Kane, J., Honigfeld, G., Singer, J., Meltzer, H.Y. & The Clozaril Collaborative Study Group (1988) Clozapine for the treatment-resistant schizophrenia: a double-blind comparison with chlorpromazine. *Archives of General Psychiatry*, **45**, 789–796.

Kane, J., Honigfeld, G., Singer, J. & Meltzer, H.Y. (1990) Is clozapine response different in neuroleptic nonresponders vs partial responders? *Archives of General Psychiatry*, **47**, 189.

Kane, J.M., Kinon, B., Perovich, R. & Johns, C. (1992) Alternative treatments for nonresponding patients. *Schizophrenia Research*, **6(2)**, 108.

Kaplan, M.J., Laff, M., Kelly, K., Lukin, R. & Garver, D.L. (1990) Enlargement of cerebral third ventricle in psychotic patients with delayed response to neuroleptics. *Biological Psychiatry*, **27**, 205–214.

Kavanagh, D.J. (1992) Recent developments in expressed emotion. *British Journal of Psychiatry*, **160**, 611–620.

Keefe, R.E., Mohs, R.C., Silverman, J.M., Losonczy, M.F., Davidson, M., Horvath, T.B. & Davis, K.L. (1990) Characteristics of Kraepelinian schizophrenia and their relationship to premorbid sociosexual functioning. In Angrist, B. & Schulz, S.C. (eds) *The Neuroleptic Nonresponsive Patient: Characterization and Treatment*, pp. 3–21. American Psychiatric Association, Washington DC.

Keith, S.J., Matthews, S.M. & Schooler, N.R. (1991) Psychosocial treatment of schizophrenia: a review of psycho-educational family approaches. In Tamminga, C.A. & Schulz, S.C. (eds) *Schizophrenia Research*, pp. 247–254. Raven Press, New York.

Kenny, J.T. & Schulz, S.C. (1993) Neuropsychological functioning in adolescent psychosis. *Schizophrenia Research*, **9**, 180.

Kolakowska, T., Williams, A.O., Ardern, M. *et al.* (1985) Schizophrenia with good and poor outcome. *British Journal of Psychiatry*, **146**, 229–246.

Kushner, I. & Dawson, N.V. (1992) Changing perspectives in the treatment of RA. *Journal of Rheumatology*, **19(12)**, 1831–1834.

Lieberman, J.A., Alvir, J.M., Woerner, M. *et al.* (1992) Prospective study of psychobiology in first-episode schizophrenia at Hillside Hospital. *Schizophrenia Bulletin*, **18**, 351–372.

Lieberman, J.A., Jody, D., Geisler, S. *et al.* (1993) Time course and biological predictors of treatment response in first-episode schizophrenia. *Archives of General Psychiatry*, **50**, 369–376.

Lieberman, J.A, Jody, D., Geisler, S. *et al.* (1989) Treatment outcome of first-episode schizophrenia. *Psychopharmacology Bulletin*, **25**, 92–96.

Loebel, A.D., Lieberman, J.A., Alvir, J.M.J., Mayerhoff, D.I., Geisler, S.H. & Szymanski, S.R. (1992) Duration of psychosis and outcome in first-episode schizophrenia. *American Journal of Psychiatry*, **149**, 1183–1188.

Losonczy, M.F., Song, I.S., Mohs, R.C. *et al.* (1986) Correlates of lateral ventricular size in chronic schizophrenia. I. Behavioral and treatment response measures. *American Journal of Psychiatry*, **143**, 976–981.

McCreadie, R.G. & McDonald, I.M. (1977) High dosage haloperidol in chronic schizophrenia. *British Journal of Psychiatry*, **131**, 310–316.

Meltzer, H.Y. (1990) Commentary: defining treatment refractoriness in schizophrenia. *Schizophrenia Bulletin*, **16(4)**, 563–565.

Meltzer, H.Y. (1992a) Treatment of the neuroleptic-nonresponsive schizophrenic patient. *Schizophrenia Bulletin*, **18(3)**, 515–542.

Meltzer, H.Y. (1992b) Dimensions of outcome with clozapine. *British Journal of Psychiatry*, **160** (Suppl. 17), 46–53.

Meltzer, H.Y. & Fang, V.S. (1976) The effect of neuroleptics on serum prolactin in schizophrenic patients. *Archives of General Psychiatry*, **33**, 279–286.

Meltzer, H.Y., Sommers, A.A. & Luchins, D.J. (1986) The effect of neuroleptics and other psychotropic drugs on negative symptoms in schizophrenia. *Journal of Clinical Psychopharmacology*, **6**, 329–338.

Miller, D.D., Flaum, M.A., Coryell, W. & Andreasen, N.C. (1991) A magnetic resonance imaging study in schizophrenia comparing treatment response. New Orleans Louisiana. *Society of Biological Psychiatry*, 43A.

Naber, D. & Hippius, H. (1990) The European experience with the use of clozapine. *Hospital and Community Psychiatry*, **41**, 886–890.

Nasrallah, H.A., Kuperman, S. & Hamra, B.J. (1983) Clinical differences between schizophrenic patients with and without enlarged cerebral ventricles. *Journal of Clinical Psychiatry*, **44**, 407–409.

Neppe, V.M. (1983) Carbamazepine as adjunctive treatment in nonepileptic chronic inpatients with EEG temporal lobe abnormalities. *Journal of Clinical Psychiatry*, **44**, 326–330.

Nimgaonkar, V.L., Wessely, S., Tune, L.E. & Murray, R.M. (1988) Response to drugs in schizophrenia: the influence of family history, obstetric complications, and ventricular enlargement. *Psychological Medicine*, **18**, 583–592.

Osser, D.N. & Albert, L.G. (1990) Is clozapine response different in neuroleptic nonresponders vs partial responders? *Archives of General Psychiatry*, **47**, 189.

Pandurangi, A.K., Goldberg, S.C., Brink, D.D., Hill, M.H., Gulati, A.N. & Hamer, R.M. (1989) Amphetamine challenge test, response to treatment, and lateral ventricle size in schizophrenia. *Biological Psychiatry*, **25**, 207–214.

Rifkin, A., Doddi, S., Karajgi, B., Borenstein, M. & Wachspress, M. (1991) Dosage of haloperidol for schizophrenia. *Archives of General Psychiatry*, **48**, 166–170.

Rosen, I. (1957) The clinical significance of obsessions in schizophrenia. *Journal of Mental Sciences*, **103**, 773–785.

Schulz, S.C., Butterfield, L., Garciano, M., Narasimhachari, N. & Friedel, R.O. (1984) Beyond the therapeutic window: a case presentation. *Journal of Clinical Psychiatry*, **45**, 223–225.

Schulz, S.C., Conley, R.R., Kahn, E.M. & Alexander, J.E. (1989) Nonresponders to neuroleptics: a distinct subtype. In Schulz, S.C. & Tamminga, C.A. (eds) *Schizophrenia: Scientific Progress*, pp. 341–350. Oxford University Press, Oxford.

Schulz, S.C., Kahn, E.M., Baker, R.W. & Conley, R.R. (1990) Lithium and carbamazepine augmentation in treatment refractory schizophrenia. In Angrist, B. & Schulz, S.C. (eds) *The Neuroleptic Nonresponsive Patient: Characterization and Treatment*, pp. 109–136. American Psychiatric Association, Washington DC.

Schulz, S.C., Sinicrope, P., Kishore, P. & Friedel, R.O. (1983) Treatment response and ventricular brain enlargement in young schizophrenic patients. *Psychopharmacology Bulletin*, **19**, 510–512.

Seibyl, J.P. & Lieberman, J.A. (1993) Substance abuse and schizophrenia. In Powchichk, P. & Schulz, S.C. (eds) *Psychiatric Clinics of North America*, pp. 123–138. WB Saunders, Philadelphia.

Shelton, R.C., Karson, C.N., Doran, A.R., Pickar, D., Bigelow, L.B. & Weinberger, D.R. (1988) Cerebral structural pathology in schizophrenia: evidence for a selective prefrontal cortical defect. *American Journal of Psychiatry*, **145**, 154–163.

Silver, H. & Nasser, A. (1992) Fluvoxamine improves negative symptoms in treated chronic schizophrenic: an add-on double-blind, placebo-controlled study. *Biological Psychiatry*, **31**, 698–704.

Silverman, J.M., Mohs, R.C., Davidson, M. *et al.* (1987) Familial schizophrenia and treatment response. *American Journal of Psychiatry*, **144**, 1271–1276.

Siris, S.G. (1991) Diagnosis of secondary depression in schizophrenia: implications for DSM-IV. *Schizophrenia Bulletin*, **17**, 75–98.

Siris, S.G., Beranzohn, P.C., Mason, S.E. & Shuwall, M.A. (1994) Maintenance imipramine therapy for secondary depression in schizophrenia. *Archives of General Psychiatry*, **51**, 109–115.

Small, J.G., Kellans, J.J., Milstein, V. & Moore, J. (1975) A placebo-controlled study of lithium combined with neuroleptics in chronic schizophrenic patients. *American Journal of Psychiatry*, **132**, 1315–1317.

Smith, M., Wolf, A.P., Bordie, J.D. *et al.* (1988) Serial (^{18}F)-N-methylspiroperidol PET studies to measure change in antipsychotic drug D2 receptor occupancy in schizophrenic patients. *Biological Psychiatry*, **23(7)**, 653–663.

Sternberg, D.E., Van Kammen, D.P., Lerner, P. & Bunney, W.E. (1982) Schizophrenia: dopamine beta-hydroxylase activity and treatment response. *Science*, **216**, 1423–1425.

Sternberg, D.E., VanKammen, D.P., Lake, C.R., Ballenger, J.C., Marder, S.R. & Bunney, W.E. (1981) The effect of pimozide on CSF norepinephrine in schizophrenia. *American Journal of Psychiatry*, **138**, 1045–1051.

Strauss, J.S. & Carpenter, W.T. (1972) The prediction of outcome in schizophrenia. 1. Characteristics of outcome. *Archives of General Psychiatry*, **27**, 734–746.

Thompson, P.A., Buckley, P.F. & Meltzer, H.Y. (1994) The brief psychiatric rating scale: effect of scaling system on clinical response assessment. *Journal of Clinical Psychopharmacology*, **14**, 344–346.

Uematsu, M. & Kaiya, H. (1988) Cerebellar vernal size predicts drug response in schizophrenic patients: a magnetic resonance imaging (MRI) study. *Progress in Neuropsychopharmacology and Biological Psychiatry*, **12**, 837–848.

Van Kammen, D.P., McAllister, C., Yao, J.K. *et al.* (1994) A clinical and biochemical model of relapse prediction in schizophrenia: a role for CSF interleukin 2? *Schizophrenia Research*, **11**, 128.

Van Putten, T., Marder, S.R., Mintz, J. & Poland, R. (1988) Haloperidol plasma levels and clinical response: a therapeutic relationship. *Psychopharmacology Bulletin*, **24**, 172–175.

Van Putten, T., Marder, S.R., Wirshing, W.C., Aravagiri, M. & Chabert, N. (1991) Neuroleptic plasma levels. *Schizophrenia Bulletin*, **17**, 197–216.

Wallace, C.J. (1986) Functional assessment in rehabilitation. *Schizophrenia Bulletin*, **12**, 604–630.

Weiden, P.J., Dixon, L., Frances, A., Appelbaum, P., Haas, G. & Rapkin, B. (1991) Neuroleptic noncompliance in schizophrenia. In Tamminga, C.A. & Schulz, S.C. (eds) *Schizophrenia Research*, pp. 285–296. Raven Press, New York.

Weinberger, D.R., Bigelow, L.B., Kleinman, J.E., Klein, S.T., Rosenblatt, J.E. & Wyatt, R.J. (1980) Cerebral ventricular enlargement in chronic schizophrenia: association with poor response to treatment. *Archives of General Psychiatry*, **37**, 11–14.

Wilson, W.H. (1993) Addition of lithium to haloperidol in non-affective, antipsychotic non-responsive schizophrenia: a double blind, placebo controlled, parallel design clinical trial. *Psychopharmacology*, **111**, 359–366.

Wolkin, A. (1990) Positron emission tomography and the study of neuroleptic response. In Angrist, B. & Schulz, S.C. (eds) *The Neuroleptic Nonresponsive Patient: Characterization and Treatment*, pp. 35–49. American Psychiatric Association, Washington DC.

Wolkin, A., Barouch, F., Wolf, A.P. *et al.* (1989) Dopamine blockade and clinical response: evidence for two biological subgroups of schizophrenia. *American Journal of Psychiatry*, **146**, 905–908.

Wolkowitz, O.M. & Pickar, D. (1991) Benzodiazepines in the treatment of schizophrenia: a review and re-appraisal. *American Journal of Psychiatry*, **48**, 714–726.

Wolkowitz, O.M., Rapoport, M.H. & Pickar, D. (1990) Benzodiazepine augmentation of neuroleptics. In Angrist, B. & Schulz, S.C. (eds) *The Neuroleptic Nonresponsive Patient: Characterization and Treatment*, pp. 87–108. American Psychiatric Association, Washington DC.

Wolkowitz, O.M., Breier, A., Doran, A. *et al.* (1988) Alprazolam augmentation of the antipsychotic effects of fluphenazine in schizophrenic patients. *Archives of General Psychiatry*, **45**, 664–671.

Wyatt, R.J. (1991) Neuroleptics and the natural course of schizophrenia. *Schizophrenia Bulletin*, **17**, 325–351.

Chapter 25
Atypical Antipsychotic Drug Therapy for Treatment-Resistant Schizophrenia

H. Y. MELTZER

Summary

Clozapine has superior efficacy for positive, negative and disorganization symptoms in treatment-resistant schizophrenic patients. Because it produces agranulocytosis in 1% of patients, weekly monitoring of white blood cell counts is required for the period of greatest risk. About 60% of treatment-resistant patients may be expected to respond favourably, with some having a nearly complete remission. Clozapine also produces fewer extrapyramidal symptoms (EPS) and has not been shown to cause tardive dyskinesia or dystonia, although it is frequently able to mask the symptoms thereof. The time course of clozapine may be delayed in some patients so that a clinical trial may need to last 6–12 months.

Risperidone and remoxipride are also atypical in that they produce fewer EPS than standard neuroleptics at clinically effective doses. Reports that risperidone at some lower dose range is more effective than haloperidol are intriguing but must be verified. There is, as yet, no evidence that risperidone is effective in treatment-resistant schizophrenia. Remoxipride does not appear to be more effective than typical neuroleptic drugs. Numerous other agents have been selected as potential atypical neuroleptic drugs based on a variety of hypotheses, mostly involving dopaminergic mechanisms.

Introduction

Until clozapine was shown to be an effective treatment for schizophrenic patients resistant to or intolerant of standard antipsychotic drugs, because of parkinsonism and tardive movement disorders, pharmacological treatments, including various types of adjunctive therapies, for these indications have generally provided modest relief at best (see Chapter 24, this volume). Clozapine, although not the first antipsychotic to be called atypical, has become the gold standard for atypical antipsychotics. Various definitions have been used to delimit this class of agents (Meltzer, 1991b). The definition employed here will be the least controversial and simplest — an antipsychotic with a clear advantage with regard to EPS. Differences or similarities with regard to overall efficacy, effect on negative symptoms or prolactin stimulation

485

are considered irrelevant for atypical classification. Other than clozapine, only two new agents, risperidone and remoxipride, available in some European countries and under review in the USA, appear to qualify as atypical. Many other putative atypical antipsychotic drugs are at various stages of development. Thioridazine, a well-studied agent, would meet this simple criterion of atypicality, but because it has been widely utilized and has no efficacy advantages for neuroleptic-resistant patients, will not be discussed here. Rather, the major focus will be on clozapine, the only agent known to be effective in at least a high proportion of treatment-resistant schizophrenic patients, and to a lesser extent, risperidone and remoxipride.

Clozapine

History

Clozapine, a dibenzazepine tricyclic chemically related to loxapine, was first synthesized in 1959. It was introduced in Europe in the late 1960s as a treatment for schizohrenia (Schmutz & Eichenberger, 1982). Consistent with preclinical studies which demonstrated that it produced no catalepsy in rodents, although it blocked amphetamine-induced locomotor activity, its main advantages compared with other antipsychotic drugs appeared to be fewer acute and subacute EPS (Hippius, 1989). The populations of the initial, relatively small-scale clinical trials of clozapine compared with antipsychotic drugs may be assumed to have included mainly those schizophrenic patients with a poor history of response to typical neuroleptic drugs. More than half these studies found clozapine to be superior to typical neuroleptic drugs, while others found no advantage with clozapine. Superiority with regards to EPS was generally found for clozapine (Baldessarini & Frankenberg, 1991).

In 1975, clozapine was implicated as the proximate cause of eight deaths due to agranulocytosis (Amsler *et al.*, 1977). These deaths occurred mainly in elderly patients who were receiving other drugs. Lack of awareness that agranulocytosis might be a consequence of clozapine administration definitely contributed to the high mortality rate. This led to its withdrawal from general use in Europe and cessation of further development in the USA because there was, at that time, no definite evidence of marked advantages over other antipsychotic drugs. Subsequently, a number of the original group of schizophrenic patients who received clozapine were allowed to receive it again because substitution of other antipsychotic drugs led to significant deterioration in clinical status (Povlsen *et al.*, 1985; Lindström, 1988). Clozapine also remained available to some clinicians in Europe and the USA for clinical research purposes, to study its mechanism of action, as well as for humanitarian purposes, to treat cases of resistant schizophrenia or severe tardive dyskinesia, which often seemed to respond better to clozapine than to other drugs (Meltzer & Luchins, 1984). Over the next decade, clinical experience with clozapine suggested that it was more effective, in some instances, than standard neuroleptic agents with regard to suppression of the symptoms of tardive dyskinesia as well as to control schizophrenia. Furthermore, during this era of restricted use, no new cases of tardive dyskinesia associated with clozapine treatment emerged, although no definitive data to establish this critical point could be obtained. In addition, clozapine was shown not to increase plasma prolactin (PRL) levels in humans (Meltzer *et al.*, 1979). This positive experience with clozapine stimulated the manufacturer to petition the US Food and Drug Administration (FDA) to approve clozapine for use in patients who had moderate−severe tardive dyskinesia. Despite the absence of controlled data, the evidence offered in support of this proposal earned the approval of the FDA Psychopharmacology Advisory Board. However, the FDA staff required controlled study data. In order to obtain these data, a double-blind study comparing clozapine and chlorpromazine in treatment-resistant schizophrenic patients was initiated. The patients to be included in this study had a history of failure to respond to three or more typical neuroleptic drugs, moderate−severe positive psychotic symptoms and poor social function for at least 2 years prior to entry. In the initial phase of the study, a 6-week open trial of haloperidol documented the neuroleptic resistance of these patients. All the non-responders to haloperidol and a few haloperidol-intolerant patients entered the double-blind phase. Of nearly 150 clozapine-treated patients, 30% responded within 6 weeks of clozapine treatment compared with only 4% of an equal number of chlorpromazine-treated patients (Kane *et al.*, 1988). The clozapine-treated patients improved on negative as well as positive symptoms and had fewer EPS. These data led to the approval of clozapine in 1989 in the USA for neuroleptic-resistant schizophrenic patients. Subsequently, clozapine has been approved for use in the UK, Canada, France, Israel and Italy, as well as a variety of Asian and South American countries.

Indications

Treatment-resistant schizophrenia

The major indication for clozapine is in the treatment of neuroleptic-resistant schizophrenia, i.e. patients who have an unsatisfactory response to typical neuroleptic drugs (Lieberman *et al.*, 1989; Meltzer, 1992). Neuroleptic-resistant patients will generally have at least moderate positive, negative or disorganization (incoherence, loose associations, inappropriate affect and poverty of thought content) symptoms (Liddle *et al.*, 1992; Thompson & Meltzer, 1993), or one of the above, and impaired social function, despite at least two adequate trials of typical antipsychotic drugs chosen from two or more different classes of these agents (Kane *et al.*, 1988). These trials should be at least 6 weeks in duration and span a range of dosages. The generally accepted norm to establish treatment resistance is at least two trials of neuroleptic drugs for at least 6 weeks each at doses equal to $10-20$ mg haloperidol per day or its equivalent (Meltzer, 1992). Lieberman *et al.* (1993) reported that 12 out of 70 (17%) first-admission schizophrenic patients had not had a complete remission by the end of 12 months of neuroleptic treatment, despite several trials of neuroleptic

drugs. Other patients first become treatment resistant at a later phase of their illness (Huber *et al.*, 1975; Ciompi, 1980; McGlashan, 1988; Brier *et al.*, 1991). However, Shaler *et al.* (1993) recently reported that with three successive trials of different neuroleptics, 57 out of 60 (95%) schizophrenic patients had at least a 30% improvement in brief psychiatric rating scale (BPRS) scores. The idiosyncratic nature of referral patterns and inclusion in trials accounts for much of the variance in these results. However, recent studies suggest that even one unsuccessful prolonged trial of a neuroleptic drug may identify neuroleptic-resistant patients. The standard for what constitutes an unsatisfactory response to neuroleptic drugs will vary widely. Return to best premorbid function should be considered as a standard (Meltzer, 1990). Patients who are unable to return to their previous level of social and intellectual function, despite control of positive, negative and disorganization symptoms, may be candidates for clozapine treatment. This may be based on cognitive dysfunction, which is sometimes helped by clozapine and not by standard neuroleptic drugs (Hagger *et al.*, 1993). It should be noted, however, that one study found no benefit of clozapine on any aspect of cognitive function studies (Goldberg *et al.*, 1993). However, this study involved only 15 subjects. Six of the patients were receiving lithium carbonate, which has been reported to have adverse neurological consequences when combined with clozapine (Blake *et al.*, 1992). Neuroleptic-intolerant patients, i.e. patients with tardive dyskinesia of at least moderate severity despite optimal adjustment of neuroleptic dosage, and patients who cannot tolerate therapeutic doses of low EPS-producing antipsychotic drugs, such as thioridazine, are also often considered as candidates for clozapine, although no FDA approval for these indications has been given. Its use in such patients seems entirely appropriate to the author once the risks, benefits and alternatives have been explained to the patients, along with significant others or guardians, and an informed consent has been obtained. As will be discussed, risperidone or remoxipride may be useful in some of these patients.

There are no known teratogenic risks of clozapine (Sandoz, personal communication). Fourteen normal births have been recorded in clozapine-treated women. Nevertheless, clozapine should be used cautiously in pregnant women, and clozapine-treated women should not nurse their children.

Clozapine has been used with generally favourable results in small numbers of psychotic children and young adolescents who are poor responders to typical neuroleptic drugs. It has been successfully used in elderly neuroleptic-resistant or intolerant schizophrenic patients, but at lower dosages.

Non-treatment-resistant schizophrenia

Twelve studies have compared the efficacy of clozapine with standard neuroleptic drugs in a broad spectrum of patients with schizophrenia, of whom at most a minority were treatment resistant. In ten of these studies, clozapine was reported to have an advantage over typical neuroleptic drugs with regard to global psychopathology or specific positive symptoms (Angst *et al.*, 1971; Ekblom & Häggström, 1974; Fischer-Cornelssen *et al.*, 1974; Gerlach *et al.*, 1974; Singer & Law, 1974; Vencovsky *et al.*, 1975; Fischer-Cornelssen & Ferner, 1976; Gelenberg & Doller, 1979; Shopsin *et al.*, 1979; Claghorn *et al.*, 1987), whereas clozapine was reported to be equal in efficacy to typical antipsychotic drugs in the other two studies (Chiu *et al.*, 1976; Guirguis *et al.*, 1977). Despite this impressive evidence, these data are still insufficient to establish the risk:benefit ratio for clozapine treatment of neuroleptic-responsive schizophrenic patients. This must be developed in controlled trials which will probably have to be of longer duration and larger sample size than for treatment-resistant patients, and balanced against the possibility that other safer antipsychotic drugs under development will have similar advantages over standard drugs. Were the risk of clozapine to be reduced by advances in prediction of agranulocytosis, the issue of clozapine as a first-line drug should be re-examined.

Other indications

There are some non-approved usages of clozapine which are being tried by clinicians: (i) treatment-resistant mood disorders, including rapid cycling mania (Calabrese *et al.*, 1991; Suppes *et al.*, 1992) and psychotic depression (Parsa *et al.*, 1991); (ii) L-dopa-induced psychosis (Friedman & Lannon, 1989); and (iii) severe, disabling akathisia (Levin *et al.*, 1992). The precept that clozapine should be tried on an experimental basis in patients with diagnoses other than schizophrenia, in which neuroleptic drugs are legitimately used and sometimes effective, e.g. severe mood disorders and organic brain disorder, but have failed to be effective, seems reasonable. Examples include organic psychoses such as Huntington's chorea (Sajatovic *et al.*, 1991) and severe head injury (Michaels *et al.*, 1993). Informed consent would be essential in such cases and side effects may be increased (Michaels *et al.*, 1993). Clozapine has also proven useful to treat polydypsia in schizophrenic patients (Lee *et al.*, 1991).

Administration

Clozapine treatment should not be initiated in patients who are receiving multiple psychotropic drugs (Meltzer, 1992). The optimal way to initiate clozapine is in patients who are not receiving other psychotropic drugs. There are two classes of reasons for this. First, many of clozapine's side effects, such as hypotension, sedation and anticholinergic effects (Baldessarini & Frankenberg, 1991), may be increased by concomitant psychotropic drugs, especially low-potency neuroleptics. Concomitant neuroleptic drugs, especially high-potency agents, would tend to cause EPS which could change a patient's perception of the advantages of clozapine and affect compliance. Second, potent D_2 dopamine-receptor blockade due to concomitant neuroleptic therapy would be predicted to prevent the limbic selective biological effects of clozapine, which may be critical to its efficacy in treatment-resistant patients. However, controlled trials of neuroleptic drugs in combination with clozapine at the outset of treatment with clozapine are needed to establish whether this combination does, in fact, delay or impair response to clozapine.

If patients have been receiving various psychotropic drugs prior to beginning clozapine treatment, it is desirable to switch to a single high-potency neuroleptic such as fluphenazine or haloperidol. These should be given at as low a dose as is consistent with safety, comfort and patient compliance, e.g. 10 mg haloperidol per day or its equivalent. Long-acting neuroleptic drugs are not a contraindication to using clozapine when initiating treatment because granulocytopaenia or agranulocytosis is very rare during the initial weeks of clozapine treatment. Withdrawal from the single neuroleptic should then precede initiation of clozapine treatment whenever possible, for the reasons discussed above. If that is not possible, clozapine should be added to the high-potency neuroleptic. As the dose of clozapine is increased to 200−300 mg/day over a 2-week period, the dose of neuroleptic should be decreased and eventually eliminated. This can usually be accomplished within another 2 weeks.

The recommended starting dose of clozapine is 12.5 mg to test for possible hypotensive reactions. It is possible to start clozapine in out-patients with close monitoring of blood pressure, pulse and sedation for the first 2−4 h after its administration. The dose of clozapine may be increased by 25 mg every other day until it reaches 100 mg. This can be done on an out-patient basis if the patient is assessed to be able to adhere to the prescribed schedule, or if there are support people who can assist the patient. It can then be increased by 50 mg every other day until a dose of 300−450 mg/day is reached, generally by 3 weeks. Twice-a-day dosage is recommended because the half-life of clozapine is 16 h (Choc *et al.*, 1987; Jann *et al.*, 1993). The dose need not exceed 450−600 mg/day in most adults ≤60 years old in the initial phase of treatment. However, if the response at 600 mg/day is unsatisfactory, the dosage should be further increased up to a maximum of 900 mg/day. The dosage of clozapine required in the elderly is usually 200−300 mg/day. There are no data available as to whether lower doses of clozapine are needed for maintenance treatment.

There are, as yet, no fixed dose studies to determine optimal dosage. In Europe, clinical practice has been to use doses of 200−300 mg/day or even lower (Naber *et al.*, 1989), while in the USA doses of 400−600 mg/day are most common. The reasons for this discrepancy require further study. There may be a relationship between dose, plasma levels and severity or duration of illness, suggesting that the European patients may, on average, be less severely ill, i.e. non-treatment-resistant (Meltzer *et al.*, in preparation). The use of concomitant neuroleptic drugs is also more common in Europe.

Clozapine improves positive symptoms, negative symptoms and disorganization (Kane *et al.*, 1988; Meltzer *et al.*, 1989b). It appears to be particularly effective in decreasing symptoms of disorganization (Fig. 25.1). It also alleviates mood symptoms in schizoaffective patients. The abilities of clozapine to improve different types of psychotic symptomatology may be independent of each other and should be evaluated separately as outcome measures. Improvement in social functioning during clozapine treatment has been reported (Meltzer *et al.*, 1990), including the quality of life scale which scored double over a 6-month period in 38 clozapine-treated patients (Heinrichs *et al.*, 1984). All aspects of social function rated by this scale, including work and activities of daily living, were found to improve. Even some previously regressed patients with marked defect symptoms have been able to return to work after receiving clozapine (Lindström, 1988; Meltzer *et al.*, 1990). The marked reduction in rehospitalization which usually results from clozapine treatment also contributes to improvement in social function (Meltzer, 1991b).

The response to clozapine in treatment-resistant schizophrenia may be delayed beyond 6 weeks but about 30% of patients will respond by 6 weeks (Meltzer, 1989b). Another 30% respond between 6 weeks and 6 months, or even longer. There are anecdotal reports that the initial improvement in positive symptoms may not be apparent in some subjects until 12 months

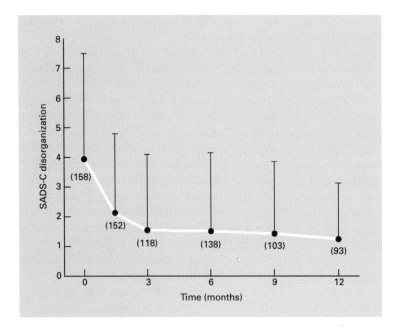

Fig. 25.1 Effect of clozapine on schedule for affective disorders and schizophrenia-change (SADS-C) disorganization subscale scores (N).

of treatment. The reasons for such a delayed response to clozapine are unknown. It could be due to fundamental changes in neural structure and functioning of a plasticity nature. Because of the frequent delay in the onset of clinical advantages over standard drugs, clozapine should probably not be discontinued for lack of apparent efficacy before less than 6 months of treatment have elapsed. Outcome measures such as fewer EPS, blockade of symptoms of tardive dyskinesia, better compliance, etc. should be considered before deciding to stop clozapine treatment in patients whose psychopathology is minimally improved. It should also be noted that the risk of agranulocytosis is highest between 4 and 18 weeks so the risk:benefit ratio improves after that time.

Clozapine may be no more effective than standard neuroleptics in treating positive symptoms in up to 25% of neuroleptic-resistant schizophrenic patients, despite a trial of adequate dose (up to 900 mg/day) or duration (up to 6 months or longer) (Meltzer *et al.*, 1989b, 1990). Addition of a low dose of a high-potency neuroleptic drug, such as haloperidol, to such patients after 6 months of clozapine alone has sometimes

been effective. Clozapine plus electroconvulsive therapy may be useful in some cases (Meltzer, 1989a). There are as yet no studies to indicate what other strategies, if any, might be helpful to supplement clozapine. It is likely that clinicians will choose to add other psychotropic drugs based upon symptomatic criteria, e.g. antidepressants or anxiolytics for patients with persistent symptomatology of either type. Specific 5-hydroxytryptamine (5-HT) uptake inhibitors, such as fluoxetine, fluvoxamine, paroxetine or sertraline, have proven to be tolerated better than tricyclic antidepressants (Cassady & Thaker, 1992).

Psychosocial treatments should be provided from the very beginning of treatment with clozapine to facilitate recovery of social function. Group, family and individual therapy, social skills training, education about the nature of schizophrenia, elements of vocational counselling, etc. are the most helpful forms of treatment. Patients who are very regressed prior to clozapine treatment, especially those who have been chronically institutionalized, will most certainly need intensive social skills training. Empathic, experienced therapists are necessary to help these patients improve their social interaction.

There is some evidence that abrupt withdrawal of clozapine, as may occur with non-compliance or because of agranulocytosis, may be associated with a severe exacerbation (Ekblom *et al.*, 1984; Alphs & Lee, 1991; Parsa *et al.*, 1993). This is a rare occurrence. Reinstating clozapine is best in cases of non-compliance. Prolonged treatment with standard neuroleptics may be necessary in cases of agranulocytosis and should be reinstituted as soon as the white blood cell count has reached 2000–3000/mm^3 to minimize the risk of a severe exacerbation.

Clinical pharmacology and plasma levels

Animal and human basic pharmacology are discussed in Chapters 21 and 18, respectively. Peak clozapine plasma levels following its oral administration are achieved in 1–4 h. The half-life after twice-a-day dosing at the steady state is about 14 h (range 6–33). Thus, steady-state levels should be achieved about 1 week after constant-dose twice-daily administration (Choc *et al.*, 1987). The major metabolites of clozapine, nor-clozapine and clozapine-*N*-oxide are, to the best of current knowledge, inactive, but given the uncertainty as to the mechanism of action of clozapine, they could be functionally important.

It seems likely that measurement of plasma levels of clozapine will be clinically useful. The optimal plasma levels for treatment-resistant schizophrenia appear to be greater than 350 ng/ml (Perry *et al.*, 1991; Hasegawa *et al.*, 1993). Plasma levels may be measured by high-pressure liquid chromatography (Lovdahl *et al.*, 1991). Plasma levels are more useful than dose *per se* as a guide to dosage. Mean plasma levels of clozapine average 200–400 ng/ml (range 60–1000 ng/ml). There is no evidence for a therapeutic window. Dosage may be guided by plasma levels as well as side effects and clinical response. Patients with poor response should definitely be checked for adequate plasma levels. Smoking may affect plasma levels in males (Haring *et al.*, 1989). It may be prudent in very carefully selected cases to exceed the recommended limit of 900 mg/day if plasma levels

are less than 450 ng/ml and there are no major cardiovascular or other side effects (Hasegawa *et al.*, 1993). Clozapine metabolism may be blocked by cimetidine (Szymanski *et al.*, 1991) and phenytoin (Miller *et al.*, 1991).

Clozapine produces electroencephalogram (EEG) abnormalities in nearly all patients (Tiihonen *et al.*, 1991). Abnormal EEGs should not preclude raising the dose of clozapine.

Prediction of response

Factors which affect the response to clozapine in treatment-resistant schizophrenic patients have received some study. There is some evidence that paranoid subtype, *more* hospitalizations and less grandiosity predict better outcome, but the predictive power is poor (Honigfeld & Patin, 1989). Prefrontal sulcal prominence as measured by computerized tomography (CT) is inversely related to the response to clozapine, but ventricular brain ratio (VBR) does not predict clinical response (Friedman *et al.*, 1991). Shorter duration of illness, females and younger age are significant demographic and historical predictors of a good outcome (Meltzer *et al.*, unpublished data). Other biological predictors of response to clozapine are currently being studied as predictors of response. The identification of effective predictors of efficacy could change the risk:benefit ratio of using clozapine more broadly.

Drug interactions

There has been considerable concern about combining clozapine and benzodiazepines because of reports of respiratory arrest. Clozapine may suppress the activity of the respiratory centre. The evidence for a negative interaction between clozapine and benzodiazepines is not strong. Benzodiazepines are sometimes useful in diminishing anxiety when initiating clozapine treatment in neuroleptic-free schizophrenic patients (Lieberman *et al.*, 1989). No adverse effects of the combination of benzodiazepines and clozapine have occurred in the author's extensive use of the combination. When the combination is first given, it may be desirable to have the patient hospitalized or observed in an out-patient setting for 2–4 h.

Clozapine and lithium have been implicated in several cases of neuroleptic malignant syndrome (Pope *et al.*, 1991) as well as other types of neurotoxicity (Blake *et al.*, 1992). These reports suggest that lithium should be used with clozapine only if hypomanic symptoms are not adequately controlled with clozapine. Valproic acid may be the safest agent to combine with lithium carbonate therapy if supplemental mood stabilization is required.

Side effects

Granulocytopaenia and agranulocytosis

The major side effect of clozapine which limits its use is the significant risk of agranulocytosis (Krupp & Barnes, 1989). Because of this, weekly total white blood cell or neutrophil counts must be carried out on an indefinite basis in the USA. However, other countries usually require only monthly monitoring after the first 4 months of treatment, since approximately 80% of cases of neutropaenia or agranulocytosis occur within the first 18 weeks of treatment. It is possible that less frequent monitoring, e.g. every 2 weeks, of the white blood cell or neutrophil count after the first 6, 12 or 18 months of clozapine treatment in the future may be authorized on the basis of risk: benefit analysis of available data. There are no proven risk factors or predictors of agranulocytosis; an early suggestion for an association between HLA-B38 DR4 DQW3 haplotype and clozapine-induced agranulocytosis in Ashkenazi Jewish individuals (Lieberman *et al.*, 1990) has not been confirmed by subsequent research (Krupp, personal communication). However, one case in a native American with the same haplotype as identified by Lieberman *et al.* (1990) has been reported (Pfister *et al.*, 1992).

The fall in white blood cell count due to clozapine may be abrupt or gradual. Steadily falling total white blood cell or neutrophil counts should increase concern, even if none are below

$3000/mm^3$. An abrupt drop of $\geq 3000/mm^3$ in a single week may signal impending agranulocytosis. Twice-weekly white blood cell counts with differentials are indicated in such patients. When the total white blood cell count falls below $3000/mm^3$ or the neutrophil count falls below $1500/mm^3$, clozapine must be discontinued and the white cell count with differential followed for 4 weeks.

The aetiology of agranulocytosis is unknown. High plasma levels of clozapine or its metabolite, norclozapine, are not related to agranulocytosis or granulocytopaenia (Hasegawa *et al.*, 1994). The possibility that a free-radical-containing metabolite of clozapine could be responsible for agranulocytosis has been proposed (Fischer *et al.*, 1991). If so, a free-radical scavenger such as vitamin C might decrease the incidence of this side effect. Management of agranulocytosis should be undertaken in conjunction with a haematologist and/or an infectious disease specialist. Hospitalization with reverse isolation on a medical unit is usually indicated. Prophylactic antibiotic treatment, if agranulocytosis develops, should be considered. Because the duration of agranulocytosis may be longer than for other drug-induced blood dyscrasias, neutropaenia fever, should it develop, is often a challenging management problem. Upon withdrawal of clozapine, the haematological status usually returns to normal within 2–3 weeks. The successful use of granulocyte colony-stimulating factor (G-CSF) to promote recovery from agranulocytosis has recently been reported (Barnas *et al.*, 1992; Weide *et al.*, 1992). Recovery time may be expected to be much more rapid with G-CSF. This is a highly promising development which may be widely adopted and should reduce morbidity and mortality associated with clozapine use. It should be used only for agranulocytosis or severe neutropaenia ($<1000/mm^3$).

Patients who have developed agranulocytosis from clozapine treatment once will experience it again within 1–4 weeks after being rechallenged (Krupp & Barnes, 1989). Thus, rechallenge with clozapine after clear granulocytopaenia agranulocytosis should not be tried. There is no evidence that the use of lithium or granulocyte-stimulating factors can protect such patients, or that lithium, which can increase white blood cell production, can prevent agranulocytosis. Patients who are withdrawn from clozapine treatment during a neutropaenic phase (white blood cell count $2000-3500/mm^3$) may be rechallenged but more intensive and differential monitoring is indicated.

Extrapyramidal reactions

The absence, or very low incidence, of EPS is a major clinical advantage associated with clozapine therapy (Meltzer, 1992). This feature of clozapine contributes significantly to patient acceptance and compliance. There have been no reported cases of dystonic reactions in patients who have not received any neuroleptics except clozapine. Clozapine rarely produces akathisia. It does not worsen parkinsonian symptoms in Parkinson's disease (Friedman & Lannon, 1989). There have been no definite reported cases of tardive dyskinesia linked to clozapine treatment alone. At the same time, clozapine is quite effective in blocking this syndrome in two-thirds of patients (Casey, 1989; Lieberman *et al.*, 1991). Approximately 30% of cases with tardive dyskinesia treated with clozapine will have a remission of the tardive dyskinesia and another 30% will have a reduction in severity (Meltzer *et al.*, in preparation). However, symptoms recur when clozapine is stopped. The lack of tardive dyskinesia or dystonia due to clozapine makes it an appealing choice for patients who appear to be developing moderate−severe tardive dyskinesia after relatively brief trials with neuroleptic drugs but who, nevertheless, require chronic neuroleptic therapy.

Other side effects

Clozapine, like other antipsychotic medications, can reduce the seizure threshold, sometimes resulting in major motor seizures or myoclonus (Devinsky *et al.*, 1991). However, a seizure history is not an absolute contraindication for the use of clozapine. The overall incidence of major motor seizures in patients receiving clozapine is estimated to be 1−2% at doses below 300 mg/day, 2−4% at doses greater than 300 mg/day and 4−6% at doses greater than 600 mg/day. In patients who develop seizures, reduction of the clozapine dosage to perhaps 50% of the dose prior to the seizure, concurrent with pharmacological management of the seizures, may be necessary. Valproate has proven to be the most useful anticonvulsant for this purpose (Haller & Binder, 1990). Phenytoin, which is also useful for seizure control, may diminish clozapine plasma levels (Miller, 1991).

There have been several reports of clozapine-induced exacerbations of obsessive−compulsive symptoms (Baker *et al.*, 1992; Patil, 1992). This may be due to $5-HT_2$-receptor blockade and should ameliorate with treatment with serotonin reuptake inhibitors such as fluoxetine.

The main cardiovascular effects of clozapine are orthostatic hypotension and tachycardia (Lieberman *et al.*, 1989). Tolerance develops in some subjects but tachycardia may be especially persistent. The ability of clozapine to antagonize α-adrenergic receptors is responsible for its orthostatic hypotension. The risk of syncope can be significantly reduced by a conservative titration procedure. In most cases, even in the presence of significant initial orthostasis, full therapeutic doses can be achieved. Hypertension may also be observed, most frequently in the first 2 weeks of treatment.

In patients receiving clozapine, tachycardia is predominantly the result of the anticholinergic effects of clozapine. The mean heart rate can increase by 20−25 beats/min and can persist for over 1 year in some patients. Similar to orthostatic hypotension, this effect is also dose dependent. Beta-adrenergic blockers have been successfully used to decrease the heart rate in some normotensive patients with clozapine-induced tachycardia.

During clozapine therapy, almost one-third of patients complain of hypersalivation. Reduction in the dosage of clozapine or treatment with an anticholinergic medication such as benztropine can prove beneficial (Lieberman *et al.*, 1989). The α-adrenergic agonist clonidine, which causes a dry mouth by suppressing sympathomimetic sialagogic mechanisms, may also be helpful (Grabowski, 1992).

Sedation and dizziness are common side effects of clozapine; approximately 40% and 20% of patients, respectively, experience symptoms of these two side effects. Both occur most frequently within the first 2 months of treatment; tolerance usually develops thereafter. Dizziness is more common in elderly patients. Sedation may limit the ability to drive or operate dangerous equipment.

Weight gain is sometimes a troublesome problem with clozapine (Lamberti *et al.*, 1992; Leadbetter *et al.*, 1992). The mean weight gain appears to be about 10% of body weight. Some gain as much as 40 kg. In a recent study, the mean clozapine-induced weight gain was 6 kg or 8.9% of body weight (Leadbetter *et al.*, 1992). The magnitude of weight gain appears to be positively correlated with clinical response (Lamberti *et al.*, 1992; Leadbetter *et al.*, 1992). Nutritional counselling is important to prevent or reverse this side effect when it occurs. Dosage reduction may be the only effective intervention in some cases. A serotonin reuptake inhibitor such as fluoxetine may also be of help. There is no evidence that limiting the weight gain would impair the clinical response, but this possibility should be considered.

Cost effectiveness

Clozapine, as the first new antipsychotic drug introduced in the USA in a decade, with a limited target population (at most 10–30% of schizophrenic patients) and special costs associated with its use (a national registry, assurance of weekly blood monitoring and education of physicians to use it appropriately and safely), is much more expensive than other, approved antipsychotic drugs. The approximate cost of clozapine at a dose of 450 mg/day for a year, excluding the weekly blood monitoring and associated expenses, is $4500 per patient. This cost has most certainly impacted on the willingness to use clozapine in public mental health systems which are responsible for providing care to most schizophrenic patients.

Two studies have examined the cost effec-

tiveness of clozapine in treatment-resistant schizophrenia. Revicki *et al.* (1990) conducted a retrospective cost-effectiveness study in 86 treatment-resistant schizophrenic patients, comparing estimated costs before and during clozapine therapy with those for a comparable group of patients who received conventional therapies. Total costs averaged $10 040 per patient (1987 dollars) more in the clozapine group than the neuroleptic group in the first year after the start of treatment. In the first year after treatment commenced, the clozapine group averaged $9011 less in costs than the neuroleptic group. By the second year, total costs in the clozapine group had decreased by more than $24 000 per patient, compared with the pretreatment year. These data suggested that clozapine could be a cost-effective treatment after at least 2 years of treatment.

In a prospective study, we compared the total costs of treatment for 2 years before and 2 years after clozapine treatment in 37 treatment-resistant schizophrenic patients (Meltzer *et al.*, 1993). The median total cost for 2 years decreased from $42 934 (1987 dollars) to $23 772, a decrease of $19 162. The median cost of hospitalization decreased from $21 700 to 0. These 37 patients had a total of 84 hospitalizations in the 2 years before clozapine treatment and only 11 hospitalizations in the 2 years after clozapine treatment (an 86.9% decrease). For comparison purposes, the costs associated with 10 patients who were treated with clozapine for relatively brief periods were examined. The median total cost increased from $35 752 to $87 725, an increase of $51 973. The median change in total costs was −$18 070 for the clozapine group compared with +$17 644 for the comparison group, a difference of $35 714. These figures do not include the cost of the index hospitalization because hospitalization was not necessarily needed to begin clozapine treatment and could often have been charged to the period prior to beginning clozapine treatment.

These studies suggest that large savings are possible with clozapine treatment for treatment-resistant schizophrenic patients who have had frequent hospitalizations. Significant savings were observed when the figures were calculated using cost data for public-sector or private-sector psychiatry only. It is possible that the cost of clozapine will decrease when patent protection expires in late 1994, especially if generic versions are introduced. There does not appear to be any reason to expect that clozapine will be a financial burden on the already financially strapped mental health system if appropriate patients are selected.

Conclusion

Clozapine provides the possibility of significant help for severely psychotic patients who fail to respond adequately to typical neuroleptics, as well as a reduced potential to cause EPS, including tardive dyskinesia. On the other hand, because of its relatively complex delivery system and high cost, and its profile of side effects, the use of clozapine has aroused considerable concern and controversy in the USA and other countries. It is currently used to treat only about 30 000 of the 2 million schizophrenic patients in the USA. This is about half its rate of use in Europe, where it has been available for much longer. There is an emerging consensus among mental health officials that it definitely is an advance in the treatment of schizophrenia (Collins *et al.*, 1992).

A reasonable conclusion is that all truly treatment-resistant schizophrenic patients should be given a trial of clozapine alone for up to 6 months. With appropriate monitoring of the neutrophil or total white blood cell count and careful attention to other side effects, the risks of clozapine are acceptable and the chances for clinically significant improvement very real. The greater effectiveness of clozapine will usually be apparent as a decrease in positive and EPS symptoms, but less disorganization, negative symptoms, improved social interaction, work function and less rehospitalization will often also occur. Although only a small number of treatment-resistant schizophrenic patients will respond to clozapine with a near-complete resolution of their manifest psychosis, the more modest improvement in many others is still of unequivocal benefit to

them since it permits patients who were previously severely disabled to function much better, albeit still at compromised levels. Clozapine is, indeed, a major advance in the treatment of schizophrenia, one which provides clinicians with a unique tool to treat some of the most difficult patients.

Risperidone (see also Chapters 18 & 21)

Risperidone is a benzisoxazole derivate, chemically unrelated to any other currently available antipsychotic drug. Risperidone, like clozapine, is a potent $5-HT_2$ and relatively weak D_2 dopamine-receptor antagonist (Leysen *et al.*, 1988). Its affinity for the D_2 receptor is similar to that of haloperidol (1−5 nmol/l). It has low potency for D_1 and D_4 dopamine receptors. It is a potent α_1-adrenergic and histamine H_1 antagonist. *In vivo*, risperidone blocks dopamine agonist-induced locomotor activity at doses which cause weak catalepsy, a profile which suggests it should produce low EPS at antipsychotic doses (Megens *et al.*, 1988). Risperidone, like clozapine, can stimulate prolactin secretion in rodents (Bowden *et al.*, 1992). However, unlike clozapine, it stimulates prolactin secretion in humans (Van den Bussche *et al.*, 1988; Mesotten *et al.*, 1989; Bersani *et al.*, 1990).

Clinical pharmacology

Risperidone is rapidly and completely absorbed following oral administration and reaches peak plasma levels within 2 h (Van den Bussche *et al.*, 1988). Risperidone is extensively metabolized in the liver; 9-hydroxyrisperidone, the major metabolite, has a half-life of 17−22 h compared with 2−4 h (mean 2−8 h) for risperidone. Thus, the pharmacologically active moiety is the sum of risperidone and 9-hydroxyrisperidone. Poor metabolizers of debrisoquine (8% of the Caucasian population) will also be unable to metabolize risperidone because the 9-hydroxylation is catalysed by CYP2 D6. Poor metabolizers of risperidone have half the active moiety of good metabolizers, because risperidone levels will be much higher in the poor metabolizers. Elimination of the active moiety is independent of metabolic phenotype, with a half-life of 20 h. There are no data about a relationship between plasma levels of the active moiety and clinical response.

Efficacy

Risperidone, in doses of 4–6 mg/day, appears to be at least equivalent to haloperidol 10–20 mg/day in decreasing positive and negative symptoms (Castelao *et al.*, 1989; Meco *et al.*, 1989; Mesotten *et al.*, 1989; Bersani *et al.*, 1990; Svestka *et al.*, 1990; Ishigooka, 1991; Borison *et al.*, 1992a,b; Claus *et al.*, 1992; Chourinard *et al.*, 1993). Risperidone has been reported to be superior to haloperidol in treating positive and negative symptoms in schizophrenia and possibly to have a faster onset of action in some cases (Svestka *et al.*, 1990; Claus *et al.*, 1992; Chourinard *et al.*, 1993). These claims, which are unique for any antipsychotic drug other than clozapine, require additional confirmation. The study by Claus *et al.* (1992) included some apparently neuroleptic-resistant schizophrenic patients, raising the possibility that risperidone might be effective in some, if not all, of the patients for whom clozapine is effective. However, no head-to-head comparisons of risperidone and clozapine have been conducted to date and until several such studies are completed it would be premature to broaden the indication for risperidone to this class of patients. Should risperidone prove equally effective to clozapine in such patients, it would strengthen the claim for its superiority to standard neuroleptic drugs in neuroleptic-responsive patients.

There is some evidence that risperidone can partially mask the symptoms of tardive dyskinesia (Chouinard *et al.*, 1993). There is no evidence yet that would suggest risperidone has a low potential to cause tardive dyskinesia or dystonia, but this possibility is worthy of further study.

Side effects

Risperidone has been reported to produce fewer EPS than haloperidol but more than placebo (Borison *et al.*, 1992a,b). However, available data suggest it is not as free of EPS as clozapine is. Consistent with this, the use of antiparkinsonian agents is less frequent with risperidone treatment but it is needed in about 20% of patients (Claus *et al.*, 1992; Chouinard *et al.*, 1993). This is a much higher proportion than with clozapine. At doses ≥10 mg/day, the incidence of EPS with risperidone might be expected to equal that of EPS with haloperidol. Therefore, in clinical practice, it will be of considerable importance to keep the dose of risperidone in the range 4–6 mg/day.

The most common adverse effects of risperidone are insomnia, anxiety, agitation, dizziness, rhinitis, hypotension, weight gain and menstrual disturbances (Borison *et al.*, 1992a,b). It may be expected to cause neuroleptic malignant syndrome and galactorrhea.

Usage

The usual starting dose of risperidone is 1 mg twice daily, increasing to 2 mg twice daily and 3 mg twice daily over the next 2 days. The mean optimal dose is 6 mg/day but higher doses may be needed to control positive symptoms. Risperidone, like clozapine, should usually be given as monotherapy to avoid EPS. However, in a recent study, risperidone was superior to placebo as an add-on therapy in mentally retarded patients with persistent behavioural disturbances (Van den Borre *et al.*, 1993).

Conclusion

Risperidone should prove useful as a first-line antipsychotic agent provided that it proves to have advantages in EPS or efficacy over standard neuroleptic drugs. Much will depend upon the ability of prescribers to obtain the desired results within a narrow therapeutic window, 4–6 mg/day or possibly 8 mg/day. At these higher doses, more complete D_2 receptor blockade may prevail. This increases EPS and may even contribute to diminished efficacy.

Remoxipride

Remoxipride is a selective D_2 dopamine-receptor antagonist which has a potentially favourable EPS profile.

Pharmacokinetics

The pharmacokinetics of remoxipride have been summarized by Von Bahr *et al.* (1992). Remoxipride is rapidly absorbed and has good bioavailability. The mean plasma half-life is $4-7$ h. It has no active metabolites. It is about 80% bound to plasma proteins.

Clinical studies

The major studies of remoxipride have involved double-blind multicentre comparisons with haloperidol. These data have been summarized by Lewander *et al.* (1990): combined analysis of nine trials, involving 667 remoxipride- and 437 haloperidol-treated patients, indicated that after $4-6$ weeks of treatment, $55-60\%$ of patients in both groups were rated as much, or very much, improved. Both agents had similar effects on positive and negative symptoms with approximately 60 and 30% improvement in each, respectively, using an intention-to-treat analysis. The dose of remoxipride in these studies ranged from 120 to 600 mg/day, while that of haloperidol ranged from 5 to 45 mg/day.

Since the major advantage of remoxipride appears to be its low EPS profile (see below), it is useful to compare remoxipride with thioridazine, the neuroleptic with the least potential to cause EPS. McCreadie *et al.* (1990) compared remoxipride and thioridazine in a total of 61 newly admitted schizophrenic patients who were matched on relevant variables. There was evidence for greater efficacy of thioridazine in the global assessment measure but not in psychopathology. Thioridazine produced more sedation, anticholinergic effects, autonomic dysfunction and weight gain. The two drugs did not differ with regard to EPS.

Side effects

In the composite summary of data from nine multicentre trials, remoxipride has clear advantages over haloperidol with regard to EPS (Lewander *et al.*, 1990). This is especially true for interference with gait, elbow rigidity, fixation of position, head dropping, tremor and salivation. However, 20% of remoxipride-treated patients required anticholinergic drugs. There is no evidence to suggest that remoxipride would not induce tardive dyskinesia if given for prolonged periods. Of remoxipride-treated patients, $10-30\%$ report drowsiness, tiredness and difficulty in concentrating; this is significantly less than with haloperidol but not dramatically so.

Remoxipride has been reported to produce aplastic anemia in about 1 per 10 000 treated patients. Because of this, it is no longer available for clinical use in any country.

Conclusion

Remoxipride appears to be an effective antipsychotic drug that could have been particularly useful in treating patients who experience significant EPS and sedation with standard neuroleptic drugs. Thioridazine is the most similar drug available in the USA, while in Europe comparisons with sulpiride and amisulpiride will be of interest. There is no evidence yet as to whether remoxipride has any advantages over these other substituted benzamides. Because of its ability to cause aplastic anemia, it is no longer in active use.

Seroquel

Seroquel is a dibenzothiazepine with clozapine-like pharmacology. Like clozapine, it has stronger affinity for the 5-HT$_{2A}$ than the D2 receptor ($IC_{50} = 148$ and 329 nM, respectively). It is a relatively potent α_1 and α_2-adrenergic antagonist ($IC_{50} = 90$ and 270 nM, respectively). These affinities are relatively low compared to those of clozapine (Saller & Salama, 1993), although the clinical dose range is comparable for the two drugs. Seroquel shows selectivity for mesolimbic DA neurons after chronic treatment (Goldstein et al., 1993). It produces low catalepsy and, at clinically relevant doses, does not elicit dyskinetic reactions in haloperidol-sensitized cebus monkeys (Migler et al., 1993). Like clozapine, it produces transient elevations of serum prolactin levels in rodents (Saller & Salama, 1993).

Early clinical trials, as yet unpublished, have been summarized by Hirsch et al. (in press). Two six-week, multicentre, randomized, placebo-controlled, double-blind trials in the United States of 109 and 286 hospitalized schizophrenic patients with an acute exacerbation, provide evidence for superiority of Seroquel over placebo on total psychopathology measures (BPRS, CGI) at day 42. There were modest differences in negative symptoms as measured by the SANS in favour of Seroquel.

Seroquel has been compared to chlorpromazine in a six week, multicentre, randomized, double-blind study using a population of patients similar to those described. Doses of both drugs ranged from 75–750 mg/day. The mean dose of Seroquel was 407 mg/day. Both drugs were equally effective. The main side effect of Seroquel was somnolence. There was little evidence of EPS and no dystonic reactions. Seroquel did not increase plasma prolactin levels.

These studies clearly indicate that Seroquel is similar to clozapine in not causing plasma or serum prolactin increases, and causing low EPS and sedation at clinically effective doses. Further study is needed to demonstrate whether or not it has superior efficacy to standard antipsychotic drugs in neuroleptic-resistant or -responsive patients.

Olanzapine

Olanzapine, a thienobenzodiazepine, like clozapine, has a higher affinity for the 5-HT_{2A}, (K_1, 4 nM) than the D_2 (11 nM) receptor. It also has a high affinity for the D_1 (31 nM), D_4 (27 nM), 5-HT_{2C} (11 nM), muscarinic (M_1) (1.9 nM), α_1-adrenergic (19 nM) and H_1 (7 nM)histamine receptors

(Moore et al., 1993). Like clozapine and Seroquel, it causes low catalepsy and is selective for mesolimbic DA neurons (Moore et al., 1993).

In a recent double-blind clinical trial, 335 chronic schizophrenic patients were randomized to three doses of olanzapine (5 ± 2.5 mg/day [OLZ-L], 10 ± 2.5 mg/day [OLZ-M], 15 ± 2.5 mg/day [OLZ-H]), haloperidol (15 ± 5 mg/day [HAL]) or placebo (Beasley et al., in press). OLZ-M, OLZ-H and HAL were superior to placebo after six weeks in an intention to treat analysis of BPRS Total and Positive symptoms. The OLZ-H group showed greater improvement in negative symptoms as assessed by the SANS. Major side effects with olanzapine were somnolence, agitation, asthenia and nervousness. EPS were less with OLZ-H than with HAL. OLZ and placebo produced comparable negligible changes in serum prolactin.

These results suggest that olanzepine is an effective atypical antipsychotic drug, e.g., low EPS at clinical doses. The results with regard to negative symptoms are encouraging but must be documented by further analyses and additional studies.

Other atypical antipsychotic drugs

There are now numerous drugs in advanced stages of clinical testing as potential atypical antipsychotic drugs (Table 25.1). It is premature to discuss any in detail because of the absence of reliable clinical data about their efficacy. Most fall into the risperidone category, having been selected on the basis of strong 5-HT_2, low D_2 receptor blockade, being available to achieve low EPS and provide superior efficacy (Meltzer et al., 1989a). This theory has not been put to a definitive test but will be by these agents. Most other drugs under investigation rely on directly or indirectly altering dopaminergic function, e.g. D_1 receptor blockade, dopamine autoreceptor agonists, partial dopamine agonists and 5-HT_3 antagonists (which inhibit dopamine release). No doubt, drugs will be developed that have selectivity as D_3 and D_4 antagonists. Other non-dopaminergic strategies are needed.

Table 25.1 Novel atypical antipsychotic drugs

5-HT$_2$/D$_2$ antagonists	*Dopamine autoreceptor agonists*
Amperozide	BHT-920
Ziprasidone	Pramipexole
Melperone	3-PPP
Org 5222	
Rilapine	*Partial dopamine agonists*
Sertindole	MER-327
SM-9018	
SND 919	
5-HT$_3$ antagonists	*Glycine agonists*
GR 68755C (Glaxo)	Milacemide
D$_1$ antagonists	*Sigma antagonists*
SCH-23390	DUP734
NO-01-0687	

5-HT, 5-hydroxytryptamine; D, dopamine.

Acknowledgements

The research reported was supported in part by USPHS MH 41684, GCRC MO1RR00080 and grants from the Elisabeth Severance Prentiss and John Pascal Sawyer foundations. The author is the recipient of a USPHS Research Career Scientist Award MH 47808. The secretarial assistance of Ms Lee Mason is greatly appreciated.

References

Alphs, L.D. & Lee, H.S. (1991) Comparison of withdrawal of typical and atypical antipsychotic drugs: a case study. *Journal of Clinical Psychiatry*, 52, 346–348.

Amsler, H.A., Teerenhovi, L., Bartha, E., Harjula, K. & Vuopio, P. (1977) Agranulocytosis in patients treated with clozapine: a study of the Finnish epidemic. *Acta Psychiatrica Scandinavica*, 56, 241–248.

Angst, J., Jaenicke, U., Padrutt, A. & Scharfetter, C.H. (1971) Ergbnisse eines Doppelblindversuches von HF-1854 (8-Chlor-11-[4-methyl-1-piperazinyl]-5-H-dibenzo[b,e] [1,4]diazepin) im Vergleich zu Levomepromazin. *Pharma-kopsychiatrie*, 4, 192–200.

Baker, R.W., Chengappa, K.N., Baird, J.W., Steengard, S., Christ, M.A. & Schooler, N.R. (1992) Emergence of obsessive–compulsive symptoms during treatment with clozapine. *Journal of Clinical Psychiatry*, 53, 439–442.

Baldessarini, R. & Frankenburg, F.R. (1991) Clozapine: a novel antipsychotic agent. *New England Journal of Medicine*, 324, 746–754.

Barnas, C., Swierzina, H., Hummer, M. Sperner-Unterweger, B., Stern, A. & Fleishchacker, W.W. (1992) Granulocyte-macrophase colony-stimulating factor (GM-CSF) treatment of clozapine-induced agranulocytosis: a case report. *Journal of Clinical Psychiatry*, 53, 245–247.

Beasley, C.M., Tollefson, G., Tran, P. *et al.* (1995) Olanzapine versus placebo and haloperidol: acute phase results of the North American double-blind olanzapine trial. *Neuropsycho-pharmacology* (in press).

Bersani, G., Bressa, G.M., Meco, G. & Pozzi, F. (1990) Mixed D$_2$ and S$_2$ antagonism in a preliminary study with risperidone (R 64 766). *Human Psychopharmacology*, 5, 225–231.

Blake, L.M., Marks, R.C. & Luchins, D.J. (1992) Reversible neuroleptic symptoms with clozapine. *Journal of Clinical Psychopharmacology*, 12, 297–298.

Borison, R.L., Diamond, B.I., Pathiragja, A. & Meibach, R.C. (1992a) Clinical overview of risperidone. In Meltzer, H.Y. (ed.) *Novel Antipsychotic Drugs*, pp. 223–239. Raven Press, New York.

Borison, R.L., Pathiragja, A.P., Diamond, B.I. & Meibach, R.C. (1992b) Risperidone: clinical safety and efficacy in schizophrenia. *Psychopharmacology Bulletin*, 28, 213–218.

Bowden, C.C., Voina, S.J., Woestenborghs, R., de Coster, R. & Hyekants, J. (1992) Stimulation by risperidone of rat prolactin secretion *in vivo* and in cultured pituitary cells *in vitro*. *Journal of Pharmacology and Experimental Therapeutics*, 262, 699–706.

Brier, A., Schreiber, J.L., Dyer, J. & Pickar, D. (1991) National Institute of Mental Health longitudinal study of chronic schizophrenia. *Archives of General Psychiatry*, 48, 239–246.

Calabrese, J.R., Meltzer, H.Y. & Markovitz, P.J. (1991) Clozapine prophylaxis in rapid cycling bipolar disorder. *Journal of Clinical Psychopharmacology*, 11, 396–397.

Casey, D.E. (1989) Clozapine: neuroleptic-induced EPS and tardive dyskinesia. *Psychopharmacology*, Suppl. 99, S47–S53.

Cassady, S.L. & Thaker, G.K. (1992) Addition of fluoxetine to clozapine. *American Journal of Psychiatry*, 149, 1274.

Castelao, J.F., Ferrerira, L., Gelders, Y.G. & Heylen, S.L.E. (1989) The efficacy of the D$_2$ and 5-HT$_2$ antagonist risperidone (R 64 766) in the treatment of chronic psychoses. An open dose finding study. *Schizophrenia Research*, 2, 411–415.

Chiu, E., Burrows, G. & Stevenson, J. (1976) Double-blind comparison of clozapine with chlorpromazine in acute schizophrenic illness. *Australian and New Zealand Journal of Psychiatry*, 10, 343–347.

Choc, M.G., Lehr, R.G., Hsuan, F. *et al.* (1987) Multiple-dose pharmacokinetics of clozapine in patients. *Pharma-ceutical Research*, 4, 402–405.

Chouinard, G., Jones, B., Remington, G. *et al.* (1993) A Canadian multicenter placebo-controlled study with risperidone and haloperidol in the treatment of chronic schizophrenic patients. *Journal of Clinical Psychopharmacology*, 13, 25–40.

Ciompi, L. (1980) Catamnestic long-term study on the course

of life and aging of schizophrenics. *Schizophrenia Bulletin*, **6**, 606–618.

Claghorn, J., Honigfeld, G., Abuzzahab, F.S. *et al.* (1987) The risks and benefits of clozapine versus chlorpromazine. *Journal of Clinical Psychopharmacology*, **7**, 377–384.

Claus, A., Bollen, J., de Cuyper, H. *et al.* (1992) Risperidone vs. haloperidol in the treatment of chronic schizophrenic inpatients: a multicenter double-blind comparative study. *Acta Psychiatrica Scandinavica*, **85**, 295–305.

Collins, E.J., Lalonde, P., Jones, B.D. *et al.* (1992) Clozapine in the treatment of refractory schizophrenia: Canadian policies and clinical guidelines. *Canadian Journal of Psychiatry*, **37**, 482–496.

Devinsky, O., Honigfeld, G. & Patin, J. (1991) Clozapine-related seizures. *Neurology*, **41**, 369–371.

Ekblom, B. & Häggström, J.E. (1974) Clozapine (Leponex) compared with chlorpromazine: a double-blind evaluation of pharmacological and clinical properties. *Current Therapeutic Research*, **16**, 945–957.

Ekblom, B., Eriksson, K. & Lindström, L.H. (1984) Supersensitivity psychosis in schizophrenic patients after sudden clozapine withdrawal. *Psychopharmacology*, **83**, 293–294.

Fischer, V., Haar, J.A., Grenier, L., Lloyd, R.V. & Mason, R.P. (1991) Possible role of free radical formation in clozapine-(Clozaril®)-induced agranulocytosis. *Molecular Pharmacology*, **40**, 846–853.

Fischer-Cornelssen, K.A. & Ferner, U.J. (1974) Multifokale Psychopharmakaprufung ('Multihospital Trial'). *Arzneimittal-Forschung*, **24**, 1706–1724.

Fischer-Cornelssen, K.A. & Ferner, U.J. (1976) An example of European multicenter trials: multi-spectral analysis of clozapine. *Psychopharmacology Bulletin*, **12**, 34–39.

Friedman, J.H. & Lannon, M.C. (1989) Clozapine in the treatment of psychosis in Parkinson's disease. *Neurology*, **39**, 1219–1221.

Friedman, L., Knutson, L., Shurell, M. & Meltzer, H.Y. (1991) Prefrontal sulcal prominence is inversely related to response to clozapine in schizophrenic patients. *Biological Psychiatry*, **29**, 865–877.

Gelenberg, A.J. & Doller, J.C. (1979) Clozapine versus chlorpromazine for the treatment of schizophrenia: preliminary results from a double-blind study. *Journal of Clinical Psychiatry*, **40**, 238–240.

Gerlach, J., Koppelhus, P., Helweg, E. & Manrad, A. (1974) Clozapine and haloperidol in a single-blind cross-over trial. Therapeutic and biochemical aspects in the treatment of schizophrenia. *Acta Psychiatrica Scandinavica*, **50**, 410–424.

Goldberg, T.E., Greenberg, R.D., Griffin, S.J. *et al.* (1993) The effect of clozapine on cognition and psychiatric symptoms in patients with schizophrenia. *British Journal of Psychiatry*, **162**, 43–48.

Goldstein, J.M., Litwin, L.C., Sutton, E.B. & Malick, J.B. (1993) Seroquel: electrophysiological profile of a potential atypical antipsychotic. *Psychopharmacology*, **112**, 293–299.

Grabowski, J. (1992) Clonidine treatment of clozapine-induced hypersalivation. *Journal of Clinical Psychopharmacology*, **12**, 69–70.

Guirguis, E., Voineskos, G., Gray, J. & Schlieman, E. (1977) Clozapine (Leponex) vs. chlorpromazine (Largactil) in acute schizophrenia (a double-blind controlled study). *Current Therapeutic Research*, **21**, 707–719.

Hagger, C., Buckley, P., Kenny, J.T., Friedman, L., Ubogy, D. & Meltzer, H.Y. (1993) Improvement in cognitive functions and psychiatric symptoms in treatment-refractory schizophrenic patients receiving clozapine. *Biological Psychiatry*, **34**, 702–712.

Haller, E. & Binder, R.L. (1990) Clozapine and seizures. *American Journal of Psychiatry*, **147**, 1067–1071.

Haring, C., Meise, U., Humpel, C., Saria, A., Fleischhacker, W.W. & Hinterhuber, H. (1989) Dose-related plasma levels of clozapine: influence of smoking behaviour, sex and age. *Psychopharmacology*, Suppl. **99**, S38–S40.

Hasegawa M., Gutierrez-Esteinou, R., Way, L. & Meltzer, H.Y. (1993) Relationship between clinical efficacy and clozapine plasma concentrations in schizophrenia: effect of smoking. *Journal of Clinical Psychopharmacology*, **13**, 383–390.

Hasegawa, M., Cola, P.A. & Meltzer, H.Y. (1994) Plasma clozapine and desmethyclozapine levels in clozapine-induced agranulocytosis. *Neuropsychopharmacology*, **11**, 45–47.

Heinrichs, D.W., Hanlon, E.T. & Carpenter, W.T. Jr (1984) The Quality of Life Scale: an instrument for rating the schizophrenic deficit syndrome. *Schizophrenia Bulletin*, **10**, 388–398.

Hippius, H. (1989) The history of clozapine. *Psychopharmacology*, Suppl. **99**, S3–S5.

Hirsch, S.R., Link, C.G.G., Goldstein, J.M. & Arvanitis, L.A. Seroquel: a new atypical antipsychotic drug. (In press.)

Honigfeld, G. & Patin, J. (1990) A two-year clinical and economic follow-up of patients on clozapine. *Hospital and Community Psychiatry*, **41**, 882–885.

Huber, G., Gross, G. & Schuttler, R. (1975). A long-term follow-up study of schizophrenia. Psychiatric course of illness and prognosis. *Acta Psychiatrica Scandinavica*, **52**, 49–57.

Ishigooka, J. (1991) Clinical experience with risperidone in Japan — a multicentre early phase II trial. In Kane, J.M. (ed.) *Risperidone: Major Progress in Antipsychotic Treatment*, pp. 40–43. Oxford Clinical Communications, Oxford.

Jann, M.W., Grimstey, S.R., Gray, E.C. & Change, W.-H. (1993) Pharmacokinetics and pharmacodynamics of clozapine. *Clinical Pharmacokinetics*, **24**, 161–176.

Kane, J., Honigfeld, G., Singer, J., Meltzer, H.Y. and the Clozaril Collaborative Study Group (1988) Clozapine for the treatment-resistant schizophrenic: a double-blind comparison with chlorpromazine. *Archives of General Psychiatry*, **45**, 789–796.

Krupp, P. & Barnes, P. (1989) Leponex-associated granulocytopenia: a review of the situation. *Psychopharmacology*, Suppl. **99**, S118–S121.

Lamberti, J.S., Bellnier, T. & Schwarzkopf, S.B. (1992) Weight gain among schizophrenic patients treated with clozapine. *American Journal of Psychiatry*, **149**, 689–690.

Leadbetter, R., Schulty, M., Pavalonis, D., Vieweg, V., Hippius, P. & Downs, P. (1992) Clozapine-induced weight gain: prevalence and clinical relevance. *American Journal of Psychiatry*, **149**, 68–72.

Lee, H.S., Kwon, K.Y., Alphs, L.D. & Meltzer, H.Y. (1991)

Effect of clozapine on psychogenic polydipsa in chronic schizophrenia. *Journal of Clinical Psychopharmacology*, **11**, 222–223.

Levin, H., Chengappa, K.N., Kambhampati, R.K., Mathdavi, N. & Ganguli, R. (1992) Should chronic treatment-refractory akathisia be an indication for the use of clozapine in schizophrenic patients. *Journal of Clinical Psychiatry*, **53**, 248–251.

Lewander, T., Westerberg, S.-E. & Morrison, D. (1990) Clinical profile of remoxipride – a combined analysis of a comparative double-blind multicentre trial programme. *Acta Psychiatrica Scandinavia*, **82** (Suppl. 358), 92–98.

Leysen, J.C., Gommeren, W., Eens, A., de Chaffoy de Courcelles, D., Stoff, J.C. & Janssen, P.A.J. (1988) Biochemical profile of risperidone, a new antipsychotic. *Journal of Pharmacology and Experimental Therapeutics*, **247**, 661–670.

Liddle, P.F., Friston, K.J., Frith, C.D., Jones, T., Hirsch, S.R. & Frackowiak, R.S.J. (1992) Patterns of cerebral blood flow in schizophrenia. *British Journal of Psychiatry*, **160**, 179–186.

Lieberman, J.A., Kane, J.M. & Johns, C.A. (1989) Clozapine: guidelines for clinical management. *Journal of Clinical Psychiatry*, **50**, 329–338.

Lieberman, J.A., Saltz, B.L., Johns, C.A., Pollack, S., Borenstein, M. & Kane, J. (1991) The effect of clozapine on tardive dyskinesia. *British Journal of Psychiatry*, **158**, 503–510.

Lieberman, J.A., Yunis, J., Egea, E., Canoso, R.T., Kane, J.M. & Yunis, E.J. (1990) HLA-B38, DR4, DQw3 and clozapine-induced agranulocytosis in Jewish patients with schizophrenia. *Archives of General Psychiatry*, **47**, 945–948.

Lieberman, J., Jody, D., Geisler, S. *et al.* (1993) Time course and biological correlates of treatment response in first episode schizophrenia. *Archives of General Psychiatry*, **50**, 369–376.

Lindström, L.H. (1988) The effect of long-term treatment with clozapine in schizophrenia: a retrospective study in 96 patients treated with clozapine for up to 13 years. *Acta Psychiatrica Scandinavica*, **77**, 524–529.

Lovdahl, M.J., Perry, P.J. & Miller, D.D. (1991) The assay of clozapine and *N*-desmethylclozapine in human plasma by high-performance liquid chromatography. *Therapeutic Drug Monitoring*, **13**, 69–72.

McCreadie, R.G., Todd, M., Livingston, M. *et al.* (1990) A double-blind comparative study of remoxipride and thioridazine in the acute phase of schizophrenia. *Acta Psychiatrica Scandinavica*, **82** (Suppl. 358), 136–137.

McGlashan, T.H. (1988) A selective review of recent North American long-term follow-up studies of schizophrenia. *Schizophrenia Bulletin*, **14**, 515–542.

Meco, G., Bedini, L., Bonifati, V. & Sonini, U. (1989) Risperidone in the treatment of chronic schizophrenia with tardive dyskinesia: a single blind crossover study versus placebo. *Current Therapeutic Research*, **46**, 876–883.

Megens, A.A., Awouters, F.H. & Niemegeers, C.J. (1988) Differential effects of new antipsychotic risperidone on large and small motor movements in rats: a comparison with haloperidol. *Psychopharmacology*, **95**, 493–496.

Meltzer, H.Y. (1989a) Clozapine and electroconvulsive therapy. *Archives of General Psychiatry*, **47**, 290–291.

Meltzer, H.Y. (1989b) Duration of a clozapine trial in neuroleptic-resistant schizophrenia. *Archives of General Psychiatry*, **46**, 672.

Meltzer, H.Y. (1990) Commentary: defining treatment refractoriness in schizophrenia. *Schizophrenia Bulletin*, **16**, 563–566.

Meltzer, H.Y. (1991a) Atypical antipsychotic drugs: a clinical update. In Meltzer, H.Y. & Nerozzi, D. (eds) *Current Practices and Future Developments in the Pharmacotherapy of Mental Disorders*, pp. 59–65. Elsevier, Amsterdam.

Meltzer, H.Y. (1991b) The mechanism of action of novel antipsychotic drugs. *Schizophrenia Bulletin*, **17**, 263–287.

Meltzer, H.Y. (1992) Treatment of the neuroleptic non-responsive schizophrenic patient. *Schizophrenia Bulletin*, **18**, 515–542.

Meltzer, H.Y. & Luchins, D.J. (1984) Effect of clozapine in severe tardive dyskinesia: a case report. *Journal of Clinical Psychopharmacology*, **4**, 286–287.

Meltzer, H.Y., Bastani, B., Ramirez, L.F. & Matsubara, S. (1989b) Clozapine: new research on efficacy and mechanism of action. *European Archives of Psychiatry and Neurological Science*, **238**, 332–339.

Meltzer, H.Y., Burnett, S., Bastani, B. & Ramirez, L.F. (1990) Effect of six months of clozapine treatment on the quality of life of chronic schizophrenic patients. *Hospital and Community Psychiatry*, **41**, 892–897.

Meltzer, H.Y., Goode, D.J., Schyve, P.M., Young, M. & Fang, V.S. (1979) Effect of clozapine on human serum prolactin levels. *American Journal of Psychiatry*, **136**, 1550–1555.

Meltzer, H.Y., Bastani, B., Kwon, K.Y., Ramirez, L.F., Burnett, S. & Sharpe, J. (1989a) A prospective study of clozapine in treatment-resistant patients. I. Preliminary report. *Psychopharmacology*, Suppl. **99**, S68–S72.

Meltzer, H.Y., Cola, P., Way, L. *et al.* (1993) Cost effectiveness of clozapine in neuroleptic-resistant schizophrenia. *American Journal of Psychiatry*, **150**, 1630–1638.

Mesotten, F., Suy, E., Pictquin, M., Burton, P., Heylen, S. & Gelders, Y. (1989) Therapeutic effect and safety of increasing doses of risperidone (R 64766) in psychotic patients. *Psychopharmacology*, **99**, 445–449.

Michaels, M.L., Crimson, M.L., Robert, S. & Childs, A. (1993) Clozapine response and adverse effects in nine brain-injured patients. *Journal of Clinical Psychopharmacology*, **13**, 192–203.

Migler, B.M., Warawa, E.J. & Malik, J.B. (1993) Seroquel: behavioral effects in conventional and novel tests for atypical antipsychotic drug. *Psychopharmacology*, **112**, 299–307.

Miller, D.D. (1991) Effect of phenytoin on plasma clozapine concentrations in two patients. *Journal of Clinical Psychiatry*, **52**, 23–35.

Miller, D.D., Sharafuddin, M.J.A. & Kathol, R.G. (1991) A case of clozapine-induced neuroleptic malignant syndrome. *Journal of Clinical Psychiatry*, **52**, 99–101.

Moore, N.A., Calligaro, D.O., Wong, D.T., Bymaster, F. & Tye, N.C. (1993) The pharmacology of olanzapine and other new antipsychotic agents. *Current Opinion in Invest*

Drug, **2**, 281–293.

Naber, D., Leppig, M., Grohmann, R. & Hippius, H. (1989) Efficacy and adverse effects of clozapine in the treatment of schizophrenia and tardive dyskinesia — a retrospective study of 387 patients. *Psychopharmacology*, Suppl. **99**, S73–S76.

Parsa, M.A., Al-Lanhram, Y., Ramirez, L.F. & Meltzer, H.Y. (1993) Prolonged psychotic relapse after abrupt clozapine withdrawal. *Journal of Clinical Psychopharmacology*, **13**, 154–155.

Parsa, M., Ramirez, L.F., Loula, E.C. & Meltzer, H.Y. (1991) Effect of clozapine on psychotic depression and parkinsonism. *Journal of Clinical Psychopharmacology*, **11**, 330–331.

Patil, J. (1992) Development of transient obsessive-compulsive symptoms during treatment with clozapine. *American Journal of Psychiatry*, **449**, 272.

Perry, P.J., Miller, D.D., Arndt, S.V. & Cadoret, R.J. (1991) Clozapine and norclozapine plasma concentrations and clinical response of treatment-refractory schizophrenic patients. *American Journal of Psychiatry*, **148**, 231–235.

Pfister, G.M., Hanson, D.R., Roerig, J.L., Landbloom, R. & Popkin, M.K. (1992) Clozapine-induced agranulocytosis in a native American: HLA typing and further support for an immune-mediated mechanism. *Journal of Clinical Psychiatry*, **53**, 242–244.

Pope, H.G. Jr, McElroy, S.L., Keck, P.E. & Hudson, J.I. (1991) Valproate in the treatment of acute mania. *Archives of General Psychiatry*, **44**, 113–118.

Povlsen, U.J., Noring, U., Fog, T. & Gerlach, J. (1985) Tolerability and therapeutic effect of clozapine: a retrospective investigation of 216 patients treated with clozapine for up to 12 years. *Acta Psychiatrica Scandinavica*, **71**, 176–185.

Revicki, D.A., Luce, B.R., Wechsler, J.M., Brown, R.E. & Adler, M.A. (1990) Cost-effectiveness of clozapine for treatment-resistant schizophrenic patients. *Hospital and Community Psychiatry*, **41**, 850–855.

Sajatovic, M., Verbanac, P., Ramirez, L.F. & Meltzer, H.Y. (1991) Clozapine treatment of psychiatric symptoms resistant to neuroleptic treatment in patients with Huntington's chorea. *Neurology*, **41**, 156.

Saller, C.F. & Salama, A.I. (1993) Seroquel: biochemical profile of a potential atypical antipsychotic. *Psychopharmacology*, **112**, 285–292.

Schmutz, J. & Eichenberger, E. (1982) Clozapine. In Bindra, J.S. & Lednicer, D. (eds) *Chronicles in Drug Discovery*, Vol. 1, pp. 39–58. Wiley, New York.

Shaler, A., Harmesh, H., Rothberg, J. & Munitz, H. (1993) Poor neuroleptic response in acutely exacerbated schizo-phrenia patients. *Acta Psychiatrica Scandinavica*, **87**, 86–91.

Shopsin, B., Klein, H., Aaronson, M. & Collora, M. (1979) Clozapine, chlorpromazine and placebo in newly hospitalized, acutely schizophrenic patients. *Archives of General Psychiatry*, **36**, 657–664.

Singer, K. & Law, S.K. (1974) A double-blind comparison of clozapine (Leponex) and chlorpromazine in schizophrenia of acute symptomatology. *Journal of Internal Medical Research*, **2**, 433–435.

Suppes, T., McElroy, S.L., Gilbert, J., Dessain, E.C. & Cole, J.O .(1992) Clozapine in the treatment of dysphoric mania. *Biological Psychiatry*, **32**, 270–280.

Svestka, J., Ceskora, E., Rysanek, R. & Obrovske, V. (1990) Double-blind clinical comparison of risperidone and haloperidol in acute schizophrenic and schizoaffective psychoses. *Activas Nervosa*, **32** (Suppl.), 237–238.

Szymanski, S., Lieberman, J.A., Picou, D., Masiar, S. & Cooper, T. (1991) A case report of cimetidine-induced clozapine toxicity. *Journal of Clinical Psychiatry*, **52**, 21–22.

Thompson, P.A. & Meltzer, H.Y. (1993) Positive, negative and disorganization factors from the Schedule of Affective Disorders and Schizophrenia-Change scale and the Present State Examination. *British Journal of Psychiatry*, **163**, 111–119.

Tiihonen, J., Nousiainen, U., Hakola, P. *et al.* (1991) EEG abnormalities associated with clozapine treatment. *American Journal of Psychiatry*, **148**, 1406.

Van den Borre, R., Vermite, R., Buttiens, M. *et al.* (1993) Risperidone as addon therapy in behavioral disturbances in mental retardation: a double-blind placebo-controlled cross-over study. *Acta Psychiatrica Scandinavica*, **87**, 167–171.

Van den Bussche, G., Heykants, J. & De Coster, R. (1988) Pharmacokinetic profile and neuroendocrine effects of the new antipsychotic risperidone. *Psychopharmacology*, **96** (Suppl.), 334.

Vencovsky, E., Peterova, E. & Baudis, P. (1975) Comparison of therapeutic effect of clozapine and chlorpromazine. *Ceskoslovenska Psychiatrie*, **71**, 21–26.

Von Bahr, C., Movin, G., Yisak, W.-A., Jostell, K.G. & Widman, M. (1992) Clinical pharmacokinetics of remoxipride. *Acta Psychiatrica Scandinavica*, **82** (Suppl. 358), 41–44.

Weide, R., Köppler, H., Heymanns, J., Pfüger, K.H. & Havemann, K. (1992) Successful treatment of clozapine-induced agranulocytosis with granulocyte-colony stimulating factor (G-CSF). *British Journal of Haematology*, **80**, 557–559.

Chapter 26
Electroconvulsive Therapy and Schizophrenia

R. B. KRUEGER AND H. A. SACKEIM

Introduction

Using intramuscular injection of camphor, Meduna was the first to deliberately induce seizures with the aim of treating schizophrenia (Meduna, 1935). Soon afterwards, Cerletti and Bini (1938) introduced the use of electricity as a method of seizure induction, again with the intent of treating schizophrenia. During the 1940s and 1950s, electroconvulsive therapy (ECT) was widely adopted and its use extended to a number of disorders. In subsequent decades, particularly in the USA, the introduction of effective pharmacological treatments for schizophrenia and mood disorders led to a sharp drop in ECT utilization (Thompson & Blaine, 1987). However, interest in ECT has increased in recent years and its use after declining markedly from the levels in the 1950s, appears to be increasing (Fink, 1987).

The efficacy of ECT in some disorders, such as major depression, is well supported (Janicak et al., 1985; Sackeim, 1989). Indeed, one can argue that in the case of major depression the evidence regarding the efficacy of ECT is among the strongest in all of medicine (Sackeim et al., 1993). However, the indications for the use of ECT and its efficacy in schizophrenia are less clear. Some authorities have dismissed or warned against the use of ECT in schizophrenia (Ottosson, 1985; Hamilton, 1986). More recently, the American Psychiatric Association (APA) Task Force on ECT stated that ECT is an effective treatment for 'psychotic schizophrenic exacerbations', particularly in the context of catatonia, when affective symptomatology is prominent, or when there is a history of a favourable response to ECT (APA, 1990). Others have more decisively advocated that ECT is indicated in schizophrenia or specific subtypes (Van Valkenburg & Clayton, 1985; Abrams, 1987; Kalinowsky, 1988; Hertzman, 1992). Here, we review the literature on the use of ECT in schizophrenia and address many issues that confront the clinician: is ECT useful in the treatment of schizophrenia? If so, for what types of schizophrenia or for what symptoms? At what point should ECT be considered? Should it be administered after neuroleptic medications have failed, or in combination with medications to enhance efficacy or to reduce neuroleptic dosage? Are there special risks in providing ECT to this population? How should ECT be administered? How many treatments should be given? How long do the beneficial and adverse effects last? Is there a place for maintenance ECT?

Current practice and recommendations

A number of surveys, in several countries, have examined the extent to which schizophrenic patients are represented among ECT recipients. The APA Task Force on ECT surveyed APA members in 1976 and estimated that 17% of patients who received ECT in the USA had diagnoses of schizophrenia (APA, 1978). Thompson and Blaine (1987), using medical record data collected by the National Institute of Mental Health (NIMH), estimated that in 1980 16.6% of the patients who received ECT in public and private in-patient facilities in the USA carried the diagnosis of schizophrenia. These patients constituted only 2.1% of those admitted to these facilities with this diagnosis. Similarly, in a survey conducted at a US teaching hospital, Tancer *et al.* (1989) found that schizophrenic patients constituted 15% in 1970 and 11% in 1980–81 of those administered ECT.

In Great Britain, Pippard and Ellam (1981) sent a questionnaire to 3221 psychiatrists, of whom 1274 reported on the use of ECT. Of 2591 treatment series identified in this survey, 83% were for patients with depressive disorders and 13% were for patients with a diagnosis of schizophrenia. In Ireland, Latey and Fahy (1988) surveyed 49 psychiatrists and found that, of 391 treatment series given, most patients had depressive disorders, but 17% had schizophrenia. Malla (1986) retrospectively examined 5729 consecutive admissions between 1975 and 1978 to three general hospitals and the mental hospital in St John's, Newfoundland, Canada; 28.8% of the admissions that received ECT had a diagnosis

of schizophrenia. In fact, of all admissions of schizophrenic patients, 36.5% went on to receive ECT. Martin *et al.* (1984), in a study of ECT administered at the Clarke Institute in Toronto, Canada, found that patients with a primary discharge diagnosis of an affective disorder received 54.3% of the courses, whereas those with schizophrenia received 36.0%. Bland and Brintnell (1985) reviewed the use of ECT over an 11-year period, from 1972 to 1982, in the University of Alberta hospitals: 5% of patients received ECT, and approximately 75% of patients so treated had a discharge diagnosis of affective psychosis and 20% had a diagnosis of schizophrenia. Smith and Richman (1984), using Medicare data, hospital discharge statistics and questionnaires in selected Canadian hospitals, found that during the years 1975–78, 8.0% of females and 6.5% of males with schizophrenia and paranoid psychoses were treated with ECT. Shugar *et al.* (1984) reviewed data from 221 hospitals in Ontario during 1980–81 and observed that of a total of 1977 courses of ECT administered, 24.3% were given to schizophrenic patients. They found great variation in the utilization of ECT between hospitals, with a range of 0.6–32.8%, with individuals with schizoaffective disorder having higher ECT rates.

In a retrospective examination of all patients treated in 1984 with ECT at the Aarhus Psychiatric Hospital in Risskov, Denmark, Strömgren (1988) found that only 2.9% had a diagnosis of schizophrenia. Shukla (1981) described the use of ECT in an Indian rural teaching hospital between 1977 and 1980. Of the 503 cases reviewed, 75% of the patients had a diagnosis of schizophrenia. In a recent national survey of psychiatrists in India, it was reported that 13.4% of psychiatric patients were administered ECT (Agarwal *et al.*, 1992). Of this group, 43% had a diagnosis of schizophrenia. Thus, there appears to be marked variability both between and within countries in the representation of schizophrenic patients among those who receive ECT. Clearly, many prescribers consider schizophrenia an indication for ECT.

This diversity of practice is reflected in current recommendations of national medical and psychiatric organizations. The APA Task Force on ECT recently recommended the treatment for psychotic schizophrenic exacerbations when catatonia or affective symptomatology were prominent, or given a history of a favourable response to ECT (APA, 1990). This group suggested that ECT is also effective in related psychotic disorders, notably schizophreniform disorder and schizoaffective disorder, and in atypical psychosis when the clinical features were similar to those of other major diagnostic indications.

In contrast, a National Institutes of Health (NIH) Consensus Development Panel stated:

> Neuroleptics are the first line of treatment for schizophrenia. The evidence for the efficacy of ECT in schizophrenia is not compelling, but is strongest for those schizophrenic patients with a shorter duration of illness, a more acute onset, and more intense affective symptoms. It has not been useful in chronically ill schizophrenic patients. Although ECT is frequently advocated for treatment of patients with schizophreniform psychoses, schizoaffective disorders, and catatonia, there are no adequate controlled studies (NIH, 1985).

The Canadian Psychiatric Association stated that ECT was useful for some patients with schizophrenia (Pankratz, 1980). Since it was felt that pharmacological agents were typically more effective, ECT should be reserved for the schizophrenic patient who had failed at least one adequate pharmacological trial. The British Royal College of Psychiatrists Memorandum on the use of ECT, citing the May (1968) study, also stated that in general the efficacy of ECT in schizophrenia was less than that of standard neuroleptic treatment (Royal College of Psychiatrists, 1977). Furthermore, this group questioned whether there are specific features of schizophrenia that are particularly responsive to ECT.

Thus, among expert groups and national psychiatric associations, there is a lack of consensus regarding the role of ECT in schizophrenia.

Efficacy

Early studies

The efficacy of ECT in schizophrenia has been the subject of several critical reviews (Staudt & Zubin, 1957; Riddell, 1963; Turek & Hanlon, 1977; Fink, 1979; Salzman, 1980; Scovern & Kilmann, 1980; Kendell, 1981; Taylor, 1981; Small, 1985; Abrams, 1992). Many of the earlier reports on this use of ECT consisted of uncontrolled case material (Guttmann *et al.*, 1939; Ross & Malzberg, 1939; Zeifert, 1941; Kalinowsky, 1943; Kalinowsky & Worthing, 1943; Danziger & Kindwall, 1946; Kino & Thorpe, 1946; Kennedy & Anchel, 1948; Miller *et al.*, 1953). Additionally, diagnostic practice preceded the introduction of operationalized criteria for schizophrenia, and often patient samples and outcome criteria were poorly characterized. International differences in the rate of diagnosis of schizophrenia have been well described, with documentation that psychiatrists in the USA, compared with British colleagues, were overinclusive in diagnosing schizophrenia, often labelling patients with affective or schizoaffective disorder as schizophrenic. Thus, earlier US studies describing samples of schizophrenic patients may have contained substantial representation of mood-disorder patients, who may be particularly likely to respond to ECT (Mowbray, 1959; Kendell, 1971; Abrams *et al.*, 1974; Abrams & Taylor, 1976b; Pope & Lipinski, 1978; Pope *et al.*, 1980).

Overall, the earlier reports on the use of ECT in schizophrenia were enthusiastic for patients with relatively recent onset of illness, with recovery or marked improvement noted in a large proportion of cases, typically in the order of 75% (Fink, 1979; Small, 1985). Historical comparisons (Ellison & Hamilton, 1949; Gottlieb & Huston, 1951; Currier *et al.*, 1952; Bond, 1954) and comparisons to psychotherapy or milieu therapy suggested that the introduction of ECT resulted in both superior short-term clinical outcome and more sustained remissions (Goldfarb & Kieve, 1945; McKinnon, 1948; Palmer *et al.*, 1951; Wolff 1955; Rachlin *et al.*, 1956). However, in this early era, the view was also expressed that ECT was considerably less effective in schizophrenic patients with insidious onset and long duration of illness (Cheney & Drewry, 1938; Ross & Malzberg, 1939; Zeifert, 1941; Chafetz, 1943; Kalinowsky, 1943; Lowinger & Huddleson, 1945; Danziger & Kindwall, 1946; Shoor & Adams, 1950; Herzberg, 1954). In addition, it was suggested that schizophrenic patients often required intensive courses of ECT, involving more frequent and closely spaced treatments (Baker *et al.*, 1960a; Kalinowsky, 1943).

Studies of sham vs. real ECT in schizophrenia

ECT is a highly ritualized treatment, involving a repeated, complex procedure. In ECT research, the sham vs. real ECT comparison is similar to the placebo-controlled trial in pharmacological research. With sham ECT, patients undergo the complete ECT procedure, including the administration of anaesthesia, but no electric current is applied. Superior response rates with 'real' ECT relative to sham conditions indicate that the passage of current and/or the production of a generalized seizure contribute to the efficacy of ECT. Table 26.1 summarizes the sham vs. real ECT studies that have included schizophrenic patients.

Miller *et al.* (1953) selected 30 chronic patients who had been diagnosed with catatonic schizophrenia. The patients were randomized to three groups: unmodified (no anaesthetic agent) bilateral ECT; sham ECT with pentothal; or pentothal plus low-intensity, non-convulsive stimulation for 5 min. All the treatment groups evidenced improvement in social performance, as evaluated by blind and non-blind raters, without group differences.

Ulett *et al.* (1954, 1956) conducted a double-blind random assignment study involving 84 patients. Four treatment groups were contrasted: sham ECT involving seconal anaesthesia, ECT, subconvulsive photoshock and convulsive photoshock. The photoshock therapy involved pretreating patients with an intravenous convulsant drug, hexazol, and then administering intermittent photic stimulation. In the subconvulsive condition, photic stimulation resulted in a few minutes of generalized myoclonic activity without evidence of a generalized seizure or loss of consciousness. All patients received intravenous seconal to induce anaesthesia before each session. The two groups who experienced full convulsions (ECT or photoconvulsive) had significantly greater improvement in symptom ratings than did the other two groups. However, the acute schizophrenic subgroup was not analysed separately.

Brill *et al.* (1957, 1959a−c) studied a heterogeneous group of 97 patients that included 67 patients diagnosed as having schizophrenic reactions, 14 with schizoaffective disorders and 16 with depressive reactions. The patients were randomized to one of five treatment groups: unmodified ECT, ECT plus succinylcholine, ECT plus thiopental, thiopental alone and nitrous oxide alone. In this double-blind study, three different methods were used to evaluate clinical outcome 1 month after the end of treatment. There were no differences among the groups in ratings of therapeutic change. In particular, among the schizophrenic patients, the differences were slight between those that had received a form of ECT and those that had not.

Heath *et al.* (1964) selected 77 patients with a diagnosis of chronic schizophrenia. This randomized, double-blind experiment was divided into two substudies. The first substudy compared the effects of four ECT treatments with four sham treatments in 45 patients. The second part involved a total sample of 32 patients, divided into four groups. One group was administered eight real treatments, a second group was administered eight sham treatments, a third group constituted an 'untreated' control and a fourth group was told that they would receive ECT but their somatic treatment was left unchanged. In both substudies, a therapeutic advantage for real ECT could not be identified. Heath *et al.* questioned whether 'the elaborate procedure involved in providing ECT was worth it'.

Taylor and Fleminger (1980) conducted a randomized, double-blind trial in a group of 20 schizophrenic patients. Of particular note, both

Table 26.1 Prospective clinical trials comparing real and sham electroconvulsive therapy (ECT) in schizophrenia

Study	Patients	Study design	Number of treatments	Results/comments
Miller *et al.* (1953)	30 chronic catatonic schizophrenics (average hospitalization 10 years)	Sham vs. subconvulsive stimulation vs. ECT	ECT given 5 days per week for 3 weeks; subconvulsive and sham given 5 days per week for 4 weeks	All groups improved, with no differences among the groups
Ulett *et al.* (1954, 1956)	20 brief schizophrenic reactions included in sample of 84 patients	Sham vs. subconvulsive photic stimulation vs. convulsive photic stimulation vs. ECT	12–15 treatments, 3 times per week	Convulsive therapies superior to sham and subconvulsive stimulation. Study hampered by inhomogeneous groups, lack of diagnostic criteria and lack of separate analysis for schizophrenia
Brill *et al.* (1957, 1959a–c)	67 of 97 patients had chronic schizophrenic reactions	Unmodified ECT vs. ECT and succinylcholine vs. ECT and thiopental vs. thiopental alone vs. nitrous oxide alone	Generally 20 treatments, 3 times per week	No difference in effectiveness among the five groups or in the pooled ECT vs. non-ECT groups; no difference in effectiveness for the 67 schizophrenics and the 30 depressives considered separately
Heath *et al.* (1964)	77 chronic schizophrenics with 5 years or greater hospitalization	Sham vs. ECT vs. 'untreated' control vs. group promised but not given ECT; many patients received phenothiazines during the trial	Sample divided into 45 patients who received real or sham ECT once a week for 4 weeks or no treatment, and 32 patients who received real or sham ECT twice a week for 4 weeks, an 'untreated' control group and a promised ECT but not delivered control group	The groups could not be distinguished in efficacy variables. Sample size was small for discrete treatment conditions
Taylor and Fleminger (1980)	20 schizophrenics by Present State Examination; both acute (<6 months) and chronic patients excluded	Sham vs. ECT; patients maintained on standard doses of neuroleptics (CPZ 300 mg/day or equivalent) for 2 weeks before entry into trial	8–12 treatments, 3 times per week; seven patients received bilateral ECT and three patients unilateral ECT	ECT superior to sham at 2, 4 and 8 weeks; no difference at 16 weeks

Continued on p. 508

Table 26.1 (*Continued*)

Study	Patients	Study design	Number of treatments	Results/comments
Brandon *et al.* (1985)	17 schizophrenics by Present State Examination	Sham vs. ECT; equivalent daily doses of neuroleptic in real and sham ECT groups	8 treatments; twice weekly for 4 weeks	ECT superior to sham at 2 and 4 weeks; no difference at 12 and 28 weeks
Abraham and Kulhara (1987)	22 schizophrenic patients by the RDC with duration of illness <2 years	Sham vs. ECT; trifluoperazine held constant, no more than 20 mg/day	8 treatments, twice weekly for 4 weeks	ECT group showed more rapid improvement than sham group; from 12 weeks to 6 months no difference

CPZ, chlorpromazine; RDC, research diagnostic criteria.

the patients with short duration of illness and the patients with chronic conditions were excluded. All patients received standard doses of neuroleptics for at least 2 weeks before and throughout the ECT trial. Both groups improved in symptom scores, but the improvement with real ECT was significantly greater after six treatments and at the end of the treatment course. However, 3 months following the treatment course, there was little difference between the groups.

Brandon *et al.* (1985) conducted a random-assignment, double-blind study with 17 patients, assigned to either real or sham ECT. Neuroleptics were restricted during the 4-week trial period in the following manner: patients were not permitted to commence a new course of neuroleptics, but if a patient was already stabilized on neuroleptic prior to starting the trial, this could be continued. At the end of the 4 weeks, the real ECT group showed significantly greater improvement in ratings of schizophrenic symptoms, depressive symptoms and global psychopathology. This difference was not maintained at 12-week and 28-week assessment points.

Abraham and Kulhara (1987) studied 22 schizophrenic patients maintained on trifluoperazine (up to 20 mg/day) and randomized to real or sham ECT. In this double-blind study, clinical outcome was superior with real ECT for up to 12 weeks after the start of treatment. Assessments conducted between 16 and 26 weeks yielded no group differences.

Summary

With the possible exception of the study of Ulett *et al.* (1956), the early studies that compared real ECT and sham ECT failed to demonstrate a therapeutic advantage for the application of electricity and seizure induction relative to administration of general anaesthesia alone (Miller *et al.*, 1953; Brill *et al.*, 1959a–c; Heath *et al.*, 1964). In contrast, at least in the short term, the three recent studies each found clinically significant therapeutic advantages for real ECT vs. sham ECT (Taylor & Fleminger, 1980; Brandon *et al.*, 1985; Abraham & Kulhara, 1987). The source of this discrepancy is unknown. The recent studies have had small sample sizes, but this factor should have limited the possibility of obtaining statistically significant findings. It is noteworthy that Taylor and Fleminger (1980) explicitly focused on a 'middle-prognostic' group, and excluded patients with chronic conditions. The representation of patients with chronic schizophrenia in some of the early studies may have mitigated against establishing an ECT advantage (e.g. Heath *et al.*, 1964). Another possibility is that in each of the recent studies, patients have been maintained on neuroleptic medications during the sham-ECT trial. As discussed below, there is reason to believe that the combination of ECT and neuroleptics is a more effective treatment than either form of monotherapy. Additive or synergistic ECT–neuroleptic interactions may have augmented the efficacy of real ECT conditions in the recent studies.

It is also noteworthy in the recent work that the advantage of real ECT relative to sham conditions only pertained to the period of time during and immediately following the active administration of ECT. Within months of trial termination, symptomatic differences between the groups were not evident. The importance of these negative findings is questionable. In each case, the treatment received following the completion of the randomized trial was uncontrolled. Indeed, in some cases, patients assigned to the sham condition went on to receive ECT. Without a more consistent approach to additional acute treatment and control over continuation therapy, it is impossible to determine whether the advantages observed in these studies for real ECT relative to sham conditions were truly short lived.

Studies comparing ECT with neuroleptics or other therapies

From a clinical vantage point, determining that ECT is more effective than sham treatment is of limited utility. A more pressing question concerns the efficacy of ECT compared with other somatic treatments, particularly the use of neuroleptic medication. Soon after the introduction of antipsychotic medications, a series of retrospective and prospective reports appeared and provided such comparisons. In general, the findings of the retrospective studies were inconclusive (e.g. DeWet, 1957; Borowitz, 1959; Ayres, 1960; Rohde & Sargant, 1961), although some contended that the combination of ECT and antipsychotic medication was particularly effective (Ford & Jameson, 1955; Rohde & Sargant, 1961; Weinstein & Fischer, 1971). Here we concentrate on the prospective investigations. This work is summarized in Table 26.2.

Baker *et al.* (1958) selected 48 chronically ill, hospitalized, female schizophrenics and assigned

18 to an ECT group, 15 to an insulin coma group and 15 to a chlorpromazine (CPZ) group. The groups were treated for different periods, ranging from 5 weeks for insulin coma to 8 weeks for CPZ. Improvement ratings were equivalent among the groups 1 week following the trial. However, relapse rates were significantly higher in the CPZ group than in the ECT or insulin coma group. This study was limited by use of low CPZ dosage. In addition, the blindness of clinical ratings was not discussed, and the length of the follow-up period for determining relapse was unspecified.

In a later report, Baker *et al.* (1960b) abandoned the CPZ group on the grounds of limited efficacy and added patients to the ECT and insulin coma conditions. The final sample of 37 ECT patients had a higher rate of treatment completion and hospital discharge than did the final sample of 36 patients assigned to insulin coma.

Langsley *et al.* (1959) randomized 106 patients with 'acute schizophrenia' or manic reactions to ECT or CPZ conditions. Ratings by blind psychiatrists demonstrated that the groups were equivalent in short-term clinical improvement. However, there were indications that the CPZ group could be discharged earlier than the ECT group. Among other problems, the findings were not reported separately for patients with manic and schizophrenic diagnoses. In addition, the entry requirement of a maximum of 3 months of psychotic symptoms suggests that the schizophrenic group may have contained a large number of patients who would now be termed schizophreniform.

King (1960) studied 84 newly admitted women with a diagnosis of schizophrenia. One group received unmodified ECT followed by maintenance CPZ (300 mg/day). The other group received CPZ in rapidly increasing doses, with each patient receiving a maximum of 1200 mg/day by day 5–7. Rates of remission were found to be equivalent in the ECT and CPZ groups. However, the CPZ group had a shorter period to remission or discharge. In addition to unclarity regarding the blindness of clinical ratings, the study was compromised by the use of ECT in some patients who had insufficient response to

Table 26.2 Prospective clinical trials comparing electroconvulsive therapy (ECT) with neuroleptics or other treatments in schizophrenia

Study	Patients	Study design	Nature of treatment	Results/comments
Baker *et al.* (1958)	48 'poor prognosis' schizophrenic females, aged 18–40 years	ECT vs. insulin coma therapy vs. CPZ; random assignment; blindness of evaluations uncertain	20 unmodified ECT at three per week; 30 insulin coma at six per week; CPZ 300 mg/day for 8 weeks	No differences among the groups in clinical outcome 1 week following acute trial; both ECT and insulin groups had lower relapse rates than the medication group; medication dosage was low
Baker *et al.* (1960b)	73 'poor prognosis' schizophrenic females, aged 18–40; 33 patients had participated in Baker (1958) in ECT or insulin conditions	ECT vs. insulin coma therapy; this study added patients to the ECT and insulin coma conditions reported by Baker *et al.* (1958)	ECT and insulin coma as in Baker *et al.* (1958)	ECT superior to insulin coma in percentage of patients who completed acute treatment and could be discharged
Langsley *et al.* (1959)	106 females (18–45) in psychotic manic or schizophrenic episode of short duration (<3 months)	ECT vs. CPZ; random assignment, single-blind	15–20 unmodified ECT at three per week; approximately 800 mg CPZ per day (range 200–2000 mg/day)	Clinical improvement was equivalent for ECT and CPZ, but the latter was associated with a shorter period to discharge
King (1960)	84 newly admitted female schizophrenic patients	ECT vs. CPZ; assigned alternately to treatments; blindness of evaluation uncertain	20 unmodified ECT at five per week; CPZ 900–1200 mg/day for 1 month	Rates of remission equivalent for ECT and CPZ; CPZ group had shorter period to remission or discharge; study contaminated by use of CPZ with some patients in the ECT group and vice versa; blindness unclear
Ray (1962)	60 schizophrenic patients with an average duration of illness 1–2 years	ECT vs. CPZ vs. ECT plus CPZ; uncertain whether treatment assignment was random and evaluations blind	ECT group given approximately 15 unmodified treatments — 3 times weekly for first 3 weeks and then tapered over 3 months; CPZ 250–300 mg/day for 10 weeks; combined group received both treatments	ECT alone and CPZ alone equivalent in rates of clinical improvement; combined treatment associated with the greatest rate of improvement. Improvement rated by clinical impression and medication dosage was low

Continued

Table 26.2 (*Continued*)

Study	Patients	Study design	Nature of treatment	Results/comments
Childers (1964)	80 newly admitted schizophrenic females, 16–55 years	ECT vs. fluphenazine vs. CPZ vs. ECT plus CPZ; sequential assignment	12 ECT at three per week; fluphenazine 20 mg/day for 30 days; CPZ 1000 mg/day for 30 days; CPZ 1000 mg/day for 30 days plus 12 ECT	Improvement rates: 55% ECT alone, 45% fluphenazine, 45% CPZ, and 80% CPZ and ECT; the combination treatment was most effective. Nature and blindness of outcome ratings not described
May and Tuma (1965), May (1968), May *et al.* (1976, 1981)	228 first-admission schizophrenic patients with 'middle prognosis' by clinical judgement, 16–45 years	ECT vs. trifluoperazine vs. psychotherapy vs. psychotherapy plus trifluoperazine vs. milieu treatment alone; random assignment, single-blind, with long follow-up period	Averaged 19 ECT for males and 25 ECT for females at variable rate; trifluoperazine-alone group had maximal dose of 25.5 mg/day	Short-term outcome was superior in groups that received medication relative to ECT, and the ECT group had superior short-term outcome compared with psychotherapy or milieu treatment. Long-term outcome (up to 5 years) was statistically equivalent in somatic treatment groups and superior to psychotherapy or milieu treatment. However, ECT group showed trends for the best long-term outcome; dosage of medication was low by modern standards and treatment following the acute phase was uncontrolled
Bagadia *et al.* (1970)	300 schizophrenic patients, with varying prognosis scores	ECT vs. insulin coma vs. CPZ vs. trifluoperazine vs. trifluperidol vs. flupenthixol; groups matched for distributions of prognosis; unclear whether assignment was random or whether evaluations were blind	Up to 10 unmodified ECT over 4 weeks; 20–30 insulin coma treatments at six treatments per week over 4 weeks. Medications administered over 3–4 weeks: CPZ up to 2400 mg/day, trifluoperazine up to 60 mg/day trifluperidol up to 6 mg/day flupenthixol up to 15 mg/day	Relative to each of the other treatments, ECT resulted in the most rapid improvement and the highest rate of complete symptomatic remission. Ratings of symptomatic improvement were impressionistic; methodological details lacking

Continued on p. 512

Table 26.2 (*Continued*)

Study	Patients	Study design	Nature of treatment	Results/comments
Murillo and Exner (1973a,b), Exner and Murillo (1973, 1977)	53 chronic 'process' schizophrenic patients	Regressive ECT vs. pharmacotherapy and psychotherapy; treatment assignment not randomized	Regressive treatment involved twice daily, bilateral ECT, 7 days per week, until regression occurred (helplessness, confusion, mutism and neurological signs); medication group received haloperidol ($n = 11$), CPZ ($n = 6$) or CPZ plus trifluoperazine ($n = 4$) in unspecified doses; nature of concomitant psychotherapy not described	Regressive ECT superior to the medication and psychotherapy condition in extent of clinical improvement at discharge and 7– 9 weeks following discharge; at 24– 30 months post discharge no differences between the groups in neuropsychological testing; study compromised by non-random assignment (medication group had refused regressive ECT) and lack of standardization of treatments
Bagadia *et al.* (1983)	38 schizophrenic patients with positive symptoms but no depressive or manic features	ECT and placebo vs. 18 sham ECT and CPZ	Six modified bilateral ECT plus placebo; six sham ECT with 400– 900 mg CPZ per day over 2–3 weeks	Clinical improvement equivalent in the two groups; 40 patients dropped out of the trial and were not included in analyses

CPZ, chlorpromazine

CPZ, and the use of CPZ in patients who did not respond to ECT, thereby contaminating the group comparisons.

Ray (1962) assigned 60 consecutively admitted schizophrenic patients to one of three groups: unmodified bilateral ECT alone, CPZ alone or combination ECT and CPZ. Outcome was grossly classified as no improvement, improvement with residual symptoms and symptom free. Ray (1962) reported that 50% of patients treated with ECT alone or CPZ showed no improvement. In contrast, this was observed in only 25% of patients who received combination treatment. Perhaps because of the small sample size per treatment condition ($n = 20$), these differences in short-term response rate were not statistically signifi-

cant. Furthermore, it was unclear whether the assignment to treatment conditions was random, and blindness of clinical evaluations was doubtful.

Childers (1964) sequentially assigned 80 newly admitted schizophrenic patients to bilateral ECT, fluphenazine, CPZ or CPZ plus bilateral ECT. Global ratings were made of clinical improvement following the acute treatment phase and the blindness of ratings was not described. Impressionistically, the findings suggested that the combination treatment was more effective than ECT alone or neuroleptic alone (Table 26.2). However, with sample sizes of 20 per group, differences among the four treatment conditions in improvement rate were of only marginal significance ($P = 0.08$), as was our explicit comparison of ECT alone and the combination treatment ($P = 0.09$).

May *et al.* conducted a landmark study in which 228 first-admission, 'middle prognosis' schizophrenics were randomized to five treatment conditions: bilateral ECT, antipsychotic medication alone, psychotherapy alone, antipsychotic medication plus psychotherapy or milieu therapy (May & Tuma, 1965; May, 1968; May *et al.*, 1976, 1981). Diagnosis of schizophrenia was based on independent interviews by six physicians. The characterization of middle prognosis was based on a clinical judgement that the patient was neither showing signs of rapid recovery during the evaluation period nor having little chance of recovery over a 2-year period.

Modified bilateral ECT (atropine, thiopental, succinylcholine) was administered at first at a rate of three treatments per week. The duration of the treatment course and the spacing of subsequent treatments was determined individually for each patient, based on clinical response and side effects. The main medication used was trifluoperazine, given orally, although intramuscular medication was also given and a few patients also received concomitant CPZ. Medication dosage was determined on an individual basis and an antiparkinsonian agent (procyclidine) was also used. The medication groups had an average daily trifluoperazine dose of approximately 20 mg/day. Psychotherapy was given for an average of not less than 2 h/week. The therapists were residents or psychiatrists of limited experience, but each was supervised by a psychoanalyst. The content of the psychotherapy was uncontrolled, but was described as generally focusing on reality testing and as ego supportive.

Across a variety of objective outcome measures, the short-term findings clearly favoured the medication conditions in terms of ratings of psychopathology, days hospitalized, discharge rate and costs. The short-term outcome results with ECT were intermediate between those of antipsychotic medications and psychological treatments (psychotherapy or milieu therapy). However, a 2- to 5-year follow-up indicated that subsequent time spent in hospital was equivalent for the medication- and the ECT-treated patients (May *et al.*, 1976). Another follow-up study showed that 3−5 years after discharge from the hospital, the medication-alone and the ECT groups tended to have the best outcome, and the psychotherapy-alone group the worst outcome (May *et al.*, 1981). Indeed, long-term outcome tended to be best in those initially assigned to ECT. May *et al.* (1981) concluded:

> Patients who had been treated with ECT fared, in the long run, at least as well as those given drug therapy, and in some respects even better, but not to a statistically significant extent. It seems that the status and role of ECT in the treatment of schizophrenia merit serious objective study.

A fundamental limitation in the interpretation of this work was the fact that the follow-up was naturalistic and treatment after the acute phase was uncontrolled. However, in a recent reanalysis of this study, Wyatt (1991) pointed out that during the follow-up period only the group treated with ECT had a statistically significant decrease in neuroleptic dosage. Despite lower neuroleptic dosage, the ECT group averaged 50 days of rehospitalization during the 2 years following discharge, compared with 70 days for neuroleptic alone, 55 days for neuroleptic and psychotherapy, 80 days for milieu therapy and 120 days for psychotherapy alone (Wyatt, 1991). Only the comparison between psychotherapy alone and ECT indicated a reliable difference.

Murillo and Exner (1973a,b; Exner & Murillo, 1973, 1977) compared a group of 32 process schizophrenic patients who were treated with 'regressive' ECT with a group of 21 similar patients treated with antipsychotic medications and psychotherapy. The patients were said to be characterized by a premorbid history of chronic disorganization, detachment, and chaotic and unpredictable behaviour. Assignment was not random, as the medication group comprised patients who had refused regressive ECT. Three different medications were used, haloperidol, CPZ and trifluoperazine, but dosage and duration were not specified. Analysis of 55 variables indicated that the groups were equivalent at study entry. At discharge, the ECT group differed significantly from the medication group in 28 of the 55 variables. All the differences favoured the ECT group, including symptomatic evaluations based on self-report and ratings by relatives and by referring physicians. Exner and Murillo (1977) conducted a long-term follow-up of a subgroup of these patients, with a minimum 24-month follow-up interval. Neuropsychological and projective testing revealed few, if any, differences between the groups. However, by family member and self-report, a significantly greater proportion of the ECT patients were working regularly in a full-time job, had taken a recent vacation, regularly drove a car and had terminated psychiatric treatment. In contrast, a higher proportion of the medication group were regularly taking medication and had recently visited physicians for problems not related to psychiatric causes. Lack of a standardized medication regimen, non-random assignment and uncertainty about the blindness of evaluations were clear limitations.

Bagadia et al. (1983) reported on 38 patients who were symptomatic for at least 1 month and manifested delusions, hallucinations or irrelevant verbal production in the context of clear consciousness and an absence of depressive or manic symptoms. Patients had not received antipsychotic medication within 3 weeks or ECT or insulin coma within 8 weeks of study entry. This double-blind, random assignment study contrasted bilateral ECT and medication placebo with sham ECT and CPZ. Real and sham ECT involved administration of atropine, thiopental and succinylcholine. CPZ was started at 200 mg/day and increased gradually to 600 mg/day, at which level it was maintained, increased or decreased after evaluation by a consultant psychiatrist, blind to the mode of treatment. An initial sample of 78 patients had been randomized, but 40 patients were excluded for irregular attendance, non-compliance or for discontinuation of treatment. Brief psychiatric rating scale (BPRS) measures showed a trend for greater improvement in the real ECT group after 7 days, but no difference between the groups in total or subscale scores after 20 days. Both samples showed marked clinical improvement. In addition to a high dropout rate, this study was limited by use of a fixed and low number of ECT treatments.

Summary

There has been a surprising paucity of prospective research contrasting ECT with pharmacological treatments of schizophrenia. The limitations of this literature in fundamental aspects of clinical trial methodology, particularly the reliability and validity of diagnosis, the nature of assignment to treatment groups, and the blindness and reliability of clinical evaluations, further underscore the need for caution in interpreting the findings. Other limitations pertain to the adequacy of treatment delivery, in terms of both ECT administration and pharmacotherapy. With these caveats, it appears that generally short-term outcome was equivalent or superior with antipsychotic medication relative to ECT (Langsley et al., 1959; King, 1960; Ray, 1962; May & Tuma, 1965; May, 1968), although even here there were exceptions (Murillo & Exner, 1973a). There is little indication from this literature about the clinical or treatment history features that might distinguish schizophrenics who preferentially respond to antipsychotic medications or ECT. In contrast, a seemingly consistent theme in this literature was the suggestion that patients who were administered ECT had superior long-term outcome compared with medication groups (Baker et al., 1958; May et al., 1976; Exner & Murillo, 1977; May et al., 1981). Similarly, in a retrospective comparison of ECT, insulin coma, CPZ and reserpine, Ayres (1960) reported that schizophrenic patients treated with ECT were the least likely to require rehospitalization. This pattern is unexpected, given the perspective that virtually all the behavioural and physiological effects of ECT are relatively short lived (Snaith, 1981; Sackeim, 1988; Sackeim et al., 1990). Furthermore, most of these studies were conducted in an era when the importance of continuation and maintenance treatment was not appreciated and none controlled treatment following resolution of the schizophrenic episode. Nonetheless, the possibility that ECT may have beneficial long-term effects merits attention.

Studies comparing combined ECT and medication treatment with medication alone or ECT alone

Two of the studies described in Table 26.2 contained comparisons of ECT administered alone with ECT administered in combination with antipsychotic medication (Ray, 1962; Childers, 1964). Both studies produced suggestive evidence that combination treatment was more effective than monotherapy with ECT or antipsychotic medications. In the real vs. sham trial by Abraham and Kulhara (1987), all patients received 20 mg trifluoperazine per day, resulting in another comparison of combination treatment with medication alone (see Table 26.1). This study found that in the short-term real ECT (combination treatment) was more effective than sham ECT (antipsychotic medication alone). Table 26.3 summarizes all the prospective clinical trials that have compared ECT combined with antipsychotic medication with ECT alone or with antipsychotic medication alone.

The trials reported by Ray (1962) and Childers (1964) were described earlier. Smith *et al.* (1967) reported on a group of 54 largely chronic schizophrenic patients. Patients assigned to a combination ECT−CPZ group ($n = 29$) comprised every fifth white-patient admission who met criteria for the NIMH-PSC Collaborative Study of Phenothiazines (NIMH-PSC, 1964). This treatment group was compared with one of the treatment conditions ($n = 25$) taken from a concurrent pharmacological trial (NIMH-PSC, 1964). The comparison group was treated only with CPZ. Clinical outcome was repeatedly evaluated with standardized scales during a 6-week acute treatment period and at 6 months and 1 year follow-up. Ratings were blind to the type of neuroleptic medication or placebo, but presumably raters were not blind to status in the ECT group. On various global and symptomatic ratings, the combination condition showed more rapid clinical improvement and superior outcome at the end of the first 6 weeks. It was noted that the combination group displayed significantly less hostility and ideas of persecution at 6 weeks, but more confusion and memory deficits. Cross-sectional

evaluation at the 6-month and 1-year follow-ups failed to distinguish the groups. However, the combination treatment was associated with significantly more rapid discharge, fewer days of hospitalization and fewer rehospitalizations during the year following admission. For example, 6 months after admission, 40% of the CPZ-alone group had not been discharged compared with 14% in the group given combination treatment. The rehospitalization rates after discharge were 33% for CPZ alone and 10% for combination treatment. While limited by failing to use random assignment and fully blinded evaluations, this study suggested that ECT combined with antipsychotic medication may be superior to antipsychotic medication alone, both in the short term and long term. As with previous studies, the lack of control over treatment received after the acute trial period was a critical limitation in interpreting the follow-up findings.

Small *et al.* (1982; Small, 1985) randomized 75 'middle prognosis' patients who met the Feighner *et al.* (1972) criteria for schizophrenia to one of four conditions: ECT combined with thiothixene, ECT and medication placebo, thiothixene alone or medication placebo. A randomization scheme was used that resulted in small sample sizes for the ECT and placebo, and placebo only groups. Both the number of ECT treatments and medication dosages were titrated with the aim of achieving maximal clinical response. Thiothixene dosage was said to be equivalent in the two groups receiving active medication, but was reported as averaging 650 mg CPZ equivalents per day in the ECT and thiothixene group and 913 mg/day in the thiothixene-alone group. Clinical outcome was assessed with a variety of standardized scales, with modified double-blind procedures. Generally, the authors stated that across rating scales there was a hierarchy of clinical response. The best outcomes were observed with the combination of ECT and thiothixene, followed by thiothixene alone, ECT alone and placebo alone. Scores on the abnormal involuntary movement scale (AIMS) indicated that patients given only thiothixene had more orofacial movements than other treatment groups. ECT is known to exert an antiparkinsonian effect, both in some forms of idiopathic Parkinson's disease, as

Table 26.3 Prospective clinical trials comparing combination treatment with electroconvulsive therapy (ECT) and antipsychotic medication with ECT alone or antipsychotic medication alone

Study	Patients	Study design	Nature of treatment	Results/comments
Ray (1962)	60 schizophrenic patients with an average duration of illness 1–2 years	ECT vs. CPZ vs. ECT plus CPZ; uncertain whether treatment assignment was random and evaluations blind	ECT group given approximately 15 unmodified treatments – 3 times weekly for first 3 weeks and then tapered over 3 months; CPZ 250–300 mg/day for 10 weeks; combined group received both treatments	ECT alone and CPZ alone equivalent in rates of clinical improvement; combined treatment associated with the greatest rate of improvement. Improvement rated by clinical impression; medication dosage was low
Childers (1964)	80 newly admitted schizophrenic females, 16–55 years	ECT vs. fluphenazine vs. CPZ vs. ECT plus CPZ; sequential assignment	12 ECT at three per week; fluphenazine 20 mg/day for 30 days; CPZ 1000 mg/day for 30 days; CPZ 1000 mg/day for 30 days plus 12 ECT	Improvement rates: 55% ECT alone, 45% fluphenazine, 45% CPZ, and 80% CPZ and ECT; the combination treatment was most effective. Nature and blindness of outcome ratings not described
Smith *et al.* (1967)	54 schizophrenic patients, with average duration of 6 years since first episode and 20 previous admissions	ECT and CPZ vs. CPZ; every fifth white patient assigned to combination treatment, CPZ cell from a pharmacological study; study personnel blind to drug or placebo in CPZ cell	12 modified ECT at three per week plus an average of 400 mg CPZ per day; CPZ alone averaged 655 mg/day during 6-week acute trial	Various standardized rating indicated that ECT and CPZ group had faster clinical response and superior outcome at end of 6-week acute trial. At 6-month and 1-year cross-sectional follow-up no differences observed. However, ECT and CPZ group had a higher discharge rate and a lower rehospitalization rate than CPZ only group
Small *et al.* (1982), Small (1985)	75 schizophrenic patients (Feighner criteria), with middle prognosis (>6 months and <2 years hospitalization)	ECT and thiothixene ($n = 25$) vs. thiothixene alone ($n = 26$) vs. ECT and placebo ($n = 16$) vs. placebo alone ($n = 8$); random assignment and modified double-blind design with standardized outcome measures	ECT groups received an average of 15 modified right unilateral treatments at three per week; thiothixene-alone group averaged 913 mg CPZ equivalents per day; thiothixene in combination group averaged 650 mg CPZ equivalents per day; considerable dropout in ECT-alone and placebo groups	Statistical findings never presented. Authors concluded that ECT and thiothixene was superior in clinical outcome to thiothixene alone, which in turn was superior to both ECT alone and placebo

Continued

Table 26.3 (*Continued*)

Study	Patients	Study design	Nature of treatment	Results/comments
Janakiramaiah *et al.* (1982)	60 schizophrenic or schizophreniform patients (RDC) with continuous illness between 2 months and 6 years	ECT and CPZ 300 mg/day vs. CPZ 300 mg/day alone vs. ECT and CPZ 500 mg/day vs. CPZ 500 mg/day alone; treatment free at study entry; random assignment; partial blindness in evaluations	Modified ECT administered at three per week; 300 mg CPZ group averaged 9.5 ECT, and 500 mg CPZ group averaged 10.4 treatments; CPZ administered for 6 weeks	At completion of acute trial (6 weeks) inferior clinical outcome in the CPZ 300 mg/day group. ECT and CPZ 500 mg/day had earliest clinical response, but no advantage to combination treatment relative to CPZ 500 mg/day alone at 6 weeks
Ungvári & Pethö (1982)	75 recently admitted schizophrenic patients (RDC) with average duration of illness of approximately 7 years	ECT and low-dose haloperidol vs. high-dose haloperidol; study duration only 6 days; assignment to group random; blind evaluation	Two modified ECTs on each of three occasions over a period of 6 days plus an average of haloperidol 6.5 mg/day; high-dose haloperidol group averaged 72 mg/day (range 50−120 mg/day)	Analyses stratified by diagnostic distinction between systematic and unsystematic schizophrenia (similar to reactive/process distinction). Treatment groups equivalent among unsystematic schizophrenics; ECT and low-dose haloperidol superior to high-dose haloperidol among systematic schizophrenics. Short duration of trial and unusual ECT schedule limit clinical relevance
Abraham and Kulhara (1987)	22 schizophrenic patients by the RDC with duration of illness <2 years	Sham ECT vs. real ECT; trifluoperazine held constant during trial, 20 mg/day to all patients; random assignment, double-blind	Eight sham or real (modified) treatments, twice weekly for 4 weeks	ECT group showed more rapid improvement than sham group; from 12 weeks to 6 months no difference
Das *et al.* (1991)	48 newly admitted schizophrenic patients; 30 described as chronic	Naturalistic comparison of patients treated with neuroleptics alone or neuroleptics and ECT; GAS completed at admission and discharge	Medications involved CPZ 500−900 mg/day, trifluoperazine 15−45 mg/day or haloperidol 15−45 mg/day; adjunctive ECT used, typically because of symptom severity, medication resistance or intolerance; ECT not described	Combined ECT and neuroleptic group more severely ill at baseline; both groups manifested strong improvement; extent of change in GAS scores greater in the combined ECT and neuroleptic group. Neuroleptic only group had half the length of stay. Nonblind, naturalistic comparison

CPZ, chloromazine; RDC, research diagnostic criteria; GAS, global assessment scale.

well as with neuroleptic-induced extrapyramidal side effects (APA, 1990).

Janakiramaiah *et al.* (1982) studied 60 patients who fulfilled modified research diagnostic criteria (RDC; Spitzer *et al.* 1978) for schizophrenia or schizophreniform illness. Patients were randomly assigned to one of four treatment groups: CPZ 300 mg/day, CPZ 300 mg/day with ECT, CPZ 500 mg/day, and CPZ 500 mg/day with ECT. Clinical assessments, conducted weekly for 6 weeks, were partially blind to treatment condition and involved global ratings, BPRS ratings and an evaluation of extrapyramidal symptoms. Consistently, from the second through sixth week, the CPZ 300 mg/day only group had inferior clinical outcome compared with the other groups. After the first week of treatment, the combined CPZ 500 mg/day and ECT group had greater improvement than the other three groups. However, at the end of the trial there was no advantage to combining CPZ 500 mg/day with ECT relative to CPZ 500 mg/day alone.

In an unusual study, Ungvári and Pethö (1982) treated 75 recently admitted patients with schizophrenia, randomizing them to either a high-dosage haloperidol group (*n* = 39) or a group that received ECT and low-dosage haloperidol (*n* = 36). The high-dosage group was administered between 50 and 120 mg haloperidol per day, with an average dose of 72 mg/day. A total of six modified seizures were elicited with ECT, two seizures in each of three sessions over 6 days. Patients in the ECT group were also administered an average of haloperidol 6.5 mg/day (range 4.5–9 mg/day). The total duration of this trial was only 6 days, suggesting that patients in the ECT group were evaluated very shortly following a multiple seizure induction. Evaluations were said to be blind, using a modified version of the BPRS. Analyses of efficacy were stratified by the diagnostic distinction of Leonhard (1979), contrasting unsystematic and systematic schizophrenia. This distinction is similar to the process/reactive dichotomy. Both forms of treatment were efficacious in each patient subgroup. However, among systematic schizophrenic patients, the ECT–haloperidol treatment was notably superior to treatment with high-dosage haloperidol.

Das *et al.* (1991) reported a naturalistic, prospective comparison of schizophrenic patients treated with medications alone or with medications combined with ECT. Over a 6-month period, 48 patients were identified who received either CPZ, trifluoperazine or haloperidol. In this relatively young sample, 23 patients were administered concurrent ECT because of severe symptomatology, medication resistance or medication intolerance. The medication-alone group had half the hospital stay compared with the ECT group (17 vs. 34 days). Using the global assessment scale (GAS), the ECT group was more impaired at admission. At discharge, the two groups had similar GAS scores, with the change significantly greater in the ECT group.

Summary

This literature is also characterized by a host of methodological difficulties. As in the comparisons of monotherapy with ECT or with antipsychotic medication, the adequacy of pharmacological treatment and ECT administration was often questionable in the studies that examined the efficacy of combined treatment. Relatively few of these studies involved random assignment, and fewer still involved fully blind outcome assessment. Nonetheless, it is noteworthy that in each of the three studies in which ECT alone was compared with ECT combined with antipsychotic medication, there were suggestions that the combination was more effective (Ray, 1962; Childers, 1964; Small *et al.*, 1982). A larger number of investigations have contrasted the combination treatment with monotherapy with an antipsychotic medication. With the exception of the study of Janakiramaiah *et al.* (1982), in each instance there was evidence that treatment with an antipsychotic medication in combination with ECT was more effective than treatment with an antipsychotic medication alone (Ray, 1962; Childers, 1964; Smith *et al.*, 1967; Small *et al.*, 1982; Ungvári & Pethö, 1982; Abraham & Kulhara, 1987; Das *et al.*, 1991). In some cases, a superior outcome was obtained despite an apparent lower average neuroleptic dose in the combination condition (Smith *et al.*, 1967; Small *et al.*, 1982; Ungvári &

Pethö, 1982). Few of these studies followed patients beyond the acute treatment period and in none was there standardization of continuation or maintenance treatments. Therefore, the relative persistence of any advantage for combination treatment is unknown. In this respect, the findings reported by Smith *et al.* (1967), suggesting a reduced rate of relapse in patients treated acutely with neuroleptics and ECT relative to neuroleptics alone, were particularly intriguing. When considered with the follow-up results of May *et al.* (1981), there is added reason to explore whether ECT, particularly in combination with antipsychotic medication, may exert a long-term beneficial effect in schizophrenia.

ECT and neuroleptic medication in medication-resistant schizophrenic patients

In general, the studies that used sham vs. real ECT designs and the studies that have contrasted ECT and traditional antipsychotic medications indicate that ECT has efficacy in the treatment of schizophrenia. In isolation, this fact is of limited clinical utility, since little has been identified about the patients most likely to benefit from ECT. Moreover, standard treatment of schizophrenia begins with trials of antipsychotic medication. A critical question is whether ECT is efficacious in patients who fail to respond to traditional neuroleptic medications. Such patients constitute 5–25% of all individuals with this diagnosis (Meltzer, 1992). Few studies have explicitly examined the use of ECT in medication-resistant schizophrenic patients. This work is summarized in Table 26.4.

The earliest study was undertaken by Childers and Therrien (1961) and involved 48 schizophrenic patients who were sequentially assigned to one of four groups: CPZ, trifluoperazine, placebo medication or no treatment. At the end of 35 days, those patients who had not received active medication and had not improved were crossed over to one of the two active medication groups. This crossover occurred in all but one of the patients initially assigned to placebo or no treatment. Patients who failed to improve with CPZ or trifluoperazine alone (initial or crossover

phase) were switched to the other medication and also received a concurrent course of ECT. Bilateral ECT was administered at a schedule of three per week for 5 weeks and patients also received concurrent CPZ or trifluoperazine. Eleven of 23 patients who had failed to respond to neuroleptic treatment were considered improved when switched to an alternative neuroleptic and ECT. In addition to non-blind evaluation, the significance of these findings was limited by the simultaneous use of an alternative neuroleptic with ECT.

Rahman (1968) reviewed the treatment of 176 schizophrenic patients admitted to a psychiatric hospital in East Pakistan during 1965. Patients were typically first treated with an antipsychotic medication (prochlorperazine, CPZ or trifluoperazine) and received ECT with antipsychotic medication only after they had failed to improve over 2–3 months. Rahman (1968) concluded that ECT combined with one of the phenothiazines produced superior results than phenothiazines alone. All 50 patients treated with combination ECT and medication were rated as either improved (48%) or remitted (52%), rates that exceeded medication comparison groups.

In another impressionistic, retrospective study, Lewis (1982) reviewed the charts of patients diagnosed as schizophrenic and who received ECT during a 4.5-year period (1974–78) at the Payne Whitney Clinic in New York. Of 29 patients identified, 23 had failed an adequate medication trial prior to receiving an average of 14 ECT treatments. The patients were relatively young, and presumably had a relatively short duration of illness. In 24 of the 29 patients, outcome was rated as good or excellent. The significance of this observation was limited by the fact that clinical outcome was not rated at the termination of ECT, but rather at discharge from the hospital. In some cases, patients received other forms of treatment following ECT and prior to discharge.

Friedel (1986) prospectively identified 21 patients meeting the *Diagnostic and Statistical Manual* DSM-III criteria for schizophrenia. These patients underwent a standardized trial with thiothixene. Neuroleptic dosage was increased until there was moderate to marked

Table 26.4 Clinical trials of electroconvulsive therapy (ECT) in medication-resistant schizophrenic patients

Study	Patients	Study design	Nature of treatment	Results/comments
Childers and Therrien (1961)	48 newly admitted schizophrenic patients (26 chronic undifferentiated, 16 paranoid, three schizoaffective, two hebephrenic and one simple)	Sequentially assigned to one of four groups: CPZ, trifluoperazine, placebo medication or no treatment. Non-responders to placebo or no treatment crossed over to one of the active medication conditions. Medication non-responders given ECT and the alternative medication at reduced dosage	Initial treatment phase involved CPZ 1000 mg/day or trifluoperazine 40 mg/day for 35 days. Medication failures received 15 ECT treatments at three per week plus either CPZ 500 mg/day or trifluoperazine 20 mg/day	23 of 48 patients failed to respond to medication alone; 11 of the 23 patients responded when ECT was combined with the alternative neuroleptic
Rahman (1968)	176 newly admitted schizophrenic patients; average age of 28.9 years with average 20 months duration of illness	Naturalistic, retrospective comparison of clinical outcome with one of three neuroleptics (prochlorperazine, CPZ, trifluoperazine) and ECT combined with neuroleptic. Patients typically received the combination after failing single neuroleptic treatment for 2−3 months	Typical neuroleptic treatment involved prochlorperazine 75 mg/day, CPZ 300 mg/day, or trifluoperazine 15 mg/day. Nature of ECT not described	All 50 patients who received combined ECT and neuroleptic treatment considered improved (48%) or remitted (52%), rates superior to neuroleptic alone. Outcome criteria impressionistic and not blindly evaluated
Lewis (1982)	29 newly admitted schizophrenic (DSM-III) patients, with an average age of 27 years	Retrospective evaluation of outcome in medication-resistant patients; 23 of 29 rated as medication resistant, with most failing neuroleptic treatment equivalent to at least 1 g CPZ per day for at least 3 weeks	Neuroleptic medication continued during ECT, but typically at reduced dosage; nature of ECT not described; average of 14 treatments administered	Outcome was rated as good or excellent in 24 of 29 patients. Outcome was assessed at time of discharge and other treatments intervened following ECT
Friedel (1986)	Nine patients with DSM-III schizophrenia and moderate to severe psychotic symptoms	Larger group of 21 patients treated with thiothixene until plasma levels exceeded 15 ng/ml or were intolerant. Nine non-responders received ECT plus thiothixene	ECT ranged from eight to 25 treatments with average of 13.6; six patients received unilateral and three patients received bilateral ECT. Thiothixene doses ranged from 30−60 mg/day during ECT	Eight of nine patients achieved complete remission and one patient had mild symptoms following ECT. Open clinical trial that used strict standards for medication resistance

Continued

Table 26.4 (*Continued*)

Study	Patients	Study design	Nature of treatment	Results/comments
Gujavarty *et al.* (1987)	Eight patients with DSM-III schizophrenia and moderate to severe symptoms	Retrospective chart review. Patients did not respond to two courses of neuroleptics, each in a generally accepted dose range for at least 6 weeks	Unilateral or bilateral ECT at three per week, with an average of 14.4 treatments; neuroleptic medication continued during ECT	Seven of the eight patients improved; this was sustained in five patients after 6 and 12 months. Five of these eight patients had a history of prominent affective symptoms
Konig and Glatter-Gotz (1990)	13 patients with ICD-9 schizophrenia	Retrospective chart review; 11 of 13 patients referred for ECT due to medication resistance, typically failing in excess of 1 g CPZ equivalents per day	Nature of ECT not described; patients received an average of 12.4 treatments; neuroleptic medication continued during ECT	Nine of the 13 patients judged to have good clinical outcome. In these patients, neuroleptic dosage was decreased by 72% following ECT
Milstein *et al.* (1990)	110 patients with DSM-III-R schizophrenia (25 schizoaffective, 39 paranoid, 46 non-paranoid)	Patients were usually referred for ECT due to medication resistance or intolerance; clinical ratings prospectively collected with standardized instruments	Unilateral and bilateral ECT given, three per week with an average of 16.8 treatments. Unilateral non-responders crossed over to bilateral ECT. 87 patients received concurrent neuroleptics	54% of sample rated as much improved or very much improved. Clinical response was independent of diagnostic subtype and categorization of concurrent neuroleptic treatment. Explicit criteria for medication resistance not used, nor internal analysis reported for resistant patients
Sajatovic and Meltzer (1993)	Nine medication-resistant schizophrenic patients	Patients failed neuroleptic treatment prior to receiving ECT and loxapine; ECT responders administered continuation ECT. Open clinical trial	Details regarding ECT and medication dosage not provided; average of eight ECT treatments	Five of nine patients had a good clinical response to combination ECT and loxapine. Of five patients given continuation ECT, three relapsed within 4 months

CPZ, chlorpromazine; DSM, *Diagnostic and Statistical Manual*; ICD, *International Classification of Disease*.

improvement, intolerable side effects or until thiothixene and desmethylthiothixene plasma levels exceeded 15 ng/ml. For 11 patients who showed no or slight clinical improvement, dosage was increased further until plasma levels were greater than 15 ng/ml. These patients were non-responders, and nine were administered ECT and also continued on thiothixene at a dose of 30–60 mg/day. Eight of the nine patients had a complete remission and one patient was significantly improved. The extent of improvement in this open clinical trial was impressive, particularly since the average patient had been continuously psychotic for over 3 years and had previously failed other neuroleptics and lithium. Friedel (1986) called for a randomized, controlled trial of ECT combined with neuroleptic medication vs. neuroleptic medication alone in a medication-resistant sample of schizophrenic patients.

Prompted by the Friedel (1986) report, Gujavarty *et al.* (1987) reviewed the records of 90 patients treated with ECT at their facility during a 2-year period. Eight patients with DSM-III diagnoses of schizophrenia were identified who had not improved after at least two trials of neuroleptic medication and had been continuously hospitalized for at least 90 days. These patients received an average of 14.4 ECT treatments. A variety of neuroleptic medications was also administered throughout the ECT course. Seven of the eight patients improved, with this improvement sustained in five patients at 6- and 12-month follow-ups. Gujavarty *et al.* (1987) noted, however, that five of the eight patients had manifested significant affective symptomatology in the past.

Konig and Glatter-Gotz (1990) conducted a retrospective survey of 13 schizophrenic patients who were treated with ECT at an Austrian hospital between 1979 and 1982. Eight cases were referred for ECT owing to neuroleptic resistance. Three other patients also were considered treatment resistant and had catatonic exacerbations while receiving neuroleptic treatment. Prior to ECT, these patients were treated with neuroleptics generally in excess of 1 g CPZ equivalents per day. One patient was medication intolerant. Nine of the 13 patients showed a good response to ECT. In these nine patients, neuroleptic dosage was reduced by 72% following ECT.

Milstein *et al.* (1990) reported on the treatment of 110 patients with DSM-III-R diagnoses of schizoaffective disorder, paranoid schizophrenia or non-paranoid schizophrenia. Patients were referred for ECT owing to a failure to respond to medications or to intolerable side effects. Systematic criteria for medication resistance were not used. Standardized rating scales were administered prior to and following the ECT course, including the BPRS and the clinical global impression (CGI). In these relatively young patients (average age of 26.4 years), 54% were rated as much improved or very much improved following ECT. Eighty-seven of the 110 patients received concurrent antipsychotic medications. Treatment outcome was independent of whether or not patients received neuroleptics during ECT or judgements of whether neuroleptic dosage was low or high. Clinical outcome was also independent of diagnostic subtyping as schizoaffective, paranoid or non-paranoid schizophrenia. Milstein *et al.* (1990) noted that the response rate was lower than that of patients with mood disorders treated at the facility. Nonetheless, in a presumably largely medication-resistant sample, this study provided additional impressionistic evidence that ECT may be efficacious in schizophrenic patients resistant to traditional antipsychotic medications.

Sajatovic and Meltzer (1993) collected nine patients with schizophrenia or schizoaffective illness who had inadequate response to prior neuroleptic treatment. These patients then received ECT combined with loxapine. Five patients were regarded as manifesting significant clinical improvement, with the beneficial effects most marked for positive, relative to negative, symptoms. Of note, the presence of affective symptoms (schizoaffective disorder) was not associated with good ECT outcome. Five of the patients were administered continuation ECT, following the acute trial. While two patients maintained improvement, three relapsed within 4 months.

Summary

We have yet to have a double-blind, random assignment study contrasting the efficacy of ECT and neuroleptic treatment with continued neuroleptic treatment alone in medication-resistant schizophrenic patients. All the information available on this issue comes from largely impressionistic observations. Nonetheless, it is evident that, starting with the report of Childers and Therrien (1961), there have been indications that some medication-resistant schizophrenic patients may benefit substantially by the addition of ECT. These indications seemingly contradict the clinical tenet that ECT is of limited value in chronic schizophrenic patients with long durations of illness (Kalinowsky & Worthing, 1943; Salzman, 1980). Our experience in treating chronically institutionalized schizophrenic patients with concurrent ECT and traditional neuroleptics has suggested that the combination may result in dramatic improvement in only a small minority of patients, and is without substantial benefit in most cases. We are left then with unanswered questions. It could be that the positive findings of Friedel (1986), Gujavarty *et al.* (1987), Milstein *et al.* (1990) and others reflect samples with high representation of patients with prominent affective symptomatology. It could be that, in the absence of affective symptoms, the combination of ECT and neuroleptic treatment is particularly valuable for medication-resistant patients who have relatively short duration of illness. Whatever the source of these discrepant impressions, it is clear that we need better information, particularly about the clinical and historical features of those medication-resistant patients who may benefit from the combination treatment.

Atypical antipsychotics and ECT

Clozapine is an effective treatment for schizophrenic patients resistant to classical neuroleptics (Kane *et al.*, 1988a; Lieberman *et al.*, 1989). Nonetheless, a substantial proportion of such patients do not respond to clozapine. There have been scattered case reports on the use of ECT in clozapine-resistant patients. Initially, there was concern about the safety of combining ECT and clozapine, due to the risk of seizures with clozapine. The concern was that, with concurrent clozapine, ECT-induced seizures would be prolonged or result in status epilepticus.

Masiar and Johns (1991) reported on a 26-year-old man with a 4-year history of chronic paranoid schizophrenia and who received up to 800 mg clozapine per day with limited response. The patient was administered bilateral ECT 4 days after discontinuing clozapine, which had been tapered over a 14-day period along with diazepam (20–5 mg/day). The patient had two spontaneous grand mal seizures, witnessed by staff on days 4 and 6 following the first and only ECT treatment. It was unknown whether the delayed seizures were due to residual effects of the clozapine, the dosage reduction of the benzodiazepine, a delayed effect of ECT or some combination of these.

Klapheke (1991a) reported on the safe use of ECT combined with clozapine in a 26-year-old woman with schizoaffective disorder who remained psychotic and combative while on clozapine (450 mg/day). Previously, she had failed to respond to regimens involving molindone, mesoridazine, thiothixene, lithium, carbamazepine, clonazepam and imipramine. She was treated with two seizure inductions per ECT session for the first five sessions and then had four more treatments, with the clozapine dosage increased from 450 to 600 mg/day during the ECT course. She tolerated ECT well and had a dramatic clinical response. A few months later the patient relapsed when clozapine was stopped owing to a drop in white blood cell count (Klapheke, 1991b). She received a second course of ECT with concurrent loxapine, involving a total of nine bilateral treatments that produced only mild to moderate improvement.

Landy (1991) reported no difficulty in treating two delusionally depressed patients with ECT and clozapine. Both patients had failed to respond to a variety of somatic treatments, including ECT combined with a traditional neuroleptic, and exhibited marked response to the combination of ECT and clozapine.

Safferman and Munne (1992) summarized a case of a patient with schizophrenia who had had a response to clozapine alone, and while on clozapine was virtually symptom free for 5 months. However, her psychosis recurred and did not improve despite continuation of clozapine (900 mg/day) for about 12 months and the addition of valproic acid, lithium and CPZ. With eight bilateral ECT treatments, concurrent with a reduced clozapine dose (400 mg/day), she manifested marked improvement.

Summary

As yet, the published literature is meagre on the use of ECT in schizophrenic patients resistant to clozapine and the more general use of combination ECT and clozapine in medication-resistant schizophrenia. Outside of what has been published, a few groups have additional experience with this combination and initial impressions have been salutary. Particularly because the schizophrenic patient who fails clozapine has very limited therapeutic options, having typically exhausted traditional pharmacological approaches, rigorous investigation of the combination of ECT and clozapine is needed. Furthermore, to our knowledge, there has yet to be any documentation of the safety or efficacy of ECT when combined with other, newer atypical antipsychotics, such as risperidone.

Prediction of outcome

With the introduction of the neuroleptics, use of ECT in schizophrenia diminished sharply. In part, this was due to the belief that ECT and antipsychotic medications overlapped in patients most responsive to treatment. ECT was believed to be particularly effective in patients with short illness duration and acute onset (Kalinowsky, 1943; Kalinowsky & Worthing, 1943; Lowinger & Huddelson, 1945; Herzberg, 1954), and relatively ineffective in chronic patients. As described earlier, since neuroleptics were generally found to be as or more effective than ECT alone in the treatment of non-chronic patients, clinicians began to favour the use of neuroleptics. Relatively little attention was devoted to the issue of whether the symptoms most responsive to ECT and medications were comparable, or whether there was equivalence in the quality of remission. The evidence suggesting that combination ECT and antipsychotic medication may be more efficacious than either form of treatment alone has had relatively little impact on practice. As we have seen, surprisingly little research has addressed the issue of whether medication-resistant patients may benefit from ECT.

Demographic and clinical predictors

This synopsis indicates that views concerning the predictors of clinical outcome have been critical in delimiting the use of ECT. Soon after the introduction of ECT, several investigators examined putative predictors. The features that were associated with positive clinical outcome in schizophrenia included being married (Herzberg, 1954), having at least a skilled or clerical occupation (Herzberg, 1954), an absence of premorbid personality disturbance and poor premorbid functioning (Wittman, 1941), manifestation of catatonic symptoms (Kalinowsky & Worthing, 1943; Hamilton & Wall, 1948; Ellison & Hamilton, 1949; Wells, 1973), affective symptoms (Folstein *et al.*, 1973; Wells, 1973) and acute onset and short illness duration (Cheney & Drewry, 1938; Ross & Malzberg, 1939; Zeifert, 1941; Kalinowsky, 1943; Lowinger & Huddleson, 1945; Danziger & Kindwall, 1946; Herzberg, 1954). It is noteworthy that many of these features have been found to predict outcome with pharmacological treatment (Leff & Wing, 1971; WHO, 1979; Watt *et al.*, 1983), and may be more general markers of prognosis. Nonetheless, the meaningfulness of these findings is questionable given that these early studies often used assessment techniques of questionable reliability and lacked standardized diagnostic criteria. Unfortunately, very few recent studies have examined predictors of ECT response in schizophrenia.

Koehler and Sauer (1983) reviewed the records of 142 first-admission schizophrenic patients treated only with ECT at the University of Heidelberg during 1948–50 and who were evaluated by Schneider. Presentation of first-rank (Schneiderian) symptoms was associated with inferior ECT outcome. Landmark *et al.* (1987) retrospectively contrasted clinical outcome predictors for fluphenazine and bilateral ECT. A group of 120 patients were followed at an outpatient clinic and received fluphenazine decanoate; 65 of these patients had been treated earlier in their history with bilateral ECT at other facilities. Landmark *et al.* (1987) claimed that fluphenazine was associated with superior clinical outcome relative to ECT. Within the ECT group, preoccupation with delusions and hallucinations was a significant predictor of positive clinical outcome, while a diagnosis of schizophrenia following the first hospitalization predicted poorer outcome. The latter was interpreted as indicating poorer ECT outcome in chronic schizophrenic patients. Of note, the presence of catatonic symptoms was non-predictive.

In recent times, there has been only one prospective study of predictors of ECT outcome in schizophrenia. Dodwell and Goldberg (1989) reported on 17 schizophrenic patients who were assessed with standardized instruments both before and following ECT. Of note, 12 of the 17 patients met the RDC for schizoaffective disorder, depressed and all patients were treated with concomitant neuroleptic medication. In this small sample, positive outcome was associated with short duration of illness (both historically and current episode), fewer schizoid and paranoid premorbid personality traits and the presence of perplexity. Catatonic and depressive symptoms were not predictive.

Symptoms responsive to ECT

As with patient features that predict outcome, in recent years little research has examined the symptoms of schizophrenia that show most benefit from the use of ECT. Basic questions, such as the relative impact of ECT on positive and negative symptoms, have not been addressed. The sham vs. real trials of Taylor and Fleminger (1980), Brandon *et al.* (1985) and Abraham and Kulhara (1987) generally found that while depressive symptoms in schizophrenic patients improved during an ECT course (combined with neuroleptic), they were not particularly responsive. Taylor and Fleminger (1980) reported that delusions of control, delusions of reference, delusional mood, thought interference and auditory hallucinations were particularly responsive. Similarly, Smith *et al.* (1967) had reported that combination ECT and CPZ resulted in particular improvement in symptoms of hostility and ideas of persecution relative to neuroleptic alone. Witton

(1962) also claimed that ideas of persecution and auditory hallucinations showed especially favourable response.

Special populations

Catatonia

It has long been contended that presentation of catonic symptoms constitutes special indication for the use of ECT (Kalinowsky & Worthing, 1943; Hamilton & Wall, 1948; Ellison & Hamilton, 1949; Wells, 1973; Fink, 1989). Part of the difficulty in evaluating this claim is the recognition that catatonia may be manifested in a variety of psychiatric disorders or as a consequence of medical illness. Abrams and Taylor (1976a) examined 55 patients with catatonic symptoms who were admitted to an in-patient psychiatric unit and found that only four satisfied research criteria for schizophrenia, with the others having a preponderance of affective disorders. Pataki *et al.* (1992) examined the records of admissions to an in-patient unit between 1985 and 1990. Of 43 cases with admission or discharge diagnoses of schizophrenia, catatonic subtype, 19 were felt to have records adequate for more detailed review. Only seven of these patients were identified as schizophrenic. Of the entire group of catatonic patients, 11 underwent ECT with excellent results being obtained in eight; 34 psychotropic medication trials were identified, with successful results in only two patients. Fink (1989) has advocated conceptualizing catatonia as a behavioural syndrome by itself, which can be associated with numerous disorders, not only schizophrenia, and for which ECT is the treatment of first choice. However, others (Fricchione, 1989; Rosebush *et al.*, 1992) have suggested use of benzodiazepines as the primary treatment for this syndrome. As indicated, the small, recent prospective study by Dodwell and Goldberg (1989) did not find catatonic symptoms to be predictive of ECT outcome. In an older sham vs. real ECT study conducted with catatonic schizophrenic patients, no effect of real ECT was discerned (Miller *et al.*, 1953). A complication here is distinguishing between the treatment of catatonic manifestations and treatment of the underlying psychosis. In our experience, ECT results in rapid and often dramatic improvement in specific catatonic features, such as mutism and motility disturbance, but more variable effects on core psychotic phenomena.

Lethal catatonia

Special consideration should be given to the syndrome of lethal catatonia. This is a life-threatening condition, characterized by stupor or excitement, hyperthermia, clouded consciousness and autonomic dysregulation (Mann *et al.*, 1986). Mann *et al.* (1986) identified 292 cases in the world literature published since 1960. In 256 (88%) cases, lethal catatonia was believed to be an outgrowth of a functional psychotic disorder, with a primary diagnosis of schizophrenia in 117 cases. Of note, 176 (60%) of the 292 cases died. The literature on this syndrome, which consists solely of case series, suggests that neuroleptic treatment is of limited efficacy. Indeed, given the difficulty in distinguishing lethal catatonia from neuroleptic malignant syndrome (NMS), escalation of neuroleptic dosage may be counterproductive. In contrast, ECT, particularly when instituted prior to a comatose stage, appears to be effective (Arnold & Stepan, 1952; Tolsma, 1967; Sedivec, 1981; Gabris & Muller, 1983; Mann *et al.*, 1990; Rummans & Bassingthwaighte, 1991).

Schizoaffective disorder

Expert groups, such as the APA Task Force on ECT, have suggested that this form of treatment is particularly valuable when schizophrenic patients present with prominent affective symptoms. Some of the early investigators found that mood disturbance was a predictor of positive ECT outcome in schizophrenic patients (Folstein *et al.*, 1973; Wells, 1973). This may not be specific to ECT as affective features may portend a better prognosis in schizophrenia, regardless of treatment (WHO, 1979). Folstein *et al.* (1973)

reviewed the charts of 118 consecutive patients who received ECT at a facility in New York. Regardless of a diagnosis of schizophrenia, mood disorder or neurosis or personality disorder, the presence of a family history of mood disorder, suicide and symptoms of hopelessness, worthlessness and guilt were associated with favourable ECT outcome. In a chart review of patients at the University of Rochester Medical Center, Wells (1973) identified 267 patients admitted between 1960 and 1969 with a diagnosis of schizophrenia and treated with ECT. Schizoaffective and catatonic subtypes, patients in their first episode of illness, and those with prominent depressive symptoms were each associated with superior outcome.

The small prospective study by Dodwell and Goldberg (1989) did not observe predictive value for the quantitative evaluations of affective symptomatology or for RDC diagnosis as schizoaffective. On the other hand, these investigators reported that perplexity was a significant symptomatic predictor. Confusion or perplexity is a common feature of 'cycloid psychoses' (Leonhard, 1961), which traditionally have been thought to be exquisitely responsive to ECT (Perris, 1974). Ries *et al.* (1981) reported the only study restricted to the use of ECT in schizoaffective disorder. They identified nine patients who met the RDC for schizoaffective, depressed ($n = 5$) or manic subtype ($n = 4$) and who had failed two different antipsychotic medications prior to ECT. All patients were young (average age 25.2 years), had paranoid delusions and six of the nine patients had intermittent catatonic symptoms. Of note, confusion was moderate to severe in eight of the nine patients. All patients manifested a strong clinical response to ECT. This case series was in line with other reports suggesting that medication-resistant patients, characterized by marked psychotic and affective symptoms and by confusion, respond rapidly to ECT (Walinder, 1972; Dempsey *et al.*, 1975).

NMS

NMS shares clinical features with lethal catatonia and has been considered an iatrogenic form of lethal catatonia induced by exposure to neuroleptics (Mann *et al.*, 1990). When the clinical community became cognizant of NMS, there was reluctance to treat these patients with ECT. This reluctance was based on the fact that NMS has similar symptoms to malignant hyperthermia, a familial syndrome provoked by exposure to general anaesthesia and depolarizing muscle relaxants, such as succinylcholine (Liskow, 1985). However, NMS and malignant hyperthermia have been shown to be unrelated syndromes (Addonizio & Sussman, 1987; Hermesh *et al.*, 1988). Indeed, several reviews have documented that ECT is an effective treatment for NMS (Casey, 1987; Devanand *et al.*, 1987; Mann *et al.*, 1990; Pearlman, 1990; Davis *et al.*, 1991). In compiling the world literature, Davis *et al.* (1991) found that mortality rates in NMS patients were equivalent with ECT compared with bromocriptine, dantrolene, L-dopa or amantidine, and averaged about half that of untreated patients. The complications and deaths that have been observed with use of ECT have been tied to continued administration of neuroleptic medication and to cardiac dysregulation. Given the marked haemodynamic alterations associated with ECT, in the NMS patient it is advisable to first use medication strategies to stabilize autonomic function, before starting ECT. Since these patients must often be discontinued from antipsychotic medication, ECT has the unique properties of treating both the NMS and the underlying psychotic condition.

Treatment technique

Since the introduction of ECT, there have been a variety of improvements in treatment administration that have reduced morbidity, mortality and cognitive side effects. These modifications include the use of general anaesthesia and muscle relaxants, more efficient electrical waveforms (i.e. brief pulse vs. sine wave stimuli), unilateral electrode placements and the titration of electrical dosage to the needs of individual patients (APA, 1990). In the area of mood disorders, the introduction of some of these modifications of treatment technique has led to a reconsideration of fundamental premises regarding the mode of action of ECT. It had long been contended that the production of a generalized seizure of adequate duration provided the necessary and sufficient conditions for antidepressant effects (Ottosson, 1960; Fink, 1979). Contradicting this view, it was recently demonstrated that generalized seizures can be reliably produced that lack antidepressant effects (Sackeim *et al.*, 1987, 1993). Rather, for major depression, it appears that there are electrical dose−response relations and efficacy is contingent on the anatomical positioning of electrodes (electrode placement) and the extent to which electrical dosage exceeds seizure threshold (Sackeim *et al.*, 1991, 1993). In depression, these findings go beyond the sham vs. real ECT trial in demonstrating that physiological events over and above the production of a generalized seizure are critical to antidepressant response. These findings are also of obvious significance in designing optimal forms of ECT administration. Unfortunately, work refining the ECT technique has concentrated almost exclusively on major depression.

Electrode placement

Whether electrodes are placed on one or both sides of the head can have marked effects on cognitive consequences (Sackeim, 1992). Generally speaking, the traditional bifrontotemporal (bilateral) placement produces more extensive and severe transient amnestic effects than does unilateral placement. Electrodes placed over the left hemisphere are associated with longer times for return of orientation and greater verbal amnestic deficits than electrodes placed over the right hemisphere. In contrast, right unilateral ECT typically results in greater amnestic deficits for non-verbal material relative to left unilateral ECT (Daniel & Crovitz, 1982, 1983; Weiner *et al.*,

1986; Sackeim, 1992). Left unilateral ECT is rarely used, although theories regarding lateralized disturbances in schizophrenia would support investigation of a therapeutic advantage (Gur, 1978; Flor-Henry, 1983). In mood disorders, there has been an ongoing debate about the relative efficacy of bilateral and right unilateral ECT, with over 40 comparative trials (Abrams, 1986; Sackeim *et al.*, 1993). Only four studies have compared unilateral and bilateral ECT in schizophrenia and these are summarized in Table 26.5.

Each of the four trials contrasting unilateral and bilateral ECT in schizophrenia failed to detect differences in efficacy. In each case, the patient samples had a relatively short duration of illness and showed a strong response to ECT. However, the conclusions that can be drawn from this work are limited. Two studies were conducted in outpatients and were characterized by inordinately high dropout (Doongaji *et al.*, 1973; Bagadia *et al.*, 1988). El-Islam *et al.* (1970) determined the side of electrode placement (left or right) based on an assessment of motoric lateralization (handedness, eyedness and footedness), an inappropriate procedure (APA, 1990). Wessels (1972) treated patients on a daily basis, using a fixed number of eight treatments. Therefore, at best, there are weak indications that right unilateral and bilateral ECT may be equivalent in efficacy when treating schizophrenia. These studies used inefficient electrical waveforms and high stimulus intensity (Wessels, 1972; Doongaji *et al.*, 1973). It is unknown whether the particular sensitivity of right unilateral ECT to electrical dosage, as seen in major depression, extends to schizophrenia (Sackeim *et al.*, 1993).

Treatment frequency

Early in the history of ECT it was contended that schizophrenic patients required more closely spaced treatments and longer treatment courses than patients with other conditions (Kalinowsky, 1943; Kennedy & Anchel, 1948; Baker *et al.*, 1960a). Kalinowsky (1943) argued that discontinuation of ECT after rapid improvement in acute schizophrenia almost invariably led to early relapse, which could be prevented by administering a more prolonged ECT course. Following this dictum, regressive forms of ECT were developed, in which multiple treatments were given on the same day, often 7 days per week, with the avowed aim of producing global disorientation and dissolution of the personality in schizophrenic patients (Glueck *et al.*, 1957; Jacoby & van Houten, 1960; Murillo & Exner, 1973a; Exner & Murillo, 1977). This view has continued into the modern era, as some experts contend that schizophrenic patients typically require 10–20 treatments, and that negative symptom manifestations (withdrawn, apathetic behaviour) may require even more treatments (Fink, 1979). Empirical evidence bearing on this position is scant. Baker *et al.* (1960a) reported superior results in chronic schizophrenics after 20 treatments relative to 12 treatments. King (1959) randomized 37 male chronic schizophrenic patients to ECT given three times per week or ECT given twice daily six times per week. Both groups received 20 treatments and there was no discernible difference in outcome.

It should be noted that the recent trials of ECT in schizophrenia (e.g. sham vs. real ECT, comparisons of electrode placements) have used relatively small numbers of treatments, generally six to 12, with positive results. It is also noteworthy that early commentators on the treatment of acute mania often stated that a large number of ECT treatments were needed in this condition, at an intensive schedule (Kalinowsky & Hippius, 1972). To the contrary, recent experience has been that, if anything, relative to depressed patients, manic patients show clinical response earlier in the treatment course and daily treatment confers no advantage over more spaced treatment schedules [see Mukherjee *et al.* (1994) for a review]. In the treatment of major depression, there was also a belief that the administration of additional treatments after achieving symptomatic remission aided in delaying relapse. In the case of depression, this view was shown to be erroneous (Snaith, 1981). Similarly, it is quite possible that beliefs that schizophrenic patients require particularly long courses of ECT to achieve response or to prevent relapse are without merit. In terms of practice,

Table 26.5 Prospective clinical trials comparing unilateral and bilateral electroconvulsive therapy (ECT) in schizophrenia

Study	Patients	Study design	Nature of treatment	Results/comments
El-Islam *et al.* (1970)	41 schizophrenic patients, aged 18–40 years, with delusions or hallucinations; schizoaffective and catatonic patients excluded	Sequential assignment to 'non-dominant' ($n = 20$) or bilateral ($n = 21$) conditions; double-blind evaluation	ECT at two per week; non-dominant hemisphere inappropriately determined; all patients received concomitant trifluoperazine 15 mg/day; patients receiving unilateral ECT averaged seven treatments; bilateral averaged 7.3 treatments	Groups equivalent in clinical outcome, assessed as the number of treatments needed to relieve delusions and hallucinations, and in total number of treatments and time to discharge; slight non-significant advantage to unilateral ECT on a memory test
Wessels (1972)	100 South Sotho males, acute schizophrenia (Bleuler criteria) first admission	Sequential assignment to right unilateral ECT ($n = 51$) vs. bilateral ECT ($n = 49$). Double-blind evaluations 14 days following ECT with BPRS and NOSIE	ECT was unmodified and given daily for eight treatments; Lancaster position for unilateral ECT; CPZ 200 mg/day during ECT course and increased to 300 mg/day until day 14 following ECT	Both forms of ECT resulted in substantial improvement, with no differences; 67% of patients rated as very much improved
Doongaji *et al.* (1973)	54 schizophrenic out-patients, aged 15–45 years; no treatment for at least 3 months prior to study. Patients with illness <1 month or >2 years excluded	Randomized to left unilateral, right unilateral and bilateral ECT. Randomization stratified by age and duration of illness; double-blind evaluation with BPRS and CGI; 32 patients initially randomized not analysed	Unmodified ECT given three per week for first 2 weeks and two per week for next 2 weeks (minimum six treatments); no concurrent medication other than chloral hydrate. Both unilateral groups averaged eight ECT, bilateral averaged 9.4	No efficacy differences among the treatment groups after six ECT, at the end of ECT or after a 3-month follow-up; no difference in number of treatments. No explanation given for 32 patients being dropped from the sample prior to six ECT
Bagadia *et al.* (1988)	40 DSM-III schizophrenic out-patients aged 18–65 years	Double-blind, random assignment to right unilateral ($n = 20$) vs. bilateral ($n = 20$) ECT; BPRS and CGI at baseline, after three treatments and after six treatments; 21 patients dropped due to non-compliance or discontinuation of treatment	Unmodified ECT given three per week for first three treatments and at 4-day intervals for next three treatments (only six treatments given); no concurrent medication other than chloral hydrate	Both groups showed substantial and equivalent clinical improvement; no attempt to account for the high dropout rate

BPRS, brief psychiatric rating scale; NOSIE, nurses' observation scale for inpatient evaluation; CGI, clinical global impression.

clinicians should be guided by manifestations of clinical improvement and side effects when determining whether to continue with ECT. Prescribing a fixed number of treatments is not appropriate.

Continuation/maintenance ECT

ECT is the only somatic treatment in psychiatry that is typically stopped once shown to be effective. A minority of patients, almost exclusively individuals with affective disorders who relapse while receiving continuation or maintenance pharmacotherapy, receive ECT as a continuation or maintenance treatment (Decina *et al.*, 1987; Kramer, 1987; Thornton *et al.*, 1990; Monroe, 1991). Interest in continuation ECT in preventing relapse in mood disorders has increased markedly in recent years. In part, this may be due to preliminary evidence that standard pharmacological strategies are ineffective in preventing relapse following response to ECT, when patients have failed those strategies during treatment of the acute affective episode (Sackeim *et al.*, 1990). Similarly, ECT is often considered an adjunctive treatment in schizophrenic patients who are resistant to traditional antipsychotic medications. In this specific population, the efficacy of traditional neuroleptics in preventing relapse is unknown.

Information on the use of ECT as a continuation or maintenance treatment in schizophrenia comes mainly from older literature (Moore, 1943; Weisz & Creel, 1948; Karliner & Wehrheim, 1965). Karliner and Wehrheim (1965) reported on maintenance convulsive treatment given to 57 patients, 12% of whom relapsed after up to 6 years of observation. Of 153 patients who refused such maintenance treatment, 79% relapsed. Diagnostically, both groups were heterogeneous, consisting of schizophrenic, schizoaffective and manic-depressive patients. Asnis and Gabriel (1976) reported that maintenance ECT was successful in controlling symptoms in a number of patients with schizophrenia. Without question, difficulties in convincing patients of the need for maintenance ECT and with compliance have limited the use of this strategy in schizophrenia. Nonetheless, particularly given its theoretical potential for medication-resistant patients and its potential for reducing concomitant neuroleptic dosage (Gardos *et al.*, 1980), investigation in this area is needed. It is noteworthy that several reviews of maintenance therapy in schizophrenia do not mention ECT (Davis, 1975; Carpenter, 1987; Schooler, 1991).

Side effects

Modern ECT is associated with low rates of morbidity and mortality. It is estimated that mortality rates are about the same as with general anaesthesia for minor surgery, involving approximately one death per 10 000 patients treated (APA, 1990; Abrams, 1992). The low incidence of major complications is particularly impressive since ECT is often used in patients with pre-existing medical complications, given the belief that it is safer than antidepressant medications. The major source of morbidity and mortality with ECT is cardiovascular complications. The risk of serious complications is increased in the elderly, particularly the oldest age groups, in those with pre-existing medical conditions, particularly cardiac illness, and in those receiving concurrent medication for medical conditions (Alexopoulous *et al.*, 1984; Burke *et al.*, 1987; Cattan *et al.*, 1990; Sackeim, 1993). Consequently, the safety of ECT is expected to be particularly high among schizophrenic patients.

Cardiovascular collapse and respiratory depression may occur when reserpine is combined with ECT, and this combination should be avoided (Foster & Gayle, 1956; Bracha & Hess, 1956; Kalinowsky, 1956; Bross, 1957). There were also some suggestions after the introduction of neuroleptics that the combination of CPZ and ECT was associated with serious hypotensive crises (Weiss, 1955; Gaitz *et al.*, 1956; Kalinowsky, 1956; Grinspoon & Greenblatt, 1963). This concern has not been substantiated by subsequent experience (Gonzalez & Imahara, 1964) and has not been raised for other antipsychotic medications.

Cognition

The cognitive effects of ECT are stereotyped and their magnitude is dependent on methods of treatment administration (Sackeim, 1992). There is no reason to suspect that the nature of ECT-induced cognitive side effects differ in schizophrenia relative to other disorders. However, the presence of baseline cognitive deficits in schizophrenia is well documented (Heaton *et al.*, 1978; Seidman, 1983; Bilder *et al.*, 1992) and there is evidence for progressive cognitive deterioration as part of the natural course of the disorder (Tsuang *et al.*, 1979; Bilder *et al.*, 1992). Given this, the question arises whether individuals with schizophrenia are at risk for more severe or persistent cognitive or other neuropsychiatric complications when treated with ECT.

Perlson (1945) conducted extensive psychological studies of a patient with chronic schizophrenia who received 248 ECT treatments over an approximately 3-year period, eventually being discharged in a remitted state. He concluded that the patient had no discernible intellectual or physical sequelae. In a long-term follow-up of schizophrenic patients treated with regressive ECT or with medications, Exner and Murillo (1977) could not detect differences in neuropsychological function or in projective test results. Buhrich *et al.* (1988) examined a group of 42 long-stay hospital patients with chronic schizophrenia. They divided this sample into two age- and sex-matched groups based on temporal disorientation. A past history of ECT, among other physical treatment variables, did not distinguish patients with and without temporal disorientation. Gureje (1988) tested 70 individuals who met the Feighner criteria for definite schizophrenia, 56% of whom had received ECT treatments with the mean number of treatments being 10.8. He found that the number of ECT treatments in the past was unrelated to objective measures of psychopathology, to performance on a variety of cognitive measures or to neurological soft signs. Devanand *et al.* (1991) compared a group of eight patients (four with a diagnosis of schizophrenia), who each had received more than 100 bilateral, modified sine wave ECT treatments, with a matched group of patients who had never received ECT. They found no difference between the groups in neuropsychological measures, suggesting that patients given many courses of ECT treatment do not manifest measurable cognitive impairment at long-term follow-up. Bagadia *et al.* (1983) randomized 38 schizophrenic patients to sham ECT plus CPZ or to real ECT and placebo. At trial completion, subjective forgetfulness was reported by 15% of the patients who received CPZ and by 40% of those who received ECT. However, no differences in objective cognitive measures were found. On the contrary, following ECT there was an improvement on almost all objective cognitive measures.

In contrast to these reports, Goldman *et al.* (1972) found that performance on the Bender–Gestalt and Benton visual retention tests was impaired in male chronic schizophrenic in-patients with a history of 50 or more ECT treatments, when compared with a control group of patients matched for age, education and race. Templer *et al.* (1973) replicated these findings in a sample of 44 hospitalized schizophrenic patients; the 22 patients in the index group had in the past received from 40 to 263 ECT treatments with a median number of 58.5. Both these studies have been criticized as suffering from non-blind evaluations of ECT patients and controls, group differences in the degree of psychopathology and for the use of inappropriate instruments for neuropsychological evaluation (Weiner, 1984; Devanand *et al.*, 1991). Overall, this is little reason to suspect that ECT results in more severe or extensive neuropsychological effects in schizophrenic patients than in other populations.

It is not uncommon to observe pronounced neuropsychological deterioration early in the course of schizophrenia (Bilder *et al.*, 1992). In our experience, when ECT is used as a treatment for acute psychotic episodes in young schizophrenic patients, occasionally patients or family membes attribute the subsequent cognitive decline to this intervention. Despite similar progression in patients treated with neuroleptics, rarely are medications viewed as contributory. Perhaps sensitized by the acute cognitive effects of ECT, or by the mythology surrounding this treatment, some patients may be sensitized to attributing cognitive changes to ECT.

Neuropathological effects

It is generally contended that modern ECT, involving generalized seizures that last approximately 1 min, under conditions of general anaesthesia, muscle relaxation and continuous oxygenation does not provide the conditions necessary for neuronal death (Weiner, 1984; Meldrum, 1986; Siesjö *et al.*, 1986). Elegant animal studies have detailed the metabolic and molecular substrate for seizure-induced cell damage. During seizures, there are marked increases in cerebral glucose utilization and oxygen consumption. However, blood supply outstrips metabolic demand. When seizures are sustained for periods of hours, as in status epilepticus, supply may fall short of demand, with consequent cellular damage. The duration of the ECT-induced seizure is orders of magnitude below the threshold for this type of effect (Ingvar 1986; Meldrum, 1986).

Weinberger *et al.* (1979) reported a significant correlation among schizophrenic patients between lateral ventricular size and previous ECT. A number of other computerized tomography (CT) and magnetic resonance imaging (MRI) studies have contrasted mood-disorder or schizophrenic patients with positive and negative histories of ECT and found no differences with respect to measures of cerebral volume and sulcal widening (e.g., Nasrallah *et al.*, 1982, 1984; Dolan *et al.*, 1985; Pearlson *et al.*, 1985, Kolbeinsson *et al.*, 1986; Andreasen *et al.*, 1990; Swayze *et al.*, 1990). CT (Bergsholm *et al.*, 1989) and MRI (Coffey *et al.*, 1988, 1991; Scott *et al.*, 1990) prospective, longitudinal, structural imaging studies of patients who have received ECT also have reported negative findings regarding treatment-associated changes. Importantly, Rabins *et al.* (1991) reported that depressed patients who were *subsequently* treated with ECT showed on MRI at pretreatment baseline greater temporal horn abnormality and

generally had evidence of greater subcortical pathology than other depressed patients. This type of finding underscores the need for caution in interpreting retrospective associations between types of treatment and evidence of structural change.

Movement disorders

The potential for acute extrapyramidal symptoms (EPS), particularly neuroleptic-induced parkinsonism (NIP), and for persistent tardive dyskinesia (TD) are major drawbacks of traditional neuroleptic treatment. EPS is a ubiquitous phenomenon, and estimates of the prevalence of TD in individuals receiving traditional neuroleptic medication typically range from 25 to 50% (APA, 1980; Kane & Smith, 1982; Lieberman *et al.*, 1984; Jeste & Kaufman, 1986; Wolf & Mosnaim, 1988). While EPS is generally considered to be reversible, prospective studies have suggested that NIP predicts the subsequent development of TD (Kane *et al.*, 1988b; Chouinard *et al.*, 1988). In elderly patients, NIP has been linked to greater cognitive impairment (Mukherjee *et al.*, 1991) and to larger lateral ventricular size (Hoffman *et al.*, 1987). NIP and akathisia may also persist following the discontinuation of neuroleptics (Melamed *et al.*, 1991; Hermesh *et al.*, 1992).

ECT has antiparkinsonian properties. In both open and sham-controlled trials, ECT has been found to improve clinical symptoms in idiopathic Parkinson's disease, at least on a short-term basis (Asnis, 1977; Andersen *et al.*, 1987; Douyon *et al.*, 1989; see Faber and Trimble (1991) for a review). Typically, L-dopa requirements are sharply reduced when patients with idiopathic Parkinson's disease receive ECT. The clinical utility of ECT as a long-term treatment for medication-resistant Parkinson's disease has yet to be tested, as the use of maintenance ECT has not been evaluated in this condition. ECT also has ameliorative effects on NIP (Gangadhar *et al.*, 1983; Goswami *et al.*, 1989). For example, Goswami *et al.* (1989) studied nine schizophrenic in-patients with a longitudinal triphasic design, first using neuroleptics, then neuroleptics and ECT and then neuroleptics.

NIP was significantly reduced in a stepwise fashion when patients were treated with ECT. Hermesh *et al.* (1992) reported a case in which NIP and akathisia continued for 3 months, despite two courses of anticholinergic treatment, a change to a low-potency neuroleptic and a neuroleptic-free period. These adverse effects responded dramatically to ECT and re-emerged 3 months after discontinuation of ECT.

Recently, Mukherjee and Debsikdar (1994) introduced the notion that ECT may protect against the later development of NIP and TD. They examined 35 DSM-III-R-classified schizophrenic patients who were on neuroleptics for at least 2 weeks. All patients received 10 mg trifluoperazine per day, 28 patients received additional neuroleptic medications, and 24 patients were also receiving concurrent anticholinergic treatment. In addition, all patients were receiving ($n = 15$) or had received during the index episode ($n = 20$) a course of unmodified bilateral ECT. Standardized scales for evaluating EPS and TD were completed. None of the 35 patients had bradykinesia, rigidity or postural instability. Two patients had mild tremor of the upper extremities. Only one patient met the research diagnosis of TD criteria (Schooler & Kane, 1982) for probable TD (mild severity). The relative absence of signs of NIP and the low prevalence of TD was unexpected. Mukherjee and Debsikdar (1994) speculated that if NIP is a risk factor in the development of TD, ECT may ultimately protect against TD by preventing initial NIP. At the neurophysiological level, there is evidence that electroconvulsive shock in rodents prevents the development of dopamine-receptor supersensitivity with exposure to dopamine antagonists (Lerer *et al.*, 1982). While intriguing, establishing such a protective role for ECT will require controlled, prospective comparison of patients exposed to neuroleptics with and without a prior history of ECT.

There is also a case-report literature that suggests that ECT may have some impact on manifestations of TD. Early reports suggested that ECT may contribute to the manifestation of persistent TD (Uhrbrand & Faurbye, 1960;

Faurbye *et al.*, 1964; Holcomb *et al.*, 1983; Flaherty *et al.*, 1984). A small series was also reported in which ECT produced no short-term change in TD severity (Asnis & Leopold, 1978). More recently, a series of case studies have linked the use of ECT with often dramatic and long-term improvement in symptoms of TD (Price & Levin, 1978; Rosenbaum *et al.*, 1980; Chacko & Root, 1983; Gosek & Weller, 1988; Malek-Ahmadi & Weddige, 1988; Hay *et al.*, 1990). With one exception (Asnis & Leopold, 1978), in the published reports the primary indication for the use of ECT was the acute psychiatric condition, with effects on TD noted incidentally. In the absence of controlled, prospective investigation, no firm conclusions can be offered regarding the value of ECT in the treatment of TD. The scattering of positive reports leave unanswered questions regarding possible effects of concomitant medications during the ECT course, improvement associated with neuroleptic withdrawal and a host of other possibilities. Nonetheless, our clinical experience suggests that the effects of ECT on manifestations of TD are variable. Some patients, often with severe forms of TD, show clinically meaningful improvement, with the diminution of TD symptoms typically occurring abruptly during the ECT course. Other patients, with seemingly similar conditions, show little benefit. It is our impression that ECT-related improvement is more likely in patients with severe TD manifestations. As in some of the positive case reports, we have observed sustained remission of TD manifestations following ECT. There are also two reports of linking ECT to amelioration of tardive dystonia, where other attempts at treatment are usually disappointing (Kwentus *et al.*, 1984; Adityanjee *et al.*, 1990).

Aside from these indications that ECT may alter manifestations of TD, there are suggestions that a history of ECT may be associated with a low prevalence or delayed development of TD. Gardos *et al.* (1980) evaluated 122 schizophrenic out-patients in Hungary and reported a striking absence of severe TD. They suggested that the low prevalence was due to the avoidance of high-dosage neuroleptic treatment. Most of these patients were treated with ECT during acute episodes and as a means of forestalling new episodes. According to Gardos *et al.* (1980), this use of ECT allowed for more moderate dosing of neuroleptics. In a US sample, Cole *et al.* (1992) recently reported that a history of previous ECT was associated with a lower risk and delayed appearance of TD. As noted, Mukherjee and Debsikdar (1994) found virtually no TD in an Indian sample, and this they also attributed to the use of ECT. Schwartz *et al.* (1993), in an Israeli sample, reported a reduced incidence of TD among male schizophrenic patients with a history of ECT. If, in fact, ECT does offer long-term protection against the iatrogenic effects of later exposure to neuroleptics, this would contradict the general impression that the behavioural and physiological effects of ECT are typically transient (Sackeim, 1988).

Mechanisms

With few exceptions (e.g. Milstein *et al.*, 1990), there is little evidence that the biochemical and neurophysiological changes produced by ECT differ in schizophrenic patients compared with other psychiatric groups. Rather, the dilemma in accounting for the efficacy of ECT in schizophrenia is the same as that faced in other conditions. The application of an electrical stimulus to the brain and the production of a generalized seizure produce a remarkable diversity of short-term biochemical and neurophysiological changes. In animal models and humans, there has been little difficulty in demonstrating consistent effects on peptide, transmitter or hormone systems or in regional patterns of cerebral perfusion, metabolism and electrical activity [see Sackeim (1988) and Nutt *et al.* (1989) for reviews]. Rather, the problem has been in discerning which of these effects is linked to efficacy in particular disorders and which are epiphenomena.

Some have contended that the search for mechanisms of action of ECT is relatively hopeless given the plethora of physiological alterations that accompany and follow seizures (Kety, 1974). However, in the case of major depression, we now

know that seizures may be reliably produced that lack therapeutic properties (Sackeim *et al.*, 1987, 1993). This has created new optimism in the search for the physiological basis of antidepressant effects, by offering the opportunity to subtract the effects of therapeutic seizures from those that lack efficacy. Basic and clinical research along these lines has recently begun (Bhattacharya *et al.*, 1991; Zis *et al.*, 1991; Nobler *et al.*, 1993). In addressing mechanisms of action in schizophrenia, it may also be helpful to better isolate the components of the ECT process that are necessary and sufficient for efficacy.

At this point, it is uncertain whether ECT exerts therapeutic action through the effects it shares with antipsychotic medication or through different means. Clinical research can aid in addressing this issue by more clearly establishing the extent to which resistance to antipsychotic medication predicts resistance to ECT (e.g. Prudic *et al.*, 1990). In large part, a high degree of correlation has been assumed, with both classes of treatment generally thought to be more effective in schizophrenic patients with acute exacerbations and short duration of illness. Indeed, this overlap has led some to question whether ECT has much of a role in the treatment of schizophrenia (Royal College of Psychiatrists, 1977; Abrams, 1992). This assumption is also reflected in the recent studies of ECT in medication-resistant schizophrenic patients. This work has examined the efficacy of ECT only when used in combination with neuroleptics (Friedel, 1986; Gujavarty *et al.*, 1987). Conceptually, this would suggest that the effects of the two approaches are additive or synergistic. In line with this view, the series of studies that contrasted combination treatment with neuroleptic treatment alone or ECT alone generally found the combination to be superior (e.g. Ray, 1962; Childers, 1964; Smith *et al.*, 1967; Small *et al.*, 1982).

One suggestion that has often been given for the apparent superiority of combination ECT and neuroleptic treatment to either of them alone is that ECT results in an increased concentration of neuroleptic medication in neural tissue (e.g. Gujavarty *et al.*, 1987). Specifically, it has been suggested that the transient disruption of the blood−brain barrier that occurs acutely with seizure induction (Bolwig *et al.*, 1977) allows neuroleptics greater entry into the brain. Aoba *et al.* (1983) found that plasma and red blood cell levels of haloperidol increased transiently by about 100% immediately after ECT in schizophrenic patients, indicating a redistribution phenomenon. However, Shibata *et al.* (1989) demonstrated a similar effect in rats, but did not find any changes in cerebral concentrations of haloperidol. They attributed the peripheral increase in plasma to a transient decrease in muscle storage during the convulsion. As reviewed here, one of the difficulties with this line of thinking is that there is substantial evidence that ECT is efficacious in the treatment of schizophrenia in the absence of concomitant neuroleptics (e.g. May, 1968). Accounts of the utility of ECT that posit only an enhancement of medication effects are out of keeping with these clinical findings.

There is little doubt at both the physiological and behavioural levels that ECT and classical neuroleptics have distinct profiles. This is illustrated by the fact that ECT has powerful antipsychotic effects across a range of psychiatric and organic conditions, and yet ECT also has antiparkinsonian effects. This would suggest that ECT and classical antipsychotic medications differ in their alterations of dopaminergic transmission. Indeed, this is the case. Microdialysis studies in rodents indicate that electroconvulsive shock acutely results in increased concentrations of dopamine and dopamine metabolites in brain, with this effect showing a regional distribution (Nutt *et al.*, 1989; Nomikos *et al.*, 1991; Zis *et al.*, 1991). Repeated treatment may produce enhanced tonic levels of dopamine or its metabolites in selective brain regions. Behavioural studies indicate that dopamine-mediated behaviours are enhanced following electroconvulsive shock. Locomotion and stereotypic behaviour provoked by apomorphine and amphetamine are increased following chronic electroconvulsive shock (Green & Deakin, 1980; Costain *et al.*, 1982; Green & Nutt, 1987). This increased dopaminergic tone is

not mediated by changes at the D_2 receptor. Most studies have found that electroconvulsive shock has little effect on D_2-receptor density or second messenger function (Bergstrom & Kellar, 1979; Atterwill, 1980; Newman & Lerer, 1989), while there is accumulating evidence that altered D_1-receptor function is responsible for enhanced behavioural responses to dopamine agonists following electro-convulsive shock (Newman & Lerer, 1989; Barkai *et al.*, 1990; Hao *et al.*, 1990; Serra *et al.*, 1990; Verma & Kulkarni, 1991). This pattern of effects is quite distinct from the profile associated with traditional neuroleptics. Furthermore, ECT also differs in important ways from atypical neuroleptics, such as clozapine. It has been suggested that clozapine's therapeutic effects are related to antagonist properties at both serotonin (5-hydroxytryptamine; 5-HT_{1C}, 5-HT_2 and 5-HT_3) and dopamine (D_2) receptors (Meltzer, 1989; Meltzer *et al.*, 1989; Owen *et al.*, 1993). In contrast, it is well established that electroconvulsive shock leads to an enhancement of serotonin-mediated behaviour and, as opposed to classical antidepressant medications, to an increased density of 5-HT_2 receptors (Green *et al.*, 1983; Kellar & Stockmeier, 1986). Therefore, the biochemical effects of electroconvulsive shock on both dopamine and serotonin systems appear to be distinct from those of either typical or atypical neuroleptics. The fact that ECT is a powerful antipsychotic treatment presents a challenge for any unified theory regarding antipsychotic mechanisms.

Conclusions

There is little consensus within the clinical community regarding the role of ECT in the treatment of schizophrenia. Expert groups differ widely in their recommendations, and surveys indicate highly disparate rates of utilization between and within countries. Despite over 55 years of continuous use of convulsive therapy in schizophrenia, this lack of consensus is tied to an inadequate research base. ECT was introduced prior to the development of modern clinical trial methodology. Many of the clinical tenets regarding the use of ECT in schizophrenia derive from this era. Some of the best information we have came from studies conducted soon after the introduction of antipsychotic medications, where ECT was used as the gold standard against which to establish the efficacy of these new agents (e.g. Childers, 1964; Smith *et al.*, 1967; May, 1968). However, since then the nature of pharmacological treatment of schizophrenia has advanced and the vast bulk of clinical research on ECT has concentrated on mood disorders.

There is little doubt that ECT is efficacious in the treatment of schizophrenia, at least in patients with acute exacerbations and/or a relatively short duration of illness. However, even in this group, the short-term benefits of ECT are likely to be equivalent to, or less than, those of monotherapy with a traditional neuroleptic. In contrast, the available evidence suggests that combination treatment of ECT and neuroleptic is superior in short-term outcome to that of ECT alone or neuroleptic alone. The consistency of this observation is surprising, since it is usually difficult to establish the superiority of a treatment combination when a primary treatment, in this case neuroleptics, exerts pronounced efficacy. The combination treatment of ECT and neuroleptics has advantages that may not be fully appreciated. In general, the work that suggested superior efficacy for the combination used lower neuroleptic doses for the combined treatment groups than for the neuroleptic-alone groups. Furthermore, the antiparkinsonian effects of ECT may aid in limiting extrapyramidal side effects and in offering greater flexibility in neuroleptic dosing. There are few concerns about the safety of this combination.

Close perusal of the literature on the use of ECT in schizophrenia produced the surprising suggestion that this treatment may exert long-term benefits. In several comparative studies, patients who received ECT, either alone or in combination with neuroleptics, had superior functioning at follow-up or were less subject to relapse than patients treated only with neuroleptics (e.g. Smith *et al.*, 1967; Exner & Murillo, 1977;

May *et al.*, 1981). This work was characterized by a variety of methodological limitations, the most important of which was lack of control over treatment following resolution of the acute episode. Nonetheless, in these studies, patients who received antipsychotic medication during the acute episode typically continued with this treatment following discharge, while ECT samples may have received less aggressive maintenance treatment (Wyatt, 1991).

Another more tentative suggestion that has emerged in recent work is that schizophrenic patients treated with ECT earlier in their history may be less likely to have or have delayed manifestation of NIP and TD (Gardos *et al.*, 1980; Cole *et al.*, 1992; Mukherjee & Debsikdar, 1994). Among the possibilities here are a selection bias, whereby schizophrenic patients who receive ECT differ in vulnerability for these movement disorders relative to those not referred for this treatment. Alternatively, as suggested by Gardos *et al.* (1980), the use of ECT may have allowed more moderate exposure to traditional neuroleptics, thereby impacting on subsequent movement disorders. Mukherjee and Debsikdar (1994) offered the novel idea that manifestation of NIP is a prerequisite for later development of TD. The acute antiparkinsonian effects of ECT and its putative protective effects against later development of NIP may be related to a reduced prevalence of TD. Regardless, given their obvious clinical importance, these suggestions that ECT may have long-term clinical benefits and protective effects against movement disorders underscore the need for additional research.

At this point, there is little information to guide the clinician in determining which schizophrenic patient will benefit most from ECT, or in optimizing specific aspects of treatment administration. The long-held view that protracted courses of ECT are required in schizophrenia has not been examined specifically in recent research, but is out of keeping with evidence that substantial response is often observed after eight to 10 treatments (Brandon *et al.*, 1985; Abraham & Kulhara, 1987; Taylor & Fleminger, 1980). It is noteworthy that the original sham vs. real ECT studies that failed to find a therapeutic effect for ECT concentrated on chronic samples (e.g. Miller *et al.*, 1953; Brill *et al.*, 1959a−c; Heath *et al.*, 1964). In contrast, the more recent positive sham vs. real ECT studies (Brandon *et al.*, 1985; Abraham & Kulhara, 1987; Taylor & Fleminger, 1980) sampled patients with a shorter duration of illness and used concomitant antipsychotic medication. Recent research has not addressed the long-held view that ECT is of limited value in schizophrenic patients with insidious symptom onset and long illness duration (Kalinowsky, 1943; Fink, 1979; Salzman, 1980; Kendell, 1981). Nonetheless, this accords with our experience that only a small minority of chronic, institutionalized schizophrenic patients show palpable benefit from ECT, even when combined with neuroleptic treatment. However, in a small minority, ECT is associated with dramatic effects and can produce the first symptomatic remission to be observed in years. Among chronic patients, one cannot predict who will benefit from ECT. It is our view that, regardless of chronicity, schizophrenic patients who have exhausted pharmacological alternatives deserve a course of ECT.

Recent reports have documented a strong response to combination ECT and traditional neuroleptic treatment in patients with a shorter illness duration who have failed traditional neuroleptics (Fredel, 1986; Gujavarty *et al.*, 1987). Such patients may constitute the prime indication for the use of ECT in schizophrenia. This area requires considerable development. It is uncertain whether these positive reports pertain only to schizophrenic patients with prominent affective symptomatology (i.e. schizoaffective patients), or whether the positive effects are more general. There is virtually no information on the utility of combining ECT with atypical neuroleptics, such as clozapine. Since the clozapine-resistant patient represents a distinctly difficult therapeutic dilemma, exploration of this combination would also seem worthwhile.

Acknowledgement

Preparation of this chapter was supported in part by grants MH35636 and MH47739 from the National Institute of Mental Health.

References

Abraham, K.R. & Kulhara, P. (1987) The efficacy of electroconvulsive therapy in the treatment of schizophrenia. A comparative study. *British Journal of Psychiatry*, **151**, 152−155.

Abrams, R. (1986) Is unilateral electroconvulsive therapy really the treatment of choice in endogenous depression? *Annals of the New York Academy of Sciences*, **462**, 50−55.

Abrams, R. (1987) ECT in Schizophrenia (editorial). *Convulsive Therapy*, **3**, 169−170.

Abrams, R. (1992) *Electroconvulsive Therapy*. Oxford University Press, New York.

Abrams, R. & Taylor, M.A. (1976a) Catatonia. A prospective clinical study. *Archives of General Psychiatry*, **33**, 579−581.

Abrams, R. & Taylor, M.A. (1976b) Mania and schizoaffective disorder, manic type: a comparison. *American Journal of Psychiatry*, **133**, 1445−1447.

Abrams, R., Taylor, M.A. & Gastanaga, P. (1974) Manic-depressive illness and paranoid schizophrenia. *Archives of General Psychiatry*, **31**, 640−642.

Addonizio, G. & Susman, V.L. (1987) ECT as a treatment alternative for patients with symptoms of neuroleptic malignant syndrome. *Journal of Clinical Psychiatry*, **48**, 102−105.

Adityanjee, Jayaswal, S.K., Chan, T.M. & Subramanaim, M. (1990) Temporary remission of tardive dystonia following electroconvulsive therapy. *British Journal of Psychiatry*, **156**, 433−435.

Agarwal, A.K., Andrade, C. & Reddy, M.V. (1992) The practice of ECT in India: issues relating to the administration of ECT. *Indian Journal of Psychiatry*, **34**, 285−297.

Alexopoulos, G.S., Shamoian, C.J., Lucas, J., Weiser, N. & Berger, H. (1984) Medical problems of geriatric psychiatric patients and younger controls during electroconvulsive therapy. *Journal of the American Geriatric Society*, **32**, 651−654.

Andersen, K., Balldin, J., Gottfries, C.G. *et al.* (1987) A double-blind evaluation of electroconvulsive therapy in Parkinson's disease with 'on-off' phenomena. *Acta Neurologica Scandinavica*, **76**, 191−199.

Andreasen, N.C., Swayze, V., Flaum, M., Alliger, R. & Cohen, G. (1990) Ventricular abnormalities in affective disorder: clinical and demographic correlates. *American Journal of Psychiatry*, **147**, 893−900.

Aoba, A., Kakita, Y., Yamaguchi, N. *et al.* (1983) Electric convulsive therapy (ECT) increases plasma and red blood cell haloperidol neuroleptic activities. *Life Sciences*, **33**, 1797−1803.

APA (Task Force on ECT) (1978) *Electroconvulsive Therapy, Task Force Report #14*. American Psychiatric Association,

Washington DC.

APA (Task Force on Tardive Dyskinesia) (1980) *Tardive Dyskinesia.* American Psychiatric Association, Washington DC.

APA (Task Force on ECT) (1990) *The Practice of ECT: Recommendations for Treatment, Training and Privileging.* American Psychiatric Press, Washington DC.

Arnold, O.H. & Stepan, H. (1952) Untersuchungen zur Frage der akuten todlichen Katatonie. *Wiener Zeitschrift fur Nervenheilkunde und Deren Grenzgebiete*, **4**, 235–258.

Asnis, F. & Gabriel, A.N. (1976) ECT as maintenance therapy in schizophrenia (letter). *American Journal of Psychiatry*, **133**, 858–859.

Asnis, G.M. (1977) Parkinson's disease, depression, and ECT: a review and case study. *American Journal of Psychiatry*, **134**, 191–195.

Asnis, G.M. & Leopold, M.A. (1978) A single-blind study of ECT in patients with tardive dyskinesia. *American Journal of Psychiatry*, **135**, 1235–1237.

Atterwill, C.K. (1980) Lack of effect of repeated electroconvulsive shock on [^{3}H]spiroperidol and [^{2}H]5-hydroxytryptamine binding and cholinergic parameters in rat brain. *Journal of Neurochemistry*, **35**, 729–734.

Ayres, C. (1960) The relative value of various somatic therapies in schizophrenia. *Journal of Neuropsychiatry*, **1**, 154–162.

Bagadia, V.N., Dave, K.P. & Shah, L.P. (1970) A comparative study of physical treatments in schizophrenia. *Indian Journal of Psychiatry*, **12**, 190–204.

Bagadia, V.N., Abhyankar, R., Pradhan, P.V. & Shah, L.P. (1988) Reevaluation of ECT in schizophrenia: right temporoparietal versus bitemporal electrode placement. *Convulsive Therapy*, **4**, 215–220.

Bagadia, V.N., Abhyankar, R.R., Doshi, J., Pradhan, P.V. & Shah, L.P. (1983) Report from a WHO collaborative center for psychopharmacology in India. 1. Reevaluation of ECT in schizophrenia. *Psychopharmacology Bulletin*, **19**, 550–555.

Baker, A.A., Game, J.A. & Thorpe, J.G. (1958) Physical treatment for schizophrenia. *Journal of Mental Science*, **104**, 860–864.

Baker, A.A., Game, J.A. & Thorpe, J.G. (1960b) Some research into the treatment of schizophrenia in the mental hospital. *Journal of Mental Science*, **106**, 203–213.

Baker, A.A., Bird, G., Lavin, N.I. & Thorpe, J.G. (1960a) E.C.T. in schizophrenia. *Journal of Mental Science*, **106**, 1506–1511.

Barkai, A.I., Durkin, M. & Nelson, H.D. (1990) Localized alterations of dopamine receptor binding in rat brain by repeated electroconvulsive shock: an autoradiographic study. *Brain Research*, **529**, 208–213.

Bergsholm, P., Larsen, J.L., Rosendahl, K. & Holsten, F. (1989) Electroconvulsive therapy and cerebral computed tomography. A prospective study. *Acta Psychiatrica Scandinavica*, **80**, 566–572.

Bergstrom, D.A. & Kellar, K.J. (1979) Effect of electroconvulsive shock on monoaminergic receptor binding sites in rat brain. *Nature*, **278**, 464–466.

Bhattacharya, S.K., Banerjee, P.K., Glover, V. & Sandler, M. (1991) Augmentation of rat brain endogenous monoamine oxidase inhibitory activity (tribulin) by electroconvulsive shock. *Neuroscience Letters*, **125**, 65–68.

Bilder, R.M., Lipschutz-Broch, L., Reiter, G., Geisler, S.H., Mayerhoff, D.I. & Lieberman, J.A. (1992) Intellectual deficits in first-episode schizophrenia: evidence for progressive deterioration. *Schizophrenia Bulletin*, **18**, 437–448.

Bland, R.C. & Brintnell, S. (1985) Electroconvulsive therapy in a major teaching hospital: diagnoses and indications. *Canadian Journal of Psychiatry*, **30**, 288–292.

Bolwig, T.G., Hertz, M.M., Paulson, O.B., Spotoft, H. & Rafaelsen, O.J. (1977) The permeability of the blood–brain barrier during electrically induced seizures in man. *European Journal of Clinical Investigation*, **7**, 87–93.

Bond, E.D. (1954) Results of psychiatric treatments with a control series. *American Journal of Psychiatry*, **110**, 561–566.

Borowitz, A.H. (1959) An investigation into combined electroconvulsive and chlorpromazine therapy in the treatment of schizophrenia. *South African Medical Journal*, **33**, 836–840.

Bracha, S. & Hess, J.P. (1956) Death occurring during combined reserpine–electroshock treatment. *American Journal of Psychiatry*, **113**, 257.

Brandon, S., Cowley, P., McDonald, C., Neville, P., Palmer, R. & Wellstood-Eason, S. (1985) Leicester ECT trial: results in schizophrenia. *British Journal of Psychiatry*, **146**, 177–183.

Brill, N.Q., Crumpton, E., Eiduson, S., Grayson, H.M. & Hellman, L.I. (1959a) Predictive and concomitant variables related to improvement with actual and simulated ECT. *Archives of General Psychiatry*, **1**, 263–272.

Brill, N.Q., Crumpton, E., Eiduson, S., Grayson, H.M., Hellman, L.I. & Richards, R.A. (1959b) An experimental study of the relative effectiveness of various components of electro-convulsive therapy. *American Journal of Psychiatry*, **115**, 734–735.

Brill, N.Q., Crumpton, E., Eiduson, S., Grayson, H.M., Hellman, L.I. & Richards, R.A. (1959c) Relative effectiveness of various components of electroconvulsive therapy. *Archives of Neurology and Psychiatry*, **81**, 627–635.

Brill, N.Q., Crumpton, E., Eiduson, S. *et al.* (1957) Investigation of the therapeutic components and various factors associated with improvement with electroconvulsive treatment: a preliminary report. *American Journal of Psychiatry*, **113**, 997–1008.

Bross, R. (1957) Near fatality with combined ECT and reserpine. *American Journal of Psychiatry*, **113**, 933.

Buhrich, N., Crow, T.J., Johnstone, E.C. & Owens, D.G.C. (1988) Age disorientation in chronic schizophrenia is not associated with pre-morbid intellectual impairment or past physical treatment. *British Journal of Psychiatry*, **152**, 466–469.

Burke, W.J., Rubin, E.H., Zorumski, C.F. & Wetzel, R.D. (1987) The safety of ECT in geriatric psychiatry. *Journal of the American Geriatric Society*, **35**, 516–521.

Carpenter, W.T. Jr, Heinrichs, D.W. & Hanlon, T.E. (1987) A comparative trial of pharmacologic strategies in schizophrenia. *American Journal of Psychiatry*, **144**, 1466–1470.

Casey, D.A. (1987) Electroconvulsive therapy in the neuroleptic malignant syndrome. *Convulsive Therapy*, **3**, 278–283.

Cattan, R.A., Barry, P.P., Mead, G., Reefe, W.E., Gay, A. & Silverman, M. (1990) Electroconvulsive therapy in octogenarians. *Journal of the American Geriatric Society*, **38**,

753–758.

Cerletti, U. & Bini, L. (1938) Un neuvo metodo di shockterapie 'L'elettro-shock'. *Bolletino Accademia Medica Roma*, **64**, 136–138.

Chacko, R.C. & Root, L. (1983) ECT and tardive dyskinesia: two cases and a review. *Journal of Clinical Psychiatry*, **44**, 265–266.

Chafetz, M.E. (1943) An active treatment for chronically ill patients. *Journal of Nervous and Mental Disease*, **98**, 464–473.

Cheney, C.O. & Drewry, P.H. (1938) Results of non-specific treatment in dementia praecox. *American Journal of Psychiatry*, **95**, 203–217.

Childers, R. (1964) Comparison of four regimens in newly admitted female schizophrenics. *American Journal of Psychiatry*, **120**, 1010–1011.

Childers, R.T. & Therrien, R. (1961) A comparison of the effectiveness of trifluoperazine and chlorpromazine in schizophrenia. *American Journal of Psychiatry*, **118**, 552–554.

Chouinard, G., Annable, L., Ross-Chouinard, A. & Mercier, P. (1988) A 5-year prospective longitudinal study of tardive dyskinesia: factors predicting appearance of new cases. *Journal of Clinical Psychopharmacology*, **8** (Suppl.), 21S–26S.

Coffey, C.E., Figiel, G.S., Djang, W.T., Sullivan, D.C., Herfkens, R.J. & Weiner, R.D. (1988) Effects of ECT on brain structure: a pilot prospective magnetic resonance imaging study. *American Journal of Psychiatry*, **145**, 701–706.

Coffey, C.E., Weiner, R.D., Djang, W.T. *et al.* (1991) Brain anatomic effects of electroconvulsive therapy. A prospective magnetic resonance imaging study. *Archives of General Psychiatry*, **48**, 1013–1021.

Cole, J.O., Gardos, G., Boling, L.A., Marby, D., Haskell, D. & Moore, P. (1992) Early dyskinesia — vulnerability. *Psychopharmacology*, **107**, 503–510.

Costain, D.W., Cowen, P.J., Gelder, M.G. & Grahame-Smith, D.G. (1982) Electroconvulsive therapy and the brain: evidence for increased dopamine-mediated responses. *Lancet*, **2**, 400–404.

Currier, G.E., Cullinan, C. & Rothschild, D. (1952) Results of treatment of schizophrenia in a state hospital: changing trends since advent of electroshock therapy. *Archives of Neurology and Psychiatry*, **67**, 80–82.

Daniel, W.F. & Crovitz, H.F. (1982) Recovery of orientation after electroconvulsive therapy. *Acta Psychiatrica Scandinavica*, **66**, 421–428.

Daniel, W.F. & Crovitz, H.F. (1983) Acute memory impairment following electroconvulsive therapy. 2. Effects of electrode placement. *Acta Psychiatrica Scandinavica*, **67**, 57–68.

Danziger, L. & Kindwall, J.A. (1946) Prediction of the immediate outcome of shock therapy in dementia praecox. *Diseases of the Nervous System*, **7**, 299–303.

Das, P.S., Saxena, S. Mohan, D. & Sundaram, K.R. (1991) Adjunctive electroconvulsive therapy for schizophrenia. *National Medical Journal of India*, **4**, 183–184.

Davis, J.M. (1975) Overview: maintenance therapy in psychiatry. I. Schizophrenia. *American Journal of Psychiatry*, **132**, 1237–1245.

Davis, J.M., Janicak, P.G., Sakkas, P., Gilmore, C. & Wang, Z. (1991) Electroconvulsive therapy in the treatment of the neuroleptic malignant syndrome. *Convulsive Therapy*, **7**, 111–120.

Decina, P., Guthrie, E.B., Sackeim, H.A., Kahn, D. & Malitz, S. (1987) Continuation ECT in the management of relapses of major affective episodes. *Acta Psychiatrica Scandinavica*, **75**, 559–562.

Dempsey, G.M., Tsuang, M.T., Struss, A. & Dvoredsky-Wortsman, A. (1975) Treatment of schizo-affective disorder. *Comprehensive Psychiatry*, **16**, 55–59.

Devanand, D.P., Sackeim, H.A. & Finck, A.D. (1987) Modified ECT using succinylcholine after remission of neuroleptic malignant syndrome. *Convulsive Therapy*, **3**, 284–290.

Devanand, D.P., Verma, A.K., Tirumalasetti, F. & Sackeim, H.A. (1991) Absence of cognitive impairment after more than 100 lifetime ECT treatments. *American Journal of Psychiatry*, **148**, 929–932.

DeWet, J.S.T. (1957) Evaluation of a common method of convulsion therapy in Bantu schizophrenics. *Journal of Mental Science*, **103**, 739–757.

Dodwell, D. & Goldberg, D. (1989) A study of factors associated with response to electroconvulsive therapy in patients with schizophrenic symptoms. *British Journal of Psychiatry*, **154**, 635–639.

Dolan, R.J., Calloway, S.P. & Mann, A.H. (1985) Cerebral ventricular size in depressed subjects. *Psychological Medicine*, **15**, 873–878.

Doongaji, D.R., Jeste, D.V., Saoji, N.J., Kane, P.V. & Ravindranath, S. (1973) Unilateral versus bilateral ECT in schizophrenia. *British Journal of Psychiatry*, **123**, 73–79.

Douyon, R., Serby, M., Klutchko, B. & Rotrosen, J. (1989) ECT and Parkinson's disease revisited: a 'naturalistic study'. *American Journal of Psychiatry*, **146**, 1451–1455.

El-Islam, M.F., Ahmed, S.A. & Erfan, M.E. (1970) The effect of unilateral E.C.T. on schizophrenic delusions and hallucinations. *British Journal of Psychiatry*, **117**, 447–448.

Ellison, F.A. & Hamilton, D.M. (1949) The hospital treatment of dementia praecox. Part II. *American Journal of Psychiatry*, **106**, 454–461.

Exner, J.E. Jr & Murillo, L.G. (1973) Effectiveness of regressive ECT with process schizophrenia. *Diseases of the Nervous System*, **34**, 44–48.

Exner, J.E. Jr & Murillo, L.G. (1977) A long term follow-up of schizophrenics treated with regressive ECT. *Diseases of the Nervous System*, **38**, 162–168.

Faber, R. & Trimble, M.R. (1991) Electroconvulsive therapy in Parkinson's disease and other movement disorders. *Movement Disorders*, **6**, 293–303.

Faurbye, A., Rasch, P.J. & Peterson, P.B. (1964) Neurological symptoms in pharmacotherapy of psychoses. *Acta Psychiatrica Scandinavica*, **40**, 10–27.

Feighner, J., Robins, E., Guze, S., Woodruff, R. Jr, Winokur, G. & Munoz, R. (1972) Diagnosis criteria for use in psychiatry research. *Archives of General Psychiatry*, **26**, 57–63.

Fink, M. (1979) *Convulsive Therapy: Theory and Practice*. Raven Press, New York.

Fink, M. (1987) Is ECT usage decreasing (editorial). *Convulsive Therapy*, **3**, 171–173.

Fink, M. (1989) Is catatonia a primary indication for ECT? (editorial). *Convulsive Therapy*, **5**, 1–4.

Flaherty, J.A., Naidu, J. & Dysken, M. (1984) ECT, emergent dyskinesia, and depression. *American Journal of Psychiatry*, **141**, 808–809.

Flor-Henry, P. (1983) *Cerebral Basis of Psychopathology*. John Wright, Boston.

Folstein, M., Folstein, S. & McHugh, P.R. (1973) Clinical predictors of improvement after electroconvulsive therapy of patients with schizophrenia, neurotic reactions, and affective disorders. *Biological Psychiatry*, **7**, 147–152.

Ford, H. & Jameson, G.K. (1955) Chlorpromazine in conjunction with other psychiatric therapies: a clinical appraisal. *Diseases of the Nervous System*, **16**, 179–185.

Foster, M.W.J. & Gayle, R.F.I. (1956) Chlorpromazine and reserpine as adjuncts in electroshock treatment. *Southern Medical Journal*, **49**, 731–735.

Fricchione, G.L. (1989) Catatonia: a new indication for benzodiazepenes? *Biological Psychiatry*, **26**, 761–765.

Friedel, R.O. (1986) The combined use of neuroleptics and ECT in drug-resistant schizophrenic patients. *Psychopharmacology Bulletin*, **22**, 928–930.

Gabris, G. & Muller, C. (1983) La catatonie dite 'pernicieuse'. *Encephale*, **9**, 365–385.

Gaitz, C.M., Pokorny, A.D. & Mills, M.J. (1956) Death following electroconvulsive therapy. *Archives of Neurology and Psychiatry*, **75**, 493–499.

Gangadhar, B.N., Roychowdhury, J. & Channabasavanna, S. (1983) ECT and drug-induced parkinonism. *Indian Journal of Psychiatry*, **25**, 212–213.

Gardos, G., Samu, I., Kallos, M. & Cole, J.O. (1980) Absence of severe tardive dyskinesia in Hungarian schizophrenic out-patients. *Psychopharmacology*, **71**, 29–34.

Glueck, B., Reiss, B.B. & Bernard, L. (1957) Regressive electric shock therapy. *Psychiatric Quarterly*, **31**, 117–136.

Goldfarb, W. & Kieve, H. (1945) The treatment of psychotic-like regressions of combat soldiers. *Psychiatric Quarterly*, **19**, 555–565.

Goldman, H., Gomer, F.E. & Templer, D.I. (1972) Long-term effects of electroconvulsive therapy upon memory and perceptual-motor performance. *Journal of Clinical Psychology*, **28**, 32–34.

Gonzalez, J.R. & Imahara, J. (1964) Electroshock therapy with the phenothiazine reserpine: a survey and report. *American Journal of Psychiatry*, **121**, 253–256.

Gosek, E. & Weller, R.A. (1988) Improvement of tardive dyskinesia associated with electroconvulsive therapy. *Journal of Nervous and Mental Disease*, **176**, 120–122.

Goswami, U., Dutta, S., Kuruvilla, K., Papp, E. & Perenyi, A. (1989) Electroconvulsive therapy in neuroleptic-induced parkinsonism. *Biological Psychiatry*, **26**, 234–238.

Gottlieb, J.S. & Huston, P.E. (1951) Treatment of schizophrenia. *Journal of Nervous and Mental Disease*, **113**, 237–246.

Green, A.R. & Deakin, J.F. (1980) Brain noradrenaline depletion prevents ECS-induced enhancement of serotonin- and dopamine-mediated behaviour. *Nature*, **285**, 232–233.

Green, A.R. & Nutt, D. (1987) Psychopharmacology of repeated seizures: possible relevance to the mechanisms of action of electroconvulsive therapy. In Inversen, L., Iversen,

S. & Snyder, S. (eds) *Handbook of Psychopharmacology*, Vol. 19, pp. 375–419. Plenum Press, New York.

Green, A.R., Heal, D.J., Johnson, P., Laurence, B.E. & Nimgaonkar, V.L. (1983) Antidepressant treatments: effects in rodents on dose-response curves of 5-hydroxytryptamine- and dopamine-mediated behaviours and 5-HT$_2$ receptor number in frontal cortex. *British Journal of Pharmacology*, **80**, 377–385.

Grinspoon, L. & Greenblatt, M. (1963) Pharmacotherapy combined with other treatment methods. *Comprehensive Psychiatry*, **4**, 256–262.

Gujavarty, K., Greenberg, L.B. & Fink, M. (1987) Electroconvulsive therapy and neuroleptic medication in therapy-resistant positive-symptom psychosis. *Convulsive Therapy*, **3**, 185–195.

Gur, R.E. (1978) Left hemisphere dysfunction and left hemisphere overactivation in schizophrenia. *Journal of Abnormal Psychology*, **87**, 225–238.

Gureje, O. (1988) Schizophrenic patients treated with electroconvulsive therapy: their demographic, clinical and cognitive features. *East African Medical Journal*, **65**, 379–386.

Guttmann, E., Mayer-Gross, W. & Slater, E.T.O. (1939) Short-distance prognosis of schizophrenia. *Journal of Neurology and Psychiatry*, **2**, 25–34.

Hamilton, D.M. & Wall, J.H. (1948) The hospital treatment of dementia praecox. *American Journal of Psychiatry*, **105**, 346–352.

Hamilton, M. (1986) Electroconvulsive therapy. Indications and contraindications. *Annals of the New York Academy of Sciences*, **462**, 5–11.

Hao, X.Z., Mathë, A.A., Mathë, J.M. & Svensson, T.H. (1990) Electroconvulsive treatment attenuates behavioral response to SKF 38393 in reserpine-treated mice. *Psychopharmacology*, **100**, 135–137.

Hay, D.P., Hay, L., Blackwell, B. & Spiro, H.R. (1990) ECT and tardive dyskinesia. *Journal of Geriatric Psychiatry and Neurology*, **3**, 106–109.

Heath, E.S., Adams, A. & Wakeling, P.L. (1964) Short courses of E.C.T. and simulated E.C.T. in chronic schizophrenia. *British Journal of Psychiatry*, **110**, 800–807.

Heaton, R.K., Baade, L.E. & Johnson, K.L. (1978) Neuropsychological test results associated with psychiatric disorders in adults. *Psychological Bulletin*, **85**, 141–162.

Hermesh, H., Aizenberg, D., Lapidot, M. & Munitz, H. (1988) Risk of malignant hyperthermia among patients with neuroleptic malignant syndrome and their families. *American Journal of Psychiatry*, **145**, 1431–1434.

Hermesh, H., Aizenberg, D., Friedberg, G., Lapidot, M. & Munitz, H. (1992) Electroconvulsive therapy for persistent neuroleptic-induced akathisia and parkinsonism: a case report. *Biological Psychiatry*, **31**, 407–411.

Hertzman, M. (1992) ECT and neuroleptics as primary treatment for schizophrenia (editorial). *Biological Psychiatry*, **31**, 217–220.

Herzberg, F. (1954) Prognostic variables for electro-shock therapy. *Journal of General Psychology*, **50**, 79–86.

Hoffman, W.F., Labs, S.M. & Casey, D.E. (1987) Neuroleptic-induced parkinsonism in older schizophrenics. *Biological Psychiatry*, **22**, 427–439.

Holcomb, H.H., Sternberg, D.E. & Heninger, G.R. (1983)

Effects of electroconvulsive therapy on mood, parkinsonism, and tardive dyskinesia in a depressed patient: ECT and dopamine systems. *Biological Psychiatry*, **18**, 865–873.

Ingvar, M. (1986) Cerebral blood flow and metabolic rate during seizures: relationship to epileptic brain damage. *Annals of the New York Academy of Sciences*, **462**, 194–206.

Jacoby, M. & van Houten, Z. (1960) Regressive shock therapy. *Diseases of the Nervous System*, **21**, 582–583.

Janakiramaiah, N., Channabasavanna, S.M. & Murthy, N.S. (1982) ECT/chlorpromazine combination versus chlorpromazine alone in acutely schizophrenic patients. *Acta Psychiatrica Scandinavica*, **66**, 464–470.

Janicak, P.G., Davis, J.M., Gibbons, R.D., Ericksen, S., Chang, S. & Gallagher, P. (1985) Efficacy of ECT: a meta-analysis. *American Journal of Psychiatry*, **142**, 297–302.

Jeste, D.V. & Kaufman, C.A. (1986) Pathophysiology of tardive dyskinesia: evaluation of supersensitivity theory and alternative hypothesis. In Casey, D.E. & Gardos, G. (eds) *Tardive Dyskinesia and Neuroleptics: From Dogma to Reason*, American Psychiatric Association, Washington DC, pp. 149–157.

Kalinowsky, L.B. (1943) Electric convulsion therapy with emphasis on importance of adequate treatment. *Archives of Neurology and Psychiatry*, **50**, 652–660.

Kalinowsky, L.B. (1956) The danger of various types of medication during electric convulsive therapy. *American Journal of Psychiatry*, **112**, 745–746.

Kalinowsky, L.B. (1988) Schizophrenia and ECT (letter). *Convulsive Therapy*, **4**, 99.

Kalinowsky, L.B. & Hippius, H. (1972) *Pharmacological, Convulsive and Other Treatments in Psychiatry*. Grune & Stratton, New York.

Kalinowsky, L.B. & Worthing, H. (1943) Results with electric convulsive therapy in 200 cases of schizophrenia. *Psychiatric Quarterly*, **17**, 144–153.

Kane, J.M. & Smith, J.M. (1982) Tardive dyskinesia: prevalence and risk factors 1959 to 1979. *Archives of General Psychiatry*, **39**, 473–481.

Kane, J.M., Woerener, M. & Lieberman, J.A. (1988b) Tardive dyskinesia: prevalence, incidence, and risk factors. *Journal of Clinical Psychopharmacology*, **8** (Suppl.), 52S–56S.

Kane, J.M., Honigfeld, G., Singer, J. & Meltzer, H.Y. (1988a) Clozapine for the treatment-resistant schizophrenic. *Archives of General Psychiatry*, **45**, 789–796.

Karliner, W. & Wehrheim, H. (1965) Maintenance convulsive treatments. *American Journal of Psychiatry*, **121**, 1113–1115.

Kellar, K.J. & Stockmeier, C.A. (1986) Effects of electroconvulsive shock and serotonin axon lesions on beta-adrenergic and serotonin-2 receptors in rat brain. *Annals of the New York Academy of Sciences*, **462**, 76–90.

Kendell, R.E. (1971) Psychiatric diagnosis in Britain and the United States. *British Journal of Hospital Medicine*, **6**, 147–155.

Kendell, R.E. (1981) The present status of electroconvulsive therapy. *British Journal of Psychiatry*, **139**, 265–283.

Kennedy, C.J. & Anchel, D. (1948) Regressive electric shock in schizophrenics refractory to other shock therapies. *Psychiatric Quarterly*, **22**, 317–320.

Kety, S.S. (1974) Biochemical and neurochemical effects of electroconvulsive shock. In Fink, M., Kety, S., McGaugh, J. & Williams, T. (eds) *Psychobiology of Convulsive Therapy*,

pp. 285–294. V.H. Winton & Sons, Washington DC.

King, P.D. (1959) A comparison of REST and ECT in the treatment of schizophrenics. *American Journal of Psychiatry*, **116**, 358–359.

King, P.D. (1960) Chlorpromazine and electroconvulsive therapy in the treatment of newly hospitalized schizophrenics. *Journal of Clinical and Experimental Psychopathology*, **21**, 101–105.

Kino, F.F. & Thorpe, T.F. (1946) Electrical convulsion therapy in 500 selected psychotics. *Journal of Mental Science*, **92**, 138–145.

Klapheke, M.M. (1991a) Clozapine, ECT, and schizoaffective disorder, bipolar type. *Convulsive Therapy*, **7**, 36–39.

Klapheke, M.M. (1991b) Follow-up on clozapine and ECT (Letter). *Convulsive Therapy*, **7**, 303–305.

Koehler, K. & Sauer, H. (1983) First rank symptoms as predictors of ECT response in schizophrenia. *British Journal of Psychiatry*, **142**, 280–283.

Kolbeinsson, H., Arnaldsson, O.S., Pëtursson, H. & Skúlason, S. (1986) Computed tomographic scans in ECT patients. *Acta Psychiatrica Scandinavica*, **73**, 28–32.

Konig, P. & Glatter-Gotz, U. (1990) Combined electroconvulsive and neuroleptic therapy in schizophrenia refractory to neuroleptics. *Schizophrenia Research*, **3**, 351–354.

Kramer, B.A. (1987) Maintenance ECT: a survey of practice (1986). *Convulsive Therapy*, **3**, 260–268.

Kwentus, J.A., Schulz, S.C. & Hart, R.P. (1984) Tardive dystonia, catatonia, and electroconvulsive therapy. *Journal of Nervous and Mental Disease*, **172**, 171–173.

Landmark, J., Joseph, L. & Merskey, H. (1987) Characteristics of schizophrenic patients and the outcome of fluphenazine and of electroconvulsive treatments. *Canadian Journal of Psychiatry*, **32**, 425–428.

Landy, D.A. (1991) Combined use of clozapine and electroconvulsive therapy. *Convulsive Therapy*, **7**, 218–221.

Langsley, D.G., Enterline, J.D. & Hickerson, G.X.J. (1959) A comparison of chlorpromazine and EST in treatment of acute schizophrenic and manic reactions. *Archives of Neurology and Psychiatry*, **81**, 384–391.

Latey, R.H. & Fahy, T.J. (1988) Some influences on regional variation in frequency of prescription of electroconvulsive therapy. *British Journal of Psychiatry*, **152**, 196–200.

Leff, J.P. & Wing, J.K. (1971) Trial of maintenance therapy in schizophrenia. *British Medical Journal*, **iii**, 599–604.

Leonhard, K. (1961) Cycloid psychoses. *Journal of Mental Science*, **107**, 633–648.

Leonhard, K. (1979) *The Classification of Endogenous Psychoses*. Irvington, New York.

Lerer, B., Jabotinsky-Rubin, K., Bannet, J., Ebstein, R.P. & Belmaker, R.H. (1982) Electroconvulsive shock prevents dopamine receptor supersensitivity. *European Journal of Pharmacology*, **80**, 131–134.

Lewis, A.B. (1982) ECT in drug-refractory schizophrenics. *Hillside Journal of Clinical Psychiatry*, **4**, 141–154.

Lieberman, J.A., Kane, J.M. & Johns, C.A. (1989) Clozapine: guidelines for clinical management. *Journal of Clinical Psychiatry*, **50**, 329–338.

Lieberman, J., Kane, J.M. & Woerner, M. (1984) Prevalence of tardive dyskinesia in elderly samples. *Psychopharmacology*

Bulletin, **20**, 22–26.

Liskow, B.I. (1985) Relationship between neuroleptic malignant syndrome and malignant hyperthermia (letter). *American Journal of Psychiatry*, **142**, 390.

Lowinger, L. & Huddleson, J.H. (1945) Outcome on dementia praecox under electric shock therapy as related to mode of onset and to number of convulsions induced. *Journal of Nervous and Mental Disease*, **102**, 243–246.

McKinnon, A.L. (1948) Electric shock therapy in a private psychiatric hospital. *Canadian Medical Association Journal*, **58**, 478–483.

Malek-Ahmadi, P. & Weddige, R.L. (1988) Tardive dyskinesia and electroconvulsive therapy. *Convulsive Therapy*, **4**, 328–331.

Malla, A. (1986) An epidemiological study of electroconvulsive therapy: rate and diagnosis. *Canadian Journal of Psychiatry*, **31**, 824–830.

Mann, S.C., Caroff, S.N., Bleier, H.R., Antelo, E. & Un, H. (1990) Electroconvulsive therapy of the lethal catatonia syndrome. *Convulsive Therapy*, **6**, 239–247.

Mann, S.C., Caroff, S.N., Bleier, H.R., Welz, W.K., Kling, M.A. & Hayashida, M. (1986) Lethal catatonia. *American Journal of Psychiatry*, **143**, 1374–1381.

Martin, B.A., Kramer, P.M., Day, D., Peter, A.M. & Kedward, H.B. (1984) The Clarke Institute experience with electroconvulsive therapy. II. Treatment evaluation and standards of practice. *Canadian Journal of Psychiatry*, **29**, 652–657.

Masiar, S.J. & Johns, C.A. (1991) ECT following clozapine. *British Journal of Psychiatry*, **158**, 135–136.

May, P.R. (1968) *Treatment of Schizophrenia: A Comparative Study of Five Treatment Methods*. Science House, New York.

May, P.R. & Tuma, A.H. (1965) Treatment of schizophrenia: an experimental study of five treatment methods. *British Journal of Psychiatry*, **111**, 503–510.

May, P.R., Tuma, A.H., Yale, C., Potepan, P. & Dixon, W. (1976) Schizophrenia — a follow-up study of results of treatment. II. Hospital stay over two to five years. *Archives of General Psychiatry*, **33**, 481–486.

May, P.R., Tuma, A.H., Dixon, W.J., Yale, C., Thiele, D.A. & Kraude, W.H. (1981) Schizophrenia. a follow-up study of the results of five forms of treatment. *Archives of General Psychiatry*, **38**, 776–784.

Meduna, L.J. (1935) Versuche über die biologische Beeinflussung des Abaufes der Schizophrenia: Camphor und Cardiozolkrampfe. *Zeitschrift Gesante für die Neurologie und Psychiatrie*, **152**, 235–262.

Melamed, E., Achiron, A., Shapira, A. & Davidoviez, S. (1991) Persistent and progressive parkinsonism after discontinuation of chronic neuroleptic therapy: an additional tardive syndrome? *Clinical Neuropharmacology*, **14**, 273–278.

Meldrum, B.S. (1986) Neuropathological consequences of chemically and electrically induced seizures. *Annals of the New York Academy of Sciences*, **462**, 186–193.

Meltzer, H.Y. (1989) Clinical studies on the mechanism of action of clozapine: the dopamine–serotonin hypothesis of schizophrenia. *Psychopharmacology*, **99** (Suppl.), S18–S27.

Meltzer, H.Y. (1992) Treatment of the neuroleptic-nonresponsive schizophrenic patient. *Schizophrenia Bulletin*, **18**, 515–542.

Meltzer, H.Y., Matsubara, S. & Lee, J. (1989) Classifications of typical and atypical antipsychotic drugs on the basis of dopamine D-1, D-2, and serotonin$_2$ pK_i values. *Journal of Pharmacology and Experimental Therapeutics*, **251**, 123–130.

Miller, D.H., Clancy, J. & Cumming, E. (1953) A comparison between unidirectional current nonconvulsive electrical stimulation given with Reiters machine, standard alternating current electroshock (Cerletti method), and Pentothal in chronic schizophrenia. *American Journal of Psychiatry*, **109**, 617–620.

Milstein, V., Small, J.G., Miller, M.J., Sharpley, P.H. & Small, I.F. (1990) Mechanisms of action of ECT: schizophrenia and schizoaffective disorder. *Biological Psychiatry*, **27**, 1282–1292.

Monroe, R.R.J. (1991) Maintenance electroconvulsive therapy. *Psychiatric Clinics of North America*, **14**, 947–960.

Moore, M.P. (1943) The maintenance treatment of chronic psychotics by electrically induced convulsions. *Journal of Mental Science*, **89**, 257–269.

Mowbray, R.M. (1959) Historical aspects of electric convulsant therapy. *Scottish Medical Journal*, **4**, 373–378.

Mukherjee, S. & Debsikdar, V. (1994) Absence of neuroleptic-induced parkinsonism in psychotic patients receiving adjunctive electroconvulsive therapy. *Convulsive Therapy*, **10**, 53–58.

Mukherjee, S., Sackeim, H.A. & Schnur, D.B. (1994) Electroconvulsive therapy of acute manic episodes: a review of 50 years of experience. *American Journal of Psychiatry*, **151**, 169–176.

Mukherjee, S., Decina, P., Scapicchio, P.L. & Caracci, G. (1991) Cognitive impairment in schizophrenic patients: relations to tardive dyskinesia and neuroleptic-induced parkinsonism. *Biological Psychiatry*, **29**, 176A.

Murillo, L.G. & Exner, J.E. Jr (1973a) The effect of regressive ECT with process schizophrenics. *American Journal of Psychiatry*, **130**, 269–273.

Murillo, L.G. & Exner, J.E. Jr (1973b) Ataractic drugs versus ECT in schizophrenia (letter). *American Journal of Psychiatry*, **130**, 1162–1163.

Nasrallah, H.A., McCalley-Whitters, M. & Jacoby, C.G. (1982) Cerebral ventricular enlargement in young manic males: a controlled CT study. *Journal of Affective Disorders*, **4**, 15–19.

Nasrallah, H.A., McCalley-Whitters, M. & Pfohl, B. (1984) Clinical significance of large cerebral ventricles in manic males. *Psychiatry Research*, **13**, 151–156.

Newman, M.E. & Lerer, B. (1989) Post-receptor-mediated increases in adenylate cyclase activity after chronic antidepressant treatment: relationship to receptor desensitization. *European Journal of Pharmacology*, **162**, 345–352.

NIH (1985) Consensus conference: electroconvulsive therapy. *Journal of the American Medical Association*, **254**, 2103–2108.

NIMH-PSC (Collaborative Study Group) (1964) Phenothiazine treatment in acute schizophrenia. *Archives of General Psychiatry*, **10**, 246–261.

Nobler, M.S., Sackeim, H.A., Solomou, M., Luber, B., Devanand, D.P. & Prudic, J. (1993) EEG manifestations during ECT: effects of electrode placement and stimulus intensity. *Biological Psychiatry*, **34**, 321–330.

Nomikos, G.G., Zis, A.P., Damsma, G. & Fibiger, H.C. (1991) Electroconvulsive shock produces large increases in interstitial concentrations of dopamine in the rat striatum: an *in vivo* microdialysis study. *Neuropsychopharmacology*, **4**, 65–69.

Nutt, D.J., Gleiter, C.H. & Glue, P. (1989) Neuropharmacological aspects of ECT: in search of the primary mechanism of action. *Convulsive Therapy*, **5**, 250–260.

Ottosson, J.-O. (1960) Experimental studies of the mode of action of electroconvulsive therapy. *Acta Psychiatrica Scandinavica*, Suppl. **145**, 1–141.

Ottosson, J.-O. (1985) Use and misuse of electroconvulsive treatment. *Biological Psychiatry*, **20**, 933–946.

Owen, R.R.J., Gutierrez-Esteinou, R., Hsiao, J. *et al.* (1993) Effects of clozapine and fluphenazine treatment on responses to *m*-chlorophenylpiperazine infusions in schizophrenia. *Archives of General Psychiatry*, **50**, 636–644.

Palmer, D.M., Sprang, H.E. & Hans, C.L. (1951) Electroshock therapy in schizophrenia: a statistical survey of 455 cases. *Journal of Nervous and Mental Disease*, **114**, 162–171.

Pankratz, W.J. (1980) Electroconvulsive therapy: the position of the Canadian Psychiatric Association. *Canadian Journal of Psychiatry*, **25**, 509–514.

Pataki, J., Zervas, I.M. & Jandorf, L. (1992) Catatonia in a university inpatient service (1985–1990). *Convulsive Therapy*, **8**, 163–173.

Pearlman, C. (1990) Neuroleptic malignant syndrome and electroconvulsive therapy (letter). *Convulsive Therapy*, **6**, 251–253.

Pearlson, G.D., Garbacz, D.J., Moberg, P.J., Ahn, H.S. & DePaulo, J.R. (1985) Symptomatic, familial, perinatal, and social correlates of computerized axial tomography (CAT) changes in schizophrenics and bipolars. *Journal of Nervous and Mental Disease*, **173**, 42–50.

Perlson, J. (1945) Psychologic studies on a patient who received two hundred and forty-eight shock treatments. *Archives of Neurology and Psychiatry*, **54**, 409–411.

Perris, C. (1974) A study of cycloid psychoses. *Acta Psychiatrica Scandinavica*, Suppl. **253**, 1–77.

Pippard, J. & Ellam, L. (1981) *Electroconvulsive Treatment in Great Britain*. Gaskell Books, Ashford.

Pope, H.G. Jr & Lipinski, J.F. (1978) Diagnosis in schizophrenia and manic-depressive illness. *Archives of General Psychiatry*, **35**, 811–827.

Pope, H.G. Jr, Lipinski, J.F., Cohen, B.M. & Axelrod, D.T. (1980) 'Schizoaffective disorder': an invalid diagnosis? A comparison of schizoaffective disorder, schizophrenia, and affective disorder. *American Journal of Psychiatry*, **137**, 921–927.

Price, T.R. & Levin, R. (1978) The effects of electroconvulsive therapy on tardive dyskinesia. *American Journal of Psychiatry*, **135**, 991–993.

Prudic, J., Sackeim, H.A. & Devanand, D.P. (1990) Medication resistance and clinical response to electroconvulsive therapy. *Psychiatry Research*, **31**, 287–296.

Rabins, P.V., Pearlson, G.D., Aylward, E., Kumar, A.J. & Dowell, K. (1991) Cortical magnetic resonance imaging changes in elderly inpatients with major depression. *American Journal of Psychiatry*, **148**, 617–620.

Rachlin, H.L., Goldman, G.S., Gurvitz, M., Lurie, A. & Rachlin, L. (1956) Follow-up study of 317 patients discharged from Hillside Hospital in 1950. *Journal of Hillside Hospital*, **5**, 17–40.

Rahman, R. (1968) A review of treatment of 176 schizophrenic patients in the mental hospital Pabna. *British Journal of Psychiatry*, **114**, 775–777.

Ray, S.D. (1962) Relative efficacy of ECT and CPZ in schizophrenia. *Journal of the Indian Medical Association*, **38**, 332–333.

Riddell, S.A. (1963) The therapeutic efficacy of ECT. *Archives of General Psychiatry*, **8**, 546–556.

Ries, R.K., Wilson, L., Bokan, J.A. & Chiles, J.A. (1981) ECT in medication resistant schizoaffective disorder. *Comprehensive Psychiatry*, **22**, 167–173.

Rohde, P. & Sargant, W. (1961) Treatment of schizophrenia in general hospitals. *British Medical Journal*, **ii**, 67–70.

Rosebush, P.I., Hildebrand, A.M. & Mazurek, M.F. (1992) The treatment of catatonia: benzodiazepines or ECT? (letter). *American Journal of Psychiatry*, **149**, 1279–1280.

Rosenbaum, A.H., O'Connor, M.K., Duane, D.D. & Auger, R.G. (1980) Treatment of tardive dyskinesia in an agitated, depressed patient. *Psychosomatics*, **21**, 765–766.

Ross, J.R. & Malzberg, B. (1939) A review of the results of the pharmacological shock therapy and the metrazol convulsive therapy in New York State. *American Journal of Psychiatry*, **96**, 297–316.

Royal College of Psychiatrists (1977) The Royal College of Psychiatrists' Memorandum on the use of electroconvulsive thearpy. Part 1. Effectiveness of ECT — a review of the evidence. *British Journal of Psychiatry*, **131**, 261–268.

Rummans, T.A. & Bassingthwaighte, E. (1991) Severe medical and neurologic complications associated with near-lethal catatonia treated with electroconvulsive therapy. *Convulsive Therapy*, **7**, 121–124.

Sackeim, H.A. (1988) Mechanisms of action of electroconvulsive therapy. In Hales, R.E. & Frances, J. (eds) *Annual Review of Psychiatry*, Vol. 7, pp. 436–457. American Psychiatric Association, Washington DC.

Sackeim, H.A. (1989) The efficacy of electroconvulsive therapy in treatment of major depressive disorder. In Fisher, S. & Greenberg, R.P. (eds) *The Limits of Biological Treatments for Psychological Distress: Comparisons with Psychotherapy and Placebo*, pp. 275–307. Erlbaum, Hillsdale.

Sackeim, H.A. (1992) The cognitive effects of electroconvulsive therapy. In Moos, W.H., Gamzu, E.R. & Thal, L.J. (eds) *Cognitive Disorders: Pathophysiology and Treatment*, pp. 183–228. Marcel Dekker, New York.

Sackeim, H.A. (1993) Use of electroconvulsive therapy in late-life depression. In Schneider, L.S., Reynolds, C.F. III, Liebowitz, B.D. & Friedhoff, A.J. (eds) *Diagnosis and Treatment of Depression in Late Life*, pp. 259–277. American Psychiatric Association, Washington DC.

Sackeim, H.A., Devanand, D.P. & Prudic, J. (1991) Stimulus intensity, seizure threshold, and seizure duration: impact on the efficacy and safety of electroconvulsive therapy. *Psychiatric Clinics of North America*, **14**, 803–843.

Sackeim, H.A., Decina, P., Kanzler, M., Kerr, B. & Malitz, S. (1987) Effects of electrode placement on the efficacy of titrated, low-dose ECT. *American Journal of Psychiatry*, **144**, 1449–1455.

Sackeim, H.A., Prudic, J., Devanand, D.P., Decina, P., Kerr, B. & Malitz, S. (1990) The impact of medication resistance and continuation pharmacotherapy on relapse following response to electroconvulsive therapy in major depression. *Journal of Clinical Psychopharmacology*, **10**, 96–104.

Sackeim, H.A., Prudic, J., Devanand, D.P. *et al.* (1993) Effects of stimulus intensity and electrode placement on the efficacy and cognitive effects of electroconvulsive therapy. *New England Journal of Medicine*, **328**, 839–846.

Safferman, A.Z. & Munne, R. (1992) Combining clozapine with ECT. *Convulsive Therapy*, **8**, 141–143.

Sajatovic, M. & Meltzer, H.Y. (1993) The effect of short-term electroconvulsive treatment plus neuroleptics in treatment-resistant schizophrenia and schizoaffective disorder. *Convulsive Therapy*, **9**, 167–175.

Salzman, C. (1980) The use of ECT in the treatment of schizophrenia. *American Journal of Psychiatry*, **137**, 1032–1041.

Schooler, N. (1991) Maintenance medication for schizophrenia: strategies for dose reduction. *Schizophrenia Bulletin*, **17**, 311–324.

Schooler, N. & Kane, J.M. (1982) Research diagnoses for tardive dyskinesia. *Archives of General Psychiatry*, **39**, 486–487.

Schwartz, M., Silver, H., Tal, I. & Sharf, B. (1993) Tardive dyskinesia in northern Israel: preliminary study. *European Neurology*, **33**, 264–266.

Scott, A.I., Douglas, R.H., Whitfield, A. & Kendell, R.E. (1990) Time course of cerebra; magnetic resonance changes after electroconvulsive therapy. *British Journal of Psychiatry*, **156**, 551–553.

Scovern, A.W. & Kilmann, P.R. (1980) Status of electroconvulsive therapy: review of the outcome literature. *Psychological Bulletin*, **87**, 260–303.

Sedivec, V. (1981) Psychoses endangering life. *Ceskoslovenska Psychiatrie*, **77**, 38–41.

Seidman, L.R. (1983) Schizophrenia and brain dysfunction: an integration of recent neurodiagnostic findings. *Psychological Bulletin*, **94**, 195–238.

Serra, G., Collu, M., D'Aquila, P.S., De, M.O.G. & Gessa, G.L. (1990) Possible role of dopamine D1 receptor in the behavioural supersensitivity to dopamine agonists induced by chronic treatment with antidepressants. *Brain Research*, **527**, 234–243.

Shibata, M., Aoba, A., Kitani, K. *et al.* (1989) Redistribution of haloperidol after electroshock: experimental evidence. *Life Sciences*, **44**, 749–753.

Shoor, M. & Adams, F.H. (1950) The intensive electric shock therapy of chronic disturbed psychotic patients. *American Journal of Psychiatry*, **107**, 279–282.

Shugar, G., Hoffman, B.F. & Johnston, J.D. (1984) Electroconvulsive therapy for schizophrenia in Ontario: a report on therapeutic polymorphism. *Comprehensive Psychiatry*, **25**, 509–520.

Shukla, G.D. (1981) Electroconvulsive therapy in a rural teaching general hospital in India. *British Journal of Psychiatry*, **139**, 569–571.

Siesjö, B.K., Ingvar, M. & Wieloch, T. (1986) Cellular and molecular events underlying epileptic brain damage. *Annals of the New York Academy of Sciences*, **462**, 207–223.

Small, J.G. (1985) Efficacy of electroconvulsive therapy in schizophrenia, mania, and other disorders. I. Schizophrenia. *Convulsive Therapy*, **1**, 263–270.

Small, J.G., Milstein, V., Klapper, M., Kellams, J.J. & Small, I.F. (1982) ECT combined with neuroleptics in the treatment of schizophrenia. *Psychopharmacology Bulletin*, **18**, 34–35.

Smith, K., Surphlis, W.R., Gynther, M.D. & Shimkunas, A.M. (1967) ECT-chlorpromazine and chlorpromazine compared in the treatment of schizophrenia. *Journal of Nervous and Mental Disease*, **144**, 284–290.

Smith, W.E. & Richman, A. (1984) Electroconvulsive therapy: a Canadian perspective. *Canadian Journal of Psychiatry*, **29**, 693–699.

Snaith, R.P. (1981) How much ECT does the depressed patient need? In Palmer, R.L. (ed.) *Electroconvulsive Therapy: An Appraisal*, pp. 61–64. Oxford University Press, New York.

Spitzer, R.L., Endicott, J. & Robins, E. (1978) Research diagnostic criteria: rationale and reliability. *Archives of General Psychiatry*, **35**, 773–782.

Staudt, V.M. & Zubin, J. (1957) A biometric evaluation of the somatotherapies in schizophrenia. *Psychological Bulletin*, **54**, 171–196.

Strömgren, L.S. (1988) Electroconvulsive therapy in Aarhus, Denmark, in 1984: its application in nondepressive disorders. *Convulsive Therapy*, **4**, 306–313.

Swayze, V.W., Andreasen, N.C., Alliger, R.J., Ehrhardt, J.C. & Yuh, W.T. (1990) Structural brain abnormalities in bipolar affective disorder. Ventricular enlargement and focal signal hyperintensities. *Archives of General Psychiatry*, **47**, 1054–1059.

Tancer, M.E., Golden, R.N., Ekstrom, R.D. & Evans, D.L. (1989) Use of electroconvulsive therapy at a university hospital: 1970 and 1980–81. *Hospital and Community Psychiatry*, **40**, 64–68.

Taylor, P.J. (1981) ECT in schizophrenia: a review. In Palmer, R.L. (ed.) *Electroconvulsive Therapy: An Appraisal*, pp. 37–54. Oxford University Press, New York.

Taylor, P.J. & Fleminger, J.J. (1980) ECT for schizophrenia. *Lancet*, **1**, 1380–1382.

Templer, D.I., Ruff, C.F. & Armstrong, G. (1973) Cognitive functioning and degree of psychosis in schizophrenics given many electroconvulsive treatments. *British Journal of Psychiatry*, **123**, 441–443.

Thompson, J.W. & Blaine, J.D. (1987) Use of ECT in the United States in 1975 and 1980. *American Journal of Psychiatry*, **144**, 557–562.

Thornton, J.E., Mulsant, B.H., Dealy, R. & Reynolds, I.I.C. (1990) A retrospective study of maintenance electroconvulsive therapy in a university-based psychiatric practice. *Convulsive Therapy*, **6**, 121–129.

Tolsma, F.J. (1967) The syndrome of acute pernicious psychosis. *Psychiatrie, Neurologie, und Neurochirurgie*, **70**, 1–21.

Tsuang, M.T., Woolson, R.F. & Fleming, J.A. (1979) Long-term outcome of major psychoses. 1. Schizophrenia and affective disorders compared with psychiatrically symptom-free surgical conditions. *Archives of General Psychiatry*, **36**, 1295–1301.

Turek, I.S. & Hanlon, T.E. (1977) The effectiveness and safety of electroconvulsive therapy (ECT). *Journal of Nervous and Mental Disease*, **164**, 419–431.

Uhrbrand, L. & Faurbye, A. (1960) Reversible and irreversible dyskinesia after treatment with perphenazine, chlorpromazine, reserpine, and ECT. *Psychopharmacologia*, **1**, 408–418.

Ulett, G.A., Smith, K. & Gleser, G. (1956) Evaluation of convulsive and subconvulsive shock therapies utilizing a control group. *American Journal of Psychiatry*, **112**, 795–802.

Ulett, G.A., Gleser, G.C., Caldwell, B.M. & Smith, K. (1954) The use of matched groups in the evaluation of convulsive and subconvulsive photoshock. *Bulletin of the Menninger Clinic*, **18**, 138–146.

Ungvári, G. & Pethö, B. (1982) High-dose haloperidol therapy: its effectiveness and a comparison with electroconvulsive therapy. *Journal of Psychiatric Treatment and Evaluation*, **4**, 279–283.

Van Valkenburg, C. & Clayton, P.J. (1985) Electroconvulsive therapy and schizophrenia. *Biological Psychiatry*, **20**, 699–700.

Verma, A. & Kulkarni, S.K. (1991) Chronic electroconvulsive shock alters hypothermic response of B-HT 920 and SKF 38393 in rats. *Journal of Pharmacy and Pharmacology*, **43**, 813–814.

Walinder, J. (1972) Recurrent familial psychosis of the schizo-affective type. *Acta Psychiatrica Sandinavica*, **48**, 274–283.

Watt, D.C., Katz, K. & Shepherd, M. (1983) The natural history of schizophrenia: a 5-year prospective follow-up of a representative sample of schizophrenics by means of a standardized clinical and social assessment. *Psychological Medicine*, **13**, 663–670.

Weinberger, D.R., Torrey, E.F., Neophytides, A.N. & Wyatt, R.J. (1979) *Lateral cerebral ventricular enlargement in chronic schizophrenia. Archives of General Psychiatry*, **36**, 735–739.

Weiner, R.D. (1984) Does ECT cause brain damage? *Behavioral and Brain Sciences*, **7**, 1–53.

Weiner, R.D., Rogers, H.J., Davidson, J.R. & Squire, L.R. (1986) Effects of stimulus parameters on cognitive side effects. *Annals of the New York Academy of Sciences*, **462**, 315–325.

Weinstein, M.R. & Fischer, A. (1971) Combined treatment with ECT and antipsychotic drugs in schizophrenia. *Diseases of the Nervous System*, **32**, 801–808.

Weiss, D.M. (1955) Changes in blood pressure with electroshock therapy in a patient receiving chlorpromazine hydrochloride (Thorazine). *American Journal of Psychiatry*, **111**, 617–619.

Weisz, S. & Creel, J.N. (1948) Maintenance treatment in schizophrenia. *Diseases of the Nervous System*, **9**, 10–14.

Wells, D.A. (1973) Electroconvulsive treatment for schizophrenia. A ten-year survey in a university hospital psychiatric department. *Comprehensive Psychiatry*, **14**, 291–298.

Wessels, W.H. (1972) A comparative study of the efficacy of bilateral and unilateral electroconvulsive therapy with thioridazine in acute schizophrenia. *South African Medical Journal*, **46**, 890–892.

WHO (1979) *Schizophrenia: An International Follow-up Study*. John Wiley & Sons, New York.

Wittman, P. (1941) A scale for measuring prognosis in schizophrenic patients. *Elgin Papers*, **4**, 20–33.

Witton, K. (1962) Efficacy of ECT following prolonged use of psychotropic drugs. *American Journal of Psychiatry*, **119**, 79.

Wolf, M.E. & Mosnaim, A.D. (1988) *Tardive Dyskinesia: Biological Mechanisms and Clinical Aspects*. American Psychiatric Press, Inc., Washington, D.C.

Wolff, G.E. (1955) Electric shock treatment. *American Journal of Psychiatry*, **111**, 748–750.

Wyatt, R.J. (1991) Neuroleptics and the natural course of schizophrenia. *Schizophrenia Bulletin*, **17**, 325–351.

Zeifert, M. (1941) Results obtained from the administration of 12 000 doses of metrazol to mental patients. *Psychiatric Quarterly*, **15**, 772–778.

Zis, A.P., Nomikos, G.G., Damsma, G. & Fibiger, H.C. (1991) *In vivo* neurochemical effects of electroconvulsive shock studied by microdialysis in the rat striatum. *Psychopharmacology*, **103**, 343–350.

Chapter 27
Neuroleptic-Induced Acute Extrapyramidal Syndromes and Tardive Dyskinesia

D. E. CASEY

Introduction

Neuroleptic (antipsychotic) drugs are the mainstay of treatment for both acute and chronic psychoses. Since they were labelled 'neuroleptic' in the 1950s to encompass the concept of 'taking control of the neurone', this terminology has remained (Deniker, 1984). Originally, it was believed that neuroleptic drugs had both their antipsychotic and extrapyramidal motor side effects develop at the same or very similar doses. Thus, this became identified as the neuroleptic threshold concept. This hypothesis was practically applied to indicate that when patients developed extrapyramidal syndromes (EPS), they were receiving an adequate antipsychotic dose. Eventually, the concept that antipsychotic and EPS effects were inextricably linked was gradually disproved. However, it is clear that most neuroleptic drugs have a very narrow therapeutic index, so that the majority of patients who do benefit from appropriate antipsychotic doses will also develop motor side effects.

Drug-induced disorders of motor function can develop along two separate general time courses. The acute EPS develop early in the course of treatment and may continue as long as neuroleptic drug therapy is prescribed. Tardive dyskinesia (TD) occurs much later during chronic neuro-

leptic therapy. Although TD is often considered to be the most serious side effect of neuroleptic drugs, the acute EPS are only considered as minor inconveniences to the patient. However, this perspective should be carefully reviewed because the majority (50–75%) of patients develop EPS and these may be an important cause of physical and mental impairment (Casey & Keepers, 1988). Additionally, patients will often discontinue their neuroleptic drugs because of the mental and physical discomfort associated with them. In contrast, TD occurs in a minority of patients (approximately 20%) and is usually of mild severity, often not noticed by the patient, and produces little or no disability or discomfort in most cases. However, the severe forms of TD, which fortunately occur only rarely, can produce substantial impairment (Gardos et al., 1987; Casey & Keepers, 1988).

This chapter reviews current knowledge about neuroleptic-induced acute EPS and TD. Information about clinical manifestations, pathophysiology, epidemiology, risk factors, outcome and treatment approaches will be reviewed. Strategies for combining patient, drug and temporal information will be used to develop clinical algorithms for maximizing the benefit and minimizing the short- and long-term detriments of these drugs.

Acute EPS

Since the initial use of neuroleptic drugs, the EPS of akathisia, dystonia and parkinsonism have been recognized. These disorders occur in most patients receiving neuroleptics and are often considered as different manifestations of the same disorder with the same underlying pathophysiology. However, since there are several important distinctions between these different syndromes, it is important to consider them as separate entities.

Clinical manifestations

Akathisia is a syndrome of subjective feelings of restlessness or distress that may be accompanied by objective signs of these feelings. Patients may describe akathisia as anxiety, loss of internal calmness, an inability to relax, feeling uptight or internal jitteriness. Objective signs of restlessness are pacing, rocking back and forth while sitting or standing, lifting the feet as if marching in place, crossing and uncrossing the legs when sitting or other repetitive, purposeless actions.

There is some debate whether patients who deny inner feelings of restlessness, yet show objective signs of restlessness, should be diagnosed as having akathisia. A strict adherence to the originally proposed definition requires that subjective discomfort be present, and that the presence of only objective signs without subjective restlessness should be called pseudoakathisia (Barnes & Braude, 1985). Yet it is not clear that this distinction has either practical or heuristic value. Many patients appear to have classic objective signs of pacing and appear to be uncomfortably restless but do not admit to these subjective experiences. For some patients, it may be that their psychosis prevents them from giving accurate reports.

Akathisia can often be misdiagnosed as psychotic agitation, which leads to a further increase in neuroleptic dose and greater aggravation of akathisia. The core problem in this issue may be that psychotic patients often have great difficulty communicating their feelings of restlessness and discomfort, and may describe their feelings with bizarre and delusional statements.

Acute dystonia is characterized by involuntary muscle spasms that produce briefly sustained or fixed abnormal postures. These can include bizarre positions of the limbs and trunk, oculogyric crises, tongue protrusion, trismus, torticollis and laryngeal−pharyngeal constriction. If these symptoms occur within the first few days of initiating or substantially increasing existing neuroleptic drug treatment, the patient should be given the benefit of the doubt and neuroleptic drug-induced dystonia should be the first item on the differential diagnosis. Because dystonia may often appear as isolated and fluctuating symptoms in the first few days, these unusual symptoms are often misdiagnosed as malingering, hysteria or seizures (Casey, 1991a).

Drug-induced and idiopathic parkinsonism are phenomenologically identical. The classic triad of tremor, rigidity and bradykinesia is present in both forms of the disorder. Tremor is a rhythmical to-and-fro motion that is usually worse at rest. Rigidity may be asymmetrical and is easily identified in the limbs as a ratchet-like or cog-wheel resistance during passive motion. Bradykinesia, also referred to as akinesia, is the reduction in spontaneous activity. Usually this is noticed as a mask-like facial expression, softening of the voice, decreased associated arm movements during walking and reduced ability to initiate movement. Neuroleptic drug-induced parkinsonism can be diagnosed when any one or more of the triad of symptoms is present. As in idiopathic parkinsonism, symptoms may be unilateral, symmetrical or asymmetrically bilateral.

It is critically important to attempt to distinguish bradykinesia from negative symptoms of psychosis, psychological withdrawal or depression. However, this is often very difficult to do and may not be fully achievable until neuroleptic drugs have been discontinued for several weeks or months.

The rabbit syndrome is an uncommon side effect characterized by perioral lip tremor (Villeneuve, 1972; Casey, 1992a). It can occur anytime during neuroleptic treatment and is most likely a variant of drug-induced parkinsonism because it has the characteristic tremor rate (3−6 Hz/cps) and responds to antiEPS drugs, as does parkinsonism.

Paradoxical TD is a seldom-reported, though probably under-recognized, disorder that symptomatically resembles TD, but it is pharmacologically similar to acute EPS. One clinical difference is that paradoxical TD often appears to have more stereotyped movements that look somewhat like, and possibly may be in part, akathisia. Paradoxical TD improves when neuroleptics are decreased or discontinued and usually responds well to antiEPS agents (Gerlach *et al.*, 1974; Casey & Denney, 1977; Casey, 1981, 1992b).

Pathophysiology

Acute EPS are widely believed to be due to the single pathophysiological mechanism of dopamine-receptor blockade in the basal ganglia. Because all commercially available neuroleptic drugs have in common the property of blocking dopamine D_2 receptors, it has been concluded that this receptor subtype mediates EPS. However, not all data are supportive of this. Animal models show that dopamine D_1-receptor antagonism can also produce dystonia and other acute EPS in monkeys (Gerlach *et al.*, 1988; Casey, 1992c). Although some neuroleptics, such as flupenthixol and clozapine, have both D_1 and D_2 antagonist properties, the absence of pure D_1 antagonists in the clinic makes it very difficult to attribute the relative contributions and interrelationships between D_1 and D_2 antagonism in neuroleptic-induced EPS. Clinically effective doses of clozapine produce receptor occupancy rates of 35–65% for the D_1 receptor and just slightly higher rates for the D_2 receptor, and patients do not have EPS. In contrast, other neuroleptics with D_2-receptor occupancy rates over 80% tend to produce EPS, whereas those drugs with D_2 occupancy rates under 80% tend to have fewer EPS (Farde *et al.*, 1989).

There are several problems with explaining all acute EPS on the basis of dopamine-receptor blockade in the basal ganglia. The major problem is the time discrepancy between drug action and symptom onset. Neuroleptics block receptors within minutes to hours, whereas acute EPS symptoms may not occur for several hours to many

days after administration (Keepers *et al.*, 1983; Casey & Keepers, 1988; Waddington, 1989; Nordström *et al.*, 1992).

Akathisia is the least well-understood EPS. There are no neuroanatomical correlates to this disorder, and typical antiEPS drug therapy is much less effective in akathisia than it is in other disorders (Casey & Keepers, 1988; Adler *et al.*, 1989). Beta-adrenergic blockers, such as propranolol, effectively treat akathisia in many, but not all, patients (Lipinski *et al.*, 1984); β-blockers that are lipophilic are more efficacious than hydrophilic agents (Adler *et al.*, 1989). The mechanism of this effect is very unclear, since neuroleptic drugs have no direct effect on β-adrenergic receptors. This implies that neuroleptic drugs induce compensatory or secondary processess that initiate akathisia.

Neuroleptic drug-induced dystonia has been hypothesized to be caused by either a hypo- or hyperdopaminergic state following the initiation of neuroleptic drug-induced blockade of dopamine receptors in the caudate, putamen and globus pallidus (Rupniak *et al.*, 1986). The observation of dystonia on the second day of treatment following a single neuroleptic dose has been difficult to interpret. On the one hand, it appears that dystonia is associated with decreasing neuroleptic blood levels several hours after peak levels have been achieved (Garver *et al.*, 1976). However, it is also possible that the data could be interpreted to account for a higher-than-baseline level of neuroleptic drug in the blood, which might produce dystonia. An additional difficulty with this model of investigation is that most patients do not get just a single dose of neuroleptic within the first 24–36 h of initiating treatment. Rather, they receive several doses within the first few days, often at 12- or 24-h intervals, so that dystonia is occurring sometime between the increasing blood levels following recent drug intake and the decreasing blood levels of the drug that is being metabolized throughout the subsequent 12–24 h. This complex situation indicates the importance of the possibility of a specific ratio between endogenous dopamine levels and the degree of receptor antagonism. The relative balance of receptor blockade induced by the neuroleptic and high levels of endogenous dopamine, which are released by the dopamine feedback system after receptors have been blocked, will be critically important to understanding the pathophysiology of dystonia. Finally, as in akathisia, other neurotransmitter mechanisms may also be involved.

Neuroleptic drug-induced parkinsonism purportedly develops from blockade of nigrostriatal dopamine systems. The delay of several days before symptom onset after neuroleptics are initiated is not compatible with the mechanism of acute receptor blockade that takes place within hours after neuroleptics are administered. One more important temporal factor to account for is the partial or complete tolerance of neuroleptic drug-induced parkinsonism that may evolve over several months, even though neuroleptic treatment remains stable. This gradual development of tolerance also indicates the importance of compensatory processes which are not well understood and may be secondary consequences to dopamine-receptor blockade (Casey, 1987, 1991b).

Epidemiology

Prevalence/incidence

EPS prevalence spans a wide range of 2−90% (Sovner & DiMascio, 1978; Casey & Keepers, 1988). Prevalence may approach 100% in highly vulnerable groups of patients (Ganzini *et al.*, 1991b). The EPS risk is strongly influenced by patient, drug and time characteristics. There has been a steady increase in the prevalence of acute EPS since neuroleptics were introduced. The most likely explanation for this observation is the greater utilization of high drug dosages with low-milligram, high-potency compounds. The incidence of dystonia was 2.3% in the late 1950s (Ayd, 1961) and gradually increased to approximately 40% in the 1980s (Keepers *et al.*, 1983). Special risk groups, such as young males receiving high doses of high-potency compounds, may develop acute dystonia in 90−100% of cases (Boyer *et al.*, 1989; Casey, 1992d).

Patient variables

Age, gender and history of EPS all influence whether a patient will develop EPS with drug treatment. Young males are the most vulnerable to acute dystonia, whereas drug-induced parkinsonism occurs more often in older patients, and akathisia is only slightly more common in middle-aged females (Ayd, 1961; Keepers *et al.*, 1983; Casey & Keepers, 1988). Age undoubtedly plays an important role in patient susceptibility to EPS. Adolescents and children are particularly vulnerable to acute dystonia, but this disorder seldom occurs in the elderly. Drugs which commonly cause dystonia in children, who present in emergency rooms when these drugs have been inadvertently taken, are the antiemetic compounds, such as prochlorperazine (Compazine), promethazine (Phenergan), metoclopramide (Reglan) or other drugs in this group, which function as dopamine-receptor antagonists. A patient's history of prior EPS is a strong predictor of vulnerability to future EPS, if a similar drug and dose are represcribed. The recurrence of these disorders can be reliably predicted with approximately 75−85% accuracy, if the EPS prior history is known (Keepers & Casey, 1987, 1991).

Drug characteristics

Correlating acute EPS with parameters of neuroleptic drug exposure is complex. The dose−response curve between drug dose and EPS is often an inverted u-shaped function. Therefore, lower doses produce fewer EPS than do moderate to high doses. However, very high doses or megadoses also produce fewer EPS than do moderate to high doses (Keepers *et al.*, 1983; Casey & Keepers, 1988).

The fact that neuroleptics affect multiple neurotransmitters also greatly influences EPS rates. The relative balance between blockade of dopamine, acetylcholine, serotonin, histamine, noradrenaline and other receptors is undoubtedly important. The most well-established and clinically relevant hypothesis is the reciprocal balance between dopamine- and acetylcholine-receptor blockade in the basal ganglia. The greater the ratio of dopamine:acetylcholine antagonism, the more likely a drug is to produce EPS (Snyder *et al.*, 1974), although other mechanisms of action have been proposed as mediators of acute EPS in drugs that do have the favourable dopamine: acetylcholine ratio (Sayers *et al.*, 1976). Low-milligram, high-potency compounds [e.g. halo-peridol (Haldol), fluphenazine (Prolixin)] have little anticholinergic activity and produce more EPS than high-milligram, low-potency com-pounds [e.g. chlorpromazine (Thorazine), thio-ridazine (Mellaril)], which have considerably more anticholinergic activity.

A recent and controversial hypothesis suggests that a favourable ratio between serotonin (5-hydroxytryptamine; 5-HT_2) and dopamine D_2-receptor antagonism will produce few or no EPS (Meltzer *et al.*, 1989). This proposal derives from a combination of behavioural studies and biochemical measures in rodents (Balsara *et al.*, 1979; Meltzer *et al.*, 1989). However, this has not been consistently shown in a series of studies with non-human primates (Korsgaard *et al.*, 1985; Povlsen *et al.*, 1986; Casey, 1989a, 1991c,d).

Rates of EPS should not be the sole determinant in deciding which neuroleptic to use. These syn-dromes can be managed quite well in most patients with antiEPS agents (Fig. 27.1). In addition, other side effects, such as hypotension, anticholinergic effects, photosensitivity and leucopoenia, must also be considered when selecting a neuroleptic. Clozapine (Clozaril), a compound used for treatment-resistant schizophrenia or neuroleptic-intolerant patients, has a very low EPS profile (Casey, 1989b) and is a high-milligram, low-potency, highly anticholinergic drug that causes agranulocytosis in approximately 1% of patients.

The relationship between neuroleptic levels and acute EPS is shown in most, but not all, studies. One study that did not find such a relationship failed to control for patient or time variables (Tune & Coyle, 1981). Other studies do find a significant positive correlation between blood levels and symptoms (Hansen *et al.*, 1981; Baldessarini *et al.*, 1988; Casey & Aaes-Jorgensen, 1988; Nordström *et al.*, 1993), and between recep-tor occupancy in positron emission studies and symptoms (Farde *et al.*, 1989; Nordström *et al.*, 1993).

Treatment

Treatment phase

Each EPS has a fairly characteristic temporal pattern. Akathisia may have its onset within a few hours to a few days of initiating neuroleptics. This best corresponds to the time course of brain−blood drug levels, as two studies have shown a correlation between peak D_2-receptor occupancy rates and akathisia (Farde, 1992; Nordström *et al.*, 1992). Acute dystonia, which has its onset within the first 96 h of beginning or rapidly increasing neuroleptic dosages, has not been con-sistently correlated with either blood levels or dopamine-receptor occupancy in the brain. Par-kinsonism may develop anywhere from a few days to a few weeks after initiating neurolepic treatment (Ayd, 1961). Since the acute EPS may spon-taneously decrease or resolve over several weeks or months of continuous neuroleptic treatment in many patients, extended antiEPS drug therapy may not be necessary for all those patients who required it within the first few weeks of initiating neuroleptic treatment.

Treatment strategies

The management of neuroleptic drug-induced EPS falls into three separate treatment strategies. These are: (i) initial prophylaxis; (ii) therapy for treatment-emergent symptoms; and (iii) extended prophylaxis. Initial prophylaxis with antiEPS drugs is controversial. Proponents argue that prophylaxis prevents dystonic episodes, which are potentially dangerous, and automatically treats subtle forms of bradykinesia or akathisia that may be unrecog-nized. Opponents argue that these drugs have their own side effects, such as autonomic nervous system dysfunction, memory impairment and the risk of delirium. Therefore, prophylaxis unnecess-arily exposes patients who would not develop acute EPS to these treatment side effects. Dogmatically applying either approach to all patients fails to achieve the maximum benefits. Instead, a well-thought-out treatment strategy that incorporates knowledge about risk factors is the most useful approach.

Treating neuroleptic-induced emergent acute EPS with antiEPS drugs is standard practice. All the anticholinergic and antihistaminic agents are more or less equally efficacious. Amantadine (Symmetrel), a prodopaminergic drug, is equally effective and has fewer anticholinergic side effects. This agent must be used with caution in patients with renal disease, as it is primarily cleared through the kidneys.

Extended prophylaxis (arbitrarily defined as continued use of antiEPS drugs for more than 3 months) is also controversial. This treatment approach can be initiated by either extending the initial prophylaxis or maintaining effective drug therapy for symptoms that were treatment emergent. This strategy requires periodic review, as many patients who develop EPS at initiation of drug treatment may eventually develop tolerance to EPS and will no longer need all or some of the antiEPS drug treatment.

Managing acute EPS

The algorithm (Fig. 27.1) identifies several choice points in managing acute EPS. After a neuroleptic has been prescribed, careful consideration of the issues related to initial prophylaxis should be considered. Obtaining a careful psychiatric and neurological evaluation prior to starting neuroleptic therapy is critically important because it serves as a reference point for the patient at this time, as well as providing documentation for potential changes that may occur later. Initial prophylaxis is justified when there is: (i) a high risk of EPS; (ii) documented predisposition to EPS; and (iii) anticipated detrimental consequences of EPS (Casey & Keepers, 1988). By considering patient characteristics (age, gender, EPS history), drug characteristics (dosage, milligram potency, intrinsic anticholinergic action) and temporal aspects, the estimated risk of developing acute EPS can be closely approximated.

Acute dystonic reactions can have important psychological consequences for future drug compliance. The paranoid patient who believes that external forces are controlling him/her may further solidify these beliefs when an acute dystonic reaction develops without warning and is beyond the patient's control.

Initial prophylaxis can be rationally employed for the first 7–10 days of neuroleptic treatment in high-risk patients. Then, the antiEPS drug may be gradually decreased and ultimately discontinued if no EPS develop. The efficacy for initial prophylaxis is well established. Several studies consistently show that antiEPS agents reduce the rates of acute dystonia and other EPS (Keepers *et al.*, 1983; Sramek *et al.*, 1986; Casey & Keepers, 1988; Boyer *et al.*, 1989). In contrast, where there is a low risk of EPS, initial prophylaxis should not be initiated in conjunction with neuroleptics because the risk of antiEPS drug side effects greatly outweighs their potential benefit.

Managing treatment-emergent EPS with antiEPS agents is well-established, standard care (Fig. 27.1). Dystonia is treated with parenteral anticholinergic [benztropine (Cogentin)] or antihistaminic [diphenhydramine (Benadryl)] agents. Within 15–45 min, most symptoms improve on the first or second drug administration. If there is no improvement after a third injection, a search for other possible causes of dystonia should be initiated.

There are several approaches for managing drug-induced parkinsonism and these follow a prioritized, step-by-step strategy. Reducing the neuroleptic dose is the preferred approach. However, for many patients experiencing a psychotic exacerbation, this approach is not practical. Therefore, adding an antiEPS agent is the next and logical alternative. Changing to a different neuroleptic with a different side-effect profile is another option, although this is usually not necessary and can delay treatment while attempting to establish equipotent doses of drugs.

Akathisia is the most difficult EPS to manage. That there are so many different drug approaches to akathisia indicates that none is truly effective for most patients. Like drug-induced parkinson-

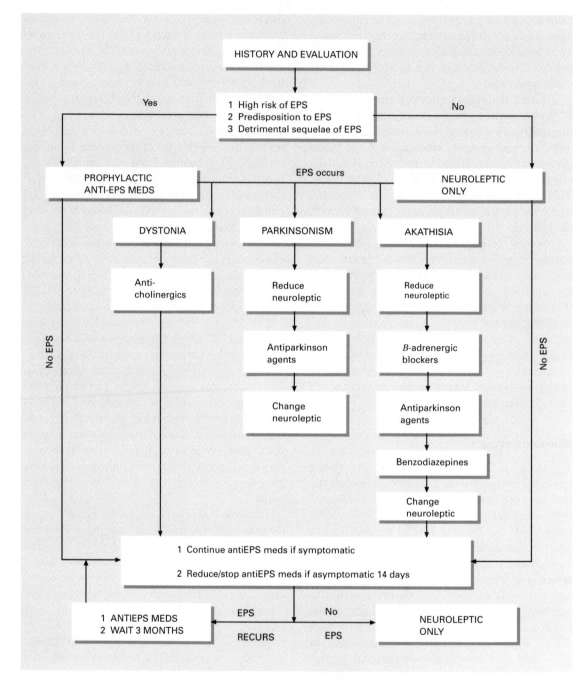

Fig. 27.1 An algorithm for managing acute extrapyramidal syndromes (EPS). (From Casey and Keepers, 1988.)

ism, the preferred strategy is to reduce the neuro-leptic dose. If this cannot be done on the basis of clinical grounds, β-adrenergic blockers which penetrate the blood−brain barrier, such as pro-pranolol (Inderal) 30−120 mg/day, are often effective (Lipinski *et al.*, 1984; Adler *et al.*, 1989). If this is not effective, one could consider using the standard anticholinergic or antihistaminic agents. Eventually, switching to benzodiazepines may be necessary and helpful for some patients. Caution is warranted in adopting this strategy since this class of drugs used on an extended basis raises the concern for potential problems of dependence and abuse. Finally, changing to a different neuroleptic always remains a choice. For patients who are not able to achieve an adequate antipsychotic dose because severe EPS limit their daily dosage, switching to clozapine (Clozaril) may be a practical alternative, although there are more limitations imposed upon the patient with this drug treatment.

Extending antiEPS treatment on an open-ended basis will be necessary for a substantial subgroup of patients. Unfortunately, many patients improve but do not have their symptoms completely resolve. Therefore, patients will need to continue both their neuroleptic and antiEPS drugs on an indefinite basis. However, if EPS are no longer present, drugs to control these symptoms should be reduced and discontinued. If EPS recur, then the antidote drug should be reinstituted. A review of extended prophylaxis studies published since 1980 found that 35−90% of patients benefited from this treatment strategy (Casey & Keepers, 1988).

Much of the debate about the appropriate indi-cations for antiEPS drugs would be much less relevant if neuroleptic drugs were prescribed in lower doses. Since there is no compelling evidence that high neuroleptic doses routinely produce more benefit than standard doses (Baldessarini *et al.*, 1988), a trend toward reduced neuroleptic dosage is encouraged. This would benefit the majority of patients, who would experience fewer acute EPS and would thus need fewer antiEPS drugs.

This algorithm for managing neuroleptic-induced EPS offers a balanced strategy to obtain the most benefit with the least risk. This approach encourages the practitioner to consider all the information available in making flexible decisions regarding treatment, rather than being locked into an inflexible all-or-none treatment approach. By considering all the information available, it is possible to predict with a reasonable degree of certainty who is likely to develop EPS and, thus, who may benefit from prophylaxis or from waiting until treatment-emergent symptoms develop.

TD

TD is characterized by involuntary hyperkinetic abnormal movements that occur in predisposed patients during or shortly after the termination of long-term neuroleptic drug treatment. The realistic concern about the potential irreversibility of TD has led to a careful reassessment about the appropriate indications for utilizing the highly efficacious neuroleptic drugs. The goal is to obtain the maximum benefits with the fewest risks. How-ever, even when all precautions have been taken, some patients will inevitably develop TD.

TD was initially described in 1957 in the German literature (Schönecker, 1957). Shortly thereafter, other cases were described in French literature (Sigwald *et al.*, 1959). A Danish group published the first English-language report in 1960 (Uhrbrand & Faurbye, 1960). In the ensuing years, several other reports substantiated these original observations. Before the term 'tardive dyskinesia' was proposed in 1964 (Faurbye *et al.*, 1964), descriptive terms such as 'bucco-linguo-masticatory syndrome' and 'terminal extrapyr-amidal insufficiency syndrome' appeared in the early literature.

Clinical manifestations

The most common forms of typical TD include repetitive, involuntary, hyperkinetic movements, such as chewing, tongue protrusion, vermicular tongue motion, lip smacking, puckering and pursing or paroxysms of rapid eye blinking. In addition, choreoathetoid movements in the limbs and trunk may occur. Abnormal stereotypic movements in the fingers may look as though the patient is playing an invisible piano or guitar. Although it is uncommon, TD may involve the respiratory system with irregular breathing or swallowing that causes aerophagia, irregular respiratory rates, belching and grunting noises (Casey, 1981).

Recent attention has focused on atypical forms of TD, though these have been described for many years in individual case reports. Tardive dystonia is a syndrome of sustained abnormal postures or positions. Symptoms include torticollis, retrocollis, anterocollis, blepharospasm, grimacing and torsion of the trunk or limbs. These symptoms may persist for months or years after neuroleptics have been discontinued (Burke *et al.*, 1982; Gardos *et al.*, 1987). If a patient has received neuroleptic drugs, it is a particularly vexing problem to decide whether abnormal dystonic symptoms are due to neuroleptics or idiopathic dystonia. Occasionally, patients present to physicians with mild symptoms of dystonia or other motor function, and they often receive neuroleptic drugs as potential treatments for these motor dysfunctions. When the histories of such patients are ambiguous as to when drug treatment began, it is very difficult to determine properly how much of the movement disorder should be attributed to drugs or to idiopathic causes. One helpful point in making this distinction is the natural course of the symptoms. When neuroleptics are discontinued, tardive dystonia should remain stable or gradually improve. In contrast, idiopathic dystonias will usually slowly progress in severity, as well as have new symptoms develop over months and years. Unfortunately, responses of tardive dystonia to pharmacological interventions do not help distinguish it from idiopathic dystonia because both syndromes do not respond well to any drug intervention. Some patients with either diagnosis may benefit from dopamine agonists, dopamine antagonists or cholinergic antagonists. At this time, it is not possible to identify in advance which patients, if any, will benefit from which medicines.

Tardive akathisia is a syndrome of persisting subjective and/or objective signs of restlessness

(Barnes & Braude, 1985). This disorder is symptomatically similar to acute akathisia but is differentiated by its persistence for months or years after neuroleptics have been discontinued. Both tardive dystonia and tardive akathisia may occur alone or in combination with the typical orofacial and choreoathetoid signs of TD. An additional complication is that any of these disorders may also occur in combination with neuroleptic-induced acute EPS if patients are concurrently receiving these drugs. It is not yet clear whether these different tardive syndromes represent unique and different pathophysiological mechanisms, or are better explained by a unitary underlying pathophysiology that is phenomenologically expressed in different symptom clusters in different patients.

TD and tardive dystonia also occur in children. In some patients there may be few or none of the typical hyperkinetic orofacial dyskinesias but, rather, patients may express a predominance of limb and truncal symptoms. However, in other patients, classic TD symptoms are similar to those typically found in adults (Campbell *et al.*, 1983; Gualtieri *et al.*, 1984).

Terminology

Carefully classifying TD incorporates temporal aspects of this disorder. Covert TD describes TD that is unmasked when neuroleptic drug therapy is reduced or discontinued. Withdrawal TD also appears when neuroleptics are reduced or discontinued but disappears spontaneously in 1–3 months. There is no uniformly agreed-upon definition of when TD should be characterized as irreversible. Twelve months has often been arbitrarily defined as the cut-off point for irreversible. However, there is no scientific basis for this arbitrary definition of irreversible. Such a characterization fails to account for symptom change, which occurs in many patients over several years. Rather, a more useful concept utilizes a time-course continuum to characterize TD along the dimension of persisting vs. resolving (Casey, 1987). Since the pathophysiology of TD is unknown, it is not yet possible to link the factors controlling outcome with the underlying physiological abnormality.

Research criteria also exist for TD (Schooler & Kane, 1982). These require at least 3 months of cumulative neuroleptic drug exposure, at least mild movements in two or more body areas or moderate symptoms in one body region for the diagnosis of presumed TD. Persisting TD requires that symptoms continue for 3 months or longer and that other conditions that might produce involuntary hyperkinetic dyskinesias have been ruled out. The abnormal involuntary movement scale (AIMS) is the most commonly used rating tool for assessing TD (Guy, 1976). It is useful to re-emphasize that rating scales have been developed to characterize the nature and severity of abnormal movements, and are not diagnostic instruments. A diagnosis requires a thorough evaluation of epidemiological, aetiological, phenomenological and temporal aspects of symptom development, and is undertaken in conjunction with a thorough medical and neuropsychiatric evaluation.

Differential diagnosis

There are many causes of abnormal movements. These include idiopathic syndromes, other drug-induced movement disorders, hereditary diseases and dyskinesias that are secondary to systemic illnesses.

Idiopathic syndromes

Long before the introduction of neuroleptic drugs, Kraepelin and Bleuler described spontaneous dyskinesias in psychotic patients (Kraepelin, 1907; Bleuler, 1950; Casey, 1985a). Both these astute observers described 'grimacing' and 'irregular movements of the tongue and lips'. Unfortunately, comparative epidemiological studies cannot be carried out with current findings because prevalence rates of these abnormalities were not recorded by Kraepelin and Bleuler at the turn of the 20th century.

Stereotypic behaviour (seemingly purposeless and meaningless actions) and mannerisms (peculiar ways of completing normal actions) are frequently associated with psychoses and must be part of a differential diagnosis of TD. Several spontaneous hyperkinetic dyskinesias have been variously identified in the literature as 'spontaneous orofacial dyskinesia', 'senile dyskinesia' and 'blepharospasm−oromandibular dystonia' (Smith & Baldessarini, 1980). These are all now generally classified as idiopathic focal dystonias. Both these dyskinesias and dystonias occur with increasing age and are also more commonly seen in patients with concomitant neuromedical conditions (Lieberman *et al.*, 1984). Tourette's syndrome, characterized by involuntary tics and vocalizations that begin before the age of 21, must also be considered. These can be differentiated by occurring early in life and by their waxing and waning course throughout a patient's lifetime. Simple tics or complex motor tics, as well as dental problems, must be carefully differentiated from TD (Casey, 1981).

Neuroleptic drug-induced acute EPS

Neuroleptic drug-induced EPS coexist with TD in approximately one-third of patients who have TD and continue neuroleptic therapy (Casey, 1981; Richardson & Craig, 1982). Therefore, some patients may have more than one neuroleptic drug-induced movement disorder at the same time, and these must be distinguished from each other. The acute EPS respond to antiEPS drugs, whereas TD usually remains unchanged or worsens with these agents. But some patients with tardive dystonia may improve with anticholinergic, antiEPS drugs (Burke *et al.*, 1982).

Other drug-induced dyskinesias

Several other drugs can produce symptoms similar to TD. There are a few compounds that, like neuroleptics, antagonize dopamine receptors but are not commonly known as neuroleptics, although they can produce TD with extended use. These include the dopamine antagonist antiemetics, prochlorperazine (Compazine), the dyspeptic drug metoclopramide (Reglan) and the antidepressant amoxapine (Asendin). Dopamine agonists, such as bromocriptine (Parlodel) and pergolide (Permax), and the dopamine precursor L-dopa/ carbidopa (Sinemet) can all produce hyperkinetic dyskinesias in patients with idiopathic parkinsonism. Chorea and stereotyped behaviour can be seen during both the acute phases of and withdrawal from amphetamine and other stimulant abuse. Chronic anticholinergic and antihistaminic use have only rarely been associated with TD-like abnormal movements. Anticonvulsant agents at therapeutic or higher levels can produce hyperkinetic dyskinesias similar to TD. Also, oral contraceptives and chloroquine-based antimalarial agents can produce chorea and hyperkinetic dyskinesias. Lithium carbonate and tricyclic antidepressants may aggravate existing TD, but there is not convincing evidence that these agents by themselves produce TD. However, they can produce rapid, fine, irregular tremors that may be superimposed on TD. This list identifies only some of the more commonly prescribed drugs that may be causes of hyperkinetic involuntary movements.

Hereditary and systemic illnesses

Huntington's disease is characterized by choreoathetosis and dementia that may be preceded or accompanied by psychotic symptoms. If patients have received neuroleptics before the onset of chorea, the differential diagnosis becomes more complicated. Then, one must rely on family history, progression of symptoms and development of dementia to help clarify the diagnosis. Wilson's disease (hepatolenticular degeneration), a disorder of copper metabolism, can be distinguished from TD on the basis of clinical signs, laboratory tests and family history. The disease of iron metabolism, Hallervorden–Spatz disease, usually has its onset during childhood and is predominated by symptoms of dystonia and bradykinesia.

Endocrinopathies of hyperthyroidism, hypoparathyroidism or severe hyperglycaemia have been infrequently associated with choreoathetosis. Chorea of pregnancy (chorea gravidarum) may be pathophysiologically linked to mechanisms in

common with oral contraceptive-induced chorea. Inflammatory or immune disorders, such as lupus erythematosus, Schönlein–Henoch purpura and Sydenham's chorea, can have dyskinesias as a component of the syndrome. Finally, inflammatory or space-occupying lesions of the central nervous system can produce dyskinesias that must be delineated from TD.

Pathophysiology

There are no consistently demonstrable abnormalities in the central nervous system to explain TD. Biochemical studies of cerebral spinal fluid or analyses of D_1 and D_2 receptors at postmortem consistently fail to show reliable abnormalities between patients with and without TD (Casey, 1987). Neuroimaging investigations with computerized tomography, positron emission tomography or magnetic resonance imaging also do not reliably identify lesions associated with TD. In spite of the lack of evidence in the human brain of the underlying pathophysiology of TD, the theory of dopamine-receptor hypersensitivity is widely used as an explanation of TD (Tarsy & Baldessarini, 1973; Baldessarini *et al.*, 1980). This hypothesis proposes that dopamine in the nigrostriatal pathways becomes functionally aberrant via unknown mechanisms that are related to increased numbers of dopamine receptors following prolonged dopamine-receptor blockade induced by neuroleptics. Though human postmortem studies do not support this hypothesis (Casey, 1987), the clinical pharmacological data do indicate a role for dopamine in TD. However, this role may be a secondary or tertiary modulatory rather than primary role. The suppressant effect of neuroleptics on TD or the aggravating effects of dopamine agonists on dyskinesias may be compatible with the modulatory role of dopamine on neurocircuitry that has its underlying primary pathophysiology in a separate neuroanatomical and biochemical system (Casey, 1987).

Animal models span a diverse approach to understanding TD. Increased behavioural responses to dopamine agonists after neuroleptic treatment of a single dose, a few doses, or treatment for several weeks or a year are seen in rodents (Klawans & Rubovits, 1972; Tarsy & Baldessarini, 1973; Christensen *et al.*, 1976; Clow *et al.*, 1979). These behaviours are uniformly reversible within a brief period of time . In addition, most, but not all, studies (Waddington *et al.*, 1983) correlate elevated D_2 receptor numbers with increased behavioural responses (Baldessarini *et al.*, 1980; Casey, 1984a, 1987). A common deficiency of these models in rodents is that they do not correspond to many of the important clinical characteristics of TD, such as symptom onset without acute agonist drug provocation, individual vulnerability, late onset and potential irreversibility. Other rodent models of TD include spontaneous vacuous chewing, central nervous system destruction with unilateral 6-hydroxydopamine lesions, and cortical ablations (Ungerstedt, 1971; Waddington *et al.*, 1983; Casey, 1987).

Non-human primate models in *Cebus* monkeys are a more proximate fit to TD because they conform to many of the clinical characteristics of this disorder, corresponding to factors of symptom similarity, individual vulnerability, causation from chronic neuroleptic treatment and a variable course that is reversible/irreversible (Casey, 1984a, 1985b, 1987, 1988a). Studies in *Cebus* monkeys are consistent with either the dopamine hypersensitivity hypothesis or the proposal that reduced gamma-aminobutyric acid (GABA) underlies TD (Gunne & Häggström, 1985; Nguyen *et al.*, 1989). Unfortunately, clinical trials with GABA agonists in patients with TD do not show consistent benefits (Jeste & Wyatt, 1982; Casey, 1987).

Noradrenergic dysfunction has also been offered as an explanation of TD. This hypothesis derives from observations of significantly greater dopamine β-hydroxylase activity in TD patients, as well as correlations between cerebrospinal fluid, norepinephrine and TD severity. Many of these theories are undoubtedly oversimplified and no one theory or set of data offers a parsimonious explanation to understanding the complex disorder of TD.

Epidemiology

There is a wide variation in the prevalence (number of existing cases) of TD, ranging from 0.5 to more than 70% (Baldessarini *et al.*, 1980; Kane & Smith, 1982; Kane *et al.*, 1984b, 1992; Casey, 1985a, 1987). This is surely due to a wide range of characteristics unique to each study, such as differences in the types of patients studied, criteria for diagnosis and year of investigation. Most studies note that TD occurs at a prevalence of 15–20%. High-risk groups such as the elderly, however, may have TD occur in up to 70% of those chronically treated with neuroleptic drugs (Casey, 1987; Toenniessen *et al.*, 1985; Saltz *et al.*, 1991). Spontaneous dyskinesias (dyskinesias that are clinically similar to TD but occur in patients who have never received neuroleptic treatment) occur at a prevalence of 1–5%. These occur at even lower rates in young, healthy individuals and are most common in older patients with coexisting neuromedical conditions (Lieberman *et al.*, 1984; Casey 1985a, 1987). The incidence (new cases per year) of TD is 3–5% (Barnes *et al.*, 1983; Kane *et al.*, 1984b; Casey & Gerlach, 1986).

Long-term outcome

Though the reversible outcome of TD has been noted since the earliest reports (Schönecker, 1957; Sigwald *et al.*, 1959; Uhrbrand & Faurbye, 1960), this more favourable scenario has been overshadowed by the cases of irreversible TD. Strictly adhering to the admonition of prohibiting neuroleptic drugs in patients with TD will lead to the inevitable and unacceptable consequence of insufficiently treated psychotic patients. The most rational and pragmatic approach is to prescribe neuroleptic drugs in the lowest possible dose to patients who benefit from them.

TD improvement rates vary widely across studies from 0 to 92% (Casey, 1985c, 1987, 1990; Casey & Gerlach, 1986). The multiple contributions of patient, drug and temporal factors undoubtedly influence this outcome range. Age is negatively correlated with TD improvement.

Younger patients are the most likely to improve, whereas elderly patients are the least likely to do so (Smith & Baldessarini, 1980; Casey, 1987; Kane *et al.*, 1992). Nevertheless, this does not exclude any patient from the possibility of symptom improvement or resolution.

Early diagnosis and treatment intervention are associated with a more favourable prognosis. Perhaps this is due to intervening when TD is early in its development course. However, for many patients, it is not possible to know when TD first developed because neuroleptic drugs have possibly been masking symptoms for an unknown period of time. Discontinuing neuroleptic drugs is positively correlated with a favourable outcome in most, but not all, studies (Quitkin *et al.*, 1977; Casey, 1985c, 1987; Casey & Gerlach, 1986; Kane *et al.*, 1986, 1992; Gardos *et al.*, 1987).

TD may also improve when neuroleptic drugs are continued, but symptom stabilization is also a common outcome. Only rarely do patients with TD continue to worsen when low to moderate doses of neuroleptics are continued. Duration of follow-up is also positively correlated with TD outcome. Since this disorder tends to be a chronic, long-term problem, the longer the follow-up, the more likely there is a chance to observe symptom change. Drug holidays of compulsory neuroleptic discontinuation are not recommended because there is no evidence that they are beneficial. There is some evidence that they might be harmful (Jeste *et al.*, 1979) and, most importantly, this strategy unnecessarily exposes patients to the high risk of psychotic relapse.

The outcome of TD raises important and puzzling questions about neuroleptic drugs. How can neuroleptic drugs cause TD, which then gradually decreases or resolves in many patients while they remain on neuroleptic treatment? In all likelihood, neuroleptics play only a part in the overall explanation of TD. Perhaps these drugs play a partial role in converting a covert vulnerability to develop movement disorders into clinically overt dyskinesias.

Risk factors

Age and sex

TD prevalence is positively correlated with increasing age. Approximately 5–10% of patients younger than 40 years develop TD, whereas elderly patients have prevalence rates of 50–70% for TD (Smith & Baldessarini, 1980; Casey, 1987; Kane *et al.*, 1992). Women have a greater risk of TD compared with men at a ratio of 1.7:1 in most, but not all, studies (Casey, 1987; Kane *et al.*, 1992).

Psychiatric diagnosis

Vulnerability to TD is influenced by psychiatric diagnosis. Relatively brief exposure to neuroleptic drugs may cause TD in patients with affective disorders, particularly depression (Casey, 1984b, 1988b; Kane *et al.*, 1984a; Davis *et al.*, 1976). By implication, patients with schizophrenia may be relatively less vulnerable to TD (Casey, 1988b). If these observations are correct, they imply that different psychiatric diagnoses instil different TD vulnerabilities, which may give important clues to the underlying pathophysiology of TD.

Patients without psychotic diagnoses are also at risk for TD if they receive extended neuroleptic treatment. Some drugs are dopamine-receptor antagonists but are not marketed as neuroleptics. These include the antiemetic prochlorperazine (Compazine), the dyspeptic agent metoclopramide (Reglan) and the antidepressant amoxapine (Asendin).

Diabetes mellitus

Diabetes mellitus (DM) is also a risk factor for TD (Ganzini *et al.*, 1991a, 1992). Both psychotic and non-psychotic patients receiving long-term neuroleptics have greater prevalence and more severe TD if they have DM. This is particularly important for elderly patients, as the risk of both TD and DM increases with age.

Neuroleptic dose and duration of treatment

The degree of exposure to neuroleptic drugs is directly associated with TD risk. The greater the total drug intake, the greater the likelihood of developing TD (Kane *et al.*, 1984b). However, studies have not yet addressed the complex issue of teasing apart the relative risks of concomitantly increasing age and total drug exposure, since these two parameters often increase concomitantly in patients with chronic illness. There are not consistent data to show a relationship between neuroleptic blood level and the onset of TD (Fairbairn *et al.*, 1983; Jeste *et al.*, 1986).

Neuroleptic drug type

An analysis of the clinical literature indicates that any one of the traditional neuroleptic drugs is more or less likely to cause TD. Similarly, there is no convincing evidence that the depot neuroleptics carry a different TD risk. Overall, it is not possible to implicate one drug or one drug class as having greater liability to cause TD. However, it does appear that clozapine has a considerably lower risk of producing TD, similar to its low acute EPS profile (Casey, 1989b).

The mechanism of action of clozapine, the only clearly atypical neuroleptic drug, is unknown, although several hypotheses have been proposed. It has weak antagonist action at both the dopamine D_1 and D_2 receptors, and has more potent antagonist activity at serotonergic, cholinergic, histaminic and adrenergic receptors. The effect of clozapine on TD is quite variable. Typical orofacial TD is less suppressed by clozapine than traditional neuroleptics. However, there is a modest dose-related TD suppression (Casey, 1989b). Many patients with tardive dystonia have substantial benefit with clozapine (Lieberman *et al.*, 1989).

AntiEPS drugs

The effect of anticholinergic or antihistaminic drugs in producing TD is controversial. There are data both for and against this hypothesis (Kane & Smith, 1982; Casey, 1987; Kane *et al.*, 1992). These drugs will often temporarily aggravate existing TD, but TD symptoms return to baseline when these drugs are discontinued. Anticholinergic drugs may appear to be associated with TD because anticholinergic drugs are associated with acute EPS. If acute EPS are the actual link to TD, then any treatment for acute EPS, such as antiEPS drugs, will also show a correlation with TD.

Organic brain factors

Early reports suggested a correlation between TD vulnerability and organic brain disease, but later reviews have questioned this (Casey, 1987; Kane *et al.*, 1992). There are also conflicting findings about the relationship between abnormalities found on computerized tomography and TD risk (Famuyiwa *et al.*, 1979; Hoffman & Casey, 1991). These studies have such methodological differences, often lack age-matched controls and may involve patients with masked TD, so that it is very difficult to compare and contrast findings across studies.

Treatment

There are no uniformly safe and effective treatments for TD. The long list of potential treatments for this disorder attests to the general ineffectiveness of any one of these agents (Jeste & Wyatt, 1982; Casey, 1987; Kane *et al.*, 1992).

Multiple assessments over an extended period are necessary to obtain an accurate picture of TD. Masking and unmasking effects of changes in drug treatment, as well as daily fluctuations in symptoms, make it necessary to have a long-term perspective. TD may appear to increase when neuroleptic dosages are decreased, when in fact the dosage reduction is probably just unmasking existing stable symptoms. Adding anticholinergic antiEPS drugs to the treatment regimen may also unmask covert TD. Conversely, TD may decrease when neuroleptics are increased or antiEPS drugs are discontinued.

In certain clinical situations, it may be necessary

to consider a specific drug therapy for moderate to severe TD. The literature is replete with small studies or brief case reports indicating that one or two patients did quite well with a particular drug, whereas the majority of patients may have little or no benefit. Unfortunately, it is not possible to know in advance which patients will benefit from which treatment. Therefore, it may be necessary to have a systematic approach of trying different drug therapies to control TD symptoms. Several different treatment approaches are listed below.

Dopamine

Suppressing or masking TD is best achieved by reducing dopaminergic activity. However, this strategy is justified only in those uncommon cases where TD is severe, debilitating or life-threatening (Casey & Rabins, 1978). Most cases of TD are not so severe that treatment with dopamine suppressants is justified solely on the basis of TD. However, many patients also have coexisting psychoses which will justify continuing neuroleptic therapy. Two strategies for reducing dopaminergic activity include presynaptic depletion with reserpine or by false neurotransmission with methyldopa (Aldomet), but these have yielded only variably beneficial results (Jeste & Wyatt, 1982; Kane *et al.*, 1992). Tetrabenazine, a compound which is still experimental in the USA, has both presynaptic depleting and postsynaptic dopamine-receptor blockade activity that has had some success in decreasing TD (Jankovic & Ford, 1983; Burke & Kang, 1988). Although these drugs have not been convincingly associated with causing TD, it should be kept in mind that compounds that decrease dopamine function should be used cautiously because of the theoretical concern that this approach, like neuroleptics, may reproduce the same biochemical pathophysiology as dopamine-receptor blockade. Also, these drugs have their own potentially troublesome side effects, and little is known about the consequences of extended high-dose use.

The theory of resetting dopaminergic hypersensitivity back to normal sensitivity with dopamine agonists has not been clinically useful.

Agents such as bromocriptine (Parlodel) and pergolide (Permax) or dopamine precursors, such as L-dopa/carbidopa (Sinemet), have not yielded consistently beneficial results (Jeste & Wyatt, 1982; Kane *et al.*, 1992).

Acetylcholine

TD is usually temporarily aggravated by anticholinergic agents; however, it may be beneficial in high doses in some patients with tardive dystonia. Clozapine has also been useful in tardive dystonia and may have benefits because of its highly anticholinergic properties. Loading the cholinergic system through precursor dietary supplements is an attractive but unsuccessful approach. Both choline and lecithin showed some initial promise, but later controlled trials were disappointing (Jeste & Wyatt, 1982; Casey, 1987; Kane *et al.*, 1992). Results with physostigmine, an acetylcholinesterase inhibitor, have been inconsistent, and the lack of an oral form of this drug makes it impractical.

Free-radical reduction

One hypothesis proposes that TD is due to structural damage from free-radical formation of catecholamine metabolism in the brain. Clinical studies with α-tocopherol (vitamin E) have yielded inconsistent results. An initial study showed some benefit (Lohr *et al.*, 1987), but other studies have found variable or no benefit (Elkashef *et al.*, 1990; Egan *et al.*, 1992; Shriqui *et al.*, 1992).

Other drugs

TD has been treated with many other drugs. Although GABA hypofunction has been proposed as part of the pathophysiology underlying TD, treatment with GABA agents has produced inconsistent results. Benzodiazepines help some patients, although it is unclear whether this is a specific or a non-specific sedative effect. Long-term use of benzodiazepines carries the potential of dependence or abuse.

Other drugs with highly variable results include the serotonergic agents tryptophan or cyproheptadine (Periactin), lithium carbonate, the β-adrenergic blocker propranolol (Inderal) and the α-adrenergic agonist clonidine (Catapres). Also, studies with neuropeptides, such as *met*-enkephalin, destyrosine-γ-endorphin and vasopressin, as well as approaches through the opiate mechanisms with morphine and naloxone (Narcan), have all been ineffective. Compounds such as oestrogen, pyridoxine, fusaric acid, manganese, phenytoin, ergoloid mesylates, papaverine and others have produced only sporadic benefit (Jeste & Wyatt, 1982; Casey, 1987; Kane *et al.*, 1992).

Managing TD

The clinical strategy for managing TD is pre-sented in the algorithm shown in Fig. 27.2 (Casey & Gerlach, 1984; Casey, 1990). The primary goal is to provide appropriate neuroleptic drug treatment for those who benefit from it and at the same time minimize the TD risk. This strategy is for patients both with and without TD.

It is important to be vigilant for the early signs of TD. Maintaining a high index of suspicion for TD will lead to early diagnosis and appropriate intervention. Informed consent is also an important aspect of neuroleptic drug use. Periodic discussions with patients and/or a concerned family member or friend should include the risks and benefits of treatment, alternative treatments and no treatment. These discussions should occur when patients can understand the information and should recur periodically throughout long-

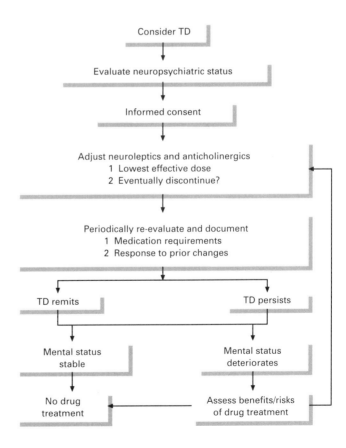

Fig. 27.2 An algorithm for managing tardive dyskinesia (TD). (From Casey, 1990.)

term therapy. Successful informed consent is more of a process than the ritualized signing of a form as a one-time event.

The American Psychiatric Association Task Force on TD advocates using neuroleptic drugs in the lowest effective dose for those patients who benefit from this treatment (Kane *et al.*, 1992). The primary indications for neuroleptics are acute and chronic schizophrenia and other psychoses, as well as some uncommon neurological disorders, such as Tourette's syndrome and Huntington's disease. Secondary indications include the treatment of acute mania, psychotic depression or unstable manic-depressive illness. Neuroleptics are not indicated for neuroses, personality disorders, insomnia or other non-psychotic conditions, although special circumstances may require considering these compounds.

Prescribing neuroleptics is not a one-time decision. Regularly reviewing the benefits as well as the risks of neuroleptic and antiEPS drugs is an important aspect of managing psychoses. Although a few patients may be able to discontinue these drugs, patients with remitting and relapsing psychoses need to continue their drugs for symptom control. Documenting these re-evaluations and discussions with patients is a valuable part of extended care.

TD will either persist or remit. The mental status may remain stable or deteriorate with an exacerbation of psychosis. If such a relapse occurs, it will once again be necessary to re-evaluate the risks and benefits of treatment with neuroleptics, and adjust the neuroleptic dose if indicated.

Acute EPS and TD are major limitations to neuroleptic drugs. Each of these disorders has its own characteristic risk profile of patient, drug and temporal considerations. These motor side effects have been a major impetus to the search for drugs that are antipsychotic but free of these side effects. Strategies and algorithms for managing acute EPS and TD are presented. These will maximize the benefits and minimize the risks of the current neuroleptic drugs until new agents are discovered.

Acknowledgements

This work was supported in part by funds from the Veterans Administration Research Program and by NIMH Grant no. 36657. Sherry Rueger prepared the typescript.

References

Adler, L.A., Angrist, B., Reiter, S. & Rotrosen, J. (1989) Neuroleptic-induced akathisia: a review. *Psychopharmacology*, **97**, 1–11.

Ayd, F.J. (1961) A survey of drug-induced extrapyramidal reactions. *Journal of the American Medical Association*, **175**, 1054–1060.

Baldessarini, R.J., Cohen, B.M. & Teicher, M.H. (1988) Significance of neuroleptic dose and plasma level in pharmacological treatment of psychosis. *Archives of General Psychiatry*, **45**, 79–91.

Baldessarini, R.J., Cole, J.O., Davis, J.M. *et al.* (1980) *Tardive Dyskinesia: A Task Force Report*. American Psychiatric Press, Washington DC.

Balsara, J.J., Jadhav, J.H. & Chandorkar, A.G. (1979) Effect of drugs influencing the central serotonergic mechanisms on haloperidol-induced catalepsy. *Psychopharmacology*, **62**, 67–69.

Barnes, T.R.E. & Braude, W.M. (1985) Akathisia variants and tardive dyskinesia. *Archives of General Psychiatry*, **42**, 874–878.

Barnes, T.R.E., Kidger, T. & Gore, S.M. (1983) Tardive dyskinesia: a 3-year follow-up study. *Psychological Medicine*, **13**, 71–81.

Bleuler, E. (1950) *Dementia Praecox or the Group of Schizophrenias*. International Universities Press, New York.

Boyer, W.F., Bakalar, N.H. & Lake, C.R. (1989) Anticholinergic prophylaxis of acute haloperidol-induced dystonic reactions. *Journal of Clinical Psychopharmacology*, **7**, 164–166.

Burke, R.E. & Kang, U.J. (1988) Tardive dystonia: clinical aspects and treatment. In Jankovic, J. & Tolosa, E. (eds) *Advances in Neurology*, Vol. 49, *Facial Dyskinesias*, pp. 199–210. Raven Press, New York.

Burke, R.E., Fahn, S., Jankovic, J. *et al.* (1982) Tardive dystonia: late-onset and persistent dystonia caused by antipsychotic drugs. *Neurology*, **32**, 1335–1346.

Campbell, M., Grega, D.M. & Green, W.H. (1983) Neuroleptic-induced dyskinesias in children. *Clinical Neuropharmacology*, **6**, 207–222.

Casey, D.E. (1981) The differential diagnosis of tardive dyskinesia. *Acta Psychiatrica Scandinavica*, **63**(Suppl. 291), 71–87.

Casey, D.E. (1984a) Tardive dyskinesia — animal models. *Psychopharmacology Bulletin*, **20**, 376–379.

Casey, D.E. (1984b) Tardive dyskinesia and affective disorders. In Gardos, G. & Casey, D.E. (eds) *Tardive Dyskinesia and Affective Disorders*, pp. 1–20. American Psychiatric Press, Washington DC.

Casey, D.E. (1985a) Spontaneous and tardive dyskinesias: clinical and laboratory studies. *Journal of Clinical Psychiatry*, **46**, 42–47.

Casey, D.E. (1985b) Behavioral effects of long-term neuroleptic treatment in cebus monkeys. In Casey, D.E., Chase, T., Christensen, A.V. & Gerlach, J. (eds) *Dyskinesia: Research and Treatment*, pp. 211–216. Springer-Verlag, Berlin.

Casey, D.E. (1985c) Tardive dyskinesia: reversible and irreversible. In Casey, D.E., Chase, T., Christensen, A.V. & Gerlach, J. (eds) *Dyskinesia: Research and Treatment*, pp. 88–97. Springer-Verlag, Berlin.

Casey, D.E. (1987) Tardive dyskinesia. In Meltzer, H. (ed.) *Psychopharmacology: The Third Generation of Progress*, pp. 1411–1419. Raven Press, New York.

Casey, D.E. (1988a) Dopamine D1 and D2 agonists and antagonists in cebus monkeys (abstract). *Proceedings of the Society of Biological Psychiatry*, 13.

Casey, D.E. (1988b) Affective disorders and tardive dyskinesia. *Encephale*, **14**, 221–226.

Casey, D.E. (1989a) Serotonergic aspects of acute extrapyramidal syndromes in nonhuman primates. *Psychopharmacology Bulletin*, **25**, 457–459.

Casey, D.E. (1989b) Clozapine: neuroleptic-induced EPS and tardive dyskinesia. *Psychopharmacology*, **99**, S47–S53.

Casey, D.E. (1990) Tardive dyskinesia. *Western Journal of Medicine*, **153**, 535–541.

Casey, D.E. (1991a) Neuroleptic-induced acute dystonia. In Lang, A.E. & Weiner, W.J. (eds) *Drug-Induced Movement Disorders*. Futura Press, New York.

Casey, D.E. (1991b) Neuroleptic drug-induced extrapyramidal syndromes and tardive dyskinesia. *Schizophrenia Research*, **4**, 109–120.

Casey, D.E. (1991c) Extrapyramidal syndromes in nonhuman primates: typical and atypical neuroleptics. *Psychopharmacology Bulletin*, **27**, 47–50.

Casey, D.E. (1991d) Serotonin and dopamine relationships in nonhuman primate extrapyramidal syndromes. *Journal of the European College of Neuropsychopharmacology*, S15–3, 351–353.

Casey, D.E. (1992a) The rabbit syndrome. In Joseph, A.B. & Young, R. (eds) *Disorders of Movement in Psychiatry and Neurology*, pp. 139–142. Blackwell Scientific Publications, Oxford.

Casey, D.E. (1992b) Paradoxical tardive dyskinesia. In Joseph, A.B. & Young, R. (eds) *Disorders of Movement in Psychiatry and Neurology*, pp. 67–69. Blackwell Scientific Publications, Oxford.

Casey, D.E. (1992c) Dopamine D1 (SCH 23390) and D2 (haloperidol) antagonists in drug-naive monkeys. *Psychopharmacology*, **107**, 18–22.

Casey, D.E. (1992d) Acute neuroleptic-induced dystonia. In Joseph, A.B. & Young, R. (eds) *Disorders of Movement in Psychiatry and Neurology*, pp. 106–110. Blackwell Scientific Publications, Oxford.

Casey, D.E. & Aaes-Jorgensen, T. (1988) Relationships between neuroleptic drug dose, blood level, and extrapyramidal symptoms in cebus monkeys (abstract). *Proceedings of the Society of Biological Psychiatry*, **250**.

Casey, D.E. & Denney, D. (1977) Pharmacological characterization of tardive dyskinesia. *Psychopharmacology*, **54**, 1–8.

Casey, D.E. & Gerlach, J. (1984) Tardive dyskinesia. In Stancer, H.C., Garkifinkel, P.E. & Rakoff, V.M. (eds) *Guidelines for the Use of Psychotropic Drugs: A Clinical Handbook*, pp. 183–203. Spectrum, Jamaica.

Casey, D.E. & Gerlach, J. (1986) Tardive dyskinesia: what is the long-term outcome? In Casey, D.E. & Gardos, G. (eds) *Tardive Dyskinesia and Neuroleptics: From Dogma to Reason*, pp. 76–97. American Psychiatric Press, Washington DC.

Casey, D.E. & Keepers, G.A. (1988) Neuroleptic side effects: acute extrapyramidal syndromes and tardive dyskinesia. In Casey, D.E. & Christensen, A.V. (eds) *Psychopharmacology: Current Trends*, pp. 74–93. Springer-Verlag, Berlin.

Casey, D.E. & Rabins, P. (1978) Tardive dyskinesia as a life-threatening illness. *American Journal of Psychiatry*, **135**, 969–971.

Christensen, A.V., Fjalland, B. & Moller Nielsen, I. (1976) On the supersensitivity of dopamine receptors induced by neuroleptics. *Psychopharmacology*, **48**, 1–6.

Clow, A., Jenner, P. & Marsden, C.D. (1979) Changes in dopamine-mediated behaviour during one year's neuroleptic administration. *European Journal of Pharmacology*, **57**, 365–375.

Davis, K.L., Berger, P.A. & Hollister, L.E. (1976) Tardive dyskinesia and depressive illness. *Psychopharmacology Communications*, **2**, 125–130.

Deniker, P. (1984) Introduction of neuroleptic chemotherapy into psychiatry. In Ayd, F.J. & Blackwell, B. (eds) *Discoveries in Biological Psychiatry*, pp. 155–164. Ayd Medical Communications, Baltimore.

Egan, M.F., Hyde, T.M., Albers, G.W. *et al.* (1992) Treatment of tardive dyskinesia with vitamin E. *American Journal of Psychiatry*, **149**, 773–777.

Elkashef, A.M., Ruskin, P.E., Bacher, N. & Barrett, D. (1990) Vitamin E in the treatment of tardive dyskinesia. *American Journal of Psychiatry*, **147**, 505–506.

Fairbairn, A.F., Rowell, F.J., Hui, S.M., Hassanych, F., Robinson, A.J. & Eccleston, D. (1983) Serum concentration of depot neuroleptics in tardive dyskinesia. *British Journal of Psychiatry*, **142**, 579–583.

Famuyiwa, O.O., Eccleston, D., Donaldson, A.A. & Garside, R.F. (1979) Tardive dyskinesia and dementia. *British Journal of Psychiatry*, **135**, 500–504.

Farde, L. (1992) Selective D1 or D2 dopamine receptor blockade induces akathisia in humans — a PET study with [^{11}C] SCH 23390 and [^{11}C] raclopride. *Psychopharmacology*, **107**, 23–29.

Farde, L., Wiesel, F.A., Nordström, A.L. & Sedvall, G. (1989) D1- and D2-dopamine receptor occupancy during treatment with conventional and atypical neuroleptics. *Psychopharmacology*, **99**, S28–S31.

Faurbye, A., Rasch, P.J., Bender Peterson, P., Brandenborg, G. & Pakkenberg, H. (1964) Neurological symptoms in the pharmacotherapy of psychoses. *Acta Psychiatrica Scandinavica*, **40**, 10–26.

Ganzini, L., Casey, D.E., Hoffman, W.F. & Heintz, R.T. (1992) Tardive dyskinesia and diabetes mellitus. *Psychopharmacology Bulletin*, **28**(3), 281–286.

Ganzini, L., Heintz, R., Hoffman, W. & Casey, D.E. (1991a)

Prevalence of tardive dyskinesia in neuroleptic-treated diabetics. *Archives of General Psychiatry*, **48**, 259–263.

Ganzini, L., Heintz, R., Hoffman, W.F., Keepers, G.A. & Casey, D.E. (1991b) Acute extrapyramidal syndromes in neuroleptic-treated elders: a pilot study. *Journal of Geriatric Psychiatry and Neurology*, **4**, 222–225.

Gardos, G., Cole, J.O., Salomon, M. & Schniebolk, S. (1987) Clinical forms of severe tardive dyskinesia. *American Journal of Psychiatry*, **144**, 895–902.

Garver, D.L., Davis, J.M., Dekirmenjian, H., Ericksen, S., Gosengeld, L. & Haraszti, J. (1976) Dystonic reactions following neuroleptics: time course and proposed mechanisms. *Psychopharmacology*, **47**, 199–201.

Gerlach, J., Reisby, N. & Randrup, A. (1974) Dopaminergic hypersensitivity and cholinergic hypofunction in the pathophysiology of tardive dyskinesia. *Psychopharmacology*, **34**, 21–35.

Gerlach, J., Casey, D.E., Kistrup, K. & Lublin, H. (1988) Dopamine D-1 and D-2 receptor functions in acute extrapyramidal syndromes and tardive dyskinesia. In Belmaker, R.H., Sandler, M. & Dahlstrom, A. (eds) *Neurology and Neurobiology*, Vol. 42C, *Progress in Catecholamine Research, Part C, Clinical Aspects*, pp. 1–4. Alan Liss, New York.

Gualtieri, C.T., Quade, D., Hicks, R.E., Mayo, J.P. & Schroeder, S.R. (1984) Tardive dyskinesia and other clinical consequences of neuroleptic treatment in children and adults. *American Journal of Psychiatry*, **141**, 20–23.

Gunne, L.M. & Häggström, J.E. (1985) Pathophysiology of tardive dyskinesia. In Casey, D.E., Chase, T., Christensen, A.V. & Gerlach, J. (eds) *Dyskinesia: Research and Treatment*, pp. 191–193. Springer-Verlag, Berlin.

Guy, W. (1976) *ECDEU Assessment Manual for Psychopharmacology* (revised 1976), pp. 534–537. United States Government Printing Office, Washington DC.

Hansen, L.B., Larsen, N.E. & Vestergard, P. (1981) Plasma levels of perphenazine (Trilafon) related to development of extrapyramidal side effects. *Psychopharmacology*, **74**, 306–309.

Hoffman, W.F. & Casey, D.E. (1991) Computed tomographic evaluation of patients with tardive dyskinesia. *Schizophrenia Research*, **5**, 1–12.

Jankovic, J. & Ford, J. (1983) Blepharospasm and orofacial-cervical dystonia: clinical and pharmacologic findings in 100 patients. *Annals of Neurology*, **13**, 402–411.

Jeste, D.V. & Wyatt, R.J. (1982) Therapeutic strategies against tardive dyskinesia. *Archives of General Psychiatry*, **39**, 803–816.

Jeste, D.V., Lohr, J.B., Kaufmann, C.A. & Wyatt, R.J. (1986) Pathophysiology of tardive dyskinesia: evaluation of supersensitivity theory and alternative hypotheses. In Casey, D.E. & Gardos, G. (eds) *Tardive Dyskinesia and Neuroleptics: From Dogma to Reason*, pp. 15–32. American Psychiatric Press, Washington DC.

Jeste, D.V., Potkin, S.G., Sinha, S., Feder, S. & Wyatt, R.J. (1979) Tardive dyskinesia — reversible and irreversible. *Archives of General Psychiatry*, **36**, 585–590.

Kane, J.M. & Smith, J.M. (1982) Tardive dyskinesia: prevalence and risk factors, 1959 to 1979. *Archives of General Psychiatry*, **39**, 473–481.

Kane, J.M., Woerner, M., Sarantakos, S., Kinon, B. & Lieberman, J. (1986) Do low-dose neuroleptics prevent or ameliorate tardive dyskinesia? In Casey, D.E. & Gardos, G. (eds) *Tardive Dyskinesia and Neuroleptics: From Dogma to Reason*, pp. 99–108. American Psychiatric Press, Washington DC.

Kane, J.M., Woerner, M., Weinhold, P., Kinon, B., Lieberman, J. & Borenstein, M. (1984a) Incidence and severity of tardive dyskinesia in affective illness. In Gardos, G. & Casey, D.E. (eds) *Tardive Dyskinesia and Affective Illness*, pp. 22–28. American Psychiatric Press, Washington DC.

Kane, J.M., Woerner, M., Weinhold, P., Wegner, J., Kinon, B. & Borenstein, M. (1984b) Incidence of tardive dyskinesia: Five year data from a prospective study. *Psychopharmacology Bulletin*, **20**, 39–40.

Kane, J.M., Jeste, D.V., Barnes, T.R.E. *et al.* (1992) *Tardive Dyskinesia: A Task Force Report of the American Psychiatric Association*. American Psychiatric Association, Washington DC.

Keepers, G.A. & Casey, D.E. (1987) Prediction of neuroleptic-induced dystonia. *Journal of Clinical Psychopharmacology*, **7**, 342–344.

Keepers, G.A. & Casey, D.E. (1991) Use of neuroleptic-induced extrapyramidal symptoms to predict future vulnerability to side effects. *American Journal of Psychiatry*, **148**, 85–89.

Keepers, G.A., Clappison, V.J. & Casey, D.E. (1983) Initial anticholinergic prophylaxis for neuroleptic-induced extrapyramidal syndromes. *Archives of General Psychiatry*, **40**, 1113–1117.

Klawans, H.L. & Rubovits, R. (1972) An experimental model of tardive dyskinesia. *Journal of Neural Transmission*, **33**, 235–246.

Korsgaard, S., Gerlach, J. & Christensson, E. (1985) Behavioral aspects of serotonin–dopamine interaction in the monkey. *European Journal of Pharmacology*, **118**, 245–252.

Kraepelin, E. (1907) *Clinical Psychiatry*. MacMillan, New York.

Lieberman, J., Kane, J.M. & Woerner, M. (1984) Prevalence of tardive dyskinesia in elderly samples. *Psychopharmacology Bulletin*, **20**, 22–26.

Lieberman, J.A., Saltz, B.L., Johns, C.A., Pollack, S. & Kane, J.M. (1989) Clozapine effects on tardive dyskinesia. *Psychopharmacology Bulletin*, **25**, 57–62.

Lipinski, J.F., Zubenko, G.S., Cohen, B.M. & Barreira, P.J. (1984) Propranolol in the treatment of neuroleptic-induced akathisia. *American Journal of Psychiatry*, **141**, 412–415.

Lohr, J.B., Cadet, J.L., Lohr, M.A., Jeste, D.V. & Wyatt, R.J. (1987) Alphatocopherol in tardive dyskinesia. *Lancet*, **1**, 913–914.

Meltzer, H.Y., Matsubara, S. & Lee, J.C. (1989) Classification of typical and atypical antipsychotic drugs on the basis of dopamine D-1, D-2 and serotonin pK_1 values. *Journal of Pharmacology and Experimental Therapeutics*, **251**, 238–246.

Nguyen, J.A., Thaker, G.K. & Tamminga, C.A. (1989) Gamma-aminobutyric acid (GABA) pathways in tardive dyskinesia. *Psychiatric Annals*, **19**, 302–309.

Nordström, A.-L., Farde, L. & Halldin, C. (1992) Time

course of D2 dopamine receptor occupancy examined by PET after single oral doses of haloperidol. *Psychopharmacology*, **106**, 433–438.

Nordström, A.-L., Farde, L., Wiesel, F.-A. *et al.* (1993) Central D2 dopamine receptor occupancy in relation to antipsychotic drug effects: a double-blind PET study of schizophrenic patients. *Biological Psychiatry*, **33**, 227–235.

Povlsen, U.J., Noring, U., Laursen, A.L., Korsgaard, S. & Gerlach, J. (1986) Effects of serotonergic and anticholinergic in haloperidol-induced dystonia in cebus monkeys. *Clinical Neuropharmacology*, **9**, 84–90.

Quitkin, F., Rifkin, A., Gochfeld, L. & Klein, D.F. (1977) Tardive dyskinesia: are first signs reversible? *American Journal of Psychiatry*, **134**, 84–87.

Richardson, M.A. & Craig, T.J. (1982) The coexistence of parkinsonism-like symptoms and tardive dyskinesia. *American Journal of Psychiatry*, **139**, 341–343.

Rupniak, N.M.J., Jenner, P. & Marsden, C.D. (1986) Acute dystonia induced by neuroleptic drugs. *Psychopharmacology*, **88**, 403–419.

Saltz, B.L., Kane, J.M., Woerner, M.G. *et al.* (1991) Prospective study of tardive dyskinesia incidence in the elderly. *Journal of the American Medical Association*, **266**, 2402–2406.

Sayers, A.C., Burki, H.R., Ruch, W. & Asper, H. (1976) Anticholinergic properties of antipsychotic drugs and their relation to extrapyramidal side effects. *Psychopharmacology*, **51**, 15–22.

Schönecker, M. (1957) Ein eigentumliches Syndrom im oralen Bereich bei Megaphenapplikation. *Nervenarzt*, **28**, 35–36.

Schooler, N.R. & Kane, J.M. (1982) Research diagnoses for tardive dyskinesia. *Archives of General Psychiatry*, **39**, 486–487.

Shriqui, C.L., Bradwejn, J., Annable, L. & Jones, B.D. (1992) Vitamin E in the treatment of tardive dyskinesia: a double-blind placebo-controlled study. *American Journal of Psychiatry*, **149**, 391–393.

Sigwald, J., Bouttier, D. & Raymondeaud, C. (1959) Quatre cas de dyskinesie facio-bucco-linguo-masticatrice a l'evolution prolongee secondaire a un traitement par les neuroleptiques. *Revue Neurologique*, **100**, 751–755.

Smith, J.M. & Baldessarini, R.J. (1980) Changes in prevalence, severity and recovery in tardive dyskinesia with age. *Archives*

of General Psychiatry, **37**, 1368–1373.

Snyder, S., Greenberg, D. & Yamamura, H. (1974) Antischizophrenic drugs and brain cholinergic receptors. *Archives of General Psychiatry*, **31**, 58–61.

Sovner, R. & DiMascio, A. (1978) Extrapyramidal syndromes and other neurological side effects of psychotropic drugs. In Lipton, M.A., DiMascio, A. & Killam, D.K. (eds) *Psychopharmacology: A Generation of Progress*, pp. 1021–1032. Raven Press, New York.

Sramek, J.J., Simpson, G.M., Morrison, R.L. & Heiser, J.F. (1986) Anticholinergic agents for prophylaxis of neuroleptic-induced dystonic reactions: a prospective study. *Journal of Clinical Psychiatry*, **47**, 305–309.

Tarsy, D. & Baldessarini, R.J. (1973) Pharmacologically induced behavioral supersensitivity to apomorphine. *Nature*, **245**, 262–263.

Toenniessen, L.M., Casey, D.E. & McFarland, B.H. (1985) Tardive dyskinesia in the aged. *Archives of General Psychiatry*, **42**, 278–284.

Tune, L. & Coyle, J.T. (1981) Acute extrapyramidal side effects: serum levels of neuroleptics. *Psychopharmacology*, **75**, 9–15.

Uhrbrand, L. & Faurbye, A. (1960) Reversible and irreversible dyskinesia after treatment with perphenazine, chlorpromazine, reserpine, and electroconvulsive therapy. *Psychopharmacologia*, **1**, 408–418.

Ungerstedt, U. (1971) Post-synaptic supersensitivity after 6-hydroxydopamine-induced degeneration of the nigrostriatal dopamine system. *Acta Physiologica Scandinavica*, **82**(Suppl. 367), 69–93.

Villeneuve, A. (1972) The rabbit syndrome: a peculiar extrapyramidal reaction. *Canadian Psychiatric Association Journal*, **17**, 69–72.

Waddington, J.L. (1989) Implications of recent research on dopamine D1 and D2 receptor subtypes in relation to schizophrenia and neuroleptic drug action. *Neurosciences and Neuropsychiatry*, **2**, 89–92.

Waddington, J.L., Cross, A.J., Gamble, S.J. & Bourne, R.C. (1983) Spontaneous orofacial dyskinesia and dopaminergic function in rats after 6 months of neuroleptic treatment. *Science*, **220**, 530–532.

Chapter 28
Non-neurological Side Effects
of Antipsychotic Agents

D. C. GOFF AND R. I. SHADER

Introduction

The non-neurological side effects of antipsychotic drugs may substantially affect clinical outcome and compliance with treatment, but have been largely overshadowed by the attention paid to extrapyramidal side effects. Because the newer atypical antipsychotics, such as clozapine and risperidone, produce substantially fewer neurological side effects, the problem of non-neurological side effects recently has been brought to the forefront of clinical practice.

Conventional antipsychotic medications are postulated to produce their therapeutic effects and extrapyramidal side effects through the antagonism of dopamine D_2 receptors (Tune et al., 1980). 'High-potency' agents (e.g. haloperidol, fluphenazine and pimozide), which display higher affinities for D_2 receptors in brain and so require lower doses than 'low-potency' agents for comparable therapeutic effects, also tend to have greater selectivity for dopamine systems. Low-potency agents (e.g. chlorpromazine and thioridazine) act on several other neurotransmitter systems as well, producing a wide range of non-

neurological side effects (Tables 28.1 & 28.2) (Richelson, 1984; Baldessarini, 1985; Kane, 1985).

Surveys of general clinical populations have suggested that non-neurological side effects, such as sedation, lassitude and weight gain, may be as common as extrapyramidal symptoms (EPS) and may be even more distressing to patients (Lingjaerde et al., 1987; Buis, 1992). 'Neuroleptic dysphoria' is also frequently cited as an important reason for patients refusing pharmacotherapy. Non-compliance rates in schizophrenic outpatients range from 24 to 63% and may in part reflect the burden of side effects (Parkes et al., 1962; Renton et al., 1963; Willcox et al., 1965; Reilly et al., 1967; McClellan & Cowan, 1970; Irwin et al., 1971; Van Putten, 1974; Buchanan, 1992). When patients and their psychiatrists were asked to rate the impact of drug side effects vs. perceived therapeutic benefit, the burden of side effects equalled or exceeded the perceived therapeutic gain from both vantage points (Finn et al., 1990). Only from the perspectives of families and society did therapeutic benefit outweigh the burden of side effects. Clearly, improved understanding and management of the side effects of

Table 28.1 Antipsychotic-induced adverse effects associated with brain-receptor affinities

Dopaminergic	*Acetylcholine*	*Other*
Dystonia	Confusion	Agranulocytosis
Parkinsonism	Dry mouth	Thrombocytopoenia
Akathisia	Constipation	Cutaneous pigmentation
Tardive dyskinesia	Blurred vision	Ocular pigmentation
Hyperprolactinaemia	Urinary retention	Pigmentary retinopathy
Gynaecomastia	Tachycardia	Cholestatic jaundice
Galactorrhoea	Retrograde ejaculation	
Amenorrhoea	Exacerbation of narrow-	
Diminished libido	angle glaucoma	
Neuroleptic malignant		
syndrome		
α-Adrenergic	*Histaminergic*	*Serotonergic*
Postural hypotension	Sedation	Weight gain
Impotence	Postural hypotension	

Table 28.2 Antipsychotic side-effect profiles in relation to clinical potency

Antipsychotic*	Anticholinergic	EPS	Sedation	Hypotension
Haloperidol (Haldol)	+	+++++	++	+
Fluphenazine (Prolixin)	++	+++++	++	++
Thiothixene (Navane)	++	++++	++	++
Trifluoperazine (Stelazine)	++	++++	++	++
Perphenazine (Trilafon)	++	+++	++	++
Molindone (Moban)	+	+++	+	++
Loxapine (Loxitane)	+++	+++	+++	++
Chlorpromazine (Thorazine)	++++	++	+++++	++++
Thioridazine (Mellaril)	+++++	++	+++++	++++
Clozapine (Clozaril)	+++++	+	+++++	++++

* Antipsychotic agents listed in descending order of clinical potency.
EPS, extrapyramidal symptoms.
(+), low rate — (+++++), high rate of occurence.

antipsychotic agents are needed if compliance rates and the quality of life for schizophrenic patients are to be improved substantially.

Mood and behavioural effects

Dysphoric response

Shortly after the introduction of chlorpromazine to clinical practice, depression was reported to be associated with its use (Fellner, 1958). The issue of treatment-emergent depression during treatment with antipsychotic agents is quite complex, since depressive symptoms may represent a specific dysphoric effect of these medications, a consequence of EPS or the recognition of concomitant depression previously obscured by psychotic symptoms. Acutely, antipsychotic agents can produce dysphoria, anxiety and panic attacks which may be dose related (Sanberg & Norman, 1989). Belmaker and Wald (1977) described apathy, profound inner restlessness, anergia and severe anxiety after they administered 5 mg haloperidol intravenously to themselves. Neither investigator was able to return to work for 36 h after this experiment. Caine and Polinsky (1979) reported dysphoria in six of 72 patients with Tourette's syndrome who received haloperidol 2.5–4.0 mg/day. These symptoms were not associated with EPS and were alleviated by dose reduction. Van Putten et al. (1984) reported a 23% incidence of dysphoria following a single dose of haloperidol 5 mg, and a 25% incidence following a dose of thiothixine 0.22 mg/kg. Onset of dysphoria did not correlate with plasma concentrations of haloperidol but did appear to relate to emergence of akathisia.

Acute dysphoric reactions to antipsychotic agents can be quite distressing. In one study, six of 14 schizophrenic patients attributed their refusal of treatment to prior experiences of neuroleptic-associated dysphoria (Van Putten et al., 1981). An early dysphoric response, which may include feelings of listlessness or tension, has also been associated with a poor antipsychotic response in several studies (May et al., 1976, 1981; Van Putten & May, 1978a; Singh & Kay, 1979; Van Putten et al., 1981, 1989; Hogan & Awad, 1992) and with subsequent poor compliance (Hogan et al., 1983; Van Putten, 1983). This reaction is not restricted to high-potency agents; in one study, chlorpromazine was associated with early dysphoria at a slightly higher frequency than haloperidol (Hogan & Awad, 1992). Early dysphoria has been associated with akathisia in some (Van Putten et al., 1980a,b), but not all, studies (Hogan & Awad, 1992).

Akinetic depression

Neuroleptic-associated dysphoria may be a manifestation of parkinsonian akinesia in some patients. Van Putten and May (1978b) reported that more than half of akinetic patients developed a modest, although significant, worsening of measures of dysphoria as their psychotic symptoms improved with antipsychotic treatment. Treatment with the anticholinergic agent trihexyphenidyl improved depression and anxiety in these patients. Marder et al. (1984) found elevated levels of depression, interpersonal sensitivity and phobic anxiety in patients treated for 1 month with conventional doses of fluphenazine decanoate (25 mg twice weekly) compared with patients treated with low doses (5 mg twice weekly). Ratings of anxiety and depression correlated with ratings of akathisia and retardation.

Postpsychotic depression

Although treatment with antipsychotic agents may be associated with dysphoric response initially and development of EPS may be linked to modest elevations of anxiety and depression, most depression experienced by patients with schizophrenia is probably unrelated to drug treatment (Barnes et al., 1989). Depressive symptoms were described following resolution of acute psychotic episodes long before the introduction of antipsychotic agents (Mayer-Gross, 1920). After reviewing 34 double-blind trials of neuroleptic drugs, Robertson and Trimble (1982) concluded that treatment with these agents is more likely to improve than to worsen depressive symptoms.

Early work attributing 'postpsychotic depression' to drug therapy has not been validated by controlled trials. Most evidence suggests that depressive symptoms usually are present at the time antipsychotic treatment is initiated, and improve during the course of treatment, although they may become more prominent as psychotic symptoms recede (Knights & Hirsch, 1981). However, in some patients postpsychotic depression may also represent a psychological response to illness as patients are newly able to assess the impact of psychotic illness upon their lives (McGlashan & Carpenter, 1976).

Behavioural toxicity

Several toxic behavioural responses have been associated with antipsychotic agents. Delirium and acute confusional states may occur early in the course of treatment, particularly in the elderly. While this probably reflects an anticholinergic toxicity in most cases, behavioural toxicity may occur in the absence of anticholinergic toxicity (Barnes & Bridges, 1980). Neuroleptic-induced behavioural toxicity, consisting of agitation, disorganization, paranoia and depersonalization, has also been described in 'borderline schizophrenics' (Steiner *et al.*, 1979). Finally, somnambulism (Huapaya, 1976), night terrors (Flemenbaum, 1976) are neuroleptic-induced Kluver−Bucy syndrome (Varga *et al.*, 1979) have also been reported with neuroleptic therapy.

Cognitive effects

The demonstration of an association between tardive dyskinesia (TD) and cognitive impairment raised the concern that antipsychotic agents might produce persistent cognitive dysfunction (Struve & Willner, 1983; Ganguli & Raghu, 1985; Spohn *et al.*, 1985; Waddington, 1987; Sorokin *et al.*, 1988). However, most evidence suggests that cognitive impairment is a pre-existent risk factor for TD, rather than the result of a shared neurotoxic process, although the mechanism of such an association remains unclear (Spohn & Strauss, 1989). At typical therapeutic doses, treatment

with these medications is most commonly associated with cognitive improvement, particularly in attention, vigilance, distractibility and idiosyncratic thinking (Spohn & Strauss, 1989; Cassens *et al.*, 1990; King, 1990). Improvement in abstraction has also been reported to accompany antipsychotic treatment (Wahba *et al.*, 1981). Conventional antipsychotic agents do not appear to improve functional 'hypofrontality' in schizophrenic patients, as Berman *et al.* (1986) reported little or no effect on activation of the dorsolateral prefrontal cortex of schizophrenic patients, as measured by regional cerebral blood flow (rCBF) during the Wisconsin card sorting test (WCST). Tomer and Flor-Henry (1989) also found no overall effect on cognition associated with treatment, but did demonstrate reversal of an asymmetry of attention.

Trials of relatively low doses (e.g. chlorpromazine 60 mg/day) have failed to demonstrate cognitive impairment in normal subjects (Liljequist *et al.*, 1975, 1978; King, 1990). However, cognitive dysfunction may occur at high doses during clinical use, often associated with a worsening of psychotic symptoms (Tune *et al.*, 1980; Cole, 1982; Spohn *et al.*, 1985). While cognitive impairment has been demonstrated in schizophrenic patients receiving relatively high doses of sedating phenothiazines, tolerance appears to develop to this effect (Kornetsky *et al.*, 1959; Judson & MacCasland, 1960; Latz & Kornetsky, 1965). Kornetsky (1972) reported that scores on the continuous performance test (CPT) improved with chronic phenothiazine administration, but showed initial impairment during testing after the first dose. Kornetsky *et al.* (1959) also found that performance of normal subjects on psychomotor tests was more negatively affected by a single dose of phenothiazine (chlorpromazine 100 and 200 mg) than was the performance of schizophrenic subjects.

Impairments of memory and the span of apprehension are common in schizophrenic patients receiving anticholinergic agents for the control of parkinsonian side effects of their antipsychotic medication. Tune *et al.* (1982) demonstrated that memory impairment in stabilized schizophrenic patients was significantly correlated with serum anticholinergic activity and was unrelated to serum levels of antipsychotic medication as measured by a radioreceptor assay.

Finally, Linnoila and colleagues (Linnoila, 1973; Linnoila & Maki, 1974) demonstrated significant impairment of driving-related psychomotor performance in normal subjects after a single 25-mg dose of thioridazine. The impact on simulated driving performance was greater than that produced by diazepam 10 mg or by haloperidol 5 mg. While most evidence suggests that antipsychotic agents do not impair cognitive function at usual clinical doses, clinicians should warn patients of the possible risks associated with driving, particularly if receiving low-potency agents early in the course of treatment. The addition of anticholinergic agents for control of EPS represents a much more serious threat to cognitive functioning (Baker *et al.*, 1983; Goff & Baldessarini, 1993).

Endocrine effects

Hyperprolactinaemia

Prolactin secretion from the lactotroph cells of the pituitary is tonically inhibited by dopamine, the putative prolactin release inhibiting factor (PRIF). Conventional antipsychotic agents elevate prolactin levels by blocking dopaminergic activity in the tuberoinfundibular system. In single-dose trials, subtherapeutic doses of antipsychotics (i.e. haloperidol 0.5–1.5 mg) produce a maximal prolactin elevation within 1–2 h, which then returns to baseline over approximately 6 h (Gruen *et al.*, 1978a,b). In one study, drug-free male schizophrenic patients demonstrated blunted prolactin responses to a single dose of haloperidol (Keks *et al.*, 1987). With repeated dosing, prolactin levels remain elevated in most patients and the degree of elevation tends to correlate with neuroleptic potency and dose. Six of 17 studies have found a correlation between prolactin levels and antipsychotic response, although this area is complicated by considerable methodological problems (Green & Brown, 1988). Additional evidence suggests that tolerance may develop to the pro-

lactin-elevating effect of antipsychotic agents, so that chronically treated patients may have prolactin levels within the normal range (Gruen *et al.*, 1978b; Laughren *et al.*, 1979; Kolakowski *et al.*, 1981; Igarashi *et al.*, 1985; Rubin, 1987).

Neuroleptic-induced hyperprolactinaemia underlies several clinical side effects. Mild elevation of prolactin may cause menstrual irregularities; higher prolactin levels may result in amenorrhoea. As many as 90% of women treated with neuroleptics report changes in their menstrual cycle (Sandison *et al.*, 1960; Ghadirian *et al.*, 1982). Elevated levels of prolactin also stimulate breast tissue, which commonly results in breast tenderness, gynaecomastia and galactorrhoea. Galactorrhoea has been reported in as many as 57% of females treated with antipsychotic agents, whereas gynaecomastia is an infrequent complication of antipsychotic therapy in men (Robinson, 1957; Plante & Roy, 1967). Hyperprolactinaemia secondary to pituitary tumours is associated with a loss of bone density (Klibanski *et al.*, 1981), although this potential adverse effect has not been established in women taking antipsychotic agents (Rogers & Burke, 1987; Ataya *et al.*, 1988). Hyperprolactinaemia increases the risk for breast tumours in laboratory animals, but exposure to antipsychotic agents does not appear to increase the risk in humans (Overall, 1978).

Hyperthyroidism

Haloperidol and perphenazine are both reported to produce a toxic state resembling either thyroid storm or neuroleptic malignant syndrome (NMS) when administered to patients with pre-existing hyperthyroidism (Weiner, 1979; Jefferson & Marshal, 1981). This neurotoxic reaction may include fever, rigidity, diaphoresis, dyspnoea and dysphagia. One fatality has been reported from this combination (Weiner, 1979). Although the frequency and mechanism of this adverse effect are unclear, animal studies have indicated that the combination of haloperidol and thyroxine may be toxic (Selye & Szabo, 1972).

Syndrome of inappropriate antidiuretic hormone

The syndrome of inappropriate antidiuretic hormone (SIADH) has been attributed to haloperidol or thiothixine administration in individual case reports (Aljouni *et al.*, 1974; Peck & Shenkman, 1979). In an additional case, SIADH was associated with fluphenazine, thiothixine and trifluoperazine, but resolved when the patient was treated with molindone (Glusac *et al.*, 1990). Inappropriate release of antidiuretic hormone (vasopressin) may produce hyponatraemia and symptoms of water intoxication (confusion, lethargy, seizures), particularly in the presence of polydipsia. However, controlled studies in schizophrenic and normal subjects have not demonstrated an elevation of antidiuretic hormone associated with administration of antipsychotic agents (Kendler *et al.*, 1978; Raskind *et al.*, 1987; Sarai & Matsunaga, 1989). In general, treatment with antipsychotic agents is more likely to normalize hyponatraemia in schizophrenic patients than to dysregulate sodium metabolism (Illowsky & Kirch, 1988).

Weight gain

Weight gain is a serious potential side effect of neuroleptics, since it contributes to noncompliance and may lead to medical morbidity. The low-potency agents have been associated with the greatest degree of weight gain. Amidsen (1964) reported that 80% of 179 patients treated with chlorpromazine experienced weight gain, which in 25% of patients was considered excessive. The average weight gain associated with chlorpromazine was 16% of maximal ideal body weight compared with 8% in patients treated with perphenazine and 7% with clopenthixol. Klett and Caffey (1960) recorded an average weight gain of 9 lb over the first 3 months of chlorpromazine treatment of male schizophrenic patients. Most of the weight gain occurred during the first few weeks of treatment and weights tended to return to baseline after discontinuing the medication. Clozapine is also associated with

excessive weight gain in as many as 75% of patients, with the average weight gain ranging from 9 to 25 lb (Cohen *et al.*, 1990; Lamberti *et al.*, 1992; Leadbetter *et al.*, 1992). Leadbetter *et al.* (1992) found that clinical improvement was greater among patients with marked weight gain. Haloperidol and other high-potency agents are reported to produce considerably less weight gain (Bernstein, 1987). However, Falloon *et al.* (1978) reported an average 10% weight gain over a 1-year period in 38 patients treated with fluphenazine decanoate or pimozide. Molindone may produce the least weight gain and in some studies has been associated with weight loss, particularly when prescribed to patients who have gained weight while receiving other antipsychotic agents (Gallant & Bishop, 1968; Kellner *et al.*, 1976; Gardos & Cole, 1977).

The mechanism of neuroleptic-induced weight gain remains unclear. Bernstein (1987) has proposed a serotonergic mechanism to explain the increased propensity for certain agents to produce weight gain. Robinson *et al.* (1975) demonstrated an increased appetite in patients started on phenothiazines and this was related to dose. Rats administered phenothiazines display increased food intake as well as increased calorie utilization (Boyd, 1960; Reynolds & Carlisle, 1961; Greenberg *et al.*, 1962; Stolerman, 1970). In addition, antipsychotic treatment may result in a dry mouth, either as a result of intrinsic anticholinergic properties of low-potency agents or from coadministration of antiparkinsonian agents. Excessive consumption of high-calorie beverages in response to a dry mouth contributes to weight gain.

Sexual dysfunction

Sexual dysfunction occurs in as many as 60% of sexually active schizophrenic patients taking antipsychotic medication, although research in this area has largely focused on male patients (Degen, 1982; Mitchell & Popkin, 1982). Ghadirian *et al.* (1982) found that 54% of male and 30% of female schizophrenic patients reported sexual dysfunction after starting neuroleptics, with changes in the quality of orgasm the most common complaint. In non-schizophrenic patients treated with fluphenazine decanoate, Bartholomew (1986) found a 71% rate of sexual dysfunction. As previously discussed, all conventional antipsychotic agents elevate prolactin levels, which may secondarily lower testosterone and leutinizing hormone levels. Low levels of gonadal hormones diminish libido in both sexes, but have not been systematically studied in patients treated with neuroleptics. A few studies have found diminished libido associated with antipsychotic treatment, although findings have been inconsistent, possibly reflecting the variable impact of schizophrenic illness on sexuality (Witton 1962; Haider, 1966; Nestores *et al.*, 1980).

Erectile dysfunction often develops shortly after initiating antipsychotic treatment, particularly with thioridazine. Kotin *et al.* (1976) found that 44% of men treated with thioridazine described difficulty in achieving an erection compared with 19% of men treated with other antipsychotic agents. Erectile dysfunction has been reported with thioridazine at relatively low daily doses (150 mg). In one case, chlorpromazine-induced dysfunction resolved after the daily dose was decreased from 1000 to 600 mg (Greenberg, 1971). Erectile dysfunction usually resolves fairly quickly after the neuroleptic is discontinued (Mitchell & Popkin, 1982). Thioridazine may also produce ejaculatory inhibition or ejaculatory delay more frequently than other neuroleptics. Ejaculatory dysfunction is described by 30–50% of men treated with thioridazine and may occur at doses as low as 30 mg/day (Heller, 1961; Shader, 1964; Blair & Simpson, 1966; Kotin *et al.*, 1976). Ejaculatory difficulties have also been reported with mesoridazine (Shader, 1972) and occur infrequently with higher potency agents (Blair & Simpson, 1966). Priapism, a prolonged, painful erection, is a rare complication of phenothiazine treatment and can require surgery and result in impotence (Dorman & Schmidt, 1976). Mitchell and Popkin (1982) found 19 published cases of neuroleptic-associated priapism. Of the cases which identified the neuroleptic, thioridazine or chlorpromazine were thought to be responsible in all but one case.

A single intramuscular injection of chlorpromazine (25 mg) was linked to priapism in one report (Merkin, 1977).

Degan (1982) described orgasmic inhibition (prolonged time for orgasm to occur) in two women treated with neuroleptics. Although orgasm is frequently unaffected in cases of ejaculatory impairment, the quality of orgasm is perceived as altered in approximately 8% of patients taking neuroleptics (Freyhan, 1961; Heller, 1961; Clein, 1962; Kotin *et al.*, 1976). Painful orgasm has also been reported with thioridazine, trifluoperazine and haloperidol (Kotin *et al.*, 1976; Berger, 1979).

Cardiovascular effects

Myocardial depression

The phenothiazines, particularly thioridazine and chlorpromazine, produce direct myocardial depressant effects which usually are manifested by benign changes on the electrocardiogram (ECG) but may rarely result in sudden death (Risch *et al.*, 1981). Thioridazine slows atrial and ventricular conduction and prolongs refractory periods (Descotes *et al.*, 1979; Yoon *et al.*, 1979). This myocardial depressant effect can produce toxicity if thioridazine is added to quinidine (Risch *et al.*, 1981). Chlorpromazine at a dose as low as 150 mg/day can also produce prolongation of the QT interval as well as depression of T waves and changes in AV conduction time (Backman & Elosuo, 1964; Ban & St Jean, 1964; Huston & Bell, 1966; Alexander *et al.*, 1967; Wendkos, 1967). Classes of antipsychotic agents other than the phenothiazines are much less likely to produce changes in the ECG (Ban & St Jean, 1964; Risch *et al.*, 1981), with the exception of pimozide which may produce clinically significant ECG changes as a result of its calcium channel blocking properties (Opler & Feinberg, 1991). It is recommended that serial ECGs be obtained when treatment with pimozide is started and the drug should be stopped if the QT interval exceeds 520 ms in adults or 470 ms in children (Baldessarini, 1985). Extremely high doses of intravenous haloperidol (up to 1000 mg in 24 h) have been administered safely in patients with cardiac disease, although rare cases of QT-interval prolongation and Torsade de Pointes have been reported at these doses (Metzger & Friedman, 1993).

Several reports of sudden death have been attributed to thioridazine or chlorpromazine therapy in young, healthy patients (Aherwadker *et al.*, 1964; Giles & Modlin, 1968). Postmortem studies have revealed intramyocardial lesions secondary to the accumulation of acid mucopolysaccharides believed to be ralated to chronic neuroleptic exposure (Richardson *et al.*, 1966). The risk of fatal arrhythmias associated with phenothiazine treatment remains difficult to determine, since some cases of sudden death may result from other causes such as aspiration or asphyxiation (Leestma & Koenig, 1968; Moore & Book, 1969). Efforts to determine whether the incidence of sudden death increased with the advent of neuroleptic treatment have produced conflicting results (Brill & Patton, 1962; Richardson *et al.*, 1966). However, thioridazine or chlorpromazine probably do rarely produce serious arrhythmias, particularly in patients with underlying cardiac disease or hypokalaemia.

Recently, cases of sudden death have been associated with the combination of clozapine and benzodiazepines. This toxic reaction has been characterized by sedation, ataxia, sialorrhoea and, in some cases, fainting, loss of consciousness and respiratory arrest (Grohmann *et al.*, 1989; Cobb *et al.*, 1991; Friedman *et al.*, 1991). If such an interaction does occur, it is quite rare, and the mechanism remains uncertain.

Orthostatic hypotension

Orthostatic hypotension is also commonly reported with low-potency neuroleptics and is believed to result from α-adrenergic blockade (Richelson, 1984). Oral administration of moderate doses of chlorpromazine (50–200 mg/day) generally do not produce significant changes in systolic blood pressure, whereas intravenous or intramuscular administration of moderate doses is associated with a high frequency of hypotensive reactions (Foster *et al.*, 1954; Bourgeois-Govardin *et al.*, 1955; Kornetsky, 1960; Blumberg *et al.*, 1964; Korol *et al.*, 1965). Silver *et al.* (1990) measured blood pressure at rest and standing in 196 medicated schizophrenic patients and found that 77% of patients displayed postural hypotension after 1 min of standing and 17% after 3 min. Although the mean systolic blood pressure drop at 1 min was 28 mmHg, patients did not report dizziness or light headedness. The degree of blood pressure drop did not correlate with dose or with age of the patient. Thioridazine affected blood pressure significantly more than did chlorpromazine or haloperidol. Surprisingly, the drop in pressure did not correlate with α_1-receptor binding activity. Clozapine frequently produces orthostatic hypotension and resting tachycardia early in the course of treatment (Baldessarini & Frankenburg, 1991). Tolerance appears to develop to the cardiovascular effects of clozapine and use of low doses at the initiation of treatment may reduce the risk of hypotension to a rate comparable with that associated with conventional neuroleptics (Ereshefsky *et al.*, 1989).

Cutaneous effects

Allergic reactions

Antipsychotic drugs can affect the skin as a result of allergic reactions, photosensitivity effects or pigmentary changes (Zelickson, 1966). Cutaneous allergic reactions to antipsychotic agents typically occur 2–10 weeks after the initiation of treatment and patients present with maculopapular rashes on the face, neck, chest or extremities. Discontinuation of the offending agent usually results in a clearing of skin lesions within a week. Cases of 'cross allergy' to other antipsychotic drugs have been reported and should be monitored when switching to a new agent. Occasionally, antipsychotic agents can produce severe cutaneous reactions, such as exfoliative dermatitis, generalized urticaria and angioneurotic oedema. Discontinuation of the drug and treatment with antihistamines or topical steroids are usually sufficient for cutaneous reactions. Desensitization protocols have been developed for antibiotics, and recently for fluoxetine, but have not been tested with antipsychotic agents (Leznoff & Binkley, 1992).

Photosensitivity

Low-potency antipsychotics (e.g. chlorpromazine and thioridazine) produce enhanced sensitivity to sunlight in about 3% of patients. Photosensitivity reactions resemble sunburn and appear on areas of the body exposed to sunlight. Although the mechanism is not well understood, photosensitivity may involve the formation of free radicals which can injure cells in the skin (Chignell et al., 1985). Patients treated with such agents should be warned about the risk of prolonged exposure to sunlight during summer months. Antipsychotic agents can also produce discolouration of exposed skin by affecting melatonin metabolism. Pigmentary changes may first appear like a dark tan and progress to blue or purple; they are frequently associated with pigmentary changes in the eye. The incidence of cutaneous pigmentation has been estimated at about 1−3% in patients treated with low-potency agents (Greiner & Berry, 1964; Ban & Lehmann, 1965; Ananth et al., 1972). Although it is generally believed that chlorpromazine is most likely to produce cutaneous pigmentation, Ban et al. (1985) reported similar rates with haloperidol in a multinational study. However, four cases have been reported of chlorpromazine-associated pigmentation which resolved when the patients were switched to haloperidol (Thompson et al., 1988).

Ocular effects

Ocular changes associated with pigmentation of the skin were first reported with chlorpromazine by Greiner and Berry (1964). As many as 79% of patients treated with chlorpromazine exhibit white or yellow−brown deposits on the cornea or lens (Siddall, 1968). Epithelial keratopathy, presenting as clouding of the anterior cornea in the area of the palpebral fissure, has also been attributed to chlorpromazine exposure. Pigmentation of the retina is reported in about 20% of chlor-

promazine-treated patients. Pigmentary changes in the eye, like cutaneous pigmentation, probably involve melanin metabolism and are related to the dose and duration of exposure to chlorpromazine. Fortunately, vision is rarely affected. Ocular pigmentation has also been reported with perphenazine, thiothixene and trifluoperazine, but is believed to occur at a much lower frequency with these agents (Prien et al., 1970; Barron et al. 1972; Fraunfelder & Meyer, 1982). Ulberg et al. (1970) reported the rare occurrence of ocular pigmentary changes in infants exposed in utero to phenothiazines.

Thioridazine appears to be unique in producing irreversible pigmentary retinopathy. While retinal toxicity has been reported at relatively low doses, it usually results from doses greater than 800 mg/day given for periods of several months or longer. Clinical manifestations include diminished visual acuity, loss of peripheral vision and scotoma. The mechanism of thioridazine-induced retinopathy remains unclear, although it may involve free-radical injury to the rods, resulting in part from a loss of the protective effect of melanin. Cases of chromatopsia have also been associated with thioridazine, in which patients describe 'yellow vision' or 'red vision'.

The low-potency neuroleptics may also impair ocular function via anticholinergic effects. Patients may complain of blurred vision, and upon examination may display mydriasis and loss of accommodation. The anticholinergic action of low-potency agents may also precipitate narrow-angle glaucoma.

Gastrointestinal and hepatic effects

Xerostomia (dry mouth) is a common anticholinergic side effect associated with low-potency neuroleptics and with antiparkinsonian agents (Sreebny & Schwartz, 1986). Xerostomia may cause difficulties with chewing, swallowing and speaking, and increases vulnerability to dental caries and candidiasis. Attempts to alleviate a dry mouth by sucking on candy or drinking sweetened beverages can further increase the risk of dental infection and obesity. Although patients may cease to complain of a dry mouth over time, studies of salivary production in patients taking nortriptyline indicate that tolerance does not develop to this side effect (Asberg *et al.*, 1970; Bertram *et al.*, 1979) and probably does not develop with antipsychotic either. Sialorrhoea occurs in approximately 23% of patients treated with clozapine (Baldessarini & Frankenburg, 1991). Patients may report soaking their pillows at night and some experience a distressing sensation of choking on their saliva. The mechanism of clozapine-induced sialorrhoea remains unclear and is paradoxical in light of its strong anticholinergic effects.

Antipsychotic agents with anticholinergic activity can also impair the gag reflex, placing patients at risk for aspiration, particularly if swallowing is already impaired. The presence of TD may be an additional factor affecting the gag reflex; Craig *et al.* (1982) found an impaired gag reflex in 74% of schizophrenic patients with TD taking anticholinergic agents vs. 30% of the remainder of schizophrenic patients. However, in one study of drug-free schizophrenic patients, half displayed abnormalities in swallowing (Husser & Bragg, 1969). Anticholinergic effects of low-potency neuroleptics can also slow gastric emptying and impair intestinal and colonic motility, producing gastroesophageal reflux, anorexia, nausea, vomiting, constipation, abdominal distention or obstruction (Warnes *et al.*, 1967; Davis & Nusbaum, 1973; Giordano *et al.*, 1975; Evans *et al.*, 1979; Kemeney *et al.*, 1980). Paralytic ileus has been reported with haloperidol (Maltbie *et al.*, 1981).

Hepatic effects

Antipsychotic agents also produce several effects on the liver, ranging from benign elevation of liver enzymes to cholestatic jaundice and hepatocellular toxicity (Leipzig, 1992). Chlorpromazine is the best studied in relation to liver function, and may be the most likely to produce toxicity. Approximately 25–60% of patients treated with chlorpromazine display mild elevation of liver enzymes during the first month of exposure (Dickes *et al.*, 1957; Shay & Siplet, 1957; Bartholomew *et al.*,

1958; Laursen & Borup Svendsen, 1959; Gupta *et al.*, 1962). These elevations of liver enzymes appear to be benign and usually return to normal despite continued treatment (Gupta *et al.*, 1962).

However, chlorpromazine has direct hepatotoxic effects which can result in subclinical cholestasis and damage to liver cells (Sherlock, 1979, 1989; Kaplowitz *et al.*, 1986). Hydroxylated metabolites of chlorpromazine may be particularly hepatotoxic, possibly as a result of the production of free radicals (Samuels & Carey, 1978; Watson *et al.*, 1988). Patients who produce higher levels of these metabolites, because of reduced sulphoxidation of the parent compound, may be at greater risk for cholestatic jaundice. Approximately 1–2% of patients treated with chlorpromazine develop cholestatic jaundice within 1–5 weeks of starting to take the drug (Ishak & Irey, 1972; Zimmerman & Ishak, 1987). This appears to be a hypersensitivity reaction as it is usually accompanied by eosinophilia, fever and rash, and rapidly recurs when the patient is rechallenged. Fortunately, most patients recover within 1 year and tolerate other classes of antipsychotics without cross-reactivity. While haloperidol has also been associated with hepatotoxicity, the risk is estimated to be quite low (approximately 0.2%) (Crane, 1967; Fuller *et al.*, 1977; Dincsoy & Saelinger, 1982; Leipzig, 1992).

Haematological effects

Agranulocytosis caused by clozapine is the most common serious haematological effect produced by antipsychotic agents. Clozapine-induced agranulocytosis occurs in approximately 1–2% of patients exposed for 1 year to the drug, with about 80% of cases occurring within the first 18 weeks of exposure (Krupp & Barnes, 1989). Ashkenazi Jews with histocompatibility antigen (HLA) types B38, DR4, DQW3 and patients of Finnish descent may be at increased risk (Amsler *et al.*, 1977; Lieberman *et al.*, 1990). The mechanism appears to be immune related, as sensitization is suggested by the more rapid relapse following rechallenge and by the presence of a distinct antibody in the immunoglobulin (Ig)M fraction of sera from patients who develop agranulocytosis (Lieberman *et al.*, 1988; Claas, 1989). Leucopoenia is much more common than agranulocytosis with clozapine and is not associated with an increased risk for agranulocytosis. Eosinophilia, leucocytosis and thrombocytopoenia have also been reported with clozapine.

Earlier surveys of patients treated with relatively high doses of phenothiazines found an incidence of agranulocytosis of about 0.5% and benign leucopoenia (white blood cell count, $2.5-4.0 \times 10^9$/l) in about 10% of patients (Pisciotta, 1969, 1992; Litvak & Kaelblin, 1971). More recent data suggest that contemporary use of moderate doses of chlorpromazine may have substantially reduced the risk of agranulocytosis, and that earlier studies may have included patients with complicating medical illnesses (Levinson & Simpson, 1987). Phenothiazine-associated agranulocytosis generally occurs between 20 and 90 days after initiating treatment and may be more common in elderly women (Mandel & Gross, 1968; Pisciotta, 1969). Unlike clozapine, the phenothiazines are believed to produce agranulocytosis via direct bone marrow toxicity (Pisciotta, 1971, 1973). Agranulocytosis secondary to both clozapine and phenothiazine exposure is generally reversible; with discontinuation of the drug and proper medical care, recovery is common (Lieberman *et al.*, 1988).

Seizures

Chlorpromazine had been marketed for less than 1 year before a case of chlorpromazine-related seizure was reported (Anton-Stephens, 1953). Logothetis (1967) studied 859 patients treated with phenothiazines over 5 years and found a 1.2% risk for seizures. The risk for seizures was strongly related to dose, as the rate of seizures approached 10% in patients treated with greater than 1000 mg chlorpromazine per day. Rapid increases in dose and the presence of organic brain disease also increased the risk for seizures. Data from the Boston Collaborative Drug Surveillance Program indicated a frequency of seizures in patients treated with chlorpromazine of only 0.22% (Jick *et al.*, 1970). Other surveys have supported a relationship between seizures and higher doses of phenothiazines (Schlichther *et al.*, 1956; Messing *et al.*, 1984). The risk of seizures is greatest with clozapine, reaching an estimated incidence of 10% in patients receiving the drug and followed for 4 years (Devinsky *et al.*, 1991). The risk of seizures also increases with dose; prophylactic treatment with an anticonvulsant has been suggested for some patients treated with clozapine at daily doses of 500 mg or greater (Baldessarini & Frankenburg, 1991). For antipsychotic agents other than clozapine, the risk of provoking seizures in patients with epilepsy appears quite small. One study of 59 patients with seizure disorders found that the addition of psychotropic medication, including antipsychotics, was generally associated with improved seizure control (Ojemann *et al.*, 1987).

The mechanism by which antipsychotic agents affect seizure threshold remains unclear. Animal studies suggest that the seizure threshold is elevated by dopamine agonists (McKenzie & Soroko, 1972; Meldrum *et al.*, 1975) and lowered by cholinergic agents (Millichap *et al.*, 1968; Arnold *et al.*, 1974). These observations led to the recommendation that highly anticholinergic agents such as thioridazine be selected for patients at risk for seizures (Remick & Fine, 1979). However, seizures are probably quite infrequent with haloperidol, an agent without appreciable anticholinergic activity (Oles, 1960; Baldessarini & Lipinski, 1976; Kaminer & Munitz, 1984). In general, the least-sedating agents may be least likely to produce seizures (Itil & Soldatos, 1980). In mice, chlorpromazine, promethazine and mepazine lower the seizure threshold, whereas trifluoperazine and prochloroperazine produce little or no effect (Tedeschi *et al.*, 1958). Animal models and *in vitro* methods for assessing relative drug effects on seizure threshold have produced complex and often conflicting results (Tedeschi *et al.*, 1958; Chen *et al.*, 1968; Oliver *et al.*, 1982). Effects on seizure threshold may follow curvilinear relationships with respect to brain concentrations for some drugs but not others (Oliver *et al.*, 1982).

NMS

NMS is a potentially lethal complication of anti-psychotic treatment, usually characterized by hyperthermia, rigidity, confusion, diaphoresis, autonomic instability, elevated creatine phospho-kinase (CPK) and leucocytosis. Most cases of NMS occur during the first 2 weeks of exposure, although it can occur at any time (Addonizio *et al.*, 1987). NMS has been viewed as a spectrum disorder, with a full syndromal incidence esti-mated at 0.02–2.4%, and with mild, subsyn-dromal cases occurring at an incidence of about 12% (Addonizio *et al.*, 1986; Adityanjee *et al.*, 1988; Keck *et al.*, 1991; Gurrera *et al.*, 1992). Because of the relative infrequency of this adverse reaction, identification of risk factors and assess-ment of treatment efficacy remain quite prelimi-nary. Possible risk factors for NMS include: male gender, the presence of organic brain disease or mental retardation, high dose or rapid escalation of neuroleptic dose, concomitant lithium adminis-tration and intramuscular administration of high-potency antipsychotic agents (Addonizio, 1985; Addonizio *et al.*, 1987; Keck *et al.*, 1987, 1989). Cases of NMS have occurred most frequently with high-potency agents, but it remains unclear whether this association merely reflects the more widespread clinical use of these agents (Levenson, 1985). The mechanism of NMS also is uncertain. Parallels have been drawn between NMS and malignant hyperthermia, largely on the basis of common clinical characteristics (Addonizio *et al.*, 1987). However, patients with a history of either NMS or malignant hyperthermia appear to be at no increased risk for developing the other syn-drome, and analysis of muscle biopsies has not consistently demonstrated a physiological link between the two conditions (Addonizio *et al.*, 1987). It has been observed that some patients with Parkinson's disease develop an NMS-like syndrome when dopamine agonists are abruptly discontinued, suggesting that dysregulation of dopaminergic function is involved in the aetiology of NMS (Friedman *et al.*, 1985).

Neuroleptic-induced heatstroke may also pre-sent with fever and elevated CPK, but can usually be distinguished from NMS by the presence of agitation, muscle flaccidity and dry skin (Lazarus, 1989). Seizures frequently occur in neuroleptic-induced heatstroke, which is reported to cause a mortality rate of 20–50%. More difficult to rule out as part of the differential diagnosis of NMS is lethal catatonia, a febrile form of catatonia associ-ated with schizophrenia and which often exhibits all the clinical signs of NMS (Mann *et al.*, 1986; Gurrera *et al.*, 1992; Weller, 1992). It is possible that some cases of NMS are actually lethal cata-tonia, or represent an interaction between lethal catatonia and dopamine blocking drugs. White and Robins (1991) observed that in five consecu-tive cases of NMS, a catatonic state preceded the administration of a neuroleptic and the subsequent onset of NMS. These authors have suggested that NMS might represent a 'neuroleptic-aggravated' form of catatonia (White & Robins, 1991; White, 1992).

If NMS develops, the offending agent should be immediately discontinued and the patient hos-pitalized for hydration, temperature control and monitoring of vital signs and renal function. Bromocriptine and dantrolene may facilitate recovery, although neither has been studied in controlled trials and data on efficacy remain unclear (Rosebush *et al.*, 1991; Sakkas *et al.*, 1991). Although a 15% mortality rate has been reported, patients with NMS usually recover within an average of 14 days or approximately 30 days if treated with depot neuroleptic at the time of onset of NMS (Addonizio *et al.*, 1987). Duration of time elapsed between the resolution of NMS and restarting antipsychotic medication appears to be an important determinant of the risk for relapse (Rosebush *et al.*, 1989). Although cases have been reported of NMS occurring in patients receiving clozapine, the risk of NMS is probably lower with clozapine than with con-ventional agents (Anderson & Powers, 1991; DasGupta & Young, 1991; Miller *et al.*, 1991).

Conclusion

Antipsychotic agents produce a diverse collection of non-neurological side effects, reflecting the large number of neurotransmitter systems affected by these drugs. Non-neurological side effects range from the common and under-recognized effects of weight gain and sexual dysfunction, which can be quite distressing to patients, to the rare but potentially lethal side effects of NMS and sudden cardiac arrhythmias. As neurological side effects become less pronounced with the newer atypical agents, attention should increasingly be paid to the non-neurological side effects which also significantly affect outcome and compliance. A broad understanding of many physiological systems is necessary to predict, diagnose and manage this wide range of adverse effects.

References

Addonizio, G. (1985) Rapid induction of extrapyramidal side effects with combined use of lithium and neuroleptics. *Journal of Clinical Psychopharmacology*, **5**, 296–298.

Addonizio, G., Susman, V.L. & Roth, S.D. (1986) Symptoms of neuroleptic malignant syndrome in 82 consecutive inpatients. *American Journal of Psychiatry*, **143**, 1587–1590.

Addonizio, G., Susman, V.L. & Roth, S.D. (1987) Neuroleptic malignant syndrome: review and analysis of 115 cases. *Biological Psychiatry*, **22**, 1004–1020.

Adityanjee, Singh, S., Singh, G. & Ong, S. (1988) Spectrum concept of neuroleptic malignant syndrome. *British Journal of Psychiatry*, **153**, 107–111.

Aherwadker, S.J., Eferdigil, M.C. & Coulshed, N. (1964) Chlorpromazine therapy and associated acute disturbances of cardiac rhythm. *British Heart Journal*, **36**, 1251–1252.

Alexander, S., Shader, R. & Grinspoon, L. (1967) Electrocardiographic effects of thioridazine hydrochloride (Mellaril). *Lakey Clinic Foundation Bulletin*, **16**, 207–215.

Aljouni, K., Kern, M.W., Tures, J.F., Theil, G.B. & Hagan, T.C. (1974) Thiothixene-induced hyponatremia. *Archives of Internal Medicine*, **134**, 1103–1105.

Amdisen, A. (1964) Drug-produced obesity: experiences with chlorpromazine, perphenazine, and clopenthixol. *Danish Medical Bulletin*, **11**, 182–189.

Amsler, H.A., Teerenhovi, L., Barth, E., Harjula, K. & Vuopio, P. (1977) Agranulocytosis in patients treated with clozapine. A study of the Finnish epidemic. *Acta Psychiatrica Scandanavia*, **56**, 241–248.

Ananth, J.V., Ban, T.A., Lehmann, H.E. & Rizvi, F.A. (1972) A survey of phenothiazine-induced skin pigmentation. *Indian Journal of Psychiatry*, **14**, 76–80.

Anderson, E.S. & Powers, P.S. (1991) Neuroleptic malignant syndrome associated with clozapine use. *Journal of Clinical Psychiatry*, **52**, 102–104.

Anton-Stephens, D. (1953) Preliminary observations on the psychiatric use of chlorpromazine. *Journal of Mental Science*, **100**, 543–547.

Arnold, P., Racine, R.J. & Wise, R. (1974) Effect of atropine, reserpine, 6-OHDA and handling on seizure development in the rat. *Experimental Neurology*, **45**, 355–363.

Asberg, M., Cronholm, B., Sjooqvist, F. & Tuck, D. (1970) Correlation of subjective side effects with plasma concentrations of nortriptyline. *British Medical Journal*, **4**, 18–21.

Ataya, K., Mercado, A., Kartaginer, J., Abbasi, A. & Moghissi, K.S. (1988) Bone density and reproductive hormones in patients with neuroleptic-induced hyperprolactinemia. *Fertility and Sterility*, **50**, 876–881.

Backman, H. & Elosuo, R. (1964) Electrocardiographic findings in connection with a clinical trial of chlorpromazine. With particular references to T-wave changes and the duration of ventricular activity. *Annals of Medicine Internal Fenn*, **53**, 1–8.

Baker, L.A., Cheng, L.Y. & Amara, I.B. (1983) The withdrawal of benztropine mesylate in chronic schizophrenic patients. *British Journal of Psychiatry*, **143**, 584–590.

Baldessarini, R. (1985) *Chemotherapy in Psychiatry: Principles and Practice*, 2nd edn. Harvard University Press, Cambridge.

Baldessarini, R.J. & Frankenburg, R. (1991) Clozapine — a novel antipsychotic agent. *New England Journal of Medicine*, **324**, 746–754.

Baldessarini, R.J. & Lipinski, J.F. (1976) Toxicity and side effects of antipsychotic, antimanic and antidepressant medications. *Psychiatry Annals*, **6**, 484–493.

Ban, T.A. & Lehmann, H.E. (1965) Skin pigmentation, a rare side effect of chlorpromazine. *Canadian Psychiatric Association Journal*, **10**, 112–124.

Ban, T.A. & St Jean, A. (1964) The effects of phenothiazines on the electrocardiogram. *Canadian Medical Association Journal*, **91**, 537–540.

Ban, T.A., Guy, W. & Wilson, W.H. (1985) Neuroleptic-induced skin pigmentation in chronic hospitalized schizophrenic patients. *Canadian Journal of Psychiatry*, **30**, 406–408.

Barnes, T. & Bridges, P.K. (1980) Disturbed behaviour induced by high-dose antipsychotic drugs. *British Medical Journal*, **281**, 274–275.

Barnes, T.R.E., Curson, D.A., Liddle, P.F. & Patel, M. (1989) The nature and prevalence of depression in chronic schizophrenic in-patients. *British Journal of Psychiatry*, **154**, 486–491.

Barron, C.N., Murchison, T.E., Rubin, M.L., Herron, W., Muscarella, M. & Birkhead, H. (1972) Chlorpromazine and the eye of the dog. VI. A comparison of phenothiazine tranquilizers. *Experimental and Molecular Pathology*, **16**, 172–179.

Bartholomew, A.A. (1986) A long-acting phenothiazine as a possible agent to control deviant sexual behavior. *American Journal of Psychiatry*, **124**, 77–83.

Bartholomew, L.G., Cain, J.G., Frazier, S. *et al.* (1958) Effect of chlorpromazine on the liver. *Gastroenterology*, **34**, 1096–1107.

Belmaker, R.H. & Wald, D. (1977) Haloperidol in normals. *British Journal of Psychiatry*, **131**, 222–223.

Berger, S.H. (1979) Trifluoperazine and haloperidol. Sources of ejaculatory pain? *American Journal of Psychiatry*, **136**, 350.

Berman, K.F., Zec, R.F. & Weinberger, D.R. (1986) Physiologic dysfunction of dorsolateral prefrontal cortex in schizophrenia. II. Role of neuroleptic treatment, attention, and mental effort. *Archives of General Psychiatry*, **43**, 126–135.

Bernstein, J.G. (1987) Induction of obesity by psychotropic drugs. *Annals of the New York Academy of Sciences*, **499**, 203–215.

Bertram, U., Kragh-Sorenson, P., Rafaelson, O.J. & Larsen, N. (1979) Saliva secretion following long-term antidepressant treatment with nortriptyline controlled by plasma levels. *Scandinavian Journal of Dental Research*, **87**, 58–64.

Blair, J. & Simpson, G. (1966) Effect of antipsychotic drugs on reproductive functions. *Diseases of the Nervous System*, **27**, 645–647.

Blumberg, A.G., Klein, D.F. & Pollack, M. (1964) Effects of chlorpromazine and imipramine on systolic blood pressure in psychiatric patients: relationship to age, diagnosis and initial blood pressure. *Journal of Psychiatry Research*, **2**, 51–60.

Bourgeois-Govardin, M., Nowill, W.K., Margolis, G. & Stephen, C.R. (1955) Chlorpromazine: a laboratory and clinical investigation. *Anesthesiology*, **16**, 829–847.

Boyd, E.M (1960) Chlorpromazine tolerance and physical dependence. *Journal of Pharmacology and Experimental Therapeutics*, **128**, 75.

Brill, M. & Patton, R.E. (1962) Clinical–statistical analysis of population changes in New York state mental hospitals since the introduction of psychotropic drugs. *American Journal of Psychiatry*, **119**, 20–33.

Buchanan, A. (1992) A two-year prospective study of treatment compliance in patients with schizophrenia. *Psychological Medicine*, **22**, 787–797.

Buis, W. (1992) Patients' opinions concerning side effects of depot neuroleptic (letter). *American Journal of Psychiatry*, **149**, 844–845.

Caine, E.D. & Polinsky, R.J. (1979) Haloperidol-induced dysphoria in patients with Tourette syndrome. *American Journal of Psychiatry*, **136**, 1216–1217.

Cassens, G., Inglis, A.K., Appelbaum, P.S. & Gutheil, T.G. (1990) Neuroleptics: effects on neuropsychological function in chronic schizophrenic patients. *Schizophrenia Bulletin*, **16**, 477–499.

Chen, G., Ensor, C.R. & Bohner, B. (1968) Studies of drug effects on electrically induced extensor seizures and clinical implications. *Archives Internationales de Pharmacodynamie et de Therapie*, **172**, 183–218.

Chignell, C.F., Motten, A.G. & Buettner, G.R. (1985) Photo-induced free radicals from chlorpromazine and related phenothiazines: relationship to phenothiazine-induced photosensitization. *Environmental Health Perspectives*, **64**, 103–110.

Claas, F.H.J. (1989) Drug-induced agranulocytosis: review of possible mechanisms, and prospects for clozapine studies. *Psychopharmacology*, **99**(Suppl.), 113–117.

Clein, L. (1962) Thioridazine and ejaculation. *British Medical Journal*, **2**, 548–549.

Cobb, C.D., Anderson, C.B. & Seidel, D.R. (1991) Possible interaction between clozapine and lorazepam (letter). *American Journal of Psychiatry*, **148**, 1606–1607.

Cohen, S., Chiles, J. & MacNaughton, A. (1990) Weight gain associated with clozapine. *American Journal of Psychiatry*, **147**, 503–504.

Cole, J.O. (1982) Psychopharmacology update: antipsychotic drugs: is more better? *McLean Hospital Journal*, **7**, 61–87.

Craig, T.J., Richardson, M.A., Bark, N.J. & Klebanov, R. (1982) Impairment of swallowing, tardive dyskinesia, and anticholinergic use. *Psychopharmacology Bulletin*, **18**, 84–86.

Crane, G.E. (1967) A review of clinical literature on haloperidol. *International Journal of Neuropsychiatry*, **3**, 110–127.

DasGupta, K. & Young, A. (1991) Clozapine-induced neuroleptic malignant syndrome. *Journal of Clinical Psychiatry*, **52**, 105–107.

Davis, J.T. & Nusbaum, M. (1973) Chlorpromazine therapy and functional large bowel obstruction. *American Journal of Gastroenterology*, **60**, 635–639.

Degen, K. (1982) Sexual dysfunction in women using major tranquilizers. *Psychosomatics*, **23**, 959–961.

Descotes, J., Lievre, M., Ollagnier, M., Faucon, G. & Evreux, J.C. (1979) Study of thioridazine cardiotoxic effects by means of his bundle activity recording. *Acta Pharmacologia et Toxicologica*, **44**, 370–376.

Devinsky, O., Honigfeld, G. & Patin, J. (1991) Clozapine-related seizures. *Neurology*, **41**, 369–371.

Dickes, R., Schenker, V. & Deutsch, L. (1957) Serial liver function and blood studies in patients receiving chlorpromazine. *New England Journal of Medicine*, **256**, 1–7.

Dincsoy, H. & Saelinger, D.A. (1982) Haloperidol-induced chronic cholestatic liver disease. *Gastroenterology*, **83**, 694–700.

Dorman, B.W. & Schmidt, J.D. (1976) Association of priapism in phenothiazine therapy. *Journal of Urology*, **116**, 51–53.

Ereshefsky, M.D., Watanabe, M.D. & Tran-Johnson, T.K. (1989) Clozapine: an atypical antipsychotic agent. *Clinical Pharmacy*, **8**, 691–709.

Evans, D.L., Rogers, J.F. & Peiper, S.C. (1979) Intestinal dilatation associated with phenothiazine therapy: a case report and literature review. *Journal of Psychiatry*, **136**, 970–972.

Falloon, I., Watt, D. & Shepard, M. (1978) Pimozide and fluphenazine decanoate in continuation therapy. *Psychological Medicine*, **8**, 59–70.

Fellner, C.H. (1958) A clinical note on drug-induced depression. *American Journal of Psychiatry*, **115**, 547–548.

Finn, S.E., Bailey, J.M., Schultz, R.T. & Faber, R. (1990) Subjective utility ratings of neuroleptics in treating schizophrenia. *Psychological Medicine*, **20**, 843–848.

Flemenbaum, A. (1976) Pavor nocturnus: a complication of single daily tricyclic or neuroleptic dosage. *American Journal of Psychiatry*, **133**, 570–572.

Foster, C.A., O'Mullane, E.J., Gaskell, P. & Churchill-Davidson, H.C. (1954) Chlorpromazine: a study of its action in man. *Lancet*, **2**, 614–617.

Fraunfelder, F.T. & Meyer, S.M. (1982) *Drug-Induced Ocular Side Effects and Drug Interactions*, 2nd edn. Lea & Febiger, Philadelphia.

Freyhan, F. (1961) Loss of ejaculation during mellaril treatment. *American Journal of Psychiatry*, **118**, 171–172.

Friedman, J.H., Feinberg, S.S. & Feldman, R.G. (1985) A neuroleptic malignant-like syndrome due to levodopa therapy withdrawal. *Journal of the American Medical Association*, **254**, 2792–2795.

Friedman, L.J., Tabb, S.E. & Sanchez, C.J. (1991) Clozapine — a novel antipsychotic agent (letter). *New England Journal of Medicine*, **325**, 518.

Fuller, C.M., Yassinger, S., Donlon, P., Imperato, T.J. & Ruebner, B. (1977) Haloperidol-induced liver disease. *Western Journal of Medicine*, **127**, 515–518.

Gallant, D.M. & Bishop, M.P. (1968) Molindone: a controlled evaluation in chronic schizophrenic patients. *Current Therapeutic Research*, **10**, 441–447.

Ganguli, R. & Raghu, U. (1985) Tardive dyskinesia, impaired recall, and informal consent. *Journal of Clinical Psychiatry*, **46**, 434–435.

Gardos, G. & Cole, J.O. (1977) Weight reduction in schizophrenics by molindone. *American Journal of Psychiatry*, **134**, 302–304.

Ghadirian, A.M., Chouinard, G. & Annable, L. (1982) Sexual dysfunction and plasma prolactin levels in neuroleptic-treated schizophrenic outpatients. *Journal of Nervous and Mental Disease*, **170**, 463–467.

Giles, T.O. & Modlin, R.K. (1968) Death associated with ventricular arrhythmias and thioridazine hydrochloride. *Journal of the American Medical Association*, **205**, 108–110.

Giordano, J., Huang, A. & Canter, J.W. (1975) Fatal paralytic ileus complicating phenothiazine therapy. *Southern Medical Journal*, **68**, 351–353.

Glusac, E., Patel, H., Josef, N.C. & Yeragani, V.K. (1990) Polydipsia and hyponatremia induced by multiple neuroleptics but not molindone. *Canadian Journal of Psychiatry*, **35**, 268–269.

Goff, D. & Baldessarini, R. (1993) Drug interactions with antipsychotic agents. *Journal of Clinical Psychopharmacology*, **13**, 57–67.

Green, A.I. & Brown, W.A. (1988) Prolactin and neuroleptic drugs. *Endocrinology and Metabolism Clinics of North America*, **17**, 213–223.

Greenberg, H. (1971) Inhibition of ejaculation by chlorpromazine. *Journal of Nervous and Mental Disease*, **152**, 364–366.

Greenberg, S.M., Ellison, T. & Mathues, J.K. (1962) Comparative studies of growth-stimulating properties of phenothiazine analogs in the rat. *Journal of Nutrition*, **76**, 302–309.

Greiner, A.C. & Berry, K. (1964) Skin pigmentation and corneal and lens opacities with prolonged chlorpromazine therapy. *Canadian Medical Association Journal*, **90**, 663–664.

Grohmann, R., Ruther, E., Sassim, N. & Schmidt, L.G. (1989) Adverse effects of clozapine. *Psychopharmacology*, **99** (Suppl.), 101–104.

Gruen, P.H., Sacher, E.J., Altman, N., Langer, G., Tabrizi, M.A. & Halpern, F.S. (1978a) Relation of plasma prolactin to clinical response in schizophrenic patients. *Archives of General Psychiatry*, **35**, 1222–1227.

Gruen, P.H., Sacher, E.J., Langer, G. *et al.* (1978b) Prolactin responses to neuroleptics in normal and schizophrenics subjects. *Archives of General Psychiatry*, **35**, 108–116.

Gupta, N.N., Pant, S.S. & Mehrotra, R.M.L. (1962) Toxic effects of chlorpromazine with special reference to jaundice. *Indian Journal of Medical Science*, **16**, 315–323.

Gurrera, R.J., Chang, S.S. & Romero, J.A. (1992) A comparison of diagnostic criteria for neuroleptic malignant syndrome. *Journal of Clinical Psychiatry*, **53**, 56–62.

Haider, I. (1966) Thioridazine and sexual dysfunction. *International Journal of Neuropsychiatry*, **5**, 255–257.

Heller, J. (1961) Another case of inhibition of ejaculation as a side effect of mellaril. *American Journal of Psychiatry*, **118**, 173.

Hogan, T.P. & Awad, A.G. (1992) Subjective response to neuroleptics and outcome in schizophrenia: a re-examination comparing two measures. *Psychological Medicine*, **22**, 347–352.

Hogan, T.P., Awad, A.G. & Eastwood, M.R. (1983) A self-report scale predictive of drug compliance in schizophrenics: reliability and discriminative validity. *Psychological Medicine*, **13**, 177–183.

Huapaya, L. (1976) Somnambulism and bedtime medication (letter). *American Journal of Psychiatry*, **133**, 1207.

Husser, A.E. & Bragg, D.G. (1969) The effect of chlorpromazine on the swallowing function in chronic schizophrenic patients. *American Journal of Psychiatry*, **126**, 570–573.

Huston, J.R. & Bell, G.E. (1966) The effect of thioridazine hydrochloride and chlorpromazine on the electrocardiogram. *Journal of the American Medical Association*, **198**, 16–20.

Igarashi, Y., Higuchi, T., Toyoshima, R., Noguchi, T. & Moroji, T. (1985) Tolerance to prolactin secretion in the long-term treatment with neuroleptics in schizophrenia. *Advances in Biochemical Psychopharmacology*, **40**, 95–98.

Illowsky, B.P. & Kirch, D.G. (1988) Polydipsia and hyponatremia in psychiatric patients. *American Journal of Psychiatry*, **145**, 675–683.

Irwin, D.S., Weitzel, W.D. & Morgan, D.W. (1971) Phenothiazine intake and staff attitudes. *American Journal of Psychiatry*, **127**, 1631–1635.

Ishak, K.G. & Irey, N.S. (1972) Hepatic injury associated with the phenothiazines. *Archives of Pathology*, **93**, 283–304.

Itil, T. & Soldatos, C. (1980) Epileptogenic side effects of psychotropic drugs. *Journal of the American Medical Association*, **244**, 1460–1463.

Jefferson, J.J. & Marshall, J.R. (1981) *Neuropsychiatric Features of Medical Disorders*, Plenum Press, New York.

Jick, O., Miettinen, O.S., Shapiro, S., Lewis, G.P., Siskind, V. & Slone, D. (1970) Comprehensive drug surveillance. *Journal of the American Medical Association*, **213**, 1455–1460.

Judson, A.M. & MacCasland, B.W. (1960) The effects of chlorpromazine on psychological test scores. *Journal of Consulting Psychology*, **24**, 192.

Kaminer, Y. & Munitz, H. (1984) Case report: psychomotor status-like episodes under haloperidol treatment. *British Journal of Psychiatry*, **145**, 87–90.

Kane, J.M. (1985) Antipsychotic drug side effects: their relationship to dose. *Journal of Clinical Psychiatry*, **46**, 16–21.

Kaplowitz, N., Aw, T.Y., Simon, F.R. & Stolz, A. (1986) Drug-induced hepatotoxicity. *Annals of Internal Medicine*, **104**, 826–839.

Keck, P.E.J., Pope, H.G.J. & McElroy, S.L. (1987) Frequency and presentation of neuroleptic malignant syndrome: a prospective study. *American Journal of Psychiatry*, **144**, 1344–1346.

Keck, P.E.J., Pope, H.G.J. & McElroy, S.L. (1991) Declining frequency of neuroleptic malignant syndrome in a hospital population. *American Journal of Psychiatry*, **148**, 880–882.

Keck, P.J., Pope, H., Cohen, B., McElroy, S. & Nierenberg, A. (1989) Risk factors for neuroleptic malignant syndrome. A case control study. *Archives of General Psychiatry*, **46**, 914–918.

Keks, N.A., Copolov, D.L. & Singh, B.S. (1987) Abnormal prolactin response to haloperidol challenge in men with schizophrenia. *American Journal of Psychiatry*, **144**, 1335–1337.

Kellner, R., Rada, R.T., Egelman, A. & Macaluso, B. (1976) Long-term study of molindone hydrochloride in chronic schizophrenia. *Current Therapeutic Research*, **20**, 686–693.

Kemeny, M.M., Martin, E.C., Lane, F.C. & Stillman, R.M. (1980) Abdominal distension and aortic obstruction associated with phenothiazines. *Journal of the American Medical Association*, **243**, 683–684.

Kendler, K.S., Weitzman, R.E. & Rubin, R.T. (1978) Lack of arginine vasopressin response to central dopamine blockade in normal adults. *Journal of Clinical Endocrinology and Metabolism*, **47**, 204–207.

King, D.J. (1990) The effect of neuroleptics on cognitive and psychomotor function. *British Journal of Psychiatry*, **157**, 799–811.

Klett, C.J. & Caffey, E.M.J. (1960) Weight changes during treatment with phenothiazine derivatives. *Journal of Neuropsychiatry*, **2**, 102–108.

Klibanski, A., Neer, R. & Beitins, I. (1981) Decreased bone density in hyperprolactinemic women. *New England Journal of Medicine*, **303**, 1511–1514.

Knights, A. & Hirsch, S.R. (1981) 'Revealed' depression and drug treatment for schizophrenia. *Archives of General Psychiatry*, **38**, 806–811.

Kolakowski, T., Braddock, L., Wiles, D., Franklin, M. & Gelder, M. (1981) Neuroendocrine tests during treatment with neuroleptic drugs. I. Plasma prolactin response to haloperidol challenge. *British Journal of Psychiatry*, **139**, 400–412.

Kornetsky, C. (1960) Alterations in psychomotor functions and individual differences in responses produced by psychoactive drugs. In Uhr, L. & Miller, I.G. (eds) *Drugs and Behavior*, pp. 297–312. Wiley, New York.

Kornetsky, C. (1972) The use of a simple test of attention as a measure of drug effects in schizophrenic patients. *Psychopharmacologia*, **24**, 99–106.

Kornetsky, C., Pettit, M., Wynne, R. & Evarts, E.V. (1959) A comparison of the psychological effects of acute and chronic administration of chlorpromazine and secobarbital (quinalbarbitone) in schizophrenic patients. *Journal of Mental Science*, **105**, 190–198.

Korol, B., Lang, W.J., Brown, M.L. & Gershon, S. (1965) Effects of chronic chlorpromazine administration on systemic arterial pressure in schizophrenic patients. Relationship of body position to blood pressure. *Clinical Pharmacology and Therapeutics*, **6**, 587–591.

Kotin, J., Wilbert, D.E., Verburg, D. & Soldinger, S.M. (1976) Thioridazine and sexual dysfunction. *American Journal of Psychiatry*, **133**, 82–85.

Krupp, P. & Barnes, P. (1989) Leponex-associated granulocytopenia: a review of the situation. *Psychopharmacology*, **99** (Suppl.), 118–121.

Lamberti, J.S., Bellnier, T. & Schwarzkopf, S.B. (1992) Weight gain among schizophrenic patients treated with clozapine. *American Journal of Psychiatry*, **149**, 689–690.

Latz, A. & Kornetsky, C. (1965) The effects of chlorpromazine and secobarbital under two conditions of reinforcement on the performance of chronic schizophrenic subjects. *Psychopharmacologia*, **7**, 77–88.

Laughren, T.P., Brown, W.A. & Williams, B.W. (1979) Serum prolactin and clinical state during neuroleptic treatment and withdrawal. *American Journal of Psychiatry*, **136**, 108–110.

Laursen, T. & Borup Svendsen, B. (1959) Glutamic pyruvic transaminase in the serum during treatment with chlorpromazine. *Danish Medical Bulletin*, **6**, 38–42.

Lazarus, A. (1989) Differentiating neuroleptic-related heatstroke from neuroleptic malignant syndrome. *Psychosomatics*, **30**, 454–456.

Leadbetter, R., Shutty, M., Pavalonis, D., Vieweg, V., Higgins, P. & Downs, M. (1992) Clozapine-induced weight gain: prevalence and clinical relevance. *American Journal of Psychiatry*, **149**, 68–72.

Leestma, J.E. & Koenig, K.L. (1968) Sudden death and phenothiazines. *Archives of General Psychiatry*, **18**, 137–148.

Leipzig, R.M. (1992) Gastrointestinal and hepatic effects of psychotropic drugs. In Lieberman, J.A. & Kane, J.M. (eds) *Adverse Effects of Pyschotropic Drugs*, pp. 408–430. Guilford Press, New York.

Levenson, J.L. (1985) Neuroleptic malignant syndrome. *American Journal of Psychiatry*, **142**, 1137–1145.

Levinson, D.F. & Simpson, G.M. (1987) Serious nonextrapyramidal adverse effects on neuroleptics-sudden death, agranulocytosis and hepatotoxicity. In Meltzer, H. (ed.) *Psychopharmacology: The Third Generation of Progress*, pp. 1431–1436. Raven Press, New York.

Leznoff, A. & Binkley, K.E. (1992) Adverse cutaneous reactions associated with fluoxetine: strategy for reintroduction of this drug in selected patients. *Journal of Clinical Psychopharmacology*, **12**, 355–357.

Lieberman, J.A., Johns, C.A., Kane, J.M. *et al.* (1988) Clozapine-induced agranulocytosis: non-cross reactivity with other psychotropic drugs. *Journal of Clinical Psychiatry*, **49**, 271–277.

Lieberman, J.A., Yunis, J., Egea, E., Canoso, R.T., Kane, J.M. & Yunis, E.J. (1990) HLA-B38, DR4, DQW 3 and clozapine-induced agranulocytosis in Jewish patients with schizophrenia. *Archives of General Psychiatry*, **47**, 945–948.

Liljequist, R., Linnoila, M. & Mattila, M.J. (1978) Effect of diazepam and chlorpromazine on memory functions in man. *European Journal of Clinical Pharmacology*, **14**, 339–343.

Liljequist, R., Linnoila, A., Mattila, M.J., Saario, I. & Seppala, T. (1975) Effects of two-weeks treatment with thioridazine, chlorpromazine, sulpiride, and bromazepam alone or in combination with alcohol. *Psychopharmacologia*, **44**, 205–208.

Lingjaerde, O., Ahlfors, U.G., Bech, P., Dencker, S.J. & Elgen, K. (1987) The UKU side effect rating scale. *Acta*

Psychiatrica Scandinavica, **334** (Suppl. 76), 1–100.

Linnoila, M. (1973) Effects of diazepam, chlorpromazine, thioridazine, haloperidol, flupenthixol, and alcohol on psychomotor skills related to driving. *Annals Medicinae Experimentacts et Biologiae Fenniae*, **51**, 125–132.

Linnoila, M. & Maki, M. (1974) Acute effects of alcohol, diazepam, thioridazine, flupenthixol, and atropine on psychomotor performance profiles. *Arzneimittel-Forschung*, **24(4)**, 565–569.

Litvak, R. & Kaelblin, G. (1971) Agranulocytosis, leukopenia and psychotropic drugs. *Archives of General Psychiatry*, **24**, 265–267.

Logothetis, J. (1967) Spontaneous epileptic seizures and electroencephalographic changes in the course of phenothiazine therapy. *Neurology*, **17**, 869–877,

McClellan, T.A. & Cowan, G. (1970) Use of antipsychotic and antidepressant drugs by chronically ill patients. *American Journal of Psychiatry*, **126**, 1771–1773.

McGlashan, T.H. & Carpenter, W.T.J. (1976) Postpsychotic depression in schizophrenia. *Archives of General Psychiatry*, **33**, 231–239.

McKenzie, G.M. & Soroko, F.E. (1972) The effects of apomorphine, (+)-amphetamine and L-dopa on maximal electroshock convulsions — a comparative study in the rat and mouse. *Journal of Pharmacy and Pharmacology*, **24**, 696–701.

Maltbie, A.A., Varia, I.G. & Thomas, N.V. (1981) Ileus complicating haloperidol therapy. *Psychosomatics*, **22**, 158–159.

Mandel, A. & Gross, M. (1968) Leukopenia and psychotropic drugs. *Archives of General Psychiatry*, **24**, 265–267.

Mann, S.C., Caroff, S.N. & Bleier, H.R. (1986) Lethal catatonia. *American Journal of Psychiatry*, **143**, 1374–1381.

Marder, S.R., Van Putten, T., Mintz, J. *et al.* (1984) Costs and benefits of two doses of fluphenazine. *Archives of General Psychiatry*, **41**, 1025–1029.

May, P.R.A., Van Putten, T., Jenden, D.J., Yale, C., Dixon, W.J. & Goldstein, M.J. (1981) Prognosis in schizophrenia: individual differences in psychological response to a test dose of antipsychotic drug and their relationship to blood and saliva levels and treatment outcome. *Comprehensive Psychiatry*, **22**, 147–152.

May, P.R.A., Van Putten, T. & Yale, C. (1976) Predicting individual responses to drug treatment in schizophrenia: a test dose model. *Journal of Nervous and Mental Disease*, **162**, 177–183.

Mayer-Gross, W. (1920) Ueber die Stellungnahme zur abgelaufenen akuten Psychose. Eine Studiueber verstandliche Zusammenhange in der Schizophrenie (The attitude towards past acute psychosis. A study on the intelligible context of schizophrenia.). *Zeitschrift für die Gesamte Neurologie und Psychiatrie*, **60**, 160–212.

Meldrum, B., Anlezark, G. & Trimble, M. (1975) Drugs modifying dopaminergic activity and behaviour, the EEG and epilepsy in *Papio papio*. *European Journal of Pharmacology*, **32**, 202–213.

Merkin, T.E. (1977) Priapism as a sequela of chlorpromazine therapy. *JACEP*, **6**, 367–368.

Messing, R.O., Closson, R.G. & Simon, R.P. (1984) Drug-

induced seizures: a 10-year experience. *Neurology*, **17**, 869–877.

Metzger, E. & Friedman, R. (1993) Prolongation of the corrected QT and Torsades de Pointes cardiac arrhythmia associated with intravenous haloperidol in the medically ill. *Journal of Clinical Psychopharmacology*, **13**, 128–132.

Miller, D.D., Sharafuddin, M.J.A. & Kathol, R.G. (1991) A case of clozapine-induced neuroleptic malignant syndrome. *Journal of Clinical Psychiatry*, **52**, 99–101.

Millichap, J.G., Pitchford, G.L. & Millichap, M.G. (1968) Anticonvulsant activity of antiparkinsonism agents. *Proceedings of the Society for Experimental Biology and Medicine*, **127**, 1187–1190.

Mitchell, J.E. & Popkin, M.K. (1982) Antipsychotic drug therapy and sexual dysfunction in men. *American Journal of Psychiatry*, **139**, 633–637.

Moore, M.T. & Book, M.H. (1969) Sudden death in phenothiazine therapy. *Psychiatric Quarterly*, **40**, 389–402.

Nestores, J.N., Lehmann, H.E. & Ben, T.A. (1980) Neuroleptic drugs and sexual function in schizophrenics. *Modern Problems in Pharmacopsychiatry*, **15**, 111–130.

Ojemann, L.M., Baugh-Bookman, C. & Dudley, D.L. (1987) Effect of psychotropic medications on seizure control in patients with epilepsy. *Neurology*, **37**, 1525–1527.

Oles, M. (1960) Klinische Erfahrungen mit dem neuroleptikum Haloperidol (R 1625). *Archives of Neurology and Psychiatry*, **60**, 100–107.

Oliver, A.P., Luchins, D.J. & Wyatt, R.J. (1982) Neuroleptic-induced seizures. An *in vitro* technique for assessing relative risk. *Archives of General Psychiatry*, **39**, 206–209.

Opler, L.A. & Feinberg, S.S. (1991) The role of pimozide in clinical psychiatry: a review. *Journal of Clinical Psychiatry*, **52**, 221–233.

Overall, J. (1978) Prior psychiatric treatment and the development of breast cancer. *Archives of General Psychiatry*, **35**, 898–899.

Parkes, C.M., Brown, G.W. & Monck, E.M. (1962) The general practitioner and the schizophrenic patient. *British Medical Journal*, **1**, 972–976.

Peck, P. & Shenkman, L. (1979) Haloperidol-induced syndrome of inappropriate secretion of antidiuretic hormone. *Clinical Pharmacology and Therapeutics*, **26**, 442–444.

Pisciotta, A.V. (1969) Agranulocytosis induced by certain phenothiazine derivatives. *Journal of the American Medical Association*, **208**, 1862–1868.

Pisciotta, A.V. (1971) Studies on agranulocytosis: a biochemical defect in chlorpromazine-sensitive marrow cells. *Journal of Laboratory and Clinical Medicine*, **78**, 435–448.

Pisciotta, A.V. (1973) Immune and toxic mechanisms in drug-induced agranulocytosis. *Seminars in Hematology*, **10**, 279–310.

Pisciotta, A.V. (1992) Hematologic reactions associated with psychotropic drugs. In Lieberman, J.A. & Kane, J.M. (eds) *Adverse Effects of Psychotropic Drugs*. Guilford Press, New York.

Plante, N. & Roy, P. (1967) Galactorrhea and neuroleptics. *Laval Medical*, **38**, 103–107.

Prien, R.F., DeLong, S.L., Cole, J.O. & Levine, J. (1970) Ocular changes occurring with prolonged high-dose chlorpromazine therapy. *Archives of General Psychiatry*, **23**, 464–468.

Raskind, M.A., Courtney, N. & Mursburg, M.M. (1987) Antipsychotic drugs and plasma vasopressin in normals and acute schizophrenic patients. *Biological Psychiatry*, **22**, 453–462.

Reilly, E.L., Wilson, W.P. & McClinton, H.K. (1967) Clinical characteristics and medication history of schizophrenics readmitted to the hospital. *International Journal of Neuropsychiatry*, **3**, 85–90.

Remick, R.A. & Fine, S.H. (1979) Antipsychotic drugs and seizures. *Journal of Clinical Psychiatry*, **40**, 78–80.

Renton, C.A., Affleck, J.W., Carstairs, G.M. & Forrest, A.D. (1963) A follow-up of schizophrenic patients in Edinburgh. *Acta Psychiatrica Scandinavica*, **39**, 548–581.

Reynolds, R.W. & Carlisle, H.J. (1961) The effect of chlorpromazine on food intake in the albino rat. *Journal of Comparative and Physiological Psychology*, **54**, 354.

Richardson, H.L., Graupner, K.I. & Richardson, M.E. (1966) Intramyocardial lesions in patients dying suddenly and unexpectedly. *Journal of the American Medical Association*, **195**, 254–260.

Richelson, E. (1984) Neuroleptic affinities for human brain receptors and their use in predicting adverse effects. *Journal of Clinical Psychiatry*, **45**, 331–336.

Risch, S.C., Groom, G.P. & Janowsky, D.S. (1981) Interfaces of psychopharmacology and cardiology — part two. *Journal of Clinical Psychiatry*, **42**, 47–57.

Robertson, M.M. & Trimble, M.R. (1982) Major tranquillizers used as antidepressants: a review. *Journal of Affective Disorders*, **4**, 173–193.

Robinson, B. (1957) Breast changes in the male and female with chlorpromazine or reserpine therapy. *Medical Journal of Australia*, **44**, 239–241.

Robinson, R.G., McHugh, P.R. & Folstein, M.F. (1975) Measurement of appetite disturbance in psychiatric disorders. *Journal of Psychiatric Research*, **12**, 59–68.

Rogers, G.A. & Burke, G. (1987) Neuroleptics, prolactin and osteoporosis. *American Journal of Psychiatry*, **144**, 388–389.

Rosebush, P.I., Stewart, T. & Mazurek, M.F. (1991) The treatment of neuroleptic malignant syndrome: are Dantrolene and Bromocriptine useful adjuncts to supportive care? *British Journal of Psychiatry*, **159**, 709–712.

Rosebush, P.I., Stewart, T.D. & Gelenberg, A.J. (1989) Twenty neuroleptic rechallenges after neuroleptic malignant syndrome in 15 patients. *Journal of Clinical Psychiatry*, **50**, 295–298.

Rubin, R.T. (1987) Prolactin and schizophrenia. In Meltzer, H. (ed.) *Psychopharmacology: The Third Generation of Progress*, pp. 803–808. Raven Press, New York.

Sakkas, P., Davis, J.M., Janicak, P.G. & Wang, Z. (1991) Drug treatment of the neuroleptic malignant syndrome. *Psychopharmacology Bulletin*, **27**, 381–384.

Samuels, A.M. & Carey, M.C. (1978) Effects of chlorpromazine hydrochloride and its metabolites on Mg^{2+} and Na^+, K^+-ATPase activities of canalicular-enriched rat liver plasma membranes. *Gastroenterology*, **74**, 1183–1190.

Sanberg, P.R. & Norman, A.B. (1989) Underrecognized and underresearched side effects of neuroleptics. *American Journal of Psychiatry*, **146**, 411–412.

Sandison, R.A., Whitelaw, E. & Currie, J.D. (1960) Clinical trials with Mellaril in the treatment of schizophrenia. *Journal of Mental Science*, **106**, 732–741.

Sarai, M. & Matsunaga, H. (1989) ADH secretion in schizophrenic patients on antipsychotic drugs. *Biological Psychiatry*, **26**, 576–580.

Schlichther, W., Bristow, M.E., Schultz, S. & Henderson, A.C. (1956) Seizures occurring during intensive chlorpromazine therapy. *Canadian Medical Association Journal*, **74**, 364–366.

Selye, H. & Szabo, S. (1972) Protection against haloperidol by catatoxic steroids. *Psychopharmacologica*, **24**, 430–434.

Shader, R. (1972) Sexual dysfunction associated with mesoridazine besylate (Serentil). *Psychopharmacologia*, **27**.

Shader, R.I. (1964) Sexual dysfunction associated with thioridazine hydrochloride. *Journal of the American Medical Association*, **188**, 1007–1009.

Shay, H. & Siplet, H. (1957) Study of Chlorpromazine jaundice, its mechanism and prevention; special reference to serum alkaline phosphatase and glutamic oxalacetic transaminase. *Gastroenterology*, **32**, 571–591.

Sherlock, S. (1979) Progress report. Hepatic reactions to drugs. *Gut*, **20**, 634–648.

Sherlock, S. (1989) Drugs and the liver. In Sherlock, S. (ed.) *Diseases of the Liver and Biliary System*, pp. 372–409. Blackwell Scientific Publications, Oxford.

Siddall, J.R. (1968) Ocular complications related to phenothiazines. *Diseases of the Nervous System*, **29** (Suppl.), 10–13.

Silver, H., Kogan, H. & Zlotogorski, D. (1990) Postural hypotension in chronically medicated schizophrenics. *Journal of Clinical Psychiatry*, **51**, 459–462.

Singh, M.M. & Kay, S.R. (1979) Dysphoric response to neuroleptic treatment in schizophrenia: its relationship to autonomic arousal and prognosis. *Biological Psychiatry*, **14**, 277–294.

Sorokin, J.E., Giordani, B., Mohs, R.C. *et al.* (1988) Memory impairment in schizophrenic patients with tardive dyskinesia. *Biological Psychiatry*, **23**, 129–135.

Spohn, H.E. & Strauss, M.E. (1989) Relation of neuroleptic and anticholinergic medication to cognitive functions in schizophrenia. *Journal of Abnormal Psychology*, **98**, 367–380.

Spohn, H.E., Coyne, L., Lacoursiere, R., Mazur, D. & Hayes, K. (1985) Relation of neuroleptic dose and tardive dyskinesia to attention, information-processing, and psychophysiology in medicated schizophrenics. *Archives of General Psychiatry*, **42**, 849–859.

Sreebny, L.M. & Schwartz, S.S. (1986) A reference guide to drugs and dry mouth. *Gerontology*, **5**, 75–99.

Steiner, M., Elizur, A. & Davidson, S. (1979) Behavioral toxicity. *Confinia Psychiatrica*, **22**, 226–233.

Stolerman, I.P. (1970) Eating, drinking, and spontaneous activity in rats after the administration of chlorpromazine. *Neuropharmacology*, **9**, 405.

Struve, F.A. & Willner, A.E. (1983) Cognitive dysfunction of tardive dyskinesia. *British Journal of Psychiatry*, **143**, 597–600.

Tedeschi, D.H., Benigni, J.P., Elder, C.J., Yeager, J.C. &

Flanigan, J.V. (1958) Effects of various phenothiazines on minimal eletroshock seizure threshold and spontaneous motor activity of mice. *Journal of Pharmacology and Experimental Therapeutics*, **123**, 35–38.

Thompson, T.R., Lal, S., Yassa, R. & Gerstein, W. (1988) Resolution of chlorpromazine-induced pigmentation with haloperidol substitution. *Acta Psychiatrica Scandinavica*, **78**, 763–765.

Tomer, R. & Flor-Henry, P. (1989) Neuroleptics reverse attention asymmetries in schizophrenic patients. *Biological Psychiatry*, **25**, 852–860.

Tune, L.E., Creese, I., DePaulo, J.R., Slavney, P.R., Coyle, J.T. & Snyder, S.H. (1980) Clinical state and serum neuroleptic levels measured by radioreceptor assay in schizophrenia. *American Journal of Psychiatry*, **137**, 187–190.

Tune, L.E., Strauss, M.E., Lew, M.F., Breitlinger, E. & Coyle, J.T. (1982) Serum levels of anticholinergic drugs and impaired recent memory in chronic schizophrenic patients. *American Journal of Psychiatry*, **139**, 1460–1462.

Ulberg, S., Linguist, N. & Sjostrand, S. (1970) Accumulation of chorio-retinotoxic drugs in the foetal eye. *Nature*, **225**, 1257.

Van Putten, T. (1974) Why do schizophrenic patients refuse to take their drugs? *Archives of General Psychiatry*, **31**, 67–72.

Van Putten, T. (1983) The clinical management of non-compliance. In Barofsky, I. & Budson, R.D. (eds) *The Chronic Psychiatric Patient in the Community: Principles of Treatment*, pp. 383–395. Spectrum, Jamaica.

Van Putten, T. & May, P.R.A. (1978a) Subjective response as a predictor of outcome in pharmacotherapy. *Archives of General Psychiatry*, **35**, 477–480.

Van Putten, T. & May, P.R.A. (1978b) 'Akinetic depression' in schizophrenia. *Archives of General Psychiatry*, **35**, 1101–1107.

Van Putten, T., May, P.R.A. & Marder, S.R. (1980b) Subjective responses to thiothixene and chlorpromazine. *Psychopharmacology Bulletin*, **16**, 36–38.

Van Putten, T., May, P.R.A. & Marder, S.R. (1984) Akathisia with haloperidol and thiothixene. *Archives of General Psychiatry*, **41**, 1036–1039.

Van Putten, T., Marder, S.R., Aravagiri, M., Chabert, N. & Mintz, J. (1989) Plasma homovanillic acid as a predictor of response to fluphenazine treatment. *Psychopharmacology Bulletin*, **25**, 89–91.

Van Putten, T., May, P.R.A., Jenden, D.J., Cho, A.K. & Yale, C. (1980a) Plasma and saliva levels of chlorpromazine and subjective response. *American Journal of Psychiatry*, **137**, 1241–1242.

Van Putten, T., May, P.R.A., Marder, S.R. & Wittam, L. (1981) Subjective response to antipsychotic drugs. *Archives of General Psychiatry*, **38**, 187–190.

Varga, E., Haher, E.J. & Simpson, G.M. (1979) Neuroleptic-induced Kluver–Bucy syndrome. *Biological Psychiatry*, **10**, 65–68.

Waddington, J.L. (1987) Tardive dyskinesia in schizophrenia and other disorders: associations with ageing, cognitive dysfunction, and structural brain pathology in relation to neuroleptic exposure. *Psychopharmacology*, **2**, 11–22.

Wahba, M., Donlon, P.T. & Meadow, A. (1981) Cognitive changes in acute schizophrenia with brief neuroleptic treatment. *American Journal of Psychiatry*, **138**, 1307–1310.

Warnes, H., Lehmann, H.E. & Ban, T.A. (1967) Adynamic ileus during psychoactive medication. *Canadian Medical Association Journal*, **96**, 1112–1113.

Watson, R.G.P., Olomu, A., Clements, D., Waring, R.H., Mitchell, S. & Elias, E. (1988) A proposed mechanism for chlorpromazine jaundice-defective hepatic sulphoxidation combined with rapid hydroxylation. *Journal of Hepatology*, **7**, 72–78.

Weiner, M. (1979) Haloperidol, hyperthyroidism, and sudden death. *American Journal of Psychiatry*, **16**, 717–718.

Weller, M. (1992) NMS and lethal catatonia. *Journal of Clinical Psychiatry*, **53**, 294.

Wendkos, M.H. (1967) Cardiac changes related to phenothiazine therapy with special reference to thioridazine. *Journal of the American Geriatrics Society*, **15**, 20–28.

White, D.A.C. (1992) Catatonia and the neuroleptic malignant syndrome — a single entity? *British Journal of Psychiatry*, **161**, 558–560.

White, D.A.C. & Robins, A.H. (1991) Catatonia: harbinger of the neuroleptic malignant syndrome. *British Journal of Psychiatry*, **158**, 419–421.

Willcox, D.R.C., Gillan, R. & Hare, E.H. (1965) Do psychiatric outpatients take their drugs? *British Medical Journal*, **2**, 790–792.

Witton, K. (1962) Sexual dysfunction secondary to Mellaril. *Diseases of the Nervous System*, **23**, 175.

Yoon, M.S., Han, J., Dersham, G.H. & Jones, S.A. (1979) Effects of thioridazine (Mellaril) on ventricular electrophysiologic properties. *American Journal of Cardiology*, **43**, 1155–1158.

Zelickson, A.S. (1966) Skin changes and chlorpromazine. Some hazards of long-term drug therapy. *Journal of the American Medical Association*, **198**, 341–344.

Zimmerman, H.J. & Ishak, K.G. (1987) Hepatic injury due to drugs and toxins. In McSween, R.N.M., Anthony, P.P. & Schever, P.J. (eds) *Pathology of the Liver*, pp. 503–576. Churchill Livingstone, Edinburgh.

PART 4
PSYCHOSOCIAL ASPECTS

Chapter 29
Schizophrenia and Psychosocial Stresses

P. E. BEBBINGTON, J. BOWEN, S. R. HIRSCH
AND E. A. KUIPERS

Domains of psychosocial stress

When normal individuals experience an increase in stress levels, they may respond by becoming worried and tense. Greater degrees of stress may lead to actual autonomic anxiety, disturbance of sleep, impairment of concentration, loss of energy and apathy. Some people respond by becoming miserable and depressed. People who have experienced a schizophrenic illness also respond to adversity in this way (Hirsch *et al.*, submitted). The interesting question is whether, in some cases, stress can exacerbate the features of the illness, in the form of either withdrawal or florid symptoms. Over the last 30 years or so, the social reactivity of schizophrenia has become virtually the accepted view in clinical psychiatry. It is probably correct, although there has been more difficulty in demonstrating the impact of life events in schizophrenia than many clinicians may realize.

Although there may have been a broad appreciation that social experiences influence the course of schizophrenia, the earliest attempts to characterize this phenomenon scientifically were concerned to establish a relationship between the poverty of the social environment and the prevalence of negative symptoms in schizophrenia (Wing & Freudenberg, 1961; Brown *et al.*, 1966; Wing, 1966; Wing & Brown, 1970). At the same time, there was an awareness that trying to overcome negative symptoms by providing a more stimulating environment carried the opposite risk: too much pressure placed on patients in rehabilitation programmes sometimes led to the re-emergence of positive, florid symptoms of schizophrenia (Wing *et al.*, 1964; Stevens, 1973; Goldberg *et al.*, 1977; Drake & Sederer, 1986).

It was against this background that Brown and Birley carried out their seminal study into the effects of life events in schizophrenia (Brown & Birley, 1968), although Kraepelin (1913) had observed long before that periods of remission were frequently terminated by major changes in patients' lives. Finally, the idea that stresses within the families of patients may provoke relapse has been tested tangentially through the expressed emotion (EE) measure. This too dates back a long way (Brown *et al.*, 1958, 1962; Brown, 1959). There has been a veritable explosion of EE research in the last 5 or 10 years, and this has provided some of the strongest evidence for the social reactivity of schizophrenia.

In this chapter, we shall concentrate on reviewing the life-event and EE literature. The findings concerning life events are much less robust than those relating to EE, and for this reason we have paid much more attention to the methodological issues of life-event research.

Life-event studies

Methodological issues

The measurement of life events

A few studies have examined responses to a single type of event. One of the neatest was that of Steinberg and Durell (1968). These authors studied the effects of recruitment into the army for purposes of National Service, following which they plotted the frequency of schizophrenic breakdown. They were able to demonstrate that the rate of breakdown was significantly higher in the few months immediately after recruitment. However, most life-event studies in schizophrenia have attempted to evaluate the response of sufferers to a wide range of life events. This inevitably brings up issues of measurement.

Once the generality of life-event stress is considered, it becomes apparent that events are not equivalent, and there has to be some way of assessing the likely impact of a given event on a subject. This depends on a large number of variables, relating to the nature both of the event and of the subject's prior experiences. Inevitably, each person's experience of events is unique, and this in turn underwrites a unique susceptibility.

Nevertheless, it is possible to make general statements about relative impact. For example, the death of a child will always be a far more serious event than a child moving out of the home to go to university or to get married. However, most events resemble the last examples more than the first, and discriminating their probable impact is difficult and heavily dependent on context. It might seem an obvious answer to the idiosyncratic perception of events to ask subjects how events did indeed affect them. However, this immediately raises the possibility of two types of bias. On the one hand, subjects unfortunately share their research hypotheses with the researcher: it is characteristic of human beings that they seek to impose meaning to their lives in terms of their experiences. This is the 'search after meaning' (Bartlet, 1932). The second bias is that the experience of mental illness itself may distort

subjects' assessments of their experiences. However, if we decline to accept a respondent's own judgements, we are faced with the difficulty of arriving at our own.

There have been two basic attempts to deal with this problem. One was to define events a priori by constructing a list of event types. This was the so-called inventory approach, exemplified by the work of Holmes and Rahe (1967). A history was then elicited from respondents by presenting them with the list, either on paper or verbally, and asking them to endorse those events they had experienced within a given period. The disadvantage of this method is that it largely delegated the judgement of deciding whether an experience matched up with an event category to the respondent. The authors of this approach dealt with the problem of the differential impact of events by getting a *sample of raters* to ascribe values to each event category. The scores of the rating sample were then averaged to give a stress rating for the event. The effect of this was to give a crude rating completely divorced from the specific circumstances that might surround an event of a given type in the individual case. It was certainly one way of stripping out the subjective evaluation of individual experience.

Event inventories are still used in psychiatric research. However, most people now acknowledge that they do represent a very insensitive methodology. Likewise, it is accepted that the alternative technique, of a semistructured interview based around role areas, offers a considerable improvement (Brown, 1974; Brown & Harris, 1978). Those using this approach have relied heavily on the development of the life events and difficulty schedule (LEDS) of Brown and colleagues, although some have modified the instrument to suit local circumstances. The subject's recent experiences are elicited, and those that may meet the technical criteria for life events are recorded by the interviewer and then presented to a rating panel, which ascribes a severity rating to them. As the interviewer is able to provide a considerable amount of context, this means that the individual circumstances of the event can be taken into account, in a way which is not feasible with the simple inventory approach. Thus, some degree of individuality of response is retained, while the subject's evaluation is removed from consideration. This represents a reasonable compromise between uncontrolled subjectivity and the crudeness of evaluating events merely by categorizing them.

A further problem in deciding how to research life events of different impact is that they may be considered along a number of dimensions. The classic dispute was between those who saw the amount of *change* connoted by an event as being crucial to its impact, and those who felt that change need not necessarily reflect the degree of *stress* occasioned by an event. Empirically, it would seem that the most predictive dimension is indeed stressfulness (Mueller *et al.*, 1977), although this raises more conceptual difficulties than measurement of mere change. The LEDS relies on measures of threat, although events can also be rated according to the degree of loss they connote. Another dimension which may have particular relevance to the re-emergence of schizophrenic symptoms is that of 'intrusiveness' (Harris, 1987). This has interesting potential relationships with some of the phenomena underlying the measure of EE.

However, there are other important issues apart from the dimensions of impact that must be considered in evaluating the causal relationship between events and any kind of psychiatric disorder. One of the problems is that it is not always possible to be absolutely sure that the temporal requirements for a causal inference have been made. In other words, for an event to be held to cause a relapse in schizophrenia, it must precede the relapse. However, relapse itself can be difficult to define and, indeed, date. In consequence, we are very often not quite sure that the identified event does in fact precede relapse. Although it might at first sight appear to do so, the event may itself have come about because of changes in the subject's behaviour, changes that were themselves occasioned by impending relapse.

In response to this problem, Brown and colleagues developed the concept of *independence* (Brown & Harris, 1978). This is a measure of the extent to which events can be seen to be independent of illness-related behaviour on the part of the subject. This rating has become increasingly complex over the years since it was introduced. However, much of the life-event research on schizophrenia depends on a threefold division of events into *independent, possibly independent* and *dependent*. Independent events are basically those for which every mechanism whereby they might be brought about by impending breakdown is extremely improbable. Possibly independent events are those where such a relationship cannot be ruled out, but where there is no actual evidence that the event in question was brought about by changed behaviour. In most cases, people either use the independent category or combine it with the possibly independent category, in order to establish those events which should be considered as possible causes of a subsequent relapse.

The sheer difficulty of achieving confident inferences that life events may be causally related to relapse in schizophrenia is underlined by the status of interpersonal events. Events concerning relationships are central to most people's lives; however, these, by their very nature, cannot be independent of the patient's influence. We are therefore faced with a dilemma, of cutting out a large amount of important experience, or of including events that we can never be quite sure about. The best we can do is to make sure that our inclusion of events in the possibly independent category is carried out as conscientiously as possible.

Eliciting a history of life events from subjects inevitably requires that they are able to recall the events in question. This assumption is certainly overoptimistic and, in some cases, perhaps wildly so. Everyone has a tendency to forget things that have happened to them, and powers of recall obviously differ between individuals. It seems likely that mental illness impairs the faculty of recall. This is particularly so when the patient is still acutely disturbed. Some authors have attempted to get round this by delaying interview until the patient has considerably recovered. However, this raises the problem that patients are consequently being asked to remember events that are more remote in time. It is likely that recall will be best when the period recalled is not very remote and the interviewers are well trained (Wittchen *et al.*, 1989). There is also evidence that, for events of moderate and marked threat at any rate, the dangers of recall are minimized by using the LEDS.

Some workers have corroborated the respondent's account with that of a close relative. However, this leaves the problem of what to do when there is a discrepancy. In most cases, this will be due to the fact that the event is private to the respondent. Corroborative accounts must therefore be evaluated carefully. The difficulties of recall are particularly significant for case-control studies where life events are usually elicited over a longer period than with prospective studies.

Research design and the inference of causality

There are several different ways in which the association between life events and relapse in schizophrenia might be tested. These include retrospective within-patient designs in which a comparison of the experience of life events is made between a defined period immediately prior to the onset of illness and a more distant period. This approach can be combined with a classic, retrospective case-control design in which the life-event experience of the patients prior to onset is compared with an equivalent period in normal controls, usually the period immediately preceding interview. The problem with both these approaches is that the length of recall differs between the period where the events are expected to be elevated and the period in which they are not. In the within-case comparison, this operates in favour of the hypothesis of an excess of events preceding onset, while in the case-control design, it works against it.

The particular methodological difficulties of the retrospective case-control design have been discussed at length elsewhere (Day, 1981, 1989; Brown & Harris, 1989; Creed, 1990; Hirsch *et al.*, 1992). It seems likely that these contribute to the inconsistencies in research findings and make comparison difficult.

There is another difficulty. It is not clear what the appropriate control group is for a group of people with schizophrenia. Such people may have attributes that affect their life-event rate. One would, perhaps, expect them to have a lowered life-event rate because their illness, and indeed their premorbid adjustment, might lead them to withdraw from certain areas of life that may be a source of events, for example intense emotional relationships or employment. However, if anything, event rates in schizophrenia may be higher than would be expected in a normal control group (Schwarz & Myers, 1977; Bebbington *et al.*, 1993; Hirsch *et al.*, submitted). As a result, the most secure evidence in support of a triggering role for life events in schizophrenic relapse may be the finding of a within-patient peaking of events before the episode.

Another problem with using the case-control design is that people with schizophrenia may be abnormally sensitive to the impact of stress. Because of this, they may respond adversely to relatively minor disturbances in their social world. In consequence, their experience of life events may be no more than would be expected. This is another reason why the within-case comparison may be the most appropriate.

It is possible to investigate the life-event hypotheses using a prospective design, i.e. prospective in the sense that the life-event history is established prior to an episode of recurrence. Thus, patients may be interviewed, say, every 2 months, at which time life events and symptom worsening are evaluated for the intervening period. Such evaluations have inevitably to be retrospective. What the researcher is left with is a continuous series of periods in which life events or exacerbations, or both, may have occurred. It is then possible to look at the experience of life events in the period *immediately preceding* that in which an exacerbation occurred. Once more, it is possible to compare such periods with dissimilar periods in the same subject, or in other subjects who did not experience exacerbations. This is quite a powerful design, but depends crucially on evaluating patients sufficiently frequently for events in one period to be not too distant in time from an exacerbation in the next period. It also requires diligent evaluation of life events and the careful definition of exacerbation or relapse.

Most studies, whether retrospective or prospective, have examined the life-event rate before relapse, i.e. they have counted events backwards from the fixed point of relapse onset. Hardesty *et al.* (1985) departed from this procedure by performing a forward count of relapse or of increased morbidity from event onset. This allows the demonstration of an increased relapse rate in proximity to events. Day (1989) has also provided an analysis of this type.

In general, little attention has been devoted to the differences in sampling procedures between studies of life events and schizophrenia. This is partly because the condition is a serious one that usually leads to specialist psychiatric contact. The sampling of patient groups has varied, but retrospective studies have generally been of hospitalized patients with first onsets or relapse. Prospective designs inevitably require that the patient already has experienced an episode of schizophrenia. Cohorts of such patients can then be followed in remission. Studying relapses rather than first onsets necessarily defines groups of patients at particularly high risk.

In addition to these administrative aspects, the phenomenological characteristics of patients have varied. Recent studies have used operationalized diagnostic criteria to determine the entry of patients. However, in many studies the sample has been of mixed clinical profile, including, for example, both first-onset and relapsing cases, or both nuclear schizophrenia and schizophreniform or schizoaffective cases. In several studies, some of the so-called relapses have merely been increases in the level of psychotic symptoms, properly an exacerbation. However, because most studies are actually of small numbers, the effect of these case differences cannot be satisfactorily examined. A lack of difference between subgroups may indicate the true state of affairs, or merely be a type-II error.

Several authors have argued that life events 'trigger' episodes of schizophrenia. This term has two separate and disconnected meanings. One is that the life-event stress merely adds the final impetus toward illness in somebody who was already strongly predisposed because of an underlying diathesis. This is another way of saying that, in relation to other factors, the role of life events is not very important. This can be tested by examining the strength of the association between events and onset or relapse.

The other meaning of the 'triggering' hypothesis concerns the length of the causal period in which life events are thought to operate. This has a methodological implication, as it is important that the antecedent period chosen for canvassing a life-event history should be at least as long as the causal period. Events would be seen as having a triggering role in this sense if they occurred in close proximity to the onset of relapse of the disorder. It is generally held that a 6-month period of study should be sufficient to cover all events that might have a role in engendering relapse, although this has recently been queried (Bebbington *et al.*, 1993; Hirsch *et al.*, submitted).

Life-event studies in schizophrenia

Sixteen systematic studies specifically examining the effect of life events on the aetiology or course of schizophrenia have been published (Table 29.1). The inaugural and still seminal study in this area is that of Brown and Birley (1968). Using careful methods, they found that there was a significantly raised rate of life events that appeared to be limited to the 3 weeks before the onset or relapse of schizophrenic illness. Among cases at least 46% had one independent event in the 3 weeks before relapse compared with around 12% in more distant periods. This finding was analysed further and interpreted as an effect of life events in precipitating, or triggering, the onset of illness which would have happened anyway, albeit a few weeks later (Brown *et al.*, 1973).

Many subsequent studies from a wide range of cultural settings have been carried out, but they provide inconsistent support for these initial findings. Most have used retrospective designs, although prospective studies have been performed recently. Some studies report statistically signifi-

Table 29.1 Studies of independent life events in schizophrenic illness

| Study | Country | Period/method | Patient sample | Number | Significant results for time period before relapse | |
					3–5 weeks	>3 months
Retrospective						
Brown and Birley (1968)	UK	12 weeks	Broad group: 30% first onset	50	Yes, for 3 weeks	Not addressed
Jacobs and Myers (1976)	UK	1 year: not LEDS	Narrow definition: all first onset	62	Not addressed	NS
Malzacher *et al.* (1981)	Germany	6 months	First onset	90	Not addressed	NS
Canton and Fraccon (1985)	Italy	6 months: not LEDS	24 first onset	54	Not addressed	Possible support
Chung *et al.* (1986)	USA	6 months	Narrow definition: some first onset	15	NS	NS
Al Khani *et al.* (1986)	Saudi Arabia	1 year	Narrow definition: recent onset	48	Yes, in small subgroups only	NS
Day *et al.* (1987)	10 centres worldwide	12 weeks	Broad definition: some first onset	13–67	Yes, for five of six analysed fully	Not addressed
Dohrenwend *et al.* (1987)	USA	6 months: not LEDS	21 first onset	66	NS	Yes, for 'non-fateful' events
Gureje and Adewumni (1988)	Nigeria	6 months: not LEDS	All first onset: RDC definition	42	NS	NS
Bebbington *et al.* (1993)	UK	6 months	Narrow definition	52	Yes	Yes, for up to 6 months
Prospective						
Leff *et al.* (1973)	UK	Clinical trial	Nine on medication relapsed	116	For medicated only (5 weeks)	NS
Hardesty *et al.* (1985)	USA	1 year	2–3 years in remission	36	NS (morbidity 3 weeks post life event)	Not addressed
Ventura *et al.* (1989)	USA	1 year on medication (see Ventura *et al.*, 1992)	*Recent onset: 11/30 relapsers		Yes, for 4 weeks	NS
Malla *et al.* (1990)	Canada	1 year	Seven relapsed	22	Not addressed	NS, unless trivial events included

Continued

Table 29.1 (*Continued*)

Study	Country	Period/method	Patient sample	Number	Significant results for time period before relapse	
					3−5 weeks	>3 months
Ventura *et al.* (1992)	USA	1 year of medication status (see Ventura *et al.*, 1989)	*Recent onset: off medication	13	NS, for those off medication status	NS
Hirsch *et al.* (submitted)	UK	1 year on/off medication status	Narrow. Relapses: off medication 21/35; on medication 5/36	71	NS for both on and off medication groups	Yes, for up to 1 year

* Recent onset: illness history <2 years.
LEDS, life events and difficulty schedule; NS, not significant; RDC, research diagnostic criteria.

cant findings of independent events occurring more frequently in the 3 or 4 weeks before relapse compared with control periods. Thus, in a multi-centre World Health Organization (WHO), study, Day *et al.* (1987) used a retrospective design and employed loglinear methods to demonstrate results similar to those of Brown and Birley (1968) in five out of six centres. Ventura *et al.* (1989) examined patients on regular neuroleptic medication and again found results which would support a triggering hypothesis.

Other studies, using widely varying methods, have found significantly increased rates of independent events during longer periods of time, up to 6 months or 1 year preceding relapse or illness onset (Dohrenwend *et al.*, 1987; Bebbington *et al.*, 1993; Hirsch *et al.*, submitted). However, several other studies yielded negative results (e.g. Jacobs & Myers, 1976; Malzacher *et al.*, 1981; Al Khani *et al.*, 1986; Chung *et al.*, 1986; Gureje & Adewumni, 1988; Malla *et al.*, 1990). A study performed in Saudi Arabia (Al Khani *et al.*, 1986), while finding no statistically significant effect overall, reported a significant difference for married females. Some of the negative studies did find non-significant patterns of elevation of life-event rates preceding illness onset [e.g. for Japan and two out of three developing countries' centres

in the WHO study (Day *et al.*, 1987)], but the methodological problems of this type of research need to be considered carefully before these trends towards significance may be interpreted as supporting the earlier findings.

Prospective life-event studies in the field of schizophrenia suffer from few of the important methodological problems of retrospectives studies but, to date, have not offered consistent support for the triggering hypothesis. One study in California found no significant change in positive symptoms in the 3 weeks after major independent events occurred (Hardesty *et al.*, 1985). The analysis in this study was limited by the small number of cases and the small number of major independent events that occurred (3% of the total number of life events occurring, so the negative findings might represent a type-II error). Two subsequent prospective studies, in Canada and in London, could find no increase in independent major events in the 4 weeks preceding relapse (Malla *et al.*, 1990; Hirsch *et al.*, submitted), while two studies in California found a significant association of events preceding illness in patients on regular neuroleptics, but not in those who had recently come off medication (Ventura *et al.*, 1989, 1992).

Two recent studies

There have been two recent British studies that have used different designs to investigate the relationship between life events and schizophrenia. The first of these is the Camberwell Collaborative Psychosis Study (Bebbington *et al.*, 1993; Jones *et al.*, 1993). This involved the collection of a range of biological and social data on a large sample of people suffering from psychosis, broadly defined. In the course of the study, 51 subjects were identified as having experienced a datable episode of schizophrenic relapse within the past year. Using the LEDS, life event histories were taken for the 6-month period immediately preceding the relapse (Brown & Harris, 1978). These were compared with equivalent histories from a psychiatrically healthy sample, obtained from a community survey carried out in the same area. There was a significant excess of life events, particularly in the 3 months before relapse (Fig. 29.1).

While the detailed analysis of the results from this study lends itself to more than one interpretation, the authors argue that the findings strongly imply that events do increase before onset, that this increase is of aetiological significance, and that it begins quite far back in time. In other words, events can exert an aetiological effect across a sizeable interval.

The second recent British study is that of Hirsch *et al.* (submitted). This involved the prospective study of 71 patients fulfilling criteria for the *Diagnostic and Statistical Manual* DSM-III-R criteria for schizophrenia, half of whom did not take regular neuroleptic medication. A subgroup of the cohort was randomized on a double-blind basis to medication or placebo. Patients were followed up for 1 year with assessment of morbidity and life events (using the LEDS) every 2 months.

During the study, 21 of the patients without medication relapsed, whereas only five of the medicated group relapsed. The life-event experience in the 4 weeks before relapse was not found to be significantly different from the experience of the same group of patients in more remote periods, whether or not they were receiving medication. Using a proportional hazards regression analysis, the cumulative experience of events for the total duration of the study before relapse was found to be significant. When relative risk and population-attributable risk were calculated for medication and for cumulative event experience, the effect of medication was found to be much larger (Fig. 29.2).

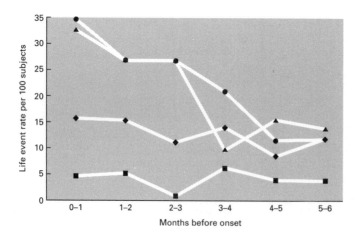

Fig. 29.1 Life events before episodes of schizophrenia. (From Bebbington *et al.*, 1993.) Schizophrenia life events rated 1 or 2 (▲), rated 3 (▼); controls rated 1 or 2 (■), rated 3 (♦).

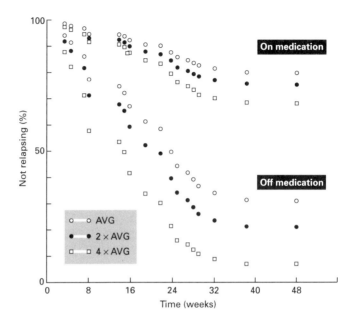

Fig. 29.2 Survival without relapse over time according to medication status and cumulative event experience. (From Hirsch *et al.*, submitted.)

For a number of reasons, it is interesting to compare this study with that of Bebbington *et al.* (1993), described above. The results are similar in that they may be interpreted as supporting an effect of events over a longer period of time than the causal period, estimated from some previous studies, of just a few weeks. Another point of interest is that each study examines a different profile of patients. Hirsch *et al.* examined patients with long-standing illness, in contrast to many studies published so far. The use of prospective methodology minimizes the problems of recall, described above. In addition, the incorporation of medication effects allows for the evaluation of interactions between medication and event status. This has only been undertaken systematically in one other study so far (Ventura *et al.*, 1992).

EE and relapse in schizophrenia

The origins of the measure of EE have been reviewed extensively (Leff & Vaughn, 1985; Kuipers & Bebbington, 1988; Lam, 1991; Kavanagh, 1992; Bebbington & Kuipers, 1994). It was developed over a period of a decade, follow-ing the observation that returning to a family home was not always associated with a good outcome in severe mental illness (Brown *et al.*, 1958; Brown, 1959) and the speculation that this might be due to aspects of the home environment.

EE is rated from an audiotape of an interview with a carer (the Camberwell Family Interview (CFI); Brown & Rutter, 1966). This has a semi-structured format that allows a flexible use of standard questions and probes and encourages the interviewer to listen to information as it emerges. It covers the onset of problems, focuses on the month prior to interview and encompasses other aspects of relationships, such as irritability and tension. The interviewer enquires after symptoms and coping responses, and probes for recent examples if the carer is reticent or vague. The interviewer also establishes a time budget for a typical week. This allows an evaluation of the amount of time that the patient and carer spend together.

The definitive ratings are then made from the audiotape of the interview, based on the content, but, more importantly, the prosodic aspects of speech. These include pitch and emphasis. This is intended to allow the rating of emotional aspects of communication regardless of specific contents. Five scales are rated from the interview. These are: frequency ratings of the number of critical comments (CCs) and positive remarks, and global ratings of hostility, warmth and emotional over-involvement (EOI). CCs, hostility and EOI have turned out to be the most predictive of relapse. High EE is defined as either criticism exceeding a cut-off of six CCs, or a moderate amount of EOI, or any degree of hostility. The consequence is that EE is probably a dimorphic rating, since hostility and criticism are clearly related to each other, but less so to overinvolvement. In the research literature the cut-off points have tended to vary somewhat. This causes problems of comparability, although as Kavanagh (1992) points out: 'The data do not support the contention that EE results are significantly affected by changing criteria.' Where the criteria for EE vary, they do not do so to a gross extent. Relative insensitivity to changes in sampling and criteria is of course in any case an indication of robust findings. However, critics have pointed out that the variation of criteria has been carried out *post hoc* in some cases, in order to ensure a significant result, thus risking spuriously positive findings.

The literature using EE as a measure predictive of relapse in schizophrenia tends to rely on rather similar research designs. Typically, a sample of patients is followed up following recovery from an episode of florid symptoms of schizophrenia. When they are well on the way to recovery, commonly at the point of discharge, carers are interviewed using the CFI to establish levels of EE. Patients are then followed up for a period of 9 months or 1 year, and evaluated for signs of relapse. The definition of relapse has typically varied, in some cases being based on symptomatic criteria and in others merely on readmission to hospital. Patients are divided into high- and low-EE groups. This may be defined either in terms of the attributes of a designated 'key' relative or on the basis that at least one relative in the immediate family is rated as high EE. Case definition has varied between different studies, in some instances being operationally defined in terms of nuclear

schizophrenia, while others include schizoaffective cases.

There are now at least 26 prospective studies of the role of EE as a risk factor for relapse in schizophrenia, although more are in progress. We have recently carried out an aggregate analysis of 25 studies of EE, described in greater detail elsewhere (Bebbington & Kuipers, 1994). Where possible, data on individual cases were obtained from the original authors (17 studies). In the remaining eight studies, published results were used to reconstruct as completely as possible data on individual cases. One study (Dulz & Hand, 1986) was omitted because a substantial proportion of subjects were not living with their EE-rated relative, and it was impossible to work out which. In the other studies, we were able to exclude subjects in this category, resulting in a reduction in numbers. As a result, the relationship between EE and relapse was different from that quoted in the published reports. Altogether, 15 studies showed an association beyond the 5% level, two just failed to reach this level, five showed a non-significant trend and three either no trend or a small trend in the reverse direction.

Based on these 25 studies, the total number of cases was 1346. The numbers are less than this in some analyses because of the problem of missing variables, particularly where the analysis involved several variables.

Worldwide, the proportion of high-EE cases is 52%. This is striking in view of the fact that the original cut-off for EE was chosen because it was a median value. In those studies where gender information was provided ($n = 855$), 60% of cases were male. However, in 48% of cases, gender was not reported. Of those cases where medication status was reported ($n = 884$), two-thirds were receiving medication. It was found that 62% of patients were in high contact with their relatives.

The overall relapse rate for high-EE cases was 50%, whereas that in low-EE cases was 21%. This result was overwhelmingly significant ($\chi^2 = 131.6$; d.f. $= 1$; $P < 0.00001$).

Hogarty (1985) made the suggestion that the evidence for the predictive capacity of EE was relatively meagre for females. Our data on the aggregate analysis (Table 29.2) suggest that although the outcome in terms of relapse is better overall in females, the strength of the association between relapse and high EE is virtually identical in the two genders.

The relationship between medication, EE and relapse rate is shown in Table 29.3. The implication of this is that the effect of EE is actually stronger than that of medication. The strength of the association of relapse with EE is virtually identical in the medicated and non-medicated groups.

In Table 29.4 we examine the relationship between the degree of contact with the relative

Table 29.2 The effect of gender on the ability of expressed emotion (EE) to predict relapse

Gender	Relapse rate
Males	
High EE	54.4% (147/270)
Low EE	21.8% (52/239)
	$\chi^2 = 56.9$; d.f. = 1; $P = 0.0001$
	Kendall's Tau B = 0.33
Females	
High EE	47.1% (74/157)
Low EE	16.9% (32/189)
	$\chi^2 = 36.8$; d.f. = 1; $P = 0.0001$
	Kendall's Tau B = 0.33

Table 29.3 The effect of medication on the ability of expressed emotion (EE) to predict relapse

Medication status	Relapse rate
On medication	
High EE	44.3% (135/305)
Low EE	18.4% (52/282)
	$\chi^2 = 45.0$; d.f. = 1; $P = 0.00001$
	Kendall's Tau B = 0.28
Not on medication	
High EE	57.7% (97/168)
Low EE	27.9% (36/129)
	$\chi^2 = 26.3$; d.f. = 1; $P = 0.00001$
	Kendall's Tau B = 0.30

Table 29.4 The association of contact with relapse according to the level of expressed emotion (EE)

Level of EE	Relapse rate
High EE	
High contact	58.8% (151/257)
Low contact	41.7% (75/180)
	$\chi^2 = 12.4$; d.f. = 1; $P = 0.0004$
	Kendall's Tau B = 0.17
Low EE	
High contact	18.3% (46/251)
Low contact	23.9% (32/134)
	$\chi^2 = 1.66$; d.f. = 1; $P = 0.197$
	Kendall's Tau B = -0.07

and the predictive capacity of EE. Face-to-fact contact was found to be a significant variable in the original British studies (Vaughn & Leff, 1976). However, later studies from elsewhere in the world have shown this less consistently. In Table 29.3 we examine the relationship between contact, EE and relapse. This analysis is based on over 800 subjects. It appears from this that the strength of association between high EE and relapse is greater where contact is high, while living in high contact with a low-EE relative is, if anything, protective.

We bring all these variables together in Fig. 29.3, which emphasizes the very high rate of relapse in patients unprotected by medication and who live in high contact with high-EE relatives.

Multivariate analyses of this dataset confirmed that the association of relapse with high EE is highly significant and unaffected by the location of the study. At one stage, it was thought that patients with schizophrenia living with low-EE relatives did not require the protection of medication. However, in this analysis medication and EE were independently related to relapse, confirming that EE status has no bearing on the decision to prescribe medication.

The acknowledgement that the family atmosphere plays a role in relapse in schizophrenia has led several authors to conduct intervention studies (Falloon *et al.*, 1982, 1985; Leff *et al.*, 1982, 1985,

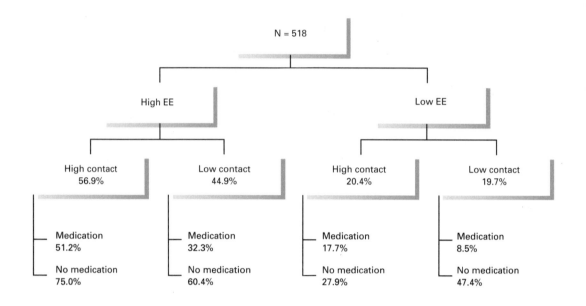

Fig. 29.3 Relapse rates according to expressed emotion (EE), contact and medication status.

1989, 1990; Hogarty *et al.*, 1986; Tarrier *et al.*, 1988; Kuipers *et al.*, 1989; McCreadie *et al.*, 1991; Vaughan *et al.*, 1992). These interventions have been successful in some, but not all, cases. This indicates that it is possible to modify family atmosphere and thus reduce relapse rates, but that this is probably dependent upon the techniques used and the expertise of the therapists using them. Intervention studies have been reviewed extensively elsewhere (Kuipers & Bebbington, 1988; Lam, 1991; Kavanagh, 1992). It is probable that the changes leading to a reduction in EE are a sufficient, but not a necessary, component of intervention (Hogarty *et al.*, 1986). These studies thus provide very good corroboration that the elements of family atmosphere detected by the EE measure are causally related to relapse in schizophrenia.

In addition to the predictive power of EE rated in relatives, high ratings in key members of professional staff may have similar consequences. Staff seem to have rates of high EE not markedly below those of family members (Watts, 1988; Herzog, 1992; Moore *et al.*, 1992). This is perhaps

not surprising as, even though their relationship is a professional one, staff share with relatives the impact of many of the behavioural problems and disturbances of clients. However, staff have much more respite (MacCarthy *et al.*, 1989). Moreover, preliminary evidence suggests that high EE in staff has an adverse effect on the course of the disorder. A prospective naturalistic study of patients in two hostels, one characterized by a majority of staff with high EE and the other by low-EE staff, found worse outcomes in the former (Ball *et al.*, 1992). The study of EE ratings in staff has implications that are at once theoretical, clinical and educational.

The EE measure uses an individual relative's behaviour in the artificial conditions of the CFI to predict the likelihood of subsequent relapse in the patient with whom the relative lives. It is presumed that it is able to do this because it reflects some significant and enduring aspect of the interplay between the patient and relatives, or the relatives' ability to cope with crises (Kuipers, 1979).

It has long been known that relatives who make frequent CCs when alone behave similarly in the presence of the patient, albeit usually more restrained (Brown & Rutter, 1966; Rutter & Brown, 1966). This view is substantiated by the work on negative affective style. This is a coding system which can be used to assess families taking part in a standardized task designed to recreate everyday interaction in a laboratory setting (Goldstein *et al.*, 1968; Doane *et al.*, 1981). Negative affective style in these direct interactions is consistently highly correlated with EE measured in the usual way (Strachan *et al.*, 1986; Miklowitz *et al.*, 1989).

However, we now have considerably more information about how high ratings on the EE measure are related to aspects of the patients' and the relatives' behaviour (Table 29.5). It can be seen from this that EE is picking up a number of different attributes of interpersonal behaviour. Some of these are not closely related conceptually, although they may well occur together in given relatives and families. Kuipers (1992) has likened the EE measure to blood pressure. The latter is an indirect way of measuring cardiovascular function, which is extremely predictive of certain outcomes. We now know that blood pressure is related to a variety of pathophysiological processes, and this increased knowledge has enhanced the range of potential palliatives and treatments. In the same way, EE has justified its use as a predictor. This does not preclude the use of other measures, nor does it prevent the emergence of richer and more sophisticated explanations of its predictiveness.

Quite early on in the history of EE research, there were concerns about the origins of the behaviours it measures. This has a theoretical implication. Could it be that the EE measure is predictive merely because relatives respond in a characteristic way to sufferers whose illness has a poor prognosis for other reasons? In the first fully worked out study of EE (Brown *et al.*, 1972), the authors did control for the extent of positive symptoms in patients, but found that EE was still predictive.

Birchwood and Smith (1987), however, have argued that high EE and the behaviours associated with it develop as the response of some relatives to the burden of living with a person with schizophrenia. They base their argument on the fact that high EE is less apparent in relatives of patients experiencing first, rather than subsequent, admissions for schizophrenia. Recent work has indeed suggested that at least some components of high EE are associated with abnormalities of various sorts in the patient (Miklowitz *et al.*, 1983; Mavreas *et al.*, 1992).

Birchwood and Smith put forward a model whereby the coping style of families develops over time. There is little to argue with in this. It is difficult to see how the characteristics of high EE might arise *except* from an interaction between the relative and the patient. However, this does not mean that maladaptive responses on the part of the relatives have no influence on the subsequent course of the disorder. This is why intervention studies have been useful whatever the origins of EE-related behaviours.

Moreover, although difficult behaviour on the part of the sufferer may cause distress to the relatives and thus lead to suboptimal responses, it is clear that these responses are not obligatory. Thus, the relatives of a given patient may differ in

Table 29.5 Behaviour and attitudes characteristic of high-expressed emotion (EE) families

Carers
Fears and anxieties (Greenley, 1986)
Negative affective style (Strachan *et al.*, 1986; Miklowitz *et al.*, 1989)
Poor listening (Kuipers *et al.*, 1983)
Non-illness attributions (Brewin *et al.*, 1991)
Attribution of negative outcomes to patient (Brewin *et al.*, 1991)
Maladaptive coping (Kuipers, 1983; Bledin *et al.*, 1990)

Patients
More critical (Brown & Rutter, 1966; Strachan *et al.*, 1989)
Less autonomous (Strachan *et al.*, 1989)

Interaction
Negative (Hooley & Hahlweg, 1986; Hubschmid & Zemp, 1989)
Rigid ⎫
Conflict-prone structure ⎭ (Hubschmid & Zemp, 1989)

their EE ratings, while Beltz *et al.* (1991) have shown that there is no consistent relationship between staff and family levels of EE. It is virtually certain that the pattern of high-EE-related behaviours and frequent relapses represent a vicious cycle rather than linear causality. It seems that if this vicious cycle is entered, high EE is often an extremely persistent characteristic of relatives. Favre *et al.* (1989) found considerable stability of EE over a 9-month period, while McCreadie *et al.* (1993) have reported that this stability extends to 5 years. In both these studies, there was an intermediate minority of relatives who moved between high- and low-EE status. Although few of the changes observed seemed to depend on the clinical state of patients, it is possible that there is a subgroup of relatives who typically become high EE under stress. It is of interest that the frequency of relapse in this fluctuating group in the study of McCreadie *et al.* resembled that in patients living with relatives rated persistently high in EE, and that they were noticeably different from the consistently low-EE group.

It is our view that the EE measure taps into the quality and style of interactions within family systems that are necessarily complex. Living with a high-EE relative probably constitutes a chronic stress. However, it is very likely that low-EE relationships are not merely neutral, in the sense of representing an absence of stress, but actually have positive and beneficial effects on patients. Thus, Hubschmid and Zemp (1989) found that low-EE relatives made significantly more emotionally positive and supportive statements in interaction with patients. This has parallels with the results of our aggregate analysis suggesting that high contact with low-EE relatives is actually protective for patients who are not on medication; in other words, vulnerable patients do better with a bigger dose of their relatives. There is some corroboration from electrophysiological studies suggesting that the presence of low-EE relatives actually serves to reduce arousal (Tarrier *et al.*, 1988; Tarrier, 1989; Hegerl *et al.*, 1990).

The large investment in EE research has established that high EE is predictive of relapse in schizophrenia, and confirms that a range of associ-

ated behaviours on the part of relatives creates an environment where relapse is considerably more likely. EE is equally predictive in males and females; greater contact between high-EE relatives and sufferers increases the risk of relapse; and medication can act as a buffer alternating the effects of EE. This is strong evidence for the importance of the social environment in schizophrenia.

The interaction of stress, medication and relapse in schizophrenia

We have already had evidence from our aggregate analysis of EE studies that medication can have an effect in protecting patients from the deleterious effects of living with high-EE relatives. There is some evidence that medication has a similar role in protecting people with schizophrenia from the effects of life-event stresses. A number of studies have addressed this issue. Birley and Brown (1970) found that the relationship between life events and relapse was weakest in those patients who had been off medication for less than 1 year. The relationship was stronger both in patients who had not taken medication for more than 1 year and for those who remained on medication. Leff *et al.* (1973) used data from a double-blind placebo-controlled trial to examine the effect of medication on the life event–relapse relationship. In a *post hoc* analysis, life events appeared to precede relapse in patients on active medication but not in those on placebo. Bartko *et al.* (1987) report similar findings from a non-randomized design. The implication is that those patients who are on medication require an event before they will relapse, while patients without medication may be so sensitive to small changes in their environment that the sorts of life event picked up in the research studies are not necessary.

However, for methodological reasons, these studies are inconclusive. More weight can be placed on the prospective studies of Ventura *et al.* (1992) and Hirsch *et al.* (submitted). Ventura *et al.* (1992), investigating patients with short histories of illness, found an excess of events in those on regular medication compared with those not receiving any medication. Hirsch *et al.* (1992) studied a population with more long-standing illness. They failed to find any differences in the experience of events prior to relapse in medicated and unmedicated groups. This is possibly a type-II error, as only five out of 36 patients on medication relapsed during the 1-year follow-up. This study is interesting because it compares the relative size of the effect of medication with that of the cumulative event rate, and found that the former was much the greater. This is an interesting contrast to the results from the aggregate analysis of EE studies described above.

Other links with the EE research have been postulated. Leff and Vaughn (1980) found that there was a much stronger event−relapse relationship in schizophrenic patients who came from low-EE families than in those who came from high-EE families. These patients were largely off medication. It seems from this as though patients required one sort of stress or the other, but either would do. People living with a high-EE relative may be so vulnerable in consequence that very small perturbations in the social environment can precipitate relapse. Leff *et al.* (1983) used results from their family intervention study to explore this issue further. They concluded that for patients off medication, relapse can be provoked by either a life event or contact with a high-EE relative.

However, for patients on medication, relapse appeared to require the presence of the two factors in combination. This idea is represented graphically in Fig. 29.4.

What can be made of these findings? If the life-event results could be taken on their own, the lack of robustness in the findings might justify the conclusion that social factors were relatively unimportant in schizophrenic relapse. However, this must be set against the EE studies which suggest a large and robust effect. It is not tenable to argue on this basis that social factors are unimportant. Why is it that the life-event research does not corroborate the EE research in a more convincing manner? One possibility is that the relatively abrupt changes represented by life events may not be so important in producing relapse as the continuing, albeit perhaps relatively low, level of stress occasioned by living with a high-EE family member. Another explanation is that the rating of life events is essentially derived from research concerned mainly with depressive disorders. In consequence, the ratings may be set at the wrong threshold for picking up the life events important in schizophrenia. If people with schizophrenia are unnaturally sensitive to life events, it is possible that the relapse is brought about by events that on the surface would seem incapable of provoking an emotional response. One study

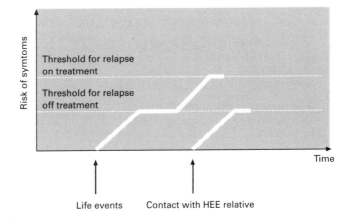

Fig. 29.4 A proposed model to describe the relationship between the effect on risk of relapse of life events and contact with a high-expressed emotion (HEE) relative, with and without the protective effect of medication. (From Leff *et al.*, 1983.)

(Malla *et al.*, 1990) only found a significant effect of events on relapse if trivial events or 'hassles' were included in the analysis. The study of Bebbington *et al.* (1993), described above, also suggested that events of mild threat were in excess in schizophrenia, as in other psychoses. This would certainly tie in with the experience of many clinicians, who, in managing people with long-standing schizophrenia, are very concerned to protect them from even minor changes in their daily routine.

References

Al Khani, M.A.F., Bebbington, P.E., Watson, J.P. & House, F. (1986) Life events and schizophrenia: a Saudi Arabian study. *British Journal of Psychiatry*, **148**, 12–22.

Ball, A., Moore, E. & Kuipers, L. (1992) Expressed emotion in community care staff. A comparison of patient outcome in a nine month follow-up of two hostels. *Social Psychiatry and Psychiatric Epidemiology*, **27**, 35–39.

Bartko, G., Maylath, E. & Herczeg, I. (1987) Comparative study of schizophrenic patients relapsed on and off medication. *Psychiatry Research*, **22**, 221–227.

Bartlet, F.C. (1932) *Remembering: A Study in Experiment and Social Psychology*. Cambridge University Press, Cambridge.

Bebbington, P.E. & Kuipers, L. (1994) The predictive utility of expressed emotion in schizophrenia. *Psychological Medicine*, **24**, 707–718.

Bebbington, P.E., Wilkins, S., Jones, P. *et al.* (1993) Life events and psychosis: initial results from the Camberwell Collaborative Psychosis study. *British Journal of Psychiatry*, **162**, 72–79.

Beltz, J., Bertrando, P., Clerici, M., Albertini, E., Merati, O. & Cazullo, C.L. (1991) *Emotive espresso e schizophrenia: Dai familiari agli operatori psichiatrici* (Symposium on expressed emotion in Latin-based languages.) Barcelona.

Birchwood, M. & Smith, J. (1987) Schizophrenia in the family. In Orford, J. (ed.) *Coping with Disorder in the Family*, Croom Helm, London.

Birley, J.L.T. & Brown, G.W. (1970) Crises and life changes preceding the onset or relapse of acute schizophrenia: clinical aspects. *British Journal of Psychiatry*, **116**, 327–333.

Bledin, K., MacCarthy, B., Kuipers, L. & Woods, B. (1990) Expressed emotion in the daughters of people with dementia. *British Journal of Psychiatry*, **157**, 221–227.

Brewin, C.R., MacCarthy, B., Duda, K. & Vaughn, C.E. (1991) Attribution and expressed emotion in the relatives of patients with schizophrenia. *Journal of Abnormal Psychology*, **100**, 546–554.

Brown, G.W. (1959) Experiences of discharged chronic schizophrenic mental hospital patients in various types of living group. *Millbank Memorial Fund Quarterly*, **37**, 105–131.

Brown, G.W. (1974) Meaning measurement and stress of life events. In Dohrenwend, B.S. & Dohrenwend, B.P. (eds) *Stressful Life Events: Their Nature and Effects*, pp. 217–243.

Wiley, New York.

Brown, G.W. & Birley, J.L.T. (1968) Crises and life changes and the onset of schizophrenia. *Journal of Health and Social Behaviour*, **9**, 203–214.

Brown, G.W. & Harris, T.O. (1978) *Social Origins of Depression*. Tavistock, London.

Brown, G.W. & Harris, T.O. (eds) (1989) *Life Events and Illness*. Unwin Hyman, London.

Brown, G., Bone, M., Dalison, B. & Wing, J. (1966) *Schizophrenia and Social Care*. Oxford University Press, London.

Brown, G.W., Birley, J.L.T. & Wing, J.K. (1972) Influence of family life on the course of schizophrenic disorders: a replication. *British Journal of Psychiatry*, **121**, 241–258.

Brown, G.W., Carstairs, G.M. & Topping, G.C. (1958) The post hospital adjustment of chronic mental patients. *Lancet*, **ii**, 685–689.

Brown, G.W., Monck, E.M., Carstairs, G.M. & Wing, J.K. (1962) Influence of family life on the course of schizophrenic illness. *British Journal of Preventive and Social Medicine*, **16**, 55–68.

Canton, G. & Fraccon, I.G. (1985) Life events and schizophrenia: a replication. *Acta Psychiatrica Scandinavica*, **71**, 211–216.

Chung, R.K., Langeluddecke, P. & Tennant, C. (1986) Threatening life events in the onset of schizophrenia, schizophreniform psychosis and hypomania. *British Journal of Psychiatry*, **148**, 680–686.

Creed, F. (1990) Life events and disorder. *Current Opinion in Psychiatry*, **3**, 259–263.

Day, R. (1981) Life events and schizophrenia: the triggering hypothesis. *Acta Psychiatrica Scandinavica*, **64**, 97–122.

Day, R. (1989) Schizophrenia. In Brown, G.W. & Harris, T.O. (eds) *Life Events and Illness*, pp. 113–137. Unwin Hyman, London.

Day, R., Neilsen, J.A., Korten, A. *et al.* (1987) Stressful life events preceding the acute onset of schizophrenia: a cross national study from the World Health Organisation. *Culture, Medicine and Psychiatry*, **11**, 123–206.

Doane, J.A., West, K.L., Goldstein, M.J., Rodnick, E.H. & Jones, J.E. (1981) Parental communication deviance and affective style: predictors of subsequent schizophrenia spectrum disorders in vulnerable adolescents. *Archives of General Psychiatry*, **38**, 679–685.

Dohrenwend, B.P., Levav, I., Shrout, P.E. *et al.* (1987) Life stress and psychopathology: progress with research begun with Barbara Snell Dohrenwend. *American Journal of Community Psychology*, **15**, 677–713.

Drake, R.E. & Sederer, L.I. (1986) The adverse effects of intensive treatment of chronic schizophrenia. *Comprehensive Psychiatry*, **27**, 313–326.

Dulz, B. & Hand, I. (1986) Short-term relapse in young schizophrenics: can it be predicted and affected by family (CFI), patient, and treatment variables? An experimental study. In Goldstein, M.J., Hand, I. & Hahlweg, K. (eds) *Treatment of Schizophrenia: Family Assessment and Intervention*, pp. 59–75. Springer-Verlag, Berlin.

Falloon, I.R.H., Boyd, J.L., McGill, C.W., Razani, J., Moss, H.B. & Gilderman, A.M. (1982) Family management in the prevention of exacerbations of schizophrenia. A controlled study. *New England Journal of Medicine*, **306**, 1437–1440.

Falloon, I.R.H., Boyd, J.L., McGill, C.W. *et al.* (1985) Family management in the prevention of morbidity of schizophrenia. Clinical outcome of a two-year longitudinal study. *Archives of General Psychiatry*, **42**, 887–896.

Favre, S., Gonzales, C., Lendais, G. *et al.* (1989) *Expressed Emotion (EE) of Schizophrenic Relatives*. Poster presented at VIIIth World Congress of Psychiatry, Athens, 12th–19th October.

Goldberg, S.C., Shooler, N.R., Hogarty, G.E. & Roper, M. (1977) Prediction of relapse in schizophrenic outpatients treated with drug and sociotherapy. *Archives of General Psychiatry*, **34**, 171–184.

Goldstein, M., Judd, L.L., Rodnick, E.H., Alkire, A. & Gould, E. (1968) A method for studying social influence and coping patterns within families of disturbed adolescents. *Journal of Nervous and Mental Disease*, **147**, 233–251.

Greenley, J.R. (1986) Social control and EE. *Journal of Nervous and Mental Disorders*, **174**, 24–30.

Gureje, O. & Adewumni, A. (1988) Life events in schizophrenia in Nigerians. A controlled investigation. *British Journal of Psychiatry*, **153**, 367–375.

Hardesty, J., Falloon, I.R.H. & Shirin, K. (1985) The impact of life events, stress and coping on the morbidity of schizophrenia. In Falloon, I.R. (ed.) *Family Management of Schizophrenia*. John Hopkins University Press, Baltimore.

Harris, T.O. (1987) Recent developments in the study of life events in relation to psychiatric and physical disorders. In Cooper, B. (ed.) *Psychiatric Epidemiology: Progress and Prospects*, pp. 81–100. Croom Helm, London.

Hegerl, U., Priebe, S., Wildgrube, C. & Muller-Oerlinghausen, B. (1990) Expressed emotion and auditory evoked potentials. *Psychiatry*, **53**, 108–114.

Herzog, T. (1992) Nurses, patients and relatives: a study of family patterns on psychiatric wards. In Cazzullo, C.L. & Invernizzi, G. (eds) *Family Intervention in Schizophrenia: Experiences and Orientations in Europe*. ARS, Milan (in press).

Hirsch, S., Cramer, P. & Bowen, J. (1992) The triggering hypothesis of the role of life events in schizoprenia. *British Journal of Psychiatry*, **161**, 84–87.

Hirsch, S., Bowen, J., Emami, J. *et al.* (1993) A 1-year prospective study of the effect of life events and medication in the aetiology of schizophrenic relapse (submitted to the *British Journal of Psychiatry*).

Hogarty, G.E. (1985) Expressed emotion and schizophrenic relapse: implications from the Pittsburg Study. In Alpert, M. (ed.) *Controversies in Schizophrenia*. Guilford Press, New York.

Hogarty, G.E., Anderson, C.M., Reiss, D.J. *et al.* (1986) Family psycho-education, social skills training and maintenance chemotherapy in the aftercare treatment of schizophrenia. I. One year effects of a controlled study on relapse and expressed emotion. *Archives of General Psychiatry*, **43**, 633–642.

Holmes, T.H. & Rahe, R.H. (1967) The social readjustment rating scale. *Journal of Psychosomatic Research*, **11**, 213–218.

Hooley, J.M. & Hahlweg, K. (1986) The marriages and interaction patterns of depressed patients and their spouses: comparison of high and low EE dyads. In Goldstein, M.J., Hand, I. & Hahlweg, K. (eds) *Treatment of Schizophrenia: Family Assessment and Intervention*, pp. 84–95. Springer-Verlag, Berlin.

Hubschmid, T. & Zemp, M. (1989) Interactions in high- and low-EE families. *Social Psychiatry and Psychiatric Epidemiology*, **24**, 113–119.

Jacobs, S. & Myers, J. (1976) Recent life events and acute schizophrenic psychosis: a controlled study. *Journal of Nervous and Mental Disease*, **162**, 75–87.

Jones, P.B., Bebbington, P.E., Foerster, A. *et al.* (1993) Premorbid social underachievement in schizophrenia: results from the Camberwell Collaborative Psychosis Study. *British Journal of Psychiatry*, **163**, 65–71.

Kavanagh, D.J. (1992) Recent developments in expressed emotion and schizophrenia. *British Journal of Psychiatry*, **160**, 601–620.

Kraepelin, E. (1913) *Clinical Psychiatry*. William Wood, New York.

Kuipers, L. (1979) Expressed emotion: a review. *British Journal of Social and Clinical Psychology*. **18**, 237–243.

Kuipers, L. (1983) *Family factors in schizophrenia: an intervention study*. PhD Thesis, University of London.

Kuipers, L. (1992) Expressed emotion research in Europe. *British Journal of Psychology*, **31**, 429–443.

Kuipers, L. & Bebbington, P.E. (1988) Expressed emotion research in schizophrenia: theoretical and clinical implications. *Psychological Medicine*, **18**, 893–910.

Kuipers, L., MacCarthy, B., Hurry, J. & Harper, R. (1989) A low-cost supportive model for relatives of the long-term adult mentally ill. *British Journal of Psychiatry*, **154**, 775–782.

Kuipers, L., Sturgeon, D., Berkowitz, R. & Leff J.P. (1983) Characteristics of expressed emotion: its relationship to speech and looking in schizophrenic patients and their relatives. *British Journal of Clinical Psychology*, **22**, 257–264.

Lam, D. (1991) Psychosocial family intervention in schizophrenia: a review of empirical studies. *Psychological Medicine*, **21**, 423–441.

Leff, J.P. & Vaughn, C.E. (1980) The interaction of life events and relative's expressed emotion in schizophrenia and depressive neurosis. *British Journal of Psychiatry*, **136**, 146–153.

Leff, J.P. & Vaughn, C. (1985) *Expressed Emotion in Families*. Guilford Press, New York.

Leff, J.P., Kuipers, L., Berkowitz, R., Eberlein-Fries, R. & Sturgeon, D. (1982) A controlled trial of social intervention in schizophrenic families. *British Journal of Psychiatry*, **141**, 121–134.

Leff, J.P., Kuipers, L., Berkowitz, R. & Sturgeon, D. (1985) A controlled trial of social intervention in the families of schizophrenic patients: two-year follow-up. *British Journal of Psychiatry*, **146**, 594–600.

Leff, J.P., Hirsch, S.R., Gaind, R., Rohde, P.D. & Stevens, B.C. (1973) Life events and maintenance therapy in schizophrenic relapse. *British Journal of Psychiatry*, **123**, 659–660.

Leff, J.P., Kuipers, L., Berkowitz, R., Vaughn, C.E. & Sturgeon, D. (1983) Life events, relatives' expressed emotion and maintenance neuroleptics in schizophrenic relapse. *Psychological Medicine*, **13**, 799–806.

Leff, J., Berkowitz, R., Shavit, N., Strachan, A., Glass, I. & Vaughn, C. (1989) A trial of family therapy v. a relatives' group for schizophrenia. *British Journal of Psychiatry*, **154**,

58−66.

Leff, J.P., Berkowitz, R., Shavit, N., Strachan, A., Glass, I & Vaughn, C. (1990) A trial of family therapy vs a relatives' group for schizophrenia: two-year follow-up. *British Journal of Psychiatry*, **157**, 571−677.

MacCarthy, B., Kuipers, L. Hurry, J., Harper, R. & Le Sage, A. (1989) Evaluation of counselling for relatives of the long-term adult mentally ill. *British Journal of Psychiatry*, **154**, 768−775.

McCreadie, R.G., Phillips, K., Harvey, J.A., Waldron, G., Stewart, M. & Baird, D. (1991) The Nithsdale Schizophrenia Surveys. VIII. Do relatives want family intervention and does it help? *British Journal of Psychiatry*, **158**, 110−113.

McCreadie, R.G., Robertson, L.J., Hall, D.J. & Berry, I. (1993) The Nithsdale Schizophrenia Surveys. XI. Relatives' expressed emotion. Stability over five years and its relations to relapse. *British Journal of Psychiatry*, **162**, 393−397.

Malla, A.K., Cortese, L., Shaw, T.S. & Ginsberg, B. (1990) Life events and relapse in schizophrenia: a one-year prospective study. *Social Psychiatry and Psychiatric Epidemiology*, **25**, 221−224.

Malzacher, M., Merz, J. & Ebnother, D. (1981) Einschneidende Lebensereignisse im Vorfeld akuter schizophrener Episoden: Erstmals erkrankte Patienten im Vergleich mit einer Normalstichprobe. *Archiv für Psychiatrie und Nervenkrankheiten*, **230**, 227−242.

Mavreas, V.G., Tomaras, V., Karydi, V., Economon, M. & Stefanis, C. (1992) Expressed emotion in families of chronic schizophrenics and its association with clinical measures. *Social Psychiatry and Psychiatric Epidemiology*, **27**, 4−9.

Miklowitz, D.J., Goldstein, M.J. & Falloon, I.R.H. (1983) Premorbid and symptomatic characteristics of schizophrenics from families with high and low levels of expressed emotion. *Journal of Abnormal Psychology*, **3**, 359−367.

Miklowitz, D.J., Goldstein, M.J., Doane, J.A. *et al.* (1989) Is expressed emotion an index of a transactional process. I. Parent's affective style. *Family Process*, **28**, 153−167.

Moore, E., Ball, R.A. & Kuipers, L. (1992) Expressed emotion in staff working with the long-term adult mentally ill. *British Journal of Psychiatry*, **161**, 802−808.

Mueller, D.P., Edwards, D.W. & Yarvis, R.M. (1977) Stressful life events and psychiatric symptomatology: change or undesirability. *Journal of Health and Social Behaviour*, **18**, 307−317.

Rutter, M.L. & Brown, G.W. (1966) The reliability and validity of measures of family life and relationships in families containing a psychiatric patient. *Social Psychiatry*, **1**, 38−53.

Schwarz, C. & Myers, J. (1977) Life events and schizophrenia. Parts I and II. *Archives of General Psychiatry*, **34**, 1238−1248.

Steinberg, H. & Durell, J. (1968) A stressful situation as a precipitant of schizophrenic symptoms: an epidemiological study. *British Journal of Psychiatry*, **114**, 1097−1105.

Stevens, B.C. (1973) Evaluation of rehabilitation for psychotic patients in the community. *Acta Psychiatrica Scandinavica*, **46**, 136−140.

Strachan, A.M., Feingold, D., Goldstein, M.J., Miklowitz, D.J. & Nuechterlein, K.H. (1989) Is expressed emotion an index of a transactional process? II. Patient's coping style. *Family Process*, **28**, 169−181.

Strachan, A.M., Leff, J.P., Goldstein, M.J., Doane, A. & Burt, C. (1986) Emotional attitudes and direct communication in the families of schizophrenics: a cross-national replication. *British Journal of Psychiatry*, **149**, 279−287.

Tarrier, N. (1989) Electrodermal activity, expressed emotion and outcome in schizophrenia. *British Journal of Psychiatry*, **155**(Suppl. 5), 51−56.

Tarrier, N., Barrowclough, C., Vaughn, C. *et al.* (1988b) The community management of schizophrenia: a controlled trial of a behavioural intervention with families to reduce relapse. *British Journal of Psychiatry*, **153**, 532−542.

Vaughn, C.E. & Leff, J.P. (1976) The measurement of expressed emotion in the families of psychiatric patients. *British Journal of Clinical and Social Psychology*, **15**, 157−165.

Vaughan, K., Doyle, M., McConathy, N., Blaszczyski, A., Box, A. & Tarrier, N. (1992) The relationship between relatives' EE and shizophrenic relapse: an Australian replication. *Social Psychiatry and Psychiatric Epidemiology*, **27**, 10−15.

Ventura, J., Nuechterlein, K.H., Hardisty, J.P. & Gitlin, M. (1992) Life events and schizophrenic relapse after withdrawal of medication: a prospective study. *British Journal of Psychiatry*, **161**, 615−620.

Ventura, J., Nuechterlein, K.H., Lukoff, D. & Hardisty, J.P. (1989) A prospective study of stressful life events and schizophrenic relapse. *Journal of Abnormal Psychology*, **98**, 407−411.

Watts, S. (1988) *A Descriptive Investigation of the Incidence of High EE in Staff Working with Schizophrenic Patients in a Hospital Setting.* Diploma in Clinical Psychology Dissertation, British Psychological Society.

Wing, J.K. (1966) Social and psychological changes in a rehabilitation unit. *Social Psychiatry*, **1**, 21−28.

Wing, J.K. & Brown, G.W. (1970) *Institutionalism and Schizophrenia. A Comparative Study of Three Mental Hospitals 1960−68.* Cambridge University Press, Cambridge.

Wing, J.K. & Freudenberg, R.K. (1961) The response of severely ill chronic schizophrenic patients to social stimulation. *American Journal of Psychiatry*, **118**, 311−322.

Wing, J.K., Bennett, D.H. & Denham, J. (1964) *The Industrial Rehabilitation of Long Stay Schizophrenic Patients.* Medical Research Council Memo No. 42. London, HMSO.

Wittchen, H.U., Essau, C.A., Hecht, H., Teder, W. & Pfister, H. (1989) Reliability of life-event assessments, test−retest reliability and fall-off effects of the Munich Interview for the assessment of life events. *Journal of Affective Disorders*, **16**, 77−92.

Chapter 30
Cognitive-Behavioural Therapies in Psychiatric Rehabilitation

R. P. LIBERMAN, W. D. SPAULDING AND P. W. CORRIGAN

Introduction

As clinical trials of pharmacological and psychosocial treatments for schizophrenia have incorporated longer term follow-ups in their design, researchers and practitioners alike have increasingly acknowledged the necessity for indefinite, continuous, maintenance treatment of persons with schizophrenia using psychosocial as well as drug therapies. Just as schizophrenic individuals are more likely to relapse when withdrawn from maintenance antipsychotic drugs, so susceptibility to stress-induced relapse increases when effective psychosocial treatments are terminated. The realization that the continuous application of biopsychosocial therapies can reduce the long-term disability and persisting or relapsing psychotic symptoms inherent in schizophrenia has given birth to the field of *psychiatric rehabilitation* (Anthony & Liberman, 1986; Liberman *et al.*, 1988).

While early and effective intervention for acute psychotic episodes is important for minimizing long-term disability, psychiatric rehabilitation emphasizes continuous, comprehensive services — linked to the phase of the person's illness — for symptom control, prevention or mitigation of relapses, and optimizing the chronically ill patient's performance in social, vocational, educational and familial roles, with the least amount of support necessary from the helping professions. The clinical practice of psychiatric rehabilitation joins together three approaches:

1 pharmacotherapy judiciously keyed to the type and severity of psychopathology with doses that do not produce sedation, neuromotor and other toxic side effects that interfere with positive and active engagement in rehabilitation;

2 development of skills in the patient that are linked to stressors and life situations, as well as personal assets and deficits, which challenge the individual's adaptation and independence; and

3 a range of supportive social services, such as case management, which offer a decent quality of life, even to individuals whose symptoms and functional disabilities persist despite our best efforts at treatment and rehabilitation.

In addition, a pillar of psychiatric rehabilitation lies on the assumption that disabled persons need empowerment to be actively involved in treatment decisions and to achieve the highest feasible quality of life in the community (Anthony *et al.*, 1988).

The challenge to psychiatric rehabilitation is of public health proportions. With the fragmented mental health service system in the USA, thousands of homeless mentally ill people live wretchedly and even more are warehoused in prisons and locked residential facilities in the community. These regressive trends, eerily reminiscent of the dark ages of pre-19th-century indifference to the mentally ill, come just at the time when internationally replicated studies have shown that substantial symptomatic and social recoveries can be achieved with more than half of chronic schizophrenics when continuous, rehabilitative services are available over a 20- to 40-year period (Harding *et al.*, 1987).

Our failure to provide high-quality, continuous psychiatric treatment is brought into bold relief by the availability of new rehabilitative technologies that, when systematically organized and delivered, have the potential for accelerating recovery by reducing morbidity, disability and handicaps. That the augmentation of our therapeutic armamentarium with more effective biobehavioural techniques can indeed accelerate remission of psychotic symptoms and recovery of social functioning is illustrated by a recent study that found an unprecedented zero relapse rate during 1 year in carefully diagnosed chronic schizophrenics — with the use of antipsychotic drug therapy, social skills training and family psychoeducation (Hogarty *et al.*, 1986).

Conceptual framework for rehabilitation

Studies in Europe, the USA and Japan that have followed up 20–40 years later persons who experienced disabling forms of schizophrenia during early adulthood have found a remarkable 50–66% functioning actively in their communities, with few symptoms, a reasonably good subjective quality of life and only limited dependence on professional caregivers. The findings from these studies have spurred interest in psychiatric rehabilitation as a means of accelerating the prospects for social and symptomatic recoveries among the seriously mentally ill. With an attachment to databased empiricism and hypothesis testing, an emerging interdisciplinary cadre of specialists in psychiatric rehabilitation have derived new assessment and intervention methods from the *stress–vulnerability–protective factors* model of psychiatric impairment, disability and

handicap. The model is depicted in Fig 30.1, where the course and outcome of major mental disorders are defined by the following.

Impairments, which are the characteristic positive and negative symptoms and associated cognitive and affective abnormalities of disorderes such as schizophrenia, autism and bipolar disorder.

Disabilities, which are the restrictions, imposed by impairments, on functional life domains such as personal hygiene, medication self-management, recreation for leisure, and family and social relationships.

Handicap, which is the disadvantage experienced by an individual having impairments and disabilities that limits or prevents the fulfilment of normal roles such as worker, student, citizen and family member.

Moving mentally disabled persons along the spectrum of impairments, disability and handicap — from poor to good outcomes — requires orchestration of *protective factors* in treatment and community support services. As long as the *psychobiological vulnerability factors* responsible for the specific syndrome are unknown, interventions cannot directly modify them. These vulnerability factors, most likely genetically mediated, are enduring and present before the manifest symptoms of the disorder emerge, as well as during periods of symptom remission and relapse. Similarly, as long as we adhere to the principles of community care of the mentally ill, it is not possible to isolate vulnerable individuals from *socio-environmental stressors*. Stressors, whether drugs of abuse or social overstimulation, are a fact of life for the mentally ill — even in the so-called asylums where privacy is nil and violence is omnipresent. Even in the absence of major life events or the noxious effects of illicit drugs and alcohol, vulnerable individuals can succumb to ambient levels of tension or conflict in their environment, or microstressors if they lack the protection conferred by medication, coping abilities and social support.

Psychiatric rehabilitation must harness the protective factors in both the treatment and natural environments to offset and buffer the adverse effects of stress superimposed upon vulnerability. These protective factors include

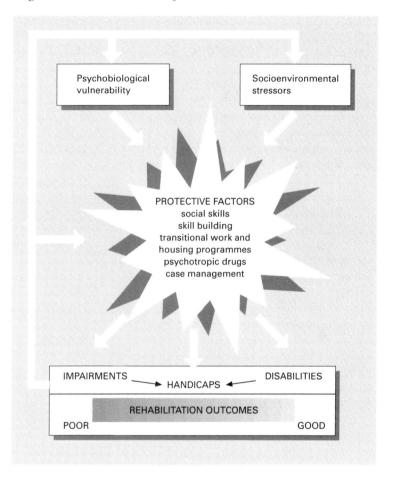

Fig. 30.1 The heterogeneity among persons with schizophrenia in cognitive impairments, symptoms, functional deficits, disabilities and social role handicaps can be viewed as an outcome of the interactions among psychobiological vulnerability, socioenvironmental stressors and protective factors within the person and his/her environment. Since there are no treatments that can directly affect the enduring vulnerabilities in the central nervous system, rehabilitative interventions must be aimed at reducing stress or strengthening protective factors. Recovery from schizophrenia is possible as protection is conferred against stress-induced relapse through continuous, comprehensive and coordinated biobehavioural services.

optimal psychopharmacological interventions that can raise the threshold at which environmental stressors precipitate symptoms in an individual with a given level of vulnerability to a serious mental disorder. But even when pharmacotherapy is prescribed with attention to the highest possible benefit:risk ratio — maximizing therapeutic effects while minimizing side effects — protection against relapse is not assured. Medications must be supplemented by psychosocial interventions that: (i) equip patients with personal, social and vocational coping and competence; and (ii) galvanize necessary social support services to compensate for the intrusion of symptoms, deficits and disabilities that even the best system of care cannot remediate.

Organization and delivery of rehabilitation

It is now widely accepted that a continuum of psychiatric, medical and social services should be available to persons with schizophrenia in the community through the operation of mobile and assertive outreach teams of clinicians (Test, 1992). This framework for delivering services is often referred to as 'intensive case management', 'training in community living' or 'assertive community treatment'. The spectrum of cognitive and behavioural therapies described in this chapter must be competently learned and used by the clinicians and case managers who indefinitely serve the needs of persons with schizophrenia in the community (Vaccaro *et al.*, 1992). While this chapter will focus primarily on modalities of cognitive and behaviour therapy, the importance of embedding such techniques within the context of continuous, comprehensive and supportive services cannot be emphasized enough. As the needs of patients change with different phases of their illness, the continuous-treatment team must offer varying degrees of case management support and appropriate forms of pharmacotherapy, family education, social service entitlements, housing, skills training and vocational rehabilitation.

Research has clearly shown that patients treated in well-administered community support programmes have better outcomes than patients who remain in hospital during the same period of time and then are released (Herz *et al.*, 1971; Mosher & Menn, 1978; Stein & Test, 1978; Test & Stein, 1978; Test, 1992). Community support programmes subsume a spectrum of services including outreach, rehabilitation, health care, crisis intervention, housing, income support, family care and advocacy (Anthony & Blanch, 1987). Case management plays a central role in coordinating services and in assuring that quality and continuity of care remain.

Specific duties of case managers include discharge planning from the in-patient setting, establishing linkages with community programmes, networking with these programmes to confirm that linkages have occurred, assurance that quality community care is proffered and advocacy for services when they are insufficient, of poor quality or not provided at all (Kanter, 1989).

An assessment of symptoms and functional status — repeatedly checked and monitored — drives the clinician's decision-making regarding the timing, intensity, form and comprehensiveness of treatments that need to be provided. If remissions of psychotic symptoms and social recoveries are to be accelerated and sustained, the treatment decisions must be guided by ongoing, periodic assessment of the individual's psychopathology, functional assets and deficits, deviant behaviours and personal and environmental resources that can be mobilized for community support. Assessment and intervention are inextri-

cably interwoven in the pursuit of realistic goals and removal of obstacles to rehabilitation. Moreover, the individual patient and his/her relatives or caregivers must be engaged collaboratively in the assessment, goal setting and treatment process from the very start. When patients and their natural support network are active partners in the clinical process, progress in rehabilitation is greatly facilitated.

The remainder of this chapter will describe the current status of cognitive and behaviour therapies for the rehabilitation of people with schizophrenia. Like the pharmacotherapies for schizophrenia, cognitive-behaviour therapies have been designed by theory-driven research and validated by empirical methods. They are considered the psychosocial treatments of choice in schizophrenia (Liberman & Bedell, 1989). Cognitive remediation will be the first modality presented, followed by behavioural management of psychotic symptoms, social skills training, token economy and social learning methods and behaviourally orientated vocational rehabilitation. These modalities should not be viewed as self-sufficient or stand-alone treatments, but rather as components in a multimodal, comprehensive and continuous service system that responds flexibly to patients' needs as determined by the phase or type of disorder.

Cognitive remediation

Abnormalities are found in schizophrenia at all levels of the cognitive system, and in all phases in the course of the disorder. Cognitive impairments are thought to play a number of roles in schizophrenia's aetiology and expression (Cromwell & Spaulding, 1978; Nuechterlein & Dawson, 1984; Nuechterlein & Asarnow, 1989). It is therefore an appealing hypothesis that remediation of such impairments might lead to improvements in personal and social functioning. Many classical treatment approaches in psychiatry have attempted to address cognitive impairments in schizophrenia, but systematic specification of procedures and evaluation of outcome began in the cognitive-behavioural era.

Early efforts to treat schizophrenic cognition directly were carried out by Meichenbaum and Cameron (1973), using a self-instructional training approach that has since become ubiquitous in cognitive-behavioural therapy. Applied to schizophrenia, the approach involves rehearsal of self-instructions designed to establish and maintain continuous attention to tasks, inhibit impulsive responses and prompt self-reinforcement. The self-instructions are rehearsed while performing various tasks, at first simple laboratory tests and later more complex *in vivo* social or work tasks. The original study (Meichenbaum & Cameron, 1973) showed beneficial treatment effects for this approach, measured by improvements in interview performance, ambient social behaviour and psychological tests. However, these findings have not always proved replicable (Margolis & Shemberg, 1976). Later studies (reviewed by Spaulding *et al.*, 1986; Bentall *et al.*, 1987) suggest that a beneficial effect can reliably be observed provided that the self-instructional training is adequately tailored to individual patients' abilities and impairments, and implemented in a context which is meaningful enough to secure the patients' interest and cooperation.

The self-instructional approach is 'cognitive' in the sense that it uses language and related processes to organize, guide and motivate behaviour. However, the approach was not developed from any model of cognitive psychopathology. As originally applied it did not explicitly address cognitive impairments associated with schizophrenia. Rather, the self-instructions are assumed to represent a general prosthetic or compensatory aid by which the effects of impairments are reduced or bypassed. In this sense, the approach is more closely related to skills training, discussed later in this chapter, than to cognitive remediation. In discussing their original results, Meichenbaum and Cameron (1973) suggested that the design of self-instructional sets for schizophrenic patients might benefit from more specific considerations of the cognitive characteristics of the disorder and its subtypes.

As interest grew in social skills training for schizophrenics, concerns were expressed that establishing or re-establishing verbal and non-verbal communication skills does not address the core problems of the disorder (Liberman *et al.*, 1982). Recently, there has been experimental verification that cognitive impairments are associated with poorer performance in skills training (Mueser *et al.*, 1991; Kern *et al.*, 1992; Bowen *et al.*, 1993; Corrigan *et al.*, 1994). One response to this has been to develop 'cognitively sensitive' methods in skills training. This includes orientating the skills trainer or therapist to be alert for attention and short-term memory problems, minimizing distraction in the training setting, employing repetition and overlearning, and carefully pacing the training procedures. Self-instructional training used as an adjunct to skills training can also serve to reduce the impact of cognitive deficits. Self-instructions and other cognitive-behavioural techniques used in skills training for schizophrenia have become more informed by close monitoring of attentional impairments and psychopathology (Bellack *et al.*, 1989; Massel *et al.*, 1991; Heinssen & Victor, 1994).

There has been no controversy about whether it is worthwhile to develop cognitively sensitive training techniques. Most widely used skills training approaches are cognitively sensitive to varying degrees. There have been no attempts to analyse the unique contributions of cognitive sensitivity to the overall outcome of skills training, nor any calls for a highly controlled outcome trial or 'horserace', between cognitively sensitive vs. insensitive skills training. However, research in this area might profitably investigate what specific characteristics of therapy and the therapist best potentiate skills acquisition for cognitively impaired subjects. This suggests a research strategy similar to those used to determine the key factors in outcome of conventional psychotherapy and behaviour therapy (Strupp & Butler, 1990; Wixted *et al.*, 1990; Spaulding, 1992). However, interest in cognitive approaches to treatment has gone beyond increasing the cognitive sensitivity of skills training, to attempting to modify directly or remediate patients' impairments.

The approach to direct remediation that is most commonly described in the literature (reviewed by

Spaulding *et al.*, 1986; Reed *et al.*, 1992) is undertaken in a dyadic format similar to that of conventional cognitive-behavioural psychotherapy. A working relationship is established between patient and therapist. Specific cognitive impairments are identified through laboratory testing, analysis of the patient's phenomenology and observation of *in vivo* behaviour. The impairments are addressed in a series of exercises, starting with simple laboratory tasks and gradually proceeding to complex *in vivo* performance of tasks which demand effective use of the impaired processes. For example, when distractibility is identified as the cognitive impairment, the patient may practise a laboratory dichotic listening task, then simple conversation with the therapist under increasingly distracting conditions, and then more complex social and work tasks in increasingly realistic environments. These procedures would typically be included in a more comprehensive regimen of skills training for personal and social competence, with all the self-instructional techniques and therapist coaching that such a regimen demands. Reports of successful cases include patients from the entire spectrum of rehabilitation candidates, from mildly to severely cognitively impaired, in settings ranging from out-patient clinics to public institutions.

Outcome studies of this approach have been limited to case studies and small-scale experiments (Spaulding *et al.*, 1986; Reed *et al.*, 1992; Spaulding & Sullivan, 1992). The required degree of idiographic assessment and treatment tailoring make large-scale outcome studies difficult. Most reported studies have used some form of multiple baseline design to show that improvements in cognitive functioning predate other improvements in a manner consistent with the hypothesis that the cognitive intervention contributes uniquely to overall outcome. An accumulation of reports over the years provides substantial evidence for effectiveness, but conclusive verification awaits large-scale, highly controlled outcome studies. The advantages of the approach are that it is fairly accessible to cognitive-behavioural therapists with background or consultant resources in experimental psychopathology and clinical neuro-

psychology, it addresses the individual variability of cognitive impairments, and it is easily incorporated in a more comprehensive rehabilitation programme.

A variation of the dyadic therapy approach includes the use of cognitive exercise programmes borrowed from neuropsychological rehabilitation (e.g. Flesher, 1990). Some such programmes are commercially available as software packages for computer administration (Skilbeck, 1991). A number of tasks are included, addressing cognitive processes ranging from simple vigilance to complex psychomotor performance and problem solving. This allows some degree of individual tailoring of the computer program, although the packages are designed to address cognitive impairment patterns more typical of acute brain trauma and progressive dementia than of chronic schizophrenia. So far, studies of this approach have been inadequately controlled small-group experiments and case studies. The cognitive treatment has not been integrated into comprehensive, individualized rehabilitation regimens. The results of neuropsychologically orientated cognitive remediation are mildly encouraging (Olbrich & Mussgay, 1990; Stuve, 1990; Burda & Starkey, 1991; Liberman & Green, 1992; Green, 1993; Goldberg, 1994; Fine, 1994; Spaulding, 1993). Patients can clearly improve their performance by practising the programmes. However, it remains unclear whether such improvement has any clinical meaning, especially in the domain of social functioning.

There have been a few more highly controlled laboratory studies of response to specific treatment procedures targeting specific cognitive impairments (Schlank, 1987; Bellak *et al.*, 1990; Green *et al.*, 1992). These were designed primarily to verify the possibility of changing cognitive functioning with psychosocial interventions, and to explore some relevant parameters, rather than to assess the impact of the improvements on overall clinical status. Schlank (1987) studied the effects of a social apperception exercise, previously reported in case studies, on progress in a problem-solving skills training group. In the exercise, patients generate alternative story scenarios to single thematic apperception test (TAT) cards, gradually increasing their ability to generate many scenarios without bizarre or perseverative content. This is thought to address the conceptual inflexibility seen in many schizophrenic patients, which in turn is thought to limit competence in social problem solving. Schlank (1987) showed that patients who practised the exercise with a therapist made better progress in the skills training group, compared with patients who received a comparable amount of individual non-directive psychotherapy. Bellak *et al.* (1989) and Green *et al.* (1990) showed that combinations of cognitive-behavioural coaching and contingent reinforcement produce improvement in patient performance on the Wisconsin card sorting test (WCST). The WCST requires use of concept formation, short-term memory and trial-and-error problem solving, all of which may be associated with a limbic—frontal brain dysfunction found in schizophrenic patients (Weinberger *et al.*, 1988).

Brenner *et al.* (Brenner, 1987; Brenner *et al.*, 1992) have developed an integrated therapy modality which incorporates a number of specific cognitive exercises in a skills training group format. The cognitive tasks are interwoven with interpersonal activities in the group, so as to maximize generalization to social functioning. For example, an exercise of the ability to systematically categorize information is built into a group parlour game of the '20 questions' type. The modality includes five subsections: the first three address cognitive skills of increasing complexity, and the last two are similar to conventional interpersonal skills training.

This approach avoids the individualization problem by using a 'shotgun' strategy, addressing a range of impairments thought to be common in schizophrenic populations. Individual patients are expected to be stronger in some areas and weaker in others. The therapist capitalizes on individual differences by encouraging patients without impairments in a particular area to help those who have them. This provides important opportunities for generalizing skills to the interpersonal context, and for increasing patient self-esteem and investment in treatment.

A number of studies [reviewed by Brenner (1987) and Brenner *et al.* (1992)] have shown that the modality as a whole produces results superior to standard hospital treatment. One study indirectly assessed the unique contribution of its cognitive components by showing that better results are produced when the cognitive subsections precede, rather than follow, the interpersonal skills subsections. However, the controlled experimental studies required to verify a unique contribution of the explicitly cognitive parts of the modality have not yet been completed. In fact, studies comparing social skills training with Brenner's integrated therapy have found similar improvements after treatment in basic cognitive and attentional functioning (Liberman & Green, 1992).

A more individualized variation of the Brenner modality has been developed and tested by van der Gaag *et al.* (van der Gaag, 1992; van der Gaag *et al.*, 1994). Their findings support the overall effectiveness of the modality, but do not address the unique contribution to outcome by the cognitive components. However, the studies by van der Gaag *et al.* do include a fine-grained analysis of what cognitive functions respond to treatment. As might be expected from the conceptual-level emphasis of the modality, conceptual-level cognitive functions show the largest treatment effects. A similar pattern of findings was obtained by Olbrich and Mussgay (1990) in a smaller scale and more focused evaluation of cognitive training.

In summary, the effectiveness of direct cognitive remediation for schizophrenia is only tentatively supported by systematic research. The most reasonable hypothesis at this time is that direct remediation may contribute a unique component to overall outcome, when included in an integrated comprehensive programme of psychosocial treatment and rehabilitation. This has created a dilemma for researchers. Verification of cognitive effects in highly controlled laboratory tests is required to justify large-scale clinical studies, yet it is unlikely that cognitive changes produced under such conditions would have meaningful generalized effects. As a result, research has proceeded from both 'top-down' and 'bottom-up' perspectives. The bottom-up perspective starts with highly specific laboratory findings and seeks to extend these to increasingly realistic clinical contexts. The top-down perspective seeks to identify the uniquely cognitive factors in comprehensive modalities of known effectiveness. One of these more 'molar' and comprehensive therapies, social skills training, will be described later in this chapter.

Symptom management

Investigators have used various cognitive-behavioural techniques to reduce directly the symptoms and behavioural deviances associated with schizophrenia. This is accomplished sometimes by directly suppressing expression of the target symptom, and sometimes by increasing other behaviours which are incompatible with the target symptom. The conceptual assumption underlying the behaviour modification of psychotic symptoms is that by weakening the environmental antecedents (discriminative stimuli) and consequences (reinforcers) of the symptoms, the individual will 'unlearn' the symptoms and 'learn' alternative, adaptive and reality-orientated behaviours. Moreover, once the functional valence of a symptom is diminished by changing its relationship with the triggering and reinforcing events that have helped to maintain it, motivation is established for developing more constructive ways to meet personal needs.

Without denying the key role of biological vulnerabilities and central nervous system dysfunctions in the aetiology of psychotic symptoms, behaviour therapists try to manipulate the environmental contributions to the evocation and maintenance of psychopathology. It is assumed that if the overt manifestations of the symptoms decrease sufficiently in frequency and intensity, then there will also be a weakening of the covert, subjective experience of the symptoms subsequently. The prerequisites for effective behaviour therapy of psychotic and other mental disorders include:
1 operational measurement and recording of the target symptoms and adaptive behavioural goals;
2 functional analysis of the controlling environmental (and biological, if possible) antecedents

and consequences of the target symptoms and adaptive behavioural goals;
3 systematic application of principles of human learning as interventions for modifying psychotic symptoms; and
4 monitoring changes in the target symptoms and adaptive goals as a function of the interventions, and using empirical eclecticism to identify effective treatments.

Treatment of hallucinations

An early study of the behavioural modification of hallucinations suggested that auditory hallucinations could be suppressed by self-administered, painful, but harmless, electric shocks to the skin of the arm (Bucher & Fabricatore, 1970). However, a subsequent controlled study demonstrated that similar results could be obtained by a procedure that employed self-monitoring of hallucinations by the subjects without aversive stimuli (Weingaertner, 1971). Based on the assumption that social attention contributed to the maintenance of chronic hallucinations, the use of brief 'time-outs' or isolation was shown to reduce reliably the frequency of hallucinations (Davis *et al.*, 1976).

Since there is no independent means of verifying the presence of hallucinations, behaviour therapists do not distinguish between self-reports of hallucinations and the hallucinations themselves. The results of these studies merely suggest that there are circumstances which may induce patients not to report their hallucinations. In many clinical and natural contexts, this is a potentially beneficial effect. Ideally, a patient discriminates between situations where reporting hallucinations is appropriate (e.g. when discussing medication changes with the psychiatrist) and when it is not.

An alternative approach to controlling hallucinations is suggested by the hypothesis that subvocal motor activity is causally related to auditory hallucinations. Electromyographically recorded muscle activity in the chin and lips are temporally associated with patient reports of hallucinations (Gould, 1948; McGuigan, 1966). Bick and Kinsbourne (1987) tested the clinical implications of this hypothesis by instructing schizophrenic subjects to perform various muscle-movement exercises when experiencing auditory hallucinations. Subjects in the subvocal-specific exercise group were instructed to open their mouths widely, while subjects in the control condition were told to close their eyes tightly or to clench their fists. Patients completing the subvocal-specific exercises reported fewer auditory hallucinations than subjects using the control exercises.

Green and Kinsbourne (1990) replicated these findings with humming as the subvocal-specific behaviour, and biting the tongue and lifting the eyebrows as the control conditions. Only humming increased subvocal electromyograms above baseline, thereby suggesting that this subvocal-specific exercise interfered with motor activity related to auditory hallucinations. However, the temporal relationship between reports of hallucinations and electromyography was weak. It is unclear whether the effect results from attentional distraction (see Margo *et al.*, 1981; Alpert, 1985) or from some form of centrally mediated response competition. Considering the frequency with which hallucinations disrupt performance, even in optimally medicated patients, there may be significant clinical potential in this technique. Further research is summarized in Chapter 31.

Reducing delusional speech

The hypothesis that operant contingencies of reinforcement can directly extinguish 'sick talk' has been examined in various studies (Wong *et al.*, 1986). Wincze *et al.* (1972) compared the efficacy of token contingencies with verbal feedback in decreasing the frequency of delusional speech in 10 paranoid schizophrenic patients. During the token-based intervention, subjects received tokens on a fixed interval schedule for not voicing delusional statements. Feedback comprised correcting delusional statements by pointing out the falsity in the statement. For example, the therapist would tell a patient who had said he was Jesus Christ, 'Your answer is incorrect, Jesus Christ lived almost 2000 years ago. Your name is Mr M and you are 40 years old.' Results of the study showed that the rate of delusional statements both within the training sessions and on the ward decreased for seven of the 10 subjects after token contingencies were implemented. Conversely, three of the subjects showed either no effects after receiving feedback or actually increased delusional speech after feedback.

In another study, delusional speech of four chronic schizophrenic patients was shaped by controlling access to social reinforcers (Liberman *et al.*, 1973). Subjects were individually paired with a favourite staff member each evening to share pleasant banter, coffee, fruit, doughnuts and other goodies. After several non-contingent meetings, subjects were told that the length of the evening chat would be proportional to the amount of delusion-free talk accumulated during four daily interviews. After 18 days of contingent social reinforcement, the frequency of delusional speech had diminished by 200–600% across the sample of patients. Social reinforcers were then slowly faded, e.g. evening chats were offered every other night. Three of the four subjects maintained rational speech after decreasing the social contingencies. One showed no return of delusional speech at 1 year follow-up in the community (Patterson & Teigen, 1973).

Interpreting the failure of feedback to produce changes in delusional behaviour, Watts *et al.* (1973) argued that challenging delusions, especially those that are self-aggrandizing, may generate reactance in patients such that they are unwilling to comply with treatment prescriptions. For this reason, clinical investigators have adopted collaborative rather than confrontive approaches to providing feedback. In a direct test of the relative effects of confrontation vs. collaboration, 16 patients were randomly assigned to either a confrontational group (in which therapists were firm but polite, using phrases like, 'You are quite wrong I'm afraid. You have no scar, therefore the device could not have been implanted,') or a belief-modification group (in which therapists avoided disagreement; rather they taught patients to search for alternative explanations of their experience to the delusion) (Milton *et al.*, 1978). Results showed that subjects from both groups decreased delusional intensity, social anxiety and overall psychopathology. Decrements in delusional intensity for the belief-modification group, however, were greater than for the confrontational group.

Lowe and Chadwick (1990) adopted a 'collaborative empirical' approach to reframing the delusions of two chronic schizophrenic patients, wherein patient and clinician jointly evaluated the evidence (and lack thereof) supporting a delusion. Results of a multiple baseline design for the first subject showed that conviction, preoccupation and anxiety regarding delusions about a factitious spouse and Jesus Christ diminished soon after being targeted. These effects generalized to reduction of a third delusion as well, a belief about Leonardo da Vinci. Three delusions of the second patient also decreased after the patient participated in collaborative challenging. Although there was much variance from one observation period to the next, trends suggested that the second patient's level of preoccupation and anxiety with each delusion was also diminished. Other, less highly controlled studies have shown similar results using gentle confrontation (Alford, 1986; Alford & Fleece, 1982).

Another example comes from the work of Perris (1992), who has adapted the cognitive-behaviour therapy techniques developed by Beck for neurotic disorders to the treatment of persons with schizophrenia and other psychotic and borderline disorders. Infusing collaborative empiricism into both scheduled and spontaneous therapeutic interactions between patients and staff in the context of small family style residential homes, Perris and his interdisciplinary treatment teams emphasize cognitive restructuring, in which patients are encouraged to test the accuracy and utility of their delusional and other reality distorting beliefs. Controlled studies of this form of cognitive-behaviour therapy will need to be conducted if Perris reports favourable follow-up results from the current demonstration project. Converging research in this area should be expected to articulate how specific cognitive impairments in individual patients can be identified and targeted for treatment, how remediation can best be achieved and how remediation strategies can best be integrated with other treatments and with comprehensive rehabilitation.

Findings from these studies are promising, suggesting that cognitive-behavioural techniques can assist patients in managing their delusions. Collaborative empiricism provides guidance for clinicians who are frustrated by delusions that are earnestly maintained by patients in the face of conflicting evidence. The cognitive requirements of these treatments seem quite demanding, however. It is unlikely that conceptually disorganized patients would be able to comply with these prescriptions for changing attributions. For example, it may be difficult for thought-disordered patients to search for explanations to their delusions in an orderly way.

In addition to targeting hallucinations and delusions, behaviour therapists have used learning-based procedures to supplant or displace a wide variety of behavioural disabilities and deviances of chronic schizophrenics. For example, a series of studies have shown that the engagement of patients in behavioural activities (such as those used in recreational therapy) can displace bizarre stereotypies and vocalizations (Corrigan *et al.*, 1993). Other research has demonstrated successful and enduring behavioural control of psychogenic polydipsia (Bowen *et al.*, 1990), psychotic aggression (Wong *et al.*, 1985), mutism (Fichter *et al.*, 1976) and self-care deficits (Liberman *et al.*, 1974; Wong *et al.*, 1986; Glynn & Mueser, 1992).

Social skills training

Over the past decade, social skills training has become the most intensively researched and widely used psychosocial modality in the treatment and rehabilitation of severe and persistent psychiatric disorders (Liberman *et al.*, 1986a). Social skills training defines a generic set of learning activities such as modelling, reinforcement, role playing and *in vivo* exercises that help patients acquire a variety of skills in verbal and non-verbal behavioural domains. Loosely considered, these domains address the interpersonal, self-care and coping needs that patients encounter as they negotiate the demands of community living. Typically, skills training is conducted as an educational class with one or two therapists as trainers and five to 10 patients as students or trainees. The sessions last 45–90 min, depending on the patients' level of concentration and agitation, and are held 1–5 times per week (Liberman, *et al.*, 1989).

One recent innovation in training for social and independent living skills is the modular approach developed by Wallace, Liberman and their colleagues at the UCLA Clinical Research Center for Schizophrenia and Psychiatric Rehabilitation. Modules have been produced for teaching an array of skills that facilitate community adjustment, for example recreation for leisure, symptom self-management, medication self-management, basic conversation skills, grooming and self-care, job finding and interpersonal problem solving. Each module is a self-contained curriculum that teaches from four to six competencies in a major domain of community functioning. For example, the medication-management module teaches five competencies: recognizing medication benefits, recognizing its side effects, monitoring these side effects, discussing medication with physicians and other caregivers and recognizing the benefits of long-acting injectable medication. Each competency is divided into the specific knowledge and skills that define the competency and are the focus of the training. For example, competently discussing medication with physicians and other caregivers is divided into pleasantly greeting the physician, describing the problem in detail (including its duration and severity), requesting that action be taken. clarifying and repeating the doctor's prescription, and pleasantly ending the interaction while maintaining appropriate eye contact, posture and paralinguistic qualities during the entire exchange.

Each competency's constituent skills are taught with the same seven instructional techniques. The first three — introduction, videotape demonstration and role-playing practice — help patients learn and practise the skills in the training sessions. The fourth and fifth techniques — solving resource-management problems and solving outcome problems — prepare participants to use their skills outside of the training sessions. The sixth and seventh activities — *in vivo* exercises and homework assignments — require that participants use the skills outside of the training session. A detailed description of the modules is given elsewhere (Wallace *et al.*, 1985).

Each module consists of a trainer's manual, participant's workbook and demonstration videotape. The manual specifies exactly what the trainer is to say and do to teach all the module's skills; the videotape demonstrates the skills; and the workbook provides participants with written material, forms and exercises that help them to learn the skills. The trainer instructs by reading scripts and asking questions written in the manual, by playing the videotape, and by evaluating the participants' role playing with checklists written in the manual. The trainer corrects inaccurate answers or role playing by using prompting, modelling, coaching and reinforcement. A training session is generally conducted with four to eight patients and one trainer, and sessions are scheduled 2 or 3 times per week for 1–1.5 h each. Approximately 13–20 weeks of twice-weekly sessions are needed to complete each module.

Research on the modules from the UCLA Social and Independent Living Skills Program has shown that clinicians can quickly acquire the facility to use the learning activities that comprise the module, implement these learning activities with a high level of fidelity, and use then to improve patients' social and coping skills (Eckman *et al.*, 1990, 1992; Wallace *et al.*, 1992; Liberman & Corrigan, 1993). Research has also shown that social skills training significantly increases patients' range of interpersonal and instrumental skills (Brown & Munford, 1983; Morrison & Bellack, 1984; Wallace & Liberman, 1985; Benton & Schroeder, 1990). Moreover, patients who complete skills training programmes show diminished psychiatric symptomatology and decreased relapses and rehospitalizations (Bellack *et al.*, 1984; Wallace & Liberman, 1985; Hogarty *et al.*, 1986, 1987).

Acquired skills have been maintained by patients from 1 month (Jaffe & Carlson, 1976; Wallace et al., 1985) to more than 2 years (Longin & Rooney, 1975; Kindness & Newton, 1984). Findings about generalization to other settings have been more equivocal, however. Active programming of generalization strategies like overlearning, homework and *in vivo* practice may improve the transfer of skills to settings outside the treatment milieu (Stokes & Baer, 1977). In addition, for knowledge and the skill to transfer from the classroom to natural environments, it is essential for case managers or other practitioners to consult with families or other caregivers to ensure that opportunities, encouragement and acknowledgement are given to patients in their homes or work settings.

The therapeutic effects of skills training may be explained by two types of model: *topographic* and *cognitive* (Corrigan *et al.*, 1992). According to the topographic model, interpersonal skills comprise a set of discrete 'micro' skills which, when combined, yield competent social behaviour (Morrison & Bellack, 1987). For example, proficient conversation skills are comprised of nonverbal signals like eye contact, facial expression, voice intonation and interpersonal distance, as well as appropriate verbal responses including relevant comments and adequate self-disclosure. Hence, patients with poor social skills have not acquired sufficient numbers of microskills and large gaps appear as social ineptness. When patients learn these discrete skills and piece them together, the appropriate 'macro' response emerges.

The topographic model of interpersonal skills has been criticized as providing a reflexive view of social interactions (Trower, 1982). In response to limitations of the topographic view, cognitive models have evolved; these describe the skill deficits of severely mentally ill patients *vis-à-vis* impaired social information processing. In particular, skills learning has been described in terms of other information-processing deficits characteristic of schizophrenia (Mueser, *et al.*, 1991; Kern *et al.*, 1992), diminished sensitivity to social cues (Corrigan & Green, 1993a), inability to comprehend interpersonal problems and generate relevant solutions (Donahoe *et al.*, 1991), lack

of comprehension of social schemata that define the rules and goals of interpersonal situations (Corrigan *et al.*, 1992; Corrigan & Green, 1993b), and unawareness of the linguistic rules that underscore conversation (Trower *et al.*, 1978). This is closely related to the development of cognitively sensitive training approaches, described earlier in this chapter. As cognitive models of skills training evolve, the boundary between cognitive remediation and behavioural skills training becomes less distinct.

Skills training methods based on cognitive models attempt to teach patients generative rules that can be adapted for use in various situations (Liberman *et al.*, 1986b). For example, a six-step problem-solving strategy has developed as an outline for helping patients to overcome interpersonal dilemmas (D'Zurilla, 1986):

1 adopt a problem-solving attitude;
2 identify the problem;
3 brainstorm potential solutions;
4 evaluate the options for problem-solving and pick one to implement;
5 plan the implementation and carry it out; and
6 evaluate the efficacy of the plan and, if not effective, pick another alternative (Hansen *et al.*, 1985).

Because family members are often involved as primary caregivers for chronic schizophrenics, skills training and educational approaches with patients and relatives together have become an important element in psychiatric rehabilitation. The educational and training sessions, starting with information about the nature of schizophrenia and the drug and psychosocial treatments available for its treatment, can be conducted in the patient's home, or in the clinic or hospital. Topics include positive and negative symptoms, effects of psychotropic medications and treatment options in psychiatric rehabilitation. Material is presented didactically, followed by guided discussion. Patients and relatives alike are considered the 'experts' at these meetings and are invited to discuss various points about symptoms and treatments in terms of their own experiences. To varying degrees, education programmes are enhanced with basic skills training of the patient and relatives in interpersonal communication, problem solving and contingency management. One approach which emphasizes these traditional cognitive-behavioural techniques is termed *behavioural family management* (Falloon *et al.*, 1984).

Several well-controlled studies (Golstein *et al.*, 1978; Falloon *et al.*, 1982, 1985; Anderson *et al.*, 1987; Tarrier *et al.*, 1988) have shown that the rate of relapse and subsequent hospitalization for patients whose families participate in skills building and educational programmes is significantly less than for customary treatments. While it is clear that patients benefit from having their families involved in treatment, the mechanisms of the treatment effects are unknown, and the critical components of the various approaches have not been identified. Acquiring communication and problem-solving skills on the part of the patient and family members have been shown to be important, but affective and social—ecological factors may also be crucial. For example, family members are typically distressed by the patient's bizarre and asocial behaviour, anxious about increased financial burdens for the patient's treatment, uncertain about future plans and isolated from their own social supports due to caregiving responsibilities, stigma and social embarrassment (Creer & Wing, 1974). In some families, these stressors produce high levels of *expressed emotion* (criticism, disappointment, hostility and overprotectiveness). Patients who return to families with high expressed emotion are more likely to relapse than are those whose families are low in expressed emotion (Brown *et al.*, 1972; Vaughn & Leff, 1976; Vaughn *et al.*, 1982; Leff & Vaughn, 1985). Changes in expressed emotion may thus be part of the beneficial effect of family education/treatment. One outcome study which showed better social and independent functioning and improved quality of life for patients in the family treatment group (Falloon *et al.*, 1985), also showed lower expressed emotion and emotional burden in the family members.

Another approach to family treatment uses long-term, process-orientated multiple family groups, and emphasizes interfamilial support (McFarlane *et al.*, 1992). The approach assumes that in a multiple family group, the isolation and stigmatization experienced by family members is greatly diminished, and therefore the burden of care grows less overwhelming. Also, the group provides opportunities for families to share helpful suggestions about specific problems.

Although the family support group approach is not a typical cognitive-behavioural modality, it may merit systematic study. Pilot studies have shown that patient relapse rates diminish and the level of community functioning improves as patients and their families participate in multiple family support groups (McFarlane *et al.*, 1992). The participants also report subjective benefits. As with the education/treatment approaches, the mechanisms of the treatment effect are obscure. Process analyses and comparative outcome studies of educational vs. supportive approaches to family treatment should be expected to reveal much about how these approaches benefit patients and their families.

Token economy and social learning

Token economies rely on laws of operant conditioning to establish contingencies of reinforcement that increase the frequency of targeted, desirable behaviours (Skinner, 1953). Hence, strategically rewarding patient behaviour increases the performance of appropriate responses. The *law of association by contiguity* states that neutral stimuli that are frequently associated with primary reinforcers become reinforcing themselves. Hence, handing out tokens (e.g. points on a patient's 'credit' card or poker chips) that can be exchanged for cigarettes, candy and privileges make tokens rewarding in themselves. Using tokens to manage behavioural contingencies provides several benefits: (i) tokens permit more immediate reinforcement of spontaneous skills by bridging the delay between target responses and back-up reinforcement; (ii) distribution of reinforcers is more flexible with behaviours being able to be rewarded at any time; (iii) new behaviours may be maintained over extended periods when back-up reinforcement is unavailable; and (iv) learning to improve one's functioning in a token economy prepares patients for living in the economy outside the hospital (Ayllon & Azrin, 1968; Kazdin & Bootzin, 1972).

Several steps must be accomplished to implement a successful token economy. First, behaviours to be targeted in the token economy must be identified. These include self-care and appropriate social behaviours, for which all patients receive tokens, and overly aggressive or hostile behaviours, which result in token 'fines'. Each behaviour needs to be sufficiently described and operationalized so that patients and staff can reliably recognize it.

Next, contingencies must be created that govern the consequences of these behaviours. Contingencies describe 'if−then' rules connecting a target behaviour with a reinforcer or fine. When setting up a token economy, payments and fines can be determined by a staff committee familiar with the patients' behavioural level of functioning, i.e. achieving a positive balance of tokens each day is desirable for motivating patients, and thus rewards must not be too difficult to obtain. As the token economy progresses, specific contingencies can be adjusted, depending on the frequency with which individual behaviours are performed by the patient group and the fluctuating rate of commodity purchases.

After target behaviours have been fully defined and reinforcers put in place, rules must be developed to designate the manner in which patients receive and exchange tokens. Administrators of token economies must define the place and time in which tokens can be exchanged for commodities and other reinforcers. Typically, treatment units dedicate one small room to store cigarettes, decaffeinated coffee, candy, soda pop and personal articles. The prices for commodities are listed next to the door of the token store. Prices for commodities vary, depending on the demand for the item and the cost of purchasing the item from outside retailers. Demand can be assessed by marking the number of purchases each time someone comes up to the door.

Token economies provide several advantages for the management of the in-patient behavioural milieu (Kazdin, 1982). Utilization of tokens permits more immediate reinforcement of spontaneous skills by bridging the delay between the target response and back-up reinforcer. Similarly, dissemination of reinforcers is more flexible, allowing behaviours to be rewarded at any time. The token economy is not affected by satiation, a common problem when specific reinforcers, such as food or ward privileges, are used. In fact, research has shown that tokens by themselves may assume a greater and more generalized incentive value than any single primary reward.

Token economies have been extensively studied in the treatment of chronic, institutionalized psychiatric patients. Results have shown that symptoms and self-care skills of subjects in these studies have significantly improved, even after other treatments were unsuccessful (Atthowe & Krasner, 1968; Ayllon & Azrin, 1968; Glynn & Mueser, 1992). In one classic study, investigators randomly assigned 84 long-term schizophrenic and other psychotic patients to state hospital units utilizing social learning, milieu therapy or traditional custodial care approaches (Paul & Lentz, 1977). A multimodal assessment battery, including reliable time-sampled behavioural observations, revealed impressive and clearcut results favouring the social learning approach. After only 14 weeks of treatment, every resident in the social learning programme showed dramatic improvements in overall functioning, regardless of the usual prognostic indicators, such as duration of hospitalization and pretreatment level of impairment. By the end of the second year of programming, fewer than 25% of residents in either experimental condition were on maintenance psychotropic drugs. Improved functioning, enabling long-term community tenure, occurred in 97% of the social learning patients. The therapeutic milieu programme was less effective, but its 71% release and community maintenance rate was still a favourable outcome compared with the 45% rate for patients released from custodial care and living in the community for 18 months or longer. Importantly, the social learning programme was clearly the most cost effective when decreased need for hospitalization was included in cost calculations.

Despite this success, the token economy is not commonly used by clinicians serving the mentally disabled (Boudewyns *et al.*, 1986; Glynn, 1990; Corrigan, 1991). Several factors have been identified that may impede using this technology; these include poor patient selection, lack of staff interest, poor collegial support and insufficient institutional support (Hall & Baker, 1973; Corrigan *et al.*, 1992). Administrators who decide to introduce the token economy into their programme must not only concern themselves with clinical issues, but also must be mindful of administrative barriers to treatment innovations.

Vocational rehabilitation

Patients with chronic psychoses and who attend work each day are less likely to suffer symptom exacerbation (Hagen, 1983) or return to hospital (Brenner, 1973). However, research shows that patients with chronic or mental disorders find employment difficult to obtain (Anthony *et al.*, 1978; Lehman, 1983). Two behaviourally orientated strategies of vocational rehabilitation have been developed for mentally ill patients who are unlikely prospects for competitive employment: *supported employment* and *job-finding training*.

Supported employment

Following its extraordinary success in securing normal employment for the mentally handicapped or retarded, supported employment has become the most important new development in the vocational rehabilitation of the severely mentally ill (Anthony & Blanch, 1987). This intervention uses a 'place-then-train' approach, instead of the traditional 'train-then-place' method which had failed miserably to obtain competitive employment for the mentally ill in the era of sheltered workshops (Bond, 1992). Rather than spending lengthy periods in preparatory, prevocational settings, participants are matched with existing jobs in the local economy and are provided with training in work skills, instruction on work habits and supportive counselling by a 'job coach' whose goal is to sustain the productive involvement of the mentally ill person at the work site.

An important element in supported employment is social skills training to equip the mentally ill person with the conversation and problem-solving skills to meet the interpersonal expectations and demands of the work culture and setting (Mueser & Liberman, 1988). Mentally ill individuals often find the person-to-person transactions in the work setting (e.g. conversation with coworkers at lunch and during coffee and tea breaks, and asking the supervisor for assistance on a task) more stressful than the actual job tasks; thus, skills training *in vivo* can protect schizophrenic individuals from stress-induced relapse. Necessary skills and social supports are developed for the schizophrenic, in consultation with the employer, to assist the mentally ill individual to meet the specific requirements of the work environment.

Much emphasis is placed on helping the individual maintain the job. When the programme participant must acquire a new work or social skill, the job coach or case manager develops and delivers a well-planned lesson, using behavioural principles such as modelling, rehearsal, prompting, cueing, fading, shaping and reinforcement. The behavioural responses required by any job are broken down by a 'task analysis' into small chunks, which are then taught to the participant, moving at the participant's own learning rate. At times, the participant might attend social skills training sessions (Mueser & Liberman, 1988), receive medication regulated by a psychiatrist or meet for crisis intervention at sites away from the job. Thus, coordination of a wide array of mental health services as well as consultation and liaison with the employer are essential components in the performance standards for job coaches and case managers.

Evaluative research has found that 74–80% of participants in supported employment are employed for at least 60 consecutive days during a year of enrollment, and 42–52% remain employed in community workplaces at the end of the year (Bond, 1992; Danley *et al.*, 1992). However, the supported employment approach has not been used long enough to generate well-controlled studies that will determine its cost effectiveness and provide answers to questions such as: What is the dropout rate? What is the average duration in each programme phase? What do the staff actually do? What are the employment and retention rates? How satisfied are participants with their jobs?

Job-finding clubs

Patients who are able to sustain daily work demands may need training in job-finding skills which can be conducted in club-like settings (Azrin & Besalel, 1980; Azrin & Phillip, 1980; Jacobs *et al.*, 1984). Basic skills taught during job-finding seminars include identifying job leads, writing résumés, filling out job applications, rehearsing interviewing skills and using public transport. Patients who demonstrate mastery of these skills are encouraged to look for work. During the job-seeking phase, the club offers resources to support the arduous search, e.g. counsellors, buddy system of mutual aid, newspapers, phones and maps. Since studies of traditional modes of vocational rehabilitation have documented that only 15% of psychotic patients are able to keep jobs for a full year (Anthony *et al.*, 1978), job-finding clubs provide continued post-employment support and services to help individuals weather work-related problems.

Research on job-finding clubs has shown them to be an effective means to help patients obtain employment. Controlled studies have found employment rates of 42–90%, compared with 10–33% employment outcome for mentally ill subjects participating in control programmes (Keith *et al.*, 1977; Azrin & Phillip, 1980; Eisenberg & Cole, 1986). In another evaluative study of the job club, 66% of the participants found work or were enrolled full time in job-training programmes, requiring on average 22 days of participation in the club. Six-month follow-up data revealed that 68% of these employed individuals were still working (Jacobs *et al.*, 1984). More recent evaluations of the job-club programme have found lower employment rates, with individuals suffering from schizophrenia or bipolar disorder doing more poorly than those with neurotic or substance-abuse disorders. Thus, the job club may be utilitarian for only a subset of persons with schizophrenia. Interestingly, while fewer schizophrenics were successful in obtaining employment, of those who succeeded the retention rates were as high as for individuals from other diagnostic categories (Jacobs *et al.*, 1990).

Future directions

There is a great discrepancy between: (i) what is known from research and demonstration studies about effective biopsychosocial treatments and rehabilitation; and (ii) what is actually implemented at the clinical level. This discrepancy between available technology and common practice prevents thousands of persons with schizophrenia from achieving more optimal states of symptomatic and social functioning. Administrative, financial, organizational and systems' obstacles confound the best efforts of practitioners and researchers to apply the state-of-the-art. In addition, reliance on publications and conferences to disseminate innovations can never succeed in producing knowledge and technology transfer from research into practice. Much more active, brokering models of dissemination — similar to those used by agricultural field agents who introduce new seeds and fertilizers, and by pharmaceutical company sales representatives who visit physicians with well-designed information resources — must be employed to overcome the professional inertia in systems of mental care (Backer *et al.*, 1986).

The following caveats can help to bridge the gap between research and practice:

engage patients in accessible services through active outreach and mobile case-management services;

provide continuous and indefinite biopsychosocial treatment and rehabilitation in the context of reliable and mutually respectful therapeutic relationships;

engage the patient's and family's self-help and active participation in rehabilitation;

assist the patient and caregivers in the delicate balancing of risk-taking with asylum to reduce stress-related relapses to a minimum; and galvanize administrative and programme support for comprehensive and coordinated services.

A number of innovations are on the horizon and can be expected to improve the prospects for psychiatric rehabilitation. These are as follows.

Illness self-management techniques, such as those found in the UCLA Social and Independent Living Skills programme, will permit patients to assume more responsibility for monitoring their psychopathology and seek early and flexible levels of intervention.

Functional assessment will become more individualized and better linked to prescriptions for rehabilitation.

Social learning and assertive community treatment proponents will consolidate and integrate their techniques and procedures so that cognitive-behaviour therapy can be used to teach patients how to adapt to community living.

Social skills training will receive an infusion of new principles and techniques from research on the cognitive sciences. Since cognitive impairments may be the rate-limiting factors in learning and rehabilitation outcomes, cognitive remediation and compensatory and prosthetic environments will be developed to spur faster and more complete rehabilitation.

Family involvement in treatment and rehabilitation, as well as in advocacy for needed services and research, will continue to grow and professionals will design services that offer education, skills training and social support to family caregivers.

Bringing these innovations into the realistic arena of clinical practice will determine just how much accelerated recovery can be achieved in the broad-spectrum, community-based treatment and rehabilitation of persons with schizophrenia.

References

Alford, B.A. (1986) Behavioral treatment of schizophrenic delusions: a single-case experimental analysis. *Behavior Therapy*, **17**, 639–644.

Alford, H., Fleece, L. & Rothblum, E. (1982) Hallucinatory-delusional verbalizations: modification in a chronic schizophrenic by self-control and cognitive restructuring. *Behavior Modification*, **6**, 412–435.

Alpert, M. (1985) The signs and symptoms of schizophrenia. In Alpert, M. (ed.) *Controversies in Schizophrenia*, pp. 255–266. Guilford Press, New York.

Anderson, C.M., Reiss, D.J. & Hogarty, G.E. (1987) *Schizophrenia and the Family*. Guildford, New York.

Anthony, W.A. & Blanch, A.K. (1987) Supported employment for persons who are psychiatrically disabled: an historical and conceptual perspective. *Psychosocial Rehabilitation Journal*, **11**, 5–23.

Anthony, W.A. & Liberman, R.P. (1986) The practice of psychiatric rehabilitation: historical, conceptual and research base. *Schizophrenia Bulletin*, **12**, 542–559.

Anthony, W.A., Cohen, M.R. & Danley, K.S. (1988) The psychiatric rehabilitation approach as applied to vocational rehabilitation. In Ciardiello, J.A. & Bell, M.D. (eds) *Vocational Rehabilitation of Persons with Prolonged Psychiatric Disorders*, pp. 224–248. Johns Hopkins University Press, Baltimore.

Anthony, W.A., Cohen, M.R. & Vitalo, R. (1978) The measurement of rehabilitation outcome. *Schizophrenia Bulletin*, **4**, 365–383.

Atthowe, J.M. & Krasner, L. (1968) Preliminary report on the application of contingent reinforcement procedures (token economy) on a 'chronic' psychiatric ward. *Journal of Abnormal Psychology*, **73**, 37–43.

Ayllon, T. & Azrin, N. (1968) *The Token Economy: A Motivation System for Therapy and Rehabilitation*. Appleton-Century Crofts, New York.

Azrin, N.H. & Besalel, V.A. (1980) *Job Club Counselor's Manual*. University Park Press, Baltimore.

Azrin, N.H. & Phillip, R.A. (1980) The job club method for the job handicapped: a comparative outcome study. *Rehabilitation Counselling Bulletin*, **23**, 144–155.

Backer, T.E., Liberman, R.P. & Kuehnel T.G. (1986) Dissemination and adoption of innovative psychosocial interventions. *Journal of Consulting and Clinical Psychology*, **54**, 111–118.

Bellack, A.S., Morrison, R.L. & Mueser, K.T. (1989) Social problem solving in schizophrenia. *Schizophrenia Bulletin*, **15**, 101–116.

Bellak, A., Mueser, K., Morrison, R., Tierney, A. & Podell, K. (1990) Remediation of cognitive deficits in schizophrenia: training on the Wisconsin Card Sorting Test. *American Journal of Psychiatry*, **147**, 1650–1655.

Bellack, A.S., Turner, S.M., Hersen, M. & Luber, R.F. (1984) An examination of the efficacy of social skills training for chronic schizophrenic patients. *Hospital and Community Psychiatry*, **35**, 1023–1028.

Bentall, R., Higson, P. & Lowe, C. (1987) Teaching self-instructions to chronic schizophrenic patients: efficacy and generalization. *Behavioral Psychotherapy*, **15**, 58–76.

Benton, M.K. & Schroeder, H.E. (1990) Social skills training with schizophrenics: a meta-analytic evaluation. *Journal of Consulting and Clinical Psychology*, **58**, 741–747.

Bick, P.A. & Kinsbourne, M. (1987) Auditory hallucinations and subvocal speech in schizophrenic patients. *American Journal of Psychiatry*, **144**, 222–225.

Bond, G.R. (1992) Vocational rehabilitation. In Liberman, R.P. (ed.) *Handbook of Psychiatric Rehabilitation*, pp. 244–

275. Macmillan, New York.

Boudewyns, P.A., Fry, T.J. & Nightengale, E. (1986) Token economy programs in VA medical centers: where are they today? *Behavior Therapist*, **6**, 126–127.

Bowen, L., Glynn, S.M., Marshall, B.D., Kurth, L. & Hayden, J.L. (1990) Successful behavioral treatment of polydipsia in a schizophrenic patient. *Journal of Behavior Therapy and Experimental Psychiatry*, **21**, 53–61.

Bowen, L., Wallace, C.J., Nuechterlein, K.H. & Lutzker J. (1993) *Relationship of Attentional Deficits to Learning Instrumental and Problem-Solving Skills.* Unpublished manuscript available from Dr Wallace at Camarillo-UCLA Research Center, PO Box 6022, Camarillo, CA 93011.

Brenner, H. (1987) On the importance of cognitive disorders in treatment and rehabilitation. In Strauss, J., Baker, W. & Brenner, H. (eds) *Psychosocial Treatment of Schizophrenia*, pp. 184–205. Huber, Bern.

Brenner, H.D., Hodel, B., Roder, V. & Corrigan, P. (1992) Treatment of cognitive dysfunctions and behavioral deficits in schizophrenia. *Schizophrenia Bulletin*, **18(1)**, 21–26.

Brenner, M.H. (1973) *Mental Illness and the Economy.* Harvard University Press, Cambridge.

Brown, G.W., Birley, J.L.T. & Wing, J.H. (1972) The influence of family life on the course of schizophrenic disorder: a replication. *British Journal of Psychology*, **121**, 241–258.

Brown, M.A. & Munford, A.M. (1983) Life skills training for chronic schizophrenics. *Journal of Nervous and Mental Disease*, **17**, 1466–1476.

Bucher, B. & Fabricatore, J. (1970) Use of patient-administered shock to suppress hallucinations. *Behavior Therapy*, **1**, 382–385.

Burda, P.C. & Starkey, T.W. (1991) *Computer-administered cognitive training of psychiatric inpatients.* Paper presented at American Psychological Association, San Francisco.

Corrigan, P.W. (1991) Strategies that overcome barriers to token economies in community programs for severe mentally ill adults. *Community Mental Health Journal*, **26**, 151–165.

Corrigan, P.W. & Green, M.F. (1993a) Schizophrenic patients' sensitivity to social cues: the role of abstraction. *American Journal of Psychiatry*, **150**, 589–594.

Corrigan, P.W. & Green, M.F. (1993b) The situational feature recognition test: a measure of schema comprehension for schizophrenia. *International Journal of Methods in Psychiatric Research*, **3**, 29–35.

Corrigan, P.W., Kwartarini, W.Y. & Pramana, W. (1992) Staff perception of barriers to behavior therapy at a psychiatric hospital. *Behavior Modification*, **16**, 132–144.

Corrigan, P.W., Liberman, R.P. & Wong, S.E. (1993) Recreational therapy and behavior management on inpatient units: is recreation therapy therapeutic? *Journal of Nervous and Mental Disease*, **181**, 644–647.

Corrigan, P.W., Schade, M.L. & Liberman, R.P. (1992) Social skills training. In Liberman, R.P. (ed.) *Handbook of Psychiatric Rehabilitation*, pp. 95–126. Macmillan, New York.

Corrigan, P.W., Wallace, C.J. & Green, M.F. (1992) Deficits in social schemata in schizophrenia. *Schizophrenia Research*, **8**, 129–135.

Corrigan, P.W., Wallace, C.J., Schade M.L. & Green, M.F. (1994) Cognitive dysfunctions and psychosocial skill learning in schizophrenia. *Behavior Therapy*, **25**, 5–15.

Creer, C. & Wing, J. (1974) *Schizophrenia at Home.* National Schizophrenia Fellowship, London.

Cromwell, R.L. & Spaulding, W. (1978) How schizophrenics handle information. In Fann, W.E., Karacan, I., Pokorny, A.D. & Williams, R.L. (eds) *The Phenomenology and Treatment of Schizophrenia*, pp. 127–162. Spectrum, New York.

Danley, K.S., Sciarappa, K. & MacDonald, K. (1992) Choose–get–keep: a psychiatric rehabilitation approach to supported employment. In Liberman, R.P. (ed.) *New Directions for Mental Health Services: Effective Psychiatric Rehabilitation*, pp. 87–96. Jossey-Bass, San Francisco.

Davis, J.R., Wallace, C.J., Liberman, R.P. & Finch, B.E. (1976) The use of isolation (time-out) to suppress delusional and hallucinatory speech. *Journal of Behavior Therapy and Experimental Psychiatry*, **7**, 269–276.

Donahoe, C.P., Carter, M.J., Bloem, W.D. & Wallace, C.J. (1991) Assessment of interpersonal problem-solving skills. *Psychiatry*, **53**, 329–339.

Eckman, T.A., Liberman, R.P., Phipps, C.C. & Blair, K. (1990) Teaching medication self-management to chronic schizophrenics. *Journal of Clinical Psychopharmacology*, **10**, 33–38.

Eckman, T.A., Tucker, D.E., Roberts, L.J. & Liberman, R.P. (1992) An integrated biobehavioral approach for training persons with chronic psychoses in social and self-management skills. In Ferrero, F. & Salvati, R. (eds) *Schizophrenia and Affective Psychoses*, pp. 64–77. John Libbey, Rome.

Eisenberg, M.G. & Cole, H.W. (1986) A behavioral approach to job seeking for psychiatrically impaired persons. *Journal of Rehabilitation*, **27**, 46–49.

Falloon, I.R.H., Boyd, J.L. & McGill, C.W. (1984) *Family Care of Schizophrenia.* Guilford Press, New York.

Falloon, I.R.H., Boyd, J.L., McGill, C.W., Razani, J., Moss, H.B. & Gilderman, A.M. (1982) Family management in the prevention of exacerbations of schizophrenia: a controlled study. *New England Journal of Medicine*, **306**, 1437–1440.

Falloon, I.R.H., Boyd, J.L., McGill, C.W. *et al.* (1985) Family management in the prevention of morbidity of schizophrenia: clinical outcome of a two-year longitudinal study. *Archives of General Psychiatry*, **42**, 887–896.

Fichter, M., Wallace, C.J., Liberman, R.P. & Davis J.R. (1976) Improving social interaction in a chronic psychotic using 'naging' (discriminated avoidance): experimental analysis and generalization. *Journal of Applied Behavior Analysis*, **9**, 377–386.

Fine, S. (1994) Reframing rehabilitation: putting skill acquisition and the mental health system in proper perspective. In Spaulding, W. (ed.) *Cognitive Technology in Psychiatric Rehabilitation*, pp. 87–114. University of Nebraska Press, Lincoln.

Flesher, S. (1990) Cognitive habilitation in schizophrenia: a theoretical review and model of treatment. *Neuropsychology Review*, **1(3)**, 223–246.

van der Gaag, M. (1992) *The Results of Cognitive Training in Schizophrenic Patients.* Eburon, Delft.

van der Gaag, M., Woonings, F., vandenBosch, R., Appelo, M., Sloof, C. & Louwerens, J. (1994) Cognitive training of schizophrenic patients: a behavioral approach based on experimental psychopathology. In Spaulding, W. (ed.) *Cognitive Technology in Psychiatric Rehabilitation*, pp. 139–158. University of Nebraska Press, Lincoln.

Glynn, S.M. (1990) Token economy approaches for psychiatric patients. *Behavior Modification*, **14**, 383–407.

Glynn, S. & Mueser, K.T. (1992) Social learning programs. In Liberman, R.P. (ed.) *Handbook of Psychiatric Rehabilitation*, pp. 127–152. Macmillan, New York.

Goldberg, J. (1994) Cognitive retraining in a community psychiatric rehabilitation program. In Spaulding, W. (ed.) *Cognitive Technology in Psychiatric Rehabilitation*, pp. 67–86. University of Nebraska Press, Lincoln.

Goldstein, M.J., Rodnick, E.H., Evans, J.R., May, P.R.A. & Steinberg, M.R. (1978) Drug and family therapy in the aftercare of acute schizophrenia. *Archives of General Psychiatry*, **35**, 1169–1177.

Gould, L.N. (1948) Verbal hallucinations and the activity of vocal musculature. *American Journal of Psychiatry*, **105**, 367–372.

Green, M.F. (1993) Cognitive remediation in schizophrenia: is it time yet? *American Journal of Psychiatry*, **150**, 149–158.

Green, M.F. & Kinsbourne, M. (1990) Subvocal activity and auditory hallucinations: clues for behavioral treatment? *Schizophrenia Bulletin*, **16**, 617–625.

Green, M.F., Ganzell, S., Satz, P. & Vaclav, J.F. (1990) Teaching the Wisconsin Card Sorting Test to schizophrenic patients (letter). *Archives of General Psychiatry*, **47**, 91–92.

Green, M.F., Satz, P., Ganzell, S. & Vaclav, J. (1992) The Wisconsin Card Sorting Test: remediation of a stubborn deficit. *American Journal of Psychiatry*, **149**, 62–67.

Hagen, D.Q. (1983) The relationship between job loss and physical and mental illness. *Hospital and Community Psychiatry*, **34**, 438–441.

Hall, J. & Baker, R. (1973) Token economy systems: breakdown and control. *Behavior Research and Therapy*, **II**, 253–263.

Hansen, D.J., St Lawrence, J.S. & Christoff, K.A. (1985) Effects of interpersonal problem-solving training with chronic aftercare patients on problem-solving component skills and effectiveness of solution. *Journal of Consulting and Clinical Psychology*, **53**, 167–174.

Harding, C.M., Brooks, G.W., Ashikaga, T. & Strauss, J.S. (1987) The Vermont longitudinal study of persons with severe mental illness. *American Journal of Psychiatry*, **144**, 718–735.

Heinssen, R. & Victor, B. (1994) Cognitive-behavioral treatments for schizophrenia: evolving rehabilitation techniques. In Spaulding, W. (ed.) *Cognitive Technology in Psychiatric Rehabilitation*, pp. 159–182. University of Nebraska Press, Lincoln.

Herz, M.I., Endicott, J., Spitzer, R.L. & Mesnikoff, A. (1971) Day versus inpatient hospitalization: a controlled study. *American Journal of Psychiatry*, **127**, 1371–1382.

Hogarty, G.E., Anderson, C.M. & Reiss, D.J. (1987) Family psychoeducation, social skills training, and medication in schizophrenia: the long and short of it. *Psychopharmacology Bulletin*, **23**, 12–13.

Hogarty, G.E., Anderson, C.M., Reiss, D.J. *et al.* (1986) Family psychoeducation, social skills training, and maintenance chemotherapy in the aftercare treatment of schizophrenia. *Archives of General Psychiatry*, **43**, 633–642.

Jacobs, H.E., Liberman, R.P., Arruda, M.J. & Mintz, J. (1990) *The Job Finding Club: Predictors of Outcome*. Presented to the 143rd Annual Meeting of the American Psychiatric Association, New York.

Jacobs, H.E., Kardashian, S., Kreinbring, P.K., Ponder, R. & Simpson, A.R. (1984) A skills-oriented model facilitating employment among psychiatrically disabled persons. *Rehabilitation Counseling Bulletin*, **28**, 87–96.

Jaffe, P.G. & Carlson, P.M. (1976) Relative efficacy of modeling and instructions in eliciting social behavior from chronic psychiatric patients. *Journal of Consulting and Clinical Psychology*, **44**, 200–207.

Kanter, J. (1989) Clinical case management: definition, principles, components. *Hospital and Community Psychiatry*, **40**, 361–368.

Kazdin, A.E. (1982) The token economy: a decade later. *Journal of Applied Behavior Analysis*, **15**, 431–445.

Kazdin, A.E. & Bootzin, R.R. (1972) The token economy: an evaluative review. *Journal of Applied Behavior Analysis*, **5**, 343–372.

Keith, R.D., Engelkes, J.R. & Winborn, B.B. (1977) Employment seeking preparation and activity. *Rehabilitation Counseling Bulletin*, **21**, 159–165.

Kern, R.S. & Green, M.F. (1994) Cognitive prerequisites of skill acquisition in schizophrenia: bridging micro- and macro-levels of processing. In Spaulding, W. (ed.) *Cognitive Technology in Psychiatric Rehabilitation*, pp. 49–66. University of Nebraska Press, Lincoln.

Kern, R.S., Green, M.F. & Satz, P. (1992) Neuropsychological predictors of skills training for chronic psychiatric patients. *Psychiatry Research*, **43**, 223–230.

Kindness, K. & Newton, A. (1984) Patients and social skills groups: is social skills training enough? *Behavioral Psychotherapy*, **12**, 212–222.

Leff, J.P. & Vaughn, C. (1985) *Expressed Emotion in Families: Its Significance for Mental Illness*. Guilford Press, New York.

Liberman, R.P. & Associates (1988) *Psychiatric Rehabilitation for Chronic Mental Patients*. American Psychiatric Press, Washington DC.

Liberman, R.P. & Bedell, J. (1989) Behavior therapy. In Kaplan, H.I. & Saddock, B.J. (eds) *Comprehensive Textbook of Psychiatry*, 5th edn, pp. 422–445. Williams & Wilkins, Baltimore.

Liberman, R.P. & Corrigan, P.W. (1993) Designing new psychosocial treatments for schizophrenia. *Psychiatry*, **56**, 238–249.

Liberman, R.P. & Green, M.F. (1992) Whither cognitive-behavior therapy for schizophrenia? *Schizophrenia Bulletin*, **18**, 27–35.

Liberman, R.P., DeRisi, W.J. & Mueser, K.T. (1989) *Social Skills Training for Psychiatric Patients*. Pergamon Press, New York.

Liberman, R.P., Mueser, K.T. & Wallace, C.J. (1986a) Social skills training for schizophrenic individuals at risk for relapse. *American Journal of Psychiatry,* **143,** 523–526.

Liberman, R.P., Nuechterlein, K.H. & Wallace, C.J. (1982) Social skills training and the nature of schizophrenia. In Curran, J.P. & Monti, P.M. (eds) *Social Skills Training: A Practical Handbook for Assessment and Treatment,* pp. 5–56. Guilford Press, New York.

Liberman, R.P., Teigen, J., Patterson, R. & Baker, V. (1973) Reducing delusional speech in chronic paranoid schizophrenics. *Journal of Applied Behavior Analysis,* **6,** 57–64.

Liberman, R.P., Wallace C., Teigen, J. & Davis, J. (1974) Interventions in psychotics. In Calhoun, K.S., Adams, H.E. & Mitchell, E.M. (eds) *Innovative Treatment Methods in Psychopathology,* pp. 323–412. Wiley, New York.

Liberman, R.P., Mueser, K., Wallace, C.J., Jacobs, H.E. & Eckman, T. (1986b) Training skills in the severely psychiatrically disabled: learning coping and competence. *Schizophrenia Bulletin,* **12,** 631–647.

Longin, H.E. & Rooney, W.M. (1975) Teaching denial assertion to chronic hospitalized patients. *Journal of Behavior Therapy and Experimental Psychiatry,* **6,** 219–222.

Lowe, C.F. & Chadwick, P.D. (1990) Verbal control of delusions. *Behavior Therapy,* **21,** 461–480.

McFarlane, W.R., Stastny, P. & Deakins, S. (1992) Family-aided assertive community treatment: a comprehensive rehabilitation and intensive case management approach for persons with schizophrenic disorders. In Liberman, R.P. (ed.) *New Directions for Mental Health Services: Effective Psychiatric Rehabilitation,* pp. 43–54. Jossey-Bass, San Francisco.

McGuigan, F.D. (1966) Covert oral behavior and auditory hallucinations. *Psychophysiology,* **3,** 73–80.

Margo, A., Hemsley, D. & Slade, P. (1981) The effect of varying auditory input on schizophrenic hallucinations. *British Journal of Psychiatry,* **139,** 122–127.

Margolis, R.B. & Shemberg, K.M. (1976) Cognitive self-instruction in process and reactive schizophrenia: a failure to replicate. *Behavior Therapy,* **7,** 668–671.

Massel, H.K., Corrigan, P.W., Liberman, R.P. & Milan, M. (1991) Conversation skills training in thought-disordered schizophrenia through attention focusing. *Psychiatry Research,* **38,** 51–61.

Meichenbaum, D.M. & Cameron, R. (1973) Training schizophrenics to talk to themselves: a means of developing attentional controls. *Behavior Therapy,* **4,** 515–534.

Milton, F., Patwa, V.K. & Hafner, R.S. (1978) Confrontation versus belief modification in persistently deluded patients. *British Journal of Medical Psychology,* **51,** 127–130.

Morrison, R.L. & Bellack, A.S. (1984) Social skills training. In Bellack, A.S. (ed.) *Schizophrenia: Treatment, Management, and Rehabilitation,* pp. 247–280.

Morrison, R.L. & Bellack, A.S. (1987) Social functioning of schizophrenic patients: clinical and research issues. *Schizophrenia Bulletin,* **13,** 715–725.

Mosher, L.R. & Menn, A.Z. (1978) Community residential treatment for schizophrenia: two-year follow-up. *Hospital and Community Psychiatry,* **29,** 715–723.

Mueser, K. & Liberman, R.P. (1988) Skills training in vocational rehabilitation. In Ciardello, J.A. & Bell, M.D. (eds) *Vocational Rehabilitation of Persons with Prolonged Psy-chiatric Disorders,* pp. 81–103. John Hopkins University Press, Baltimore.

Mueser, K.T., Bellack, A.S., Douglas, M.S. & Wade, J. (1991) Predictions of social skill acquisition in schizophrenia and major affective disorder patients from memory and symptomatology. *Psychiatry Research,* **37,** 381–396.

Nuechterlein, K.H. & Asarnow, R.F. (1989) Cognition and perception. In Kaplan, H.I. & Sadock, B.J. (eds) *Comprehensive Textbook of Psychiatry,* 5th edn, pp. 241–256. Williams & Wilkins, Baltimore.

Nuechterlein, K.H. & Dawson, M.E. (1984) Information processing and attentional functioning in the developmental course of schizophrenic disorders. *Schizophrenia Bulletin,* **10,** 106–143.

Olbrich, R. & Mussgay, L. (1990) Reduction of schizophrenic deficits by cognitive training: an evaluative study. *European Archives of Psychiatry and Neurological Sciences,* **239,** 366–369.

Patterson, R.L. & Teigen, J.R. (1973) Conditioning and post-hospital generalization of non-delusional response in a chronic psychotic patient. *Journal of Applied Behavior Analysis,* **6,** 65–70.

Paul, G.L. & Lentz, R.J. (1977) *Psychosocial Treatment of Chronic Mental Patients: Milieu versus Social-Learning Programs.* Harvard University Press, Cambridge.

Perris, C. (1992) A cognitive-behavioral treatment program for patients with a schizophrenic disorder. In Liberman, R.P. (ed.) *New Directions for Mental Health Services: Effective Psychiatric Rehabilitation,* pp. 21–32. Jossey-Bass, San Francisco.

Reed, D., Sullivan, M., Penn, D., Stuve, P. & Spaulding, W. (1992) Assessment and treatment of cognitive impairments. In Liberman, R.P. (ed.) *New Directions for Mental Health Services: Effective Psychiatric Rehabilitation,* pp. 7–20. Jossey-Bass, San Francisco.

Schlank, A. (1987) *Effects of a conceptual processing exercise on progress in interpersonal problem solving training.* Masters Thesis, University of Nebraska.

Skilbeck, C. (1991) Microcomputer-based cognitive rehabilitation. In Ager, A. (ed.) *Microcomputers and Clinical Psychology: Applications and Future Developments,* pp. 247–274. Wiley, New York.

Skinner, B.F. (1953) *Science and Human Behavior.* MacMillan, New York.

Spaulding, W. (1992) Design prerequisites for research on cognitive therapy for schizophrenia. *Schizophrenia Bulletin,* **18(1),** 39–42.

Spaulding, W. (1993) Spontaneous and induced changes in cognition during psychiatric rehabilitation. In Cromwell, R.L. (ed.) *Schizophrenia: Innovations in Theory and Treatment,* pp. 299–312. Oxford Press, New York.

Spaulding, W. & Sullivan, M. (1992) From laboratory to clinic: psychological methods and principles in psychiatric rehabilitation. In Liberman, R.P. (ed.) *Handbook of Psychiatric Rehabilitation,* pp. 30–55. MacMillan, New York.

Spaulding, W.D., Storms, L., Goodrich, V. & Sullivan, M. (1986) Applications of experimental psychopathology in psychiatric rehabilitation. *Schizophrenia Bulletin,* **12(4),** 560–577.

Stein, L.I. & Test, M.A. (1978) *Alternatives in Mental Hospital*

Treatment. Plenum Press, New York.

Stokes, T.F. & Baer, D.M. (1977) An implicit technology of generalization. *Journal of Applied Behavior Analysis*, **10**, 349–367.

Strupp, H. & Butler, S. (1990) Psychotherapy. In Bellak, A. & Hersen, M. (eds) *Handbook of Comparative Treatments of Adult Disorders*, pp. 262–294. Wiley, New York.

Stuve, P. (1990) *An examination of computer-assisted cognitive rehabilitation for schizophrenia*. PhD Thesis, University of Nebraska.

Tarrier, N., Barrowclough, C., Vaughn, C. *et al.* (1988) The community management of schizophrenia: a controlled trial of a behavioral intervention with families to reduce relapse. *British Journal of Psychiatry*, **153**, 532–542.

Test, M.A. (1992) Training in community living. In Liberman, R.P. (ed.) *Handbook of Psychiatric Rehabilitation*. Macmillan, New York.

Test, M.A. & Stein, L.I. (1978) Community treatment of the chronic patient: research overview. *Schizophrenia Bulletin*, **4**, 350–364.

Trower, P. (1982) Toward a generative model of social skills: a critique and synthesis. In Curran, J.P. & Monti, P.M. (eds) *Social Skills Training: A Practical Handbook for Assessment and Treatment*, pp. 399–428. Guilford Press, New York.

Trower, P., Bryant, B. & Argyle, M. (1978) *Social Skills and Mental Health*. Methuen, London.

Vaccaro, J.V., Liberman, R.P., Wallace, C.J. & Blackwell, G. (1992) Combining social skills training and assertive case management: the Social and Independent Living Skills Program of the Brentwood Veterans Affairs Medical Center. In Liberman, R.P. (ed.) *New Directions for Mental Health Services: Effective Psychiatric Rehabilitation*, pp. 33–42. Jossey-Bass, San Francisco.

Vaughn, C.E. & Leff, J.P. (1976) The influence of family and social factors on the course of psychiatric illness: a comparison of schizophrenia and depressed neurotic patients. *British Journal of Psychiatry*, **129**, 125–137.

Vaughn, C.E., Snyder, K.S., Freeman, W., Jones, S., Falloon, I.R.H. & Liberman, R.P. (1982) Family factors in schizophrenic relapse: a replication. *Schizophrenia Bulletin*, **8**, 425–444.

Wallace, C.J. & Liberman, R.P. (1985) Social skills training for patients with schizophrenia: a controlled clinical trial. *Psychiatry Research*, **15**, 239–247.

Wallace, C.J., Boone, S.E., Donahoe, C.P. & Foy, D.W. (1985) The chronically mentally disabled: independent living skills training. In Barlow, D. (ed.) *Clinical Handbook of Psychological Disorders: A Step-by-Step Treatment Manual*, pp. 147–168. Guilford Press, New York.

Wallace, C.J., Liberman, R.P., MacKain, S.J., Blackwell, G. & Eckman, T.A. (1992) Effectiveness and replicability of modules for teaching social and instrumental skills to the severely mentally ill. *American Journal of Psychiatry*, **149**, 654–658.

Watts, F.N., Powell, E.G. & Austin, S.V. (1973) The modification of absurd beliefs. *British Journal of Medical Psychology*, **46**, 359–363.

Weinberger, D.R., Berman, K.F. & Illowsky, B.P. (1988) Physiological dysfunction of dorsolateral prefrontal cortex in schizophrenia. *Archives of General Psychiatry*, **45**, 609–615.

Weingaertner, A.H. (1971) Self-administered aversive stimulation with hallucinating hospitalized schizophrenics. *Journal of Consulting and Clinical Psychology*, **36**, 422–429.

Wincze, J.P., Leitenberg, H. & Agras, W.S. (1972) The effect of token reinforcement and feedback on delusional verbal behavior of chronic paranoid schizophrenics. *Journal of Applied Behavior Analysis*, **5**, 247–262.

Wixted, J., Bellak, A. & Hersen, M. (1990) Behavior therapy. In Bellak, A. & Hersen, M. (eds) *Handbook of Comparative Treatments of Adult Disorders*, pp. 202–235. Wiley, New York.

Wong, S.E., Massel, H.K., Mosk, M.D. & Liberman, R.P. (1986) Behavioral approaches to the treatment of schizophrenia. In Burrows, G.D., Norman, T.R. & Rubinstein, G. (eds) *Handbook of Studies on Schizophrenia*, pp. 79–100. Elsevier, Amsterdam.

Wong, S., Slama, K. & Liberman, R.P. (1985) Behavioral analysis and therapy for aggressive psychiatric and developmentally disabled patients. In Roth, L. (ed.) *Clinical Treatment of the Violent Person*, pp. 22–56. NIMH Monograph, Publication No. (ADM) 85–1425. US Dept of Health and Human Services, Washington DC.

Chapter 31
Psychotherapy for Schizophrenia

K. T. MUESER AND A. S. BELLACK

Introduction

Psychotherapy for schizophrenia has long been recognized to be an uphill battle, with as much debate focused on its feasibility as on the benefits it might confer. Kraepelin (1919) and his predecessors made few recommendations on this topic. Bleuler (1911), on the other hand, devoted a significant part of the chapter on 'Therapy' in his book *Dementia Praecox or The Group of Schizophrenias* to discussion of the influence of psychosocial factors on the illness and its treatment. Bleuler wrote:

> At the present time, the only type of therapy that can seriously be considered for schizophrenia as a whole is the psychic method. Unfortunately, however, we have barely passed the empirical stage in this field. Since the symptomatology of the disease is dominated by the complexes and since these often offer a starting point for us from which to penetrate the patient's psyche, it might also be expected that the disease could be influenced from this angle. Indubitably,

improvements in response to psychic treatment occur, but we are at a loss to state what must be done in each individual case in order to bring about the improvement. Therefore, we are forced to grope in the dark; indeed, it might be said that the only way is to offer chance itself a great many opportunities, so that it might seize one of them. If this is done at the right moment, a good deal can often be accomplished. (Bleuler, 1911.)

Clearly, Bleuler believed that psychotherapy for schizophrenia could be clinically efficacious, although this optimism was tempered by his frank acknowledgement that little was known as to how the treatment should be conducted. Following Bleuler's writings, a split emerged in the academic psychiatry community as to whether schizophrenia could be treated with psychotherapy. Although Freud did not rule out the possibility of psychotherapy for schizophrenia in his early writings, over time he grew more pessimistic and adamant that successful therapy could not be carried out (Arieti, 1974).

626

Despite Freud's influence and a general consensus that (psychoanalytical) psychotherapy could not be conducted with schizophrenia patients, dissent was evident from early on and a variety of approaches was developed over the following years. One of the first, and the most influential dissenter from Freud, was Sullivan (1962), who in the 1920s developed an in-patient treatment unit specializing in the intensive treatment of young men with schizophrenia. Sullivan viewed schizophrenia as a return to earlier childhood forms of comunication resulting from problematic relationships, and he developd psychotherapeutic interventions designed to correct these relationships. Sullivan, followed by Fromm-Reichman (1950), strongly maintained that schizophrenia patients retain some capacity to relate to others interpersonally, setting the stage for therapeutic work based on psychodynamic principles, but differing from traditional psychoanalysis.

Some dissenters from Freud argued that even traditional psychoanalytical approaches were appropriate for the treatment of schizophrenia, most notably Klein (1948) and her students, such as Bion (1967) and Winnicott (1965). More often, modifications were proposed in the psychoanalytical method to accommodate the unique problems posed by the schizophrenia patient, reflected in the work of innovators such as Rosen (1953) and Searles (1965). Still others (e.g. Sechehaye, 1956; Laing, 1960) proposed even more radical departures from psychoanalytical methods based partly on the therapist's ability to 'share' the patient's psychotic experience while maintaining a supportive relationship with the patient.

Ultimately, controlled research on psychodynamic interventions for schizophrenia has failed to support its efficacy (reviewed later in this chapter). However, the early work in this area was important because of the essential premise that patients with this illness could be gainfully engaged in psychotherapy. In this respect, psychodynamically orientated therapists stood apart from the rest of the field by their insistence that the severity of schizophrenia could be improved through psychotherapeutic means. Although current methods of psychotherapy for schizophrenia differ markedly from earlier approaches, they share a basic optimism that such interventions can improve symptoms and enhance patients' quality of life.

In this chapter we first make the case for the importance of psychotherapy based on our current understanding of the disorder. Next, we discuss the specific needs and liabilities of schizophrenia patients relevant to their ability to benefit from psychotherapy. In the core of the chapter we review different psychotherapeutic approaches to schizophrenia (individual, group, family) and the research supporting their efficacy. We conclude with a discussion of remaining questions and future directions for psychotherapy for schizophrenia.

The case for psychotherapy

The accumulation of evidence over the last several decades has led to a general consensus that schizophrenia is a brain disease (or set of diseases) caused by genetic and/or prenatal and perinatal insult (Weinberger, 1987; Roberts, 1991). This consensus, even in the absence of the discovery of specific biological markers for the illness, has led to the incorrect assumption that schizophrenia is not responsive to psychosocial interventions, and that progress is solely dependent upon breakthroughs in drug therapy for the illness. It is true that no psychotherapeutic intervention by itself is sufficient to treat schizophrenia. However, there is compelling evidence pointing to the impact of psychosocial factors on the course and outcome of the illness.

Ambient stressors, such as life events (Brown & Birley, 1968; Ventura *et al.*, 1989) and a negative affective climate in the family (Brown *et al.*, 1972; Kavanagh, 1992), can precipitate relapses, while environmental modification, such as the token economy (Paul & Lentz, 1977; Glynn, 1990) and family intervention (Leff *et al.*, 1985; Mueser & Glynn, 1993), can substantially improve functioning. Furthermore, even severely impaired schizophrenia patients are capable of acquiring new skills for improving their social functioning and the quality of their lives (Paul & Lentz, 1977; Wong & Woolsey, 1989).

If the goals of psychotherapy are narrowly defined in terms of the reduction of psychopathology and the complete prevention of all relapses, then failure is inevitable. But if a broader view is taken that appreciates the complex, chronic and multiply handicapping nature of the illness, an important role for psychotherapy is evident. Multiple, integrated treatments are currrently required for the long-term management of schizophrenia (Ciompi, 1987; Bellack, 1989), and it is doubtful whether significant improvements in the overall level of functioning can be achieved without psychosocial intervention. Although clinical experience and the research literature support our optimism about psychological interventions, we are acutely aware of the limitations of the extant psychosocial technologies, and the need to develop more effective interventions. We believe that continued research on the cognitive substrates of schizophrenia and associated impairments in the experience of emotion and social behaviour will lead to further innovations and even more effective psychotherapeutic treatments for the disorder.

Special needs and liabilities

Researchers, clinicians and family members are often disappointed by the relatively modest gains achieved by schizophrenia patients in psychotherapy. On the one hand, small gains may reflect the limitations of currently available treatments. On the other hand, a poor understanding of the special needs and liabilities of schizophrenia patients may lead to unrealistic expectations for success, and disappointment when expectations are not met. Four factors need to be taken into account when implementing psychotherapeutic interventions and evaluating the results:

1 the need for comprehensive and long-term treatment;
2 individual differences in treatment needs;
3 the role of the patient in treatment; and
4 the limitations imposed by cognitive deficits.

Comprehensive and long-term treatment

Since the earliest descriptions of schizophrenia, its pervasive and chronic nature have been understood to be an integral part of the illness. The symptoms of the illness affect all aspects of functioning, including social relationships, work and self-care, and some degree of chronicity is required in order to diagnose the illness (e.g. the *Diagnostic and Statistical Manual* DSM-III-R). Although longitudinal data have challenged the assumption that schizophrenia necessarily has a deteriorating course (Harding *et al.*, 1987a,b), the illness characteristically is life-long and severe. The net result is that patients often need assistance in meeting a wide variety of needs, ranging from learning how to handle the tasks of day-to-day living to engaging in social interactions, coping with depression and the management of psychotic symptoms.

The need for extended, comprehensive treatment of schizophrenia has long been recognized (Ciompi, 1987; Wing, 1987). Despite this, much research on psychotherapy has focused on short, time-limited, circumscribed interventions. The development of more effective psychotherapies has also been hampered by an overemphasis on the management and prevention of symptom recrudescences, at the cost of less work orientated towards improving the quality of life and subjective distress. A related problem has been the lack of attention paid to the timing, sequencing and integration of psychotherapy with other treatment modalities. For example, it is now clear that schizophrenia patients with substance-use disorders require integrated programmes to deal with both disorders, rather than separate and sequenced treatments (Minkoff & Drake, 1991).

The importance of long-term treatment does not negate the potential benefits of time-limited interventions. Brief treatments, such as 3- to 6-month social skills training (SST) programmes, may be useful for reducing stress or teaching patients how to handle specific problems (e.g. discussing medication issues with a physician). In addition, research indicates that gains in brief therapy can be maintained over time (Bellack *et al.*, 1984; Eckman *et al.*, 1992). It is unlikely, however, that brief psychotherapies will result in permanent changes in vulnerability to relapse. Some patients may benefit from long-term psychosocial interventions throughout their lives, while others may require more limited therapy. Clinical expectations need to take into account the limitations of brief psychotherapy.

Individual differences in treatment needs

The heterogeneity of schizophrenia has often been interpreted as reflecting either multiple aetiologies or multiple disease entities (Tsuang *et al.*, 1990; Carpenter *et al.*, 1993). Despite this heterogeneity, the search has continued for a unitary model of psychotherapy for all patients. One negative consequence of this search has been that many individual needs go unmet. Another consequence is that interventions which are effective for some patients may be prematurely abandoned if their effects are not sufficiently robust for the whole group.

Evidence of heterogeneity in areas commonly assumed to be impaired in schizophrenia underscores the importance of individual differences. For example, significant variability has been found on the Wisconsin card sorting test (WCST; Heaton, 1981), which reflects prefrontal cortical functioning. Although schizophrenia patients have repeatedly been found to perform more poorly on the WCST (Berman *et al.*, 1986; Weinberger *et al.*, 1986), the performance of many patients is in the normal range (Bellack *et al.*, 1990b; Braff *et al.*, 1991). Also, among patients with impairments on the WCST, there is considerable variability in the extent to which they can be taught to improve their performance (Goldberg *et al.*, 1987; Bellack *et al.*, 1990b).

Similar evidence of heterogeneity exists in social skills. Mueser *et al.* (1991b) found that 50% of schizophrenia patients had persistent deficits in social skills over a 1-year period, while 11% did not differ from non-patient controls, and the remainder showed variable performance. Thus, the common assumption that patients with schizophrenia have deficits in their social skills is true for many, but not for all patients.

In addition to the variability between patients, significant changes occur within patients over time and these have a bearing on their treatment needs. Young patients need special help in dealing with the fact that they have a serious illness which may interfere with their personal goals and their ability to achieve independence, a problem which may contribute to their high vulnerability to suicide and substance abuse (Test *et al.*, 1989; Caldwell & Gottesman, 1990).

Older patients may adjust to the difficulties of the illness through withdrawal or positive coping strategies (Wing, 1987; Strauss, 1989), but they face unique problems of their own. For example, parents are unable to continue caring for an offspring with schizophrenia as the patient grows older, necessitating a shift in caretaking responsibility to either siblings (Horwitz *et al.*, 1992) or the mental health system. A survey of the needs of schizophrenia patients in regular contact with their families indicated that concern over what happens when a parent dies was ranked fourth highest out of 45 topics (parents ranked this concern fifth) (Mueser *et al.*, 1992b).

In order for psychotherapy to meet the real needs of patients, between-patient differences and changes over time need to be taken into account. Clinical practice must attempt to distinguish between shared and individual needs in the provision of psychotherapy. Research is sorely needed that addresses which patients will profit from which interventions.

The role of the patient

The problems of psychosis experienced by schizophrenia patients, combined with negative symptoms (e.g. apathy, anhedonia) have often led to the false assumption that patients are not capable of actively participating in their own treatment. Indeed, many patients seem unmotivated and are uncooperative with their treatment. Such apparent disinterest and passivity, however, should not be interpreted as immutable traits.

Negative symptoms are not always stable over time and they may be secondary to demoralization, psychotic symptoms, medication side effects and other factors that vary over time (Carpenter *et al.*, 1988; McGlashan & Fenton, 1992). Paul and Lentz (1977) have shown that even extremely withdrawn, chronic schizophrenia patients can be motivated by a systematic incentive programme. In addition, there is a growing body of evidence that schizophrenia patients actively employ coping strategies to manage persistent symptoms and share these strategies with one another (Boker, 1987; Carr, 1988; Wiedl & Schottner, 1991).

Strauss (1989) has argued that it is important to view schizophrenia patients as having an active 'will', and that their behaviour is goal directed and reflects an attempt to cope with the illness as best they can. Several implications follow this assumption. First, if patients are actively trying to cope, they may benefit from learning basic information about their illness and factors that may influence vulnerability to relapse. Over the past decade there has been a trend towards educating patients about schizophrenia and its management to enable them to become more active participants in the treatment of their own illness (Pilsecker, 1981; Bisbee & Lee, 1988; Ascher-Svanum & Krause, 1991). Nevertheless, patient education is far from the norm, and little research has addressed the question of what should be taught, when and how.

A second implication of Strauss' (1989) contention is that patients are capable of learning specific strategies for coping with psychotic symptoms. Persistent psychotic symptoms are present in a substantial proportion of patients in the post-acute stage of their illness (Harrow & Silverstein, 1977; Silverstein & Harrow, 1978) and are associated with high levels of distress (Falloon & Talbot, 1981). There are numerous case reports describing the successful use of behaviour modification techniques to control psychotic symptoms (Bellack, 1986; Tarrier, 1992), but few guidelines exist regarding which patients are most likely to benefit. Although these techniques are not likely to produce enduring, fundamental changes in the illness, they may reduce the subjective distress associated with chronic psychotic symptoms and better enable patients to pursue personal goals.

A third implication of viewing the patient as actively coping with the illness is the need to involve him or her in goal setting and treatment planning. Treatments are too often imposed on patients by the treatment team and family members, with little consideration of the patient's own desires. As a consequence, patients often fail to adhere to treatment recommendations, increasing their risk of relapse and creating tensions in their relationships with family members and treatment providers. To be sure, engaging the patient to establish treatment goals can be a long, arduous process. Failure to do so, however, courts the larger risk of undermining the very purpose of treatment.

Impairments in information processing

Schizophrenia is characterized by a wide variety of impairments in information processing, including memory, attention, speed of processing, abstract reasoning and sensorimotor integration (Nuechterlein & Dawson, 1984b; Bilder & Goldberg, 1987; Braff, 1991). Despite the voluminous literature on cognitive deficits in schizophrenia, its impact on psychosocial treatment has been limited primarily to presenting information more slowly and repeatedly. This strategy is insufficient to address the range of cognitive impairments that affect how information is acquired and utilized by these patients.

Two issues need to be addressed in order to improve existing psychotherapy technologies that take into account the cognitive impairments of the illness. First, the influence of cognitive deficits on learning and retention in treatment must be determined so that treatments can be modified accordingly. For example, Mueser *et al.* (1991b) found that poor memory had a deleterious effect on learning in social skills training (SST), but that pretreatment symptomatology was unrelated to social skills acquisition. Kern *et al.* (1992) also found that memory impairment, as well as poor sustained attention (on the continuous performance test), was related to poorer learning in SST. It remains to be determined how SST strategies need to be adapted in light of the effects of cognitive impairments on learning.

The second issue is the impact of cognitive deficits on the generalization of treatment effects. A basic pretext of all psychotherapy is that information learned in the session must be generalized to the patient's natural environment. Yet, such generalization is contingent upon cognitive processes that are often disrupted in schizophrenia. Research should be conducted that identifies the specific cognitive abilities that affect the generalization of learning, and to develop strategies that either overcome or compensate for these impairments.

In recent years there has been a growth in interest of the use of cognitive rehabilitation methods in schizophrenia to improve attention, memory and reasoning (e.g. Brenner *et al.*, 1990). Although the effects of these interventions remain to be demonstrated (Bellack, 1992; Hogarty & Flesher, 1992), there is also a need to examine how the information-processing load or demands can be reduced on patients. For example, schizophrenia patients are vulnerable to stress, which further decreases their already limited information-processing capacity (Nuechterlein & Dawson, 1984a). This vulnerability might be reduced by teaching patients stress-reduction techniques, social skills for managing unavoidable stressful social situations, and how to avoid other stress. Similarly, patients may benefit from learning how to use environmental supports to compensate for their impairments, similar to strategies employed in the head injury patients (Butler & Namerow, 1988; Benedict, 1989).

Individual and group psychotherapy

A wide variety of individual and group-based psychotherapy approaches has been advocated for schizophrenia and it is beyond the scope of this chapter to review them all. In this section, we focus on those approaches which have been examined in controlled research (i.e. research designs with random assignment to treatment groups, systematic and objective assessment of outcome variables).

Psychodynamic approaches

As reviewed earlier in this chapter, psychodynamic (or psychoanalytical) approaches were the dominant psychotherapy model for schizophrenia for more than half of the 20th century. Although the popularity of these approaches has waned in recent years, they continue to be applied in spite of the limited evidence supporting their efficacy (Mueser & Berenbaum, 1990).

Four controlled studies have examined the effects of psychodynamic psychotherapy for schizophrenia: May (1968); Grinspoon *et al.* (1972); Gunderson *et al.* (1984) and Stanton *et al.* (1984); and Karon and VandenBos (1972, 1975). Three of the four studies found no beneficial effects for psychodynamic therapy, when provided either alone or in combination with neuroleptic medication (May, 1968; Grinspoon *et al.*, 1972; Gunderson *et al.*, 1984). Each of these studies is unique and has its own methodological limitations. May's study examined first-break patients but used inexperienced therapists [for comments, see Karon and VandenBos (1970) and Tuma and May (1974)]. The study of Grinspoon *et al.* did not randomly assign patients to all groups. Rather, chronically ill patients who consented to treatment were transferred to another hospital and randomly assigned to either psychodynamic treatment alone or psychodynamic treatment plus drugs, and these two groups were compared with the other patients who had not consented to therapy. The study by Gunderson *et al.* and Stanton *et al.* compared psychodynamic treatment with a comparison treatment ('reality-adaptive-supportive therapy') of unknown efficacy (both groups received drugs), so it is unclear whether both groups of patients improved or not.

Karon and VandenBos (1972, 1975) reported the remarkable result that psychodynamic psychotherapy, both with and without drugs, was superior to neuroleptic treatment alone. A complex interaction was also found between therapist experience and outcome, with concomitant medication interfering with the effects of psychodynamic therapy for inexperienced, but not experienced, therapists. However, several methodological flaws limit the generalizability of these results. First, patients who received the drug-only treatment were transferred to another hospital, which could have resulted in less effective pharmacological treatment or case management than that for patients who received therapy. Second, there was a confound between therapist experience and treatment modality. Half the patients who received only psychodynamic treatment were treated by one experienced therapist, and half the patients who received psychodynamic treatment plus drugs were treated by a different experienced therapist, with the remaining patients receiving treatment from inexperienced therapists. Thus, the interaction between therapist experience and concomitant drug treatment may simply reflect differences between these therapists, rather than therapy experience. Furthermore, the type of psychodynamic therapy differed between the no-drug group ('active psychoanalytical psychotherapy') and the drug group ('ego-analytical psychoanalytical psychotherapy'). Overall, it is impossible to determine whether positive results of this study resulted from differences in treatment facilities, therapists or psychodynamic treatment approaches. Perhaps most important, no replication of these results has been reported in the 20 years since the study was conducted.

In addition to the meagre support for psychodynamic treatment based on controlled studies, naturalistic studies shed further doubt on the efficacy of these approaches. Stone (1986) followed up 72 schizophrenia patients who had received an average of 12.3 months of intensive psychodynamic therapy. Ten to 20 years later, more than half the patients were substantially dysfunctional, and 20% had committed suicide, approximately twice the rate of suicide in the population of schizophrenia patients (Drake & Cotton, 1986). McGlashan's (1984a,b) follow-up of schizophrenia patients who received long-term, intensive psychodynamic treatment at Chestnut Lodge found that two-thirds of the patients were functioning marginally or worse 15 years later, leading him to conclude: 'Unfortunately, we still have not improved much on Kraepelin's work' (McGlashan, 1984b).

No outcome study of psychotherapy is perfect, as is evident from the studies reviewed above. However, the strong trends in the data suggest few, if any, benefits of psychodynamic psychotherapy. These findings, particularly considering the more positive effects found for other approaches (reviewed below), suggest that psychodynamic therapy does not have a role in the treatment of schizophrenia (Mueser & Berenbaum, 1990).

Social skills training (SST)

Social dysfunction is a defining characteristic of schizophrenia that is semi-independent of other domains of the illness (Strauss *et al.*, 1974; Lenzenweger *et al.*, 1991). Social functioning is also predictive of the course and outcome of the illness (McGlashan, 1986; Johnstone *et al.*, 1990). According to the expanded stress-vulnerability-coping skills model of schizophrenia (Liberman *et al.*, 1986b), both social support and coping skills mediate the noxious effects of stress on patients, protecting them from stress-induced relapses.

Social skills are specific response capabilities necessary for effective performance. These skills tend to be stable over time and make a unique contribution to the performance of social roles and quality of life (Bellack *et al.*, 1990a; Mueser *et al.*, 1991a). Over the past several decades an extensive technology of SST has been developed and empirically tested as a strategy for teaching social skills to psychiatric patients and improving their social adjustment (Liberman *et al.*, 1989). SST is described in greater detail elsewhere (Chapter 30, this volume).

A large number of single-case studies and small group designs have demonstrated the efficacy of SST for teaching a wide range of skills, including conversational skill, assertiveness and medication management (Hersen & Bellack, 1976; Wallace *et al.*, 1980). Over the past decade, six larger group studies have been conducted, with findings consistent with previous research and indicating that effects of SST are maintained for at least 6–12 months (Brown & Munford, 1983; Spencer *et al.*, 1983; Bellack *et al.*, 1984; Liberman *et al.*,

1986a; Hogarty *et al.*, 1986, 1991; Eckman *et al.*, 1992; Marder *et al.*, 1993).

Four of the six studies examined the effects of SST on symptoms, relapse and social adjustment with mixed results. Bellack *et al.* (1984) compared 3 months of group-SST in a day hospital with day hospital treatment alone. At the 6-month follow-up, patients who received SST were less symptomatic and had better social adjustment, but there were no differences in relapse at the 1-year follow-up. Liberman *et al.* (1986a) compared 2 months of intensive SST with 'holistic health' treatment for long-term residents of a state hospital awaiting discharge. At the 2-year follow-up, the SST patients were better on several symptom measures and social adjustment, but relapse rates did not differ significantly. Eckman *et al.* (1992; Marder *et al.*, 1993) compared 1 year of intensive group-SST with a supportive group. At the 2-year follow-up, patients who had received SST had better social adjustment, although their relapse rates did not differ from those of the control group.

In the only study to examine individual-SST, Hogarty *et al.* (1986, 1991) compared SST, family psychoeducation, SST plus family psychoeducation and medication only. All patients were living with, or were in contact with, high expressed emotion (EE) family members. SST, alone and in combination with family therapy, was associated with reduced relapse rates throughout the first 21 months of the study. By the 24th month, however, the effect of SST was no longer significant, due to several relapses in the last 3 months for this group. Follow-up data on social adjustment were collected only for non-relapsed patients, so the effect of SST on social functioning in this study is unclear.

Several trends emerge from these studies. There is a tendency for SST to improve social functioning, which is the primary focus of the treatment. However, it is unclear exactly which dimensions of social functioning are affected by SST, and the extent to which learning in the clinic generalizes to improved role functioning in the community. The effect of SST on relapse rate and symptoms appears to be negligible, although this is not surprising given the focus of the intervention. Despite these generally favourable findings, many questions remain about the clinical utility of SST (Benton & Schroeder, 1990; Halford & Hayes, 1991). Some of the most critical questions include: What is the optimal frequency of sessions? How long should treatment be provided? At what stage of the illness should SST be initiated? Which patients benefit the most from SST?

Although new approaches to psychotherapy for schizophrenia continue to be developed, the pace is slow and the results are unclear. The positive results of research on SST and its growing popularity among treatment providers suggest that this approach will continue to be a useful psychotherapeutic intervention for schizophrenia in the future.

Neuropsychological rehabilitation

We previously discussed the prominent information-processing impairments characteristic of schizophrenia (e.g. memory, attention, abstract reasoning). Traditional SST procedures (the 'motor skills model') have attempted to circumvent these problems by minimizing cognitive demand and repeatedly practising simple response repertoires so that the overlearned responses can be emitted in a relatively automatic fashion. There are several limitations with this strategy. Most social encounters, especially extended interactions, do not follow a script that can be prepared in advance. Effective social performance often requires cognitive skills, including accurate perception of social cues, generation of response options, evaluation of possible responses and choosing the best option (McFall, 1982; Bellack *et al.*, 1989). Patients with significant cognitive deficits may have difficulty in learning with the motor skills model, which deals primarily with response execution.

One strategy to overcome the limitations of the motor skills model of SST and improve generalization has been to embed the training of motor skills within a broader training in social problem-solving skills (Liberman *et al.*, 1986b). Patients are taught the steps of problem solving identified by D'Zurilla and Goldfried (1971); these are then practised when anticipating problems that might occur when attempting to manage one type of situation (e.g. medication management). The problem-solving method of SST has been used in several studies which reported clinical improvements (Liberman *et al.*, 1986a,b). However, it is not clear whether patients actually used the problem-solving strategies outside of the clinic or whether clinical improvements were related to improved information processing (Bellack *et al.*, 1989).

A different approach to the management of cognitive deficits has been to attempt remediation of specific information-processing deficits (e.g. attention) before training in motor skills or problem solving (Brenner *et al.*, 1992; Spring & Ravdin, 1992). Remediation strategies have been drawn from clinical work with patients with traumatic brain injury or stroke; these strategies include repeatedly practising computer-driven tasks that load on attention, memory and reasoning (Penn, 1991; Stuve *et al.*, 1991). Clinical demonstrations and small group studies have been conducted with schizophrenia patients that have shown modest gains on targeted tasks, but the ability to generalize these skills and their impact on social functioning has not been established (Penn, 1991; Bellack, 1992; Hogarty & Flesher, 1992).

Several studies have shown that performance on the WCST, a putative measure of frontal lobe functioning, can be improved by reinforcement and specific instructions (Bellack *et al.*, 1990b; Green *et al.*, 1990; Summerfelt *et al.*, 1991). However, these demonstrations were not conducted as a clinical intervention and their generalizability and durability have not been evaluated.

The most comprehensive programme for cognitive rehabilitation is integrated psychological therapy (IPT) (Brenner *et al.*, 1990). This programme first focuses on the remediation of basic cognitive capacities (e.g. concept formation, memory) before training in problem solving and social skills. Cognitive training proceeds on tasks adapted from neuropsychological test procedures (e.g. a card sorting task) and word games (e.g.

finding synonyms and antonyms). Two controlled trials of IPT reported modest gains in social skills but not only minimal improvement in cognitive functioning (Brenner *et al.*, 1990). A small replication study on chronic schizophrenia patients found limited effects of IPT on social skills and cognitive functioning (Reed, 1991).

A limitation of the work on cognitive rehabilitation is that the role of information-processing deficits in producing the social impairments of schizophrenia remains unknown. Since patients tend to have a broad array of cognitive deficits, the selection of which deficits to target for rehabilitation is arbitrary. In addition, the method employed to improve performance relies primarily on repeatedly practising cognitive skills and the use of complex mnemonics, although neither approach has been successful in producing significant gains in brain-injured patients (Schacter & Glisky, 1986; Butler & Namerow, 1988; Benedict, 1989). A more fruitful avenue to explore for the management of cognitive deficits may be to focus on environmental change, compensatory strategies and coping skills until there is a better understanding of the factors underlying the poor social performance of schizophrenia patients. For further discussion of neuropsychological rehabilitation see Chapter 30.

Cognitive interventions*

The use of cognitive behavioural therapy as one element of the comprehensive management of schizophrenia has been considered for some years. Fifteen years ago, Aaron Beck *et al.* reported a cognitive intervention for delusions (Hole *et al.*, 1979). Some clinicians have successfully incorporated cognitive and behavioural techniques into their everyday clinical practice. Notable examples include Perris' group in Sweden (Perris, 1989) and Brenner's in Switzerland (Brenner *et al.*, 1992). More recently, a number of open studies have reported success in managing persistent

---

* The following two paragraphs are by Dr T. Sensky, Charing Cross and Westminster Medical School, London.

positive symptoms of schizophrenia using cognitive techniques. Kingdon and Turkington (1991) demonstrated benefits to 64 patients with schizophrenia treated with cognitive therapy in addition to routine clinical management. Fowler and Morley (1989) described the successful use of cognitive therapy to manage hallucinations and delusions. Cognitive interventions have been shown to reduce conviction in beliefs about hallucinations and even a reduction in voice activity (Chadwick & Birchwood, 1994). Similarly, Chadwick and Lowe (1994) have reported that some individuals with delusions report a reduction in conviction about their delusions, and in preoccupation with them, following a cognitive intervention.

The rapid development of this work is highlighted by the recent publication of a comprehensive treatment manual of cognitive-behavioural therapy for schizophrenia (Kingdon & Turkington, 1994). The potential benefits of cognitive interventions and their mechanisms are now becoming clearer with the publication of the first controlled trials. Garety *et al.* (1994) have reported a pilot study of 12 patients with medication-resistant persistent positive psychotic symptoms compared with a waiting list control group receiving only routine clinical treatment. While the control group showed no significant changes, the intervention group showed reductions in their symptoms, in their conviction about their symptoms, and in affective disturbance. In a carefully conducted comparison of two interventions (coping strategy enhancement versus problem solving), Tarrier and his colleagues (Tarrier *et al.*, 1993) demonstrated significant improvements in patients with persistent delusions or hallucinations. These improvements were sustained at six months' follow up. Clearly, it will be necessary to demonstrate benefits over longer follow up periods, but the signs are encouraging that these early benefits can be sustained.

Other psychotherapy approaches

A variety of other individual interventions for schizophrenia have been evaluated in controlled studies. Rogers *et al.* (1967) examined the effects of client-centred therapy provided to chronic schizophrenic in-patients over long periods of time, up to 2 years. At the follow-up assessment, the patients who had received therapy showed only minimal improvements compared with patients who received standard treatment. However, the experience of the therapists varied widely, and pharmacological treatment was not standardized across the treatment groups.

Two studies conducted by Hogarty *et al.* have examined the effects of major role therapy, an approach involving individual case-work and vocational counselling, in combination with different pharmacological treatments for stabilized schizophrenia out-patients. In the first study, patients were randomly assigned to receive neuroleptic medication alone, therapy alone, both treatments or neither treatment over a 2-year period (Hogarty & Goldberg, 1973; Hogarty *et al.*, 1974a,b). Neuroleptic medications significantly reduced relapses, both alone and in combination with major role therapy, which did not differ. Among patients who did not receive neuroleptics, major role therapy did not lower the risk of relapse compared with patients who received no social therapy. Overall, major role therapy did not reduce relapses. Among non-relapsed patients there was a puzzling interaction between therapy and medication. Non-relapsed patients who received both therapy and medication or who received neither treatment had better social functioning than non-relapsed patients who received either medication or therapy. This interaction is difficult to interpret since data on non-relapsed patients were not available.

In the second study, Hogarty *et al.* (1979) evaluated the effects of major role therapy on patients receiving either oral neuroleptic medication or injectable depot neuroleptics over a 2-year period. There were no differences between the two drug treatments nor was the effect of having social therapy with either of the two drug treatments significantly different.

A recently completed study by Tarrier *et al.* (1993) compared the effects of training schizophrenia patients with persistent psychotic symptoms in coping strategies ('coping strategy enhancement') with problem-solving training. The patients who were taught the coping strategies experienced significantly greater reductions in persistent symptoms than patients who received training in problem solving, and these effects were maintained at a 6-month follow-up.

In summary, with the exception of the intriguing study of Tarrier *et al.* (1993), controlled research on other approaches to individual psychotherapy for schizophrenia has produced few encouraging results. The variety of different methods of psychotherapy not found to be beneficial to schizophrenia patients, including psychodynamic psychotherapy, client-centred therapy and major role therapy, suggests that there is little 'placebo response' to therapy in these patients. Further research is needed to replicate the findings of Tarrier *et al.* (1993) and to characterize which patients are most likely to benefit from training in coping skills.

Family therapy

Over the past several decades the mental health profession has undergone an evolution in its attitude toward relatives of schizophrenia patients. Until the 1960s and 1970s, family members of patients were typically viewed by professionals as either culprits for causing schizophrenia or, more benignly, irrelevant to the treatment of the illness. The confluence of several factors has resulted in a shift to the current view of families as important allies of professionals in the management of schizophrenia. These factors include: (i) research documenting that negative familial affect is predictive of symptom relapses; (ii) recognition of the heavy burden of caring for an ill relative; and (iii) the strong dissatisfaction expressed by family members over their treatment by professionals.

EE research

In a series of now classic studies, Brown, Vaughn, Leff and their colleagues showed that high levels of criticism, hostility or emotional overinvolvement (e.g. extreme self-sacrificing behaviour, dramatic displays of emotion) in the relatives of schizo-

phrenia patients, referred to as high EE, predicted psychotic relapses during the 9 months following a symptom exacerbation (Brown *et al.*, 1972; Vaughn & Leff, 1976). Since this early research, over 20 studies conducted on more than 1000 schizophrenia patients have replicated the essential findings that EE, assessed in individual interviews with each relative, is associated with a higher risk of relapse (Kavanagh, 1992). The importance of these findings is amplified by the fact that similar results have been found across different cultures, EE ratings appear to be independent of patient psychopathology and chronicity, and behavioural observation research of family interactions supports the construct validity of EE (Miklowitz *et al.*, 1984; Mueser *et al.*, 1993a).

Although many studies have replicated the finding that patients living with high-EE families are at increased risk for relapse, a few studies have not found these results (e.g. MacMillan *et al.*, 1986; Parker *et al.*, 1988; Stirling *et al.*, 1991). A variety of factors can be identified which may account for different findings across studies, such as whether both relatives were interviewed, patient selection criteria (e.g. not selecting patients with persistent psychotic symptoms), and the stage of the illness in which EE was assessed (e.g. following an acute exacerbation or during symptom stabilization). Furthermore, many EE studies have been conducted on relatively small sample sizes, which have low statistical power to detect effects of moderate magnitude. Additional support for the validity of EE assessments is provided by the positive effects of family therapy for families containing high-EE relatives of schizophrenia patients (reviewed below).

The EE construct has generated considerable debate among both family members and professionals (Hatfield, 1987; Kanter *et al.*, 1987; Jenkins & Karno, 1992; Mueser *et al.*, 1993b). At least some of this controversy reflects the concerns of family members that the EE construct harks back to a previous era where families were blamed for causing schizophrenia (e.g. Fromm-Reichmann, 1950). These concerns are justified, yet the data pointing to a relationship between family EE and relapse cannot be ignored. A major limitation of most theories about EE has been the tendency to focus on a unidirectional model of the influence of negative family affect on patient symptoms. This simplistic model fails to consider the social context in which negatively charged family interactions occur and the impact of the psychiatric illness on caretaking relatives of the patient (Mueser & Glynn, 1995; see also Chapter 29).

Family burden

The family members of schizophrenia patients often report significant levels of subjective distress, economic burden, risks to their personal safety and social isolation (Vine, 1982; Noh & Turner, 1987; Lefley, 1989). In response to the burden, some family members attempt to exert greater control over their ill relative's disruptive behaviour through critical or intrusive interactions (Greenley, 1986). For example, Jackson *et al.* (1990) found that family burden correlated with EE.

The available research suggests that EE and family burden are best conceptualized as interactive, rather than unidirectional, processes. Disruptive and symptomatic patient behaviours increase the chance that relatives will respond with stressful (high EE) communications, which in turn may worsen the patient's symptoms, leading to a vicious circle (Mueser & Glynn, 1990). Relatives' attitudes about whether the problem behaviours are under the patient's control may contribute to the conflict (Brewin *et al.*, 1991), increasing overall stress in the family. In contrast, an affectively benign or socially reinforcing family environment may encourage gradual improvement in patient functioning and provide a buffer against stress. One goal of family interventions is to foster the development of such a mutually supportive family environment.

The family advocacy and consumer movement

In addition to EE research and recognition of the burden of caring for an ill relative, the family advocacy movement and mental health con-sumerism have played a vital role in establishing a more collaborative relationship between families and professionals. Family members of schizophrenia patients have articulated their dissatisfaction with how they are treated by mental health professionals and the quality of their relative's treatment (Hatfield & Lefley, 1987; Lefley & Johnson, 1990). Families have grown tired of the stigma of mental illness in the general public and the negative attitudes of professionals towards relatives. To overcome these problems, families have begun to educate the public and dispel myths about mental illness, and to demand more information, respect and cooperation from professionals.

The vitality of the consumer movement is evident from the numerous organizations of family members and consumers that have formed in recent years to advocate for the needs of the mentally ill and their relatives. Their message has been loud and clear: (i) families are not to blame for mental illness; (ii) relatives and patients have the right to basic information about psychiatric illness and its treatment; and (iii) resources and treatment standards for the mentally ill are inadequate. A consequence of this movement has been the surge in books published recently for families about psychiatric illness (e.g. Torrey, 1988) and for professionals about working with families of the mentally ill (e.g. Marsh, 1992). In sum, the family advocacy movement and recognition of the interaction between family stress and patient functioning have been driving forces behind the development of family interventions to improve the outcome of schizophrenia (see also Chapters 29 & 30).

Research on family therapy

As mental health professionals have begun to view relatives as allies in the treatment of schizophrenia, there has been a proliferation of programmes aimed at educating families about the illness and improving their ability to manage difficult behaviours. These programmes can be broadly divided into short-term (i.e. less than 3 months) or long-term interventions.

Short-term family therapy

Among empirical trials of short-term family interventions, several approaches have focused primarily on providing education to relatives alone (Cozolino *et al.*, 1988; Smith & Birchwood, 1987; Abramowitz & Coursey, 1989; Sidley *et al.*, 1991; Birchwood *et al.*, 1992; Vaughn *et al.*, 1992), while others have included the patient in the family sessions and broadened the scope of therapy objectives to include both education and improved family functioning (Goldstein *et al.*, 1978; Glick *et al.*, 1985, 1990; Haas *et al.*, 1988; Spencer *et al.*, 1988; Mills & Hansen, 1991).

The controlled research on short-term family therapy for schizophrenia indicates that these programmes: (i) improve the understanding of family members about their relative's illness and that this knowledge is maintained for at least brief follow-up periods; (ii) produce modest improvements in family burden, although it is unclear how long these improvements last; and (iii) have limited effects on the social adjustment, symptomatology and relapse rate of patients. These studies support the feasibility of brief interventions for families with a schizophrenia patient, but also suggest that longer treatment durations are necessary for patients to achieve significant clinical improvements.

Long-term family therapy

In contrast to short-term family therapy programmes, controlled research on most long-term programmes lasting at least 9 months has provided strong support for their clinical efficacy. The single exception to this trend has been the only study to examine the efficacy of a psychodynamically orientated intervention (Kottgen *et al.*, 1984). This study found no differences in relapse rates between patients who were assigned to the family treatment and patients who received customary treatment. However, the interpretation of these findings is limited by the small sample size and the fact that the therapy groups were poorly attended (e.g. less than half the relatives and patients attended at least 75% of the scheduled sessions).

Several different long-term family therapy models have been developed, empirically tested and found to produce beneficial clinical effects at 2-year follow-ups. These models include: Falloon *et al.* (1984) behavioural family therapy model (Falloon *et al.*, 1985, 1987; Falloon & Pederson, 1985; Cardin *et al.*, 1986), Tarrier and Barrowclough's (1990) behavioural approach (Tarrier *et al.*, 1989, 1991; Barrowclough & Tarrier, 1992); Leff *et al.* (1985) psychoeducational method; Anderson, *et al.* (1986) psychoeducational method (Hogarty *et al.*, 1986, 1991); and McFarlane's (1990) multiple family group support model (McFarlane *et al.*, 1993). The core components of each of these models are summarized in Table 31.1.

Although the specific clinical strategies employed across different family therapy models are not identical, they share more in common than they differ. Lam (1991) identified seven common ingredients of effective family interventions for schizophrenia:

1 a positive approach and genuine working relationship between the therapist and family;
2 the provision of family therapy in a stable, structured format with additional contacts with therapists if necessary;
3 a focus on improving stress and coping in the 'here and now' rather than dwelling on the past;
4 encouragement of respect for interpersonal boundaries within the family;
5 the provision of information about the biological nature of schizophrenia, so as to reduce blaming the patient and family guilt;
6 the use of behavioural techniques, such as breaking down goals into manageable steps; and
7 improving communication between family members.

Control studies have been conducted comparing customary treatment with long-term family therapy using the models of Falloon *et al.* (1985), Leff *et al.* (1985), Tarrier *et al.* (1989) and Hogarty *et al.* (1991). In addition, Randolph *et al.* (1994) recently replicated the effects of family therapy (vs. customary treatment) using the model of Falloon *et al.* The 2-year relapse rates for these studies are summarized in Table 31.2. These

Table 31.1 Components of long-term psychoeducational family therapy models

Leff et al. (1985)
Assessment
Education
Relatives group
Individual family sessions to reduce expressed emotion patient-relative contact

Falloon et al. (1984)
Assessment
Education
Communication skills training
Problem-solving training
Special problems

Anderson et al. (1986)
Joining with the family
Education
Re-entry of patient into family
Enhancing work and social adjustment
Maintenance of gains

McFarlane's (1990) multiple family group
Joining with the family
Education
Relapse prevention
Improved psychosocial functioning (via problem solving)
Creation of a social network (via socialization)

Barrowclough and Tarrier (1992)
Assessment
Education
Stress-management training
Training in goal setting and attainment

studies indicate that family therapy has a significant effect on reducing relapse rates to an average of about 50% of standard (no family therapy) treatment. Furthermore, those studies which have assessed other dimensions of functioning have generally reported positive effects of treatment on patient social adjustment and reduced family burden (e.g. Falloon & Pederson, 1985; Falloon et al., 1987; Tarrier et al., 1989). There is also some evidence that long-term family intervention for schizophrenia may be cost effective because it reduces the number of days patients spend in hospital (Cardin et al., 1986; Tarrier et al., 1991).

These studies indicate that family therapy is one of the most potent interventions known for schizophrenia.

Two controlled studies have also been conducted that compared the efficacy of individual family therapy with therapy provided in multiple family groups (Leff et al., 1990; McFarlane et al., 1993). The results of these comparisons are also summarized in Table 31.2. Two trends are notable from these two studies. First, relapse rates over 2 years are relatively low for both individual and multiple family group formats, as compared with the relapse rates of other studies that used customary care as a control group. Second, the differences in relapse rates between the individual and multiple family group formats are small, although the difference approached significance ($P < 0.06$) for the McFarlane et al. (1993) study. These studies suggest that multiple family therapy may be of comparable efficacy to individual family therapy, which would make it a more economical treatment of choice. However, this conclusion awaits research that compares individual family therapy and multiple family therapy with customary care.

The treatment strategies for schizophrenia (TSS) study

TSS was a large (over 300 patients) multisite study, involving five hospitals, of pharmacological and family treatment strategies for schizophrenia that has recently been completed by the National Institute of Mental Health (Keith et al., 1989; Schooler et al., 1989, 1993). This study examined three different pharmacological management strategies — standard-dose fluphenazine decanoate, low dose and 'targeted' dose, i.e. medication was given only when symptoms worsened — and two different family treatment strategies — 'supportive' vs. 'applied' treatment — in a factorial design. Patients were randomized to one of the three medication groups after a 4- to 6-month stabilization period, with medication provided in a double-blind fashion for an additional 2 years. Psychiatrists were free to medicate with open-label medication if early warning signs appeared or a symptom exacerbation occurred. For the

Table 31.2 Two-year relapse rates for schizophrenia patients who received long-term family therapy

Reference	Theoretical orientation	Sample size	Single family therapy*	Multiple family therapy*	Routine treatment
Falloon *et al.* (1985)	Behavioural	32	17	–	83
Leff *et al.* (1985)	Supportive	24	14	–	78
Tarrier *et al.* (1989)	Behavioural	42	33	–	59
Leff *et al.* (1990)†	Supportive	23	33	36	–
Hogarty *et al.* (1991)	Family systems	57	32	–	67
McFarlane *et al.* (1993)‡	Supportive	172	42	28	–
Randolph *et al.* (1994)	Behavioural	41	10	–	40
Schooler *et al.* (1993)‡	Single family: behavioural§ Multiple family: supportive	313	29	35	–

* Single family therapy refers to family treatment provided to one family at a time; multiple family therapy refers to family treatment provided to more than one family simultaneously.
† Patients were excluded from multiple family groups.
‡ Patients were included in multiple family groups.
§ Families who received single behavioural family therapy also participated in the multiple family support groups.
‖ Based on rehospitalization rates.

supportive family treatment condition, relatives were provided with an educational workshop patterned after the 'survival skills workshop', developed by Anderson *et al.* (1986), followed by multiple family support–education groups held monthly for the approximate 2.5 years of the study, and case management as needed. For the applied family treatment condition, families received all the treatments provided to the supportive condition (i.e. the educational workshop, monthly multiple family groups and case management) as well as approximately 1.5 years of home-based behavioural family therapy (initiated at the beginning of the study), based on the behavioural family therapy model of Falloon *et al.* (1984).

The data for the TSS study are in the process of being analysed, but several clear effects have emerged. First, patients in families who received the supportive treatment did as well over the study as did patients in families who received the applied treatment, suggesting little added effect for behavioural family therapy to the supportive family treatment condition. Second, rehospitalization rates were low for both family interventions (41% cumulative rehospitalization rate over

2 years for the applied treatment, 43% for the supportive treatment), suggesting that combined family and pharmacological treatment were beneficial. Third, there were no interactions between pharmacological and family treatment conditions.

Although the results of this study require further explication, they appear to be in line with the studies of Leff *et al.* (1990) and McFarlane *et al.* (1993), who found similar effects for single and multiple family interventions for schizophrenia. Falloon *et al.* (1985) and Randolph *et al.* (1994) both reported that behavioural family therapy reduced relapse rates when compared with a standard treatment which involved no family intervention. The TSS study did not include a no-family intervention group, so it is unclear whether both interventions were effective. In addition, the TSS study design precluded the measurement of relapse rates across all patients. Since the beneficial effects of family intervention are most evident in the reduction of relapse rates, the lack of relapse data in the TSS study makes it difficult to compare with other studies of family therapy for schizophrenia. Research is needed that compares the effects of single family therapy and multiple family therapy approaches with no (or minimal) family intervention for schizophrenia.

Future directions for family therapy

The encouraging results of research on family therapy for schizophrenia raise many questions about how these interventions can be optimally applied. With the variety of different family therapy models that have been developed, it would be useful to know whether any family or patient characteristics are predictive of a differential response to treatment. For example, do socially isolated families benefit more from a multiple family group approach? Are behavioural family interventions more effective when strong negative affect is present in the family?

Another unresolved issue is the durability of family therapy. The intervention study of Tarrier *et al.* (1989) lasted for 9 months, and assessments at 2 years indicated some maintenance of effects, but most other studies provided family therapy for 2 years. McFarlane (1990) has argued against limiting the duration of family therapy. As we have discussed previously in this chapter, the expectation that time-limited psychosocial interventions will have long-lasting effects on schizophrenia may be inconsistent with the chronic nature of the illness, yet there are often practical limitations to how much therapy can be offered. The ultimate resolution probably lies somewhere between the two poles of time-limited or indefinite family therapy. Some families who either are living with a severely ill relative or face multiple hardships (e.g. poverty, substance abuse) may require ongoing family therapy as a social prosthesis against high levels of stress. Other families may need therapy for only a limited period, providing they have access to a therapist for booster sessions. Future research is needed to establish clinical guidelines regarding how often and over what duration family therapy sessions should be conducted.

A final set of remaining questions about family therapy pertains to the timing of the intervention. Tarrier (1991) has suggested that families are more amenable to intervention when the patient is in the acute stage of the illness, and most studies have initiated therapy at this time. However, this remains untested. A related issue is whether the provision of family therapy soon after the illness has developed might improve its overall chronic trajectory. Research conducted to date on family therapy has focused mainly on patients who have had the illness for many years. Family treatment provided at an earlier stage of the illness might prevent relatives and patients from adopting maladaptive strategies for coping with stress (e.g. high-EE behaviours, social withdrawal), strategies that have negative long-term consequences. Some of these negative coping styles may account for the worsening in negative symptoms found during the first few years after schizophrenia has developed (Fenton & McGlashan, 1992).

Additional considerations

Psychotherapy for schizophrenia cannot operate in a vacuum, but rather requires continuity and integration with other treatment services. The trend towards community based treatment for seriously impaired psychiatric patients underscores the need for multifaceted, long-term interventions. If the goals of treatment are to be achieved, including improved social functioning, enhanced quality of life and the reduction of relapse rates, then individual, group and family psychotherapy must be available and coordinated on a continuing basis. Stein and Test's (1985) Programme for Assertive Community Treatment (PACT) is one method for coordinating an array of treatments in the community and providing case management. Treatment team members in PACT have a high level of contact with their patients and detailed information concerning the functioning of patients in the community. This arrangement may provide a unique opportunity for increasing the availability of psychotherapy to patients who have traditionally been difficult to engage. Furthermore, treatment team members may be able to prompt patients to use specific skills in their natural environment and give valuable information to therapists regarding patient functioning in the community.

Research on the pharmacological treatment of schizophrenia has continued to make advances and there is a need to understand how to integrate medication with psychotherapy. Low doses of neuroleptics are as effective as standard doses in preventing relapses (Van Putten & Marder, 1986; Johnson *et al.*, 1987) and there is hope that improving the patient's interpersonal skills, reducing negative family affect and increasing social support will permit further dosage reductions. The potent effects of clozapine on treatment-resistant schizophrenia (Kane *et al.*, 1988) have had a major impact on many patients. After years of psychosis, clozapine responders re-establish their contact with reality and become amenable to psychotherapy, but the specific needs of these patients and their relatives have not been determined. Last, there is hope that novel neuroleptics (e.g. risperidone) with more benign side-effect profiles (Gratz & Simpson, 1992) will enable some patients to do so in psychotherapy who have been unable to do so in the past because of the side effects of conventional neuroleptics. Patients are often disturbed and distracted by side effects of neuroleptics such as akathisia (Van Putten, 1975); and anticholinergic medications used to treat side effects can interfere with learning (Strauss *et al.*, 1990). These new medications may thus facilitate learning in psychotherapy.

A final area in need of special consideration for psychotherapy is the problem of comorbid substance abuse (Mueser *et al.*, 1992). Patients with schizophrenia are at increased risk for substance abuse (Regier *et al.*, 1991), which can precipitate symptom relapses and rehospitalizations (Drake *et al.*, 1989). The clinical management of these patients is further complicated by their tendency to 'fall between the cracks' of the mental health and substance-abuse treatment systems. There is at present a paucity of controlled research on the treatment of dual diagnosis psychiatric patients. However, specialized treatment programmes that incorporate the principles of psychotherapy for both disorders have been recently developed (Minkoff & Drake, 1991), and are currently being evaluated.

Conclusions

After years of unsuccessful attempts at psychotherapy for schizophrenia, the field has at last progressed to the point where cautious optimism is merited. As evidence has accumulated supporting the efficacy of psychotherapy, so too has the realization that the benefits of treatment may be temporary and that many patients require ongoing intervention to maintain improvements. This understanding is compatible with the recognition that schizophrenia is a life-long disability, and promotes more realistic expectations on the part of treatment providers, patients and their relatives.

The absolute clinical gains resulting from family and individual psychotherapy tend to be modest. However, these positive results should be taken as encouragement by practitioners in the field, especially considering how rapid the progress has been over the past 20 years. Prior to the 1970s, there was little evidence from controlled research that any models of psychotherapy could be beneficial to schizophrenia. Now there is evidence, replicated across studies, supporting the efficacy of a variety of different family therapy models and SST; other approaches to psychotherapy continue to be developed and tested. Much work remains to be done in understanding how to better deliver existing psychotherapies, identifying which patients will benefit from which treatments and developing more effective interventions. The success achieved in recent years bodes well for continuing progress in psychotherapy for schizophrenia.

Acknowledgements

Preparation of this review was supported by NIMH grants 38636, 39998 and 41577 to A.S. Bellack.

References

Abramowitz, I.A. & Coursey, R.D. (1989) Impact of an educational support group on family participants who take care of their schizophrenia relatives. *Journal of Consulting and Clinical Psychology*, **57**, 232–236.

Anderson, C.M., Reiss, D.J. & Hogarty, G.E. (1986) *Schizophrenia and the Family.* Guilford Press, New York.

Arieti, S. (1974) *Interpretation of Schizophrenia,* 2nd edn. Basic Books, New York.

Ascher-Svanum, H. & Krause, A.A. (eds) (1991) *Psychoeducational Groups for Patients with Schizophrenia: A Guide for Practitioners.* Aspen, Gaithersburg.

Barrowclough, C. & Tarrier, N. (1992) *Families of Schizophrenic Patients: Cognitive Bahavioural Intervention.* Chapman & Hall, London.

Bellack, A.S. (1986) Schizophrenia: behavior therapy's forgotten child. *Behavior Therapy,* **17**, 199–214.

Bellack, A.S. (1989) A comprehensive model for the treatment of schizophrenia. In Bellack, A.S. (ed.) *A Clinical Guide for the Treatment of Schizophrenia,* pp. 1–22. Plenum Press, New York.

Bellack, A.S. (1992) Cognitive rehabilitation for schizophrenia: Is it possible? Is it necessary? *Schizophrenia Bulletin,* **18**, 43–50.

Bellack, A.S., Morrison, R.L. & Mueser K.T. (1989) Social problem solving in schizophrenia. *Schizophrenia Bulletin,* **15**, 101–116.

Bellack, A.S. Morrison, R.L., Wixted, J.T. & Mueser, K.T. (1990a) An analysis of social competence in schizophrenia. *British Journal of Psychiatry,* **156**, 809–818.

Bellack, A.S., Mueser, K.T., Morrison, R.L., Tierney, A. & Podell, K. (1990b) Remediation of cognitive deficits in schizophrenia. *American Journal of Psychiatry,* **147**, 1650–1655.

Bellack, A.S., Turner, S.M., Hersen M. & Luber, R.F. (1984) An examination of the efficacy of social skills training for chronic schizophrenic patients. *Hospital and Community Psychiatry,* **35**, 1023–1028.

Benedict, R.H. (1989) The effectiveness of cognitive remediation strategies for victims of traumatic head-injury: a review of the literature. *Clinical Psychology Review,* **9**, 605–626.

Benton, M.K. & Schroeder, H.E. (1990) Social skills training with schizophrenics: a meta-analytic evaluation. *Journal of Consulting and Clinical Psychology,* **58**, 741–747.

Berman, K.F., Zec, R.F. & Weinberger, D.R. (1986) Physiological dysfunction of dorsolateral prefrontal cortex in schizophrenia. II. Role of nueroleptic treatment, attention, and mental effort. *Archives of General Psychiatry,* **43**, 126–135.

Bilder, R.M. & Goldberg, E. (1987) Motor perseverations in schizophrenia. *Archives of Clinical Neuropsychology,* **2**, 1–20.

Bion, W.R. (1967) *Second Thoughts.* Heinemann, London.

Birchwood, M., Smith, J. & Cochrane, R. (1992) Specific and non-specific effects of educational intervention for families living with schizophrenia. *British Journal of Psychiatry,* **160**, 806–814.

Bisbee, C.C. & Lee, L.N. (1988) *Patient Education in Psychiatric Illness: A Practical Program Guide.* Bryce Hospital, Tuscaloosa.

Bleuler, E. (1911) *Dementia Praecox or the Group of Schizophrenias.* Translated by Zinkin, J. (1950). International Universities Press, New York.

Boker, W. (1987) On the self-help among schizophrenics: problem analysis and empirical studies. In Strauss, J.S., Boker, W. & Brenner, H.D. (eds) *Psychosocial Treatment of Schizophrenia: Multidimensional Concepts, Psychological, Family, and Self-Help Perspectives,* pp. 167–179. Hans Huber, Toronto.

Braff, D.L. (1991) Information processing and attentional abnormalities in the schizophrenic disorders. In Magaro, P.A. (ed.) *Cognitive Bases of Mental Disorders,* pp. 262–307. Sage Publications, Newbury Park.

Braff, D.L., Heaton R., Kuck, J. *et al.* (1991) The generalized pattern of neuropsychological deficits in outpatients with chronic schizophrenia with heterogeneous Wisconsin Card Sorting Test results. *Archives of General Psychiatry,* **48**, 891–898.

Brenner, H.D., Hodel, B., Roder, V. & Corrigan, P. (1992) Treatment of cognitive dysfunction and behavioral deficits in schizophrenia. *Schizophrenia Bulletin,* **18**, 21–26.

Brenner, H.D., Kraemer, S., Hermanutz, M. & Hodel, B. (1990) Cognitive treatment in schizophrenia. In Straube, E. & Hahlweg, K. (eds) *Schizophrenia: Models and Interventions,* pp. 161–191. Springer-Verlag, New York.

Brenner, H.D., Hodel, B., Genner, R., Roder, V. & Corrigan, P.W. (1992) Biological and cognitive vulnerability factors in schizophrenia: implications for treatment. *British Journal of Psychiatry,* **161** (suppl 18), 154–163.

Brewin, C.R., MacCarthy, B., Duda, K. & Vaughn, C.E. (1991) Attribution and expressed emotion in the relatives of patients with schizophrenia. *Journal of Abnormal Psychology,* **100**, 546–554.

Brown, G.W. & Birley, J.L.T. (1968) Crisis and life changes and the onset of schizophrenia. *Journal of Health and Social Behaviour,* **9**, 203–214.

Brown, G.W., Birley, J.L.T. & Wing, J.K. (1972) Influence of family life on the course of schizophrenic disorders: a replication. *British Journal of Psychiatry,* **121**, 241–258.

Brown, M.A. & Munford, A.M. (1983) Life skills training for chronic schizophrenics. *Journal of Nervous and Mental Disease,* **17**, 466–470.

Butler, R.W. & Namerow, N.S. (1988) Cognitive retraining in brain-injury rehabilitation: a critical review. *Journal of Neuropsychology and Rehabilitation,* **2**, 97–101.

Caldwell, C.B. & Gottesman, I.I. (1990) Schizophrenics kill themselves too: a review of risk factors for suicide. *Schizophrenia Bulletin,* **16**, 571–589.

Cardin, V.A., McGill, C.W. & Falloon, I.R.H. (1986) An economic analysis: costs, benefits and effectiveness. In Falloon, I.R.H. (ed.) *Family Management of Schizophrenia,* pp. 115–123. Johns Hopkins University Press, Baltimore.

Carpenter, W.T., Heinrichs, D.W. & Wagman, A.M.I. (1988) Deficit and nondeficit forms of schizophrenia: the concept. *American Journal of Psychiatry,* **145**, 578–583.

Carpenter, W.T., Buchanan, R.W., Kirkpatrick, B., Tamminga, C. & Wood, F. (1993) Strong inference, theory testing, and the neuroanatomy of schizophrenia. *Archives of General Psychiatry,* **50**, 825–831.

Carr, V. (1988) Patient's techniques for coping with schizophrenia: an exploratory study. *British Journal of Medical Psychology,* **61**, 339–352.

Chadwick, P.D. & Birchwood, M. (1994) The omnipotence of

voices. A cognitive approach to auditory hallucinations. *British Journal of Psychiatry*, **164**, 190–201.

Chadwick, P.D. & Lowe, C.F. (1994) A cognitive approach to measuring and modifying delusions. *Behaviour Research and Therapy*, **32**, 355–367.

Ciompi, L. (1987) Toward a coherent multidimensional understanding and therapy of schizophrenia: converging new concepts. In Strauss, J.S., Boker, W. & Brenner, H.D. (eds) *Psychosocial Treatment of Schizophrenia: Multidimensional Concepts, Psychological, Family, and Self-Help Perspectives*, pp. 48–62. Hans Huber, Toronto.

Cozolino, I.J., Goldstein, M.J., Nuechterlein, K.H., West, K.I. & Snyder, K.S. (1988) The impact of education about schizophrenia on relatives' expressed emotion. *Schizophrenia Bulletin*, **14**, 675–687.

Drake, R.E. & Cotton, P.G. (1986) Depression, hopelessness and suicide in chronic schizophrenia. *British Journal of Psychiatry*, **148**, 554–559.

Drake, R.E., Osher, F.C. & Wallach, M.A. (1989) Alcohol use and abuse in schizophrenia: a prospective community study. *Journal of Nervous and Mental Disease*, **177**, 408–414.

D'Zurilla, T.J. & Goldfried, M.R. (1971) Problem solving and behavior modification. *Journal of Abnormal Psychology*, **78**, 107–126.

Eckman, T.A., Wirshing, W.C., Marder, S.R. *et al.* (1992) Technology for training schizophrenics in illness self-management: a controlled trial. *American Journal of Psychiatry*, **149**, 1549–1555.

Falloon, I.R.H. & Pederson, J. (1985) Family management in the prevention of morbidity of schizophrenia: the adjustment of the family unit. *British Journal of Psychiatry*, **147**, 156–163.

Falloon, I.R.H. & Talbot, R.E. (1981) Persistent auditory hallucinations: coping mechanisms and implications for management. *Psychological Medicine*, **11**, 329–339.

Falloon, I.R.H., Boyd, J.L. & McGill, C.W. (1984) *Family Care of Schizophrenia*. Guilford Press, New York.

Falloon, I.R.H., McGill, C.W., Boyd, J.L. & Pederson, J. (1987) Family management in the prevention of morbidity of schizophrenia: social outcome of a two-year longitudinal study. *Psychological Medicine*, **17**, 59–66.

Falloon, I.R.H., Boyd, J.L., McGill, C.W. *et al.* (1985) Family management in the prevention of morbidity of schizophrenia: clinical outcome of a two-year longitudinal study. *Archives of General Psychiatry*, **42**, 887–896.

Fenton, W.S. & McGlashan, T.H. (1992) Testing systems for assessment of negative symptoms in schizophrenia. *Archives of General Psychiatry*, **49**, 179–185.

Fowler, D. & Morley, S. (1989) The cognitive-behavioural treatment of hallucinations and delusions: a preliminary study. *Behavioural Psychotherapy*, **17**, 267–282.

Fromm-Reichmann, F. (1950) *Principles of Intensive Psychotherapy*. University of Chicago Press, Chicago.

Garety, P.A., Kuipers, L., Fowler, D., Chamberlain, F. & Dunn, G. (1994) Cognitive behavioural therapy for drug-resistant psychosis. *British Journal of Medical Psychology*, **67**, 259–271.

Glick, I., Clarkin, J., Spencer, J. *et al.* (1985) A controlled evaluation of inpatient family intervention. I. Preliminary results of a 6-month follow-up. *Archives of General Psychiatry*, **42**, 882–886.

Glick, I., Spencer, J., Clarkin, J. *et al.* (1990) A randomized clinical trial of inpatient family intervention. IV. Follow-up results for subjects with schizophrenia. *Schizophrenia Research*, **3**, 187–200.

Glynn, S.M. (1990) Token economy approaches for psychiatric patients: progress and pitfalls over 25 years. *Behavior Modification*, **14**, 383–407.

Goldberg, T.E., Weinberger, D.R., Berman, K.F., Pliskin, N.H. & Podd, M.H. (1987) Further evidence for dementia of the prefrontal type in schizophrenia? *Archives of General Psychiatry*, **44**, 1008–1014.

Goldstein, M., Rodnick, E., Evans, J., May P. & Steinberg, M. (1978) Drug and family therapy in the aftercare of acute schizophrenics. *Archives of General Psychiatry*, **35**, 1169–1177.

Gratz, S.S. & Simpson, G.M. (1992) Psychopharmacology. In Hsu, L.K.G. & Hersen, M. (eds) *Research in Psychiatry: Issues, Strategies, and Methods*, pp. 309–329. Plenum Press, New York.

Green, M.F., Ganzell, S., Satz, P. & Vacav, J.F. (1990) Teaching the WCST to schizophrenic patients. *Archives of General Psychiatry*, **47**, 91–92.

Greenley, J.R. (1986) Social control and expressed emotion. *Journal of Nervous and Mental Disease*, **174**, 24–30.

Grinspoon, L., Ewalt, J.R. & Shader, R.I. (1972) *Schizophrenia: Pharmacotherapy and Psychotherapy*. Williams & Wilkins, Baltimore.

Gunderson, J.G., Frank, A., Katz, H.M., Vannicelli, M.L., Frosch, J.P. & Knapp, P.H. (1984) Effects of psychotherapy in schizophrenia. II. Comparative outcome of two forms of treatment. *Schizophrenia Bulletin*, **10**, 564–598.

Haas, G., Glick, I., Clarkin, J. *et al.* (1988) Inpatient family intervention: a randomized clinical trial. II. Results at hospital discharge. *Archives of General Psychiatry*, **48**, 217–224.

Halford, W.K. & Hayes, R. (1991) Psychological rehabilitation of chronic schizophrenic patients: recent findings on social skills training and family psychoeducation. *Clinical Psychology Review*, **11**, 23–44.

Harding, C.M., Brooks, G.W., Ashikaga, T., Strauss, J.S. & Breier, A. (1987a) The Vermont longitudinal study of persons with severe mental illness. I. Methodology, study sample, and overall status 32 years later. *American Journal of Psychiatry*, **144**, 718–726.

Harding, C.M., Brooks, G.W., Ashikaga, T., Strauss, J.S. & Breier, A. (1987b) The Vermont longitudinal study of persons with severe mental illness. II. Long-term outcome of subjects who retrospectively met DSM-III criteria for schizophrenia. *American Journal of Psychiatry*, **144**, 727–735.

Harrow, M. & Silverstein, M.L. (1977) Psychotic symptoms in schizophrenia after the acute phase. *Schizophrenia Bulletin*, **3**, 608–616.

Hatfield, A.B. (1987) The expressed emotion theory: why families object. *Hospital and Community Psychiatry*, **38**, 341.

Hatfield, A.B. & Lefley, H.P. (eds) (1987) *Families of the Mentally Ill: Coping and Adaptation*. Guilford Press, New York.

Heaton, R.K. (1981) *Wisconsin Card Sorting Test Manual*.

Psychological Assessment Resources, Odessa.

Hersen, M. & Bellack, A.S. (1976) Social skills training for chronic psychiatric patients: rationale, research findings, and future directions. *Comprehensive Psychiatry*, **17**, 559–580.

Hogarty, G.E. & Flesher, S. (1992) Cognitive remediation in schizophrenia: proceed ... with caution! *Schizophrenia Bulletin*, **18**, 51–57.

Hogarty, G.E. & Goldberg, S.C. (1973) Drug and sociotherapy in the aftercare of schizophrenic patients. III. Adjustment of non-relapsed patients. *Archives of General Psychiatry*, **28**, 609–618.

Hogarty, G.E., Goldberg, S.C. & Schooler, N.R. (1974a) Drug and sociotherapy in the aftercare of schizophrenic patients. *Archives of General Psychiatry*, **31**, 609–618.

Hogarty, G.E., Goldberg, S.C., Schooler, N.R. & Ulrich, R.F. (1974b) Drug and sociotherapy in the aftercare of schizophrenic patients. II. Two-year relapse rates. *Archives of General Psychiatry*, **31**, 603–608.

Hogarty, G.E., Schooler, N.R., Ulrich, R., Mussare, F., Ferro, P. & Herron, E. (1979) Fluphenazine and social therapy in the aftercare of schizophrenic patients. *Archives of General Psychiatry*, **36**, 1283–1294.

Hogarty, G.E., Anderson, C.M., Reiss, D.J. *et al.* (1986) Family psychoeducation, social skills training, and maintenance chemotherapy in the aftercare treatment of schizophrenia. I. One-year effects of a controlled study on relapse and expressed emotion. *Archives of General Psychiatry*, **43**, 633–642.

Hogarty, G.E., Anderson, C.M., Reiss, D.J. *et al.* (1991) Family psychoeducation, social skills training, and maintenance chemotherapy in the aftercare treatment of schizophrenia. II. Two-year effects of a controlled study on relapse and adjustment. *Archives of General Psychiatry*, **48**, 340–347.

Hole, R.W., Rush, A.J. & Beck, A.T. (1979) A cognitive investigation of schizophrenic delusions. *Psychiatry*, **42**, 312–319.

Horwitz, A.V., Tessler, R.C., Fischer, G.A. & Gamache, G.M. (1992) The role of adult siblings in providing social support to the severely mentally ill. *Journal of Marriage and the Family*, **54**, 233–241.

Jackson, H.J., Smith, N. & McGorry, P. (1990) Relationship between expressed emotion and family burden in psychotic disorders: an exploratory study. *Acta Psychiatrica Scandinavia*, **82**, 243–249.

Jenkins, J.H. & Karno, M. (1992) The meaning of expressed emotion: theoretical issues raised by cross-cultural research. *American Journal of Psychiatry*, **149**, 9–21.

Johnson, D.A.W., Ludlow, J.M., Street, K. & Taylor, R.D.W. (1987) Double-blind comparison of half-dose and standard-dose flupenthixol decanoate in the maintenance treatment of stabilised out-patients with schizophrenia. *British Journal of Psychiatry*, **151**, 634–638.

Johnstone, E.C., Macmillan, J.F., Frith, C.D., Benn, D.K. & Crow, T.J. (1990) Further investigation of the predictors of outcome following first schizophrenic episodes. *British Journal of Psychiatry*, **157**, 182–189.

Kane, J., Honigfeld, G., Singer, J. & Meltzer, H. (1988) Clozapine for the treatment-resistant schizophrenic.

Archives of General Psychiatry, **45**, 789–796.

Kanter, J., Lamb, H.R. & Loeper, C. (1987) Expressed emotion in families: a critical review. *Hospital and Community Psychiatry*, **38**, 374–380.

Karon, B.P. & VandenBos, G.R. (1970) Experience, medication and the effectiveness of psychotherapy with schizophrenia: a note on Drs. May and Tuma's conclusions. *British Journal of Psychiatry*, **116**, 427–428.

Karon, B.P. & VandenBos, G.R. (1972) The consequences of psychotherapy for schizophrenic patients. *Psychotherapy: Theory, Research and Practice*, **9**, 111–119.

Karon, B.P. & VandenBos, G.R. (1975) Issues in current research on psychotherapy vs. medication in treatment of schizophrenics. *Psychotherapy: Theory, Research and Practice*, **12**, 143–148.

Kavanagh, D.J. (1992) Recent developments in expressed emotion and schizophrenia. *British Journal of Psychiatry*, **160**, 601–620.

Keith, S.J., Bellack, A., Frances, A., Mance, R. & Matthews, S. (1989) The influence of diagnosis and family treatment on acute treatment response and short-term outcome in schizophrenia. *Psychopharmacology Bulletin*, **25**, 336–339.

Kern, R.S., Green, M.F. & Satz, P. (1992) Nueropsychological predictors of skills training for chronic psychiatric patients. *Psychiatry Research*, **43**, 223–230.

Kingdon, D.G. & Turkington, D. (1991) The use of cognitive behavior therapy with a normalizing rationale in schizophrenia. Preliminary report. *Journal of Nervous and Mental Disease*, **179**, 207–211.

Kingdon, D. & Turkington, D. (1994) *Cognitive-Behavioural Therapy of Schizophrenia*, Lawrence Erlbaum, Hove, Sussex.

Klein, M. (1948) *Contributions to Psycho-analysis*. Hogarth, London.

Kottgen, C., Sonnichsen, I., Mollenhauer, K. & Jurth, R. (1984) Group therapy with the families of schizophrenic patients: results of the Hamburg Camberwell-Family-Interview Study III. *International Journal of Family Psychiatry*, **5**, 83–94.

Kraeplin, E. (1919) *Dementia Praecox and Paraphrenia*. Translated by Barclay, R.M. 1971. Robert E. Krieger, New York.

Laing, R.D. (1960) *The Divided Self*. Tavistock, London.

Lam, D.H. (1991) Psychosocial family intervention in schizophrenia: a review of empirical studies. *Psychological Medicine*, **21**, 423–441.

Leff, J., Berkowitz, R., Shavit, N., Strachan, A., Glass, I. & Vaughn, C. (1989) A trial of family therapy vs. a relatives group for schizophrenia. *British Journal of Psychiatry*, **154**, 58–66.

Leff, J.P., Berkowitz, R., Shavit, N., Strachan, A., Glass, I. & Vaughn, C. (1990) A trial of family therapy versus a relatives' group for schizophrenia. Two-year follow-up. *British Journal of Psychiatry*, **157**, 571–577.

Leff, J., Kuipers, L., Berkowitz, R. & Sturgeon, D. (1985) A control trial of social intervention in the family of schizophrenic patients; two-year follow up. *British Journal of Psychiatry*, **146**, 594–600.

Lefley, H.P. (1989) Family burden and family stigma in major mental illness. *American Psychologist*, **44**, 556–560.

Lefley, H.P. & Johnson, D.L. (eds) (1990) *Families as Allies in Treatment of the Mentally Ill. New Directions for Mental Health*

Professionals. American Psychiatric Press, Washington DC.

Lenzenweger, M.F., Dworkin, R.H. & Wethington, E. (1991) Examining the underlying structure of schizophrenic phenomenology: evidence for a three-process model. *Schizophrenia Bulletin*, **17**, 515–524.

Liberman, R.P., DeRisi, W.D. & Mueser, K.T. (1989) *Social Skills Training for Psychiatric Patients*. Allyn & Bacon, Needham Heights.

Liberman, R.P., Mueser, K.T. & Wallace, C.J. (1986a) Social skills training for schizophrenic individuals at risk for relapse. *American Journal of Psychiatry*, **143**, 523–526.

Liberman, R.P., Mueser, K.T., Wallace, C.J., Jacobs, H.E., Eckman, T. & Massel, H.K. (1986b) Training skills in the psychiatrically disabled: learning, coping and competence. *Schizophrenia Bulletin*, **12**, 631–647.

McFall, R.M. (1982) A review and reformulation of the concept of social skills. *Behavioral Assessment*, **4**, 1–33.

McFarlane, W.R. (1990) Multiple family groups and the treatment of schizophrenia. In Herz, M.I., Keith, S.J. & Docherty, J.P. (eds) *Handbook of Schizophrenia*, Vol. 4, *Psychosocial Treatment of Schizophrenia*, pp. 167–189. Elsevier, Amsterdam.

McFarlane, W.R., Dunne, E., Lukens, E. *et al.* (1993) From research to clinical practice: dissemination of New York State's family psychoeducation project. *Hospital and Community Psychiatry*, **44**, 265–270.

McGlashan, T.H. (1984a) The Chestnut Lodge follow-up study. I. Follow-up methodology and study sample. *Archives of General Psychiatry*, **41**, 575–585.

McGlashan, T.H. (1984b) The Chestnut Lodge follow-up study. II. Long-term outcome of schizophrenia and the affective disorders. *Archives of General Psychiatry*, **41**, 586–601.

McGlashan, T.H. (1986) The prediction of outcome in chronic schizophrenia. IV. The Chestnut Lodge follow-up study. *Archives of General Psychiatry*, **43**, 167–175.

McGlashan, T.H. & Fenton, W.S. (1992) The positive–negative distinction in schizophrenia: review of natural history validators. *Archives of General Psychiatry*, **49**, 63–72.

MacMillan, J.F., Gold, A., Crow, T.J., Johnson, A.L. & Johnstone, E.C. (1986) The Northwick Park study of first episodes of schizophrenia. IV. Expressed emotion and relapse. *British Journal of Psychiatry*, **148**, 133–143.

Marder, S.R., Wirshing, W.C., Eckman, T. *et al.* (1993) Psychosocial and pharmacological strategies for maintenance therapy: effects on two-year outcome. *Schizophrenia Research*, **9**, 260.

Marsh, D.T. (1992) *Families and Mental Illness: New Directions in Professional Practice*. Praeger, New York.

May, P.R.A. (1968) *Treatment of Schizophrenia: A Comparative Study of Five Treatment Methods*. Science House, New York.

Miklowitz, D.J., Goldstein, M.J., Falloon, I.R.H. & Doane, J.A. (1984) Interactional correlates of expressed emotion in the families of schizophrenics. *British Journal of Psychiatry*, **144**, 482–487.

Mills, P.D. & Hansen, J.C. (1991) Short-term group interventions for mentally ill young adults living in a community residence and their families. *Hospital and Community Psychiatry*, **42**, 1144–1149.

Minkoff, K. & Drake, R.E. (eds) (1991) *Dual Diagnosis of Major Mental Illness and Substance Disorder*. New Directions for Mental Health Services, No. 50. Jossey-Bass, San Francisco.

Mueser, K.T. & Berenbaum, H. (1990) Psychodynamic treatment of schizophrenia: Is there a future? *Psychological Medicine*, **20**, 253–262.

Mueser, K.T. & Glynn, S.M. (1990) Behavioral family therapy for schizophrenia. In Hersen, M., Eisler, R.M. & Miller, P.M. (eds) *Progress in Behavior Modification*, Vol. 26, pp. 122–149. Sage, Newbury Park.

Mueser, K.T. & Glynn, S.M. (1993) Efficacy of psychotherapy for schizophrenia. In Giles, T.R. (ed.) *Handbook of Effective Psychotherapy*, pp. 325–354. Plenum Press, New York.

Mueser, K.T. & Glynn, S.M. (1995) *Behavioral Family Therapy for Psychiatric Disorders*. Allyn & Bacon, Boston.

Mueser, K.T., Bellack, A.S. & Blanchard, J.J. (1992a) Comorbidity of schizophrenia and substance abuse implications for treatment. *Journal of Consulting and Clinical Psychology*, **60**, 845–856.

Mueser, K.T., Gingerich, S.L. & Rosenthal, C.K. (1993b) Familial factors in psychiatry. *Current Opinion in Psychiatry*, **6**, 251–257.

Mueser, K.T., Bellack, A.S., Douglas, M.S. & Morrison, R.L. (1991a) Prevalence and stability of social skill deficits in schizophrenia. *Schizophrenia Research*, **5**, 167–176.

Mueser, K.T., Bellack, A.S., Douglas, M.S. & Wade, J.H. (1991b) Prediction of social skill acquisition in schizophrenic and major affective disorder patients from memory and symptomatology. *Psychiatry Research*, **37**, 281–296.

Mueser, K.T., Bellack, A.S., Wade, J.H., Haas, G. & Sayers, S.L. (1993a) Expressed emotion, social skill, and response to negative affect in schizophrenia. *Journal of Abnormal Psychology*, **102**, 339–351.

Mueser, K.T., Bellack, A.S., Wade, J.H., Sayers, S.L. & Rosenthal, C.K. (1992b) An assessment of the educational needs of chronic psychiatric patients and their relatives. *British Journal of Psychiatry*, **160**, 674–680.

Noh, S. & Turner, R.J. (1987) Living with psychiatric patients: implications for the mental health of family members. *Social Science and Medicine*, **25**, 263–271.

Nuechterlein, K.W. & Dawson, M.E. (1984a) A heuristic vulnerability/stress, model of schizophrenic episodes. *Schizophrenia Bulletin*, **10**, 300–312.

Nuechterlein, K.W. & Dawson, M.E. (1984b) Information processing and attentional functioning in the developmental course of schizophrenic disorders. *Schizophrenia Bulletin*, **10**, 160–203.

Parker, G., Johnston, P. & Hayward, L. (1988) Parental 'expressed emotion' as a predictor of schizophrenic relapse. *Archives of General Psychiatry*, **45**, 806–813.

Paul, G.L. & Lentz, R.J. (1977) *Psychosocial Treatment of Chronic Mental Patients: Milieu Versus Social-Learning Programs*. Harvard University Press, Cambridge.

Penn, D.L. (1991) Cognitive rehabilitation of social deficits in schizophrenia: a direction of promise or following a primrose path? *Psychosocial Rehabilitation Journal*, **15**, 27–41.

Perris, C. (1989) *Cognitive Therapy with Schizophrenic Patients*.

Guilford, New York.

Pilsecker, C. (1981) Hospital classes educate schizophrenics about their illness. *Hospital and Community Psychiatry*, **32**, 60–61.

Randolph, E.T., Eth, S., Glynn, S. *et al.* (1994) Behavioral family management in schizophrenia: outcome of a clinic-based intervention. *British Journal of Psychiatry*, **64**, 501–506.

Reed, D.D. (1991) *Effects of Cognitive Therapy on Social Functioning for Persons with Chronic Schizophrenia and other Severe Psychiatric Disorders.* PhD Thesis, University of Nebraska.

Regier, D.A., Farmers, M.E., Rae, D.S. *et al.* (1991) Comorbidity of mental disorders with alcohol and other drug abuse. *Journal of the American Medical Association*, **264**, 2511–2518.

Roberts, G.W. (1991) Schizophrenia: a neuropathological perspective. *British Journal of Psychiatry*, **158**, 8–17.

Rogers, C.R., Gendlin, E.G., Kiesler, D.J. & Traux, C.B. (1967) *The Therapeutic Relationship and its Impact: Study of Psychotherapy with Schizophrenics.* University of Wisconsin Press, Madison.

Rosen, J.N. (1953) *Direct Analysis: Selected Papers.* Grune & Stratton, New York.

Schacter, D.L. & Glisky, E.L. (1986) Memory remediation: restoration, alleviation, and the acquisition of domain-specific knowledge. In Uzzell, B.P. & Gross, Y. (eds) *Clinical Neuropsychology of Intervention*, pp. 257–282. Martinus Nijhoff, Boston.

Schooler, N.R., Keith, S.J., Severe, J.B. & Matthews, N.R. (1989) Acute treatment response and short-term outcome in schizophrenia. *Psychopharmacology Bulletin*, **25**, 331–335.

Schooler, N.R., Keith, S.J., Severe, J.B. & Matthews, N.R. (1993) Treatment strategies in schizophrenia: effects of dosage reduction and family management on outcome. *Schizophrenia Research*, **9**, 260.

Searles, H. (1965) *Collected Papers on Schizophrenia and Related Subjects.* International Universities Press, New York.

Sechehaye, M.A. (1965) *A New Psychotherapy in Schizophrenia.* Grune & Stratton, New York.

Sidley, G.L., Smith, J. & Howells, K. (1991) Is it ever too late to learn? Information provision to relatives of long-term schizophrenia suffers. *Behavioural Psychotherapy*, **19**, 305–320.

Silverstein, M.L. & Harrow, M. (1978) First rank symptoms in the post acute schizophrenic: a follow-up study. *American Journal of Psychiatry*, **135**, 1418–1486.

Smith, J. & Birchwood, M. (1987) Specific and non-specific effects of educational interventions with families of schizophrenic patients. *British Journal of Psychiatry*, **150**, 645–652.

Spencer, J., Glick, I., Haas, G. *et al.* (1988) A randomized clinical trial of inpatient family intervention. III. Effects at 6-month and 18-month follow-ups. *American Journal of Psychiatry*, **145**, 1115–1121.

Spencer, P.G., Gillespie, C.R. & Ekisa, E.G. (1983) A controlled comparison of the effects of social skills training and remedial drama on the conversational skills of chronic schizophrenic inpatients. *British Journal of Psychiatry*, **143**, 165–172.

Spring, B.J. & Ravdin, L.R. (1992) Cognitive remediation in schizophrenia: should we attempt it? *Schizophrenia Bulletin*, **18**, 15–20.

Stanton, A.H., Gunderson, J.G., Knapp, P.H. *et al.* (1984) Effects of psychotherapy in schizophrenia. I. Design and implementation of a controlled study. *Schizophrenia Bulletin*, **10**, 520–563.

Stein, L.I. & Test, M.A. (eds) (1985) *The Training in Community Living Model: A Decade of Experience* New Directions for Mental Health Services, No. 26. Jossey-Bass, San Francisco.

Stirling, J., Tantam, D., Thomas, P. *et al.* (1991) Expressed emotion and early onset schizophrenia: a one-year follow-up. *Psychological Medicine*, **21**, 675–685.

Stone, M.H. (1986) Exploratory psychotherapy in schizophrenia-spectrum patients. *Bulletin of the Menninger Clinic*, **50**, 287–306.

Strauss, J.S. (1989) Subjective experiences of schizophrenia: toward a new dynamic psychiatry II. *Schizophrenia Bulletin*, **15**, 179–187.

Strauss, J.S., Carpenter, W.T. Jr & Bartko, J.J. (1974) The diagnosis and understanding of schizophrenia. Part III. Speculations on the processes that underlie schizophrenic symptoms and signs. *Schizophrenia Bulletin*, **11**, 61–69.

Strauss, M.E., Reynolds, K.S., Jayaram, G. & Tune, L.E. (1990) Effects of anticholinergic medication on memory in schizophrenia. *Schizophrenia Research*, **3**, 127–129.

Stuve, P., Erickson, R.C. & Spaulding, W. (1991) Cognitive rehabilitation: the next step in psychiatric rehabilitation. *Psychosocial Rehabilitation Journal*, **15**, 9–26.

Sullivan, H.S. (1962) *Schizophrenia as a Human Process.* WW Norton & Company, New York.

Summerfelt, A.T., Alphs, L.D., Wagman, A.M.I., Funderbunk, F.R., Hierholzer, R.M. & Strauss, M.E. (1991) Reduction of perseverative errors in patients with schizophrenia using monetary feedback. *Journal of Abnormal Psychology*, **100**, 613–616.

Tarrier, N. (1991) Some aspects of family interventions in schizophrenia. I. Adherence to intervention programmes. *British Journal of Psychiatry*, **159**, 475–480.

Tarrier, N. & Barrowclough, C. (1990) Family interventions for schizophrenia. *Behavior Modification*, **14**, 408–440.

Tarrier, N., Lowson, K. & Barrowclough, C. (1991) Some aspects of family interventions in schizophrenia. II. Financial considerations. *British Journal of Psychiatry*, **159**, 481–484.

Tarrier, N., Barrowclough, C., Vaughan, C. *et al.* (1989) Community management of schizophrenia: a two-year follow-up of a behavioral intervention with families. *British Journal of Psychiatry*, **154**, 625–628.

Tarrier, N., Beckett, R., Harwood, S. *et al.* (1993) A trial of two cognitive behavioral methods of treating drug-resistant residual psychotic symptoms in schizophrenic patients. I. Outcome. *British Journal of Psychiatry*, **162**, 524–532.

Test, M.A., Wallish, L.S., Allness, D.J. & Ripp, K. (1989) Substance use in young adults with schizophrenia disorders. *Schizophrenia Bulletin*, **15**, 465–476.

Torrey, E.F. (1988) *Surviving Schizophrenia: A Family Manual* (Revised). Harper & Row, New York.

Tsuang, M.T., Lyons, M.J. & Faraone, S.V. (1990) Heterogeneity of schizophrenia: conceptual models and analytic strategies. *British Journal of Psychiatry*, **156**, 17–26

Tuma, A.H. & May, P.R.A. (1974) Psychotherapy, drugs and therapist expertise in the treatment of schizophrenia: a critique of the Michigan State project. *Psychotherapy: Theory, Research and Practice*, **12**, 138–142.

Van Putten, T. (1975) The many faces of akathisia. *Comprehensive Psychiatry*, **16**, 43–47.

Van Putten, T. & Marder, S.R. (1986) Low-dose treatment strategies. *Journal of Clinical Psychiatry*, **47**, (Suppl. 5), 12–16.

Vaughn, C.& Leff, J. (1976) The influence of family and social factors on the course of psychiatric illness. *American Journal of Psychiatry*, **129**, 125–137.

Vaughn, K., Doyle, M., McConaghy, A., Blaszczynski, A., Fox, A. & Tarrier, N. (1992) The Sydney intervention trial. A controlled trial of relatives' counselling to reduce schizophrenic relapse. *Social Psychiatry and Psychiatric Epidemiology*, **27**, 16–21.

Ventura, J., Nuechterlein, K.H., Lukoff, D. & Hardesty, J.P. (1989) A prospective study of stressful life events and schizophrenic relapse. *Journal of Abnormal Psychology*, **98**, 407–411.

Vine, P. (1982) *Families in Pain*. Pantheon Books, New York.

Wallace, C.J., Nelson, C.J., Liberman, R.P. *et al.* (1980) A review and critique of social skills training with schizophrenic patients. *Schizophrenia Bulletin*, **6**, 42–63.

Weinberger, D.R. (1987) Implications of normal brain development for the pathogenesis of schizophrenia. *Archives of General Psychiatry*, **44**, 660–669.

Weinberger, D.R., Berman, K.F. & Zec, R.F. (1986) Physiologic dysfunction of dorsolateral prefrontal cortex in schizophrenia. I. Regional cerebral blood flow evidence. *Archives of General Psychiatry*, **43**, 114–124.

Wiedl, K.H. & Schottner, B. (1991) Coping with symptoms of schizophrenia. *Schizophrenia Bulletin*, **17**, 525–538.

Wing, J.K. (1987) Psychosocial factors affecting the long-term course of schizophrenia. In Strauss, J.S., Boker, W. & Brenner, H.D. (eds) *Psychosocial Treatment of Schizophrenia*, pp. 13–29. Hans Huber, Toronto.

Winnicott, D.W. (1965) *The Maturational Processes and the Facilitating Environment*. International Universities Press, New York.

Wong, S.E. & Woolsey, J.E. (1989) Re-establishing conversational skills in overtly psychotic, chronic schizophrenic patients: discrete trials training on the psychiatric ward. *Behavior Modification*, **13**, 431–447.

Chapter 32
Community Care: Parts and Systems

M. MUIJEN AND T. HADLEY

Community care: developments and challenges

One could argue that the debate on the implementation of community care was concluded several decades ago. Since then, major and irreversible shifts in service provisions have taken place in the Western world and it may appear that community care has already taken over from the more traditional forms of hospital care. The number of hospital beds for the mentally ill was reduced from 560 000 to 100 000 in the USA and from 155 000 to 59 000 in the UK between 1955, when numbers were at their maximum, and 1991.

Community care is based on a combination of human liberal concerns about the freedom of the individual and the right to be part of society. Legislation has supported the development of community services by requiring the implementation of approaches aimed at supporting individuals at the place of the least restrictive environment. The relative spending on community resources has increased considerably, although mental hospital care is still using a large proportion of resources.

In the USA, there has been a consistent effort since the 1960s by all kinds of government to create community care systems with the enactment of Community Mental Health Centre legislation in 1963 at a federal level, and followed locally by legislation in at least 45 states. By 1988, state mental health authorities were spending over $1.6 billion on community care, and through the federally supported Medicaid and Medicare programmes another $1.9 billion were devoted to community care (Hadley *et al.*, 1992). In recent years in the USA there has been another phase of state hospital closures and bed reductions. In all cases, there have been dramatic reductions of long-term census and substitution of various services for state hospital bed-days. In some states, such as Vermont and Philadelphia, total long-term beds have been reduced to less than 10% of previous levels (Hadley *et al.*, 1992).

In the UK, the move towards community care is evident in the number of community psychiatric nurses (CPNs); which quadrupled in the 1980s to reach 5000 (White, 1991); about 500 community mental health teams have been established; day services and residential homes have increased considerably and hospital beds have continued to decline. Community legislation introduced in the early 1990s has obliged health services to offer coordinated and comprehensive health care to all patients with severe mental health problems, involving all relevant parties. A key worker from any one of the agencies has to be appointed to monitor the care. More drastic changes have been made to the role of social services. They have been made lead agents for community care of the mentally ill, including the responsibility for assessments, providing or purchasing social care and monitoring all elements of social care. The important distinction between health and social care has not been centrally defined, but the overall policy implication towards greater involvement of social services with community care is quite clear.

Many other countries have seen at least similar, and often more forward-looking, developments. In the Netherlands, regional community units have been established, offering a comprehensive range of care, varying from psychotherapy to rehabilitation, to the whole population. Italy has been most radical with its well-publicized legal reforms, outlawing readmissions of former long-stay patients, and requiring the creation of integrated community networks.

However, all these developments towards community care hide reservations, contradictions and interim policy shifts. In the USA the Community Mental Health Centre Act in the 1960s led to a shift of care towards people with relatively minor mental health problems at the expense of the severely mentally ill (Brown, 1985). Similar experiences have been reported in the UK (Patmore & Weaver, 1991). In Italy, the development of new community services has been very patchy, possibly benefiting patients in the richer north, while patients in the deprived south may have suffered neglect since their discharge from mental institutions. In the UK and the USA, large proportions of the homeless appear to be suffering from schizophrenia, unable to access the services they require and lost to the supposedly well-coordinated aftercare (Bachrach, 1992; Scott, 1993).

It is essential in the debate on the benefits of community care vs. hospital care to keep the issues in clear perspective. Community care advocates argue that most people can be treated at home or in hostels with minimal use of hospital beds, with a gain in quality of life and at no higher, if not lower, cost. The disadvantages of a hospital-centred service are depicted as: the excessive emphasis on psychopathology with a

medicalization of psychosocial problems; the poverty of the environment leading to negative symptoms over time; the inability to teach people skills in the environment where they will have to be applied, i.e. in the community; and the stigmatization of 'mental illness' (Wing & Brown, 1970; Marx *et al.*, 1973; Stein & Test, 1980; Hoult & Reynolds, 1983).

The critics of community care emphasize: the neglect suffered in the community when hospitals are closed without the provision of a comprehensive range of community services; the misery imposed on patients and their carers; trans-institutionalization towards poor-quality hostels and prisons; the increasingly inadequate resources; the deprofessionalization of staff; and the lack of valid evaluations (Hawks, 1975; Bassuk & Gerson, 1978; Weller, 1989).

Much publicity has been created by isolated examples of human tragedies which have been attributed fully to failures of either hospital or community care, simplifying the complex problems of institutional abuse vs. neglect in the community (Martin, 1984; Ramon, 1992). It is all too easily disregarded that the concepts of community care and hospital care in isolation are a caricature of real services. Moreover, such simplifications of services tend to idealize models of care. For example, the neglect of psychiatric patients in the community can be attributed not to the failure of community care, but often to a failure to provide adequate resources. In 1966, when 120 000 beds for the mentally ill were available in the UK (compared with 57 000 in 1990), a study in east London found that only 54% of patients with schizophrenia discharged to known addresses could be traced after 1 year, and only about one-third of these lived in satisfactory circumstances and one-third neglected themselves (Rollin, 1977). More recently, in equally deprived parts of London, 140 patients with schizophrenia were followed up after discharge from an acute unit. After 1 year, only a single patient had been lost, but four had died, three of probable suicide; about half could be diagnosed as psychotic and functioned poorly; two-thirds of the people had moved at least twice during the year; many lived in deprived circumstances and only 10% were employed; little coordination of services was found (Meltzer *et al.*, 1991; see also Chapter 33, this volume). It is somewhat futile to pursue the theoretical point whether these two examples represent the weaknesses of a hospital-based system of care, with its inherent neglect of aftercare, or the failure of community care. What is obvious is that the system failed, in both 1966 and 1991, because the services provided little beyond hospital care, and the available community services were poorly organized. Clearly, no service component, whatever its quality, can provide acceptable care in isolation. Community care will only be able to offer satisfactory services if some form of intensive 24-h care can be offered. In contrast, hospital-centred care will be ineffective if no form of aftercare is established.

Relative need for services

The crucial question for planners, managers and clinicians is the relative need for any provision. In practice, the issue is mostly to what extent community services can substitute for beds. Theoretically, there can be complete replacement of intermediate and long-term beds, but the complexity of this question in the context of a comprehensive mental health service is related to the range of alternative provisions that need to be considered, either individually or in combination, including day care, home care, crisis intervention, case management and hostels, encompassing health and social care, housing and education. The evidence of community services to provide alternatives to standard hospital services with at least equal outcomes will be considered in this chapter, including the methodological implications of model programmes on which much of the evidence is based.

The role of hospital care

Since the standard form of care for many practitioners is still hospital-based care, any evaluation of alternatives needs to explore the strengths and weaknesses of this model of care which it aims to replace. The three important issues are: to what extent hospital care improves the quality of life of patients in the community after discharge as a consequence of its interventions; whether improved results could be achieved by different interventions in hospital; and whether alternative forms of care could achieve better outcome or the same outcome more efficiently. It also has to be considered what is meant by outcome. Traditionally, the disappearance of symptoms on discharge and the reduction of relapse rates have been used, but increasingly the emphasis is placed on improved community adjustment and the user's and carer's satisfaction, i.e. a shift from deficits to strengths.

Studies evaluating the efficacy of hospital care can be categorized into three groups: evaluations of ward programmes; studies contrasting long vs. short admissions; and comparisons of hospital admissions with alternative forms of care.

Ward programmes

Often major differences can be found in practices on the various wards of the same hospital, based on the ideologies of staff, even when similar patient groups are being treated, and no doubt care procedures are even more diverse across different countries. Surprisingly little is known about the effectiveness of varying models of standard hospital care, although the relatively random distribution of patients to a range of treatments is a good set-up for controlled studies. This may be an indication of unquestioned habits based on tradition and routine, and the emergence of audit could challenge some of these practices.

These research findings of ward programmes consistently reveal that any reasonable innovation leads to improvement (Erickson, 1975). An important study was a comparative study across three mental hospitals with changing quality of care over time (Wing & Brown, 1970). It showed an association between environmental poverty, consisting of amount of activity, contact with the outside world and interaction with staff, and social poverty, which included social withdrawal, flatness of affect and poverty of speech. When environmental factors changed, social factors changed in the same direction, strongly suggesting that at least a proportion of the negative symptoms of these long-stay patients was due to social factors rather than the illness process. Other studies consistently found that any form of increased attention and motivation, regardless of the ideological origin, application or therapist's expertise, produced a better outcome. Outcome is mainly defined as ward functioning in these studies, and the effect of ward programmes on quality of life after discharge is largely unknown. There is evidence, however, that hospital treatment and improved ward adjustment are not associated with better community functioning (Ellsworth *et al.*, 1971; Anthony *et al.*, 1978). The existing research on the effectiveness of ward programmes was succinctly summarized by Erickson (1975): 'There is little order and virtually no replication.'

The conclusion that any form of intervention and attention improves ward functioning needs to be put in perspective, since the baseline, as provided by the regular ward care, may well have been less than exemplary. The pertinence of the assumed role of the hospital as a therapeutic environment has often been questioned with regard to contemporary in-patient care (Martin, 1984; Perring, 1992), and accounts from patients are invariably scathing (Chamberlin, 1977; Perring, 1992). Ironically, the gradual shift towards community care will often have led to a deterioration of in-patient care. The funding of community services required a reduction in bed and staff numbers. Community care can be expected to raise the threshold of hospital admission, concentrating on the ward patients with the most severe symptomatology and social problems (Fagin, 1985). Simultaneous with the shift to community care, there is a partial closure of wards and the transfer of a proportion of the staff, leaving the care of the most difficult patients in the hands of even fewer. Moreover, with the concept of community care being strongly promoted and hospital care considered as backward looking and oppressive, innovative and enthusiastic staff tend to apply for posts in the community. This leaves the 'institutionalized' staff on the wards, if they have not decided to leave the

system altogether. The negative effect on staff morale and quality of care seems self-evident, although only anecdotal. Studies have indicated that staff can adjust well to the shift away from hospital care, but the new role for staff in hospital settings and its training implications have not been adequately addressed. Unless this is done with some urgency, a real danger of a divisive system with components within the mental health service unable, or even unwilling, to communicate may emerge.

Length of stay

In contrast to the dearth of controlled studies on the type of care offered in hospitals, several controlled studies have evaluated the effectiveness of different lengths of stay (Glick *et al.*, 1975, 1976; Hargreaves *et al.*, 1977; Herz *et al.*, 1977; Mattes *et al.*, 1977; Hirsch *et al.*, 1979).

All studies have reported the same findings: short stay does not affect outcome negatively. It appears that the hospital duration can be shortened without any untoward impact on patient functioning, but several provisos need to be made. First, none of these studies used similar durations for mean 'brief' and 'standard' admission. These varied from 80 vs. 180 days (Mattes *et al.*, 1977) to 22 vs. 28 days (Hirsch *et al.*, 1979) and 11 vs. 60 days (Herz *et al.*, 1977). This means that the standard care in some studies was substantially longer than brief admissions in other studies, making cross-study comparisons haphazard. Second, patient groups differed, although all studies included a large proportion of patients with psychotic disorders. One project addressed subgroups (Glick *et al.*, 1975; Hargreaves *et al.*, 1977), finding inconclusive results for patients with schizophrenia, but showing persuasively that patients with neurosis do not require extended hospitalization.

Third, differences in the number of therapy sessions, medication dosages and quality of aftercare confounded many of these studies. Rather than invalidating this area of research, it points towards an important conclusion: the consistent association of any advantages in either treatment group with more care, similar to the conclusion of ward care. Glick *et al.* (1976) found that on discharge the brief-admission group functioned better than the standard-admission group assessed at the same time, but the brief-admission group had received more crisis intervention and discharge planning. At the later point of discharge of the standard group, they in turn performed better than the short-stay group, but standard-group patients had by then obtained four times the amount of interventions received by the short-stay group. Mattes *et al.* (1977) reported that during the year after discharge, standard admissions required more and longer readmissions, but brief admissions had received more medication at higher dosages. Caffey *et al.* (1971), in a complex study, controlling for aftercare and length of admission, found that the level of symptomatology on discharge was related to the intensity of care on the ward, but after 1 year follow-up symptomatology was related to the amount of aftercare, independent of the length of index admission.

Jointly, these studies suggest that hospital care achieves good outcome on discharge, but long-term benefit is related to the provision of aftercare services. Three important issues are unanswered by these studies. First, to what extent can we reduce the length of hospital care without a negative impact on the quality of life? The reviewed projects determined in advance the limits of duration of stay for brief and long admissions, allowing a conclusion only for such lengths of stay. Nevertheless, it is worth noting that in practice both brief and standard stays tended to decrease over the years, indicating the general acceptance that long admissions have no place in routine care.

The next remaining question concerns the subgroups which would benefit most from a certain type of care. Ignoring the confounding variables confusing this field, the single finding that neurotic patients benefit little from long admissions (Hargreaves *et al.*, 1977) is well overtaken by clinical practice, which these days tends to exclude this group altogether from admission, with the exception of the most extreme sufferers and private clinics.

Finally, can other service components further reduce the need for or replace hospital admission

altogether? To answer some of these questions, 'model services' have been developed; these aim to compare a range of alternative services with standard hospital care under controlled conditions. Several such projects have been evaluated, and their results will be presented.

Home care

The attempt to offer people individualized care at their own residence, and to minimize, if not displace altogether, the need for in-patient care, is the essence of community care. The transfer of former long-stay patients to hostels in the community has proven to be possible, with no decline in functioning or quality of life, provided that equivalent resources are provided (e.g. Leff, 1993). Equally important are the attempts to provide psychiatric care with the minimum use of hospital admissions to people suffering from severe mental illness, who require intensive ongoing care and in the past would have been at risk of becoming long-stay patients. This is based on the evidence that many of the skills taught in hospital do not generalize after discharge (Ellsworth *et al.*, 1971; Anthony *et al.*, 1972; Marx *et al.*, 1973; Erickson, 1975).

The contrast between community care and standard hospital care cannot simply be reduced to differing treatment locations, but the respective approaches are underpinned by incompatible models of care (Marx *et al.*, 1973; Zwerling, 1976). Zwerling states three objectives that differentiate community mental health from standard practice.

1 The potential target group is the whole population, rather than persons identified as 'patients'.
2 It seeks to maintain and promote health rather than only to treat illness.
3 It aims to understand the family, community, social-class and cultural sources of human disturbance in addition to the biological and psychological sources; in turn, it aims to promote mental health by intervention in all these structures.
This definition encompasses the strengths as well as the weaknesses of community care. It could be argued that the objectives are too ambitious, and that such a wide target group with a lack of focus

and overinclusive care aims, addressing all of society's wrongs, have been responsible for the shift towards treating the worried well at the expense of people with severe mental health problems (Stern & Minkoff, 1979; Langsley, 1980; Brown, 1985).

This problem has been addressed by obliging community teams to target patients with severe mental illness, with the objective of maximizing their functioning in the community and minimizing the use of hospital care. This was operationalized by the National Institute for Mental Health in the USA for their community support programmes, which were required to include specified components in the care of people with persistent and severe mental health problems living in the community (Turner & Ten Hoor, 1978). These components are as follows.

1 Identification of the target population and outreach that can offer appropriate services to those willing to participate.

2 Assistance in applying for benefits.

3 Crisis intervention, with hospital beds available as a last resort. The priority is to help patients and their carers cope in their own environment, with the aim of preventing future admissions by teaching the necessary skills. If the situation is so severe that people are put at risk, admission is indicated. Community care does not aim to eliminate hospital beds altogether.

4 Psychosocial rehabilitation.

5 Supportive services of indefinite duration, including employment and housing.

6 Medical and mental health care.

7 Support to relatives, friends and others.

8 Involvement of concerned community members in order to optimize support networks for patients.

9 Patient advocacy.

10 Case management.

To these points can be added the following.

11 Services need to be available 24 h a day, 7 days a week.

12 The range and intensity of interventions require input from a multidisciplinary team.

13 A high staff:patient ratio is important (between 1:8 and 1:15). The intensity and duration of care

will vary for each patient and over time, as discussed later in this chapter.

14 The team is responsible for a well-delineated sector or catchment area.

Few community services are able to comply with all these points (Bachrach, 1981), and considerable variation exists across services in approaches, staff numbers, skill mix, management structures, availability of community and hospital resources, and size and sociodemographic characteristics of the population. This is often used as an argument against the implementation of community services, based on the potential danger of generalizing services which cannot be transferred in an identical fashion. This argument would be valid if it could be supported by data suggesting that the non-transferable characteristics are likely to have influenced the outcome, or if vital differences are reported in evaluations of community care without clear explanations. The experimental evidence for and against models of community care as an alternative to hospital care for those requiring acute care therefore needs to be considered.

Community care: model programmes studies

Model programmes are often set up to test the feasibility of new approaches to care. For example, the project by Pasamanick *et al.* (1967) was remarkable in foreshadowing future developments, both in service ideology and study design, by about 20 years. It was planned in 1957, but patient intake started in Louisville only 4 years later. The delay was due to the reluctance of state hospitals to cooperate, and the originators even had to move states to gain a reluctant acceptance for the project. Unfortunately, the evaluation was flawed, emphasizing the comparison between the placebo-treated community group and the drug-treated community group; assessments of the hospital care group were discontinued after 3 months (the placebo group did particularly poorly!). Moreover, patients were included who, by modern standards, would not have been considered for hospital care; all those with any potentially complicating factor for home care, such as living alone, suicidal ideas or violence, were excluded. In addition, outcome measures were unreliable. Equally flawed were studies by Langsley *et al.* (1969, 1971), Polak and Kirby (1976) and Pai and Kapur (1982), all offering vague entry criteria, poorly specified interventions and weak evaluation methods, and not allowing any generalization. None of these studies will be further considered. This leaves four controlled studies of home care which have an acceptable rigour in both research and practice. These studies will be compared, and implications for the feasibility of home care for those with severe mental illness will be considered.

A study undertaken in Montreal (Fenton *et al.*, 1982b) used narrow entry criteria (Table 32.1). Only 19% of all hospital admissions were eventually randomized to home or hospital treatment. The main reasons for exclusion were time of admission more than 24 h before screening (20%), brain damage (19%), suicidal or violent behaviour (16%) and living alone (9%). The home care team was small in number with a low staff:patient ratio (Table 32.2). On average, patients were visited 17 times during the 1 year of follow-up, most of these contacts taking place in the first month.

The most comprehensive studies were conducted in Madison, Wisconsin (Stein & Test, 1980), Sydney (Hoult & Reynolds, 1983) and London (Muijen *et al.*, 1992). The studies in Sydney and London replicated the Madison one, with many features in common. Inclusion criteria were broad (see Table 32.1). Patients presenting with aggression, no fixed abode or no social support were accepted, and only those with brain damage or primary addition were excluded. Staff numbers and staff:patient ratios were similar (Table 32.2). The clinical approach of these projects was similar; patients were visited as often as required during the year of follow-up. The care offered was comprehensive, ranging from crisis intervention and rehabilitation to employment, housing problems and carers' support. Table 32.2 shows the socio-demographic characteristics of these four studies. Globally, patient groups appear similar, but a greater proportion of patients in London were first admissions, especially in the home care group, and more patients in Montreal were employed or married, all predictors of good outcome (the 0% of patients in Montreal living alone was due to entry criteria).

The key question is what differences in the care model relate to outcome; Table 32.3 suggests that the various programmes made a differential impact on hospital use, but were remarkably similar in clinical and social outcome 1 year after patient entry. All programmes reduced hospital use considerably. In relative terms, savings of about 80% in bed-days were consistently achieved by home care compared with hospital care, but proportions of patients admitted in the home care group differed greatly, varying from 18% in Madison to

Table 32.1 Staffing levels and contacts

Reference	Staff wte	Home care patient number	Psychiatrists wte	Nurses wte	Contacts yearly
Pasamanick *et al.* (1967)	7*	57	1	5	30
Fenton *et al.* (1982)	2	76	0.5	1	16.5
Stein and Test (1980)	10	60	1	4	80†
Muijen *et al.* (1992)	10	92	1	7	90
Hoult and Reynolds (1983)	7.5	65	0.5	3	80†

* Also involved in ratings.
† Estimated.
wte, whole time equivalent.

Table 32.2 Sociodemographic characteristics for the studies of Fenton *et al.* (1982b), Stein and Test (1980), Hoult and Reynolds (1983) and Muijen *et al.* (1992)

Characteristic	Fenton Exp.	Contr.	Stein Exp.	Contr.	Hoult Exp.	Contr.	Muijen Exp.	Contr.
Number	58	62	65	65	60	60	92	97
Mean age (years)	35*	37*	31	31	35*	35*	33	35
Male (%)	42	38	55	57	45	47	52	47
Married (%)	43	41	23	27	20	17		
Live, alone (%)	0	0	?	?	19	20	36†	45†
Employed (%)	44	42	?	?	22	22	ca. 20	ca. 20
First admission (%)	43	37	17	17	23	27	73	57
Schizophrenia (%)	41	41	ca. 50	ca. 50	57	65	49	49
Mania (%)					9	9	15	19
Depression (%)					12	13	23	25
Affective psychosis (%)	32	30			21	22	38	34
Neurosis (%)	28	30			7	5	10	14
Others (%)					16	9	3	2

* Estimated from data in papers.
† No home support.
Exp., experimental; Contr., control.

Table 32.3 The 12-month outcome of home care studies by Fenton *et al.* (1982b), Stein and Test (1980), Hoult and Reynolds (1983) and Muijen *et al.* (1992)

Characteristic	Fenton Exp.	Contr.	Stein Exp.	Contr.	Hoult Exp.	Contr.	Muijen Exp.	Contr.
Dropout (%)	28	38		15	12	20	28	33
Patients admitted (%)	38	100	18	89	40	96	84	100
Patients readmitted (%)	24	23	3	52	8	51	28	23
Mean admission duration (days)	15	42	2	29	8	54	18	87
Admission duration for those admitted only	39	42	11	33	12	56	21	87
Improved clinical symptoms	Equal		Exp. > contr.		Exp. > contr.		Exp. > /contr.	
Improved social functioning	Exp. > contr.		Equal		Equal		Exp. > /contr.	
Improved family burden	Equal				Exp. > contr.		Exp. > contr.	
Patient satisfaction					Exp. > contr.		Exp. > contr.	

> significant *P* < 0.05; >/ trend.
Exp., experimental; Contr., control.

84% in London. The number of readmissions and length of stay correlated with the proportion of admissions, especially when the Montreal study with its different entry criteria is ignored. The length of admission, but not proportion of readmissions, also correlates with the equivalent variable in the standard hospital care groups. This suggests that the teams in Madison and Sydney were more successful than the London project in keeping patients out of hospital, but that the length of stay once admission was unavoidable may have been related to local practice. On its own, this is an unsatisfactory explanation, since many factors may have contributed to the relative inability of the London team to avoid admissions or to discharge patients as rapidly as the Madison and Sydney teams achieved. Possible reasons include lower team motivation to keep patients out of hospital, more disturbed patients requiring longer and more frequent admissions, less integration between hospital wards and community services, differences in deprivation in London vs. that in Sydney and Madison and resource limitations, i.e. fewer support services, such as day hospitals, drop-in centres and respite care, in London. None of these factors is likely to exist in isolation, and it is impossible to interpret these differences conclusively.

Outcome comparisons

Although the reduction of bed usage is important in terms of resources and cost effectiveness (see below), equally important is the impact that community care makes on a range of outcome variables. The findings are relatively consistent (Table 32.3) in that all studies find some advantages for home care in clinical and social outcome, but these differences reach statistical significance only in Madison. On no variable in any of the studies does hospital care show even trends in its favour. The magnitude of the advantages of home care over standard hospital care is about 25% in both Sydney and London, but variances are so large that statistical differences are rarely found. The area in which community care is invariably superior is patient and carer satisfaction. The

exception is in Montreal, and this might be explained by the limited number of contacts offered (see Table 32.1). It appears that both patient and relatives satisfaction is strongly associated with care, rather than the type of care. In Philadelphia, Madison, Sydney and London, patients and relatives strongly preferred community care at the 12-month follow-up. After 1 month no difference was recorded for family burden in Madison and Sydney, and after 4 months community care was marginally preferred by those questioned on all sites. Apparently, the satisfaction with community care gradually increased, but this may not be the whole story. The increasing relative preference for community care was at least as much due to decreasing satisfaction with standard care, while the degree to which home care was liked increased only marginally. This suggests that the essential component of satisfaction is continuing care, which differentiates the two forms of care. Standard care provides intensive care during admission, concentrated within the initial period of entry into these studies, when types of care are equally valued. Follow-up in standard care following hospital discharge is often very limited (Meltzer *et al.*, 1991), whereas community care continues to offer relatively large amounts of input throughout the year. Reports from users and carers support the notion that the ongoing input is highly valued (Grella & Grusky, 1989).

However, the amount of benefit over time is not simply related to the amount of input in these studies. Irrespective of the treatment model, most of the clinical gains are achieved within the initial 3−4 months, after which only marginal further improvements are made, despite the major differences in amount of aftercare. Moderate advances in social functioning continue over time, favouring community care only slightly. This is surprising, particularly since the conclusion from studies comparing differing lengths of hospital admission seemed to be that aftercare was the key explanatory variable in good outcome. A possibility is that the home care studies address patient groups of such severity that gains of a magnitude which would achieve statistical significance are unrealistic. The consistent trend favouring community care may hide subgroups benefiting greatly, but subgroup analyses did not show any major differential benefits for diagnostic or acute vs. chronic subgroups. This could be due to reduced power. Discontinuation studies of home care showed that patients (Davis *et al.*, 1972; Stein & Test, 1980) lost any of the gains they had made with community care over standard care. Some demoralization after the loss of their close relationship with the community team may have contributed, but it suggests some therapeutic benefit from home care.

The conclusion of studies evaluating assertive community care shows that a large reduction in bed needs can be anticipated. Clinical and social outcome tends to favour home care somewhat, but patients and carers strongly prefer home care, especially over time. The findings of these model programmes should be related to their context, however. More often than not, the initiators are charismatic innovators who strongly believe in new models of care, and invest great amounts of time and energy to convince others around them of the merits. Their duration is short, and no studies have evaluated their sustainability over 5–10 years. Despite these doubts, model programmes have made a great impact, helped by policy changes which encouraged community support systems for people with severe and persistent mental illness. Most services differ from the above model programmes in their objective to support people with known severe disabilities and multiple service use, rather than aiming to prevent hospital admission for a mixture of presenting patients. Therefore, such case-management services may allow a better insight into the effectiveness of continuity of care for specific patient groups.

Cost of community care vs. hospital care

In the present economic climate, efficiency is a priority. Although the optimal potential for quality of care is important as an ideal to aim for, the main day-to-day concern of health service managers and clinicians is to develop a service which offers most for a determined amount of money. More precisely, what change from a hospital to a community service can be afforded within the existing budget, how effective will this service be in terms of outcome and where will the money come from within the present service?

Several of the model programmes incorporated costing into their designs, and community care was invariably reported to cost less than hospital care. Costings can be difficult to interpret, however, owing to different approaches, different assumptions and varying inclusions of direct costs (of treatment) and indirect costs (a wide range of non-treatment costs generated by the illness, potentially including areas such as benefits and costs to relatives owing to working hours missed). For example, the Madison study performed a cost:benefit analysis, including many direct and indirect costs during the 12 months after entry into the project (Weisbrod *et al.*, 1980). The conclusion was that community care offers slight savings of about 5%. The analysis shows that such a conclusion was based on several assumptions. Direct treatment costs to the health service, including hospital and community services, worked out at 25% more expensive for community care. This included an opportunity cost of 8% on capital. This has been considered as high (McGuire, 1991), since the market value was steady with little cost of depreciation. If the capital cost had been chosen at 4%, the direct community care cost would have showed a relative increase of 20%, and community care would have been 49% more expensive than hospital care. Weisbrod *et al.* also included societal costs, earnings lost to carers and patients' employment earnings, even though most of the money was earned in sheltered workshops. In the original model the earnings in the community group just tipped the overall balance in favour of community care. A less comprehensive cost-effectiveness analysis was undertaken in Sydney (Hoult & Reynolds, 1983), where only treatment costs were considered. Capital costs were excluded. Community care worked out as 10% cheaper for the service as a whole. If the cost per patient is considered, savings of community care might be as high as 22%, because the hospital group contained 49 patients and the community group 56 patients. A costing that compared only direct treatment costs of hospital and community care reported a saving of as much as 61% favouring community care (Fenton *et al.*, 1982a).

The most thorough and comprehensive analysis produces the least savings with community care, and may even suggest somewhat higher costs. The widespread belief that home care is cheaper than hospital care is rather more complex in reality, depending on the variables included in the conception of costs for which the health services are accountable, the way such costs are calculated and the role and responsibilities of the health service as part of the 'caring society'. In practice, the extrapolation of costs from model services needs to take into account several factors. First, the largest cost-saving component in each of the community studies was the vast difference in hospital use between the services. The 80% bed-saving may be consistent across programmes, but this does not imply that every community service will be able to achieve similar savings. For example, the London study reported a mean stay per patient in the hospital group of 53 and 83 days during the 3 and 9 months, respectively, following entry. Mean stays in other hospitals in the UK are far shorter for similar patients, probably about half or less. This means that bed-savings would have been reduced from 80 to 55%, assuming unchanged hospital use for the community group. In addition, the enthusiasm of staff might gradually be eroded, and the amount of hospital use for patients in community services could creep up, thereby increasing costs.

Second, start-up investment is necessary, not only for bridging loans in order to develop the new services while the old are gradually being run down, but also for staff training and small-scale community developments. Community services can also be very expensive during the first year of operation, since a large staff group will look after a gradually increasing number of patients (Muijen *et al.*, 1992).

Third, savings in hospital expenditure can lead to higher use of other resources such as hostels, bed-and-breakfast places and day centres,

increasing the costs to primary care, social services and the voluntary sector (Borland *et al.*, 1989); this has an unpredictable overall effect. A fourth obstacle is marginal costs: closure of half a ward of half a hospital does not save half the costs, because of fixed overheads. If the planning objective is to achieve a better balance between community and hospital, wholesale closure of hospitals may be difficult to achieve. Initially, it may be possible to amalgamate several wards, but overheads which cannot be reduced to the same degree, such as meals, laundry, cleaning, administration and many other core hospital tasks, are still required. It also has to be realized that it is a false economy if hospitals again become a place of cheap care with resulting poor quality and bad outcome. Good community care requires a balance and integration across its components, and any weak link will affect the whole system.

Case-management services for the long-term mentally ill

The essence of case-management teams for the long-term mentally ill is to provide continuity of care (Bachrach, 1992). The core task is to offer assessment, coordinate a comprehensive range of care, take responsibility for its provision and monitor the quality (Intagliata, 1982). Case management can be positioned along a number of axes. One is the brokerage vs. clinical model. The brokerage model stands for purchasing and coordination of services by a case manager who is responsible for the assessment and monitoring of patients, but does not offer clinical interventions. The clinical model puts the care element centrally, with the case manager offering a range of interventions, and coordinating care required from other services. Obviously, the choice of model has implications for staff:patient ratios and resources. Most case-management services have adopted the clinical model, and at its extreme is the assertive outreach programmes described earlier. Social services in the UK have adopted a brokerage model, although this is increasingly diluted and moving towards a more clinical model. The other dimension is individual vs. team case management, implying an individual and team responsibility, respectively, for the care. The individual model is most prevalent, and provides the individual relationship that is so important to this model of care (Harris & Bergman, 1988). The team model also has its strong advocates (Bond *et al.*, 1988), however, and a claimed advantage is the reduced pressure on individual staff, leading to lower burn-out.

The need for case-management services is based on the lack of comprehensive and well-coordinated aftercare services provided to patients with a large number of unmet needs, particularly in inner cities (Witheridge *et al.*, 1982; Goering *et al.*, 1984; Wasylenki *et al.*, 1985; Meltzer *et al.*, 1991). It has generally been reported that aftercare was centred around medical follow-up, with a neglect of social and housing problems. In Toronto, a team consisting of eight case managers was allocated 92 patients selected for chronic illness, poor employment, social isolation and residential instability. These patients were matched with patients receiving standard aftercare (Goering *et al.*, 1988). After 2 years, patients in the case-management programme did better in occupational functioning, housing status and social involvement. This was associated with the greater use by case-management patients of services addressing those areas. No difference was found after either 6 or 24 months in the number of admissions or length of hospital stay. This study did not perform a cost analysis, but the case-management service was probably considerably more expensive. Another problem with this study is that matching was used, which does raise the question whether the patients admitted to the case-management programme had a better prognosis than control patients who had received standard aftercare in the past.

A true randomized design was used in Houston where 417 patients, who had been admitted at least twice, were allocated to either a team of seven case managers plus supervisor or the regular aftercare services. After 1 year, no differences were found in the quality of life, but the case-management team admitted about twice as many patients who stayed longer in hospital than the control group. The case-management group also used consistently more other community services, although the proviso needs to be made that only about 50% of patients were interviewed. Again, case management was more expensive. The reasons for this pessimistic result suggesting a potential lack of effectiveness of case management are unclear and could be any of the following: the staff:patient ratio was low (1:30); there was a relative emphasis on brokerage; there was possibly too brief a period of follow-up; a lack of good and varied community resources; or the provision of good care for the control group. However, case management cannot have it both ways, explaining its negative findings as a consequence of either poorly or too well-developed complementary community support resources. It may well be that such resources are a more important predictor of good outcome than case management on its own, and that case management ought to be considered as a procedure to optimize the use and efficiency of such resources.

This conclusion is supported by studies which place less emphasis on the case-management aspect and concentrate on direct care, and which tend to be more successful. These include the assertive outreach services described earlier, which aim to avoid admissions. Other services offer assertive care after discharge from hospital. The Bridge project in Chicago provided intensive direct care and significantly reduced, hospital use, although little change on overall functioning was achieved (Witheridge *et al.*, 1982; Bond *et al.*, 1990). A Dutch study that randomized patients with schizophrenia offered a comprehensive programme of psychosocial community care to the experimental group, while the control group received out-patient care for 15 months (Vlaminck, 1989). The mean number of contacts was 31 and 16, respectively. Significantly fewer patients in the community care group were admitted (20%) compared with the out-patient group (49%), but no differences were found in psychopathology and social functioning between the groups. The costs of the community group were 40% lower, although only direct treatment costs were considered.

Very few studies have compared different models of continuity of care services. The likelihood is that few, if any, significant differences would be found unless very large patient numbers were included or either service was found to be very poor, since the small differences and large variances would produce studies with low power. If differences were to be found, many confounding variables might obscure any conclusion. An example of this was a comparison across three day centres using assertive case management based on the team sharing the case load. One did not adhere to these shared case loads, and did perform worst. However, there were many other differences, such as patient characteristics, and organizational and treatment variables. A particularly important issue is the optimal staff:patient ratio, since this has important implications for the intensity of care and costs. It may be possible to reduce the amount of support offered after stabilization has been achieved, since patients whose care was transferred after 5 years of care in a case-management programme that had a staff:patient ratio of 1:8, to a community mental health centre with a ratio of about 1:50 remained relatively well (McRae *et al.*, 1990). However, hospital use almost doubled, but the increased efficiency achieved by the change in staff:patient ratio offset the higher hospital costs. Staff:patient ratios depend on so many variables, such as therapeutic objectives, patients' disabilities, staff skills and resources, that a simplistic generalized solution is unrealistic (Sacks, 1992). Despite the doubt about the precise effect of case management, many reports attest to its popularity and perceived effectiveness, particularly in reducing hospitalization (Wright *et al.*, 1989; Bush *et al.*, 1990). A wide variety of models has arisen, including user-led services (Nikkel & Smith, 1992). This variety shows that flexibility and local initiative have taken over from rigid models, but it also means that any specific components of care, apart from the broadest concepts, will be difficult to evaluate for their effectiveness.

Towards a model of services

Most evaluations compare components of a com-prehensive service, i.e. a community team vs. hospital care, or day care vs. hospital care. In practice, the situation is a lot more complex, with the health, social, voluntary and private sectors each contributing a network of services. Little is known about system changes, however. For example, important for planning are the added benefits of day care in addition to home care as compared with standard care, which in itself is a varied range of services. Ideally, the effectiveness of comprehensive service models are evaluated, but methodologically a definite conclusion is unlikely to emerge, due to the large number of uncontrolled variables. This makes a simple answer to the question 'Is community care better than hospital care?' impossible to answer. It obviously depends, and it depends on an immeasurable number of factors. This does not imply that planning nihilism is a valid way of thinking, since some conclusions are consistent. Good community services can reduce the number of hospital admissions and length of stay, and are preferred by users and carers, although expectations regarding clinical and social improvements need to be cautious. Direct clinical input is more important than case management. Aftercare needs to be long term for people with severe and persistent mental health problems. How these conclusions are to be implemented depends on local needs, resources and imagination. In one important aspect the literature is very positive: almost any new community service shows some advantages over traditional hospital care, provided that entry criteria are adhered to, training has been given, care is relatively comprehensive and enthusiasm and resources can be sustained. That, however, is not a small challenge for planners and clinicians alike, and its success is likely to determine whether community care will be judged in the future as having been an inspired innovation or a model of care leading to neglect of precisely those people most dependent on society's protection.

References

Anthony, W.A., Buell, G.J., Sharratt, S. & Althoff, M.E.

(1972) The efficacy of psychiatric rehabilitation. *Psychological Bulletin*, **78**, 447–456.

Anthony, W.A., Cohen, M.R. & Vitalo, R. (1978) The measurement of rehabilitation outcome. *Schizophrenia Bulletin*, **4**, 365–383.

Bachrach, L.L. (1981) Continuity of care for chronic mental patients: a conceptual analysis. *American Journal of Psychiatry*, **138**, 1449–1455.

Bachrach, L.L. (1992) What we know about homelessness among mentally ill persons: an analytical review and commentary. *Hospital and Community Psychiatry*, **43**, 453–464.

Bassuk, E.L. & Gerson, S. (1978) Deinstitutionalization and mental health services. *Scientific American*, **238**, 46–53.

Bond, G.R., Miller, R.D. & Krumwied, R.D. (1988) Assertive casemangement in 3 CMHC's: a controlled study. *Hospital and Community Psychiatry*, **39**, 411–418.

Bond, G.R., Witheridge, T.F., Wasmer, D. *et al.* (1990) Assertive community treatment for frequent users of psychiatric hospitals in a large city: a controlled study. *American Journal of Community Psychology*, **18**, 865–892.

Borland, A., McRae, J. & Lycan, C. (1989) Outcomes of five years of continuous intensive case management. *Hospital and Community Psychiatry*, **40**, 369–376.

Brown, P. (1985) *The Transfer of Care. Psychiatric Deinstitutionalization and Its Aftermath*. Routledge, London.

Bush, C.T., Wayne Langford, M., Rosen, P. & Gott, W. (1990) Operation outreach: intensive case management for severely psychiatrically disabled adults. *Hospital and Community Psychiatry*, **41**, 647–651.

Caffey, E.M., Galbrecht, C.R., Klett, C.J. & Point, P. (1971) Brief hospitalization and aftercare in the treatment of schizophrenia. *Archives of General Psychiatry*, **24**, 81–86.

Chamberlin, J. (1977) *On Our Own*. Mind, London.

Davis, A.E., Dinitz, S. & Pasamanick, B. (1972) The prevention of hospitalisation in schizophrenia: five years after an experimental program. *American Journal of Orthopsychiatry*, **42**, 375–388.

Ellsworth, R., Maroney, R., Klett, W., Gordon, H. & Gunn, R. (1971) Milieu characteristics of successful psychiatric treatment programs. *American Journal of Orthopsychiatry*, **41**, 427–440.

Erickson, R.C. (1975) Outcome studies in mental hospitals: a review. *Psychological Bulletin*, **82**, 519–540.

Fagin, L. (1985) Deinstitutionalization. *Bulletin of the Royal College of Psychiatrists*, **9**, 11–12.

Fenton, F.R., Tessier, L., Contandriopoulos, A.P., Nguyen, H. & Struening, E.L. (1982a) A comparative trial of home and hospital psychiatric treatment: financial costs. *Canadian Journal of Psychiatry*, **27**, 177–187.

Fenton, F.R., Tessier, L., Struening, E.L., Smith, F.A. & Benoit, C. (1982b) *Home and Hospital Psychiatric Treatment*. Croom Helm, London.

Glick, I.D., Hargreaves, W.A., Drues, J. & Showstack, J.A. (1976) Short versus long hospitalization: a prospective controlled study. IV. One year follow-up results for schizophrenic patients. *American Journal of Psychiatry*, **133**, 509–514.

Glick, I.D., Hargreaves, W.A., Raskin, M. & Kutner, S.J.

(1975) Short versus long hospitalization: a prospective controlled study. II. Results for schizophrenic inpatients. *American Journal of Psychiatry*, **132**, 385–390.

Goering, P.N., Wasylenki, D.A., Farkas, M., Lancee, W.J. & Ballantyne, R. (1988) What difference does case management make? *Hospital and Community Psychiatry*, **39**, 272–276.

Goering, P., Wasylenki, D., Lancee, W. & Freeman, S.J.J. (1984) From hospital to community. Six-month and two-year outcomes for 505 patients. *Journal of Nervous and Mental Disease*, **172**, 667–672.

Grella, C.E. & Grusky, O. (1989) Families of the seriously mentally ill and their satisfaction with services. *Hospital and Community Psychiatry*, **40**, 831–835.

Hadley, T.R., Culhane, D.P. & Snyder, F.J. (1992) Expenditure and revenue patterns of State Mental Health Agencies, from 1981 to 1987. *Administration and Policy in Mental Health*, **19**(4), 213–234.

Hargreaves, W.A., Glick, I.D., Drues, J., Showstack, J.A. & Feigenbaum, E. (1977) Short versus long hospitalization; a prospective controlled study. VI. Two-year follow-up results for schizophrenics. *Archives of General Psychiatry*, **34**, 305–311.

Harris, M. & Bergman, H.C. (1988) Clinical case management for the chronically mentally ill: a conceptual analysis. In Harris, M. & Bachrach, L. (eds) *Clinical Case Management*. New Directions for Mental Health Services. Fossey-Bass, San Francisco.

Hawks, D. (1975) Community care: an analysis of assumptions. *British Journal of Psychiatry*, **127**, 276–285.

Herz, M.I., Endicott, J. & Spitzer, R.L. (1977) Brief hospitalization: a two-year follow-up. *American Journal of Psychiatry*, **134**, 502–507.

Hirsch, S.R., Platt, S., Knights, A. & Weyman, A. (1979) Shortening hospital stay for psychiatric care: effect on patients and their families. *British Medical Journal*, **1**, 442–446.

Hoult, J. & Reynolds, I. (1983) *Psychiatric Hospital Versus Community Treatment: A Controlled Study*. Department of Health, New South Wales.

Intagliata, J. (1982) Improving the quality of community care for the chronically mentally disabled: the role of case management. *Schizophrenia Bulletin*, **8**, 655–674.

Langsley, D.G. (1980) The community mental health center: does it treat patients? *Hospital and Community Psychiatry*, **31**, 815–819.

Langsley, D.G., Flomenhaft, K. & Machotka, P. (1969) Follow-up evaluation of family crisis therapy. *American Journal of Orthopsychiatry*, **39**, 753–759.

Langsley, D.G., Machotka, P. & Flomenhaft, K. (1971) Avoiding mental hospital admission, a follow-up study. *American Journal of Psychiatry*, **127**, 1391–1394.

Leff, J. (ed.) (1993) The TAPS project: evaluating community placement of long-stay psychiatric patients. *British Journal of Psychiatry*, **162** (Suppl. 19).

McGuire, T.G. (1991) Measuring the economic costs of schizophrenia. *Schizophrenia Bulletin*, **17**, 375–388.

McRae, J., Higgins, M., Lycan, C. & Sherman, W. (1990) What happens to patients after five years of intensive case management stops? *Hospital and Community Psychiatry*, **41**, 175–179.

Martin, J.P. (1984) *Hospitals in Trouble*. Basil Blackwell, Oxford.

Marx, A.J., Test, M.A. & Stein, L.I. (1973) Extrahospital management of severe mental illness. *Archives of General Psychiatry*, **29**, 505–511.

Mattes, J.A., Rosen, B., Klein, D.F. & Milan, D. (1977) Comparison of the clinical effectiveness of 'short' versus 'long' stay psychiatric hospitalization. II. Results of a 3-year posthospital follow-up. *Journal of Nervous and Mental Disease*, **165**, 395–402.

Meltzer, D., Hale, A.S., Malik, S.H., Hogman, G.A. & Wood, S. (1991) Community care for patients with schizophrenia one year after hospital discharge. *British Medical Journal*, **303**, 1023–1026.

Muijen, M., Marks, I., Connolly, J. & Audini, B. (1992) Home-based care and standard hospital care for patients with severe mental illness: a randomised controlled trial. *British Medical Journal*, **304**, 749–754.

Nikkel, R.E. & Smith, G. (1992) A consumer-operated case management project. *Hospital and Community Psychiatry*, **43**, 577–579.

Pai, S. & Kapur, R.L. (1982) Impact of treatment intervention on the relationship between dimensions of clinical psychopathology, social dysfunction and burden on the family of psychiatric patients. *British Journal of Psychiatry*, **12**, 651–658.

Pasamanick, B., Scarpitty, F.R. & Dinitz, S. (1967) *Schizophrenics in the Community*. Appleton-Century Crofts, New York.

Patmore, C. & Weaver, T. (1991) *Community Mental Health Teams: Lessons for Planners and Managers*. Good Practices in Mental Health, London.

Perring, C. (1992) The experience and perspectives of patients and care staff on the transition from hospital to community-based care. In Ramon, S. (ed.) *Psychiatric Hospital Closure: Myths and Realities*, pp. 122–164. Chapman and Hall, London.

Polak, P.R. & Kirby, M.W. (1976) A model to replace psychiatric hospitals. *Journal of Nervous and Mental Disease*, **162**, 13–22.

Ramon, S. (1992) The workers' perspective: living with ambiguity, ambivalence and challenge. In Ramon, S. (ed.) *Psychiatric Hospital Closure: Myths and Realities*, pp. 85–118. Chapman and Hall, London.

Rollin, E.R. (1977) Editorial: Deinstitutionalization and the community: fact and theory. *Psychological Medicine*, **7**, 181–184.

Sacks, M.H. (1992) Considerations in determining staff–patient ratios. *Hospital and Community Psychiatry*, **43**, 309.

Scott, J. (1993) Homelessness and mental illness. *British Journal of Psychiatry*, **162**, 314–324.

Stein, L.J. & Test, M.A. (1980) Alternative to mental hospital treatment. 1. Conceptual model, treatment program and clinical evaluation. *Archives of General Psychiatry*, **37**, 392–397.

Stern, R. & Minkoff, K. (1979) Paradoxes in programming for chronic patients in a community clinic. *Hospital and Community Psychiatry*, **30**, 613–617.

Turner, J.C. & Ten Hoor, W.J. (1978) The NIMH support program: pilot approach to a needed social reform. *Schizophrenia Bulletin*, **4**, 319–349.

Vlaminck, P. (1989) *Psychose Preventie Project*. Eburon, Delft.

Wasylenki, D., Goering, P., Lancee, W., Fischer, L. & Freeman, S.J.J. (1985) Psychiatric aftercare in a metropolitan setting. *Canadian Journal of Psychiatry*, **30**, 329–336.

Weisbrod, B.A., Test, M.A. & Stein, L.I. (1980) Alternative to mental hospital treatment. 2. Economic benefit–cost analysis. *Archives of General Psychiatry*, **37**, 400–405.

Weller, M.P.I. (1989) Mental illness — who cares? *Nature*, **339**, 249–252.

White, E. (1991) *The 3rd Quinquennial National Community Psychiatric Nursing Survey*. University of Manchester.

Wing, J.K. & Brown, G.W. (1970) *Institutionalism and Schizophrenia*. Cambridge University Press, Cambridge.

Witheridge, T.F., Dincin, J. & Appleby, L. (1982) Working with the most frequent recidivists: a total team approach to assertive resource management. *Psychosocial Rehabilitation Journal*, **5**, 9–11.

Wright, R.G., Heiman, J.R., Shupe, J. & Olvera, G. (1989) Defining and measuring stabilization of patients during 4 years of intensive community support. *American Journal of Psychiatry*, **146**, 1293–1298.

Zwerling, I. (1976) The impact of the community mental health movement on psychiatric practice and training. *Hospital and Community Psychiatry*, **27**, 259–263.

Chapter 33
Homelessness and Schizophrenia

T. K. J. CRAIG AND P. W. TIMMS

Introduction: what is homelessness?

Many conceptual and methodological difficulties confront the epidemiologist in the effort to study homeless populations. First among these is the lack of any clearly agreed definition of the phenomenon. The term 'homeless' has been used to describe a continuum of unsatisfactory housing conditions ranging from cardboard boxes and park benches to night shelters, bed and breakfast accommodation or even sleeping on friends' floors (Austerberry & Watson, 1986). In the widest sense, it includes not only those without access to a conventional dwelling but also those who are precariously housed, persons who have very tenuous claims to a conventional dwelling and those who lack basic financial resources and community ties (Lipton et al., 1983; Milburn & Watts, 1986; Rossi et al., 1987). As with any continuum, efforts to demarcate a core population are necessarily arbitrary and potentially contentious. Contemporary surveys of the homeless have attempted to deal with this ambiguity by adopting pragmatic, if limited, definitions according to simple descriptive typologies. For example, some investigators have adopted classifications based on demographic characteristics of age or marital status (Bhugra, 1991); others attempt to distinguish the literal homeless (who have no fixed abode or night-time shelter) from the transiently housed (Rossi et al., 1987); and others have adopted typologies based on temporal patterns of chronic, episodic and transient homelessness (Arce et al., 1983). Although each definition has proved useful in the context of a particular study, no single classification is entirely satisfactory and none has been universally adopted. It is quite unlikely that any single definition will ever suffice. Each step on the accommodation ladder encompasses several different subpopulations with varying characteristics and needs. For instance, the needs of homeless families placed in bed and breakfast hotels are very different from those of the single men and women who also use these institutions (Wall, 1991), and while plausible distinctions are sometimes made between 'rough sleepers' and other groups, it has to be acknowledged that the people who sleep rough on the street are neither a static population nor a homogeneous one.

In addition to these conceptual problems, epidemiological studies are faced with the methodological challenge of enumerating a mobile and transient population. While domiciled populations can be counted over a specified period, it is extremely difficult to obtain reliable counts of the number of people sleeping in outdoor locations, abandoned buildings and parked cars. In one of the most comprehensive efforts to obtain nation-wide estimates the US Department of Housing and Urban Development (1984) adopted four approaches which rely on a variety of information sources: (i) estimates taken from the highest pub-lished counts in 37 urban centres; (ii) a telephone interview with a nationwide sample of 60 metro-politan areas to elicit an estimate of the number of homeless people in the area; (iii) a similar estimate based on current shelter users; and (iv) street counts taken from the 1980 census and local surveys carried out in three major cities. While each method has drawbacks, the spread of approaches allowed upper and lower limits of the population to be estimated for the country as a whole. The highest estimate, derived from the first of these procedures, suggested a total of 586 000 homeless people nationwide. The lowest estimate, based on the shelter population and the local area street counts, suggested a total of 192 000 people. Taken as a whole, the survey suggests that there were, on average, 250 000–350 000 homeless people in the USA in 1984.

Since the publication of these data, there have been a number of efforts to improve census counts of street homeless people. For example, Rossi *et al.* (1987) combined a shelter survey with a street enumeration to provide a relatively unbiased estimate of the literal homeless of Chicago. For the shelter survey, they identified all shelters in the city that provided sleeping accom-modation, and interviewing teams counted all persons present in these shelters over two survey waves spanning the autumn of 1985 and March 1986. In parallel, teams of interviewers, accompanied by police, searched all places where homeless people might be found between the hours of midnight and 6 a.m. within a stratified random sample of 168 city blocks in the autumn and 245 city blocks in the winter, drawn from the 19 409 blocks within the city limits. The estimated numbers of homeless persons each night was 2344 ± 735 in autumn 1985 and 2022 ± 275 in winter 1986. This difference in figures was not statistically significant, suggesting no seasonal variation in homelessness rates.

The majority of estimates of the number of homeless people in Britain are based on local surveys and generalizations of statistics collected by a variety of statutory and voluntary organizations that provide services for homeless people. A street survey of 17 London boroughs in 1989 found 751 people sleeping on the streets or in railway stations on a single night (Canter *et al.*, 1989) and the 1991 census enumerated 2703 people sleeping rough in England and Wales, of which 1275 were in London (OPCS, 1991). However, these figures are based on surveys of a single night, carried out at sites known to be popular with rough sleepers and it is likely that significant numbers of people sleeping in abandoned buildings or less accessible sites were missed. Furthermore, a one-off census cannot deal adequately with the large numbers of people who sleep rough from time-to-time but who spent the census night in a hostel, shelter or some other temporary accommodation. Crude estimates of the numbers who might be involved in this more mobile population suggest that as many as 500 000 people in Britain sleep rough at some time during the course of a year (Matthews, 1986).

The official figures on hostel occupancy are somewhat more reliable than those of rough sleepers, although even these are subject to errors of classification and of missing data. In answer to a parliamentary question in February 1991, the Department of the Environment (DoE) reported a total of 22 383 hostel bed spaces for single people in London and a further 37 759 in the rest of England (Dorrell, 1991). Finally, data provided by the Department of Social Security (DSS) and reported by Randall (1992) indicate that in 1990 there were some 76 000 single claimants in board and lodgings in Britain, of which some 11 694 were resident in London. Nationally, the number of households placed in temporary accommodation by local authorities virtually doubled from 23 000 in 1986 to 40 000 in 1989 (Central Statistics Office, 1991).

Although the estimates of absolute numbers of homeless people vary according to whether they are taken solely from the official statistics or from the generalizations of surveys carried out by the charitable organizations which provide front-line services, there is broad agreement that the number of homeless people has grown dramatically during the past decade, in both Britain and the USA. There are, as yet, no epidemiological studies that have adequately addressed these time trends, despite evidence that these may hold vital clues as to the causes and possible solutions to the problem. In New York City shelters, there has been a shift towards more youthful populations over the past three decades (Susser *et al.*, 1989c) and there is said to be a similar growth in the number of homeless young people, women, families and ethnic minorities in Britain (e.g. Randall, 1988, 1989). There are no adequate explanations for these secular changes, although speculations include the general scarcity of low-cost housing, the erosion of traditional family networks in Western urban areas and changes in the organization and delivery of supportive (including psychiatric) services (e.g. Bachrach, 1984).

Schizophrenia among homeless populations

The observation of high rates of mental illness among homeless populations goes back a long way. The wandering lunatic is said to have been a common feature of Elizabethan and Stuart England (Beier, 1987), and in perhaps the earliest attempt to legislate the management of these cases, an Act of Parliament in 1714 empowered Justices of the Peace to confine and then return to their home parish, 'Persons of little or no Estates, who, by Lunacy or otherwise, are furiously mad, and too dangerous to be permitted to go abroad' (Alldridge, 1979).

From then to the latter half of the 20th century, very little seems to have been written on the subject of mentally ill homeless people. One of the first systematic studies was reported at the beginning of the century in Germany. At this time, vagrancy was an offence and those who could not demonstrate that they had a home to go to could be arrested and confined in the police workhouse. Wilmanns (1906) noted that many of these vagrants were subsequently transferred to

his hospital, and in a survey of 120 of these referrals, he found that the majority were suffering from schizophrenia. Early sociological investigations of the associations of social deprivation and mental illness fuelled further interest. For example, Bogue (1963), an American sociologist, in a study of alcoholism among skid row populations, found that one in five of the men he interviewed were suffering from mental illness. He commented: 'from a sociological viewpoint, Skid Row is a combination poor farm and asylum with freedom of movement where the 'patients' are all regarded as incurable and hence are fed, clothed and housed but not given curative treatment' (Bogue, 1963).

More recent studies have been concerned with establishing the rates of various forms of mental illness in the homeless population. In Britain (Table 33.1), most studies have focused on the problems of residents of hostels (Crossley & Denmark, 1969; Lodge-Patch, 1970; Marshall, 1989; Timms & Fry, 1989; Marshall & Reed, 1992), reception centres (Edwards *et al.* 1968; Tidmarsh & Wood, 1972), lodging houses (Laidlawm, 1956; Priest, 1970, 1971) and soup kitchens or night shelters (Edwards *et al.*, 1966; Weller *et al.*, 1987). Reflecting the setting of these surveys, subjects are typically male, in their late 40s and a high proportion are unemployed and few have family or friendship ties. Several of these studies have employed standardized research interviews and well-defined diagnostic criteria. Mental illness is found in 30–50% of the shelter population, with schizophrenia the most common diagnosis. Most of these schizophrenics have had previous episodes of care, typically as in-patients, and the majority are severely disabled with psychotic symptoms which are of an intensity similar to that seen in patients in the back wards of psychiatric institutions (Marshall, 1989; Stark *et al.*, 1989).

Timms and Fry (1989) surveyed a representative sample of men newly arriving at a Salvation Army hostel and compared these with a sample of men who had been resident in the hostel for longer than 1 year. In all, 124 men were interviewed using an expanded version of the *Present*

Table 33.1 Summary of UK studies of mental illness among homeless adults

Study	Location of sample	Number of subjects	Data collection methods	Schizophrenia (%)	Affective disorder (%)	Alcohol abuse (%)	Drug abuse (%)	Personality disorder (%)	Other disorder (%)	Past contact with services (%)
Crossley and Denmark (1969)	Hostel	55 men	CI	19	–	–	–	64	6	62
Priest (1976)	Hostel	77 men	SSI	32	5	18	–	12–18	2–5	14
Timms and Fry (1989)	Hostel	124 men	PSE	31	6	8	1	6	–	90 (of psychotics)
Marshall and Reed (1992)	Hostel	70 women	PSE	64	3	10	6	–	7	–
Lodge-Patch (1970)	Hostel	130 men	CI	15	8	21	–	50	13	78 (of psychotics)
Edwards et al. (1968)	Reception centre	279 men	CI	–	–	25	–	–	–	24
Tidmarsh and Wood (1972)	Reception centre	359 men	CI	30	–	33	–	11	–	29
Stark et al. (1989)	Resettlement unit	110 men	GHQ, CAGE, CI	25	5	50	3	–	39	63
Whiteley (1955)	NFA admissions	130 men	CI	32	14	14	2	19	21	–
Berry and Orwin (1966)	NFA admissions	140 men and women	CI	49	13	–	–	28	10	73
Herzberg (1987)	NFA admissions	110 men and women	CN	32	9	36	–	29	5	83

CI, clinical interview; SSI, symptom–sign inventory; PSE, *Present State Examination*; GHQ, general health questionnaire; CAGE, alcohol screening; CN, case note review; NFA, no fixed abode.

State Examination (PSE). Over half were found to be suffering from mental disorder. Schizophrenia was the most common single diagnosis, present in 25% of the new arrivals and 37% of the long-term hostel residents. Both groups reported lengthy histories of illness with short periods of in-patient care at some point during their illness.

In one of the very few British studies of female hostel populations, Marshall and Reed (1992) interviewed 70 residents of two direct-access hostels which cater specifically for homeless women. Mental state was assessed by a modified PSE. The duration of stay in the hostel varied from 1 week to 50 years, with a median stay of 2 years. Twenty-seven of the women had moved to their present accommodation from other hostels and eight had come directly from psychiatric hospitals. Forty-five women met the *Diagnostic and Statistical Manual* DSM-III criteria for schizophrenia and a further 18 suffered from other psychiatric disorders. Two-thirds of the women had seen a psychiatrist and 45 of the women reported at least one previous psychiatric admission (median 2; range 1–30), with five subjects having been in hospital during the previous 12 months. At least 15 had been detained formally in the past under mental health legistation.

The results of recent US surveys are broadly in line with their UK counterparts (Table 33.2). Between 10 and 36% of shelter and street homeless people report histories of previous hospitalizations, severe mental illness is present in 30–50%, and high rates of anxiety and depression are also recorded where appropriate questions have been asked. Of these studies, perhaps the most important is that reported by Breakey *et al.* in Baltimore. In this investigation, 289 men and 230 women were randomly selected from missions, shelters and jails in the Baltimore area. A subsample of 203 was assessed by research interviews, which included an extended PSE, the Eysenck personality inventory and the Michigan alcohol screening test (MAST). Subjects were also physically examined and a number of investigations, including breath alcohol, were carried out. Men had on average eight medical problems and women nine medical problems per person that were thought sufficient to warrant primary care treatment. Two-thirds of women had gynaecological problems and a third were anaemic. A fifth of the men were hypertensive. Cardiac arrhythmias were recorded in 15% of both men and women, and 10% had sexually transmitted diseases. Schizophrenia was diagnosed in 12% of the males and 17% of the females, and taken together with other psychoses, major depression and bipolar disorders, major mental illness was recorded in 42% of the men and 49% of the women. Three-quarters of the men reported a substance-abuse problem, as did 38% of the women. Less severe problems of anxiety and depression were particularly prevalent, so that combined with major mental disorders over 80% of the sample suffered from at least one *Diagnostic and Statistical Manual* DSM-III axis 1 mental health problem; in addition, almost half the sample were classified as suffering from a personality disorder (Breakey *et al.*, 1989).

In another recent US study that utilized sophisticated sampling methods and structured assessment interviews, Koegal *et al.* (1988) recorded lifetime and current prevalence of diagnostic interview schedule (DIS) DSM-III disorders among 328 homeless adults in the Skid Row area of Los Angeles and contrasted these estimates with prevalence data collected in the Los Angeles arm of the epidemiological catchment area (LAECA) household survey. Prevalence rates among the homeless sample were substantially higher than those recorded in the LAECA survey for every mental disorder assessed. The difference in rates was particularly striking for major mental illnesses. Schizophrenia was diagnosed in 13% of the homeless sample but in less than 1% of the household sample. While substance-use disorders were the most prevalent conditions among the homeless, they were also very common among householders (31 vs. 12%). It was estimated that over a quarter of the homeless sample were chronically mentally ill, and rates of schizophrenia were greatest among those with the longest histories of homelessness or who had been homeless many times.

Finally, Susser *et al.* compared social adjustment and mental illness rates among new and long-stay residents of New York City shelters

Table 33.2 Summary of USA studies of mental illness among homeless adults

Study	Location of sample	Number of subjects	Data collection methods	Schizophrenia (%)	Affective disorder (%)	Alcohol abuse (%)	Drug abuse (%)	Personality disorder (%)	Other disorder (%)	Past contact with services (%)
Arce et al. (1983)	Shelters	141 men; 52 women	CI/DSM-III	37	6	25		7	5	37
Bassuk et al. (1986)	Shelters	65 men; 131 women	CI	3	9	9		71	5	28 hospitalized
Kroll et al. (1986)	Shelters	60 men; 8 women	CI	40 (psychotic)		61	2			41
Morse and Calsyn (1986)	Shelters	126 men; 122 women	CI/BSI/ CAGE	47 (psychotic)		36	21	–	–	25
Susser et al. (1989c)	Shelters	223 men	SCID/MAST/ CES-D	8 (17 probable)	33	35	38	–	–	15 hospitalized
Koegal et al. (1988)	Shelter/mission	313 men; 15 women	DIS	12	21	27	10	17	14	–
Breakey et al. (1989)	Shelter/ mission/jail	289 men; 230 women	PSE/MAST	15	24	54	20	45	36	–
Lipton et al. (1983)	NFA admissions	68 men; 22 women	CN	72	9	5	–	12	–	97 hospitalized
Linn et al. (1990)	NFA at clinic	132 men; 82 women	CI	31		43	46	–	–	29 hospitalized

CI, clinical interview; DSM, *Diagnostic and Statistical Manual*; CN, case notes; BSI, Brief Symptom Inventory; CAGE/MAST, alcohol screening; DIS, Diagnostic Interview Schedule; SCID, Structured Clinical Interview for DSM-III; PSE, *Present State Examination*; CES-D, Center for Epidemiological Studies–Depression Scale.

(Susser *et al.*, 1989a,c). A random sample of 223 new arrivals to the shelters was chosen, of which 177 were successfully interviewed using the structured clinical interview for DSM-III-R (SCID), the MAST and the Center for Epidemiologic Studies of Depression scale. The majority of men had a history of mental disorder, 17% had a definite or probable diagnosis of psychosis and a further 8% had a possible history of psychosis. A confident diagnosis of schizophrenia was made in 8%. Alcohol and substance abuse were recorded in over 50% of the sample, cocaine being the drug of choice, with 27% of the sample having used it more than 50 times. In addition, 695 of 4000 long-term residents were examined using a screening questionnaire and observational rating scale. Men under 30 years were overrepresented in the new entrants to shelters, and non-whites overrepresented in both samples relative to the general population. More of the long-term homeless reported a history of psychosis than did the new entrants. A quarter of the latter had a history of probable or possible psychosis and schizophrenia was diagnosed in 18%.

In parallel with these surveys of homeless populations, studies of mental hospital admissions since the mid-1950s have reported that as many as 10% are of people with 'no fixed abode' (Whiteley, 1955; Berry & Orwin, 1966). These patients make higher demands on hospital in-patient services than do the domiciled population (Herzberg, 1987; Glover, 1989), and as many as half suffer from schizophrenia, often with lengthy histories of illness but with poor compliance with treatment, higher rates of discharge against medical advice and, consequently, a history of repeated brief hospitalizations and discharge to unsatisfactory living circumstances (Berry & Orwin, 1966; Whitly *et al.*, 1985; Herzberg, 1987).

Although the bulk of the research literature quoted has originated from Britain and the USA, it is worth noting that similar rates have been observed in studies in Australia (Herrman *et al.*, 1989), Norway (Noreik, 1965), Denmark (Nordentoft *et al.*, 1992) and Portugal (Bento & Marmeleiro, 1986). French workers have been concerned more with philosophical and psycho-logical issues, attempting to clarify a typology of homelessness and to identify a specific psycho-pathology of vagrancy, in which Balint's concept of philobatism or affinity for open spaces has been invoked to explain the behaviour of those who appear to wander with no fixed abode (e.g Mouren *et al.*, 1979).

Despite evidence that homeless populations are becoming younger, there are very few studies which have set out to examine mental illness rates among homeless youths. The few studies that have been carried out suggest a rather different profile of disorder characterized by depression, anxiety and substance abuse. For example, Shaffer and Caton (1984) found that young shelter users had psychiatric profiles largely indistinguishable from those of adolescents attending psychiatric clinics: 30% were depressed, 18% had antisocial personality disorder and 41% were both depressed and antisocial. A quarter of the sample had attempted suicide and an additional 25% had 'actively contemplated' suicide in the previous year. Psychotic symptoms have also been recorded in surveys of these populations. Mundy *et al.* (1990) found that 29% of a sample of 91 homeless adolescents in Los Angeles reported at least four psychotic symptoms on the DIS and 46% reported an attempted suicide at least once in their lives. No attempt at psychiatric diagnosis was reported.

In conclusion, regardless of how homelessness is defined, it seems certain that these populations experience a much higher prevalence of schizophrenia and other serious mental illnesses than would be expected from generalizations from the general population. The considerable variation in actual rates reported between studies reflects different methods of sample selection, measurement of symptoms and definition of caseness (Susser *et al.*, 1989a; Eagle & Caton, 1990).

Pathways to homelessness

Demographic associations

Early studies in both the UK and USA found that homeless mentally ill individuals were typically single, white, male and middle-aged (e.g. Priest, 1976; Freeman *et al.*, 1979). However, more recent evidence suggests that the average age of mentally ill homeless people is falling and is now in the mid-30s (Fischer *et al.*, 1986; Rossi *et al.*, 1987; Marshall, 1989; Stark *et al.*, 1989). There also appears to be a rise in the number of homeless mentally ill women (Burt & Cohen, 1989; George *et al.*, 1991) and of ethnic minorities (Kroll *et al.*, 1986; Burt & Cohen, 1989; Stark *et al.*, 1989). Most are single or divorced (Burt & Cohen, 1989) and fewer than a third of hostel residents have ever been married (Kroll *et al.*, 1986; Stark *et al.*, 1989), although women residents are more likely than their male counterparts to have married (Burt & Cohen, 1989; Marshall & Reed, 1992).

Over half the homeless population remain in a single city for more than 1 year (Kay, 1985; Snow *et al.*, 1986). Geographical mobility seems greater in the young (Fisher & Breakey, 1986) and, contrary to popular belief, the severely mentally ill as a group are rather less mobile than 'healthy' homeless people, tending to lack the organizational capacity and drive that high mobility demands (Snow *et al.*, 1986).

General social factors contributing to homelessness

Unemployment, poverty and the lack of cheap housing contribute significantly to homelessness in both the UK and USA (Rossi *et al.*, 1987; SHELTER, 1989; Cohen & Thompson, 1992). Few homeless people have regular paid work, though up to a quarter have had casual (and often exploitative) jobs at some time in the recent past (Stark *et al.*, 1989). Mentally ill homeless people are more likely than other homeless groups to remain without secure accommodation for longer, to have less contact with families or friends, experience more barriers to employment and have higher rates of contact with the legal system (Cohen & Thompson, 1992).

In both Britain and the USA, the past 15 years has been characterized by a substantial decline in low-cost housing, a shrinking of the job market and a tightening of the targeting of social welfare benefits. Not only are such benefits harder to obtain, but evidence suggests that homeless people may have particular problems accessing information that would help meet some of their needs. Recent British surveys suggest that less than a third of homeless people are in receipt of their entitled welfare benefits and up to two-thirds have no idea where to seek the appropriate advice or help (Stark *et al.*, 1989). In the Chicago study of urban homelessness referred to earlier (Rossi *et al.*, 1987), homeless people clustered at the extreme lower boundary of the American poverty population. Incomes were, on average, four times lower than the official poverty level for single persons under the age of 65, and approximately one in five reported having received no income at all in the previous month. Affordable housing at such income levels was virtually non-existent. The literal homeless not only were poor themselves, but came from families that already lived close to the breadline with very little capacity to provide additional financial assistance. Many were isolated from family and friends and many reported high levels of mental and physical disability which made ordinary participation in everyday social life extremely difficult, if not impossible. Similar observations have been made in a number of social surveys in Britain, which record comparable levels of extreme poverty (SHELTER, 1989) and evictions following failure to keep up with rent payments (Central Statistics Office, 1989). In the USA, the percentage of non-whites in extremely poor districts rose from 25% in the 1960s to 40% in the mid-1980s, reflecting a similiar rise in the number of homeless blacks (US Department of Housing and Urban Development, 1984). Studies examining the reasons for the loss of accommodation among the mentally ill homeless directly mirror reasons given by non-mentally ill respondents: evictions because of urban development projects; victimization by unscrupulous landlords; and an inability to afford rising rent prices.

Homeless people also frequently cite family breakdown as a significant milestone on the way to the loss of their accommodation. Several studies have found associations between homelessness and previous episodes of running away from home, difficulties at school, family disorganization and violence. Susser *et al.* (1991) reported findings from three samples of homeless populations in which they examined the relationship between childhood experiences, homelessness and mental illness. They compared childhood histories of 512 homeless patients with 271 patients who had never been homeless. In the homeless samples, 15% had a history of foster care, more than one in 10 had a history of group home placement, and one in five had a history of running away from home during childhood. These proportions compared with 2, 1 and 5% in those who had never been homeless, and the lifetime prevalence of homelessness in patients with any one of these factors was three times that of other patients. Similarly, Bassuk *et al.* (1986) found that a third of the women resident in shelters had been abused in childhood, and two-thirds reported family disruption. The proportions described by these studies are considerably higher than those found in the general population and somewhat higher than in the non-mentally ill homeless, although the latter also include a high proportion with childhood histories of being in care or separated from their parents through abuse, neglect or family breakdown. Powers *et al.* (1990) compared the make-up of families of 223 homeless adolescents with a representative sample of under-18-year-olds in the general population. Less than a quarter of the sample of homeless youths was found to come from 'intact' families compared with 68% of the general youth sample; 15% of the homeless youths had been living without either parent, compared with 2% of American youths as a whole. Of the sample, 60% had experienced physical abuse, 42% emotional abuse, 48% neglect and 21% sexual abuse. Youths in the maltreated sample were more likely to be female and to have engaged in suicidal behaviour. Such high proportions of parenting problems reflect equally elevated prevalences of parental psychiatric disorder. So, for example, Stiffman (1989) found that 141 of 291 adolescents seeking shelter at homes for runaway youths had been sexually or physically abused. One in five of the non-abused and one in three of the abused youths reported having a parent who had a problem with alcohol or exhibited behaviour consistent with an antisocial personality disorder. Overall, one in three reported that a parent had a problem with alcohol or was depressed, and one in five reported that a parent had attempted suicide. Similarly, Shaffer and Caton (1984) found that as many as 60% of homeless youths reported a parental history of substance abuse or criminality, and up to 50% described parental physical abuse to such a degree that injuries were sustained.

Although the overall impression of these studies is that childhood experiences strongly predict later homelessness, it seems likely that the actual causal pathway is complex and involves the interplay of many different factors. The majority of studies note the presence of a broad range of social and interpersonal difficulties which antedate homelessness by many years and which persist subsequently. Very few homeless people have had more than a basic education (Fischer *et al.*, 1986; Burt & Cohen, 1989; Stark *et al.*, 1989) and many report difficulties in educational settings. For example, Shaffer and Caton (1984) found that approximately 50% of their sample of homeless youths had experienced educational problems and that 71% of boys and 44% of girls had been suspended or expelled from school. Interpersonal problems, rows and antisocial behaviour may be reflected in the observation that homeless men and women have restricted social contacts (Fischer *et al.*, 1986; Marshall, 1989) and most have no close confidant (Breakey *et al.*, 1989). Among the mentally ill in this population, social networks are even more restricted — up to 90% are without regular social contacts, including their family (Bassuk *et al.*, 1986). Criminal activity, typically of a relatively minor nature or involving offences against property rather than people, is high in both male and female homeless populations and this seems to be greater among the homeless mentally ill (Lamb, 1984; Weller *et al.*, 1987; Stark *et al.*, 1989). Put together, a vulnerability to homelessness is perhaps most closely tied to a lack of adequate kin support, which itself may be determined by factors as diverse as poverty, secular changes in family structure, mental illness or dysfunction in one or more parent and the manifestation of these in a variety of deficiencies of parental care.

Is there a unique pathway to homelessness among the mentally ill?

To summarize thus far, although there are some broad differences in demographic profiles between mentally ill and mentally 'healthy' homeless people, there are rather more similarities than differences. It seems unlikely that the mentally ill members of the homeless population have followed any unique pathway to their homeless status, although two possibilities remain to be explored. First, that the nature of their illness has resulted in some degree of incompetence in goal planning, organizational functioning and hence to a chaotic drift into the homeless state; and second, that coupled to these core disabilities, the existing care system which might prevent such a social decline has at best failed to halt it, and at worst, may have spurred it along through precipitious discharge from care and inadequate attention to follow-up and supervision.

Mental illness increases the risk of homelessness

Few would doubt that severe mental illness can increase the risk of homelessness. For example, a quarter of all severely mentally ill people seen by clinical teams in the current London-wide Homeless Mental Health Initiative had lost their permanent accommodation following eviction for disturbed behaviour or non-payment of rent that was the direct result of their mental illness.

In addition to these 'obvious' examples, there is also a considerable body of evidence that suggests that a social decline (and perhaps therefore homelessness) may precede tha first manifestation of florid symptoms by several years. The high prevalence of schizophrenia among homeless populations echoes similar findings in other socially and economically deprived populations. In the Great Depression of the 1930s, the American sociologists Robert Faris and Warren Dunham found that the highest rates for treated schizo-

phrenia in Chicago were concentrated in delapidated slum areas in the centre of the city and decreased towards more affluent peripheral areas (Faris & Dunham, 1939). This increase in prevalence in economically deprived areas has since been observed repeatedly in many US and European cities (Schroeder, 1942; Clarke, 1948; Hare, 1956; Sundby & Nyhus, 1963; Gardner & Babigian, 1966) and has been further refined through a number of studies which explained the association in terms of links with low income or low-status occupations (Odegard, 1956; Hollingshead & Redlich, 1958; Turner *et al.*, 1967; Wiersma *et al.*, 1983).

These observations (and many others concerning elevated risks of schizophrenia among migrant populations, certain ethnic minority groups and the occupationally disadvantaged) have been put forward as suggestive of a causal relationship between psychosocial stressors and schizophrenia. However, many of these relationships appear to be the result, rather than the cause, of schizophrenia and current theories are more concerned with the influence of non-psychosocial environmental risk factors, such as exposure to fetal viral infection during the second gestational trimester and perinatal obstetric complications (see Chapters 12 & 13, this volume). Although the issue is not entirely resolved, it seems reasonable to conclude that the majority of the associations between schizophrenia and macrosocial indices of poverty and deprivation arise because people in the prodromal stage of the illness drift into lower status occupations and deprived inner city locations as a result of their poor premorbid level of functioning. This social drift theory was first proposed by Goldberg and Morrison (1963), who showed that the occupational status of male schizophrenics was lower than that of their fathers, who were comparable with the general population. Although this has been broadly confirmed in several later studies (Turner *et al.*, 1967; Wiersma *et al.*, 1983), a number of interesting caveats to the social drift theory have emerged. For example, Turner *et al.* (1967) noted that most of the observed discrepancy between fathers' and childrens' occupational levels was due to the latter never achieving the status of the father, rather than the result of an actual drift down the social ladder, an observation which was also made in a later Dutch cohort study (Wiersma *et al.*, 1983). It appears, therefore, that for some, the process is more one of social stagnation rather than drift. In the most recent study to examine these issues, Jones *et al.* (1993) investigated the timing and precursors of social decline in schizophrenia and affective psychosis among 195 admissions to three London hospitals. Comparison of the fathers' occupations and the probands best premorbid occupational level indicated occupational under-achievement was confined to schizophrenic patients. These underachievers had poorer edu-cational qualifications than those who equalled or bettered their parental social class, despite having a similar age of onset and premorbid intelligence quotient (IQ). A *decline* in social status was also seen in some patients after their florid illness had begun (i.e. a change from a higher to a lower occupational level). This post-onset decline was found in both schizophrenic and affective psy-choses, indicating a non-specific effect of illness on occupational and social role performance. Put together, these results support other suggestions of subtle abnormalities of cognition and person-ality in schizophrenia that antedate the onset of florid symptoms by years and may well represent a brain lesion dating from early in development (Aylward *et al.*, 1984; Murray & Lewis, 1987; see Chapter 12, this volume).

It appears, therefore, that homelessness can occur both as a direct consequence of established mental illness and as a result of defects in coping, social withdrawal and poor occupational perform-ance that characterize the prodromal phase of the illness.

The existing care system may precipitate homelessness

Closure of the asylum. Regardless of the importance of social factors in the aetiology of the disease, it also seems clear that homelessness among the severely mentally ill is related in part to the failure to provide adequate care outside of institutional or hospital settings.

The number of patients in psychiatric hospitals in England and Wales has declined steadily from 148 100 in 1954 to 97 064 in 1986 (DoH, 1990), and although there are no official statistics for the years 1990–93, a reply to a parliamentary question (Dorrell, 1991) suggested that the number of mental illness beds continued to fall to 59 290 in 1990, of which 37 350 were occupied by patients staying longer than 1 year or in secure facilities. Thirty mental hospitals closed between 1980 and 1989 and a further 38 (amounting to 12 500 beds) are scheduled for closure before 1995 (National Schizophrenia Fellowship, 1989).

A similar, and perhaps even more dramatic, picture is seen in the USA. As in Britain, the number of patients in state and county hospitals declined, from 560 00 in 1955 to 116 000 in 1987, and continues to fall (Eagle & Caton, 1990). According to one report, some 300 000 chronic mental patients reside in a variety of board and care homes, of which at least 60% are suffering from schizophrenia (Warner, 1985). A further 60 000 schizophrenics live in nursing homes and there are tens of thousands of schizophrenics who are homeless or in jails or other 'inappropriate' institutional settings. Rather fewer than half of all people with schizophrenia live in anything approaching a family home or their own domestic environment (Warner, 1985).

It is widely believed that the current crisis of street homelessness among the mentally ill is a direct result of the rundown and closure of psy-chiatric hospital accommodation, particularly that which formerly dealt with the long-stay population. There have consequently been calls to halt this process before further damage is done (Arce *et al.*, 1983; Weller, 1989). But such calls may be mis-guided. In Britain, long-stay patients discharged from mental hospitals as part of a planned closure programme have typically been accommodated in supported housing schemes, with residential care staff and specialized continuing care or rehabili-tation community teams. A very small number of these patients subsequently become homeless. In the longitudinal study of the closure of Friern Barnet Hospital, only 2% of the 278 patients were thought to have been lost to follow-up because of becoming homeless (TAPS, 1990; Leff, 1991), and in a contemporaneous study of the closure of Cane Hill Hospital, none of the 103 patients followed up 1 year after discharge to community based facilities had become homeless (Pickard *et al.*, 1991).

Part of the misunderstanding may have arisen through the injudicious use of incomplete data collected by earlier studies of homeless populations. The majority of early studies of homeless users of shelters and day-care facilities which noted the similarity of the mentally ill users to patients in the back wards of mental hospitals did not include detailed questioning about the pathways to homelessness and, particularly, the nature of prior contact with the mental health services. For example, Crossley and Denmark (1969) found that two-thirds of the 55 men in their shelter study had a past history of admission to a mental hospital; Tidmarsh and Wood (1972) in their survey of the Camberwell Reception Centre found that 29% of 359 men had been admitted to a mental hospital at some time in their life (9% within the previous 12 months); and Lodge-Patch (1970) noted that although 14 out of 18 schizophrenic men had previously been hospitalized, only three continued to receive any psychiatric care. These studies are often quoted by experts as evidence to back up claims that these patients would ordinarily have been inmates of an asylum, had such facilities not been closed. However, none of these studies report adequate details of the length and form of previous treatment on which to base such assertions.

Recent studies which have paid more attention to the details of past care suggest that relatively few of the homeless mentally ill have ever experienced prolonged hospitalization. For example, in the study of Timms and Fry (1989), although all the schizophrenic patients suffered from chronic disorders in the sense that their illness had begun more than 5 years previously, the majority had spent less than 2 years in hospital in their lifetime. Only seven of the 123 men had ever been continuously hospitalized for more than 1 year. Data on prior psychiatric treatment were also collected in the context of an experimental case-management

service for homeless mentally ill people. In the course of a year, the psychiatric team for homeless people (Brent-Smith & Dean, 1990) received 94 referrals of the most disabled or disturbed clients resident in hostels or using a variety of day services. All the patients suffered from chronic illnesses. Two-thirds had a DSM-III diagnosis of schizophrenia and four-fifths were severely socially disabled, predominantly by 'negative' symptoms of withdrawal and apathy. Despite the severity of their illness, 15 had never been admitted to hospital, and among the remainder the most common pattern of hospitalization reported was one of multiple brief admissions — with no subsequent improvement in accommodation. During the entire course of their illness, these patients had an average of 6.4 admissions to hospital with a mean length of stay of 7 months. Only two patients reported previous hospitalization for 1 year or longer. Finally, current data from the first year of the London Homeless Mentally Ill Initiative confirm the low proportion of ex-long-stay patients in the hostel or street homeless population. In the first year of this study, three clinical teams providing services to street homeless, hostel residents and users of day centres and soup kitchens assessed a total of 800 homeless people, of which 544 were found to be suffering from severe mental illness (over 60% with a diagnosis of schizophrenia). Of these, only three have been found whose longest continuous hospitalization was greater than 5 years. The great majority of cases with histories of previous hospitalization report multiple brief admissions.

In conclusion, these recent studies suggest that the homeless mentally ill are not those who have been discharged as part of the planned closure of the large mental hospital. Most have not spent long periods in hospital, but appear instead to have experienced many brief hospitalizations over a number of years interspersed with periods where psychiatric care has been virtually non-existent. A significant number have found a niche within an institutional setting which is very similar in many respects to the old asylum. Typical old-fashioned, direct-access hostels provided low-key, non-interfering environments in which it was possible to stay for many months, or even years, with only a minimum requirement of social interaction with other residents or staff. Bizarre behaviour was usually ignored and residents were not subjected to medical or social work demands to make changes in their lives, take medication or participate in rehabilitation programmes (Timms & Fry, 1989).

Failures in community care. While there is little direct evidence to support the belief that in the UK the rise in homeless mentally ill people directly mirrors the rundown of the asylum, there can be little doubt that deinstitutionalization in a wider sense plays a very important role (Lamb, 1984; Bachrach, 1992). Follow-up studies of the aftercare of schizophrenics suggest a large gap between objective disability and the provision of services, with significant numbers of recently discharged schizophrenics leading isolated and unoccupied existences, often without adequate contact with either primary or secondary health-care resources (Meltzer *et al.*, 1991). Similarly, the current London-wide homelessness service recorded that 93% of people with a diagnosis of schizophrenia, who had received psychiatric care at some time during the course of their illness, had subsequently lost contact with statutory agencies. The reasons for this loss could be directly attributed to a service failure in almost half these instances — follow-up appointments promised but never sent, the closure of community clinics and the 'loss' of the case in a tangle of interagency bureaucracy. Similarly, in a state-wide study of homelessness in Ohio, Roth and Bean (1986) estimated that only about one in five of those with severe mental illness were actually receiving care. And in another study, fewer than one in 10 of Los Angeles Skid Row *habitués* had professional out-patient mental health care, even though more than a third had spent some time in psychiatric hospitals in the past (Farr *et al.*, 1986).

Such deficiencies in the implementation of community care have been well documented (Bachrach, 1984; Lamb, 1984; Thornicroft & Bebbington, 1989; Wing, 1990; Sayce *et al.*, 1991; Marks, 1992; see also Chapter 32), and it appears that in both Britain and the USA a relatively small number of factors crop up time and again to explain this depressing observation. First, the emphasis on brief and intensive in-patient care. Surveys around London suggest that acute in-patient units now operate at very high occupancy levels, often exceeding 100% (Hollander *et al.*, 1990), and in such a climate it is not unusual for patients to be discharged prematurely in order to admit another whose problems appear more pressing or dangerous (Patrick *et al.*, 1989). Few patients can remain in hospital once the acute illness has subsided, and there is a reluctance to continue expensive hospital treatment beyond the point of medical necessity, regardless of whether or not there are adequate aftercare or housing facilities available.

Second, the current fashion of organizing psychiatric services around specific geographical sectors serves to disrupt the continuity of care for people who move between catchment areas, and is particularly problematic for the homeless person who moves between the streets and a variety of temporary accommodation, is not registered with primary care services or involved with social care agencies. Disputes between services about who 'owns' the case are compounded by splits in the organization and funding of social and health care.

Third, recent decades have seen a falling-off of commitment to people whose disorders cannot be cured. This problem has many sources and includes factors as diverse as the expansion in community services for patients with acute neurotic illnesses and transient stress reactions (Sayce *et al.*, 1991); the ethical dilemmas of 'forcing' treatment on people who appear reluctant to accept it; and the sheer complexity of arranging and delivering effective care when the organizations providing such care are not contained within a single service but are scattered around a community, operating in isolation and complete ignorance of each other (Clifford & Craig, 1989).

Finally, the prejudices of some health professionals may make services unacceptable to homeless mentally ill people (Stern & Stilwell, 1989); the emphasis on treatment and active involvement is often at odds with the client's primary needs of food, shelter and security (Bachrach, 1987).

Perhaps even more important than these problems in community care is the fact that in the last 15 years there has been a dramatic reduction in the number of beds in reception centres, Salvation Army hostels, Rowton houses and night shelters. In Britain, the number of such units has fallen steadily from 215 in 1948 to only 21 in 1970 (Hewettson, 1975). In 1985, it was decided that all remaining resettlement units should close to be replaced by smaller and more appropriate accommodation provided by local authorities and the voluntary sector. There was to be no overall reduction in funding, but potential service providers were slow in coming forward and wider changes in the funding of local authorities further conspired to reduce the likelihood that any would in fact take up the burden of reprovision. Five years later, only eight schemes had been approved and none of these provided sufficient bed spaces to replace the units that were already scheduled for closure (Central Office of Information, 1991). There has also been a loss of direct-access hostel accommodation. In 1981, there were 9751 bed spaces in direct-access hostels in London, 6000 of which were in large, traditional hostels for the homeless. By 1990, the number of these places had declined to 2000 (Harrison *et al.*, 1992). Furthermore, despite the well-documented similarity between patients in long-stay wards and mentally ill residents of these hostels, the financial allowances available for closure of these beds are vastly inferior to those available for the hospital reprovision programme, sometimes five times less than that available to develop supported accommodation for the patients of long-stay hospital wards (SHIL, 1986).

A somewhat similar decline in low-cost housing has been documented in the USA. In New York City, more than 110 000 single-room occupancy hotel spaces were lost between 1970 and 1982 (a staggering 82% of the total supply in the city), while in the same period nationwide, 1.116 million spaces were lost — almost half the total provision registered in 1971. This loss has been paralleled by a corresponding growth of places in shelters, to

the extent that the larger of these have been dubbed 'warehouses of the homeless' to which 'some ex-patients have come full circle back to the institution that had originally discharged them — this time for shelter not treatment' (Baxter & Hopper, 1982).

A conceptual model of the pathways to homelessness

In Fig. 33.1, we attempt to draw together the material reviewed to this point. In this model, the event of becoming homeless is linked to one of several other severe life crises, such as marital separation, loss of employment or a financial crisis. However, the loss of accommodation itself may be rather less important than the ability of the individual to escape from the condition once it has arisen. In this model, the likelihood of reversing a housing crisis can be seen to be dependent on the interplay of the environment ('external factors') and on psychological and coping skills ('internal factors'). Internal factors include cognitive sets of helplessness, low self-esteem and dependency. They reduce the individual's capacity to make constructive use of external resources, the ability to identify opportunities and to carry through cogent plans for the future. External factors include the lack of alternative accommodation, a meagre disposable income, unemployment and low kinship support. Such chronic difficulties give rise to severe events which, in turn, are causally linked to psychological vulnerability (helplessness, low self-esteem) and depression (Brown & Harris, 1978, 1989), and thus impede restitution by directly reducing the level of available resources as well as indirectly through their impact on psychological adjustment.

Both strands may have their origin early in life. Brown and Harris (1989), describing the social antecedents of depression in women, comment on a similar 'conveyor belt' of adversity in which severe events in adulthood arise out of chronic economic and interpersonal difficulties which can be traced to social deprivations that had been endured for years. In their studies of depression, they outline a sequence in which women moved

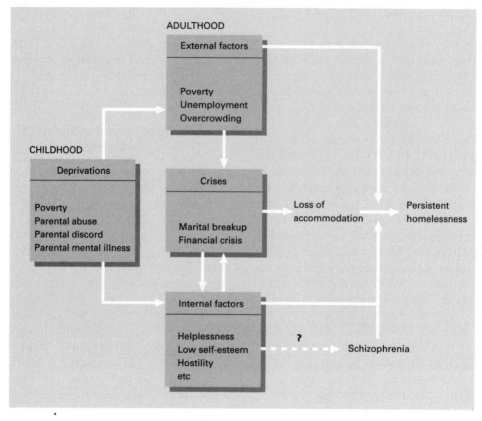

Fig. 33.1 Pathways to persistent homelessness.

from one crisis to another, starting with a lack of adequate parenting in childhood and passing through to premarital pregnancy, which trapped women in relationships that they might not otherwise have chosen and that subsequently contributed to the occurrence of severe events and difficulties, such as housing and financial problems or marital conflict with undependable spouses. Women caught on this conveyor belt were less upwardly mobile in terms of social class and emerged with fewer resources than their peers (Brown, 1989). These childhood deprivations were also linked to internal aspects of the individual — helplessness, low self-esteem and chronic subclinical symptoms of mood disorder which, as we have seen, may well contribute to an increased risk of adversity as helpless individuals fail to extricate themselves from situations that

precipitate crises (Brown & Harris, 1989).

The contribution of schizophrenia to this model is now seen to boil down to a special instance of the general effects described earlier. Leaving aside the question whether adversity, and hence homelessness itself, has a causal role in such illnesses, it is clear that mental illness contributes to the persistence of homelessness, both by impairing general coping and problem solving and by creating even more social adversity as the sufferer is less likely to gain or maintain employment or stable accommodation without assistance, and is shunned or even persecuted for displays of odd and eccentric behaviour. An insensitive, rigid organization of social and medical care compounds these personal difficulties by creating further obstacles that must be overcome.

Treatment: how then can we deliver services to this population?

There are few well-controlled experimental evaluations of services for the homeless mentally ill and even fewer that attempt to address both the mental health and social care needs of the sufferer. In keeping with current thinking on the organization of community care, most of the better interventions have included multidisciplinary approaches with assertive outreach and continuing case management, expending a great deal of effort on the task of coordinating the many service inputs that this population requires (Bachrach, 1984; Lipton *et al.*, 1988; Brent-Smith & Dean, 1990; Caton *et al.*, 1990; see also Chapter 32, this volume).

Caton *et al.* (1990) used a before-and-after study design to evaluate a day-treatment programme for 32 mentally ill homeless men. The subjects were interviewed concerning their housing stability, treatment compliance, hospitalization and involvement with the criminal justice system 6 months before and 6 months after allocation to the day-care programme. In the follow-up phase, street homelessness was virtually eliminated and shelter use decreased sevenfold. Contacts with the criminal justice system were halved, but psychiatric service attendance tripled. There were no measures of psychopathology or more subtle indices of social disability, although the impression is that these patients continued to be severely disabled by their psychiatric problems.

In Toronto, Wasylenki *et al.* (1993) also used a pre−post treatment design to examine the impact of an assertive case-management programme for 59 psychiatrically disabled homeless people (34 men and 25 women). Subjects were assessed on measures of psychiatric disorder, housing status, social functioning and social networks for the 9 months preceding entry to the study and at a 9-month follow-up interview. At the 9-month follow-up, hostel use had diminished markedly and the number of weeks spent in permanent accommodation, excluding hospital, increased substantially. Psychiatric symptoms decreased significantly and social functioning improved between baseline and follow-up, the greatest change

occurring in personal care and social acceptability. Total social contacts, number of supportive relationships and number of confidants also increased significantly between baseline and follow-up.

Lipton *et al.* (1988) randomly allocated 49 homeless chronically mentally ill in-patients to two groups. On discharge, 26 patients were assigned to an experimental residential treatment programme, while the remaining 23 received 'standard' aftercare. All subjects were interviewed at 4-month intervals during the subsequent year. Subjects in the experimental group spent significantly more nights in adequate shelter, fewer nights in hospital and were more satisfied with their living arrangements. Both groups showed similar levels of psychiatric symptoms at each time-point during follow-up.

In St Louis, Morse *et al.* (1992) compared the effectiveness of an assertive outreach case-management service to a daytime drop-in centre and a traditional out-patient clinic. Local shelters were screened by the research team to identify homeless people who were suffering severe psychiatric disorders. A total of 178 of these subjects were randomly allocated to one of the three interventions and followed up over 12 months. Clients who refused the offer of services or who were lost to the study within 1 month of screening were replaced by a further random allocation from the larger pool of eligible subjects. A total of 52 subjects participated in the case-management service, 62 were assigned to the day centre programme, and 64 received out-patient clinic care. Outcome measures were assessed at baseline and at 12-month follow-up. These measures included a count of the number of days spent homeless in the preceding month, current income, psychological distress, alcohol consumption, subjective self-esteem, alienation and interpersonal adjustment. In addition, at the 12-month follow-up only, a questionnaire was used to assess client satisfaction with the services, and a record was made of contact with the treatment programme and with other local social care, employment and legal advice agencies. At the 12-month follow-up, clients in all three services had spent less time homeless, had fewer psychiatric symptoms and reported an improved income, self-esteem and interpersonal adjustment. No changes were noted in alcohol consumption or subjective alienation. The clients who received the intensive case-management service showed only modest gains over the other treatment approaches. However, they had the lowest dropout rate (29 vs. 52% from the day-centre programme and 45% from the out-patient clinic service), were more satisfied with the care they received, used more community facilities and spent the least number of days homeless.

Finally, Brent-Smith and Dean (1990) reported a random allocation trial of case-management services for single homeless men in south London. A total of 95 men were recruited from homeless shelters and hostels and randomly allocated to clinical case management or an advice-brokerage comparison intervention. Schizophrenia was the main clinical diagnosis in two-thirds of the men. Subjects randomized to the clinical case-management service were allocated a named team member who provided a focused intervention based on an individualized, problem-orientated care plan. Subjects in the advice group were similarly assessed concerning care needs, and arrangements were made through consultation with hostel workers and existing statutory services to meet these, the team continuing to act as a service broker throughout the study but offering no direct care. Subjects were assessed at entry and 3-month intervals using multiple measures of mental state, social functioning, quality of life and service uptake. Case-managed clients had significantly lower dropout rates and higher uptake of appropriate statutory and voluntary services. At the 1-year follow-up, over a third of the advice group had lost contact with services compared with 17% of the case-management group. Differences in engagement with services emerged early in the course of the intervention, so that by 3 months the case-management subjects were more likely to be engaged with appropriate housing agencies, to report a relationship with a named mental health worker and to be attending mental health day-treatment facilities. Both groups showed an overall improvement in mental state and social functioning. The lack of differences in clinical and social outcome between groups reflects the high dropout rate among patients who received the advice-brokerage intervention and possible biases in recruitment (the advice-brokerage group comprised subjects who were somewhat younger, had less stable life styles and had received less treatment in the past, despite equally severe mental illness). It also seems likely that the two interventions were insufficiently distinct: both offered comprehensive needs assessment, care planning and service brokerage; both were provided by the same clinical team; and both were provided in hostel settings that had a long-standing working relationship with the clinical team. Nevertheless, the study provides data that underscore the importance of the individual relationship as a key factor in maintaining engagement with services.

These studies identify a number of common themes which need to be addressed by any intervention for mentally ill homeless people. For the majority, the basic necessities of daily living take first priority — more stable or permanent accommodation, food, clothing and safety (Ball, 1984). Only then can patients be engaged in medical care and treatments delivered successfully (Goldfinger & Chaftez, 1984). The sorts of accommodation required include a large number of residential places offering continuing support, and it is these that are in most short supply. In Britain, the majority of 'rehabilitation' homes which offer both day and night support are linked to the closure and reprovision of the old asylums and are seldom accessible to the homeless population who enter treatment. Recent initiatives for the homeless mentally ill emphasize the importance of transitional or 'move-on' accommodation, but few clinicians are surprised to learn that the available resources are fast silting up and that an actual 'move-on' to less intensively supported accommodation may take a very long time indeed (Leach & Wing, 1978).

Summary and conclusions

To conclude, it is clear that a sizeable proportion of homeless adults suffer from severe mental illness. Depression and anxiety are near universal, and functional psychoses, particularly schizophrenia, are greatly overrepresented. Despite levels of disability similar to those seen in the long-stay wards of psychiatric hospitals, the majority have not experienced prolonged hospitalization and are not in receipt of any regular medical or social care. There is some evidence to suggest that, in line with homeless populations in general, the mentally ill homeless now involve rather younger, more chaotic individuals with multiple disabilities and a significant comorbidity with substance abuse. This more youthful group shares other characteristics with other severely mentally ill young people from disenfranchised and disaffiliated sectors of society: a reluctance to engage with services, significant non-compliance with treatment and a history of minor infringements of the law.

Homelessness is essentially an issue of the availability of low-cost housing and there is little evidence to suggest that the pathway to homelessness among mentally ill people differs substantially from that for the remaining homeless population. However, it is also clear that once mentally ill, homeless people are much less likely to escape deprivation by their own efforts. In part, this can be attributed to the well-documented impairments of problem-solving skills, motivation and social interactions that characterize the diseases from which they suffer. But it is also apparent that a significant responsibility must rest with the poor quality of organization and focus of psychiatric and social services. In priciple, enough is known to put this right. Effective services for chronic disabilities need to be continuous, delivered where sufferers congregate and assertive in their efforts to reach people who are too disorganized to attend appointments regularly. It is also quite clear that however 'good' the outreach, progress is unlikely without adequate provision of accommodation; this is an essential first step in achieving engagement and care.

References

Allderidge, P. (1979) Hospitals, madhouses and asylums: cycles in the care of the insane. *British Journal of Psychiatry*, **134**, 321–333.

Arce, A.A., Tadlock, M., Vergare, M.J. & Shapiro, S.H. (1983) A psychiatric profile of street people admitted to an emergency shelter. *Hospital and Community Psychiatry*, **34**, 812–817.

Austerberry, H. & Watson, S. (1986) *Housing and Homelessness*. Routledge & Kegan Paul, London.

Aylward, E., Walker, E. & Bettes, B. (1984) Intelligence in schizophrenia: meta-analysis of the research. *Schizophrenia Bulletin*, **10**, 430–459.

Bachrach, L. (1984) The homeless mentally ill and the mental health services. In Lamb, H.R. (ed.) *The Homeless Mentally Ill*, pp. 11–54. American Psychiatric Association, Washington DC.

Bachrach, L.L. (1987) Issues in identifying and treating the homeless mentally ill. *New Directions in Mental Health Services*, **35**, 43–62.

Bachrach, L.L. (1992) What we know about homelessness among mentally ill persons: an analytical review and commentary. *Hospital and Community Psychiatry*, **43**, 453–464.

Ball, J. (1984) A survey of the problems and needs of homeless consumers of acute psychiatric services. *Hospital and Community Psychiatry*, **35**, 917–921.

Bassuk, E.L., Rubin, L. & Laurait, A. (1986) Characteristics of sheltered homeless families. *American Journal of Public Health*, **76**, 1097–1102.

Baxter, E. & Hopper, K. (1982) The new mendicancy: homeless in New York City. *American Journal of Orthopsychiatry*, **52**, 393–408.

Beier, A.L. (1987) *Masterless Men: The Vagrancey Problem in England 1560–1640*. Methuen, London.

Bento, A. & Marmeleiro, C. (1989) Doentes mentais sem casa em Lisboa. *Hosp. Julio de Matos*, **2**, 11–21.

Berry, C. & Orwin, A. (1966) No fixed abode: a survey of mental hospital admissions. *British Journal of Psychiatry*, **112**, 1019–1025.

Bhugra, D. (1991) *Psychiatric Care of the Homeless Mentally Ill*. Report of a Working Party of the Royal College of Psychiatrists. Royal College of Psychiatrists, London.

Bogue, D.J. (1963) *Skid Row in American Cities*. Community and Family Study Centre. University of Chicago, Chicago.

Breakey, W., Fischer, P., Kramer, M. *et al.* (1989) Health and mental health problems of homeless men and women in Baltimore. *Journal of the American Medical Association*, **262**, 1352–1357.

Brent-Smith, H. & Dean, R. (1990) *Plugging the Gaps*. Lewisham and North Southwark Health Authority, London.

Brown, G.W. (1989) Causal paths, chains and strands. In Rutter, M. (ed.) *The Power of Longitudinal Data: Studies of Risk and Protective Factors for Psychosocial Disorders*. Cambridge University Press, Cambridge.

Brown, G.W. & Harris, T.O. (1978) *The Social Origins of Depression*. Tavistock, London.

Brown, G.W. & Harris, T.O. (1989) *Life Events and Illness*. Guilford Press, London.

Burt, M.R. & Cohen, B.E. (1989) Differences among homeless single women, women with children and single men. *Social Problems*, **36**, 508–524.

Canter, D., Drake, M., Littler, T., Moore, J., Stockley, D. & Ball, J. (1989) *The Faces of Homelessness in London: Interim Report to the Salvation Army Department of Psychology*. University of Surrey, Guildford.

Caton, C., Wyatt, R.J., Grunberg, J. & Felix, A. (1990) An evaluation of a mental health program for homeless men. *American Journal of Psychiatry*, **147**, 286–289.

Central Office of Information (1991) *The Resettlement Units Executive Agency. Annual Report and Financial Statement 1990/91*. HMSO, London.

Central Statistics Office (1989) *Social Trends*. HMSO, London.

Central Statistics Office (1991) *Social Trends*. HMSO, London.

Clarke, R.E. (1948) Psychoses, income, and occupational prestige. *American Journal of Sociology*, **54**, 433–440.

Clifford, P. & Craig, T.K.J. (1989) *Case Management for People with Severe Mental Illness*. Research and Development for Psychiatry, London.

Cohen, C.I. & Thompson, K.S. (1992) Homeless mentally ill or mentally ill homeless? *American Journal of Psychiatry*, **149**, 816–823.

Crossley, B. & Denmark, J.C. (1969) Community care: a study of the psychiatric morbidity of a Salvation Army hostel. *British Journal of Sociology*, **20**, 443–449.

DoH (1990) *Health and Personal Social Services Statistics for England*. HMSO, London.

Dorrell, S. (1991) *Written Reply to Early Day Motion 298*. Hansard, London.

Eagle, P.F. & Caton, C.L.M. (1990) Homelessness and mental illness. In Caton, C. (ed.) *Homelessness in America*, pp. 59–75. Oxford University Press, Oxford.

Edwards, G., Hawker, A., Williamson, V. & Hensman, C. (1966) London's Skid Row. *Lancet*, **1**, 249–252.

Edwards, G., Williamson, V., Hawker, A., Hensman, C. & Postoyan, S. (1968) Census of a reception centre. *British Journal of Psychiatry*, **116**, 1031–1059.

Faris, R.E. & Dunham, H.W. (1939) *Mental Disorders in Urban Areas. An Ecological Study of Schizophrenia and Other Psychoses*. Hafner, New York.

Farr, R.K., Koegal, P. & Burnam, A. (1986) *A Study of Homelessness and Mental Illness in the Skid Row Area of Los Angeles*. Los Angeles County Department of Mental Health, Los Angeles.

Fischer, P.J., Shapiro, S., Breakey, W.R., Anthony, J.C. & Kramer, M. (1986) Mental health and social characteristics of the homeless: a survey of mission users. *American Journal of Public Health*, **76**, 519–524.

Fisher, P.J. & Breakey, W.R. (1986) Homelessness and mental health: an overview. *International Journal of Mental Health*, **14**, 6–41.

Freeman, S., Formo, A. & Alampur, A. (1979) Psychiatric disorder in a skid-row mission population. *Comprehensive Psychiatry*, **32**, 454–461.

Gardner, E.A. & Babigian, H.M. (1966) A longitudinal comparison of psychiatric service to selected socioeconomic areas of Monroe County, New York. *American Journal of Orthopsychiatry*, **36**, 818–828.

George, S., Shanks, N. & Westlake, L. (1991) Census of homeless people in Sheffield. *British Medical Journal*, **302**, 1387–1389.

Glover, G. (1989) The official data available on mental health. In Jenkins, R. & Griffiths, S. (eds) *Indicators for Mental Health in the Population*, pp. 18–24. HMSO, London.

Goldberg, E.M. & Morrison, S.L. (1963) Schizophrenia and social class. *British Journal of Psychiatry*, **109**, 785–802.

Goldfinger, S.M. & Chaftez, L. (1984) Developing a better service delivery system for the homeless mentally ill. In Lamb, H.R. (ed.) *The Homeless Mentally Ill*, pp. 91–108. American Psychiatric Association, Washington DC.

Hare, E.H. (1956) Mental illness and social conditions in Bristol. *Journal of Mental Science*, **102**, 349–357.

Harrison, M., Chandler, R. & Green, G. (1992) *Hostels in London: A Statistical Overview*. Resource Information Service.

Herrman, H., McGorry, P., Bennett, P., Van Riel, R. & Singh, B. (1989) Prevalence of severe mental illness in disaffiliated and homeless people in inner Melbourne. *American Journal of Psychiatry*, **146**, 1179–1184.

Herzberg, J.L. (1987) No fixed abode: a comparison of men and women admitted to an East London psychiatric hospital. *British Journal of Psychiatry*, **150**, 621–627.

Hewettson, J. (1975) Homeless people as an at-risk group. *Proceedings of the Royal Society of Medicine*, **68**, 9–13.

Hollander, D., Tobiansky, R. & Powell, R. (1990) Crisis in admission beds. *British Medical Journal*, **301**, 664.

Hollingshead, A.B. & Redlich, F.C. (1958) *Social Class and Mental Illness*. Wiley, New York.

Jones, P.B., Bebbington, P., Foerster, A. *et al.* (1993) Premorbid social underachievement in schizophrenia. Results from the Camberwell Collaborative Psychosis Study. *British Journal of Psychiatry*, **162**, 65–71.

Kay, R. (1985) *The Homeless Mentally Ill*. US Department of Health and Human Sciences, Washington DC.

Koegal, P., Burnam, M.A. & Farr, R.K. (1988) The prevalence of specific psychiatric disorders among homeless individuals in the inner city of Los Angeles. *Archives of General Psychiatry*, **45**, 1085–1092.

Kroll, J., Carey, K., Hagedorn, D., Fire Dog, P. & Benavides, E. (1986) A survey of homeless adults in urban emergency shelters. *Hospital and Community Psychiatry*, **37**, 283–286.

Laidlaw, S.I.A. (1956) *Glasgow Common Lodging Houses and People Living in Them*. Corporation of Glasgow.

Lamb, H.R. (1984) Deinstitutionalization and the homeless mentally ill. *Hospital and Community Psychiatry*, **35**, 899–907.

Leach, J. & Wing, J.K. (1978) The effectiveness of a service for helping destitute men. *British Journal of Psychiatry*, **133**, 481–492.

Leff, J. (1991) Evaluation of the closure of mental hospitals. In Hall, P. & Brockington, I. (eds) *The Closure of Mental Hospitals*, pp. 25–32. Gaskell Press, London.

Linn, L., Gelberg, L. & Leake, B. (1990) Substance abuse and mental health status of homeless and domiciled low-income users of a medical clinic. *Hospital and Community Psychiatry*, **41**, 306–310.

Lipton, F.R., Nutt, S. & Sabatini, A. (1988) Housing the homeless mentally ill: a longitudinal study of a treatment approach. *Hospital and Community Psychiatry*, **39**, 40–45.

Lipton, F.R.M., Sabatini, A. & Katz, S.E. (1983) Down and out in the city: the homeless mentally ill. *Hospital and Community Psychiatry*, **34**, 817–821.

Lodge-Patch, I. (1970) Homeless men: a London survey. *Proceedings of the Royal Society of Medicine*, **63**, 437–441.

Marks, I. (1992) Innovations in mental health care delivery. *British Journal of Psychiatry*, **160**, 589–597.

Marshall, E.J. & Reed, J.L. (1992) Psychiatric morbidity in homeless women. *British Journal of Psychiatry*, **160**, 761–768.

Marshall, M. (1989) Collected and neglected: are Oxford hostels filling up with disabled psychiatric patients? *British Medical Journal*, **229**, 706–709.

Matthews, P. (1986) Doctors for the homeless and rootless. *British Medical Journal*, **292**, 1672–1674.

Meltzer, D., Hale, A.S., Malik, S.J., Hogman, G. & Wood, S. (1991) Community care for patients with schizophrenia one year after hospital discharge. *British Medical Journal*, **303**, 1023–1026.

Milburn, N.G. & Watts, R.J. (1986) Methodological issues in research on the homeless and the homeless mentally ill. *International Journal of Mental Health*, **14**, 42–60.

Morse, G.A. & Calsyn, R.J. (1986) Mentally disturbed homeless people in St Louis: needy, willing but underserved. *International Journal of Mental Health*, **14**, 74–94.

Morse, G.A., Calsyn, R.J., Allen, G., Tempelhoff, B. & Smith, R. (1992) Experimental comparison of the effects of three treatment programs for homeless mentally ill people. *Hospital and Community Psychiatry*, **43**, 1005–1010.

Mouren, M.-C., Rajaona, F.-R., Thiebaux, M. & Tatossian, A. (1979) Le vagabondage: aspects psychologiques et psychopathologiques. *Annales Medico-Psychologiques*, **135**, 415–447.

Mundy, P., Robertson, M., Robertson, J. & Greenblatt, M. (1990) The prevalence of psychotic symptoms in homeless adolescents. *Journal of the American Academy of Child and Adolescent Psychiatry*, **29**, 724–731.

Murray, R.M. & Lewis, S. (1987) Is schizophrenia a neurodevelopmental disorder? *British Journal of Psychiatry*, **295**, 681–682.

National Schizophrenia Fellowship (1989) *Mental Hospital Closures — News Update*. National Schizophrenia Fellowship, London.

Nordentoft, M., Knudsen, H.C. & Schulsinger, F. (1992) Housing conditions and residential needs of psychiatric patients in Copenhagen. *Acta Psychiatrica Scandinavica*, **85**, 385–389.

Noreik, K. (1965) Hospitalised psychoses among wandering people in Norway. *Acta Psychiatrica Scandinavica*, **41**, 157–176.

Odegard, O. (1956) The incidence of psychosis in various occupations. *International Journal of Social Psychiatry*, **2**, 85–104.

Office of Population Census and Surveys (1991) *The 1991 Census. Preliminary Report for England and Wales, Supplementary Monitor on People Sleeping Rough.* HMSO, London.

Patrick, M., Higgit, A., Holloway, F. & Silverman, M. (1989) Changes in an inner city psychiatric inpatient service following bed losses: a follow up of the East Lambeth 1986

Survey. *Health Trends*, **21**, 121–123.

Pickard, L., Proudfoot, R. & Wolfson, P. (1991) *The Closure of Cane Hill Hospital: Report of the Cane Hill Evaluation Team.* Research and Development for Psychiatry, London.

Powers, J.L., Eckenrode, J. & Jakutsch, T. (1990) Maltreatment among runaway and homeless youth. *Child Abuse and Neglect*, **14**, 87–89.

Priest, R.G. (1970) Homeless in Chicago and Edinburgh. *Proceedings of the Royal Society of Medicine*, **63**, 441–445.

Priest, R.G. (1971) The Edinburgh homeless. *American Journal of Psychotherapy*, **25**, 194–213.

Priest, R.G. (1976) The homeless person and the psychiatric services: an Edinburgh survey. *British Journal of Psychiatry*, **128**, 128–136.

Randall, G. (1988) *No Way Home*. Centrepoint, London.

Randall, G. (1989) *Homeless and Hungry*. Centrepoint, London.

Randall, G. (1992) *Counted Out: An Investigation into the Extent of Single Homelessness Outside London*. CRISIS, London.

Rossi, P.H., Wright, J.D., Fisher, G.A. & Willis, G. (1987) The urban homeless: estimating composition and size. *Science*, **234**, 1336–1341.

Roth, D. & Bean, G. (1986) New perspectives on homelessness: findings from a statewide epidemiological study. *Hospital and Community Psychiatry*, **37**, 712–719.

Sayce, L., Craig, T.K.J. & Boardman, A.P. (1991) The development of community mental health centres in the UK. *Social Psychiatry and Psychiatric Epidemiology*, **26**, 14–20.

Schroeder, C.W. (1942) Mental disorders in cities. *American Journal of Sociology*, **48**, 40–48.

Shaffer, D. & Caton, C.L.M. (1984) *Runaway and Homeless Youth in New York City: A Report to the Ittleston Foundation.* New York State Psychiatric Institute, New York.

SHELTER (1989) *Raise the Roof Campaign*. SHELTER Publications, London.

SHIL (1986) *Single Homeless in London: A Report by the Single Homeless in London Working Party*. SHIL, London.

Snow, D.A., Baker, S.G. & Anderson, L. (1986) The myth of pervasive mental illness among the homeless. *Social Problems*, **33**, 415–423.

Stark, C., Scott, J. & Hill, M. (1989) *A Survey of the Long Stay Users of DSS Resettlement Units: A Research Report*. Department of Social Security. HMSO, London.

Stern, R. & Stilwell, B. (1989) Treadmill on trial. *Health Service Journal*, **99**, 1100–1103.

Stiffman, A.R. (1989) Physical and sexual abuse in runaway youth. *Child Abuse and Neglect*, **13**, 417–426.

Sundby, P. & Nyhus, P. (1963) Major and minor psychiatric disorders in males in Oslo: an epidemiological study. *Acta Psychiatrica Scandinavica*, **38**, 519–547.

Susser, E., Conover, M. & Struening, E. (1989a) Problems of epidemiologic method in assessing the type and extent of mental illness among homeless adults. *Hospital and Community Psychiatry*, **40**, 261–265.

Susser, E., Lovell, A. & Conover, S. (1989b) Unravelling the causes of homelessness — and of its association with mental illness. In Cooper, B. & Helgason, T. (eds) *Epidemiology and the Prevention of Mental Disorders*, pp. 228–239. Routledge & Kegan Paul, London.

Susser, E., Struening, E.L. & Conover, S. (1989c) Psychiatric problems in homeless men: lifetime psychosis, substance abuse and current desires in new arrivals at New York City shelters. *Archives of General Psychiatry*, **46**, 845–850.

Susser, E.S., Lin, S.P., Conover, S.A. & Struening, E.L. (1991) Childhood antecedents of homelessness in psychiatric patients. *American Journal of Psychiatry*, **148**, 1026–1030.

TAPS (1990) *Better Out Than In?* North-East Thames Regional Health Authority, London.

Thornicroft, G. & Bebbington, P. (1989) Deinstitutionalisation — from hospital closure to service development. *British Journal of Psychiatry*, **155**, 739–753.

Tidmarsh, D. & Wood, S. (1972) Psychiatric aspects of destitution. In Wing, J.K. & Hailey, A.M. (eds) *Evaluating a Community Psychiatric Service*, pp. 327–340. Oxford University Press, Oxford.

Timms, P.W. & Fry, A.H. (1989) Homelessness and mental illness. *Health Trends*, **21**, 70–71.

Turner, R.J., Morton, O. & Wagenfeld, M.O. (1967) Occupational mobility and schizophrenia. An assessment of the social causation and social selection hypotheses. *American Psychological Review*, **32**, 104–113.

US Department of Housing and Urban Development (1984) *A Report to the Secretary on the Homeless and Emergency Shelters*. Office of Policy Development and Research, Washington DC.

Wall, P. (1991) Health and Homelessness. *Health Service Journal*, **101**, 16–17.

Warner, R. (1985) *Recovery from Schizophrenia: Psychiatry and Political Economy*. Routledge & Kegan Paul, London.

Wasylenki, D.A., Goering, P.N., Lemire, d., Lindsey, S. & Lancee, W. (1993) The Hostel Outreach Program: assertive case management for homeless mentally ill persons. *Hospital and Community Psychiatry*, **44**, 848–853.

Weller, B.G.A., Weller, M.P.I., Coker, E. & Mahomed, S. (1987) Crisis at Christmas 1986. *Lancet*, **1**, 553–554.

Weller, M.P.I. (1989) Mental illness — who cares? *Nature*, **339**, 249–252.

Whiteley, J.S. (1955) Down and out in London: mental illness in the lower social groups. *Lancet*, **2**, 608–610.

Whitly, M.D., Osborne, C.H., Godfrey, M.A. & Johnston, K. (1985) A point-prevalence study of alcoholism and mental illness among downtown migrants. *Social Science and Medicine*, **20**, 579–583.

Wiersma, D., Giel, R., De Jong, A. & Sloof, C.J. (1983) Social class and schizophrenia in a Dutch cohort. *Psychological Medicine*, **13**, 141–150.

Wilmanns, K. (1906) Zur Psychopathologie des Landstreichers: eine klinische Studie. Barth, Leipzig.

Wing, J.K. (1990) The functions of asylum. *British Journal of Psychiatry*, **157**, 822–827.

APPENDICES

Appendix 1
DSM-IV Diagnostic Criteria
for Schizophrenia (APA, 1994)

A Characteristic symptoms of schizophrenia: at least two of the following, each present for a significant portion of time during a 1-month period (or less if successfully treated).

1 Delusions.

2 Hallucinations.

3 Disorganized speech (e.g. frequent derailment or incoherence).

4 Grossly disorganized or catatonic behaviour.

5 Negative symptoms, i.e. affective flattening, alogia or avolition.

Note Only one A symptom is required if delusions are bizarre or hallucinations consist of a voice keeping up a running commentary on the person's behaviour or thoughts, or two or more voices conversing with each other.

B Social/occupational dysfunction: for a significant portion of the time since the onset of the disturbance, one or more major areas of functioning, such as work, interpersonal relations or self-care, is markedly below the level achieved prior to the onset (or, when the onset is in childhood or adolescence, failure to achieve the expected level of interpersonal, academic or occupational achievement).

C Duration: continuous signs of the disturbance persist for at least 6 months. This 6-month period must include at least 1 month of symptoms that meet criterion A (i.e. active-phase symptoms), and may include periods of prodromal or residual symptoms. During these prodromal or residual periods, the sign of the symptoms listed in criterion A present in an attenuated form (e.g. odd beliefs or unusual perceptual experiences).

D Schizoaffective and mood disorder exclusion: schizoaffective disorder and mood disorder with psychotic features have been ruled out because either: (i) no major depressive or manic episodes have occurred concurrently with the active-phase symptoms; or (ii) if mood episodes have occurred during active-phase symptoms, their total duration has been brief relative to the duration of the active and residual periods.

E Substance/general medical condition exclusion: the disturbance is not due to the direct effects of a substance (e.g. drugs of abuse or medication) or a general medical condition.

References

APA (1994) *Diagnostic and Statistical Manual of Mental Disorders*, 4th edn. American Psychiatric Association, Washington DC.

Appendix 2
F20−F29 Schizophrenia, Schizotypal and Delusional Disorders

F20 Schizophrenia

A Either at least one of the syndromes, symptoms and signs listed below under 1, or *at least two* of the symptoms and signs listed under 2, should have been present for most of the time during an episode of psychotic illness lasting for *at least 1 month*.

1 At least one of the following.

(a) Thought echo, thought insertion or withdrawal and thought broadcasting.

(b) Delusions of control, influence or passivity, clearly referred to body or limb movements or specific thought, actions or sensations and delusional perception.

(c) Hallucinatory voices giving a running commentary on the patient's behaviour, or discussing the patient between themselves or other types of hallucinatory voices coming from some part of the body.

(d) Persistent delusions of other kinds that are culturally inappropriate and completely impossible, such as religious or political identity, superhuman powers and ability (e.g. being able to control the weather, or being in communication with aliens from another world).

2 *Or* at least two of the following.

(e) Persistent hallucinations in any modality, when accompanied by either fleeting or half-formed delusions without clear affective content, or by persistent overvalued ideas or when occurring every day for weeks or months on end.

(f) Breaks or interpolations in the train of thought, resulting in incoherence or irrelevant speech, or neologisms.

(g) Catatonic behaviour, such as excitement, posturing or waxy flexibility, negativism, mutism and stupor.

(h) 'Negative' symptoms such as marked apathy, paucity of speech, and blunting or incongruity of emotional responses (these usually result in social withdrawal and lowering of social performance). It must be clear that these are not due to depression or to neuroleptic medication.

In evaluating the presence of these abnormal subjective experiences and behaviour, special care should be taken to avoid false-positive assessments, especially where culturally or subculturally influenced modes of expression and behaviour, or a subnormal level of intelligence, are involved.

B If the patient also meets criteria for manic episode (F30) or depressive episode (F32), the criteria listed under 1 and 2 above must have been met before the disturbance of mood developed.

C The disorder is not attributable to organic brain disease (in the sense of F0), or to alcohol- or drug-related intoxication, dependence or withdrawal.

Author Index

Subject Index